RADIOLOGY OF SKELETAL TRAUMA

Third Edition

Lee F. Rogers, MD

Isadore Meschan Distinguished Professor of Radiology
Department of Radiology
Wake Forest University School of Medicine
Winston-Salem, North Carolina

Editor-in-Chief, American Journal of Roentgenology

with contributions by 29 authors

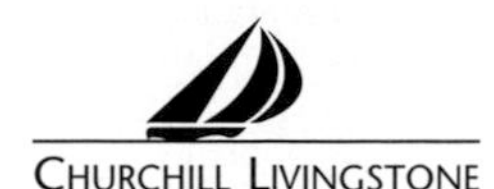

CHURCHILL LIVINGSTONE
A Harcourt Health Sciences Company
New York Edinburgh London Philadelphia

To my father, the late Doctor Watson F. Rogers, of Vienna, West Virginia, a true physician; loved by his family, admired by his patients, and respected by his colleagues. Born in St. Albans, Vermont, raised in Vergennes, Vermont, and educated at the University of Vermont, he practiced medicine in Underhill, Vermont, and Vienna and Parkersburg, West Virginia.

And to the memory of our medical heritage, all physicians, all Vermonters: my grandfather, Doctor Frank Matthew Rogers of St. Albans and Vergennes, Vermont; my great uncle, Doctor Daniel Lee Rogers of Bolton Landing, New York; my great uncle, Doctor Sam Rogers of Proctor, Vermont; my uncle, Doctor Samuel Rogers of Stowe, Vermont; and to all those who may have suffered as we learned.

And to my grandchildren, Dean, Garrison, Megan, Westin, and John, in the fond hope that whatever they may become and wherever that might be, they too find something as rewarding and meaningful to do with their lives as those of us who have preceded them.

CONTRIBUTORS

Carol J. Ashman, MD
Assistant Professor of Radiology, Musculoskeletal Imaging Section, Ohio State University College of Medicine, Columbus, Ohio
The Hip and Femoral Shaft

Sam T. Auringer, MD
Associate Professor of Radiology and Pediatrics, Wake Forest University School of Medicine, Winston-Salem, North Carolina
Special Considerations in Children

Diane Bergin, MB
Department of Radiology, Mater Misericordiae Hospital, Dublin, Ireland
The Wrist

Carol A. Boles, MD
Assistant Professor of Radiology, Associate Professor in Surgical Sciences—Orthopaedic Surgery, Wake Forest University School of Medicine; Wake Forest University Baptist Medical Center, Winston-Salem, North Carolina
Complications of Fracture; The Hand

Eric Brandser, MD
Associate Professor, University of Iowa College of Medicine; Director, Musculoskeletal Imaging, Department of Radiology, University of Iowa Hospitals and Clinics, Iowa City, Iowa
The Pelvis

Felix S. Chew, MD
Professor of Radiology, Section Head of Musculoskeletal Radiology, Vice-Chair of Education, Wake Forest University School of Medicine, Winston-Salem, North Carolina
Imaging of Fractures: Detection and Description

Mark S. Cohen, MD
Associate Professor of Orthopedic Surgery, Director of Orthopedic Education, Rush Medical College; Director, Hand and Elbow Section, Department of Orthopedic Surgery, Rush-Presbyterian-St. Luke's Medical Center, Chicago, Illinois
The Hand

T. David Cox, MD
Assistant Professor of Radiology and Pediatrics, Wake Forest University School of Medicine, Winston-Salem, North Carolina; Staff Radiologist, St. Paul Children's Hospital, St. Paul, Minnesota
The Elbow and Forearm

Richard H. Daffner, MD, FACR
Professor of Radiologic Sciences, MCP Hahnemann University School of Medicine; Senior Attending Radiologist, Allegheny General Hospital, Pittsburgh, Pennsylvania
The Thoracic and Lumbar Spine

Stephen Eustace, MB
Lecturer in Radiology, University College Dublin; Director of Radiology, Cappagh National Orthopaedic Hospital, Dublin, Ireland
The Wrist

Curtis A. Given II, MD
Department of Neuroradiology, Wake Forest University School of Medicine, Winston-Salem, North Carolina
The Skull

Clyde A. Helms, MD
Professor of Radiology and Surgery, Duke University Medical Center, Durham, North Carolina
The Knee and Shafts of the Tibia and Fibula

Ronald W. Hendrix, MD
Associate Professor of Radiology, Northwestern University Medical School; Director of Radiology, Rehabilitation Institute of Chicago, Northwestern Memorial Hospital, Chicago, Illinois
Imaging of Fractures: Detection and Description; Fracture Treatment; Fracture Healing; Complications of Fracture

Eric K. Hoffer, MD
Assistant Professor of Radiology, University of Washington School of Medicine; Director of Angio/Interventional Radiology, Harborview Medical Center, Seattle, Washington
The Thoracic Cage

David Karasick, MD
Department of Radiology, Thomas Jefferson University Hospital, Philadelphia, Pennsylvania
The Foot

Ciaran Keogh, MB
Musculoskeletal Fellow, Cappagh National Orthopaedic Hospital, Dublin, Ireland
The Wrist

Leon Lenchik, MD
Assistant Professor of Musculoskeletal Imaging, Wake Forest University School of Medicine, Winston-Salem, North Carolina
Epidemiology of Fractures; The Shoulder and Humeral Shaft

Nancy M. Major, MD
Assistant Professor, Duke University Medical Center, Durham, North Carolina
The Knee and Shafts of the Tibia and Fibula

Stuart E. Mirvis, MD
Professor of Radiology, University of Maryland School of Medicine; Director of Radiology, Maryland Shock-Trauma Center, Baltimore, Maryland
Polytrauma: The Multiple-Injury Patient

Mark E. Mullins, MD
Resident in Radiology, Harvard Medical School; Massachusetts General Hospital, Boston, Massachusetts
The Face

Robert A. Novelline, MD
Professor of Radiology, Harvard Medical School; Chief, Emergency Radiology Division, Massachusetts General Hospital, Boston, Massachusetts
The Face

Diego Nuñez Jr., MD, MPH
Visiting Professor of Radiology, Harvard Medical School; Director of Emergency Radiology, Brigham and Women's Hospital, Boston, Massachusetts
The Cervical Spine

James T. Rhea, MD
Associate Professor of Radiology, Harvard Medical School; Radiologist, Massachusetts General Hospital, Boston, Massachusetts
The Face

Mark E. Schweitzer, MD
Professor of Radiology and Orthopedic Surgery; Director, General Diagnostic Radiology, Vice-Chair, Clinical Practice Affairs, Thomas Jefferson University Hospital, Philadelphia, Pennsylvania
The Foot

Andrew Sonin, MD
Clinical Assistant Professor of Radiology, University of Maryland School of Medicine, Baltimore, Maryland; Musculoskeletal Radiologist, Radiology Imaging Associates, Denver, Colorado
The Elbow and Forearm

Eric J. Stern, MD
Professor of Radiology, University of Washington School of Medicine; Director of Thoracic Imaging, Director of Faculty Development, Harborview Medical Center, Seattle, Washington
The Thoracic Cage

Daniel W. Williams III, MD
Department of Radiology, Wake Forest University School of Medicine, Winston-Salem, North Carolina
The Skull

Anthony J. Wilson, MB, ChB
Professor of Radiology, University of Washington School of Medicine; Director of Radiology, Harborview Medical Center, Seattle, Washington
The Ankle

Joseph S. Yu, MD
Associate Professor of Radiology, Musculoskeletal Imaging Section, Ohio State University College of Medicine; Chief of Musculoskeletal Imaging, Ohio State University Medical Center, Columbus, Ohio
The Hip and Femoral Shaft

FOREWORD TO THE FIRST EDITION

It is of interest to correlate the career of the author of this text—Lee Rogers, MD—with the ever-expanding field of radiology of skeletal trauma. Dr. Rogers received his training in radiology during a period in which skeletal trauma was inherently important, but in no way reflected at that time the maturing of and interest in the field that would later be shown; nor at that time had radiology benefited from the extraordinary talents that scientists and scholars such as Dr. Rogers developed. It was not uncommon in the early periods of the growth of training programs in diagnostic radiology that cases of skeletal trauma be shunted to the junior radiologists and resident physicians working in the department. As the years went on Dr. Rogers associated himself more and more with the fascinating subject of skeletal trauma just as others developed an interest and expertise in subsections of diagnostic radiology other than skeletal radiology (e.g., neuroradiology, radiology of the chest, gastrointestinal radiology). Dr. Rogers' work and study in this discipline has culminated in the preparation of this superb text, as he has become recognized nationally and internationally as an outstanding authority on the subject.

We live in a time of violence; probably of most significance in the production of skeletal trauma are motor vehicle accidents (MVAs). Injuries are now recognized as the leading cause of death in persons aged 3 to 34 years. In this connection it is difficult to believe that almost 150,000 Americans die each year as a result of trauma, of which one third are caused by MVAs. The role of diagnostic radiology is vital in establishing the correct diagnosis and the preliminary care of the injured patient immediately following trauma.

This remarkable work of approximately 1500 pages in two volumes is almost twice as large as the first edition, published in 1982. Included in this second edition are approximately 3000 illustrations and 4000 references. The illustrations and references are plentiful, timely, and carefully selected, reflecting the high level of the entire work.

Also of interest is the ratio of the number of plain films to special modalities (i.e., computed tomographs [CTs] and magnetic resonance images [MRIs]) appearing as illustrations. Plain films make up approximately 40% of the entire number of illustrations—an interesting statistic.

The book is presented on a regional basis in separate chapters, including both the axial skeleton and the peripheral skeleton. Dr. Rogers begins each chapter with a discussion of the relevant radiographic anatomy of the region. Other chapters and sections are included in appropriate areas.

Of inordinate value is an early chapter on skeletal biomechanics, dealing with the mechanics of skeletal trauma. The treatment of skeletal trauma in biomechanical terms is included in this highly informative chapter. As Dr. Rogers astutely states, "Reduction of fractures should reverse the mechanism of injury." He includes data showing that the musculoskeletal system is a composite structure of macroscopic and microscopic levels. Macroscopic structures include bones, joints, ligaments, and so on, and microscopic levels consist of haversian canals, osteons, periosteum, and the like. Other invaluable material, including the roles of direct and indirect forces in trauma, is included in this chapter on skeletal biomechanics.

The statistical frequency of injuries is considered and the mechanics of the skeletal trauma stressed. Soft tissue involvement is included. Not only is the general anatomy incorporated within each area but the vascular supply of bone is also discussed at relevant sites. The various centers of ossification, both primary and secondary, are described. Also included is a discussion of the different types of joints and their histologic composition, including ligaments and tendons when and where important.

A chapter on the epidemiology of fractures is incorporated early in the work. The patient and the nature and number of fractures are considered and the relationship of the type of skeletal injury to different activities are stressed. Data dealing with the age of the patient are described and the varying effects of skeletal trauma on different areas of the skeleton are considered. As an example, the consequences of a fall on the outstretched hand are described for different age groups. The subject of osteoporosis is discussed in detail, particularly as related to trauma. Various types of radiographic measurements of osteoporosis to estimate bone loss are presented. Included is an excellent section on the description and classification of various special fractures (e.g., chondral, osteochondral, stress, pathologic).

A section on the special considerations of skeletal trauma in childhood is invaluable. Included is a discussion in depth of the various injuries to the growing skeleton. In addition, considerable data are provided on skeletal injuries easily missed.

The multiply injured patient is described in another

chapter; this is particularly important today with the high incidence of MVAs.

Treatment of various fractures is considered and the fundamental issues involved are discussed (e.g., postreduction films). Healing and complications of fractures are excellently described. A section on up-to-date radiographic techniques is included in a typically precise but highly informative fashion. The use of special modalities (i.e., CT, MRI) is considered in each appropriate area. Additional sections deal with trauma to the skull; consideration of the differential diagnosis, particularly as related to congenital anomalies, is stressed. Of particular importance is the presentation of the effects of trauma to the face, which is included with a description of a beautifully precise and easy-to-understand section on LeFort fractures.

A chapter on spinal trauma is admirably concise yet pragmatically informative. Many important concepts are presented and discussed in this section. The capacity to be concise yet fully informative is nowhere better demonstrated than in this excellent section on spinal trauma.

Although the first edition of this work was published ten years ago, its importance has increased as the violence innate to our society and indeed throughout the world grows apace. The basic excellence of the work is inherent in the importance and quality of what Dr Rogers has to say. No longer can departments of radiology and indeed radiologists of both academic and community-oriented departments afford to examine patients after skeletal trauma without utilizing a meaningful amount of the information that Dr. Rogers imparts in this work. Skeletal radiology has become a major discipline, and although other fine works on trauma to the skeleton exist, this book by Dr. Rogers certainly deserves top rating. This tome has been produced in a timely fashion by a man who has been trained in and retains interest in most of the subdisciplines of diagnostic radiology. Dr. Rogers thus brings to bear on this effort a thorough understanding not only of the radiologic aspects of trauma to the skeleton, but also more than a passing interest in other similarly important subdisciplines in diagnostic radiology, such as radiology of the central nervous system.

It is of interest to note that skeletal trauma comprises perhaps as much as one-third of all the referrals to the radiologist (e.g., emergency room, academic departments, community hospitals, and private practitioners of radiology). With such a very large volume of skeletal trauma it must be apparent that a copy of Dr. Rogers' work should always be at hand. The complications that ensue and the damage that is inflicted with an incorrect diagnosis in skeletal trauma are most serious.

The preparation of this work by an authority with Dr. Rogers' impeccable credentials provides a unique opportunity to share with Dr. Rogers his extensive experience and expertise in the radiologic manifestations of skeletal trauma.

This major contribution to the literature incorporates important points carefully discussed and beautifully illustrated by the author. Dr. Rogers deserves gratitude and thanks from all radiologists, orthopedic clinicians, residents in training, and medical students for creating this unsurpassed effort. This book will stand as a landmark on one of the most important subjects of the day.

I would like to express my appreciation and gratitude for being invited to prepare the Foreword to this second edition.

Harold G. Jacobson, MD
Professor Emeritus and Chairman—
Distinguished University Professor
Department of Radiology
Albert Einstein College of Medicine/
Montefiore Medical Center
Bronx, New York

PREFACE

Ten years went by between the first and second editions of this book and now another 10 years has passed. Ten years between editions is a long time, but it has gone by quickly and much has happened. Among other things, I am no longer a departmental chairman. I am now an editor. I no longer live in Chicago. I have moved from Northwestern University to Wake Forest University School of Medicine here in Winston-Salem, North Carolina.

Not only have things changed for me personally during the same 10 years but also there have been enormous changes in the imaging of skeletal trauma, largely the result of faster and more efficient computed tomography (CT) produced by helical CT and continued refinements in magnetic resonance imaging (MRI).

The role of CT and MRI in the assessment of trauma, in general, and skeletal trauma, in particular, continues to evolve, principally expanding and increasing in importance to the point that the availability of CT and MRI are now considered essential to the care of the seriously injured.

At the time of the first edition, in the early 1980s, CT was in its infancy, and radiography was the principal means of imaging skeletal trauma, augmented, on occasion, by planar tomography and skeletal scintigraphy. The objective was to identify or exclude skeletal fractures and dislocations.

At the time of the second edition, in the early 1990s, CT had achieved a central role in the assessment of intracerebral trauma and had shown promise in the evaluation of visceral injuries. The place of CT in the assessment of spinal, facial, and pelvic skeletal injuries had only just emerged.

Since the second edition, the implementation of helical CT has made CT essential in the evaluation of visceral injuries. And in that same period, MRI has been shown to accurately identify injuries of the soft tissue components of the musculoskeletal system: ligaments, tendons, muscles, menisci, and joint cartilage. Therefore, the role of radiology and imaging has expanded beyond bone to include all anatomic components of the musculoskeletal system.

Even more recently, MRI has been found to be able to identify subtle and otherwise obscure fractures and other traumatically induced abnormalities of bone—injuries that cannot be seen, even in retrospect, by radiography. Although the role of MRI in identifying occult hip fractures in the elderly is now generally accepted, the use of MRI in disclosing equally obscure fractures and other injuries elsewhere in the skeletal system is now under investigation and likely to emerge in the not too distant future.

No portion of the musculoskeletal system is blind to the probing eye of MRI. Not only can MRI identify obscure bony injuries but it also is able to suggest alternative diagnoses as the source of the patient's complaint. MRI can disclose fractures or bone bruises at sites other than that suspected clinically or demonstrate injuries of adjacent ligaments, tendons, muscles, or cartilaginous joint surfaces as the true source of the patient's problem.

This third edition had to reflect the reality of this imaging revolution. How best to do that posed a problem for me. As a result of all these advances in skeletal imaging, it is difficult for any one individual to have the necessary expertise in all areas; some degree of subspecialization is now required. Even given the time, it is unlikely that I could complete a timely and authoritative revision by myself.

Reluctantly, but wisely, I came to the conclusion that I must enlist some help, in fact, lots of it. And I did. I sought the aid and assistance of acknowledged experts, 29 in all, for the most part specialists in musculoskeletal imaging, to serve as coauthors for 21 of the book's 23 chapters. By far the majority of those selected are friends of long acquaintance whom I know well and admire, both personally and professionally, people who I was confident would provide the excellent, insightful, authoritative, up-to-date revision that I desired. None has failed me. All have made superb contributions, for which I am most grateful.

There have been other significant changes between this and the previous two editions, the most obvious of which is the color of the cover; green is gone, replaced by red. Red is a bold color denoting a sense of urgency. I am forever searching about the film reading rooms and the radiology section of the emergency department for misplaced copies of my book. Maybe the red cover will make them easier to find.

Writing a book is a lot of work and all authors require a lot of help. This book is no exception. My thanks to all who assisted in this effort.

First, to those at my publisher: to Lisette Bralow, Executive Editor, Medical Books, in particular for her constant encouragement, support, and willingness to listen; to Jennifer Shreiner, Developmental Editor, for her guidance through the entire process; to Rita Martello, Illustration Specialist, for her hard work on the figures; and to Mary Stermel, Production Manager, for the intelligence, craftsmanship, and attention to detail that she and her staff displayed in formatting and bringing to life the work of all these fine authors. The end result is superb!

Second, my thanks go to those who assisted me personally here in Winston-Salem. First and foremost, to Julianne Berckmann in the *AJR* editorial office who organized the entire effort, making it possible for me to keep track of all the authors and the whereabouts and status of all manuscripts—no small task, but one which she discharged with good humor and utmost efficiency. She made it seem so easy. My thanks also go to Debbie O'Rourke of the *AJR* editorial offices for her assistance with all the packaging and mailings required, to Carole Carr of the Department of Radiology at Wake Forest University School of Medicine for her secretarial assistance, and, lastly, to Ellen Henson, the photographer in the Department of Radiology, who produced so many fine illustrations for this edition.

Although I make specific mention of those who have helped me here in the Department of Radiology at Wake Forest University School of Medicine and in the editorial offices of the *American Journal of Roentgenology*, it should be realized that similarly dedicated people assisted all authors in their clerical, secretarial, and photographic needs. Collectively, this book has been a major undertaking that could not have been accomplished without the benefit of their assistance. My hat is off to all these fine people everywhere who pitched in to see that this edition came to fruition.

And last, but certainly not least, my thanks again to my wife, Donna B., for her continued support and forbearance, and particularly for her tolerance of my preoccupations. She is certainly the better half. It is hard for me to imagine being able to complete this task without her love, encouragment, and support.

It is said that the third time is a charm: I trust that will be the case with this, the third edition of *Radiology of Skeletal Trauma*.

Lee F. Rogers, MD
Winston-Salem, North Carolina

CONTENTS

Volume 1

INTRODUCTION 1

1 *GENERAL ANATOMY* 6

2 *SKELETAL BIOMECHANICS* 17

3 *EPIDEMIOLOGY OF FRACTURES* 26
with Leon Lenchik, MD

4 *IMAGING OF FRACTURES: DETECTION AND DESCRIPTION* 41
with Felix S. Chew, MD, and Ronald W. Hendrix, MD

5 *SPECIAL CONSIDERATIONS IN CHILDREN* 111
with Sam T. Auringer, MD

6 *POLYTRAUMA: THE MULTIPLE-INJURY PATIENT* 145
with Stuart E. Mirvis, MD

7 *FRACTURE TREATMENT* 180
with Ronald W. Hendrix, MD

8 *FRACTURE HEALING* 203
with Ronald W. Hendrix, MD

9 *COMPLICATIONS OF FRACTURE* 231
with Ronald W. Hendrix, MD, and Carol A. Boles, MD

10 *THE SKULL* 272
with Curtis A. Given II, MD, and Daniel W. Williams III, MD

11 *THE FACE* 315
with James T. Rhea, MD, Mark E. Mullins, MD, and Robert A. Novelline, MD

12 *THE CERVICAL SPINE* 376
with Diego Nuñez Jr., MD, MPH

13 *THE THORACIC AND LUMBAR SPINE* 453
with Richard H. Daffner, MD, FACR

14 *THE THORACIC CAGE* 541
with Eric J. Stern, MD, and Eric K. Hoffer, MD

INDEX

Volume 2

15 *THE SHOULDER AND HUMERAL SHAFT* 593
with Leon Lenchik, MD

16 *THE ELBOW AND FOREARM* 683
with T. David Cox, MD, and Andrew Sonin, MD

17 *THE WRIST* 779
with Ciaran Keogh, MB, Diane Bergin, MB, and Stephen Eustace, MB

18 *THE HAND* 874
with Carol A. Boles, MD, and Mark S. Cohen, MD

19 *THE PELVIS* 930
with Eric Brandser, MD

20 *THE HIP AND FEMORAL SHAFT* 1030
with Carol J. Ashman, MD, and Joseph S. Yu, MD

21 *THE KNEE AND SHAFTS OF THE TIBIA AND FIBULA* 1111
with Clyde A. Helms, MD, and Nancy M. Major, MD

22 *THE ANKLE* 1222
with Anthony J. Wilson, MB, ChB

23 *THE FOOT* 1319
with Mark E. Schweitzer, MD, and David Karasick, MD

INDEX

INTRODUCTION

Trauma can occur to anyone at any time. No one is immune, irrespective of age, gender, activity, or state of health. The occurrence of trauma is generally unexpected, and the recipient is often unprepared, without forewarning or premonitory sign. The individual may have been in excellent health and in every way normal immediately before the event, and in the next moment life may hang in the balance because of the injuries sustained. Injuries and death associated with high-speed auto travel have reached plaguelike proportions. Criminal activities, assaults, and beatings account for a significant proportion of all skeletal injury.[38, 44] Traumatic injuries, however, may result from all forms of human activity, including those in the home, at work, and at play.[27, 31, 36, 45, 52] Practically every human activity has a defined risk for accidental injury.[40, 48, 61, 67] Some situations leading to injury, particularly those in the industrial setting,[32, 35, 39, 54, 57, 59] lend themselves to analysis, and preventive measures can be taken to significantly reduce their occurrence. In other situations, such as auto travel, although significant factors have been defined, the preventive measures have been only partially accepted[42] (e.g., use of seat belts, reduction in speed of travel, and refraining from driving while under the influence of alcohol[34, 37, 46, 56, 60]); therefore, reduction of the injury rate has not been as dramatic as possible.

At worst an injury may result in death or in the threat of death. This fact is the tragedy of trauma. At best, the injury may cause no more than some degree of inconvenience. With modern techniques of emergency care, if the victim is in a decent state of health and survives the initial injury, there is every reason to expect survival and in most cases a return to former activities without undue limitation or restriction. This type of recovery is the expectation of the injured and the goal of the physician.

Injuries are now recognized as the leading cause of death in the United States for more than half of the human life span, from ages 1 to 43 (Fig. I–1). Motor vehicle accidents are the leading cause of death from ages 1 to 34 years.[12, 44, 53, 56, 60, 65] Injuries alone outnumber all other causes of death among children and young adults.[19] Trauma is the fourth most common cause of death, following heart disease, cancer, and stroke.[29, 30] Approximately 150,000 Americans of all ages (Fig. I–2) die from trauma each year, and about one third of these deaths occur as a result of motor vehicle accidents.[12, 13, 44, 51, 66] Thus, each year the number of deaths from motor vehicle accidents approaches the number of Americans killed during the Vietnam War.

Long the stepchild of medical interests and held in low regard in medical academic circles, trauma has only recently begun to receive the attention it deserves.[13, 15–17] Since the publication of the landmark white paper, *Accidental Death and Disability: The Neglected Disease of Modern Society,*[22] by the National Academy of Sciences in 1966, dramatic changes have occurred in the level of attention that is paid to trauma. In collaboration with others, the American College of Surgeons, Committee on Trauma devised plans and published guidelines for the establishment and regionalization of trauma care,[26] which now have been adopted in part, if not completely, by 20 or more states. In the states that have adopted the guidelines, there has been a significant impact on the care of the injured.* There is growing awareness of the need for more formal research in trauma,[64] particularly in view of its impact on the quality of life and its high cost,[21] exceeding $20 billion per annum.[24] There is some sentiment for the establishment of an Institute for Trauma at the National Institutes of Health (NIH).[20, 25] Accident prevention and minimization and the proper care of the injured are now recognized as an important contribution to life.

*See references 28, 33, 41, 43, 47, 49, 50, 55, 58, 62, 63, 64.

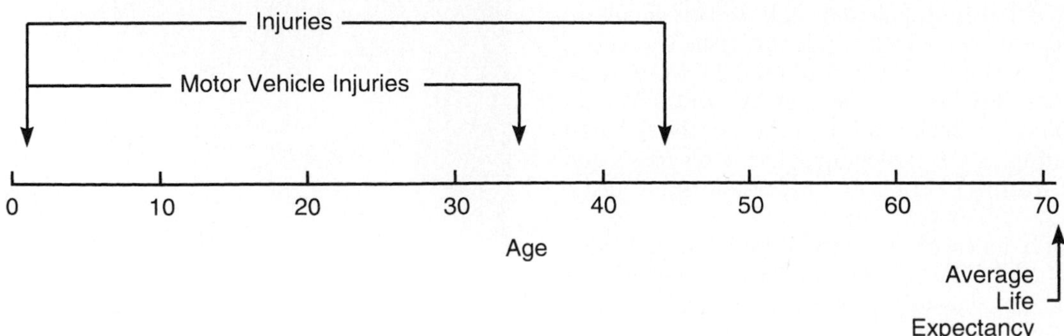

Figure I–1. The portion of the average life span during which injuries are the leading cause of death in the United States. (From Baker, S.P. [1987]. Injuries: The neglected epidemic. Stone Lecture, 1985 American Trauma Society Meeting. J. Trauma, 27:343, with permission.)

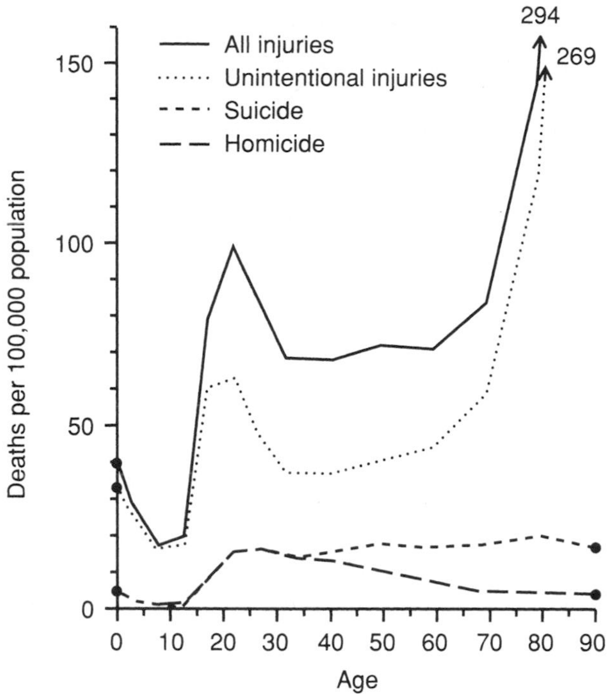

Figure I–2. Death rates in the United States for injuries by age, 1930–1980. (From Baker, S.P. [1987]. Injuries: The neglected epidemic. Stone Lecture, 1985 American Trauma Society Meeting. J. Trauma, 27:343, with permission.)

Role of Radiology

Radiographs have been used in the assessment of trauma for almost 100 years. Roentgen's discovery of the x-ray and its application to the study of the human body, particularly the skeletal system, was enthusiastically embraced by some, observed skeptically by many, and actively opposed by a few. By and large, however, the x-ray's potential in the evaluation of fractures, dislocations, and war wounds was recognized and received immediate attention.[18, 23] The discovery was made in November of 1895, reported on December 28, 1895, and published the first week of 1896. Public and professional reaction and recognition were instantaneous. The news spread rapidly and the technique was widely adopted. In 1896 alone, 1044 scientific books and articles dealing with the discovery and its uses were published. The first case of alleged malpractice for failure to take a radiograph in the evaluation of a fracture was filed in Denver on April 14, 1896.[23] X-ray equipment was dispatched with British forces to Egyptian Sudan in April 1896, and with Italian forces to Ethiopia in May 1896, and it was used in the Greco-Turkish War of 1897 and the Spanish-American War of 1898. In 1900, Carl Beck published the first book based upon the routine use of radiographs in the diagnosis and treatment of fractures.[14] In 1901, Roentgen received the Nobel Prize.

A radiograph, however, is not the most important thing in the evaluation of trauma. The initial steps in the care of the injured are a carefully performed physical examination and determination of the mechanism of the injury whenever possible. Under no circumstance is a radiograph examination to be considered a substitute for taking a history and performing a physical examination. Serious injuries commonly exist in the absence of radiographic findings. It is essential that there be careful evaluation of the airway, of the presence of shock or hemorrhage, and of open wounds. Corrective measures must be taken in each of these areas immediately. Fractures or sites of possible fracture should be noted, and splints should be applied (Figs. I–3 and I–4). Splints greatly assist in the handling of the patient and reduce morbidity in those who are seriously injured. Furthermore, they serve as an obvious expression of concern for the welfare of the patient who is less seriously injured. To the patient in an emergency room, it often seems that the prime interest is in paperwork, proof of insurance, and many other things unrelated to the injury or complaint. Every professional should be concerned about the interposition of these administrative matters between the physician and the patient. It is essential that preliminary evaluation and initial treatment, including splinting, be performed before the patient undergoes any prolonged administrative interrogation or radiographic examination.

Successful treatment of skeletal trauma begins with accurate diagnosis, which requires a well-performed and accurately interpreted radiographic examination. To plunge headlong into treatment without accurate assessment is to jump into trouble. The physician should be familiar with the common patterns of injury. Certain activities result in specific forms of injury, and certain skeletal injuries often are associated with underlying visceral

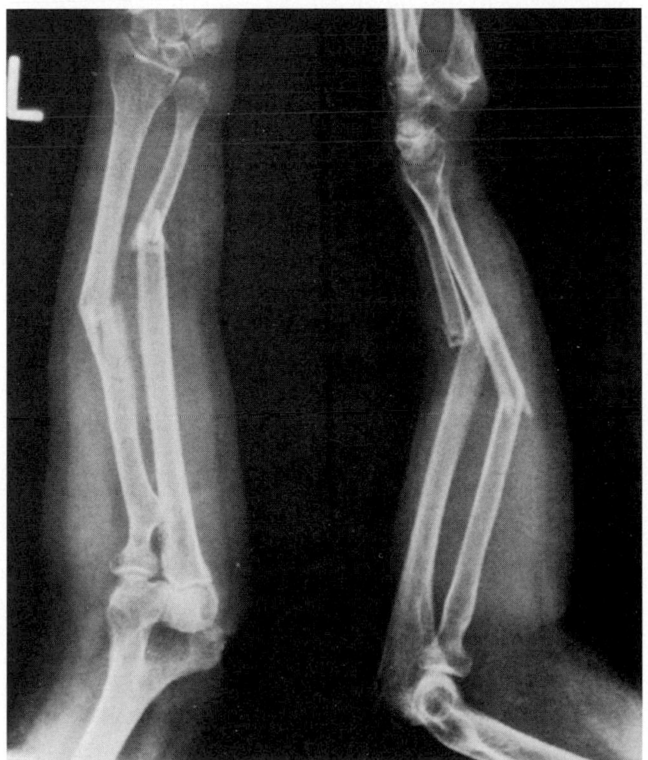

Figure I–3. Markedly angulated, minimally comminuted fracture of both bones of the forearm in an elderly woman. The examination was performed without a splint, which is regrettable. A splint would have greatly comforted the patient but certainly would not have interfered with the radiographic examination.

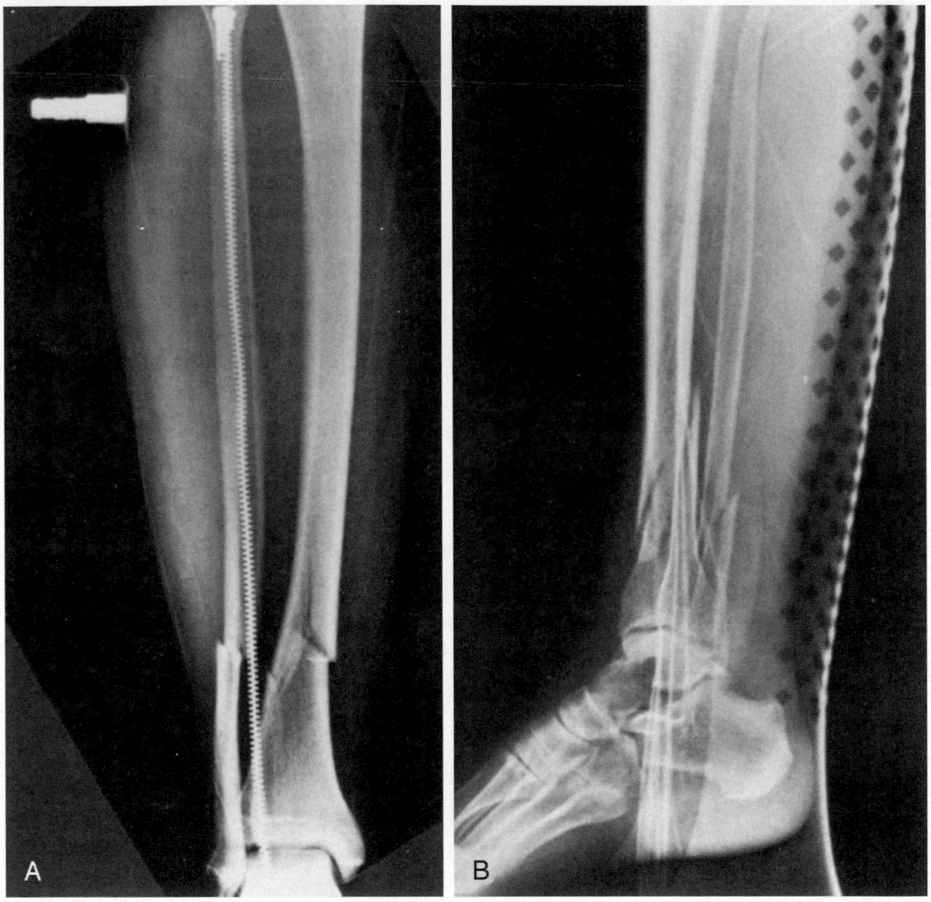

Figure I–4. Patients properly splinted prior to radiographic examination. *A,* This patient with a fracture of the distal third of the tibia and fibula was maintained in an air bag. The zipper and valve are components of the splint. *B,* Another patient with a fracture of the distal third of the tibia and fibula has been placed in a posterior aluminum molded splint. Splints that are basically radiolucent rarely interfere with demonstration of significant skeletal injuries.

injury or other skeletal injuries at remote sites, and the physician should be aware of these associations.

The initial radiographic examination should include the standard views used within the department for evaluation of the part in question. These standards have been developed because they were found to demonstrate most abnormalities. To do less than department standards would compromise the evaluation. Under no circumstances should a radiograph ever be obtained of any part in a single plane. Radiographs in two planes at right angles are the minimum, and the evaluation of bone ends and the joints often requires additional oblique views.

This book stresses the value of a directed search in the radiographic analysis of skeletal trauma. Many injuries can, of course, be identified by a simple viewing of the radiographs. The fracture or dislocation is obvious, and a diagnosis is readily established. At other times, however, the radiographic evidence of injury is subtle and may easily be overlooked. It is much more productive to look for specific features on the radiograph, to look at specific areas, and to determine the presence or absence of specific injuries than to depend on a general viewing. The search is improved by knowledge of the mechanism and circumstances of injury. This information should be available when the radiograph is being interpreted, which implies, of course, that the interpreter has some knowledge of what injuries to expect under the circumstances. Patterns of injury tend to be repetitive. Some injuries are much more common than others. Knowledge of these patterns and of the statistical frequency of injury allows a search for specific injuries—for those that are most common and therefore most likely. There are radiographic changes within the soft tissues, usually centered about joints, that serve as clues to the presence of underlying skeletal injury. The nature and reliability of these findings vary from joint to joint. However, their presence and identification may lead to the recognition of significant, though subtle injuries. A directed search in the interpretation of radiographs obtained in the evaluation of skeletal trauma leads to easier recognition, confident interpretation, and, more importantly, a correct diagnosis.

Organization of the Book

The organization of this book is regional. The basic components of the axial skeleton are discussed in separate chapters. The peripheral skeleton is organized in chapters centering on the major joints. Most trauma occurs at the end of a bone, and radiographs centered on the adjacent joint are obtained. Thus, it was thought best to discuss all of the injuries that might be disclosed by this radiograph rather than to limit the discussion to one bone or the other. Therefore, the injuries to the distal and proximal shaft as well as the joint surfaces of a bone are discussed in relation to the joint with which it is associated. Soft tissue clues to injury generally center on the joint and are equally useful for injuries to any bone encompassed by

the joint. By convention, shaft fractures are discussed in the chapter covering the proximal joint; that is, femoral shaft fractures are discussed in the same chapter as the hip.

Each chapter begins with a discussion of the pertinent radiographic anatomy of the region in question. The statistical frequency of injuries is given, and the mechanisms of injury are reviewed. The soft tissue clues to underlying bone and joint injury are presented, then each specific injury is discussed. Each chapter concludes with presentation of a systematic approach to the radiographic analysis of trauma in the region: the pitfalls, where to look if there is no obvious injury, and what else to look for if an injury is obvious. Treatment is not discussed except in very broad, general terms. Radiographic findings having therapeutic and prognostic implications are presented.

In specific skeletal injuries for which skeletal scintigraphy, computed tomography, and/or magnetic resonance imaging play a vital role, the imaging techniques are described and illustrated following a discussion of the radiographic findings. It should be recognized that the principal focus of this book is on the bony skeleton; therefore, the role of imaging in the assessment of acute skeletal injury is emphasized. No attempt is made to describe or illustrate the full range of acute and chronic injuries occurring in the supporting ligaments, tendons, joint capsules, and menisci.

In general, the use of eponyms is avoided because of the confusion surrounding their use. Many result from clinical descriptions of injuries prior to Roentgen's discovery of the x-ray in 1896. Although they were often quite accurate, they were frequently incomplete. Similarly, there are numerous classifications of almost all types of fracture in the literature. Some are used more than others, but very few are universal. Many of the original articles proposing classification are cited as references, but the fracture classifications per se are not given. Accepted classifications change with time. Most are based in part on the radiographic findings. These findings are discussed under the injury in question, although the exact classification is not used. The use of such classifications in the reporting of fractures and dislocations should be carried out with some caution. First, one is obliged to be accurate, and second, the physician who receives the report must also be fully conversant with the classification. This is not always the case, and confusion may easily result. Furthermore, one should be aware that there is considerable interobserver variability in the classification of the same injuries by multiple observers. Such studies of injuries at various sites commonly report interobserver variability in the range of 25% to 35%. This degree of variation seriously questions the day-to-day usefulness of classification systems. An exception to this general rule is the use of the Salter-Harris classification for epiphyseal injuries. This system has broad application, is generally accepted, and is therefore a convenient shorthand.

In the first section of the references to this introduction (references 1 through 11) are general texts in skeletal trauma that have been of value to me in both my education and the preparation of this book. Specific chapters from these texts are cited as references throughout the book. They represent a basic resource for anyone involved in the diagnosis and treatment of skeletal trauma.

References

1. Ballinger, W.F. II, Rutherford, R.B., & Zuidema, G.D. (1985). The Management of Trauma. 4th Ed. W.B. Saunders Co., Philadelphia.
2. Berquist, T.H. (1992). Imaging of Orthopedic Trauma and Surgery. 2nd Ed. W.B. Saunders Co., Philadelphia.
3. Gossling, H.R., & Pillsbury, S.L. (1984). Complications of Fracture Management. J.B. Lippincott Co., Philadelphia.
4. Harris, J.H., & Harris, W.H. (2000). The Radiology of Emergency Medicine. 4th Ed. Williams & Wilkins, Baltimore.
5. Heppenstall, R.B. (1980). Fracture Treatment and Healing. W.B. Saunders Co., Philadelphia.
6. Mattox, K.L., Moore, E.E., & Feliciano, D.V. (2000). Trauma. 4th Ed. Appleton & Lange, Norwalk, CT.
7. Rang, M. (1966). Anthology of Orthopaedics. Churchill Livingstone, Edinburgh.
8. Rang, M. (1983). Children's Fractures. 2nd Ed. J.B. Lippincott Co., Philadelphia.
9. Rockwood, C.A. Jr., & Green, D.P. (1990). Fractures. 3rd Ed. J.B. Lippincott Co., Philadelphia.
10. Swischuk, L.E. (1994). Emergency Radiology of the Acutely Ill or Injured Child. 3rd Ed. Williams & Wilkins, Baltimore.
11. Tachdjian, M.O. (1990). Pediatric Orthopedics. 2nd Ed. W.B. Saunders Co., Philadelphia.
12. Baker, S.P. (1987). Injuries: The neglected epidemic. Stone Lecture, 1985 American Trauma Society Meeting. J. Trauma, *27*:343.
13. Baker, S.P. (1989). Injury science comes of age. J.A.M.A., *262*:2284.
14. Beck, C. (1900). Fractures: With an Appendix on the Practical Use of the Roentgen Rays. W.B. Saunders Co., Philadelphia.
15. Cales, R.H., & Trunkey, D.D. (1985). Preventable trauma deaths: A review of trauma care systems development. J.A.M.A., *254*:1059.
16. Foege, W.H. (1987). Highway violence and public policy. N. Engl. J. Med., *316*:1407.
17. Foege, W.H., & Committee on Trauma Research. (1985). Injury in America: A Continuing Public Health Problem. National Academy Press, Washington, DC.
18. Glasser, O. (1934). Wilhelm Conrad Roentgen and the Early History of the Roentgen Rays. Charles C. Thomas, Springfield, IL.
19. Haller, J.A. Jr. (1983). Pediatric trauma: The no. 1 killer of children. J.A.M.A., *249*:47.
20. Holden, C. (1983). Pressure for trauma institute. Science, *222*:307.
21. MacKenzie, E.J., Shapiro, S., & Siegel, J.H. (1988). The economic impact of traumatic injuries. One-year treatment-related expenditures. J.A.M.A., *260*:3290.
22. National Research Council (U.S.). (1966). Accidental Death and Disability: The Neglected Disease of Modern Society. National Academy of Sciences, Washington, DC.
23. Peltier, L.F. (1953). The impact of Roentgen's discovery upon the treatment of fractures. Surgery, *33*:579.
24. Rice, D.P., Hodgson, T.A., & Kopstein, A.N. (1985). The economic costs of illness: A replication and update. Health Care Financing Review, *7*:61.
25. Roye, W.P. Jr., Dunn, E.L., & Moody, J.A. (1988). Cervical spinal cord injury: A public catastrophe. J. Trauma, *28*:1260.
26. Task Force of the Committee on Trauma. (1976). Optimal hospital resources for care of the seriously injured. Bull. Am. Coll. Surg., Sept., p. 15.
27. Saul, F.P., & Saul, J.M. (1989). Osteobiography: A Maya Example. p. 287. In Reconstruction of Life from the Skeleton. Alan R. Liss, Inc., New York.
28. West, J.G., Williams, M.J., Trunkey, D.D., & Wolferth, C.C. Jr. (1988). Trauma systems: Current status, future challenges. J.A.M.A., *259*:3597.
29. Will, G.F. (1990). The trauma in trauma care. Newsweek, March 12, p. 98.
30. Wright, F.H. (1982). Trauma research. Science, *218*:328.
31. American Academy of Pediatrics. (2000). Committee on Sports Medicine and Fitness. Pediatrics, *105*:659.
32. Brezler, G.D. (1999). Injuries in adolescent workers: Health promotion and primary prevention. AAOHN J., *47*:57.
33. Browner, B.D., Alberta, F.G., & Mastella, D.J. (1999). A new era in orthopedic trauma care. Surg. Clin. North Am., *79*:1431.
34. Butchart, A., Kruger, J., & Lekoba, R. (2000). Perceptions of injury causes and solutions in a Johanesburg township: Implications for prevention. Soc. Sci. Med., *50*:331.
35. Chen, G.X., Johnston, J.J., Alterman, T. et al. (2000). Expanded analysis of injury mortality among unionized construction workers. Am. J. Ind. Med., *37*:364.
36. Cheng, T.L., Fields, C.B., Brenner, R.A. et al. (2000). Sports injuries: An important cause of morbidity in urban youth. Pediatrics, *105*:E32.
37. Cherpitel, C.J., Giesbrecht, N., & Macdonald, S. (1999). Alcohol and injury: A comparison of emergency room populations in two Canadian provinces. Am. J. Drug Alcohol Abuse, *25*:743.
38. Cohen, L.R., & Potter, L.B. (1999). Injuries and violence: Risk factors and opportunities for prevention during adolescence. Adolesc. Med., *10*:125.

39. Conway, G.A., Lincoln, J.M., Husberg, B.J. et al. (1999). Alaska's model program for surveillance and prevention of occupational injury deaths. Public Health Rep., *114*:550.
40. Cubbin, C., LeClere, F.B., & Smith, G.S. (2000). Socioeconomic status and the occurrence of fatal and nonfatal injury in the United States. Am. J. Public Health, *90*:70.
41. Dodek, P., Herrick, R., & Phang, P.T. (2000). Initial management of trauma by a trauma team: Effect on timeliness of care in a teaching hospital. Am. J. Med. Qual., *15*:3.
42. Durbin, D.R. (1999). Preventing motor vehicle injuries. Curr. Opin. Pediatr., *11*:583.
43. Dyas, J., Ayres, P., Airey, M., & Connelly, J. (1999). Management of major trauma: Changes required for improvement. Qual. Health Care, *8*:78.
44. Gomberg, B.F., Gruen, G.S., Smith, W.R., & Spott, M. (1999). Outcomes in acute orthopaedic trauma: A review of 130,506 patients by age. Injury, *30*:431.
45. Hag, S.M., & Haq, M.M. (1999). Injuries at school: A review. Tex. Med., *95*:62.
46. Hargarten, S.W. (2000). Alcohol-related injuries: Do we really need more proof? [editorial; comment]. Ann. Emerg. Med., *33*:699.
47. Hulka, F. (1999). Pediatric trauma systems: Critical distinctions. J. Trauma, *47*:S85.
48. Judd, M.A., & Roberts, C.A. (1999). Fracture trauma in a medieval British farming village. Am. J. of Physical Anthrop., *109*:229.
49. Kivell, P., & Mason, K. (1999). Trauma systems and major injury centres for the 21st century: An option. Health Place., *5*:99.
50. Kortbeek, J.B. (2000). A review of trauma systems using the Calgary model. Can. J. Surg., *43*:23.
51. Kozik, C.A., Suntayakorn, S., Vaughn, D.W. et al. (1999). Southeast Asian J. Trop. Med. Public Health, *30*:129.
52. Lam, L.T., Ross, F.I., & Cass, D.T. (1999). Children at play: The death and injury pattern in New South Wales, Australia, July 1990–June 1994. J. Paediatr Child Health, *35*:572.
53. Li, G. (2000). Child injuries and fatalities from alcohol-related motor vehicle crashes. J.A.M.A., *283*:2291.
54. Lowery, J.T., Glazner, J., Borgerding, J.A. et al. (2000). Analysis of construction injury burden by type of work. Am. J. Ind. Med., *37*:390.
55. Mann, N.C., Mullins, R.J., MacKensie, E.J. et al. (1999). Systematic review of published evidence regarding trauma system effectiveness. J. Trauma, *47*:S25.
56. Margolis, L.H., Foss, R.D., & Tolbert, W.G. (2000). Alcohol and motor vehicle-related deaths of children as passengers, pedestrians, and bicyclists. J.A.M.A., *283*:2245.
57. McGwin, G. Jr., Scotten, S., Aranas, A. et al. (2000). The impact of agricultural injury on farm owners and workers in Alabama and Mississippi. Am. J. Ind. Med., *37*:374.
58. Nathens, A.B., Jurkovich, G.J., Rivara, F.P., & Maier, R.V. (2000). Effectiveness of state trauma systems in reducing injury-related mortality: A national evaluation. J. Trauma, *48*:25.
59. Pugh, J.K., Pienkowski, D., & Gorczyca, J.T. (2000). Musculoskeletal trauma in tobacco farming. Orthopedics, *23*:141.
60. Quinlan, K.P., Brewer, R.D., Sleet, D.A., & Dellinger, A.M. (2000). Characteristics of child passenger deaths and injuries involving drinking drivers. J.A.M.A., *283*:2249.
61. Rice, M.R., Alvanos, L., & Kenney, B. (2000). Snowmobile injuries and deaths in children: A review of national injury data and state legislation. Pediatrics, *105*:615.
62. Rogers, F.B., Shackford, S.R., Osler, T.M. et al. (1999). Rural trauma: The challenge for the next decade. J. Trauma, 47:802.
63. Sanchez, J.I., & Paidas, C.N. (1999). Childhood trauma: Now and in the new millennium. Surg. Clin. North Am., *79*:1503.
64. Templeton, J. (2000). Watson Jones Lecture. The organization of trauma services in the UK. Ann. R. Coll. Surg. Engl., *83*:49.
65. Thurman, D.J., Alverson, C., Dunn, K.A., et al. (1999). Traumatic brain injury in the United States: A public health perspective. J. Head Trauma Rehabil., *14*:602.
66. Watson, W.L., & Ozanne-Smith, J. (2000). Injury surveillance in Victoria, Australia: Developing comprehensive injury incidence estimates. Accid. Anal. Prev., *32*:277.
67. Young, C.C., & Niedfeldt, M.W. (1999). Snowboarding injuries. Am. Fam. Physician, *1*:131. (Published errata appear in Am. Fam. Physician, *59*:786 and *60*:404.)

Chapter 1
GENERAL ANATOMY

The skeleton is the hard, bony framework of the body. It is commonly divided into two components, the appendicular (the skeleton of the limbs) and the axial (the skeleton of the head and trunk). The skeleton is usually studied in the dried state, which in many ways can be misleading, because the drying process eliminates the marrow content and many of the mechanical properties of living bone. Furthermore, all of the associated nonosseous components are removed—cartilage, ligaments, muscles, and joints. When the skeleton is studied in its disjointed dried state, the full integration of the locomotor components of the body and their functional nature are difficult to conceive.

Bone is the only tissue in the body that differentiates continuously, remodels internally, and regenerates completely after injury. A coherent picture of the physiologic regulation of bone formation is lacking, so how these processes are accomplished at the molecular, cellular, and tissue levels is not yet entirely known.[1, 15]

In the living state bone is a blend of hard inorganic salts and resilient organic components.[12] The inorganic salts represent a mineral reservoir for the metabolic pathways of the body. The combination of the two components gives the body a structure that can withstand tension and compression and at the same time offers sufficient rigidity to allow locomotion. The marrow contained within the bone serves as the source of the cellular elements of the circulatory system. The skeleton, therefore, is in reality far removed from what it seems on initial examination in the anatomy laboratory. In the laboratory it is difficult to imagine the skeleton's viability, its actual mechanical properties, and its vital role in metabolism and hematopoiesis.

The radiographic examination of the skeleton in many ways can produce the same misconceptions obtained in the anatomy laboratory. A radiograph of a bone is a static image chiefly of the inorganic salts the bone contains. Although a radiograph gives an excellent representation of a bone's morphology, it gives little or no hint of its physiology or of the nature of its internal contents. Furthermore, there is only a very rudimentary outline of the associated muscles, tendons, ligaments, joint cartilage, and other significant soft tissue components of the skeletal system. Although these soft tissues, as well as cartilage, are visualized by computed tomography (CT) (see Fig. 1–2*B*) and magnetic resonance imaging (MRI) (see Fig. 1–12), they remain as static images of morphology and are largely "silent" as to the physiology of the musculoskeletal structures displayed.

Classification of Bone

All bones consist of an outer shell of compact bone. The space within the shell is the medullary cavity. The medullary cavity is filled with bony trabeculae interspersed with marrow. Bones may be conveniently divided into three types[4, 6, 17]: long, flat, and irregular. *Long bones* (Fig. 1–1) have an elongated tubular shaft containing a central medullary cavity and expanded articular ends. The shaft of the bone is the *diaphysis,* the flared or expanded portion of the shaft is the *metaphysis,* and the end of the bone is the *epiphysis.* The bony cortex is thickest in the

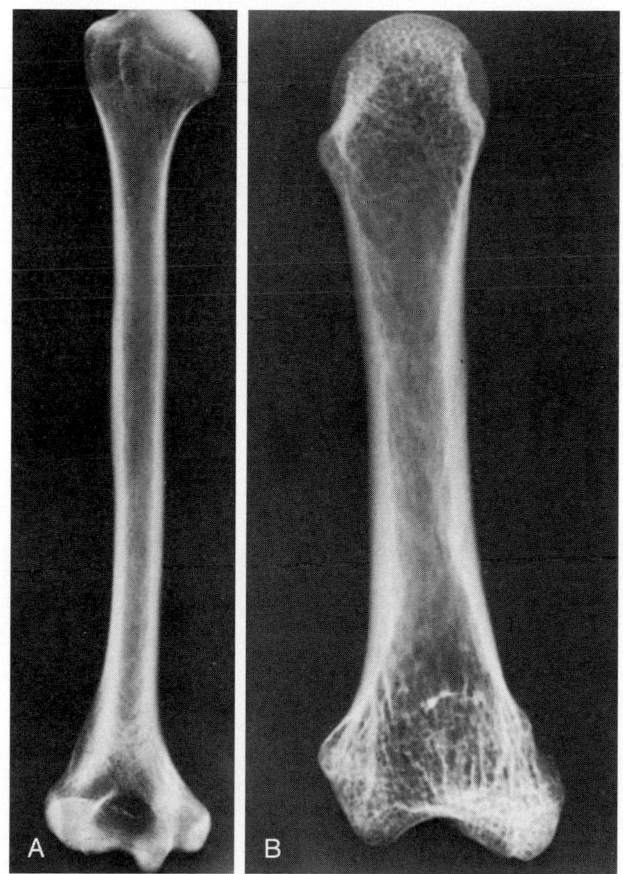

Figure 1–1. Long bones. These are characterized by elongated tubular shafts containing a central medullary cavity and expanded articular ends. The cortex is thickest in the midshaft, or diaphysis, and thinnest in the metaphysis and articular margins. Bony trabeculae are more prominent in the end of the bone than in the diaphysis. *A,* Humerus. *B,* Second metacarpal. Although the second metacarpal is shorter, the overall configuration is strikingly similar to that of the humerus.

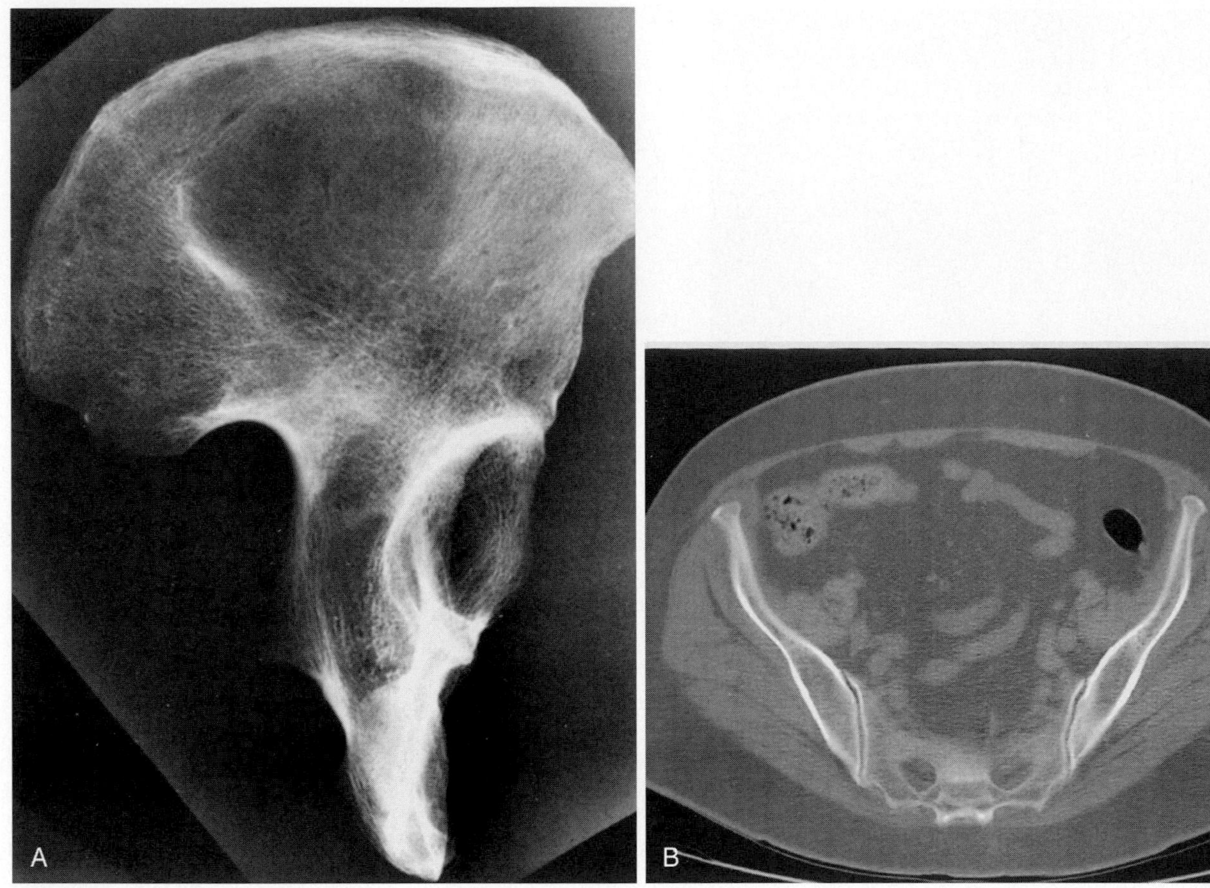

Figure 1–2. Flat bones. The innominate bone of the pelvis consists of two closely apposed sheets of cortical bone separated by a thin medullary cavity composed of spongy bone. *A,* On a radiograph the trabeculae of the medullary cavity are clearly visualized, but the cortex appears thin. *B,* On CT scan the soft tissues are clearly depicted. Note the sacroiliac joints.

diaphysis, and it gradually tapers in the metaphysis. The cortical bone in the epiphysis is characteristically thin. Generally, more bony trabeculae are found in the end of the bone than in the diaphysis. These bony trabeculae form a crisscrossing network and are thought to be aligned along the lines of stress in accordance with Wolff's law, which states that anatomic form follows function.

Long bones might be better described as tubular bones because the category includes not only the obvious bones, such as the femur and the humerus (see Fig. 1–1*A*), but also the metacarpals (see Fig. 1–1*B*) and the phalanges. Although short by comparison, these bones have the same general outline as their longer counterparts.

The *flat bones* (Fig. 1–2) generally consist of curved sheets of two apposed layers of cortical bone separated by a thin medullary cavity composed of spongy bone. Flat bones include the skull, the scapula, and the pelvis. These bones are not actually flat; platelike or sheetlike is a more appropriate description.

Irregular bones (Fig. 1–3) are bones that do not fit into either of the previous categories. They include chiefly the carpal and tarsal bones. Irregular bones are obviously irregular in outline and are composed of a cortex of more or less uniform thickness with a central medullary cavity of spongy bone. The sesamoid bones are classified as irregular bones. Sesamoid bones are somewhat irregular, more or less circular, or ovoid nodules. Most measure a few millimeters in their greatest diameter, but the largest, the patella, measures several centimeters. Sesamoids are almost always contained within tendons in close relation to articular surfaces. The surface of the sesamoid is covered with articular cartilage, as is the surface of the apposing bone.

Composition of Bone

Bone tissue consists of a ground substance or matrix in which there are embedded fibers impregnated with bone salts.[4, 12] In mature bone tissue, approximately 20% of the weight of the matrix is water. Organic materials form one third and mineral salts form two thirds of the dry weight of bone. The main organic component (90% to 95%) is collagen, a mucopolysaccharide, in combination with protein. The water content decreases and the mineralization increases with age, up to the sixth or seventh decade. The organic content remains unchanged. Organic matrix that is as yet uncalcified is known as osteoid matrix.

Mature bone is composed of two kinds of tissue: *compact bone,* which is dense in texture like ivory; and *trabecular, spongy,* or *cancellous bone,* which consists of a meshwork of trabeculae in which intercommunicating spaces are easily visible (Fig. 1–4). The compact bone is always

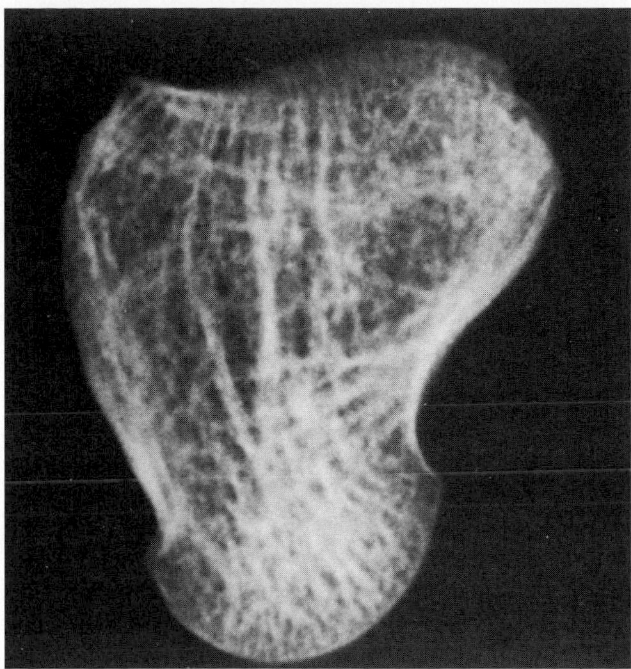

Figure 1–3. Irregular bone. The capitate of the carpus is irregular in outline, the cortex is thin, and the trabeculae within the medullary cavity are clearly visible.

on the exterior surrounding the spongy bone. Relative quantities and architecture characteristically vary for each bone. The cylinder of compact bone forming the shaft encloses a large central medullary or marrow cavity that communicates freely with the intertrabecular spaces of the expanded bone ends. These spaces are lined in their entirety by a highly vascular tissue, the endosteum, and are filled with bone marrow, either hematopoietic or adipose, with the character of the marrow varying with the age and region of the bone concerned. Compact bone is permeated by many blood vessels and, except for its cartilage-covered articular surfaces, is enclosed in a mem-

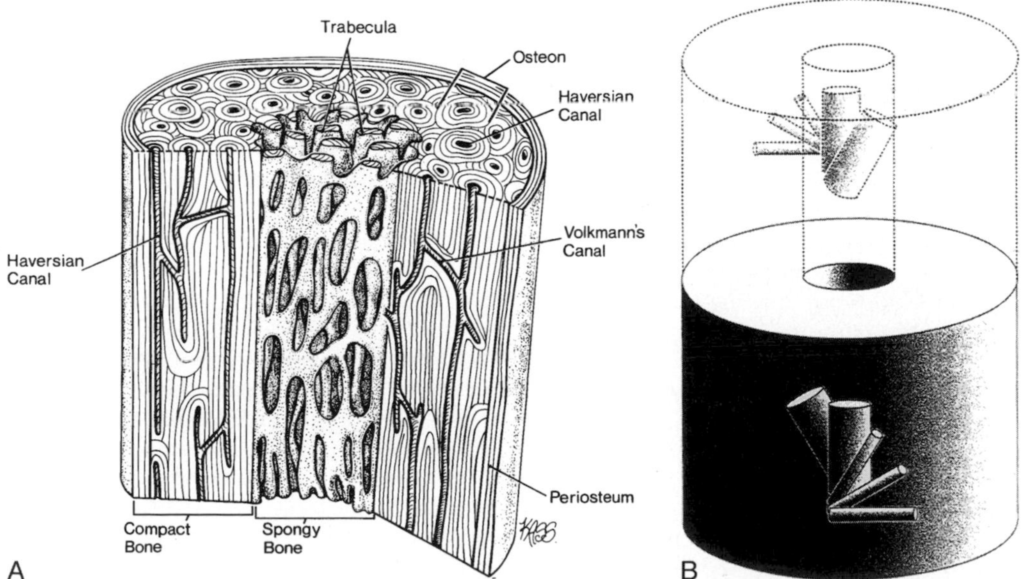

Figure 1–4. *A,* Mature bone. Compact or cortical bone encircles a central cavity, the medullary cavity, consisting of spongy or cancellous bone made up of bony trabeculae interspersed with marrow. The compact bone consists of a number of irregular cylindrical units termed the *haversian system.* A central haversian canal contains the neurovascular bundle and is surrounded by concentric lamellae of bone tissue. Each haversian canal and its lamellae are termed *osteon*. The haversian canals are interconnected by small channels, Volkmann's canals. The osteocytes reside in lacunae between the lamellae but are not depicted here. The periosteum covers the surface of the bone. *B,* Schematic of a single osteon showing the changing direction of the fibrils in successive lamellae about the central haversian canal. (*A,* Adapted from Warwick, R., & Williams, P.L. [1973]. Gray's Anatomy. 35th British Ed. W.B. Saunders Co., Philadelphia, with permission. *B,* From Liu, D., Wagner, H.D., & Weiner, S. [2000]. Bending and fracture of compact circumferential and osteonal lamellar bone of the baboon tibia, Journal of Material Science: Materials in Medicine, *4d*:60, with permission.)

brane, the periosteum. In young bones the periosteum is thick and very vascular; in older bones it is thin and less vascular.

Compact bone consists of a number of somewhat irregular cylindrical units termed the *haversian system.* This system consists of a central haversian canal containing a neurovascular bundle; the canal is surrounded by concentric lamellae of bony tissue.[5, 9] Each lamella is composed of parallel mineralized collagen fibrils. The orientation of the fibrils changes in each successive lamellae about the haversian canal (see Fig. 1–4*B*). The collagen fibrils within the lamellae are mainly longitudinal and form a spiral about the haversian canal. The pitch of the spiral differs in successive lamellae. The resultant layering and varied directions of the fibrils have been compared to plywood.[16] Between these lamellae are small spaces termed *lacunae,* which are in turn connected with each other and with the central haversian canal by many fine radiating channels called *canaliculi.* The lacunae contain the osteocytes, and the canaliculi contain the fine cytoplasmic extension of these bone cells. Because of this regular structure, normal adult bone is termed *lamellar bone.*

Vascular Supply of Bone

The vascular supply[6, 8, 14] of a long bone (Fig. 1–5) consists of several discrete points of arterial inflow that feed variable networks within the bone. These networks in turn drain into venous channels that leave the bone through all its surfaces except those covered by articular

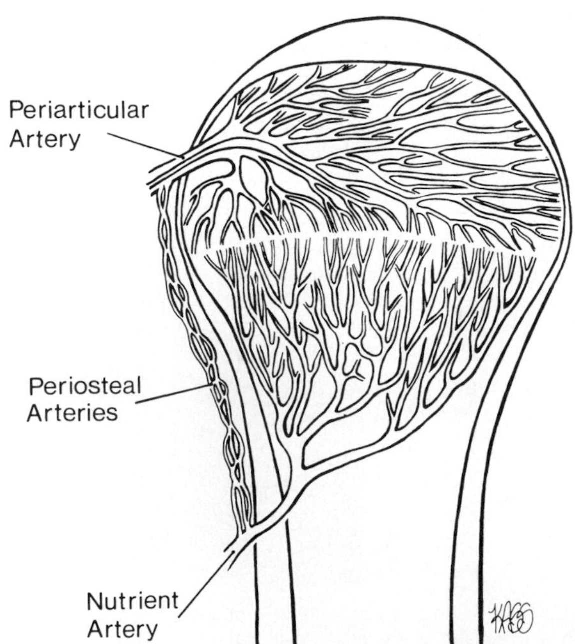

Figure 1–5. Vascular supply of mature bone. The end of the bone is supplied by numerous small periarticular arteries arising about the joint. One or more nutrient arteries pierce the cortex to supply the diaphysis and metaphysis. Usually additional metaphyseal arteries arise from systemic arteries at the end of the bone. (Adapted from Warwick, R., & Williams, P.L. [1973]. Gray's Anatomy. 35th British Ed. W.B. Saunders Co., Philadelphia, with permission.)

cartilage. One or two principal nutrient arteries course through the shaft of the long bone obliquely. Their sites of entry and angulation are very constant, and characteristically the vessels point away from the dominant growing end of the bone. There are exceptions, however. Once within the bone, the nutrient artery extends into ascending and descending branches within the medullary cavity. Near the ends these branches are joined by numerous metaphyseal arteries. The metaphyseal arteries pass directly into the bone from systemic vessels. Epiphyseal arteries arise from periarticular vessels and supply the end of the bone. There are numerous vascular foramina near the bone ends through which these arteries may enter. Most foramina contain thin-walled veins, however. The epiphyseal and metaphyseal nutrient arteries are quantitatively much more important than the diaphyseal supply in most bones. Short bones receive numerous fine blood vessels from their periosteum.

Large, irregular, flat bones, such as the scapula, receive a superficial blood supply from the periosteum and are also provided with large nutrient arteries that penetrate directly into the cancellous bone. Both systems anastomose freely. The flat bones of the skull are supplied by numerous vessels from the periosteal layers.

Ossification

Bone is formed by two principal methods[3, 4, 6, 10, 11]: intramembranous and endochondral or intracartilaginous ossification. In the *intramembranous* method, ossification is preceded by formation of a fibrocellular model of the future bone. Ossification then occurs by direct differentiation of the mesenchymal cells into osteoblasts, which lay down a network of bone trabeculae. The bone deposition expands centrifugally to replace the original fibrous model.

In *endochondral* or *intracartilaginous* ossification, the bones are preceded by formation of rods or masses of cartilage. Within these preformed cartilaginous masses an orderly sequence of changes occurs with the appearance of centers of ossification. There are two types of centers of ossification: primary and secondary.

Primary Centers of Ossification

Primary centers of ossification appear within the center of the future diaphysis during fetal development. In the fetus the ends of most long bones and the small irregular bones of the tarsus and carpus remain in the cartilaginous state. Endochondral ossification begins in the center of the preformed cartilaginous bone. The cartilaginous cells first become enlarged and vacuolated, and the intervening matrix becomes thin. The cells then undergo progressive degenerative changes and die. Their thin-walled remnants become calcified. The area is then invaded by osteoblasts, which line the calcified matrix with osteoid, the uncalcified precursor to bone. The osteoid in turn becomes calcified, and the calcified cartilage is resorbed. This process of ossification proceeds centrifugally from the primary center. The perichondrium around the periphery

of the cartilage mold is transformed into periosteum. The deep layer of the periosteum proceeds to form bone by direct osteogenesis of the intramembranous variety. This periosteal ossification accounts for the increase in the cortical thickness of bone.

The bone first laid down[6] is spongy in texture and contains a continuous labyrinth of large vascular spaces; the lacunae are irregularly scattered, and there is no lamellation. The collagen fiber bundles in the matrix are randomly arranged and form a network. This type of bone is called *woven bone* or *fibered bone.* It is found in young fetal bone and during repair of fractures. These concentric layers of nonlamellated parallel woven bone are termed *atypical haversian systems* or *primary osteons.* As the bone matures, the woven bone is replaced by typical haversian systems or secondary osteons. Their formation is always preceded by erosion. A fundamental feature of bone growth is that it proceeds exclusively by appositional mechanisms in which new layers of bony tissue are simply added sequentially to preexisting surfaces.

Secondary Centers of Ossification

Secondary centers of ossification occur within the cartilage at each end of long bones, but usually they occur only at one end of a short bone. At birth only the distal femoral and occasionally the proximal tibial ossification centers are present. The remaining ossification centers appear in chronologic sequence, depending on the sex of the individual and on hormonal and nutritional influences. Growth ceases, and the growth plates of the appendicular skeleton are closed in most bones by 20 years of age in

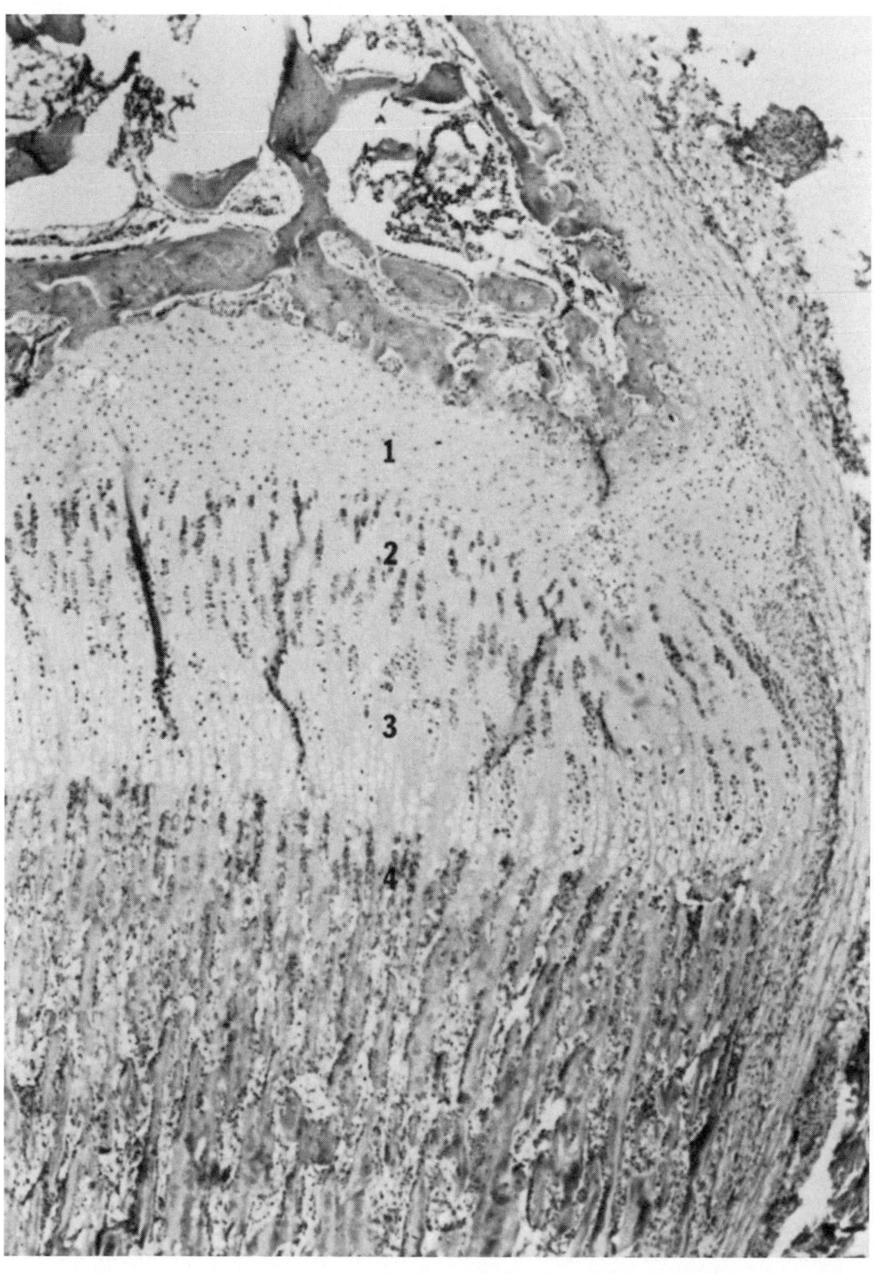

Figure 1–6. Cartilaginous growth plate of the distal ulna of a rabbit. A growth plate or physis consists of four zones of cartilage: the resting zone (1), immediately adjacent to the epiphysis; the zone of proliferation (2), consisting of flat cells arranged in columns; the hypertrophic zone (3), consisting of vesicular or vacuolated cells; and the zone of provisional calcification at the metaphysis (4).

the male and 17 years of age in the female. The last ossification center to close is the medial clavicular epiphysis. This center closes between 20 and 25 years of age in men and women. A fine sclerotic line, the epiphyseal scar, remains as evidence of the epiphyseal line for varying periods after its closure.

Ossification in the secondary centers proceeds by endochondral ossification. The cartilage between the secondary and primary centers of ossification is known as the cartilaginous growth plate or epiphyseal line (Fig. 1–6). It is this structure that is responsible for the longitudinal growth of bone. It consists of four distinct zones of cartilaginous tissue in longitudinal secretion. The first zone, adjacent to the ossification center, is a zone of small resting or mother cells. The second is a zone of flat cells arranged in columns, the proliferating cells. The third zone consists of vesicular or hypertrophic cells, and it is a zone of swollen vacuolated cells maintaining the columnar arrangement. The fourth zone is that of provisional calcification at the metaphysis.

The blood supplies of the metaphysis and epiphysis in growing bone are separate (Fig. 1–7). The metaphysis is centrally supplied by branches of the nutrient artery and numerous small branches of periosteal arteries originating from the diaphysis at its periphery. The vascular supply of the epiphysis consists of several periosteal vessels that arise from larger arteries around the joint. Thus, with this dual arrangement the epiphyseal arteries supply nourishment for cartilaginous growth, whereas the metaphyseal arteries nourish ossification.

The dual blood supply of the epiphysis is present at all secondary ossification centers with the exception of those at the proximal femur and possibly those at the proximal radius. In these situations the entire ossification center and distal metaphysis are intracapsular in location. Thus, the periarticular arteries, which under normal circumstances pass directly into the epiphysis, are forced to course along the metaphysis and cross the growth plate before entering the epiphysis. Although there is an arterial supply furnished through the ligamentum teres in the hip, this supply alone is insufficient to sustain growth in the ossification center and the adjacent growth plate.

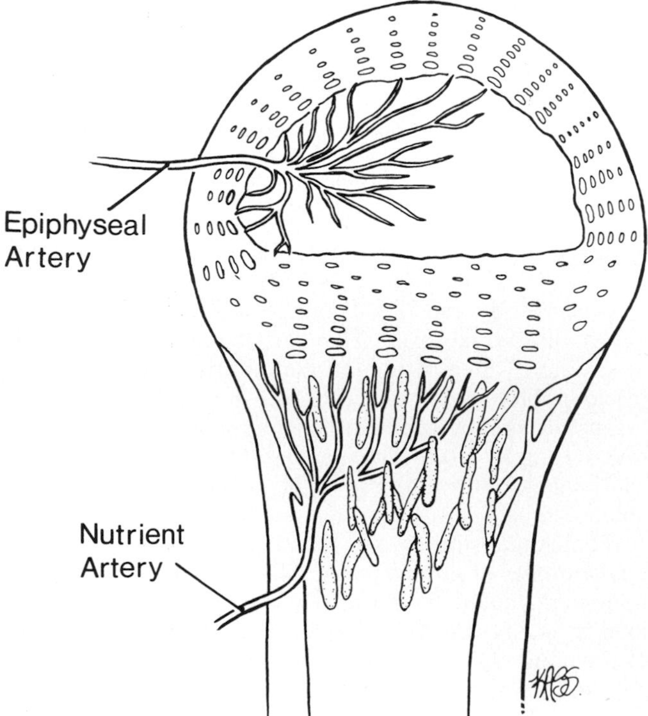

Figure 1–7. Vascular supply of growing bone. The epiphysis and metaphysis are supplied separately. Epiphyseal arteries arise about the joint and nourish cartilaginous growth, whereas metaphyseal arteries arise from the nutrient artery and nourish ossification within the metaphysis.

New cartilage is formed in the primary zone adjacent to the ossification center,[6] and each cell passes through the orderly sequence of the zonal arrangement to ultimately die and have its remnants calcified in the zone of provisional calcification. A layer of primary osteons on this calcified shell forms woven bone. These osteons are subsequently partially resorbed or in part incorporated into primary haversian systems or secondary osteons, the basic structural element in mature bone. All remodeling of bone is dependent on an ordered balance between bone deposition on some surfaces and bone removal from others. The overall shape of the bone is maintained by a delicate balance between periosteal and endosteal deposition and resorption.

There is a wide range in appearance times[7] of the secondary ossification centers, depending on sex, race, and nutrition. Furthermore, there may have been a significant change in the appearance times over the past 70 years in the United States, which may be related to changes in nutrition. In any event, the standards that are used must be applicable to the population under examination. The times of appearance and fusion of secondary ossification centers as determined by Hansman[7] of the Child Research Council are charted in Figure 1–8. Based on a study of Americans in 1960, Hansman's results form an acceptable American standard.

In the context of trauma the concern is not so much the appearance time of the secondary ossification centers as the sequence of their appearance. Despite the variability in the appearance time of the centers, the sequence of appearance is constant: The distal femoral secondary ossification center is always the first to appear and is followed by the proximal tibial secondary ossification center. In the complex epiphyseal sequence at the elbow, the capitellum is always the first to appear, followed by the medial epicondylar ossification center. It is this sequence and the general contour of the secondary ossification centers that concern those who interpret radiographs obtained for the evaluation of trauma in children and adolescents.

The secondary ossification centers may represent only a small portion of the skeletal structure at the end of the bone. The secondary center appears within a mold of cartilage, and cartilage is radiolucent and therefore not visualized on the radiograph (Fig. 1–9). This fact is particularly important at the elbow because of the frequency of injury at that joint in young children, in whom a considerable portion of the distal humerus is still in the cartilaginous state.

At birth there are no ossification centers present at the end of the bone, with the exception of the distal femur

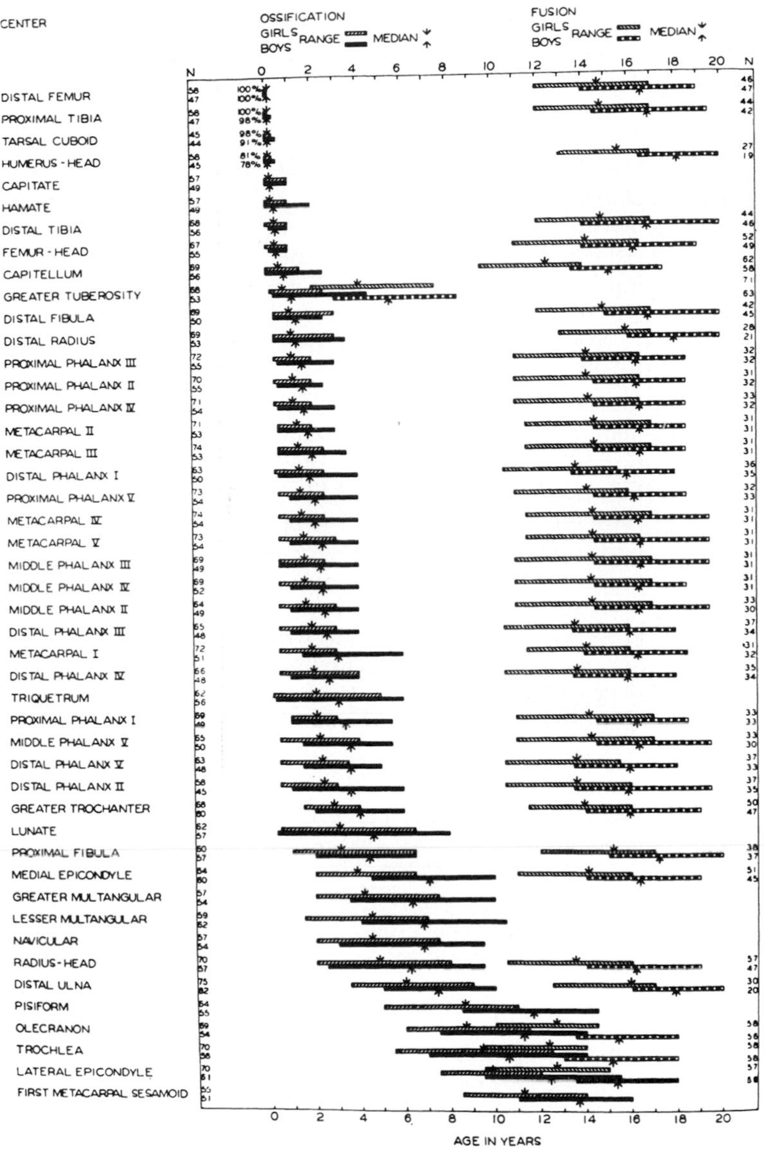

Figure 1–8. Ages at ossification and fusion of secondary skeletal centers. Bar diagrams represent the ranges over which the skeletal ossification centers appeared and fused. Shown are the range for girls (*upper bar*), the range for boys (*lower bar*), and the median age of ossification or fusion of each center (*arrows*). The centers are listed in order of the median age of appearance in girls. The figures at the beginning or end of each bar are the number of children in that group. (From Hansman, C.F. [1962]. Appearance and fusion of ossification centers in the human skeleton. A.J.R. Am. J. Roentgenol., 88:476, with permission. © [1962] American Roentgen Ray Society.)

or occasionally the proximal tibia[7]; therefore, the entire end of most bones is cartilaginous. This fact is important to keep in mind when interpreting radiographs of newborns who may have sustained birth injuries.

There are two basic types of epiphyses or secondary ossification centers: the pressure epiphysis and the traction epiphysis or apophysis (see Fig. 1–9*B*). *Pressure epiphyses* are located at the ends of long bones, and their apposing surfaces serve as the articulation for joints. The associated epiphyseal plates contribute to the longitudinal growth of long bones. It is the growth plate of cartilaginous tissue, and not the secondary ossification center at the end of the bone, that is responsible for longitudinal growth. *Traction epiphyses* or *apophyses* are nonarticular centers of ossification that serve as attachments for tendons and ligaments, and they are particularly common in the pelvis and at the hip. Growth of the traction apophysis contributes to the shape of the bone but not to the length of the bone. Apophyseal centers follow an orderly sequence of appearance and fusion times, just as the pressure epiphyses do.

Joints

Joints are the functional connections between different bones of the skeleton. They are commonly classified[4] according to their structural composition and degree of motion: fibrous joints (synarthroses; Fig. 1–10), which are essentially immovable; cartilaginous joints (amphiarthroses; see Fig. 1–10), which are slightly movable; and synovial joints (diarthroses; Fig. 1–11), which are freely movable.

The cranial sutures (see Fig. 1–10) are the most obvious examples of *fibrous joints.* The margins of the cranial bones are united by a thin layer of fibrous tissue. The joint is made essentially immobile by the interdigitation of the apposing margins of bone that essentially locks the adjacent bones together. The cranial sutures do vary, however, from the interdigitation seen in the parietal sutures to the fine serrated margins of the coronal suture and the oblique, roughened margins of the squamosal suture. The inferior tibiofibular articulation is another example of a fibrous joint. The two bones are united by

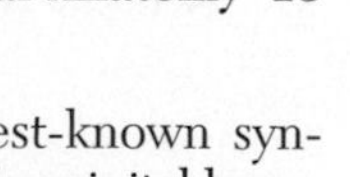

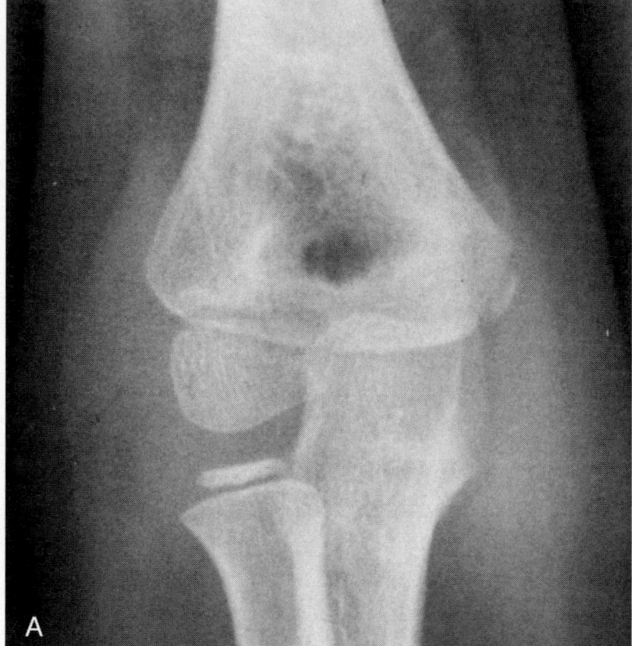

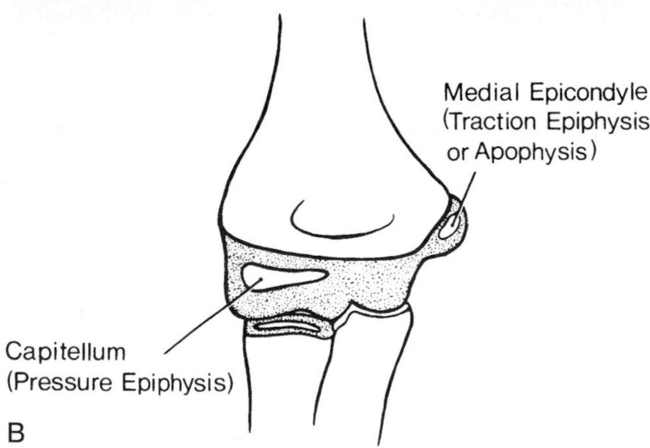

Figure 1–9. *A,* Radiograph of the elbow of a 6-year-old boy. *B,* Diagram of the radiograph in *A.* Most of the distal joint margin of the humerus consists of cartilage (*stippled area*), which can be seen by comparing the diagram with the radiograph. The largest secondary ossification center is the capitellum, which apposes the ossification center for the radial head. These centers are both pressure epiphyses. The medial epicondylar ossification center represents a traction epiphysis or apophysis. It does not participate in the formation of the joint surface but serves as the attachment of the pronator-flexor tendon of the forearm musculature and the ulnar collateral ligament of the elbow joint.

interosseous ligaments. This form of articulation is termed a *syndesmosis.*

Cartilaginous joints (see Fig. 1–10) are a form of articulation in which the contiguous bony surfaces are united by cartilage. The most common form is a *symphysis,* in which the contiguous bony surfaces are connected by a flattened disc of fibrocartilage, as in the articulation between the bodies of the vertebrae (the intervertebral disc) or the two pubic bones (the pubic symphysis). A *synchondrosis* is a temporary cartilaginous union between two bones that is later converted into bone. The junction between the secondary and primary ossification centers of a long bone is a synchondrosis. The best-known synchondrosis is between the sphenoid bone and occipital bone. Another is between the petrous portion of the temporal bone and the jugular process of the occipital bone.

Most of the joints of the body are *diarthrodial* (see Fig. 1–11) or *synovial joints* allowing free movement of the apposing surfaces. In this form of articulation, the apposing margins of the bone are covered with articular cartilage, connected by ligaments, and lined by a synovial membrane. The joint may be partially or completely divided by an articular disc or meniscus (Fig. 1–12). A complete articular disc creates two joints in series. The peripheral margin of the disc is attached to the joint capsule. A complete fibrocartilaginous disc occurs in the sternoclavicular and the inferior radioulnar joint. The term *meniscus* should be reserved for an incomplete disc, such as what occurs in the knee and occasionally in the acromioclavicular joint. The disc in the temporomandibular joint may be complete or incomplete.

A *labrum* is a fibrocartilaginous annular lip, usually triangular in cross section, attached to the margin of an articular surface. Labra are found in the glenoid fossa and in the acetabulum. They tend to deepen the socket of the joint, thus adding to the area of contact between the articulating bony surfaces.

The bones of a synovial joint are held together by a fibrous capsule consisting of connective tissue. There are frequently two or more localized thickenings in which the constituent fibrous bundles are generally parallel to one another. These thickenings are the ligaments of the joints, and they are named according to their position or attachment. In some joints the capsule is reinforced or partially replaced by the tendons or by expansions from the tendons of neighboring muscles. In some joints there are accessory ligaments located outside the capsule or intracapsularly within the joint.

The synovial membrane lines all of the nonarticular parts of synovial joints. The membrane secretes the synovial fluid, which lubricates the joint surfaces. This fluid superficially resembles egg white.

The articulating ends of the bone are covered[6, 13] by hyaline cartilage (Fig. 1–13), which provides an extremely smooth, wear-resistant surface when bathed with synovial fluid. The cartilage varies from 1 to 7 mm thick, with smaller joints having thinner cartilage. The deep surface of the cartilage is molded to the shape of the underlying bone, and the free surface is smooth and modifies the general surface geometry of the bone. The articular cartilage shows a gradual zonal variation in its microscopic structure. In the first, or superficial, zone the cells are small and more or less parallel to the surface. The cells of the second zone are larger and more rounded. In the third zone the cells are larger, rounded, and arranged in columns perpendicular to the surface. In the fourth zone the deepest part of the cartilage forms a calcified stratum that abuts cortical bone. The junction between the third and fourth zones, or between noncalcified and calcified cartilage, is known as the *tidemark.*[2] The tidemark is not present in children, but it is found in those of advanced age. The articular cartilage lacks intrinsic vascularity and derives its nutrients by diffusion from the vessels of the synovial membrane, the synovial fluid, and blood vessels

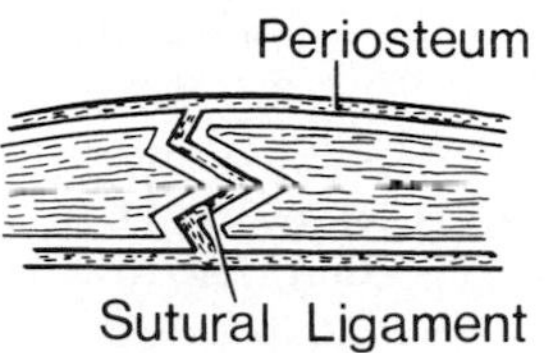

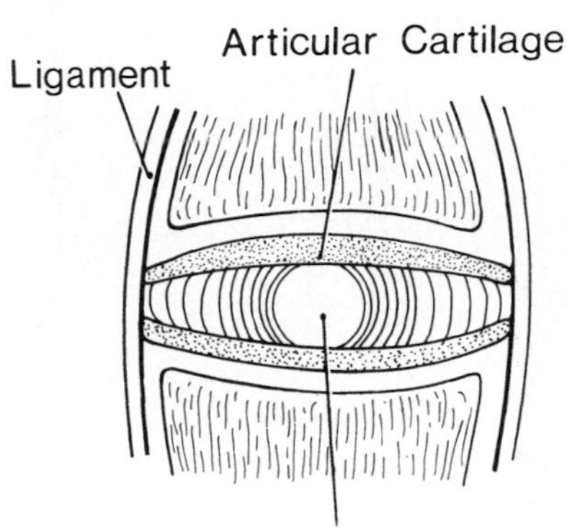

Figure 1–10. Synarthrodial and amphiarthrodial joints. A synarthrodial joint is a fibrous joint—two bones united by intervening fibrous tissue, such as the cranial sutures. An amphiarthrodial joint is a cartilaginous joint—two bones united by cartilage, such as the intervertebral disc and the pubic symphysis. (Adapted from Goss, C.M., Ed. [1995]. Gray's Anatomy. 38th American Ed. Lea & Febiger, Philadelphia, with permission.)

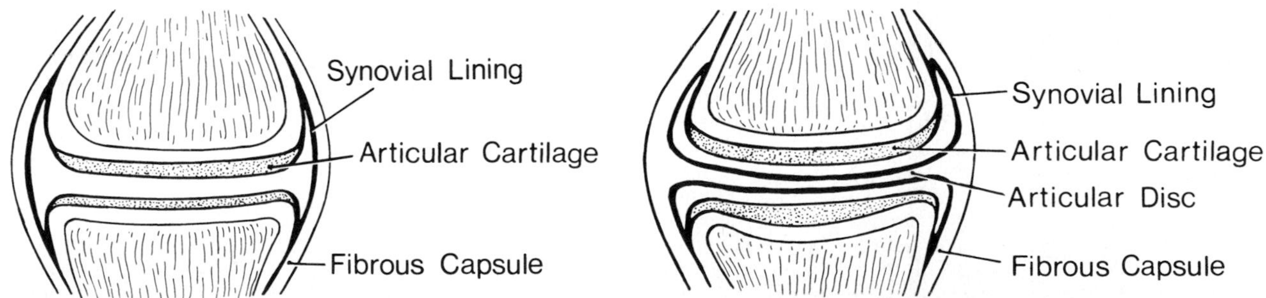

Figure 1–11. Diarthrodial or synovial joints. The apposing margins of the joint are covered by articular cartilage; the joint space is lined by a synovial membrane and surrounded by a fibrous capsule. Some diarthrodial joints are divided by an articular disc of fibrocartilage. (Adapted from Goss, C.M., Ed. [1995]. Gray's Anatomy. 38th American Ed. Lea & Febiger, Philadelphia, with permission.)

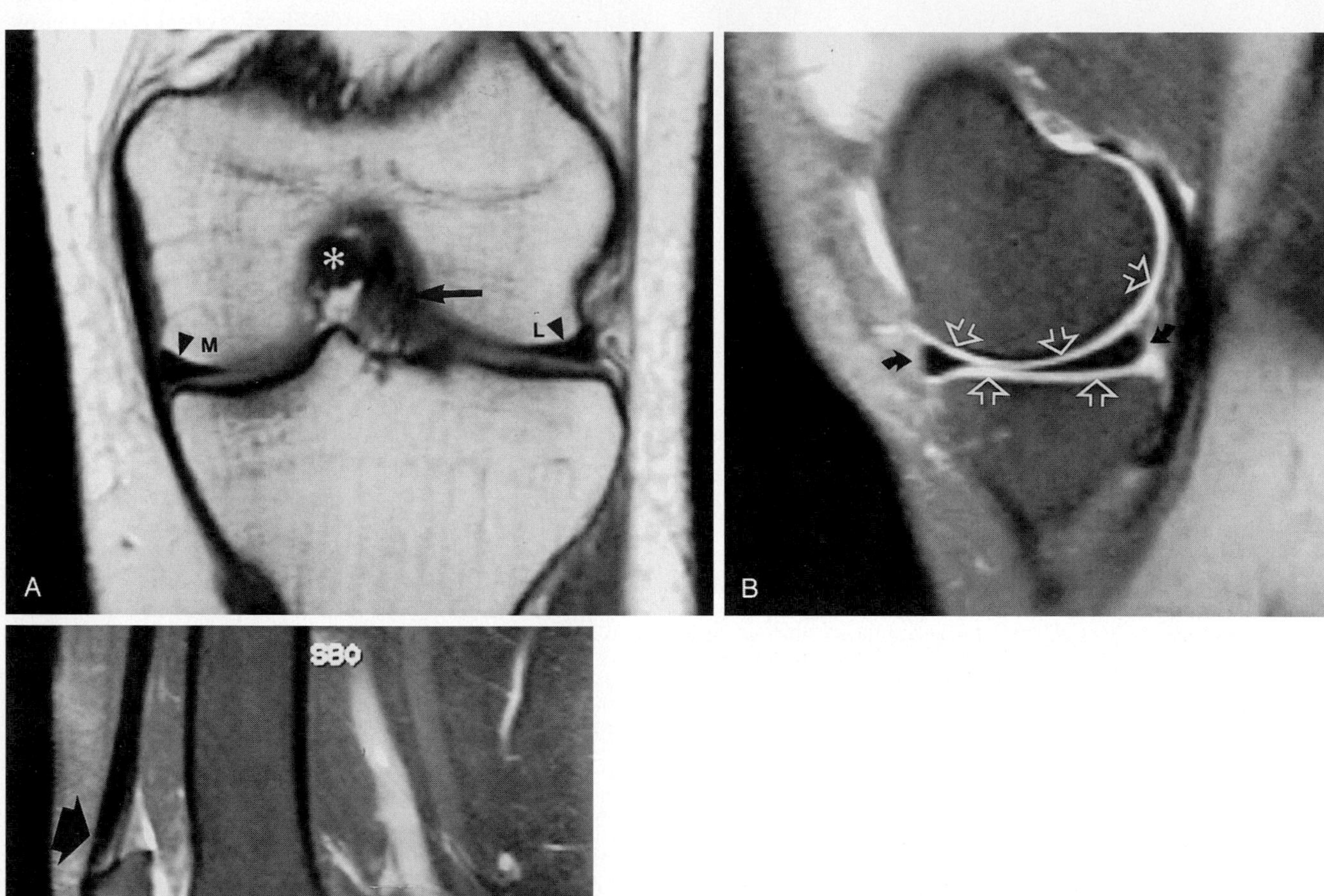

Figure 1–12. Magnetic resonance imaging of the left knee. *A,* Coronal, T_1-weighted image showing medial (M) and lateral (L) menisci (*arrowheads*) and posterior (*asterisk*) and anterior (*arrow*) cruciate ligaments. *B,* Sagittal proton density image showing medial meniscus (*dark arrows*) and bright signal of articular cartilage (*open arrows*). *C,* Sagittal proton density image showing quadriceps (*dark arrow*) and infrapatellar tendons (*open arrow*).

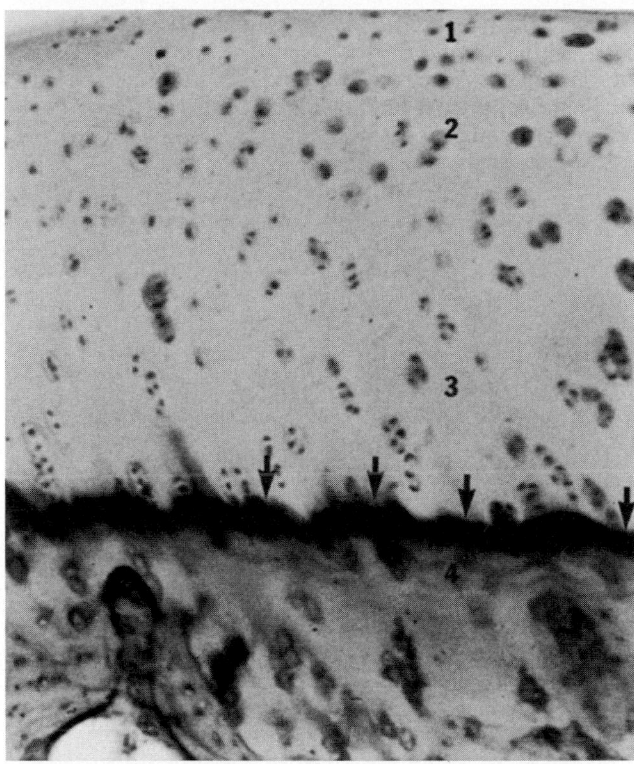

Figure 1–13. Photomicrograph of joint cartilage in an adult. In the superficial zone (1) the cells are small and parallel to the surface. The underlying cells in the second zone (2) are larger and more rounded. The cells of the third zone (3) are arranged perpendicularly to the surface. In the fourth zone (4) the cells are calcified and abut on cortical bone. The junction between the third and fourth zones—between noncalcified and calcified cartilage—is the tidemark (*arrows*).

underlying the marrow cavity. Most nutrients are derived from synovial fluid, with the joint cartilage functioning as a sponge. Fluid is squeezed from the cartilage when the cartilage is compressed and absorbed when the cartilage is released. Cyclic pressure is applied and released during joint motion. Thus, motion is required to maintain the nutritional status of joint cartilage. Growth potential of hyaline cartilage is limited.[13] Mitotic figures are infrequently identified even in young skeletons. The articular cartilage is free of nerve endings and therefore is insensitive, an important consideration in shearing injuries of the joint surface. Furthermore, there is very little capacity to repair injury,[13] which, in part, accounts for the seriousness of fractures that involve the joint surfaces. The articular cartilage appears to atrophy throughout life, and its surface becomes slightly irregular with some shredding of the superficial layer.

Ligaments and Tendons

Ligaments and tendons are attached to bone at their origins and insertions by an interweaving of their collagenous fibrils with those of the periosteum. This attachment is strengthened further by fibrils termed *Sharpey's fibers,* which extend from the ligaments and tendons through the periosteum into the substance of the underlying cortical bone. It is likely that avulsions of cortical bone accompanying injuries to tendons and ligaments are due to the firm anchorage provided by Sharpey's fibers. Tendons most commonly tear at their insertions, and tears are often accompanied by an avulsion of a small portion of the adjacent cortex; less commonly they tear at the musculotendinous junction, but rarely do they tear within the substance of the tendon itself. Similarly, ligaments may tear at their origin or insertion, and these tears may be associated with the avulsion of a variably sized fragment of adjacent bone. Unlike tendons, however, ligaments are equally likely to tear within the substance of the ligament itself.

References

1. Bilezikian, J.P., Raisz, L.G., & Rodan, G.A. (1996). Principles of Bone Biology. Academic Press, San Diego.
2. Bullough, P.G., & Jogannath, A. (1983). The morphology of the calcification front in articular cartilage. Its significant in joint function. J. Bone Joint Surg. [Br.], *65*:72.
3. Crelin, E.S. (1981). Development of the musculoskeletal system. Clin. Symp., *33*:2.
4. Goss, C.M., Ed. (1995). Gray's Anatomy. 38th American Ed. Lea & Febiger, Philadelphia.
5. Hall, B.K. (1992). Bone: Volume 1, The Osteoblast. p. 351. CRC Press, Boca Raton.
6. Ham, A.W. (1987). Histology. 9th Ed. J.B. Lippincott Co., Philadelphia.
7. Hansman, C.F. (1962). Appearance and fusion of ossification centers in the human skeleton. A.J.R. Am. J. Roentgenol., *88*:476.
8. Hughe, S.P.F., McCarthy, I.D., & Hooper, G. (1986). The vascular system in bone: Its importance and relevance to clinical practice. Clin. Orthop., *210*:31.
9. Parfitt, A.M. (1994). Osteonal and hemi-osteonal remodeling: The spatial and temporal framework for signal traffic in adult human bone. J. Cell Biochem., *55*:273.
10. Raisz, L.G., & Kream, B.E. (1983). Regulation of bone formation. (First of two parts). N. Engl. J. Med., *309*:29.
11. Raisz, L.G., & Kream, B.E. (1983). Regulation of bone formation. (Second of two parts). N. Engl. J. Med.,*309*:83.
12. Report of the Task Group on Reference Man. (1975). III. Skeleton, cartilage, nonskeletal dense connective tissue (tendons, fascia, periarticular tissue) and teeth. I.C.R.P. Publication 23. p. 62. Pergamon Press, Oxford.
13. Simon, W.H., Friedenberg, S., & Richardson, S. (1973). Joint congruence. J. Bone Joint Surg. [Am.], *55*:1614.
14. Trueta, J., & Cavadias, A.X. (1955). Vascular changes caused by the Küntscher type of nailing. J. Bone Joint Surg. [Br.], *37*:492.
15. Urist, M.R., DeLange, R.J., & Finerman, G.A.M. (1983). Bone cell differentiation and growth factors. Science, *220*:680.
16. Weiner, S., Traub, W., & Wagner, H.D. (1999). Lamellar bone: Structure-function relations. J. Struct. Biol., *126*:241.
17. Williams, P.L., & Bannister, L.H. (1995). Gray's Anatomy. 38th British Ed. Churchill Livingstone, New York.

Chapter 2

SKELETAL BIOMECHANICS

From a medical viewpoint a fracture is defined as a disruption in the continuity of bone. From a mechanical viewpoint a fracture is defined as a failure in structure resulting from excessive loading and energy absorption. A study of biomechanics is very helpful in understanding the underlying biologic and mechanical factors involved in the production of a traumatic injury to the skeletal system. The biologic factors are related to the various gross and microscopic components of the system, whereas mechanical factors are related to the various forces and their resolution. It is the result of the interplay between and the resolution of these two factors that is encountered in the clinical setting as traumatic injury. As physicians, we do not view the actual interplay; instead we are presented with the end result of this interaction. Knowledge of the components in the system and their reaction to forces allows one to reconstruct the mechanism of injury. This reconstruction is helpful not only in the diagnosis or in the determination of the full extent of the injury but in the treatment of injury. An adage states that reduction of a fracture should reverse the mechanism of injury. The adage might be expressed algebraically as: Skeletal Structure × Mechanism of Injury (Forces) = Injury. Knowledge of any two components in this equation allows prediction of the third.

The musculoskeletal system is a composite structure at both the macroscopic and microscopic levels, as are all biologic systems. Macroscopically it is composed of bone, joints, ligaments, muscle, and tendons, and it is encased in skin. The architecture, or manner in which the structures are assembled, varies greatly according to position within the body. Microscopically the system is composed of haversian systems, osteons of various types, periosteum, endosteum, and marrow. These structures or components vary in their characteristics with age.[11, 13, 39] To view a single structure in isolation without consideration of other components could be misleading. However, it is quite instructive to view each structure in the abstract to determine its particular characteristics and to recognize its contributions to and the interplay between the components to build an understanding of the whole.

Mechanical Factors in Fracture

When a force is applied to an object, the object changes or distorts.[12, 14, 18, 20, 25, 27, 40] Such a force is termed a *stress,* which is measured as load per unit area. The change or distortion is termed a *strain,* which is the ratio of the change in the dimension in question (e.g., length, width, or angulation) relative to the original dimension. Strain is a dimensionless quantity. This stress-strain relationship[12, 14, 35] may be expressed graphically (Fig. 2–1). Initially, the resultant strain is directly proportional to the force applied; thus, the initial portion of the curve forms a straight line. This zone of proportionality is the *zone of elastic deformation.* In this region, when the load is removed, both the stress and the strain disappear and the object immediately returns to its original dimension. The object is said to be elastic, and the strain is termed an *elastic strain.* The slope of this straight portion (σ/E) is called the *elastic modulus*. It is a measure of the quality of stiffness. The more stress required to deform an object, the greater the degree of stiffness.

Beyond the straight portion the curve begins to bend. The point at which the bending occurs is the yield stress and yield strain of the object. Beyond this point the stress is no longer proportional to the resultant strain; a relatively small degree of stress, or small force, results in a larger degree of strain or deformity than was present previously. Furthermore, in this portion of the curve, when the stress is removed the object is unable to return to its initial shape, and there is a residual deformity or strain. This type is a *plastic strain,* and this portion of the curve is termed the *zone of plastic deformation.* It is a measure of the quality of hardness. The greater the force required to deform an object, the greater the degree of hardness. With continued application of stress a point is reached beyond which the object can no longer withstand

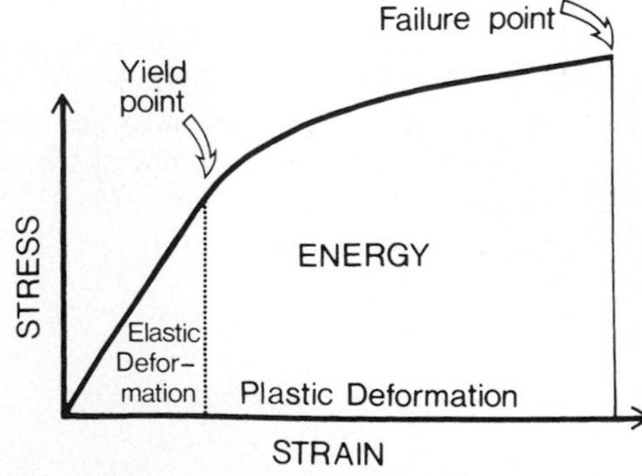

Figure 2–1. Stress-strain curve. Initially, the resultant strain is directly proportional to the force or stress applied. This is the zone of elastic deformation. Beyond the yield point the stress is no longer proportional to the resultant strain. This is the zone of plastic deformation. At the failure point the object can no longer withstand the strain, and a fracture occurs. (Adapted from Renner, R.R., Mauler, G.G., & Ambrose, J.L. [1978]. The radiologist, the orthopedist, the lawyer, and the fracture. Semin. Roentgenol., *13*:7, with permission.)

the effect of the resultant strain, and the object is disrupted or fractured. This is termed the *failure point.* The point at which failure occurs defines the ultimate stress to which the object can be subjected and the ultimate strain that it can withstand. The area under the curve up to a particular strain is a measure of the work required to achieve that strain or deformity. The area under the entire curve is a measure of the energy that may be absorbed before fracture or failure occurs.

Elastic behavior results from the straining of bonds between atoms of the object or material, whereas plastic behavior results from slippage between layers of atoms and molecules within the object or material. The character of the response divides materials into two classes: brittle and ductile.[14] *Brittle materials* break in or just beyond the zone of elastic deformation, whereas *ductile materials* exhibit considerable plastic deformation before failure or fracture occurs.

The effect that a force has on an object depends on the manner in which the force is applied. There are five major types of force to be considered (Fig. 2–2). *Tension* or *tensile* forces tend to stretch an object. *Compression* or *compressive* forces tend to compact an object. *Shear* or *shearing* forces slide one portion of an object over another. *Rotation* or *torsion* forces twist an object. *Angulation* or *bending* forces tend to curve or increase the curve of an object; bending places the convex side of the object in tension and the concave side in compression.

Most materials respond differently to each type of force.[29] This property is referred to as anisotropy. Bone is strongly anisotropic; therefore, the stress-strain curve in bone varies according to the nature of the force applied. Brittle materials, such as concrete, ceramic, or bone salts, are able to withstand greater compressive forces than tensile forces by a factor of more than 2.[12] Ductile materials, such as copper, plastic, or collagen, by contrast, are much stronger in tension than in compression.

Almost all biologic materials exhibit differences in deformity based on the rate at which the deforming force is applied.[1–3, 25, 27, 43] The differences are reflected in the stress-strain curve for each force, depending on the rate of application. This characteristic is termed *viscoelasticity,* and materials having this property are said to be *viscoelastic.*[10, 12, 27] More energy can be absorbed at a higher rate of application, which generally appears as increased tolerance to stresses with only a slight increase in tolerance to strain; that is, there is relatively a much greater increase in ultimate stress than ultimate strain at the point of fracture or failure on the stress-strain curve. Another characteristic of viscoelastic properties is the dissipation of energy with each cycle of stress.[27] There is a difference in shape between the loading and unloading phases of a stress-strain curve (Fig. 2–3). The loading curve is convex upward, and the unloading curve is convex downward. This property is known as *hysteresis*. The area between the two curves represents an energy loss with each cycle, with the energy presumably dissipated in the form of heat. The practical importance of this finding is unknown in relation to the single application of a force to the musculoskeletal system, but it could conceivably be a factor in the production of failure when considering cyclic or repeated application of stress,[9, 12, 43] which is the case in stress or fatigue fractures (see Fig. 4–26).

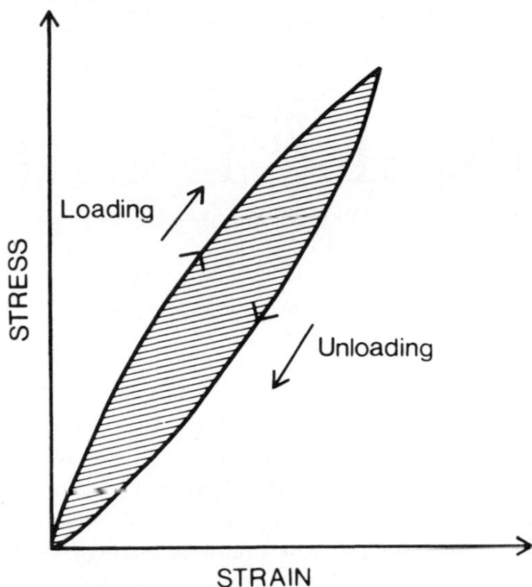

Figure 2–3. Hysteresis, a characteristic of viscoelastic materials. The energy between the loading and unloading curves is lost, presumably dissipated in the form of heat. This loss is probably of importance in cyclical stresses resulting in stress or fatigue fractures. (Adapted from Currey, J.D. [1970]. The mechanical properties of bone. Clin. Orthop., 73:210, with permission.)

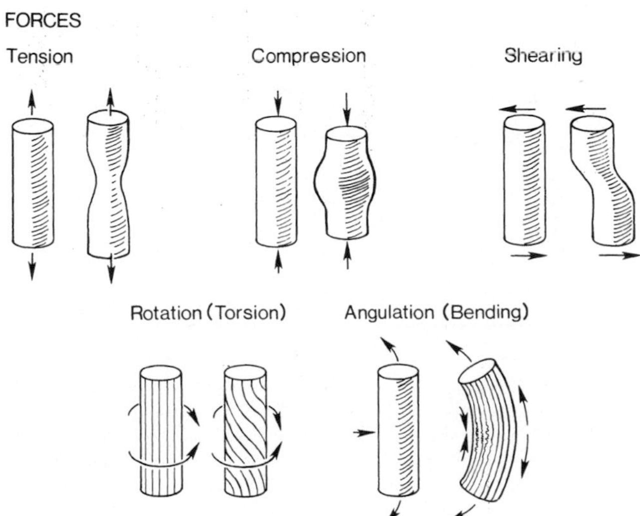

Figure 2–2. Five major types of force involved in fracture production.

Microcracking and Fatigue Phenomena. Bone, like many other materials, is subject to the phenomenon of fatigue: gradual deterioration and eventual failure when subjected to periodic or cyclical stresses. Fatigue damage in the form of microcracking is a normal phenomenon, the result of physiologic loading conditions in normal life, which leads to bone remodeling and adaption.[24, 31, 38] Fatigue strength decreases significantly with age,[37, 39] and this loss of strength plays a role in the increased incidence of fractures in those with osteoporosis.

When bone is repetitively loaded, with loads within the preyield region of the stress-strain curve, its mechanical properties gradually degrade over time[40] (see Fig. 4–26). This degradation is fatigue. The reduction in mechanical

properties is attributed to the formation of small cracks within the bony structure. As loading continues these cracks grow and coalesce until, ultimately, the bone fails catastrophically (i.e., the bone fractures). The fatigue strength of bone, as for most composite materials, is far less than its static strength, allowing failure to occur at loads far below those that would normally cause fracture. For materials that cannot repair themselves, unlike bone, the resistance to fatigue failure is a function of resistance to crack initiation and resistance to crack growth. Materials that resist the initiation of microcracks often cannot effectively resist the growth or extension of cracks, whereas those in which cracks start easily usually are more resistant to crack growth. Many highly fatigue-resistant materials derive their properties from their resistance to crack growth rather than their resistance to crack initiation. Bone is one such material. The lamellar structure of bone gives it a "grain" similar to wood,[23, 40] and the lamellar structure of bone has been likened to plywood[42] (Fig. 2–4). Cement lines around osteons are known to promote crack arrest, and crack propagation is inhibited by increased numbers of osteons.

During cyclic loading of bone, initially there is a loss of stiffness coincident with the appearance of microcracks.[36] Within the first 25% of bone's fatigue life, stiffness loss stabilizes, and no further loss occurs until just before failure. Crack growth generally does not cause immediate deterioration in the properties of the bone because crack branching and secondary cracking ahead of the front of main crack growth relieve stress concentrations at the crack tip and extend the fatigue life.[38] This stress relief occurs because of the larger surface area of the primary crack and because the crack tends to be blunted by plastic flow at its tip. In the last 10% of bone's fatigue life, stiffness decreases rapidly as the growing cracks reach critical size and coalesce, resulting in catastrophic failure, a frank fracture.[36]

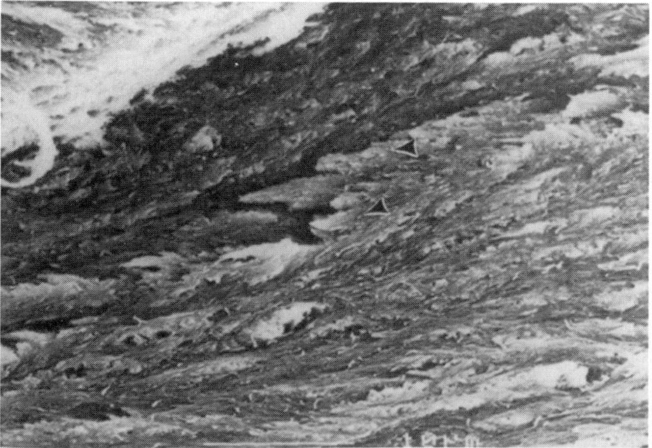

Figure 2–4. Scanning electron micrograph of the fracture surface of a cortical lamellar bone specimen. Several layers of differently aligned mineralized collagen fibril arrays are seen (*arrowheads* point to two layers). (From Liu, D., Wagner, H.D., & Weiner, S. [2000]. Bending and fracture of compact circumferential and osteonal lamellar bone of the baboon tibia. Journal of Materials in Medicine, *11*:49, with permission.)

Biologic Factors in Fracture

The shape of the stress-strain curve for any composite structure is determined by the sum total or combination of the response of each of its component parts.[12] In bone this is essentially the combination of the response of the mineral substance (a brittle material) and collagen (a ductile material). The resultant composite curve is dependent on the relative amounts of each of these components, and it has been found to vary not only with the age[11, 13] of an individual but from bone to bone[7] within the same skeleton. There is also a variation in response to different stresses between bones[17, 44]; that is, a bone such as the femur reacts differently to compression than it does to tension. Specimens taken from the human femur have been found to be weaker in tension than specimens from the tibia and fibula. Ko[21] determined that the tensile strengths in different bones from strongest to weakest were radius, fibula, tibia, humerus, and femur, with the tensile strength of the tibia being 17% higher than that of the femur. Almost the reverse sequence was reported by Yokoo[44] for compression strength, with the femur being strongest, followed by the tibia, fibula, humerus, radius, and ulna. There are even small differences depending on the site within the bone from which the specimen was taken. Additionally, it must be recognized that most of these studies were performed on thin, machined specimens[8, 11, 26] of a given dimension and not to whole bone[28, 32] with its surrounding supporting structures, as is encountered in the clinical situation. Furthermore, there is variation in response depending on whether the bone was wet or dry, live or embalmed, and because of other variables in the experimental model. Nevertheless, information derived does lend considerable understanding to the factors existing in the clinical setting.

In vitro experiments using machined specimens of cortical bone suggest that bone strength is partly related to the ratio of primary to secondary osteons[12] it contains; the larger the proportion of secondary osteons, the weaker the bone. This larger proportion of secondary osteons is the result of continued remodeling of bone throughout life and a real increase in the total number of osteons, all of the additional ones being secondary osteons by definition. There is evidence of a slight decrease in bone strength in specimens of human cortical bone older than 60 years of age.[4, 13] It should be kept in mind that these determinations are based on examination of a machined specimen of cortical bone a few millimeters thick. The results do not take into account the known decrease in cortical thickness resulting from osteoporosis. Thus, age appears to effect a qualitative change in bone as well as a quantitative change from osteoporosis that contribute to weakening of the bone. The magnitude of the loss in strength occasioned by the quantitative loss of bone as a result of osteoporosis far outweighs the contribution of any qualitative change of aging in the decreased strength of bone with aging. There are other significant changes, such as diminished agility, coordination, and strength of the supporting tissues, that add significantly to the increased susceptibility to fracture in the older population.

Production of Fracture

The site of initiation of a line of fracture is determined by the distribution of the applied forces[12] and by factors in the bone itself that are as yet not precisely determined.[15, 22] It is known from studies of nonbiologic materials that surface defects tend to serve as a focus for stresses and for the initiation of lines of failure that then extend or propagate through the material as a fracture. There are naturally occurring defects in the surface of bone—the vascular canals—that could conceivably serve as this point of focus, but that idea is conjectural. Following the initiation of a fracture it is propagated along the lines of stress imposed by the applied forces. The course of the resultant fracture is then dependent on the type and magnitude of the applied forces. Thus, in the clinical setting, the type, direction, and magnitude of a fracturing force can be inferred from the radiographic appearance of the resultant fracture (Fig. 2–5).

The forces creating a fracture may be directly applied to the bone at the site of fracture, or they may be transmitted indirectly by forces applied to some portion of the body, resulting in a fracture at a point in the skeleton remote from the site of application. These forces are termed, respectively, direct and indirect.

Indirect Forces

Most fractures are caused by indirectly applied forces acting at some point remote from the ultimate site of fracture.[12, 30] Furthermore, a combination of forces are usually at work simultaneously. The course of the fracture line, therefore, reflects the type and magnitude of force or combination of forces. In addition to tension, rotation, or bending there is usually a compressive force of weight bearing or axial loading present that to some extent modifies the fracture line from that encountered in the laboratory situation.

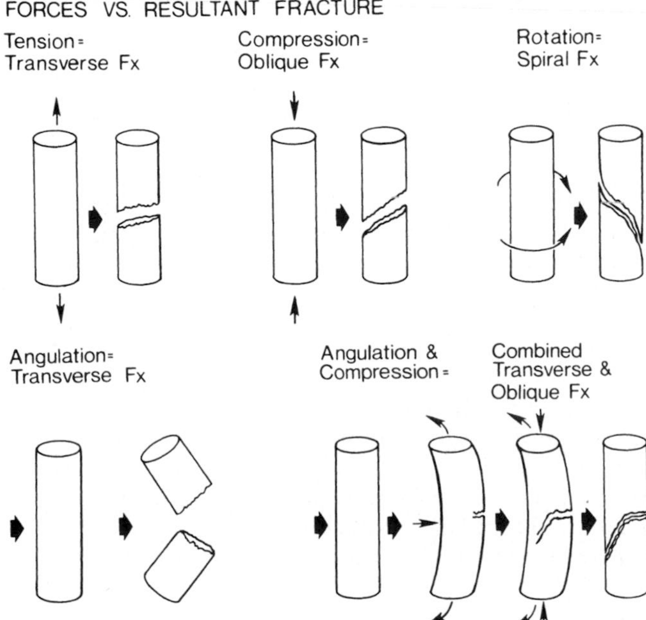

Figure 2–5. Characteristic lines of fracture created by specific types of force. Fx, fracture.

Fractures sustained by tension forces (see Fig. 2–5) are characteristically transverse. These forces are most frequently operative in ankle injuries. Because the ankle is either inverted or everted, tension is created by the pull of the lateral or medial ligaments, resulting in a transverse fracture of either the lateral or medial malleolus. Pull or traction of the quadriceps mechanism may result in sufficient tension to create a transverse fracture of the patella. Similarly, the triceps may cause a transverse fracture of the olecranon. It is difficult to generate sufficient traction or tension on the shaft of a long bone to result in a fracture; therefore, pure tensile forces are infrequently operative in shaft fractures.

Fractures sustained by rotational forces (see Fig. 2–5) are characteristically spiral. Such fractures are frequent in the long bones, particularly the humerus and femur. The torque or torsion placed on the shaft generates a complex of tensile, compressive, and shear stresses and strains.[5] The tensile stresses are oriented at 45 degrees from the long axis of the shaft and are greatest at the surface and zero at the long axis. Compressive stresses are greatest at 180 degrees to the tensile stresses and are also greatest at the surface and zero at the long axis. Both longitudinal and transverse stresses are created. The resultant fracture therefore is spiral oriented at approximately 45 degrees to the long axis of the bone.

Fractures of the shaft in long bones are rarely the result of pure compressive force as generated by axial loading. When bone is loaded in this manner the hard shaft of the bone is driven into the cancellous end of the bone, resulting in comminuted fractures of the metaphysis and joint surface. If a column or pillar[41] is loaded in this manner it fails by a linear fracture at an angle of approximately 45 degrees. The axial compressive forces are resolved into tangential shearing forces, and the shear stresses are maximized at this angle.

Fractures sustained by angulation or bending of bone (see Fig. 2–5) result in transverse fractures of the shaft. As the bone is angulated or bent, tension stress is placed on the convex side and compressive stress is placed on the concave side. A neutral plane of zero stress occurs at some level between the two. Bone is more resistant to compression than tension[12]; therefore, a fracture (crack) appears in the part under the greatest tensile stress on the surface of the convex side. The initial crack diminishes the cross-sectional area, increasing the tensile stress on the remainder, and thus the fracture spreads across the bone, resulting in a transverse fracture. In practice there may be some degree of splintering of the bone on the compression side before the transverse fracture is completed.

Fractures sustained by a combination of angulation and compression (see Fig. 2–5) result in a fracture line composed of two components, a transverse and an oblique fracture of approximately 45 degrees; the extent or contribution of each component relates to the magnitude of the forces involved. The resultant fracture may be considered curved. The compression force may have been insufficient by itself to cause failure but is amplified

by angulation. Bending diminishes the compression forces on the convex side but increases them on the concave side. Simultaneously it places the convex side in tension. The initial failure is likely due to tension creating a transverse fracture of crack on the convex side. The cross-sectional area is reduced and the compression forces are magnified, and the fracture is completed by an oblique line of fracture as a result of the shearing stresses generated by compression. The proportion of the transverse to the oblique component of the fracture line is determined by the relative magnitude of the tension and compression forces. As the axial loading or compression is increased, so is the oblique component of the fracture line at the expense of the transverse, until the fracture is entirely oblique. Often a butterfly fragment is formed. Compression force results in shearing stresses in the oblique projection that create a secondary oblique fracture line, thus creating the butterfly fragment. This second fracture line probably occurs after the primary failure and is due to movement of the fragments against each other.

Fractures sustained by a combination of rotation and angulation or bending are the equivalent of angulation about an oblique axis. The resultant fracture lies in an oblique plane of 45 degrees. In the forearm or leg both bones are fractured in the same oblique plane, thus the fracture lines are not at the same level; rather, one lies proximal to the other.

Indirect forces as well as direct crushing injuries may cause multiple fracture lines, or comminution of a fracture. This situation results from the absorption of relatively large amounts of energy, which is usually achieved by the rapid application of forces. Under these circumstances it may be difficult to resolve the major forces at play in the creation of the injury.

Direct Forces

The type of fracture created by direct forces is related to the magnitude of the applied force. Forces of low magnitude result in transverse or slightly oblique fractures. These have been termed *tapping fractures* and are the result of a direct blow to the bone. Characteristically, they are found in the ulna (Fig. 2–6*A*) and tibia. Those in the ulna are called *nightstick* or *parry* fractures, because they result from a direct blow to the forearm as it

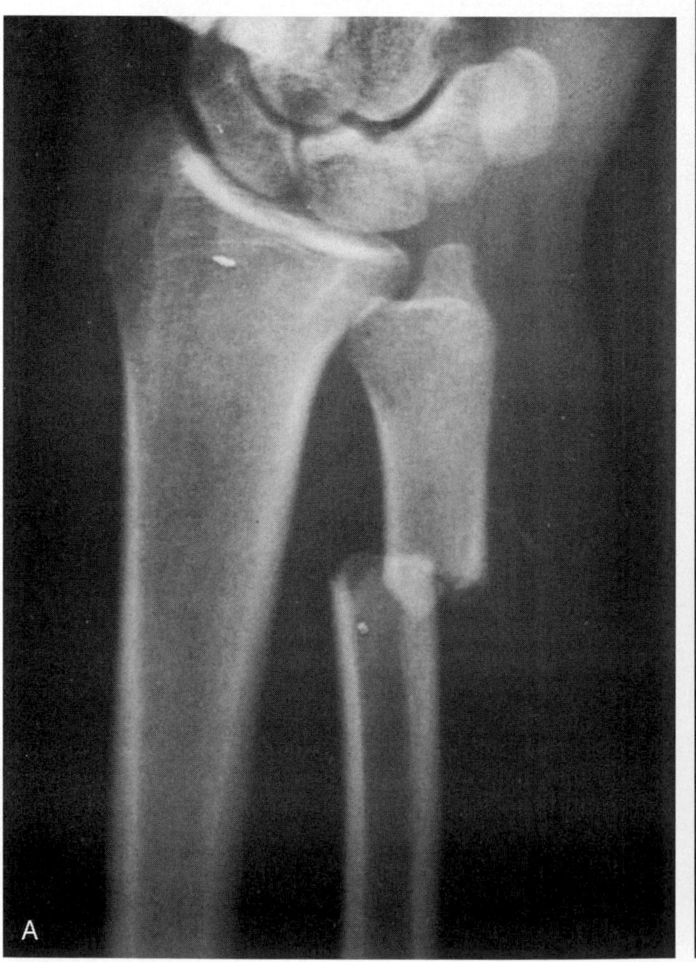

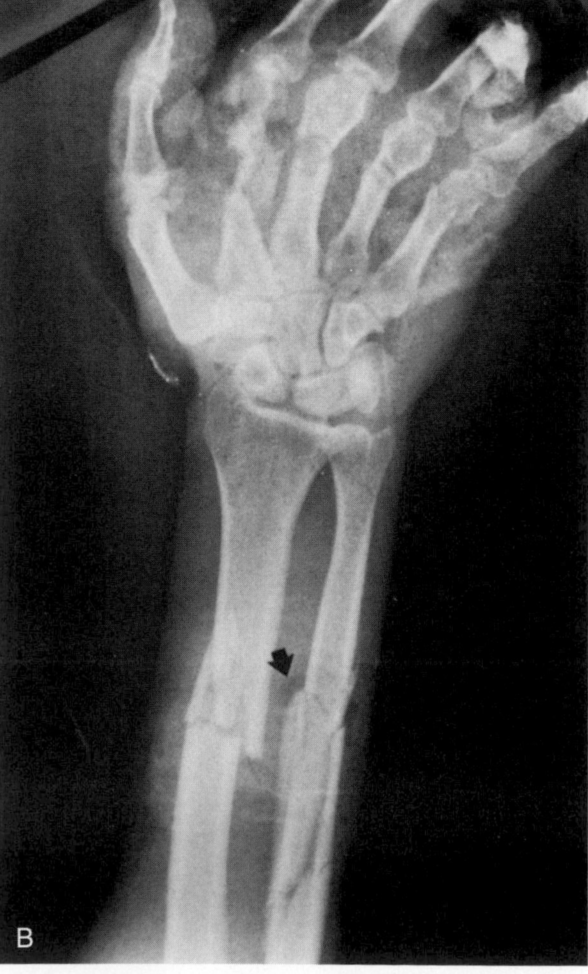

Figure 2–6. Fractures caused by direct forces. *A,* A nightstick fracture of the distal ulna in a 20-year-old man, caused by a direct blow by a hard object. The fracture line is transverse. The radius is intact. *B,* An open, comminuted fracture of both bones of the forearm and multiple metacarpals in a 52-year-old man, sustained in an auto accident. Note the air within the soft tissues (*arrow*) at the ulnar fracture site and within the palm, indicating an open wound.

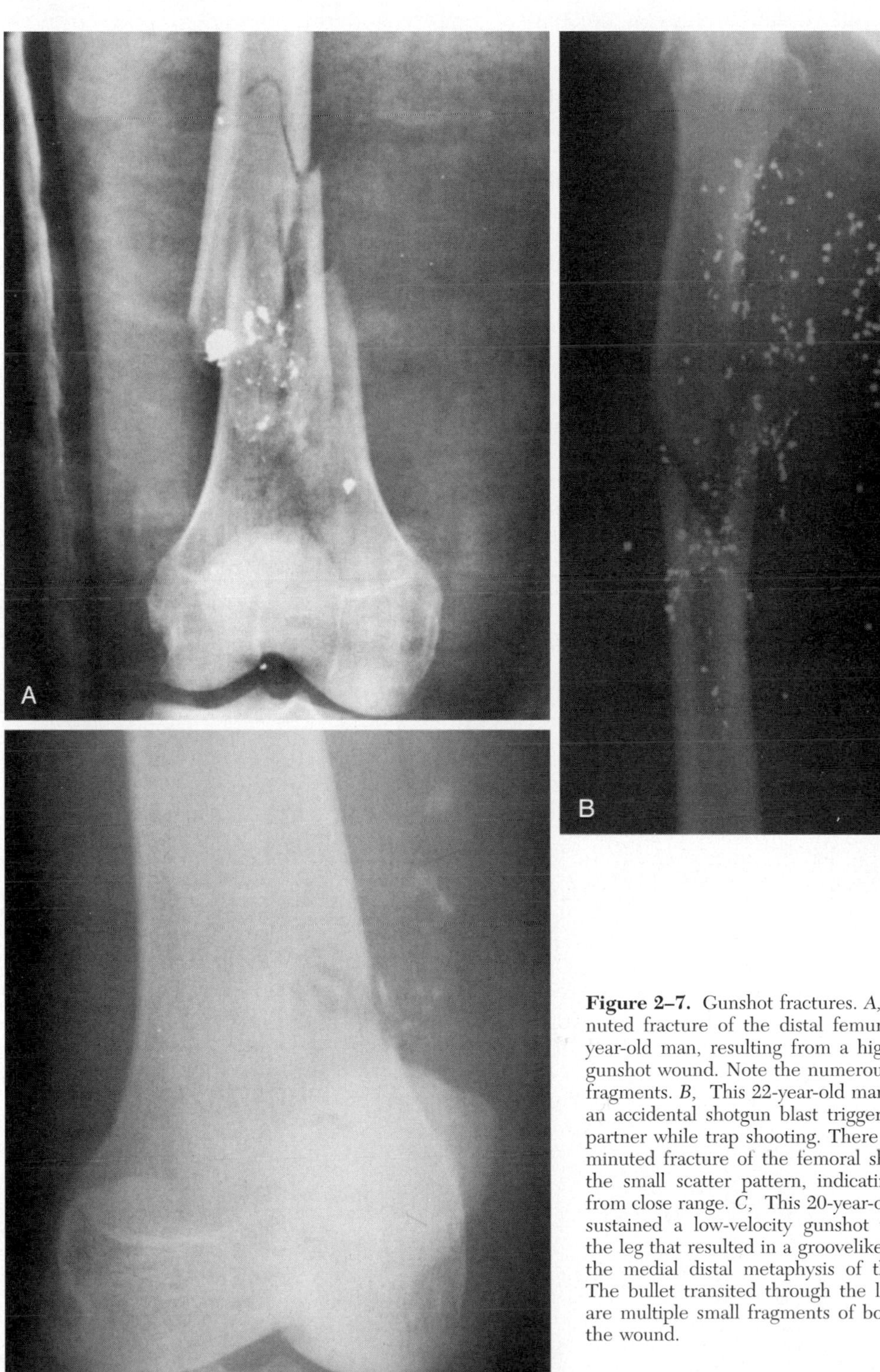

Figure 2–7. Gunshot fractures. *A,* Comminuted fracture of the distal femur in a 34-year-old man, resulting from a high-velocity gunshot wound. Note the numerous metallic fragments. *B,* This 22-year-old man received an accidental shotgun blast triggered by his partner while trap shooting. There is a comminuted fracture of the femoral shaft. Note the small scatter pattern, indicating a shot from close range. *C,* This 20-year-old patient sustained a low-velocity gunshot wound in the leg that resulted in a groovelike defect of the medial distal metaphysis of the femur. The bullet transited through the leg. There are multiple small fragments of bone within the wound.

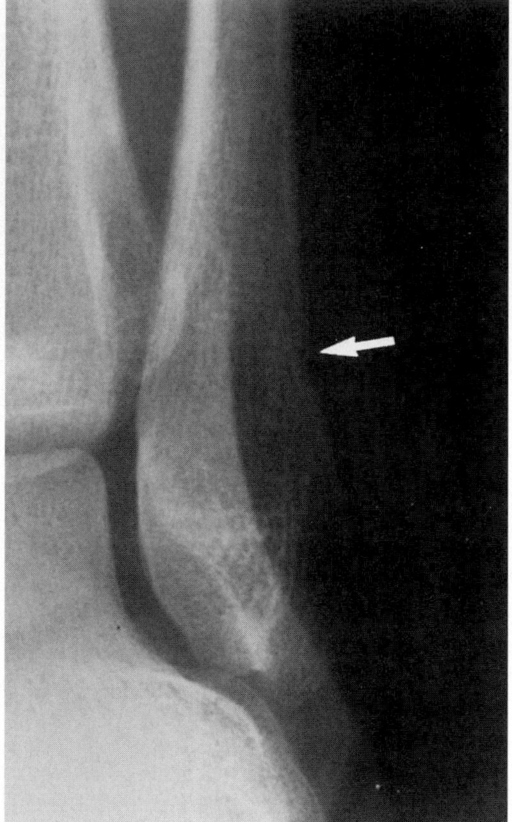

Figure 2–8. This 34-year-old man was hit in the lateral aspect of his ankle by the edge of a piece of sheet metal that had fallen from the back of a truck. He sustained a divet-like depression fracture of the lateral cortex (*arrow*) and an overlying soft tissue laceration.

is raised to protect against the blow. The transverse fracture of the tibia is usually the result of a direct blow, particularly a kick on the shin. Characteristically, the adjacent radius or fibula remains intact with these forces of low energy.

Crushing injuries of higher energy result in fragmentation of bone (see Fig. 2–6*B*), with the degree of fragmentation and extent of the associated soft tissue injury varying directly with the magnitude of the forces involved. When either the forearm or leg is involved, both bones are broken at the same level.

Gunshot wounds create distinctive fractures depending on the velocity and to a lesser extent the size of the bullet.[16, 17, 19] Low-velocity wounds are associated with comparatively little soft tissue injury and comminution of bone. High-velocity wounds characteristically have extensive soft tissue damage and considerable comminution of bone (Fig. 2–7).

Other forms of penetrating injury rarely result in fracture. Divots or grooves limited to the cortex may be created by wounds inflicted by metal objects such as sheet metal (Fig. 2–8), shovels (Fig. 2–9*A*), saws, swords, knives, or machetes.[33, 34] Complete lacerations or transections also may occur (see Fig. 2–9*B*). An unusual example

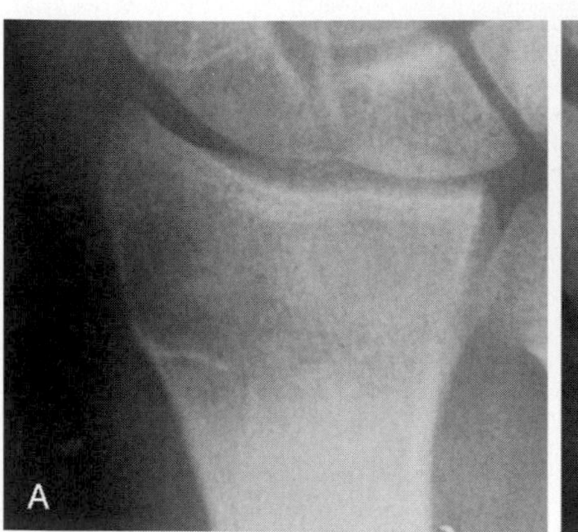

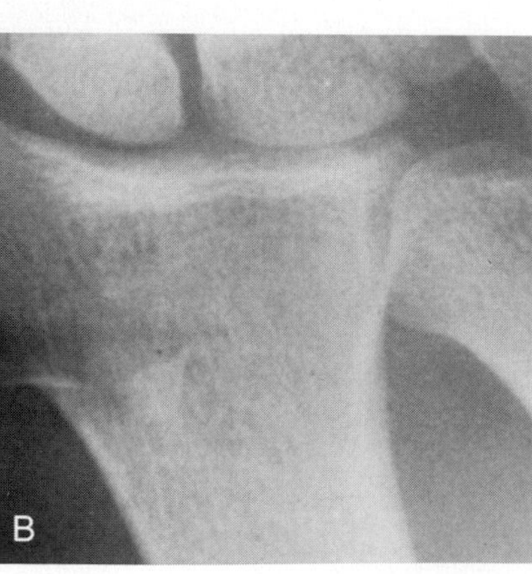

Figure 2–9. Laceration of the distal radius sustained by a 47-year-old patient who was hit with the edge of a snow shovel. *A,* The posteroanterior view demonstrates an obvious laceration of the soft tissues. There is a slightly undulant thin line of cortical bone within the distal radius underlying the soft tissue laceration. The origin of this density is not obvious. *B,* The hyperpronated oblique view reveals that the density in question represents a laceration of bone. A layer of bone is peeled away from the dorsal cortex.

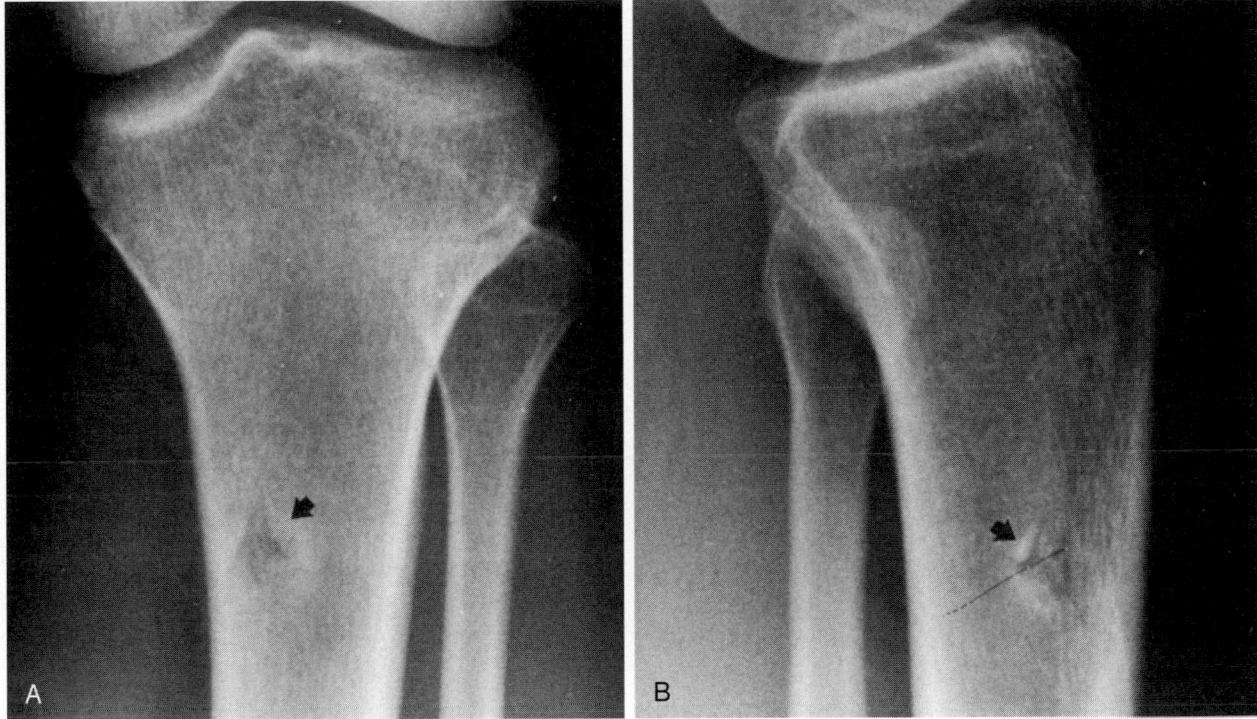

Figure 2–10. Puncture wound with depressed fracture of the proximal tibial shaft sustained in an auto accident by a 28-year-old woman. *A,* The posteroanterior view demonstrates an area of lucency surrounded by a poorly defined margin of increased bone density (*arrow*). *B,* The lateral view shows that depressed fragments of bone are more sharply defined (*arrow*). (The diagonal black line is an artifact on the original film.)

of a punctate, depressed fracture of the tibial shaft sustained from penetration of a small, pointed metallic object is shown in Figure 2–10. Such fractures occur much more commonly in the skull (see Figs. 10–18 and 10–22).

References

1. Behiri, J.C., & Bonfield, W. (1980). Crack velocity dependence of longitudinal fracture in bone. J. Mater. Sci., *15*:1841.
2. Behiri, J.C., & Bonfield, W. (1984). Fracture mechanics of bone—The effects of density, specimen thickness and crack velocity on longitudinal fracture. J. Biomech., *17*:25.
3. Bonfield, W. (1987). Advances in the fracture mechanics of cortical bone. J. Biomech., *20*:1071.
4. Bonfield W., Behiri, J.C., & Charalambides, B. (1985). Orientation and age-related dependence of the fracture toughness of cortical bone. p. 185. In Perren, S.M., & Schneider, E. Eds.: Biomechanics: Current Interdisciplinary Research. Martinus Nijhoff, Dordrecht.
5. Bonfield, W., & Grynpas, M.D. (1982). Spiral fracture of cortical bone. J. Biomech., *8*:555.
6. Brooks, D.B., Burstein, A.H., & Frankel, V.H. (1970). The biomechanics of torsional fractures. J. Bone Joint Surg. [Am.], *52*:507.
7. Brown, C.U., Yeni, Y.N., & Norman, T.L. (2000). Fracture toughness is dependent on bone location: A study of the femoral shaft and the tibial shaft. J. Biomed. Mater. Res., *49*:380.
8. Burstein, A.H., Zika, J.M., Heople, K.G., & Klein, L. (1975). Contribution of collagen and mineral to the elastic-plastic properties of bone. J. Bone Joint Surg. [Am.], *57*:956.
9. Chamay, A. (1970). Mechanical and morphological aspects of experimental overload and fatigue in bone. J. Biomech., *3*:236.
10. Currey, J.D. (1999). What determines the bending strength of compact bone? J. Exp. Biol., *202*:2495.
11. Currey, J.D., & Butler, G. (1975). The mechanical properties of bone tissue in children. J. Bone Joint Surg. [Am.], *57*:810.
12. Currey, J.D. (1970). The mechanical properties of bone. Clin. Orthop., *73*:210.
13. Evans, F.G. (1976). Mechanical properties and histology of cortical bone from younger and older men. Anat. Rec., *185*:1.
14. Frankel, V.H., & Burstein, A.H. (1970). Orthopaedic Biomechanics. Lea & Febiger, Philadelphia.
15. Frost, H.L. (1960). Presence of microscopic cracks *in vivo* in bone. Henry Ford Hosp. Bull., *8*:27.
16. Hollerman, J.J., Fackler, M.L., Coldwell, D.M., & Ben-Menachem, Y. (1990). Gunshot wounds: 1. Bullets, ballistics, and mechanisms of injury. A.J.R. Am. J. Roentgenol., *155*:685.
17. Hollerman, J.J., Fackler, M.L., Coldwell, D.M., & Ben-Menachem, Y. (1990). Gunshot wounds: 2. Radiology. A.J.R. Am. J. Roentgenol, *155*:691.
18. Holt, J.E., & Schoorl, D. (1984). Fracture in potatoes and apples. J. Irreproducible Results, *29*:3.
19. Hughes, J.L., Griend, R.V., & Bennett, T.L. (1986). Gunshot fractures. Unfallchirurg, *89*:515.
20. Kabel, J., Rietbergen, B., Odgaard, A., & Huiskes, R. (1999). Constitutive relationships of fabric, density, and elastic properties in cancellous bone architecture. Bone *25*:481.
21. Ko, R. (1953). The tension test upon compact substance in the long bone of human extremities. J. Kyoto Pref. Med. Univ., *53*:503.
22. Lakes, R., & Saha, S. (1979). Cement line motion in bone. Science, *204*:501.
23. Liu, D., Wagner, H.D., & Weiner, S. (2000). Bending and fracture of compact circumferential and osteonal lamellar bone of the baboon tibia. Journal of Materials in Medicine, *11*:49.
24. Martin, R.B., & Burr, D.B. (1982). A hypothetical mechanism for the stimulation of osteonal remodelling by fatigue damage. J. Biomech., *15*:137.
25. Melvin, J.W. (1993). Fracture mechanics of bone. J. Biomech. Eng., *115*:549.
26. Moyle, D.D., & Gavens, A.J. (1986). Fracture properties of bovine tibial bone. J. Biomech., *19*:919.
27. Natali, A.N., & Meroi, E.A. (1989). A review of the biomechanical properties of bone as a material. J. Biomed. Eng., *11*:266.
28. Oni, O.O.A., Gregg, P.J., Morrison, C., & Ponter, A.R.S. (1988). An investigation of the fracture characteristics of the tibia of mature rabbits. Injury, *19*:172.
29. Pietruszczak, S., Inglis, D., & Pande, G.N. (1999). A fabric-dependent fracture criterion for bone. J. Biomech., *32*:1071.
30. Pope, M.H., & Outwaters, J.O. (1972). The fracture characteristics of bone substance. J Biomech., *5*:457.
31. Prendergast, P.J., & Taylor, D. (1994). Prediction of bone adaptation using damage accumulation. J. Biomech., *27*:1067.
32. Pugh, J.W., Rose, R.M., & Radin, E.L. (1973). A possible mechanism of Wolff's law: Trabecular microfractures. Arch. Int. Physiol. Biochim., *81*:27.
33. Rose, S.C., Fujisaki, C.K., & Moore, E.E. (1988). Incomplete fractures associated with penetrating trauma: Etiology, appearance, and natural history. J. Trauma, *28*:106.
34. Rymaszewski, L.A., & Caullay, J.M. (1984). Bony lacerations caused by assault. J. Bone Joint Surg. [Br.], *66*:89.

35. Saha, S., & Hayes, W.C. (1976). Tensile impact properties of human compact bone. J. Biomech., 9:243.
36. Schaffler, M.B., Radin, E.L., & Burr, D.B.(1990). Long-term fatigue behavior of compact bone at low strain magnitude and rate. Bone *11*:321.
37. Schnitzler, C.M. (1993). Bone quality: A determinant for certain risk factors for bone fragility. Calcif. Tissue Int., 53:S27.
38. Tanabe, Y., & Bonfield, W. (1999). Effects of initial crack length and specimen thickness on fracture toughness of compact bone. J.S.M.E. International Journal, *42*:532.
39. Taylor, D., O'Brien, F., Prina-Mello, A. et al. (1999). Compression data on bovine bone confirms that a "stressed volume" principle explains the variability of fatigue strength results. J. Biomech., *32*:1199.
40. Turner, C.H., & Burr, D.B. (1993). Basic biomechanical measurements of bone: A tutorial. Bone, *14*:595.
41. Walker, J. (1979). The amateur scientist: Strange to relate, smokestacks and pencil points break in the same way. Sci. Am., *240*:158.
42. Weiner, S., Traub, W., & Wagner, H.D. (1999). Lamellar bone: Structure-function relations. J. Struct. Biol., *126*:241.
43. Wright, T.M., & Hayes, W.C. (1976). The fracture mechanics of fatigue crack propagation in compact bone. J. Biomed. Mater. Res. Symp., *7*:637.
44. Yokoo, S. (1952). The compression test upon the diaphysis and the compact substance of the long bones of human extremities. J. Kyoto Pref. Med. Univ., *51*:291.

Chapter 3

EPIDEMIOLOGY OF FRACTURES

with Leon Lenchik, MD

Skeletal injuries occur during the course of all human activity, with expectation and risk of injury varying with the nature of each endeavor. Simple movement or ambulation has an attendant risk of injury that is increased by the use of transportation of various forms. Injuries occur during participation in sports and at play. Various occupations carry with them peculiar hazards that could result in injury. The specific purpose of fighting is to inflict injury. In addition, osteoporosis is a major cause of fractures in the elderly.

Frequency Factors and Distribution of Fractures

The location, nature, and number of fractures are dependent on the age, gender, and race of an individual, the activity in which the person is engaged when injury occurs, and the status of the person's skeletal system during injury.[1, 2, 13, 16, 22, 128, 174, 184, 199]

Age, Gender, and Race

The skeleton is weak when immature, at maximum strength when mature, and weakened with age. Population studies in developed countries show that fracture incidence is bimodal, with peaks in the young and in the elderly (Fig. 3–1).[11, 13, 31] During infancy, adolescence, and early adult life, the most commonly fractured sites are the skull, the long bones, and the hands and feet, respectively.[11, 13, 31] In contrast, after age fifty, there is a precipitous rise in the incidence of fractures of the proximal femur,[11, 13, 21, 31, 122, 195] the pelvis,[2, 11, 13, 31, 195] the proximal humerus,[6, 11, 13, 29, 31, 195] the distal radius,[7, 11, 13, 23, 27, 31, 33, 195] and vertebral bodies (Figs. 3–2 and 3–3).[12, 24, 25, 31, 121, 195]

Fractures occur chiefly at the ends of the bone in the young and in the elderly, whereas fractures are more likely to involve the diaphysis in those between 20 and 50 years of age.[11, 13, 31, 195] The location of skeletal injury in the elderly reverts to the pattern of childhood. In people between the ages of 10 and 16 epiphyseal injuries are most likely. The epiphysis at this stage is the weakest part of bone and therefore the most common site of injury. The increased incidence of metaphyseal fractures in children younger than 10 years of age and the sparing of the epiphysis is a recognized fact, but the reasons are obscure. Fractures at the ends of bone in the elderly are due to the weakening effects of osteoporosis. In fact, the preferential loss of cancellous bone in people with osteoporosis may explain the increasing ratio of metaphyseal to diaphyseal fractures in those of advanced age.[117, 128, 174, 184, 193]

For most skeletal sites, there is a significant difference between men and women in the incidence rates of fracture (see Fig. 3–1).[1, 2, 11, 13, 31] In men, the incidence rate

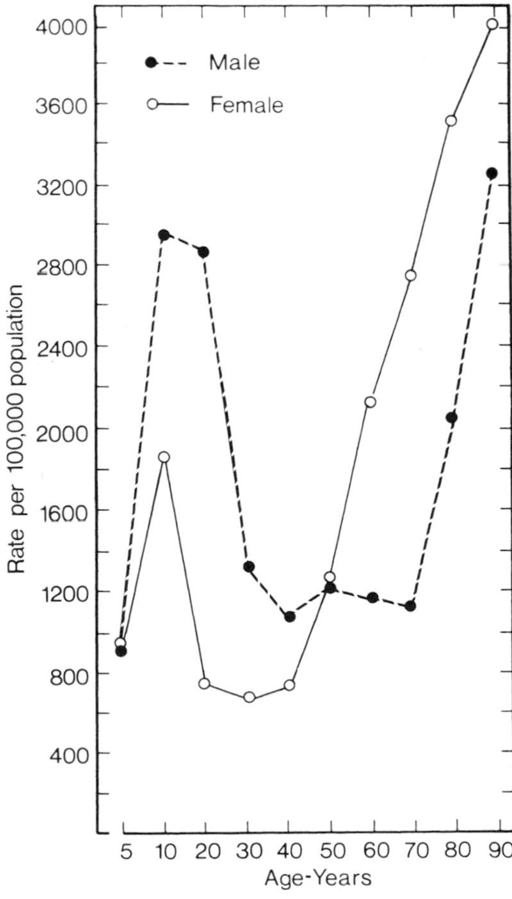

Figure 3–1. Age-specific and sex-specific incidence rates of limb fractures. (Adapted from Garraway, W.M., Stauffer, R.N., Kurland, L.T., & O'Fallon, W.M. [1979]. Limb fractures in a defined population. I. Frequency and distribution. Mayo Clin. Proc., *54*:701, with permission.)

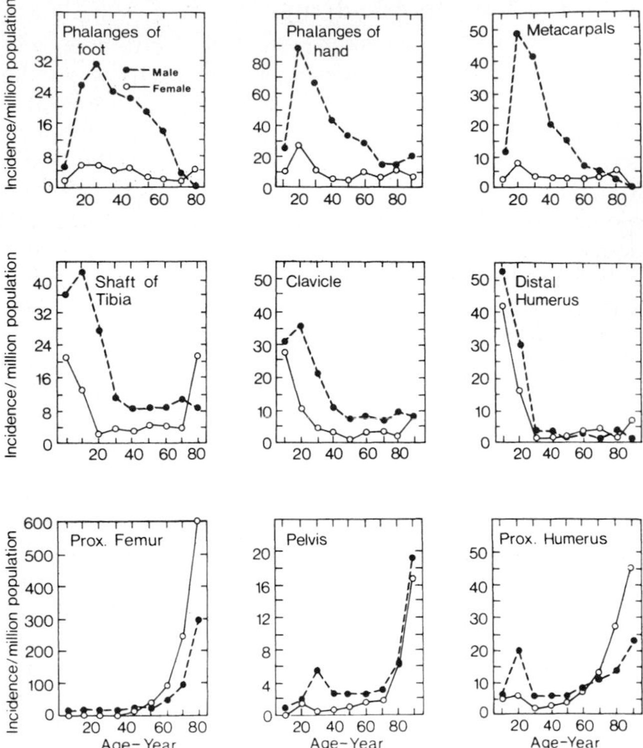

Figure 3–2. Age-specific and sex-specific incidence rates of fractures in England and Wales in 1954. (Adapted from Buhr, A.J., & Cooke, A.M. [1959]. Fracture patterns. Lancet, *1*:531, with permission.)

for extremity fractures peaks in the second and third decades, decreases by age 45 to a relatively low rate, is maintained until age 65, and increases thereafter.[11, 13, 31] In women, the incidence rate peaks in the second decade, decreases and remains low until age 45, and increases considerably thereafter.[11, 13, 31] In general, the age-adjusted incidence rates are higher in men than in women before age 50 and higher in women than in men after age 50.[11, 13, 31] The shift toward a female preponderance in fractures with increasing age is best explained by the effects of osteoporosis and falls, both occurring more commonly in women than in men.[141, 164, 193, 199, 201]

It is instructive to compare the incidence of fracture at various skeletal sites by age and gender. Each skeletal site has a particular distribution and pattern of injury (see Figs. 3–2 and 3–3). Fractures of the phalanges of the foot and hand and fractures of the metacarpals demonstrate a striking difference between men and women.[2, 13, 31] The higher incidence in men compared with the incidence in women is noted early in childhood and persists throughout adult life. The higher incidence may reflect men's participation in aggressive play and sports in childhood and their exposure to occupational hazards during adult years. After 60 years of age, the male and female incidence rates are approximately equal.[2, 13, 31]

Fractures of the tibia, clavicle, and distal humerus are common in the young and in young adults, but the incidence rates for these sites decline and level off in those older than 30 years of age.[2, 13, 31] Again, men are more frequently affected than women, which may reflect men's play and work habits.

Fractures of the proximal femur are quite rare until age 50. After age 50, the incidence of hip fracture rises exponentially; 90% of hip fractures occur in people older than 50 years of age.[21, 174] In the United States, white women younger than 35 years of age have a hip fracture incidence of 2 per 100,000 person-years.[22, 120, 174] The incidence rises to 3000 per 100,000 person-years in women older than 85 years of age.[22, 120, 174] Because the incidence rates are higher in women than in men and because women live longer, 80% of hip fractures occur in women.[119] In developed countries, the average age for hip fracture is 80.[140]

Fractures of the distal forearm are common in both adolescents and the elderly (see Fig. 3–3).[2, 23, 27, 33, 185, 195] In those younger than age 25, these fractures are more common in men than in women, and they are usually related to athletic activity. In women, there is a linear increase in the incidence rate between ages 40 and 65, but the rate plateaus after age 65.[2, 23] This plateau may reflect an age-related change in the pattern of falls.[185] Before age 65, people generally fall forward on an outstretched hand and generally fracture the forearm.[185] After age 65, people tend to fall to one side and generally fracture the hip.[185] The incidence rates in men are fairly constant throughout life.[2, 23] Fractures of the distal forearm are approximately six times more common in elderly women than in elderly men (see Fig. 3–3).[2, 23]

The epidemiology of vertebral fractures is less certain because of inconsistent definitions of fracture.[12, 24, 25, 119, 121] In population studies, fractures may be defined clinically[121] or radiologically.[25] Moreover, radiologic diagnosis may be based on a qualitative impression or on a quantitative measurement of vertebral dimensions (e.g., vertebral

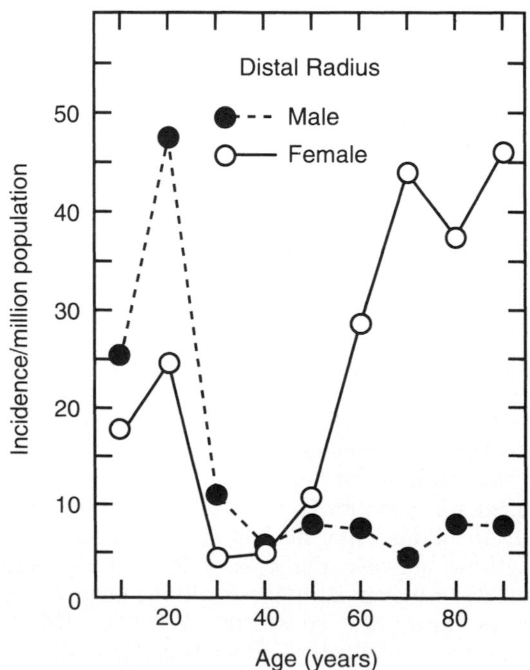

Figure 3–3. Age-specific and sex-specific incidence rates of fracture of the distal forearm in England and Wales in 1954. (Adapted from Buhr, A.J., & Cooke, A.M. [1959]. Fracture patterns. Lancet, *1*:531, with permission.)

morphometry).[24, 25] Regardless of the diagnostic method used, the incidence rates increase with age for both men and women.[12, 24, 25, 119, 121] In the United States, the incidence rate for clinical vertebral fractures in white women younger than age 45 is 20 per 100,000 person-years.[22, 121, 174] In those older than age 85, the incidence rate increases to 1200 per 100,000 person-years.[22, 121, 174] In the elderly, the female-to-male ratio of age-adjusted incidence rates is approximately 2:1.[121] Only about one third of all vertebral fractures is clinically apparent.[121] The incidence and prevalence of radiographic fracture are variable because of different diagnostic criteria. Based on radiographic surveys, 19% to 26% of postmenopausal white women have vertebral deformities.[24, 134]

The effect of race on fracture incidence has been best studied for hip fractures. In the United States, the incidence of hip fractures in men and women of all races increases exponentially with age.[184] For those between the ages of 65 and 95, the highest age-adjusted incidence rates are seen in white women, followed by white men, African American women, and African American men.[184] The incidence rate for Asians falls somewhere between that for whites and African Americans.[184]

For fractures other than the hip the data on individuals of color are limited. In the United States, vertebral fractures are four times more common in elderly whites than in African Americans.[184] The prevalence of vertebral fractures in Asians is similar to that of whites.[184] The prevalence in Mexican Americans is somewhat lower.[184] In most parts of the world, distal forearm fractures are less frequent in African Americans and Asians than in whites.[184]

Although varying patterns of fracture in men and women of different races suggest a genetic determinant for fracture risk, the role of environment cannot be ignored.[32, 149] For some fractures, the geographic differences in fracture rates among groups of similar race are compelling. In Europe, for example, there is a 7- to 12-fold variation in the age-adjusted incidence rate of hip fractures, whereas vertebral fractures have a 4-fold variation between countries.[17, 25, 133] When comparing different geographic regions, fracture rates at different skeletal sites appear to correlate. For example, both hip and forearm fracture rates in the United Kingdom are 30% lower than those in the United States.[174]

Activity

The activity in which a person is engaged when an injury occurs is in great measure predicated on age. The young are likely to be injured in the course of play or during sports activities.[41] Almost half of the deaths of American children are the result of trauma.[40] Mature adults, those between the ages of 20 and 50 years, are more likely to sustain an injury while traveling in a motor vehicle or during the course of work. The elderly are often injured in a fall[11, 45, 141, 185] while walking, descending stairs, stepping from a curb, or while in the bathroom. Fractures in the elderly may also occur in the absence of falls while bending, reaching, coughing, or doing other daily activities.[28, 184]

Motor Vehicle Accidents

In the United States, motor vehicle accidents represent the leading cause of death in individuals between the ages of 5 and 34 (see Fig. I–1).[37, 38, 42, 44] The mortality rate is highest in low population density areas in the west and lowest in high population density areas in the east.[35] Many factors account for the difference, including higher speeds in rural areas, poorer roads, less seat belt use, and poorer access to trauma care.[37] Mandating seat belt use[34, 36, 39, 42] and lowering speed limits have reduced mortality. There is also a clear association between the seriousness of the crash and alcohol.[46] Alcohol consumption has been implicated in more than half of fatal crashes, and it increases vulnerability to injury in any crash, regardless of severity.

Falls

Falls are a major source of traumatic injury and fractures throughout life (Fig. 3–4). Simple falls, that is, falls from a standing height, are the principal source of fractures and injury in the elderly.[45, 57–70, 141, 185] Almost one third of elderly men and women fall annually. About 5% of falls in the elderly result in fracture. Although only 1% of falls results in a hip fracture, most hip fractures are caused by a fall.[141, 185] Falls from greater heights commonly result in multiple injuries. These falls are common among persons in such occupations as construction work, roofing, tree trimming, and logging.[43] Falls from heights are also a source of multiple injuries in urban children, who may fall from windows or fire escapes in multistory dwellings.[47–56]

A common mechanism of injury is a fall on the outstretched hand. There is striking age dependence in the location of the resultant fracture. In a child younger than age 5, a supracondylar fracture of the humerus is likely; in a child between ages 5 and 10, a transverse fracture of the metaphysis of the distal radius occurs; in a young person between ages 10 and 16, an epiphyseal separation of the distal radius is likely; in someone between ages 15 and 35, a fracture of the scaphoid or other carpal injury is most common; in an adult older than age 40, a Colles' fracture or other fracture of the distal radius and ulna is usual; and in an elderly person older than age 70, a fracture of the proximal humerus, particularly of the surgical neck, is likely. These differences are dictated by variations in anatomic structure, the forces involved, and the individual's ability to modify the impact. Admittedly, there is some overlap in these injuries, but the general pattern holds.

Seizures

The severe, violent, and uncontrolled muscular contractions that occur with seizures may result in fractures and dislocations. Seizures are an uncommon source of fractures, but certain injuries are so distinctive that they suggest this etiology. In fact, the presence of fracture may be the first evidence of a seizure disorder. This situation is particularly true of posterior dislocation of the shoulder; when bilateral, such dislocation is virtually diagnostic of a seizure disorder.[71, 72, 74, 77] Fractures of the upper thoracic spine are also characteristic of seizure etiology.[75] Unilat-

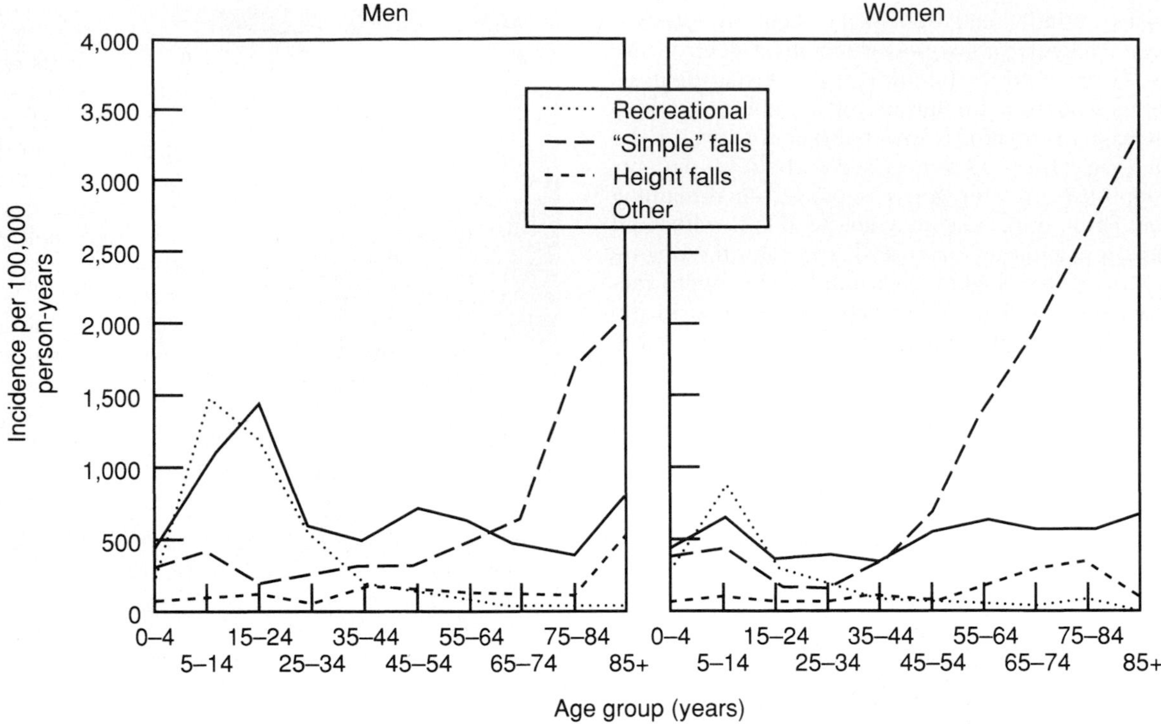

Figure 3–4. Causes of limb fractures. Age-specific and sex-specific incidence rates among residents of Rochester, Minnesota, 1969–1971. (From Melton, L.J. III, & Riggs, B.L. [1985]. Risk factors for injury after a fall. Clin. Geriatr. Med., *1*:525, with permission.)

eral and bilateral central fracture-dislocations of the hip[76, 78, 79] and the manubriosternal joint are also described.[73]

The etiology of the seizure may be epilepsy, eclampsia, electric shock, electroconvulsive therapy, hyponatremia, or severe tetanus.[73] Skeletal injuries associated with seizures are often unrecognized. Delayed diagnosis of posterior dislocations of the shoulder is especially common. Care should be taken to exclude musculoskeletal complications in any patient who has experienced a seizure.

Status of the Skeletal System

Regardless of age, gender, or race, the strength of the skeleton is diminished by disease. Common disorders such as osteoporosis, metastasis, myeloma, rheumatoid arthritis, hyperparathyroidism, osteomalacia, rickets, Cushing's disease, hyperthyroidism, diabetes, and exogenous steroids often result in fracture. Immobilization and disuse also may weaken the skeleton; indeed, there is no disease of the skeleton that increases its strength. The radiographic appearance of the bone in osteopetrosis and Paget's disease is misleading because despite the thickening of the cortex and the increased density of bone, the structure is actually weaker than normal and more susceptible to fracture.

Osteoporosis

Osteoporosis is a systemic skeletal disorder characterized by compromised bone strength predisposing to an increased risk of fracture.[114] Diminished strength results from reduced bone mass and microarchitectural deterioration of bone.[114] Osteoporosis is mostly a loss of bone mass (Fig. 3–5); the composition and the percentage distribution of mineral salt, organic substances, and water content are essentially unchanged.[5, 91, 117] The changes are predominantly quantitative; qualitative changes are considered to be much less important, and at present their role is poorly defined.

During childhood and adolescence, bone modeling takes place. Linear growth, cortical apposition, and cancellous modification characterize this process, which is responsible for skeletal growth.[117, 136] After skeletal maturity, bone modeling stops and bone remodeling, a process by which bone resorption and bone formation is coupled, becomes dominant.[117, 136] In the young adult bone remodeling ensures that the amount of bone formed is equal to the amount of bone resorbed.[117, 136] With aging, bone resorption exceeds bone formation, which causes a net loss of bone mass and eventually results in osteoporosis.[117, 136]

In patients with osteoporosis, bone resorption at the endosteal surface results in thinning of the cortex. There is little bone resorption at the periosteal surface so that the overall width of the bone is maintained. In fact, the width of bone may increase slightly because of continued (although minimal) appositional periosteal bone formation.[4] Resorption in the haversian canals results in increased porosity of the cortex. Resorption of intramedullary bone manifests as thinning of the trabeculae, trabecular perforations, and loss of the finer trabeculae.[101, 103, 105] The rate of bone resorption depends on the surface area, and because there is greater surface area in trabecular bone than in cortical bone, the loss of the trabecular bone is more apparent.[117]

Fractures of individual trabeculae occur in osteoporotic bone.[10, 65] Under a low-power scanning electron microscope (Fig. 3–6) trabecular fractures appear as rounded swellings on the surface of a trabecula, which represent callus formation surrounding a fracture of the trabecula (Fig. 3–7). As bone is resorbed in patients with osteoporosis, greater stress is placed on remaining trabeculae. Some trabeculae may not be able to withstand the added stress and thus fracture. The greater the degree of osteoporosis, the higher the number of microfractures.[10] Microfractures of trabeculae may be seen in the spine[10] and in other weight-bearing bones, such as the femoral neck.

Osteoporosis is usually classified as either primary or secondary.[186, 190] Primary osteoporosis is further subdivided into type 1 (postmenopausal) or type 2 (age related).[186, 190] Postmenopausal osteoporosis is largely dependent on loss of estrogen stimulation in women at menopause.[117, 137, 190] A similar condition can be prematurely initiated by oophorectomy. Patients with secondary osteoporosis have an identifiable cause for low bone mass, other than menopause and aging. Examples include congenital disorders such as osteogenesis imperfecta, Ehlers-Danlos syndrome, and systemic mastocytosis; endocrine conditions such as hypogonadism, hyperparathyroidism, hyperthyroidism, diabetes mellitus, and pregnancy; nutritional causes such as calcium deficiency, vitamin D deficiency, alcoholism, and malnutrition; and pharmacologic therapy such as glucocorticoids, anticonvulsants, and heparin.[186] Compared with postmenopausal women, younger women and men with osteoporosis are more likely to have secondary causes for low bone mass.[186]

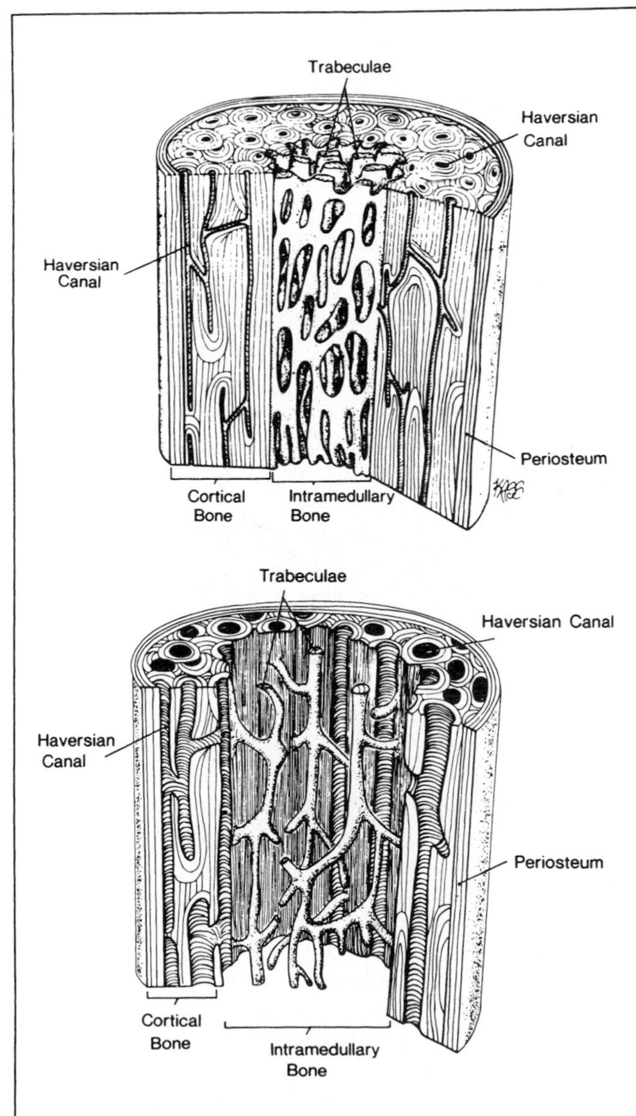

Figure 3–5. Comparison of mature (*top*) and osteoporotic (*bottom*) bone. Note thinning of cortex by endosteal resorption and widening of haversian canals. Bony trabeculae in intramedullary canal are resorbed. (From Rogers, L.F. [1985]. Skeletal trauma in the elderly: Diagnostic and epidemiologic considerations. Arch. Clin. Imag., *1*:122, with permission.)

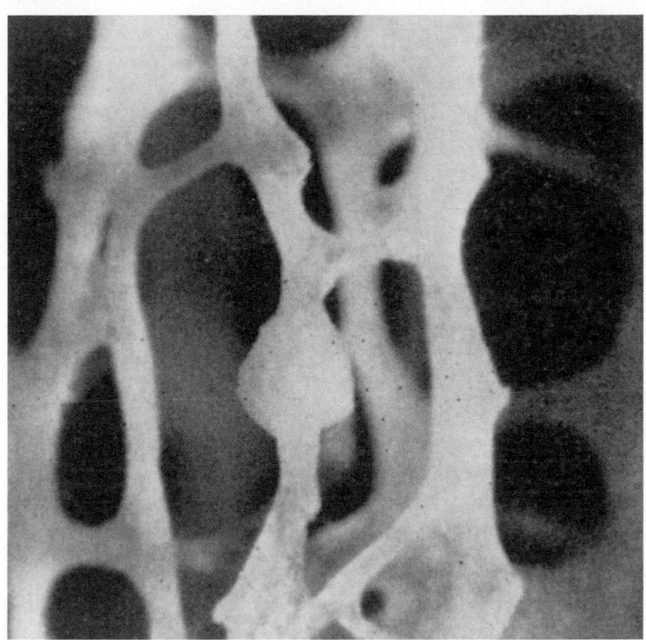

Figure 3–6. Trabecular microfracture. Under scanning electron microscope trabecular microfractures appear as well-rounded or fusiform swellings up to 0.5 mm in diameter surrounding the affected trabecula. (From Vernon-Roberts, B., & Pirie, C.J. [1973]. Healing trabecular microfractures in the bodies of lumbar vertebrae. Ann. Rheum. Dis., 32:406, with permission.)

The principal result of the bone loss in osteoporosis is an increase in bone fragility.[1, 3, 5, 86, 90, 100, 109] However, distinguishing osteoporotic from nonosteoporotic fractures may be difficult.[30, 179, 195] One approach considers fractures that occur with minimal trauma (e.g., a fall from standing position) as osteoporotic.[197] Another approach considers fractures that are associated with low bone mass and whose incidence increases in those older than age 50 as osteoporotic.[195] Complicating the issue further is recent evidence that osteoporotic individuals are more likely to fracture from high-energy injuries (e.g., motor vehicle accidents) than are normal individuals.[30]

After age 50 there is an exponential increase in the number of fractures in men and in women.[2, 13, 31, 128] The

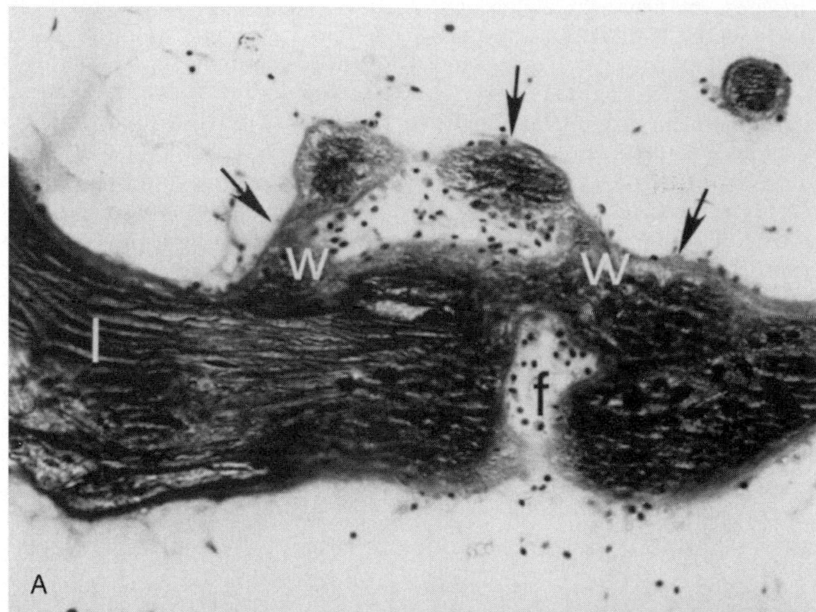

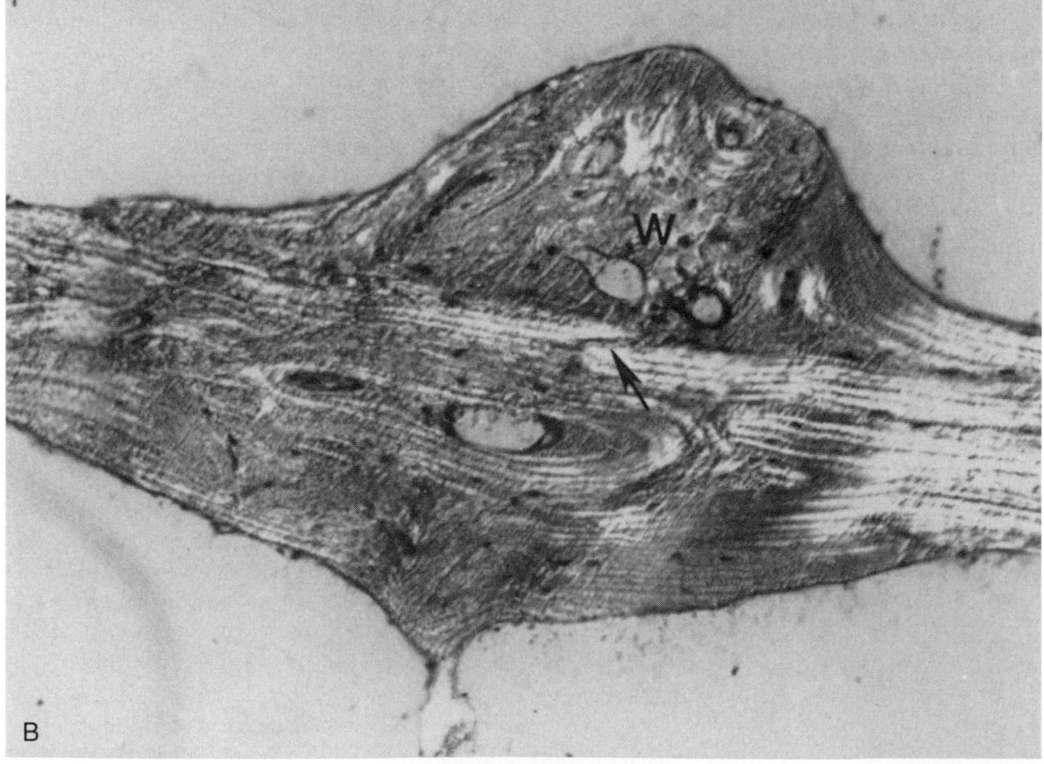

Figure 3–7. Histologic appearance of trabecular microfractures. *A,* Recent microfracture (f) with surrounding active woven bone (W) and osteoid (*arrows*); l, lamellar bone. (Fixed embedded 5-μm section stained with toluidine blue; ×500.) *B,* Old microfracture (*arrow*) overlaid with woven bone (W) showing very little cellular activity. (Fixed embedded 5-μm section stained with toluidine blue; partially polarized light × 500.) (From Wong, S.Y.P., Kariks, J., Evans, R.A. et al. [1985]. The effect of age on bone composition in viability in the femoral head. J. Bone Joint Surg. [Am.], 67:274, with permission.)

proximal femur,* distal radius,† proximal humerus,[6, 11, 13, 29, 31, 110, 195] pelvis,[2, 11, 13, 31, 99, 195] and thoracolumbar spine[12, 24, 25, 31, 121, 195] are the most common sites of fracture. Most fractures at these skeletal sites are associated with low bone mass.[195] For these reasons, the fractures are usually categorized as osteoporotic.[179] In the United States, osteoporosis results in over 1.5 million fractures each year, including approximately 300,000 proximal femur fractures, 200,000 distal radius fractures, and 700,000 spine fractures.[114, 179] There are other fractures associated with low bone density, including those of the humerus, ribs, tibia, pelvis, and femur (other than hip).[184, 195] These are sometimes categorized as osteoporotic.

Combinations of fractures involving these principal sites[5, 6] are common (Fig. 3–8). The most frequent is a fracture of the proximal femur associated with a fracture of the distal radius, occurring in 24% of hip fractures. In 16% there is a history of a previous fracture of the forearm, usually within the preceding 10 years, and in 8% there is a coincident fracture of the forearm. Fractures of the proximal humerus are combined with fractures of the proximal femur in approximately 9% of cases,[6] somewhat less than half of which are coincident. Fifteen percent of fractures of the proximal humerus[6] are combined with fractures of the distal radius. Certainly, the combination of injuries in the elderly is frequent. When an elderly individual sustains a fall, all sites should be examined clinically. If there is any suspicion of fracture, radiographic examination should be performed.

Patients who have one osteoporotic fracture have an increased risk of additional fractures later in life.[113, 156, 157, 166, 172, 178, 193] For example, having one clinically diagnosed vertebral fracture increases the risk of future vertebral

*See references 11, 13, 21, 31, 82, 83, 94–96, 98, 112, 122, 195.
†See references 7, 11, 13, 23, 27, 31, 33, 85, 87, 195.

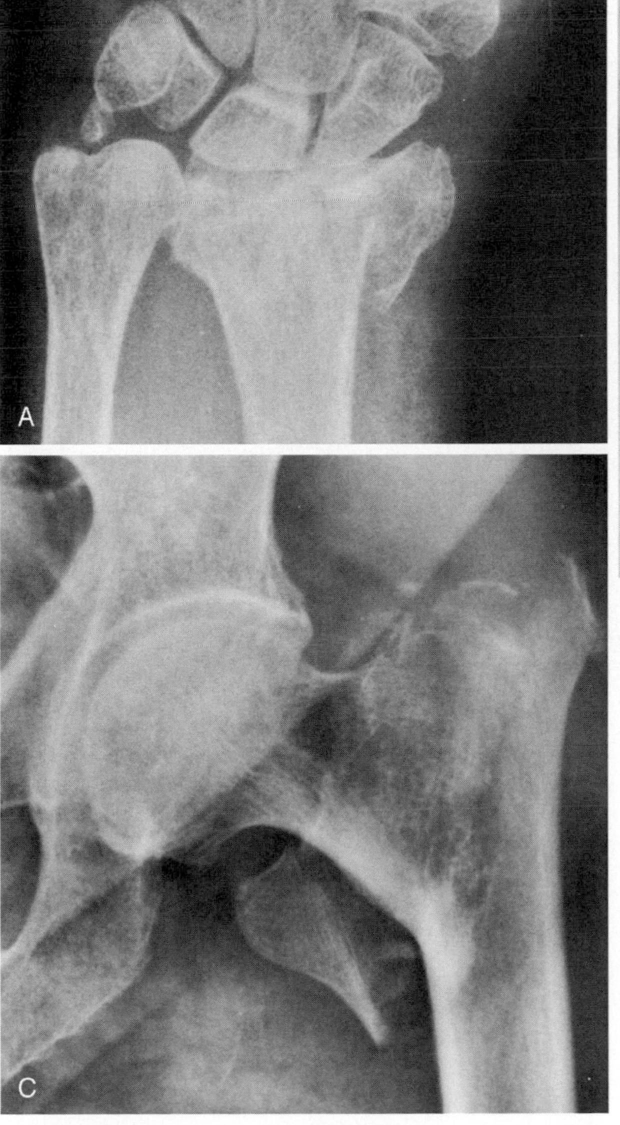

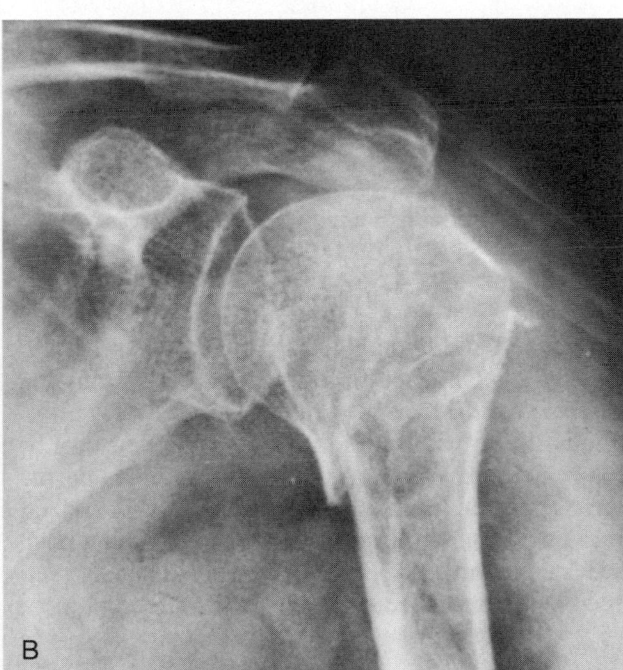

Figure 3–8. Simultaneous fractures at three sites in a 75-year-old woman, sustained in a fall. *A,* Comminuted fracture of distal end of the right radius and associated avulsion of the ulnar styloid, a Colles' fracture. *B,* Impacted fracture of the surgical neck of the left humerus. *C,* Comminuted intertrochanteric fracture of the left hip.

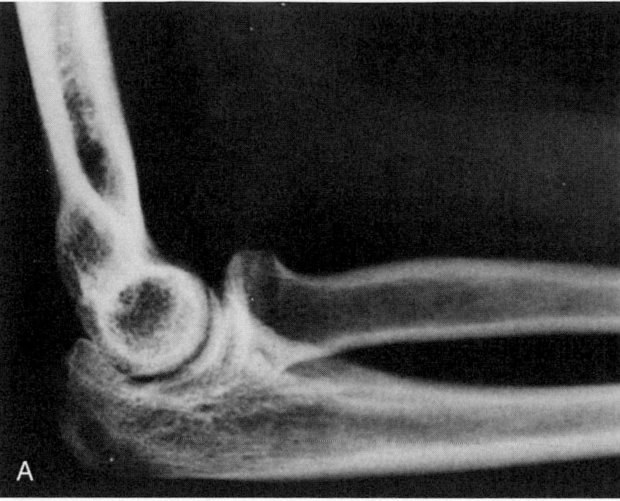

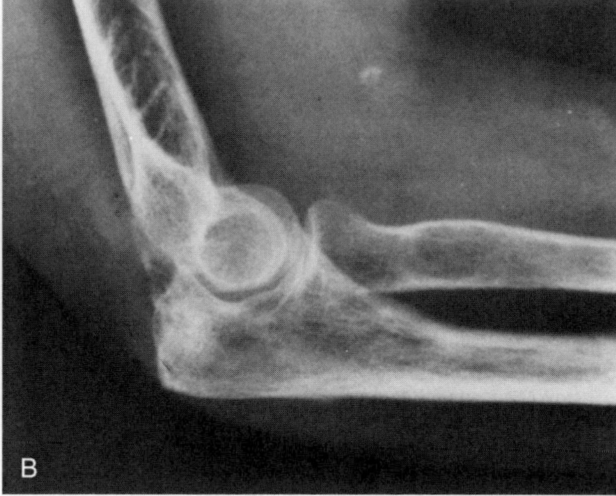

Figure 3–9. Comparison of the radiographic appearance of bone in two adult women, showing the changes of osteoporosis. *A,* In this lateral view of the elbow in a 27-year-old woman, note the cortical thickness and the indistinct appearance of the trabeculae of intramedullary bone. *B,* Compare this lateral view of the elbow in a 62-year-old woman with *A.* Note the relative thinness of the cortex and coarse trabecular pattern of intramedullary bone.

fracture by 12.6 times and of hip fracture by 2.3 times.[156] Having a hip fracture increases the risk of a second hip fracture by 10 to 12 times.[157, 172, 178]

Diagnosis

Clinical history and physical examination allow diagnosis of osteoporosis in its advanced stages, usually in the setting of a fracture caused by minimal trauma. Other findings of advanced osteoporosis may include loss of height, kyphosis, respiratory difficulties, gastrointestinal complaints, and depression. Often, patients are asymptomatic.

Requiring a fragility fracture before making a diagnosis of osteoporosis was routine ten years ago, but this is no longer considered the standard of care. Because the first osteoporotic fracture greatly increases the risk of subsequent fractures, current emphasis is on diagnosing osteoporosis before the first fracture occurs. To accomplish this, diagnostic thresholds have been developed based on results of bone densitometry examinations that allow diagnosis of osteoporosis in individuals who are asymptomatic.[154]

Conventional Radiography

The extent of bone loss can only be grossly estimated by the radiographic appearance of the skeleton.[9, 135, 169] The most common finding in patients with osteoporosis is generalized osteopenia. The cortex of the affected bone is thinned, and the trabecular pattern is coarsened (Fig. 3–9). The diagnosis is subjective and very dependent on variables such as body weight and radiographic technique.[169] It has been estimated that at least a 30% loss of bone mass must occur before osteopenia can be identified radiographically. The differential diagnosis of generalized osteopenia should include osteomalacia, hyperparathyroidism, and multiple myeloma. The combination of indistinct trabeculae and Looser's zones is diagnostic of osteomalacia. Another common radiographic finding in patients with osteoporosis is fracture. For the diagnosis and follow-up of osteoporotic fractures, conventional radiography remains unchallenged.

Bone Densitometry Overview

Bone densitometry allows diagnosis of osteoporosis in asymptomatic individuals by providing accurate, reproducible measurement of bone mineral density (BMD).* Measurement of BMD has become paramount to clinical practice for several reasons.[138, 160, 161, 182, 183] First, it allows diagnosis of osteoporosis prior to fracture. Second, the strength of bone is related to bone mass, which in turn is related to mineral content. In individual patients, BMD is the best predictor of fracture risk. Third, serial BMD measurements allow identification of individuals who are not responding to pharmacologic intervention.

Clinical indications for bone densitometry accepted in most parts of the world include estrogen deficiency, prolonged glucocorticoid therapy, radiologic osteopenia or fractures, primary hyperparathyroidism, and monitoring of therapy.[140, 146, 152, 155, 161, 182] Currently, the National Osteoporosis Foundation of the United States recommends bone densitometry for all postmenopausal white women younger than age 65 who have at least one additional risk factor to menopause and for all white women age 65 or older, regardless of other risk factors. Whether bone densitometry should be used for case finding or for population screening continues to be debated.†

Bone Densitometry Techniques

When measuring bone density, there are two distinct compartments of bone to consider, cortical and trabecular.

*See references 118, 139, 140, 152, 154, 159, 161, 181, 182, 183, 200.

†See references 115, 140, 146, 152, 155, 168, 177, 182, 194, 197, 200.

Cortical bone, predominately found in the shafts of long bones, represents 80% of bone mass. Trabecular bone, located in the ends of long bones and vertebral bodies, represents 20% of bone mass. Trabecular bone plays a major role in maintaining the strength of the ends of long bones and vertebral bodies, the sites affected by osteoporotic fractures. The relative amounts of cortical and trabecular bone vary at each site within the skeleton: at the midradius more than 95% of bone is cortical; at the distal radius 75% is cortical and 25% is trabecular.[107, 108]

Techniques used for bone mass measurement are usually divided into central and peripheral methods.[139, 150, 159, 161] Central methods allow measurement of the spine and/or hip and include dual x-ray absorptiometry (DXA) and quantitative computed tomography (QCT).[139, 150, 159, 161] Peripheral methods allow measurement of the phalanges, forearm, or calcaneus and include peripheral dual x-ray absorptiometry (pDXA), peripheral quantitative computed tomography (pQCT), and quantitative ultrasound (QUS).[139, 150, 159, 161]

Although BMD measurement of any portion of the skeleton is possible using DXA, in clinical practice the posteroanterior (PA) lumbar spine and the proximal femur are typically measured.[160] DXA integrates cortical and cancellous bone and all calcium encountered in the scan path; therefore, it results in falsely elevated values in patients with scoliosis, compression fractures, degenerative disease, and vascular calcifications.[160] In these patients, measurement of the lateral lumbar spine, distal radius, or total body may be useful.[160]

QCT is a method of BMD measurement readily adapted to conventional computed tomography (CT) scanners; however, a special software package and a calibration phantom are usually required.[84, 88, 89, 139, 159] QCT is based on the measurement of photon absorption in a volume of interest compared with that of a known reference standard in a calibrated phantom containing varying amounts of H_2HPO_4.[139] QCT has the unique advantage of selectively measuring trabecular bone and providing a volumetric density in g/cm^3.[139] Although it is used chiefly for the spine (Fig. 3–10), it can be used for the hip.

Peripheral devices provide greater portability, ease of use, and a lower radiation dose at a lower cost than do central devices.[150, 159, 161, 168] Generally, precision and accuracy are comparable to that of central devices.[150, 159, 161] Peripheral QCT is mostly used to measure BMD in the forearm. Peripheral DXA has been used to measure the forearm, phalanges, or calcaneus. QUS may be used to measure the calcaneus, forearm, or phalanges. QUS is different from other densitometric methods because it does not measure BMD.[142, 143] Instead, speed of sound and/or broadband ultrasound attenuation is usually measured.[142, 143] On some devices, additional parameters such as stiffness or quantitative ultrasound index (QUI) are calculated.[142, 143] In general, parameters measured with QUS are lower in patients with osteoporosis than in those in control groups.[142, 143] Prospective data of elderly women indicate that QUS parameters may be used to predict the risk of hip fracture.[142]

Bone Mineral Density for Diagnosis of Osteoporosis

For postmenopausal white women, the World Health Organization (WHO) has defined osteoporosis as BMD 2.5 standard deviations or more below the mean for young adult women.[140, 154, 176, 200] Using this definition, 30% of postmenopausal white women in the United States have osteoporosis at the PA spine, hip, or forearm.[176] The prevalence of osteoporosis defined with BMD increases with age.[164, 176, 200] For example, the prevalence of osteoporosis at the femoral neck in British women increases from 4% in those between the ages of 50 and 59 to 48% in those at age 80.[200]

When measured with DXA, peak BMD at the spine is achieved between ages 25 and 30[88, 89, 106] (Figs. 3–11 and 3–12; see Fig. 3–10). After this, there is a gradual loss of bone related to age. In women, this loss is accelerated in early postmenopausal years and reverts to a slower rate about a decade later. In men, the loss does not become accelerated until after age 65.

There are some unresolved issues in the use of BMD thresholds for the diagnosis of osteoporosis. For example, the rate at which BMD is accrued in childhood, the age at which peak BMD is reached, and the rate of subsequent loss of BMD is in part determined by the densitometric method used (e.g., DXA, QCT), the skeletal site measured (e.g., spine, hip), and the population studied (e.g., gender, ethnicity).[142, 164, 192, 200] Consequently, the WHO threshold should be used only in postmenopausal white women measured with DXA of the PA spine, hip, and forearm. At present, there is considerable controversy regarding appropriate diagnostic thresholds in men, younger women, individuals of color, and those measured with densitometric techniques other than DXA.[140, 142, 164]

In most populations studied, African Americans have the highest BMD, whites have the lowest BMD, and Asians have an intermediate BMD.[164, 184] Within racial groups, men have larger skeletons than do women, so men's BMD is higher than that of women using some densitometric methods but not others.[184] Measured with DXA, men's BMD is higher than women's BMD because DXA measurement is affected by bone size.[184] In contrast, men have similar BMD to women when measured with QCT, because QCT is not affected by bone size.[184]

Despite these uncertainties, bone densitometry is widely used for the diagnosis of osteoporosis. Undoubtedly, as more data become available, the controversy surrounding appropriate diagnostic thresholds will be settled. Because bone densitometry is the only way to make the diagnosis of osteoporosis in individuals prior to fracture, its use in clinical practice will continue.

Bone Mineral Density and Risk of Fracture

In clinical practice, bone densitometry is used not only to diagnose osteoporosis but also to assess the severity of disease, thereby determining prognosis. Prognosis, in turn, is inevitably linked to risk of fracture. A significant correlation between BMD and fracture risk has been demonstrated at biomechanical testing[123, 173, 196] and in epidemiologic trials.* Most biomechanical studies have shown that BMD accounts for approximately 70% to 90% of bone strength.[123, 173, 196] A recent meta-analysis[167] of 11 prospective fracture studies in women conducted in the

---

*See references 97, 124, 125, 130, 131, 148, 158, 167, 175, 193, 198, 200.

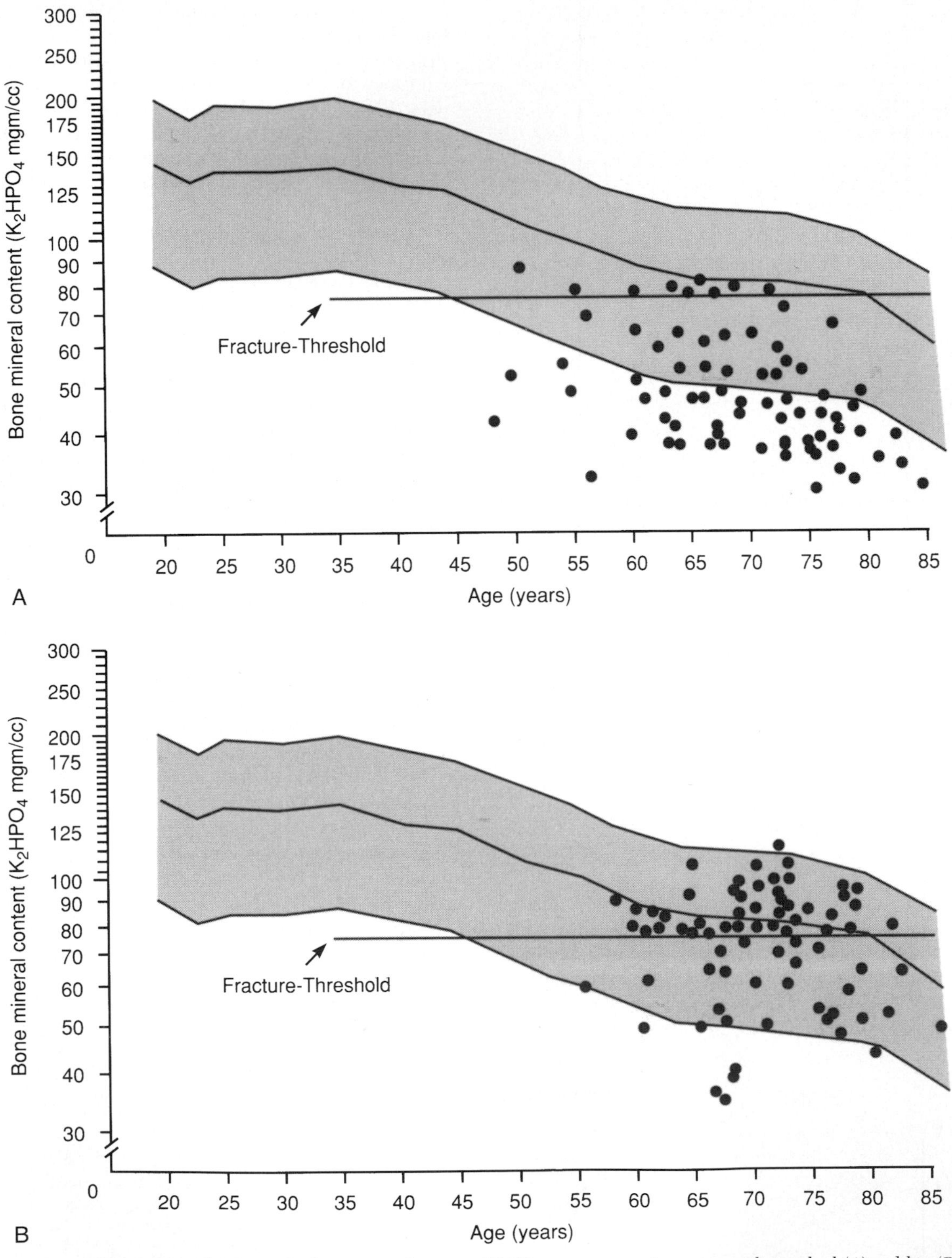

Figure 3–10. Quantitative computed tomography bone mineral content (BMC) measurements in women with vertebral (*A*) and hip (*B*) fractures. *A*, Scatter diagram of BMC measurements in 74 osteoporotic women with vertebral fractures (*black dots*). The *center line* within the shaded area depicts the age-adjusted mean spinal BMC in 419 normal women at 90% confidence limits. *B*, Scatter diagram of BMC measurements in 83 osteoporotic women with hip fracture (*black dots*). The *center line* within the shaded area depicts the age-adjusted mean spinal BMC in 419 normal women at 90% confidence limits. Note that the spinal BMC correlates sharply with the presence of spinal fracture, as depicted in *A*, but there is poor correlation between spinal BMC and fracture of the hip, as depicted in *B*. (From Firooznia, H., Rafii, M., Golimbu, C. et al. [1986]. Trabecular mineral content of the spine in women with hip fracture: CT measurement. Radiology, *159*:737, with permission.)

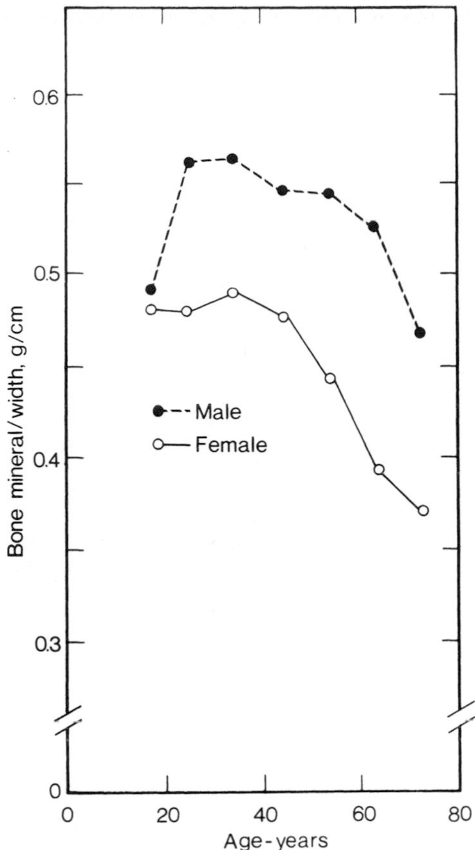

Figure 3–11. Variations with age of bone mineral content/width (g/cm^2) at the distal end of the radius of men and women, using the ^{125}I photon absorption method. Note that in both sexes, mineral content/width reaches a peak between 25 and 35 years, declining precipitously for women after 45 years and for men after 65 years. (Adapted from Goldsmith, N.F., & Johnston, J.O. [1973]. Mineralization of the bone in an insured population: Correlation with reported fractures and other measures of osteoporosis. Int. J. Epidemiol., 2:311, with permission.)

United States, Europe, and Australia concluded that for every standard deviation decrease in BMD, the risk of fracture doubles. Although the evidence in men, younger women, and individuals of color is less robust, cross-sectional data appear to support the relationship between BMD and fracture risk in these groups as well.[130, 131, 158]

Although there is a positive correlation between BMD at various sites, assessment of fracture risk is best achieved by direct measurements of the sites at risk rather than extrapolation from a different site[80, 106, 125, 167] (see Fig. 3–10). For example, the risk of hip fracture increases 2.6 times for every standard deviation decrease in femoral neck BMD, whereas the risk increases only 1.5 times for every standard deviation decrease in calcaneal BMD.[167]

Determining prognosis of osteoporosis requires a more global assessment of an individual's risk factors for fracture.[113, 129, 146, 193] Many risk factors, including female gender, increased age, estrogen deficiency, white or Asian ethnicity, family history of osteoporosis, calcium deficiency, vitamin D deficiency, low body weight, prior fracture, and smoking, are strongly associated with low BMD.[113, 129, 184] Among these, there are risk factors that predict fracture independently of BMD. For example, after controlling for BMD, advanced age and previous fracture remain powerful predictors of future fractures.[129, 156] Equally important is the fact that some risk factors for osteoporotic fracture are completely unrelated to BMD. These include propensity to fall, low physical function, impaired vision, impaired cognition, and environmental hazards.[141]

Although the osteoporotic skeleton is weak, most fractures do not occur spontaneously.[28] Hip fractures, in particular, generally require a fall.[108, 28] The risk of falling in one year increases from 1 in 5 for women ages 35 to 49 to 1 in 2 for women age 85 or older.[199] The risk of falling increases with the number of comorbid conditions present.[141] Chronic illnesses and the medications used to treat them are especially important in the pathophysiology of falls. The elderly sustain loss of agility and coordination, reduction in the sense of equilibrium, and general slowing of reaction time. These factors are frequently compounded by medications, particularly hypnotics, antidepressants, and polypharmacy, and they are further complicated by chronic illnesses, including cardiovascular disease and neurologic disorders such as Alzheimer's disease, urinary incontinence, and depression.[60, 62, 63, 141] When coupled with a decrease in muscular strength and impaired vision and hearing, these factors lead to an increased number of falls. Various hazards found in the homes of patients with osteoporosis, including loose rugs, slippery

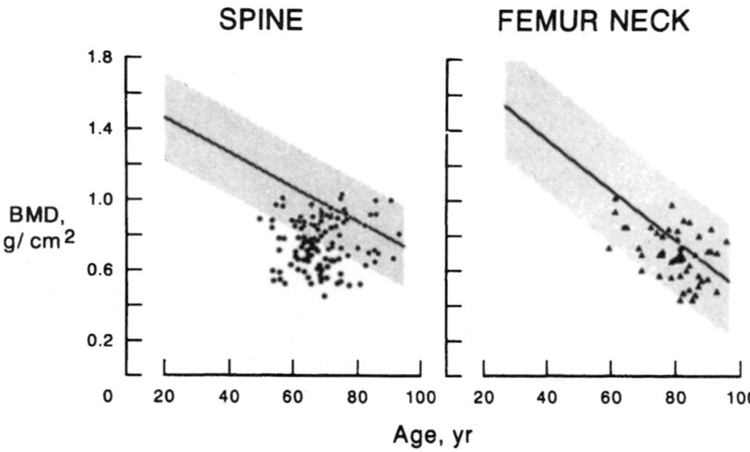

Figure 3–12. Bone mineral density (BMD) measurements of lumbar spine and femoral neck plotted as a function of age for 111 patients with vertebral fractures (*dots*) and 49 patients with hip fractures (*triangles*). The *line* represents the regression on age; the *stippled area* shows the 90% confidence limits for 166 normal women. Note that the fracture threshold (90th percentile of the measurements for patients with fractures) is about 1.0 g/cm^2 and is independent of age. (From Riggs, B.L. & Melton, L.J. III. [1986]. Involutional osteoporosis. N. Engl. J. Med., *314*:1676, with permission.)

floors, exposed electrical cords, unstable furniture, and poor lighting, contribute to the propensity of falls in these patients.[141] Certainly, the more severe the degree of osteoporosis and the greater the number of falls, the greater the likelihood of fracture. Mortality rate within 6 months of hip fracture increases by a factor of 2.5.[14, 20, 62] Thus, the older a person is, the more likely the person is to fall, to fracture a hip, and to die of the injury.[14, 20, 62]

Undoubtedly, BMD is an important contributor to fracture risk. In fact, BMD measurements are better correlated with risk of fracture than serum cholesterol measurements are with risk of cardiovascular disease.[167] However, clinicians must look beyond BMD when counseling individual patients with osteoporosis about their overall risk of fracture.

Bone Mineral Density and Monitoring of Therapy

Treatment of patients with osteoporosis with estrogens,[81, 92, 93, 101, 111, 151, 163, 171] selective estrogen receptor modulators,[127, 134, 165, 180, 191] calcitonin,[187] and bisphosphonates* has been shown to either forestall or reverse the progression of osteoporosis and thereby reduce the risk of fracture. Clinicians often use serial BMD measurements to identify patients who are not responding to pharmacologic intervention.[132, 183] Because options for medical treatment of osteoporosis will undoubtedly increase in the future, BMD testing will continue to be widely used to help patients and their doctors select the best treatment option.

Impact

The impact of all other skeletal diseases now and in the predictable future will remain relatively small compared with the problems posed by osteoporosis. Osteoporosis affects approximately 75 million people in the United States, Europe, and Japan.[140] In the United States and Europe alone it results in 2.3 million fractures annually.[140] In the future, the number of osteoporotic fractures will increase substantially due to increasing life expectancy and the resultant increase in the number of elderly people.[15, 21, 122] For example, in 1990 there were approximately 1.5 million hip fractures worldwide; by the year 2025, 3 million hip fractures per year are expected.[15, 122] Surprisingly, in some countries the age-adjusted fracture rates increased in the second part of the 20th century compared with the first part.[12, 22, 23, 26] Explanations for the increase include decreased physical activity of urban populations, increased hardness of surfaces on which people fall, and increased frailty of the elderly. Whatever the cause, secular trends may increase future fracture rates beyond what is expected from demographic shifts.

Even today, the lifetime risk of having an osteoporotic fracture is far from trivial. In the United States, the lifetime risk of hip fracture is 18% for white women and 6% for white men.[184, 200] In Britain, the risk is 14% for white women and 3% for white men.[184, 200] In the United States, the lifetime risk of hip fracture exceeds the combined lifetime risk of breast, endometrial, and ovarian cancer for women and prostate cancer for men.[184, 200] The lifetime risk of clinical vertebral fracture in the United States is 16% for white women and 5% for white men.[184, 200] In Britain, the risk is 11% for white women and 2% for white men.[184, 200] The lifetime risk of forearm fracture in the United States is 16% for white women and 3% for white men.[184, 200] In Britain, the risk is 13% for white women and 2% for white men.[184, 200] In general, the age-adjusted and sex-adjusted incidence rates of fracture are higher in whites than in African Americans or in Asians.[184, 200] The lifetime risk of hip fracture is 6% for African American women and 3% for African American men.[184, 200]

The human cost of fractures is often summarized using figures relating to mortality and morbidity. Hip fractures, in particular, have an unacceptably high mortality and morbidity.[20, 140] Up to 20% of patients die within 1 year of hip fracture and another 20% require long-term nursing home care.[14, 20] With vertebral fractures, there is no early excess mortality seen with hip fractures, but survival does worsen with increasing time from injury.[18] However, vertebral fractures result in tremendous morbidity, with marked reduction in the patient's ability to perform activities of daily living. Forearm fractures do not result in any excess morbidity, but they may result in poor functional outcome or reflex sympathetic dystrophy syndrome.[19] Psychosocial consequences of fractures in the elderly are difficult to measure, but they certainly contribute greatly to a diminished quality of life for those affected.

The cost[102, 104, 140, 189, 194, 197] of skeletal trauma in the elderly is enormous, and in light of current population trends will certainly become more so. In the United States, direct cost of all fractures is $35 to $41 billion per year.[189] Osteoporotic fractures cost the health care system $10 to $15 billion per year, with approximately 80% owing to hip fractures. Thus, osteoporotic fractures have a large impact on individual patients as well as on our society.

Fortunately, there are densitometric techniques available to identify individuals with osteoporosis who are at risk for fractures. Ultimately, early diagnosis and treatment should improve the quality of life of the elderly.

*See references 116, 126, 136, 144, 145, 147, 153, 162, 163, 170, 188.

References

General

1. Bauer, G.C.H. (1970). Epidemiology of fractures. p. 153. In Barzel, U.S. Ed.: Osteoporosis. Grune & Stratton, New York.
2. Buhr, A.J., & Cooke, A.M. (1959). Fracture patterns. Lancet, *1*:531.
3. Gallagher, J.C., Aaron, J., Horsman, A. et al. (1973). The crush fracture syndrome in postmenopausal women. Clin. Endocrinol. Metab., *2*:293.
4. Garn, S.M., Rohmann, C.G., Wagner, B., & Ascoli, W. (1967). Continuing bone growth throughout life: A general phenomenon. Am. J. Phys. Anthropol., *26*:313.
5. Goldsmith, N.F., & Johnston, J.O. (1973). Mineralization of the bone in an insured population: Correlation with reported fractures and other measures of osteoporosis. Int. J. Epidemiol., *2*:311.
6. Horak, J., & Nilsson, B.E. (1975). Epidemiology of fracture of the upper end of the humerus. Clin. Orthop., *112*:250.
7. Nilsson, B.E., & Westlin, N.E. (1974). The bone mineral content in the forearm of women with Colles fracture. Acta Orthop. Scand., *45*:836.
8. Nilsson, B.E., & Westlin, N.E. (1977). Bone mineral content and fragility fractures. Clin. Orthop., *125*:196.
9. Siegelman, S.S. (1970). The radiology of osteoporosis. p. 68. In Barzel, U.S. Ed.: Osteoporosis. Grune & Stratton, New York.

10. Vernon-Roberts, B., & Pirie, C.J. (1973). Healing trabecular microfractures in the bodies of lumbar vertebrae. Ann. Rheum. Dis., *32*:406.
11. Garraway, W.M., Stauffer, R.N., Kurland, L.T., & O'Fallon, W.M. (1979). Limb fractures in a defined population. I. Frequency and distribution. Mayo Clin. Proc., *54*:701.

Fracture Incidence

12. Bengner, U., Johnell, O., & Redlund-Johnell, I. (1988). Changes in incidence and prevalence of vertebral fractures during 30 years. Calcif. Tissue Int., *42*:293.
13. Donaldson, L.J., Cook, A., & Thomson, R.G. (1990). Incidence of fractures in a geographically defined population. J. Epidemiol. Community Health, *44*:241.
14. Forsen, L., Sogaard, A.J., Meyer, H.E. et al. (1999). Survival after hip fracture: Short- and long-term excess mortality according to age and gender. Osteoporos. Int., *10*:73.
15. Gullberg, B., Johnell, O., & Kanis, J.A. (1997). World-wide projections for hip fracture. Osteoporos. Int., *7*:407.
16. Johnasen, A., Harding, K., Evans, R., & Stone, M. (1999). Trauma in elderly people: What proportion of fractures are a consequence of bone fragility. Arch. Gerontol. Geriatr., *29*:215.
17. Johnell, O., Gullberg, B., Allander, E., & Kanis, J.A. (1992). The apparent incidence of hip fracture in Europe: A study of national register sources. MEDOS Study Group. Osteoporos. Int., *2*:298.
18. Kado, D.M., Browner, W.S., Palermo, L. et al. (1999). Vertebral fractures and mortality in older women. Arch. Intern. Med., *159*:1215.
19. Kaukonen, J.P., Karaharju, E.O., Porras, M. et al. (1988). Functional recovery after fractures of the distal forearm: Analysis of radiographic and other factors affecting the outcome. Ann. Chir. Gynaecol., *77*:27.
20. Keene, G.S., Parker, M.J., & Pryor, G.A. (1993). Mortality and morbidity after hip fractures. B.M.J., *307*:1248.
21. Melton, L.J. (1996). Epidemiology of hip fractures: Implications of the exponential increase with age. Bone, *18*:121S.
22. Melton, L.J., Crowson, C.S., & O'Fallon, W.M. (1999). Fracture incidence in Olmsted County, Minnesota: Comparison of urban and rural rates and changes in urban rates over time. Osteoporos. Int., *9*:29.
23. Melton, L.J. III, Amadio, P.C., Crowson, C.S., & O'Fallon, W.M. (1998). Long-term trends in the incidence of distal forearm fractures. Osteoporos. Int., *8*:341.
24. Melton, L.J. III, Lane, A.W., Cooper, C. et al. (1993). Prevalence and incidence of vertebral deformities. Osteoporos. Int., *3*:113.
25. O'Neill, T.W., Felsenberg, D., Varlow, J. et al. & the European Vertebral Osteoporosis Study Group. (1996). The prevalence of vertebral deformity in European men and women: The European Vertebral Osteoporosis Study. J. Bone Miner. Res., *11*:1010.
26. Obrant, K.J., Bengnér, U., Johnell, O. et al. (1989). Increasing age-adjusted risk of fragility fractures: A sign of increasing osteoporosis in successive generations? Calcif. Tissue Int., *44*:157.
27. Owen, R.A., Melton, L.J. III, Johnson, K.A. et al. (1982). Incidence of Colles' fracture in a North American community. Am. J. Public Health, *72*:605.
28. Parker, M.J., & Twemlow, T.R. (1997). Spontaneous hip fractures. Acta Orthop. Scand., *68*:325.
29. Rose, S.H., Melton, J. III, Morrey, B.F. et al. (1982). Epidemiologic features of humeral fractures. Clin. Orthop. Rel. Res., *168*:24.
30. Sanders, K.M., Pasco, J.A., Ugoni, A.M. et al. (1998). The exclusion of high trauma fractures may underestimate the prevalence of bone fragility fractures in the community: The GEELONG Osteoporosis Study. J. Bone Miner. Res., *13*:1337.
31. Sanders, K.M., Seeman, E., Ugoni, A.M. et al. (1999). Age- and gender-specific rate of fractures in Australia: A population-based study. Osteoporos. Int., *10*:240.
32. Schwartz, A.V., Kelsey J.L., Maggi, S. et al. (1999). International variation in the incidence of hip fractures: Cross-national project on osteoporosis for the world health organization program for research on aging. Osteoporos. Int., 9:242.
33. Solgaard, S., & Petersen, V.S. (1985). Epidemiology of distal radius fractures. Acta. Orthop. Scand., *56*:391.

Motor Vehicle Accidents

34. Agran, P.F., Dunkle, D.E., & Winn, D.G. (1987). Injuries to a sample of seatbelted children evaluated and treated in a hospital emergency room. J. Trauma, *27*:58.
35. Baker, S.P., Whitfield, R.A., & O'Neill, B. (1987). Geographic variations in mortality from motor vehicle crashes. N. Engl. J. Med., *316*:1384.
36. Chorba, T.L., Reinfurt, D., & Hulka, B.S. (1988). Efficacy of mandatory seat-belt use legislation: The North Carolina experience from 1983 through 1987. J.A.M.A., *260*:3593.
37. Council on Scientific Affairs. (1983). Automobile related injuries: Components, trends, prevention. J.A.M.A., *249*:3216.
38. Fife, D., Barancik, J.I., & Chatterjee, B.J. (1984). Northeastern Ohio Trauma Study. II. Injury rates by age, sex, and cause. Am. J. Public Health, *74*:473.
39. Foege, W. (1987). Highway violence and public policy. N. Engl. J. Med., *316*:1407.
40. Haller, J.A. Jr. (1983). Pediatric trauma: The no. 1 killer of children. J.A.M.A., *7*:47.
41. Kramhoft, M., & Bodtker, S. (1988). Epidemiology of distal forearm fractures in Danish children. Acta Orthop. Scand., *59*:557.
42. Orsay, E.M., Turnbull, T.L., Dunne, M. et al. (1988). Prospective study of the effect of safety belts on morbidity and health care costs in motor-vehicle accidents. J.A.M.A., *260*:3598.
43. Payne, S.R., Waller, J.A., Skelly, J.M., & Gamelli, R.L. (1990). Injuries during woodworking, home repairs and construction. J. Trauma, *30*:276.
44. Runyan, C.W., & Gerken, E.A. (1989). Epidemiology and prevention of adolescent injury: A review and research agenda. J.A.M.A., *262*:2273.
45. Smith, H.T. (1974). Fractures seen in a rural community hospital. Texas Med., *70*:65.
46. Waller, J.A. (1985). Injury Control: A Guide to the Causes and Prevention of Trauma. Lexington Books, D.C. Heath and Company, Toronto, Canada.

Falls

In Children

47. Barlow, B., Niemirska, M., Gandhi, R.P., & LeBlanc, W. (1983). Ten years of experience with falls from a height in children. J. Pediatr. Surg., *18*:509.
48. Bergner, L., Mayer, S., & Harris, D. (1971). Falls from heights: A childhood epidemic in an urban area. Am. J. Public Health, *61*:90.
49. Ramos, S.M., & Delany, H.M. (1986). Free falls from heights: A persistent urban problem. J. Natl. Med. Assoc., *78*:111.
50. Reynold, B.M., Balsano, N.A., & Reynolds, F.X. (1971). Falls from heights: A surgical experience of 200 consecutive cases. Ann. Surg., *174*:304.
51. Roshkow, J.E., Haller, J.O., Hotson, G.C. et al. (1990). Imaging evaluation of children after falls from a height: Review of 45 cases. Radiology, *175*:359.
52. Scalea, T., Goldstein, A., Phillips, T. et al. (1986). An analysis of 161 falls from a height: The Jumper Syndrome. J. Trauma, *26*:706.
53. Sieben, R.L., Leavitt, J.D., & French, J.H. (1971). Falls as childhood accidents: An increasing urban risk. Pediatrics, *47*:866.
54. Smith, M.D., Burrington, J.D., & Woolf, A.D. (1975). Injuries in children sustained in free falls: An analysis of 66 cases. J. Trauma, *15*:987.
55. Spiegel, C.N., & Lindaman, F.C. (1977). Children can't fly: A program to prevent childhood morbidity and mortality from window falls. Am. J. Public Health, *67*:1143.
56. Velcek, F.T., Weiss, A., DiMaio, D. et al. (1977). Traumatic death in urban children. J. Pediatr. Surg., *12*:375.

In the Elderly

57. Baker, S.P., & Harvey, A.H. (1985). Fall injuries in the elderly. Clin. Geriatr. Med., *1*:501.
58. Blake, A.J., Morgan, K., Bendall, M.D. et al. (1988). Falls by elderly people at home: Prevalence and associated factors. Age Ageing, *17*:365.
59. Boyce, W.J. (1987). Osteoporosis, falls, and age in fracture of the proximal femur. Br. Med. J., *295*:444.
60. Buchner, D.M., & Larson, E.B. (1987). Falls and fractures in patients with Alzheimer-type dementia. J.A.M.A., *257*:1492.
61. Cooper, C., Barker, D.J.P., Morris, J., & Briggs, R.S.J. (1987). Osteoporosis, falls, and age in fracture of the proximal femur. Br. Med. J., *295*:13.
62. Evans, J.G. (1988). Falls and fractures. Age Ageing, *17*:361.
63. Evans, J.G., Prudham, D., & Wandless, J.A. (1979). A prospective study of fractured proximal femur: Factors predisposing to survival. Age Ageing, *8*:246.
64. Gaerdsell, P., Johnell, O., Nilsson, B.E., & Nilsson, J.A. (1989). The predictive value of fracture, disease and falling tendency for fragility fractures in women. Calcif. Tissue Int., *45*:327.
65. Melton, L.J. III, & Riggs, B.L. (1985). Risk factors for injury after a fall. Clin. Geriatr. Med., *1*:525.
66. Peck, W.A. (1986). Falls and hip fracture in the elderly. Hosp. Pract., December 15, p. 72.
67. Prudham, D., & Evans, J.G. (1981). Factors associated with falls in the elderly: A community study. Age Ageing, *10*:141.
68. Tinetti, M.E., Speechley, M., & Ginter, S.F. (1988). Risk factors for falls among elderly persons living in the community. N. Engl. J. Med., *319*:1701.
69. Winner, S.J., Morgan, C.A., & Evans, J.G. (1989). Perimenopausal risk of falling and incidence of distal forearm fracture. Br. Med. J., *298*:1486.
70. Zylke, J.W. (1990). As nation grows older, falls become greater source of fear, injury, death. J.A.M.A., *263*:2021.

Seizures

71. Brown, R.J. (1984). Bilateral dislocation of the shoulders. Injury, *15*:267.
72. Coover, C. (1983). Double posterior luxation of the shoulder. Penn. Med. J., *35*:566.
73. Dastgeer, G.M., & Mikolich, D.J. (1987). Fracture-dislocation of manubriosternal joint: An unusual complication of seizures. J. Trauma, *27*:91.
74. Karpinski, M.R.K., & Porter, K.M. (1984). Bilateral posterior dislocation of the shoulder. Injury, *15*:274.
75. Kelly, J.P. (1954). Fractures complicating electro-convulsive therapy and chronic epilepsy. J. Bone Joint Surg. [Br.], *36*:70.
76. Lovelock, J.E., & Monaco, L.P. (1983). Central acetabular fracture dislocations: An unusual complication of seizures. Skeletal Radiol., *10*:91.
77. Paton, D.F. (1979). Posterior dislocation of the shoulder: A diagnostic pitfall for physicians. Practitioner, *233*:111.

78. Remec, P.T., & McCollister Evarts, C. (1983). Bilateral central dislocation of the hip: A case report. Clin. Orthop., *181*:118.
79. Varma, A.N., Seth, S.K., & Verma, M. (1981). Simultaneous bilateral central dislocation of the hip: An unusual complication of eclampsia. J. Trauma, *21*:499.

Osteoporosis

80. Barth, R.W., & Lane, J.M. (1988). Osteoporosis. Orthop. Clin. North Am., *19*:845.
81. Barzel, U.S. (1988). Estrogens in the prevention and treatment of postmenopausal osteoporosis: A review. Am. J. Med., *85*:847.
82. Boyce, W.J., & Vessey, M.P. (1985). Rising incidence of fracture of the proximal femur. Lancet, *1*:150.
83. Campion, E.W., Jette, A.M., Cleary, P.D., & Harris, B.E. (1987). Hip fracture: A prospective study of hospital course, complications, and costs. J. Gen. Intern. Med., *2*:78.
84. Cann, E.C. (1988). Quantitative CT for determination of bone mineral density: A review. Radiology, *166*:509.
85. Dias, J.J., Wray, C.C., & Jones, J.M. (1987). Osteoporosis and Colles fractures in the elderly. J. Hand. Surg. [Br.], *12*:57.
86. Dickenson, R.P., Hutton, W.C., & Stott, J.R.R. (1981). The mechanical properties of bone in osteoporosis. J. Bone Joint Surg. [Br.], *63*:233.
87. Eastell, R., Riggs, B.L., Wahner, H.W. et al. (1989). Colles fracture and bone density of the ultradistal radius. J. Bone Mineral Res., *4*:607.
88. Firooznia, H., Rafii, M., Golimbu, C. et al. (1986). Trabecular mineral content of the spine in women with hip fracture: CT measurement. Radiology, *159*:737.
89. Genant, H.K., Block, J.E., Steiger, P. et al. (1987). Quantitative computed tomography in assessment of osteoporosis. Semin. Nucl. Med., *17*:316.
90. Heaney, R.P. (1989). Osteoporotic fracture space: An hypothesis. Bone Mineral, *6*:1.
91. Kaplan, F.S. (1983). Osteoporosis. Clin. Symp., *35*:2.
92. Kelsey, J., & Hoffman, S. (1987). Risk factors for hip fracture. N. Engl. J. Med., *316*:404.
93. Kiel, D.P., Felson, D.T., Jennifer, M.P.H. et al. (1987). Hip fracture and the use of estrogens in postmenopausal women: The Framingham Study. N. Engl. J. Med., *317*:1169.
94. Lewinnek, G.E., Kelsey, J., White, A.A., & Kreiger, N.J. (1980). The significance and a comparative analysis of the epidemiology of hip fractures. Clin. Orthop., *152*:35.
95. Lizaur-Utrilla, A., Orts, A.P., Del Campo, F.S. et al. (1987). Epidemiology of trochanteric fractures of the femur in Alicante, Spain, 1974–1982. Clin. Orthop., *218*:24.
96. Makin, M. (1987). Osteoporosis and proximal femoral fractures in the female elderly of Jerusalem. Clin. Orthop., *218*:19.
97. Melton, L.J., Kan, S.H., Wahner, H.W., & Riggs, B.L. (1988). Lifetime fracture risk: An approach to hip fracture risk assessment based on bone mineral density and age. J. Clin. Epidemiol., *41*:985.
98. Melton, L.J. III, O'Fallon, W.M., & Riggs, B.L. (1987). Secular trends in the incidence of hip fractures. Calcif. Tissue Int., *41*:57.
99. Melton, L.J. III, Sampson, J.M., Morrey, B.F., & Ilstrup, D.M. (1981). Epidemiologic features of pelvic fractures. Clin. Orthop., *155*:43.
100. Mensforth, R.P., & Latimer, B.M. (1989). Hamann-Todd collection aging studies: Osteoporosis fracture syndrome. Am. J. Phys. Anthropol., *80*:461.
101. Meuleman, J. (1989). Osteoporosis and the elderly. Med. Clin. North Am., *73*:1455.
102. Owen, R.A., Melton, L.J. III, Gallagher, J.C., & Riggs, B.L. (1980). The national cost of acute care of hip fractures associated with osteoporosis. Clin. Orthop., *150*:172.
103. Parfitt, A.M. (1987). Trabecular bone architecture in the pathogenesis and prevention of fracture. Am. J. Med., *82*:68.
104. Phillips, S., Fox, N., Facobs, J., & Wright, W.E. (1988). The direct medical costs of osteoporosis for American women aged 45 and older, 1986. Bone, *9*:271.
105. Raisz, L.G. (1988). Local and systemic factors in the pathogenesis of osteoporosis. N. Engl. J. Med., *318*:818.
106. Riggs, B.L., & Melton, L.J. III. (1986). Involutional osteoporosis. N. Engl. J. Med., *314*:1676.
107. Riggs, B.L., Wahner, H.W., Dunn, W.L. et al. (1981). Differential changes in bone mineral density of the appendicular and axial skeleton with aging: Relationship to spinal osteoporosis. J. Clin. Invest., *67*:328.
108. Riggs, B.L., Wahner, W., Seeman, E. et al. (1982). Changes in bone mineral density of the proximal femur and spine with aging. J. Clin. Invest., *70*:716.
109. Rogers, L.F. (1985). Skeletal trauma in the elderly: Diagnostic and epidemiologic considerations. Arch. Clin. Imag., *1*:122.
110. Rose, S.H., Melton, L.J. III, Morrey, B.F. et al. (1982). Epidemiologic features of humeral fractures. Clin. Orthop., *168*:24.
111. Weiss, N.S., Ure, C.L., Ballard, J.H. et al. (1980). Decreased risk of fractures of the hip and lower forearm with postmenopausal use of estrogen. N. Engl. J. Med., *303*:1195.
112. Zetterberg, C., Elmerson, S., & Andersson, G.B.J. (1984). Epidemiology of hip fractures in Goeteborg, Sweden, 1940–1983. Clin. Orthop., *191*:43.

Bone Density and Risk of Fracture in Osteoporosis

113. Allolio, B. (1999). Risk factors for hip fracture not related to bone mass and their therapeutic implications. Osteoporos. Int., *2*:S9.
114. Anonymous. (1993). Consensus Development Conference: Diagnosis, prophylaxis, and treatment of osteoporosis. Am. J. Med., *94*:646.
115. Black, D. (1995). Why elderly women should be screened and treated to prevent osteoporosis. Am. J. Med., *98*(suppl 2A): 67S.
116. Black, D.M., Cummings, S.R., Karpf, D.B., et al. (1996). Randomized trial of effect of alendronate on risk of fracture in women with existing vertebral fractures. Lancet, *348*:1535.
117. Broadus, A.E. (1999). Mineral balance and homeostasis. p. 74. In Favus, M.J. Ed.: Primer on the Metabolic Bone Diseases and Disorders of Mineral Metabolism. 4th Ed. Lippincott Williams & Wilkins, Philadelphia.
118. Compston, J.E., Cooper, C., & Kanis, J.A. (1995). Bone densitometry in clinical practice. B.M.J., *310*:1507.
119. Cooper, C. (1999). Epidemiology of osteoporosis. Osteoporos. Int., *2*:S2.
120. Cooper, C. et al. (1992). Fracture Incidence in Osteoporosis. Trends Endocrine Metab., *3*:224.
121. Cooper, C., Atkinson, E.J., O'Fallon, W.M., & Melton, L.J. III. (1992). Incidence of clinically diagnosed vertebral fractures: A population-based study in Rochester, Minnesota. J. Bone Miner. Res., *7*:221.
122. Cooper, C., Campion, G., & Melton, L.J.(1992). Hip fractures in the elderly: A world-wide projection. Osteoporos. Int., *2*:285.
123. Courtney, A.C., Wachtel, E.F., Myers, E.R., & Hayes, W.C. (1995). Age-related reductions in the strength of the femur tested in a fall-loading configuration. J. Bone Joint Surg., *77A*:387.
124. Cummings, S.R., Black, D.M., & Nevitt, M.C. (1990). Appendicular bone density and age predict hip fracture in women. J.A.M.A., *263*:665.
125. Cummings, S.R., Black, D.M., & Nevitt, M.C. (1993). Bone density at various sites for prediction of hip fractures. Lancet, *341*:72.
126. Cummings, S.R., Black, D.M., Thompson, D.E. et al. (1998). Effect of alendronate on risk of fracture in women with low bone density but without vertebral fractures: Results from the Fracture Intervention Trial. J.A.M.A., *280*:2077.
127. Cummings, S.R., Eckert, S., Krueger, K.A. et al. (1999). The effect of raloxifene on risk of breast cancer in postmenopausal women: Results from the MORE randomized trial. Multiple Outcomes of Raloxifene Evaluation. J.A.M.A., *16*:281:2189.
128. Cummings, S.R., Kelsey, J.L., & Nevitt, M.C. (1985). Epidemiology of osteoporosis and osteoporotic fractures. Epidemiol. Rev., *7*:178.
129. Cummings, S.R., Nevitt, M.C., Browner, W.S. et al. (1995). Risk factors for hip fracture in white women. N. Engl. J. Med., *332*:767.
130. DeLaet, C.E.D., van Hout, B.A., Burger, H. et al. (1997). Bone density and risk of hip fracture in men and women: Cross sectional analysis. Br. Med. J. *315*:221.
131. DeLaet, C.E.D, van Hout, B.A., Burger, H. et al. (1998). Hip fracture prediction in elderly men and women: Validation in the Rotterdam Study. J. Bone Miner. Res., *13*:1587.
132. Eastell, R. (1998). Treatment of postmenopausal osteoporosis. N. Engl. J. Med., *338*:736.
133. Ellfors, L., Allander, E., & Kanis, J.A. (1994). The variable incidence of hip fracture in Southern Europe: The MEDOS Study. Osteoporos. Int., *4*:253.
134. Ettinger, B., Black, D.M., Mitlak, B.H. et al. (1999). Reduction of vertebral fracture risk in postmenopausal women with osteoporosis treated with raloxifene: Results from a 3-year randomized clinical trial. Multiple Outcomes of Raloxifene Evaluation (MORE) Investigators. J.A.M.A., *282*:637.
135. Finsen, V., & Anda, S. (1988). Accuracy of visually estimated bone mineralization in routine radiographs of the lower extremity. Skeletal Radiol., *17*:270.
136. Fleisch, H. (2000). Bone and mineral metabolism. p. 1. In Bisphosphonates in Bone Disease: From the Laboratory to the Patient. 4th Ed. Academic Press, New York.
137. Frost, H.M. (1999). On the estrogen-bone relationship and postmenopausal bone loss: A new model. J. Bone Miner. Res., *14*:1473.
138. Garton, M.J., Cooper, C., & Reid D., (1997). Perimenopausal bone density screening: Will it help prevent osteoporosis? Maturitas, *26*:35.
139. Genant, H.K., Cann, C.E., & Ettinger, B. (1982). Quantitative computed tomography of vertebral spongiosa: A sensitive method for detecting early bone loss after oophorectomy. Ann. Intern. Med., *97*:699.
140. Genant, H.K., Cooper, C., Poor, G. et al. (1999). Interim report and recommendations of the World Health Organization Task-Force for Osteoporosis. Osteoporos. Int., *10*:259.
141. Gibson, M.J. (1987). The prevention of falls in later life. Dan. Med. Bull., *34*(Suppl 4):1.
142. Gluer, C.C. (1997). Quantitative ultrasound techniques for the assessment of osteoporosis: Expert agreement on current status. The International Quantitative Ultrasound Consensus Group. J. Bone Miner. Res., *12*:1280.
143. Gonnelli, S., Cepollaro, C., & Agnusdei, D. (1995). Diagnostic value of ultrasound analysis and bone densitometry as predictors of vertebral deformity in postmenopausal women. Osteoporos. Int., *5*:413.
144. Harris, S.T., Watts, N.B., Genant, H.K. et al. (1999). Effects of risedronate treatment on vertebral and nonvertebral fractures in women with postmenopausal osteoporosis. J.A.M.A., *282*:1344.
145. Harris, S.T., Watts, N.B., Jackson, R.D. et al. (1993). Four-year study of intermittent cyclic etidronate treatment of postmenopausal osteoporosis:

Three years of blinded therapy followed by one year of open therapy. Am. J. Med., *95*:557.
146. Hodgson, S.F., & Johnston, C.C. (1996). AACE clinical practice guidelines for the prevention and treatment of postmenopausal osteoporosis. Endocrine Practice, *2*:155.
147. Hosking, D., Chilvers, C.E., Christiansen, C. et al. (1998). Prevention of bone loss with alendronate in postmenopausal women under 60 years of age. N. Engl. J. Med., *338*:485.
148. Hui, S.L., Slemenda, C.W., & Johnston, C.C. Jr. (1989). Baseline measurement of bone mass predicts fracture in white women. Ann. Intern. Med., *111*:355.
149. Jacobsen, S.J., Goldberg, J., Miles, T.P. et al. (1990). Regional variation in the incidence of hip fracture: U.S. white women aged 65 years and older. J.A.M.A., *264*:500.
150. Jergas, M., & Genant, H.K. (1993). Current methods and recent advances in the diagnosis of osteoporosis. Arthritis Rheum., *36*:1649.
151. Kanis, J.A. (1998). Are oestrogen deficiency and hormone replacement a distraction to the field of osteoporosis? Osteoporos. Int., *1*:S51.
152. Kanis, J.A., Devogelaer, J.P., & Gennari, C. (1996). Practical guide for the use of bone mineral measurements in the assessment of treatment of osteoporosis: A position paper of the European Foundation for Osteoporosis and Bone Disease. Osteoporos. Int., *6*:256.
153. Kanis, J.A., Johnell, O., Gullberg, B. et al. (1992). Evidence for efficacy of drugs affecting bone metabolism in preventing hip fracture. B.M.J., *305*:1124.
154. Kanis, J.A., Melton, L.J. III, & Christiansen, C. (1994). The diagnosis of osteoporosis. J. Bone Miner. Res., *9*:1137.
155. Kanis, J.A., Torgerson, D., & Cooper, C. (1999). Comparison of the European and U.S. practice guidelines for osteoporosis. Trends Endocrinol. Metab., *11*:28.
156. Klotzbuecher, C.M., Ross, P.D., Landsman, P.B. et al. (2000). Patients with prior fractures have an increased risk of future fractures: A summary of the literature and statistical synthesis. J. Bone Miner. Res., *15*:721.
157. Kotowicz, M.A., Melton, L.J., Cooper, C. et al. (1994). Risk of hip fracture in women with vertebral fracture. J. Bone Miner. Res., *9*:599.
158. Kroger, H., Huopio, J., Honkanen, R. et al. (1995). Prediction of fracture risk using axial bone mineral density in a perimenopausal population: A prospective study. J. Bone Miner. Res., *10*:302.
159. Lang, P., Steiger, P., & Faulkner, K. (1991). Osteoporosis: Current techniques and recent developments in quantitative bone densitometry. Radiol. Clin. North Am., *29*:49.
160. Lenchik, L., Rochmis, P., Sartoris, D.J. (1998). Optimized interpretation and reporting of dual X-ray absorptiometry (DXA) scans. A.J.R. Am. J. Roentgenol., *171*:1509.
161. Lenchik, L., & Sartoris, D.J. (1997). Current concepts in osteoporosis. A.J.R. Am. J. Roentgenol., *168*:905.
162. Liberman, U.A., Weiss, S.R., Broll, J. et al. (1995). Effect of oral alendronate on bone mineral density and the incidence of fractures in postmenopausal osteoporosis. N. Engl. J. Med., *333*:1437.
163. Lindsay, R., Cosman, F., Lobo, R.A. et al. (1999). Addition of alendronate to ongoing hormone replacement therapy in the tratement of osteoporosis: A randomized, controlled clinical trial. J. Clin. Endocrinol. Metab., *84*:3076.
164. Looker, A.C., Orwoll, E.S., Johnston, C.C. et al. (1997). Prevalance of low femoral bone density in older U.S. adults from NHANES III. J. Bone Miner. Res., *12*:1761.
165. Lufkin, E.G., Whitaker, M.D., Nickelsen, T. et al. (1998). Treatment of established postmenopausal osteoporosis with raloxifene: A randomized trial. J. Bone Miner. Res., *13*:1747.
166. Mallmin, H., Ljunghall, S., & Persson, I. (1993). Fracture of the distal forearm as a forecaster of subsequent hip fracture: A population based cohort study with 24 years of follow-up. Calcif. Tissue Int., *52*:269.
167. Marshall, D., Johnell, O., & Wedel, H. (1996). Meta-analysis of how well measures of bone mineral density predict occurrence of osteoporotic fractures. B.M.J., *312*:1254.
168. Martin, J.C., & Reid, D.M. (1996). Appendicular measurements in screening women for low axial bone mineral density. Br. J. Radiol., *69*:234.
169. Mayo-Smith, W., & Rosenthal, D.I. (1991). Radiographic appearance of osteopenia. Radiol. Clin. North Am., *29*:37.
170. McClung, M., Clemmesen, B., Daifotis, A. et al. (1998). Alendronate prevents postmenopausal bone loss in women without osteoporosis. Ann. Intern. Med., *128*:253.
171. McClung, M.R. (1999). Therapy for fracture prevention. J.A.M.A., *282*:687.
172. Melton, L.J., Atkinson, E.J., Cooper, C. et al. (1999). Vertebral fractures predict subsequent fractures. Osteoporosis. Int., *10*:214.
173. Melton, L.J., Chao, E.Y.S., & Lane, J. (1988). Biomechanical aspects of fractures. p. 111. In Riggs, B.L., & Melton, L.J. Eds.: Osteoporosis: Etiology, Diagnosis, and Management. Raven Press, New York.
174. Melton, L.J. III. (1995). Epidemiology of fractures. p 225. In Riggs, B.L., & Melton, L.J. III Eds.: Osteoporosis: Etiology, Diagnosis, and Management. 2nd Ed. Lippincott-Raven Publishers, Philadelphia.
175. Melton, L.J. III, Atkinson, E.J., & O'Fallon, W.M. (1993). Long-term fracture prediction by bone mineral assessed at different skeletal sites. J. Bone Miner. Res., *8*:1227.
176. Melton, L.J. III, Chrischilles, E.A., Cooper, C. et al. (1992). Perspective: How many women have osteoporosis? J. Bone Miner. Res., *7*:1005.
177. Melton, L.J. III, Eddy, D.M., & Johnston, C.C. Jr. (1990) Screening for osteoporosis. Ann. Int. Med., *112*:516.
178. Melton, L.J. III, Ilstrup, D.M., Beckenbaugh, R.D., & Riggs, B.L. (1981). Hip fracture recurrence: A population-based study. Clin Orthop., *167*:131.
179. Melton, L.J. III, Thamer, M., Ray, N.F. et al. (1997). Fractures attributable to osteoporosis: Report from the National Osteoporosis Foundation. J. Bone Miner. Res., *12*:16.
180. Meunier, P.J., Vignot, E., Garnero, P. et al. (1999). Treatment of postmenopausal women with osteoprosis or low bone density with raloxifene. Osteoporos. Int., *10*:330.
181. Miller, P.D. (1995). Guidelines for the clinical utilization of bone mass measurement in the adult population. Calcif. Tissue Int., *57*:251.
182. Miller, P.D., Bonnick, S.L., & Rosen, C.J. (1996). Consensus of an international panel on the clinical utility of bone mass measurement in the detection of low bone mass in the adult population. Calcif. Tissue Int., *58*:207.
183. Miller, P.D., Zapalowski, C., Kulak, C.A., & Bilezikian, J.P. (1999). Bone densitometry: The best way to detect ostoeporosis and to monitor therapy. J. Clin. Endocrinol. Metab., *84*:1867.
184. Nevitt, M.C. (1994). Epidemiology of osteoporosis. Rheum. Dis. Clin. North Am., *20*:535.
185. Nevitt, M.C., & Cummings, S.R. (1993). The Study of Osteoporotic Fractures Research Group. Type of fall and risk of hip and wrist fractures: The study of osteoporotic fractures. J. Am. Geriatr. Soc., *41*:1226.
186. Orlic, Z.C., & Raisz, L.G. (1998). Causes of secondary osteoporosis. J. Clin. Densitom., *2*:79.
187. Overgaard, K., Hansen, M.A., Jensen, S.B., & Christiansen, C. (1992). Effect of salcalcitonin given intranasally on bone mass and fracture rates in established osteoporosis: A dose-response study. B.M.J., *305*:556.
188. Pols, H.A., Felsenberg, D., Hanley, D.A. et al. (1999). Multinational, placebo-controlled, randomized trial of the effects of alendronate on bone density and fracture risk in postmenopausal women with low bone mass: Results of the FOSIT Study. Osteoporos. Int., *9*:461.
189. Ray, N.F., Chan, J.K., Thamer, M. & Melton, L.J. III. (1997). Medical expenditures for the treatment of osteoporotic fractures in the United States in 1995: Report from the National Osteoporosis Foundation. J. Bone Miner. Res., *12*:24.
190. Riggs, B.L., Khosla, S., & Melton, L.J. III. (1998). A unitary model for involutional osteoporosis: Estrogen deficiency causes both type I and type II osteoporosis in postmenopausal women and contributes to bone loss in aging men. J. Bone Miner. Res., *13*:763.
191. Riggs, B.L., Melton, L.J. III. (1992). The prevention and treatment of osteoporosis. N. Engl. J. Med., *327*:620.
192. Rizzoli, R., & Bonjour, J.P. (1999). Determinants of peak bone mass and mechanisms of bone loss. Osteoporos. Int., *2*:S17.
193. Ross, P.D., Davis, J.W., & Vogel, J.M. (1990). A critical review of bone mass and the risk of fractures in osteoporosis. Calcif. Tissue Int., *46*:149.
194. Ross, P.D., Wasnich, R.D., Maclelan, C.J. et al. (1988). A model for estimating the potential costs and savings of osteoporosis prevention strategies. Bone, *9*:337.
195. Seeley, D.G., Browner, W.S., Nevitt, M.C. et al. (1991). Which fractures are associated with low appendicular bone mass in elderly women? Ann. Intern. Med., *115*:837.
196. Spadaro, J.A., Werner, F.W., Brenner, R.A. et al. (1994). Cortical and trabecular bone contribute strength to the osteopenic distal radius. J. Orthop. Res., *12*:211.
197. Torgerson, D.J., & Reid, D.M. (1997). The economics of osteoporosis and its prevention: A review. Pharmacoeconomics, *11*:126.
198. Wasnich, R.D., Ross, P.D., & Heilbrun, L.K. (1985). Prediction of postmenopausal fracture risk with use of bone mineral measurements. Am. J. Obstet. Gynecol., *153*:745.
199. Winner, S.J., Morgan, C.A., & Evans, J.G. (1989). Perimenopausal risk of falling and incidence of distal forearm fracture. B.M.J., *298*:1486.
200. World Health Organization. (1994). Assessment of Fracture Risk and its Application to Screening for Postmenopausal Osteoporosis. Technical Report Series 843. World Health Oganization, Geneve.
201. Zimmerman, S.I., Girman, C.J., Buie, V.C. et al. (1999). The prevalence of osteoporosis in nursing home residents. Osteoporos. Int., *9*:151.

Chapter 4

IMAGING OF FRACTURES: DETECTION AND DESCRIPTION

with Felix S. Chew, MD, and Ronald W. Hendrix, MD

The Language of Fractures

The specific medical vocabulary used to describe fractures relies mostly on common, familiar words that have other meanings in other settings. When used in the context of fracture description, these words have precise, specific meanings.[11] Some of these meanings predate the discovery of x-rays, and their application to the description of diagnostic images is not always without ambiguity. Fractures are generally described and classified[3, 8, 9, 11, 12] by the location, extent, direction, position, and number of fracture lines and resultant fragments, as well as the integrity of the overlying skin. Each region of the skeleton has its own unique fracture characteristics and systems of fracture classification (see subsequent chapters).

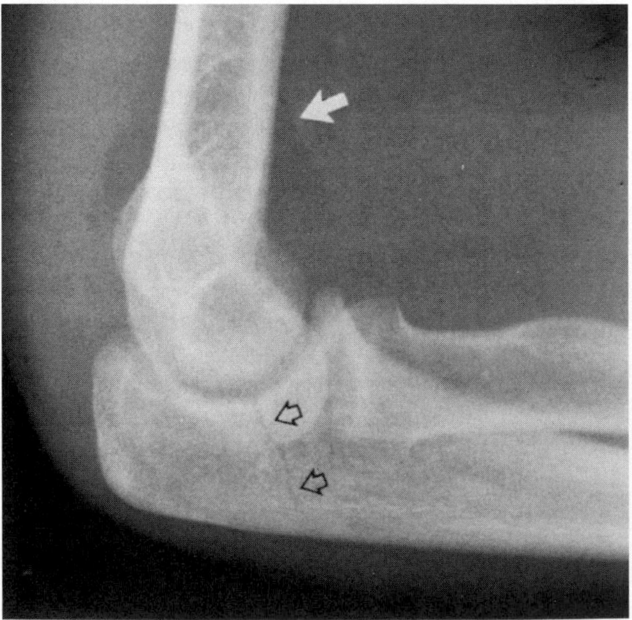

Figure 4–1. Incomplete fracture of the olecranon with joint effusion manifested by displacement of fat pads. The anterior fat pad (*solid arrow*) is lifted and the posterior fat pad is displaced by hemorrhage within the joint. A linear, nondisplaced, incomplete fracture (*open arrows*) extends from the trochlear notch of the ulna. The posterior cortex remains intact; therefore, this fracture is, by definition, an incomplete fracture.

A fracture that results in discontinuity between two or more fragments is *complete*. A fracture that results in only partial discontinuity, in which a portion or segment of the cortex remains intact, is *incomplete* (Fig. 4–1). Incomplete fractures are common in children but less common in adults.

A *comminuted fracture* is one that has two or more fracture lines and three or more fragments (Fig. 4–2). The degree of comminution is often related to the magnitude of the energy that caused the fracture. Larger forces tend to result in greater numbers of fragments, and the qualifying terms *slightly, moderately* (see Fig. 4–2), *markedly*, and *severely* (see Fig. 4–2*B*) are often used to denote the relative number of the fragments, *slightly* implying few and *markedly* implying many. Both direct and indirect forces may result in comminution.

If the overlying skin is intact, the fracture is said to be *closed*. If the overlying skin is disrupted and the fracture site is or can be exposed to the environment, the fracture is *open* (Fig. 4–3). Such fractures were formerly termed *simple* and *compound* fractures, respectively, but these terms have been generally superseded. Air in the soft tissues about the fracture site on immediate postinjury examination is highly suggestive of an open fracture, particularly if the air is in immediate contact with or in proximity to the bone fragments (see Fig. 4–3*B*). Air may become trapped in soft tissue injuries nearby but may be unrelated to the fracture; therefore, clinical inspection is better than radiographs for identifying open fractures. Open fractures may result from puncturing of the skin from the inside by a sharp bone fragment or from penetrating trauma from the outside. Fractures caused by gunshot wounds or shrapnel are always open fractures (Fig. 4–4). Traumatic amputations are also always open fractures (Fig. 4–5). The bone most frequently involved in an open fracture is the tibia (46%), followed by the femur (12.5%) and then the radius and ulna (11%).[2]

Fractures of Long Bones

Long bones are bones whose length is much greater than their width. Typically they have a shaft and a medul-

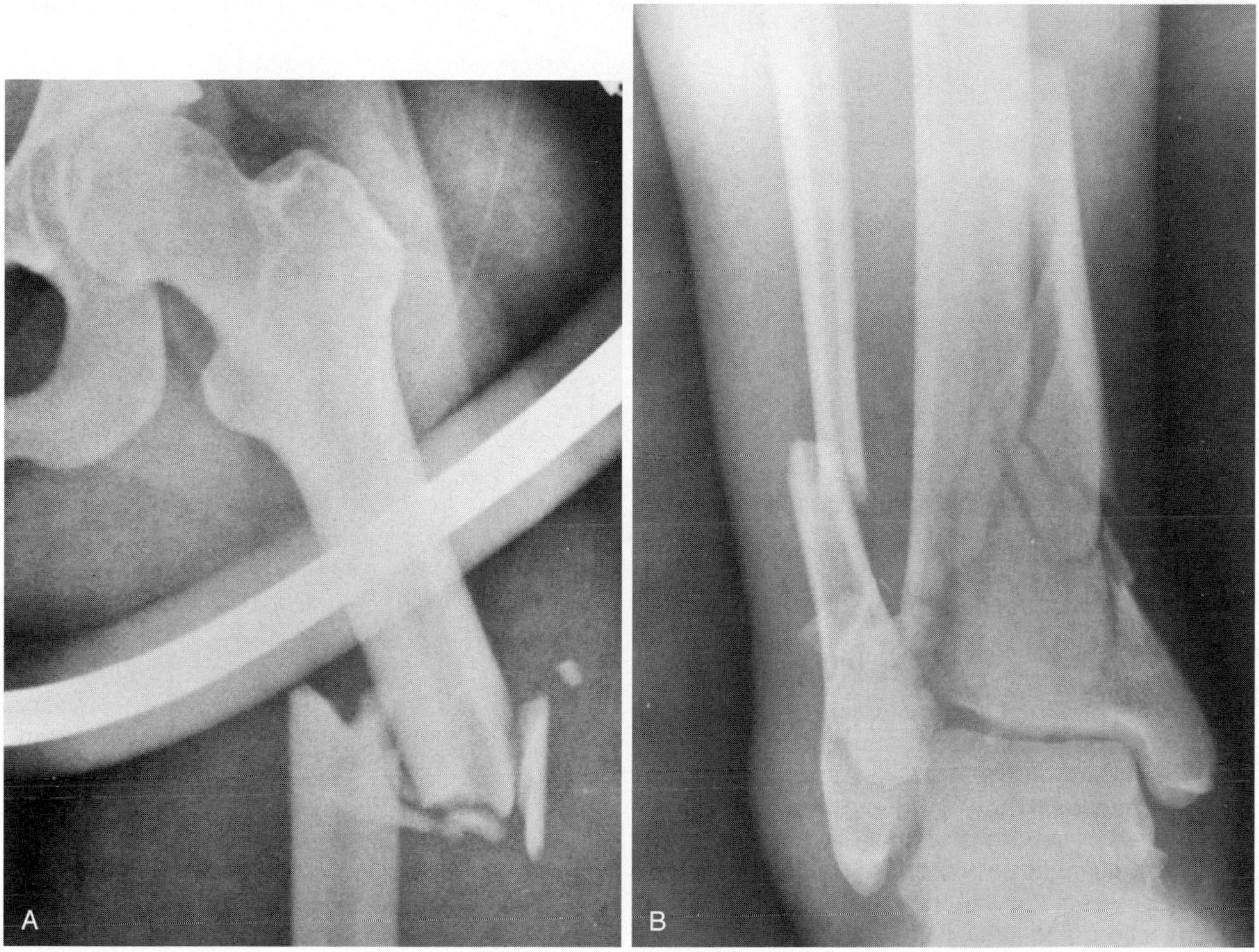

Figure 4–2. Comminuted fractures. *A*, Moderately comminuted, slightly oblique fracture of the proximal third of the femoral shaft. The proximal fragment is abducted, as is typical of a femoral shaft fracture. There is approximately 3 cm of overriding of the medially displaced distal fragment. Several fragments of bone are noted about the margin of the principal fragment. *B*, Severely comminuted fracture of the distal tibia extending into the ankle mortise with associated transverse fracture of the distal third of the fibula. All fractures occurring at the distal end of the bone should be examined closely for extension into the adjacent joint. In this case the severity of the comminution and joint extension are obvious.

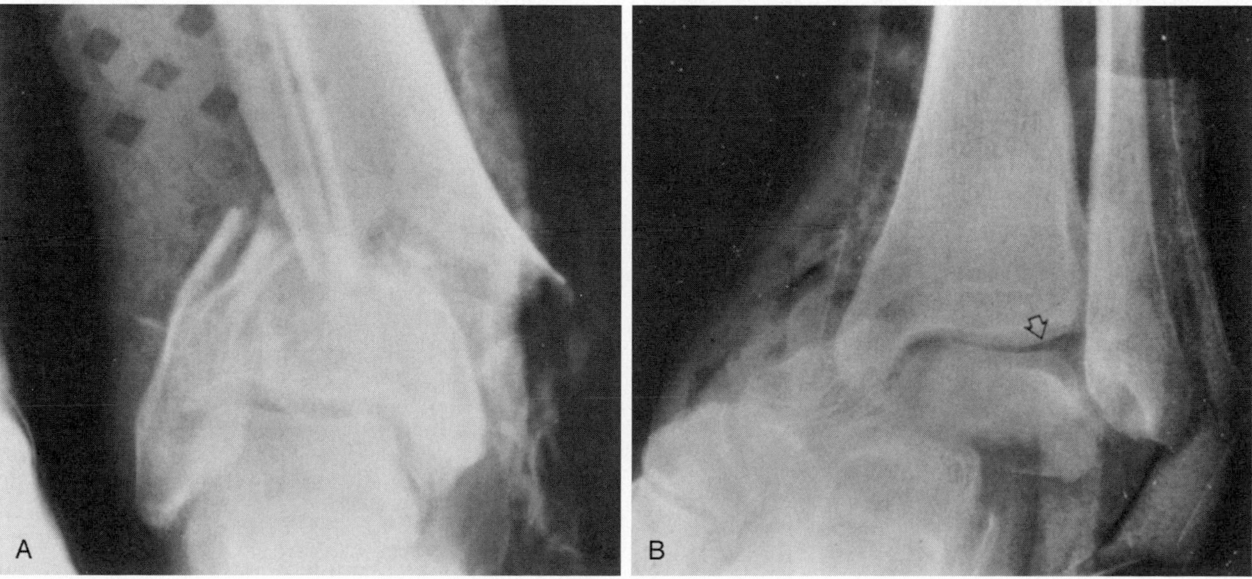

Figure 4–3. Open fractures. *A*, Open transverse fracture of distal tibia and fibula. Note that the medial corner of the proximal fragment protrudes through the skin, identifying this as an open fracture. A small amount of air is present within the soft tissues, just lateral to the distal fibular fragment. *B*, Open medial subtalar fracture dislocation of the ankle. A fracture extends through the neck of the talus, with medial dislocation of the foot. Air is present within the soft tissues medial to the tibia, identifying this as an open injury. There is also a small amount of air within the ankle mortise (*arrow*).

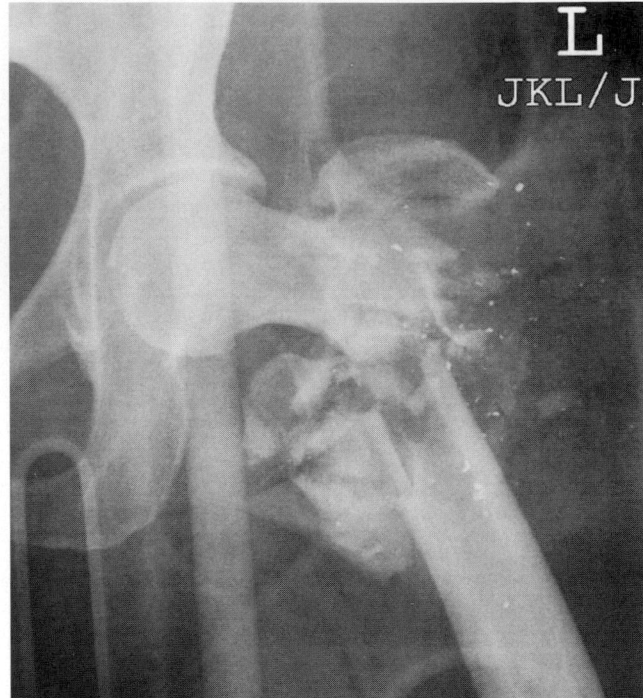

Figure 4–4. Open fracture from gunshot wound. This anteroposterior radiograph of the hip on a trauma board shows a comminuted fracture of the proximal femur with multiple small metallic fragments. Gas is present in the soft tissues. The bulk of the projectile is absent, having passed completely through the patient's body.

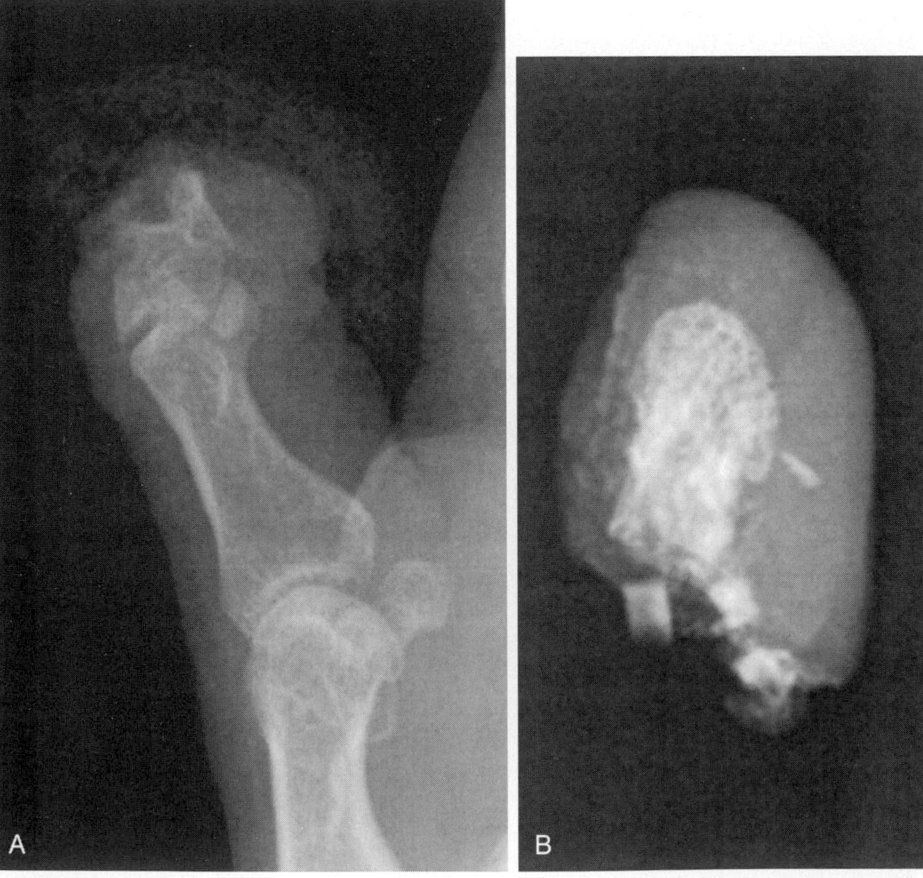

Figure 4–5. Open fracture from traumatic amputation of the thumb. *A*, The tip of the thumb has been amputated, with severe comminution. *B*, The amputated part was recovered for possible replantation.

lary space, with a joint on at least one end. The location of a fracture may be stated in terms of its relationship to or the involvement of anatomic points of reference, such as the tibial plateau, malleolus, or surgical neck. For describing fractures located within the shaft of a long bone (a region that is relatively free of anatomic detail), it is conventional to divide the length of the shaft into thirds: proximal, middle, and distal. Shaft fractures may then be described as being in the proximal, middle, or distal third or at the junction between the proximal and middle or middle and distal thirds. A fracture at the midpoint of the shaft may be described as a midshaft fracture.

The direction of a fracture line is determined by its relationship to the long axis of a long or a short bone and to the longest axis of an irregularly shaped bone such as the talus or the scaphoid. Fractures are therefore said to be transverse, longitudinal, oblique, or spiral. In certain cases, particularly with injury to the spine or patella, a fracture may be described as vertical or horizontal, depending upon its relationship to the long axis of the entire body. The direction and shape of a fracture line may be related to the location, direction, and magnitude of the forces that caused it.

A *transverse* fracture line (Fig. 4–6) runs perpendicularly to the long axis of a bone. Transverse fractures may result from direct loading or from indirect, tensile loading. Transverse fractures of the shaft of long bones may occur as the result of direct blows, particularly to bones that have little soft tissue covering such as the ulna or tibia (Fig. 4–7). Indirect bending forces frequently create transverse fractures of the midshaft of the humerus and femur, but transverse fractures are rarely found toward the ends of these bones. More often, there is an accompanying vertical load that results in some angulation of the fracture line. Transverse fractures are more commonly encountered in irregular bones such as the scaphoid or in bony projections such as the malleoli of the ankle (see Fig. 4–6*B*). Tension in ligaments or tendons may create sufficient tensile forces within the bony projections or prominences to which they are attached to result in a transverse fracture. Such fractures are commonly referred to as avulsion fractures. Fracture lines that result from direct trauma tend to be jagged and irregular, whereas fracture lines that result from indirect trauma tend to be smooth.

An *oblique* fracture line (Fig. 4–8) runs along a course that angles approximately 30 to 60 degrees to the long axis of the bone. The fracture is the result of compressive forces applied along the long axis of the bone, often combined with bending. Because this mode of injury is very frequent, the oblique fracture is very common. When bending forces have been applied during the traumatic event, a variable portion of the fracture line may be transverse (see Fig. 4–8*B*), because the bending forces that place one side of the bone under compression also place the opposite side under tension.

A *spiral* fracture line (Fig. 4–9) spirals around the shaft, encircling it once. The ends of the spiral are connected by a vertical component. A spiral fracture is created by torsional forces, but it is rare for torque to be applied in the absence of some degree of axial compres-

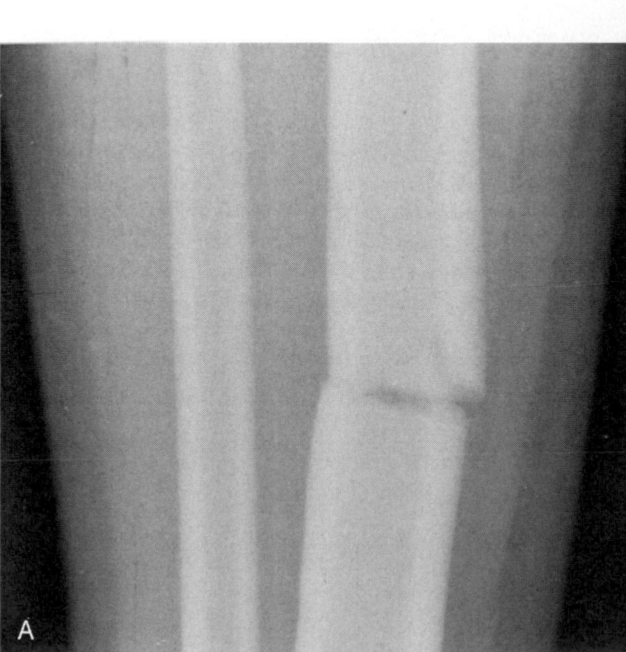

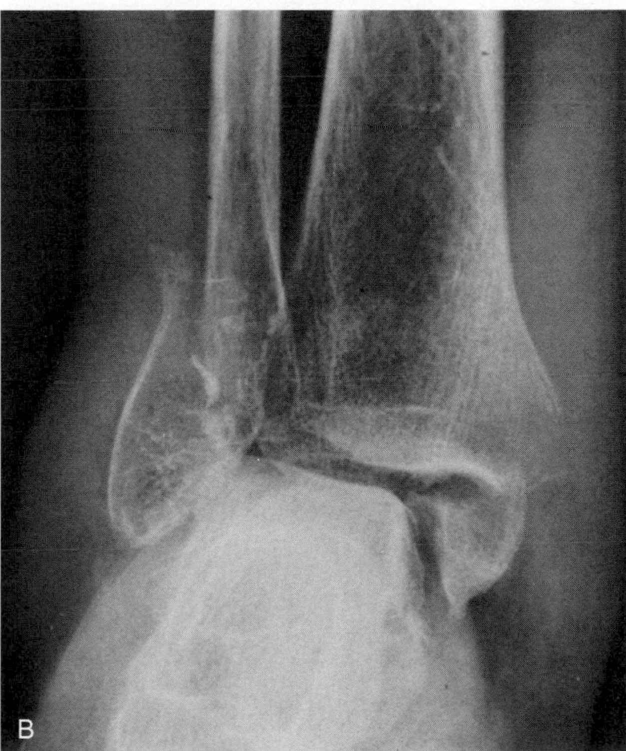

Figure 4–6. Transverse fracture. *A*, Transverse fracture of the midshaft of the tibia, due to a direct blow. The fracture line is perpendicular to the longitudinal axis of the shaft. There is a slight angulation at the fracture site and a minimal lateral offset of the distal fragment. *B*, Fracture-dislocation of the ankle. There is a transverse fracture of the medial malleolus and an oblique fracture of the lateral malleus. The talus and foot are displaced laterally. The transverse fracture of the medial malleolus is due to avulsion by the intact deltoid ligament.

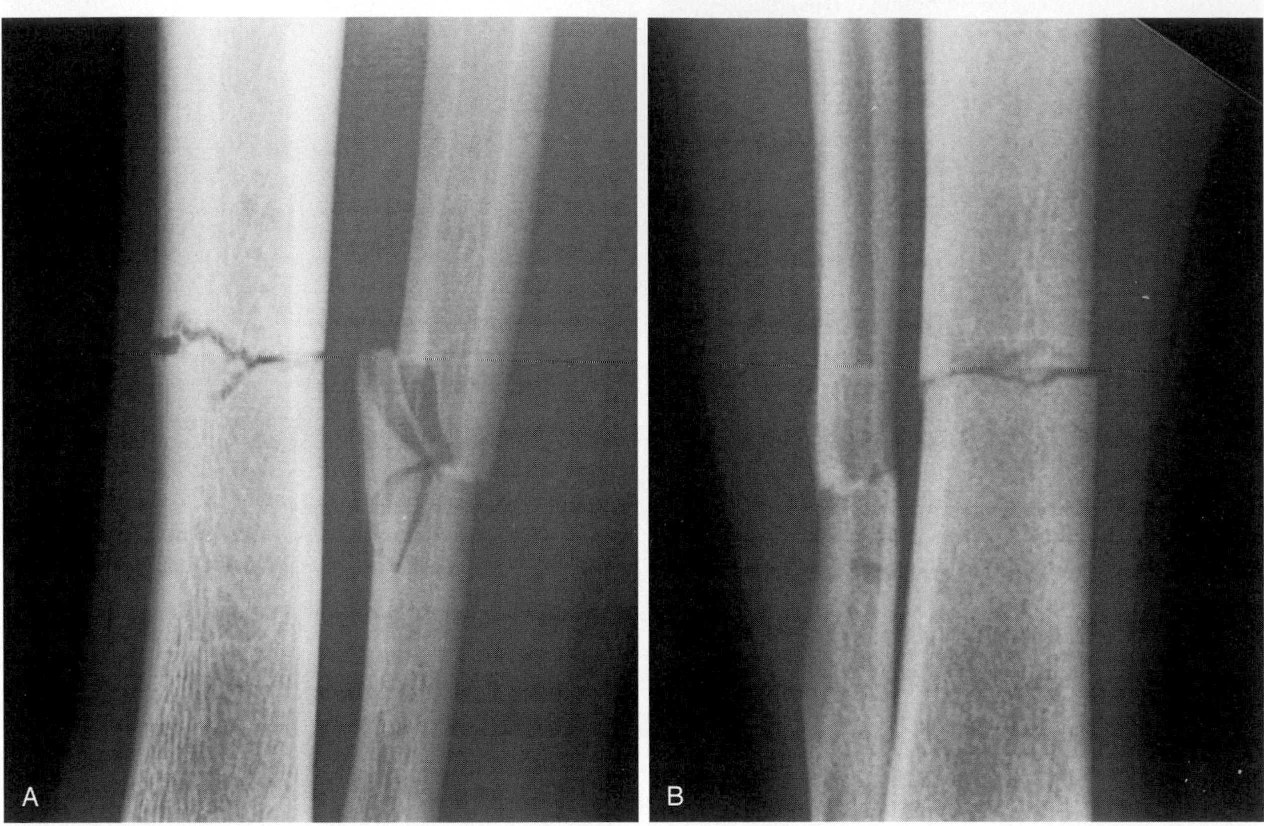

Figure 4–7. Transverse fractures. *A*, Lateral radiograph of the lower leg shows a transverse fracture of the tibia and a transverse fracture with butterfly fragment of the fibula. *B*, Anteroposterior radiograph of the lower leg shows minimal displacement and normal alignment.

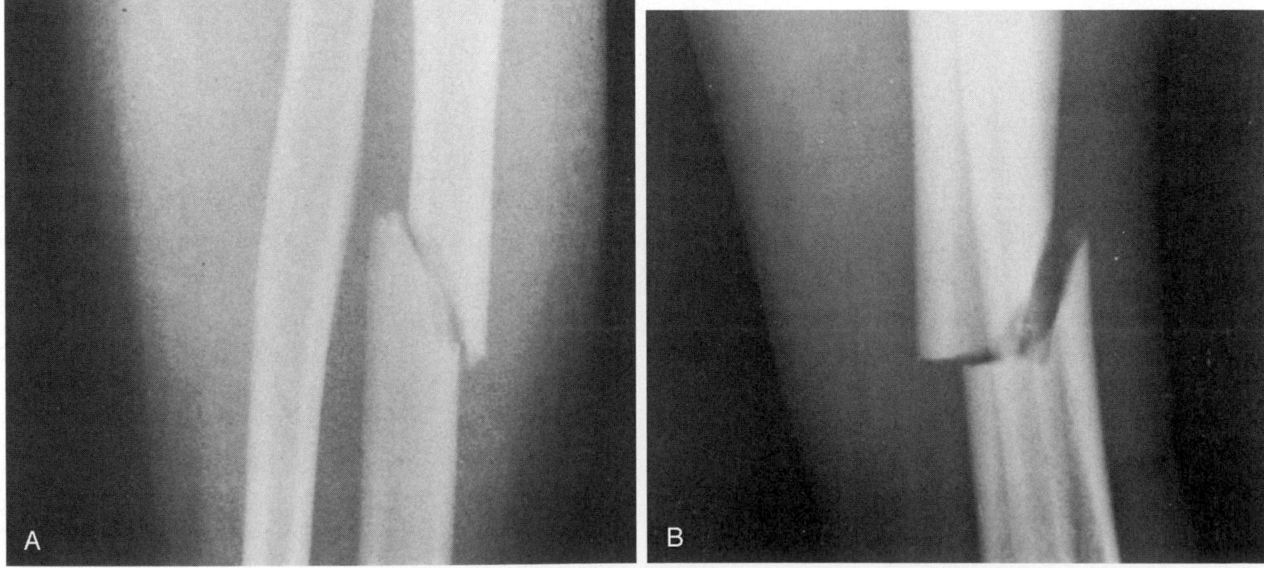

Figure 4–8. Oblique fractures. *A*, Oblique fracture of the midshaft of the ulna. The fracture crosses the longitudinal axis of the ulna at approximately 45 degrees. The fragments are slightly separated and are offset by the width of the cortex without angulation at the fracture site. *B*, An oblique fracture of the distal third of the tibia. The fracture is offset by the width of the cortex anteriorly. Note that the anterior portion of the fracture line is oblique at approximately 45 degrees. The posterior of the fracture line is transverse. This type of fracture is due to a combination of angulation and compression forces.

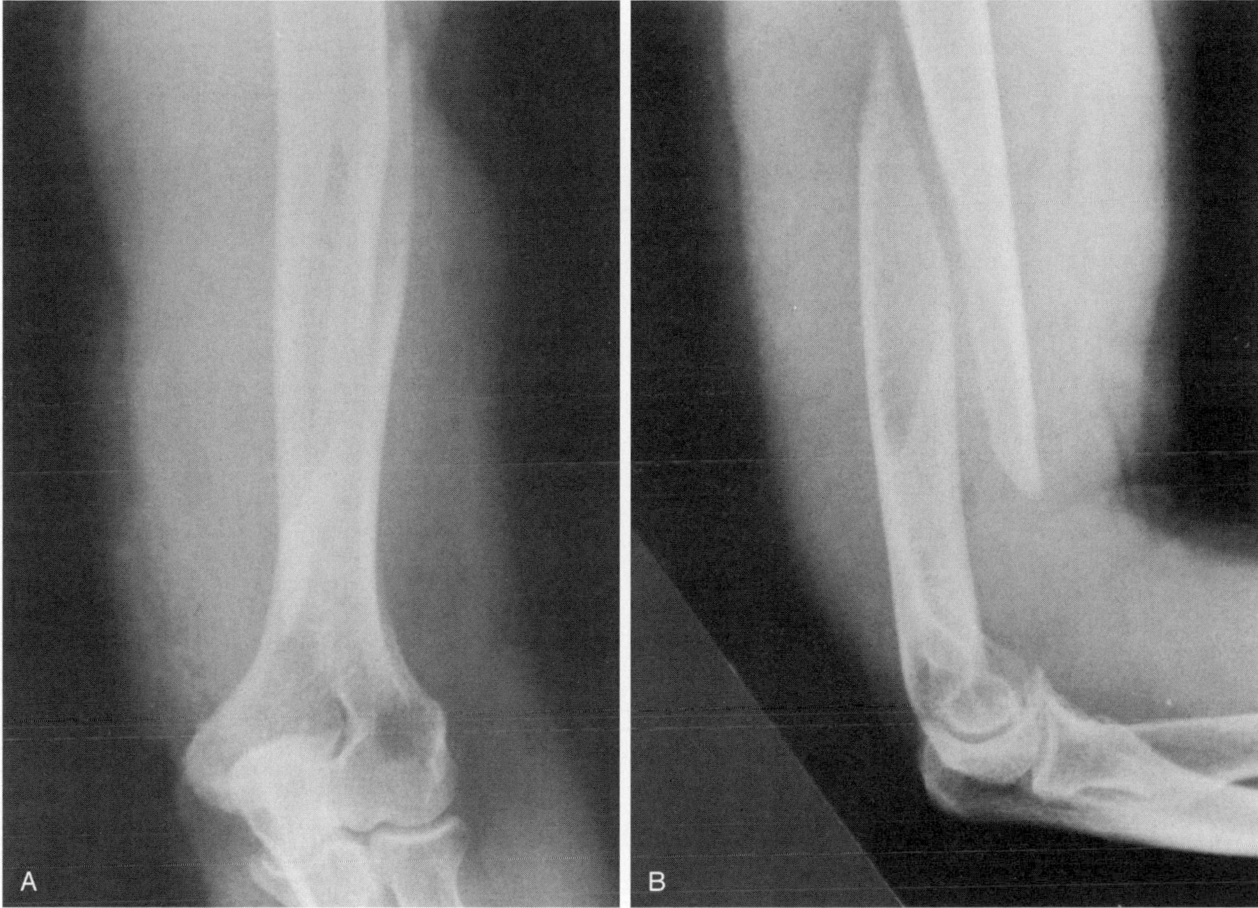

Figure 4–9. Spiral fracture of the distal humerus. *A*, The anteroposterior projection demonstrates the long spiral nature of the fracture. The overlap of the fragments on this view could be mistaken for evidence of comminution. *B*, Lateral view clearly demonstrates, however, that this is a spiral fracture without comminution. Note the characteristic pointed end of the fracture fragment. The fracture fragments are unapposed; there is clear separation. The overriding of the fracture fragments is best appreciated in *A*.

sion or angulation or both. These additional forces modify the fracture line, tending to decrease the length of the spiral and giving it a more nearly oblique course. It has been noted that the ends of a spiral fracture are pointed, like a pen point, whereas the ends of an oblique fracture are more blunt, like the end of a trowel or shovel. A spiral fracture may be mistaken for a comminuted fracture (see Fig. 4–9*A*) on the radiograph when there is a pronounced spiral with overlap of the fracture ends. The diagnosis is usually clarified by a view obtained at 90 degrees (see Fig. 4–9*B*). Spiral fractures are seen only in long bones. Depending on the direction of the spiral fracture line, these fractures may be left-handed or right-handed, and the "handedness" correlates with the direction of force.[314]

Chisel-like compression forces are generated when the end of one bone is driven into the other and may result in an incomplete *vertical fracture*. Isolated vertical fractures paralleling the long axis of the shaft are unusual. One form, aptly termed the *teacup fracture*, is an incomplete nondisplaced fracture encountered in the distal end of the tibia (Fig. 4–10). Direct blows can result in a vertical fracture of the distal phalanx (Fig. 4–11). Such an injury may also occur in the proximal phalanx of the thumb in baseball players as the tip of the thumb is hit by a ball when the player is attempting to field a bad pitch or grounder. Vertical or longitudinally oriented fractures of the shaft are much more commonly found as a component of comminuted fracture. They are important to recognize in this situation if the placement of an intramedullary nail or rod is being considered. When intramedullary fixation is used in the presence of vertical fracture lines, the fractures are frequently extended by the impact of the intramedullary device, and further comminution and instability result.

Avulsion fractures (Fig. 4–12) are generally smaller fragments pulled off (avulsed) from bony prominences by the tension in the attached ligaments or tendons. The larger avulsion fracture fragments circumscribe the entire cortex of a bony projection. The small, flakelike fracture fragments may contain only a portion of one cortex. These are related to the presence of Sharpey's fibers, which extend from the ligament or tendon into the bone perpendicular to the axis of the bone to fix a tendon or ligament to bone. This bond is sufficiently strong that a portion of the cortical bone itself may yield before the tendon or its union with the surface of the bone yields. Injuries in which small fragments are avulsed by the direct blow of a hard object, generally at the end of a long bone, are also referred to as avulsion fractures. Avulsion fractures, irrespective of size, are much more frequently the result

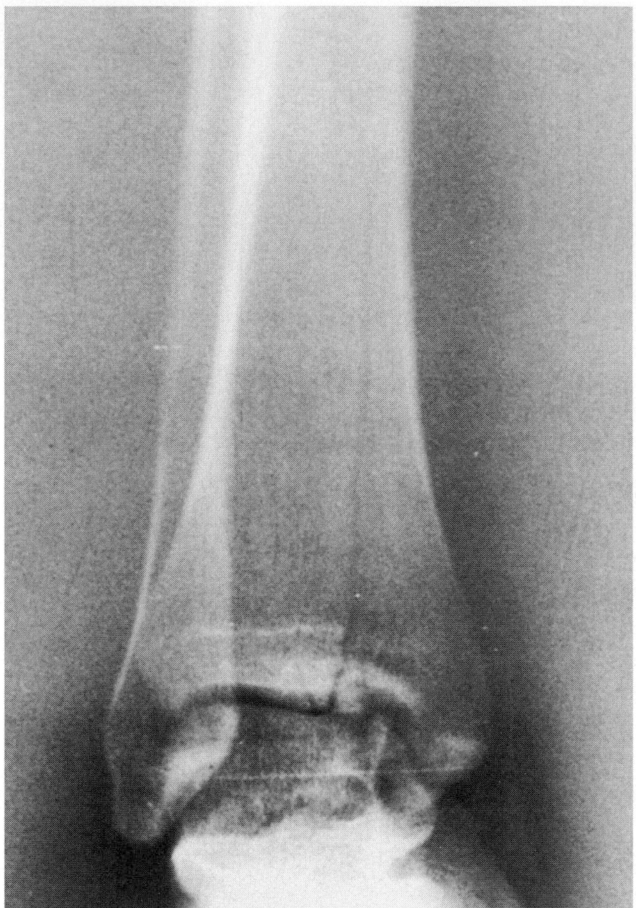

Figure 4–10. Vertical nondisplaced fracture of the distal tibia extending into the ankle joint. This type of nondisplaced incomplete fracture has been called a teacup fracture. It is due to a vertical, chisel-like force.

of indirectly applied tension forces within ligaments and tendons than of direct blows; therefore, the presence of small avulsion fragments is probably an indication of a serious soft tissue injury of ligaments or tendons rather than of a trivial fracture of bone. Avulsion fractures are sometimes referred to as "chip fractures," a term that suggests a different mechanism of injury and should be avoided.

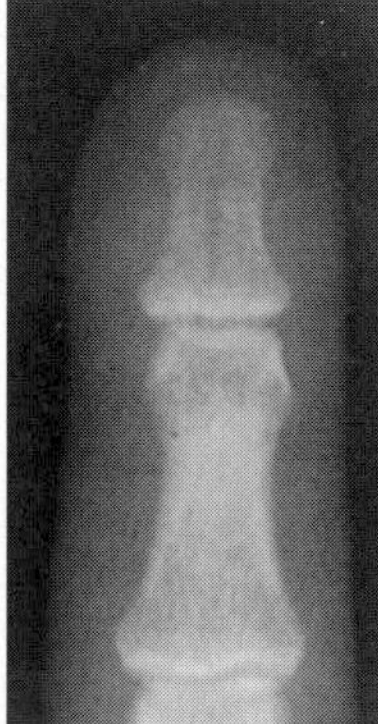

Figure 4–11. Vertical fracture of the distal phalanx sustained by a 20-year-old man who caught his finger in a punch press. Note the nondisplaced vertical fracture extending to the joint surface.

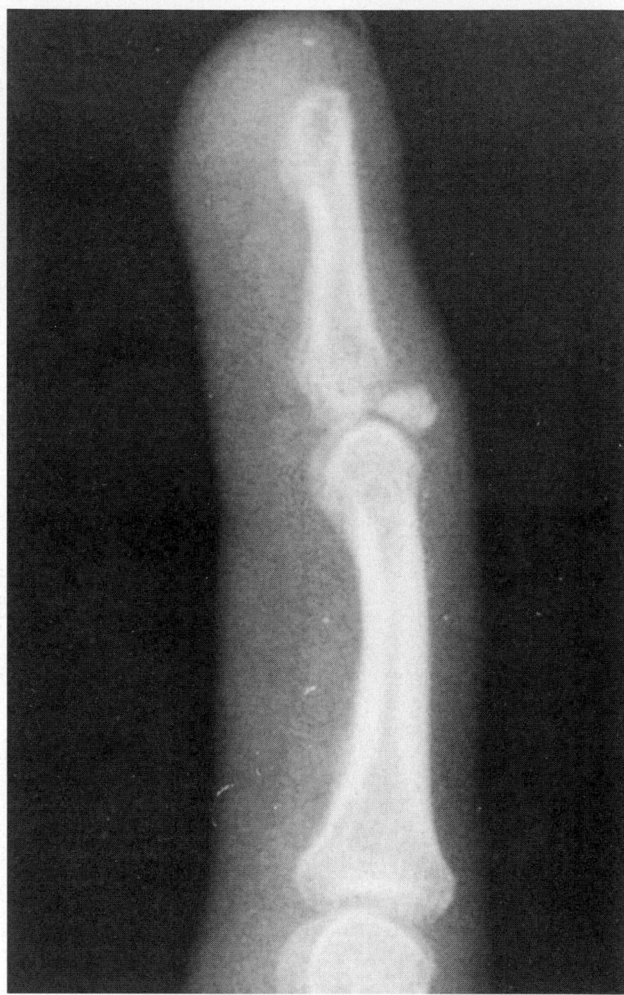

Figure 4–12. Avulsion fracture of the distal phalanx. There is a small cortical avulsion from the dorsal surface of the distal phalanx at the interphalangeal joint. This is a hyperflexion injury, and the avulsion is caused by a pull of the extensor tendon. A finger with this injury is termed a baseball or mallet finger.

Fractures of long bones may be comminuted. Specific terminology has been developed to designate common patterns of comminution in long bones. A *butterfly fragment* (Fig. 4–13*A*; see also Fig. 4–7*A*) is an elongated triangular fragment of cortical bone generally detached from two other larger fragments of a long bone. This occurs on the concave side of an angulation injury. In *segmental fracture* (Fig. 4–14; see also Fig. 4–13*B*) a segment of the shaft is isolated by a proximal and a distal line of fracture. There may be multiple segments or small fragments at the sites of the major fracture lines. A floating knee,[231, 340] elbow,[10, 304] or hip[295] is the result of an injury in which there are fractures both proximal and distal to the joint; for example, a floating elbow[10] results from concomitant ipsilateral fractures of the humerus and forearm, and a floating knee, from concomitant ipsilateral fractures of the femur and tibia. Identification of a floating joint is important because such injuries are particularly unstable; treatment is made more complex by intra-articular extension of fractures[224] or by dislocation or other injury of the floating joint itself.[250, 318, 339] A comminuted fracture occurring at the end of a long bone from

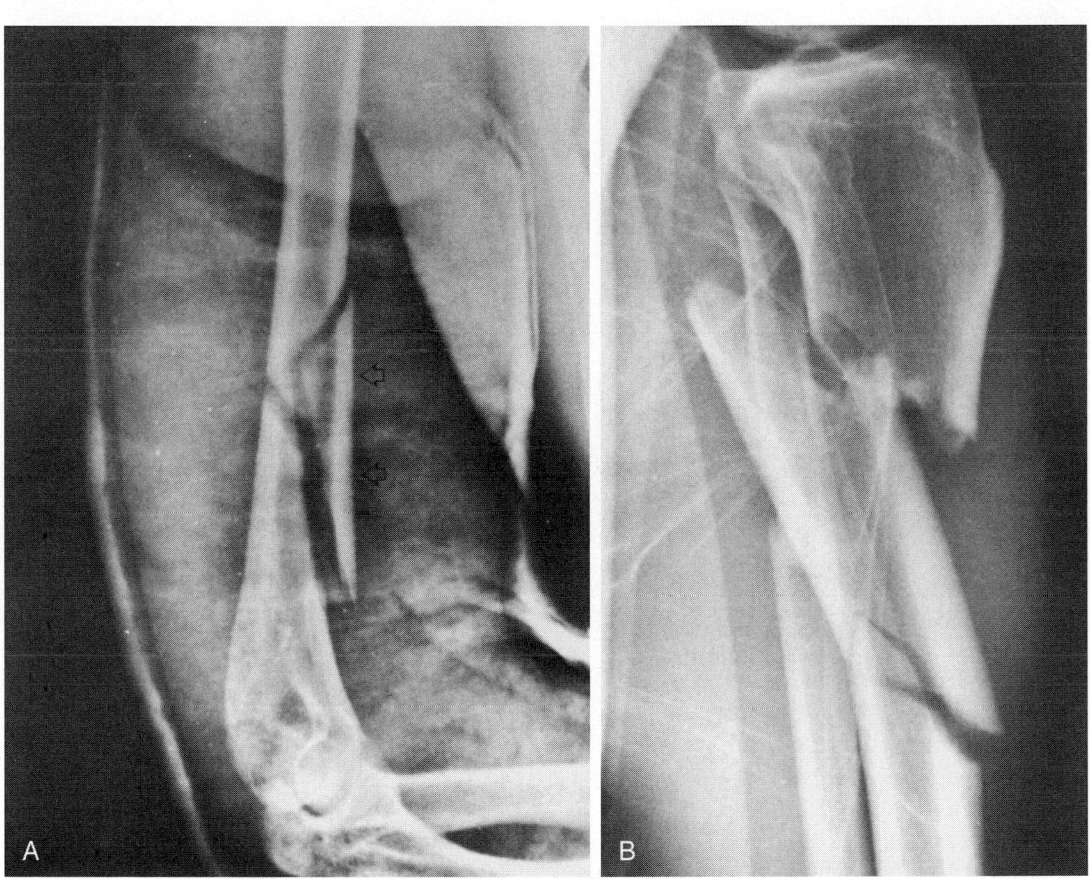

Figure 4–13. Special forms of comminution. *A*, Comminuted fracture of the distal shaft of the humerus with a butterfly fragment (*arrows*). The triangular shape identifies it as a butterfly fragment. The patient's arm is in a hanging cast. The fracture occurred in a 23-year-old man during an attempt to throw a softball. This is a "thrower's fracture," a form of stress fracture in normal bone resulting from a single, violent muscular contraction. *B*, Segmental fracture of the proximal third of the tibia. The lateral view demonstrates two oblique fractures of the shaft, which create the segmental fracture. The segment is angulated dorsally. It remains apposed at the distal fracture site but is offset slightly by more than half the width of the shaft posteriorly at the proximal fracture site. There is also an associated transverse fracture of the shaft of the fibula. The multiple linear densities overlying the bone and soft tissue represent bandages.

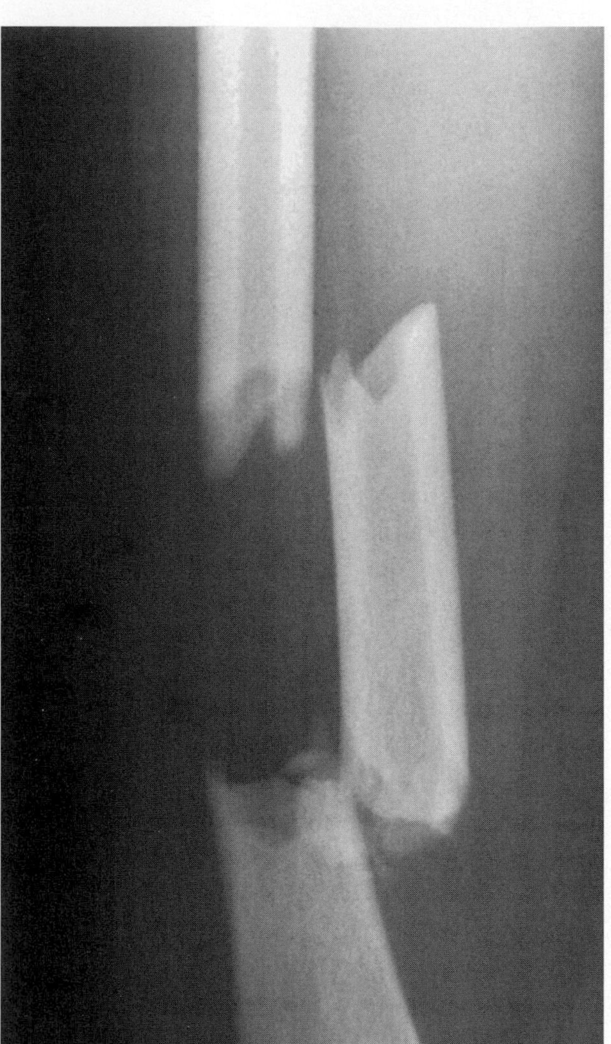

Figure 4–14. Segmental fracture of the femoral shaft. (From Chew, F.S. [1997]. Skeletal Radiology: The Bare Bones. 2nd Ed. p. 17. Williams & Wilkins, Baltimore, with permission.)

compressive forces frequently consists of three major fragments, the largest fragment being the shaft and the other two consisting of the split end of the bone. This injury is common at the distal end of the humerus or femur. Such fractures are termed either T or Y *fractures*. The vertical portion of the designating letter is formed by a vertical fracture component that splits the end of the bone. The course of the contiguous fracture line across the shaft is either transverse or V-shaped and determines the designation as either T or Y (see Fig. 4–15).

An *intra-articular fracture* is one in which the fracture line extends into a joint. The fracture may extend from the shaft into the joint, or it may involve the joint surface primarily. Intra-articular fractures may involve bone and cartilage, only bone, or only cartilage. Whenever a fracture of the metaphysis or end of the diaphysis is encountered, the adjacent end of the bone should be examined closely to rule out vertical extension into the joint (Fig. 4–16). Such extension is not always obvious. Shearing or rotational impaction forces create chondral or osteochondral fractures. The fragment may consist entirely of cartilage and be visualized only on magnetic resonance imaging (MRI). If the fragment contains a small flake of articular bone, it may be easily overlooked on radiographs but will be more apparent on computed tomographic images.

Fractures of Other Bones

Morphologic types of bones other than long bones include short bones (cuboidal bones found in the carpus and tarsus), flat bones (usually from intramembranous formation and surrounding a body cavity, such as ribs and calvaria), irregular bones (of mixed shape, such as pelvic bones and vertebrae), sesamoid bones, and accessory bones or ossicles. Many fractures of these bones are amenable to terminology used for long bones. Additional terminology is required for certain other fractures. Many of these terms are introduced and described in subsequent chapters.

Fractures resulting from the forces generated in driving one bone against the other may be described by three specific terms: A *compression fracture* occurs in the vertebral body (Fig. 4–17) as a result of flexion of the spine. The superior end plate is driven into the medullary portion, and the cortical margins fold like an accordion in response to the stress, resulting in a wedge-shaped deformity of the vertebral body. *Impaction fracture* of the humeral head may occur in association with dislocation of the shoulder, or much less commonly, the femoral head may sustain such a fracture in a dislocation of the hip. The fracture results from impaction of the displaced humeral or femoral head against the hard bony edge of the glenoid or acetabulum. This impact creates a characteristic troughlike depression in the humeral or femoral head. A *depressed fracture* describes the situation in which one or more significant fracture fragments are displaced downward relative to an anatomic plane of reference. Such descriptions are commonly applied in the skull, relative to the outer surface, or at joints, relative to the joint surface.

Chondral and Osteochondral Fractures

Shearing, rotary, or tangentially aligned impaction forces generated by abnormal joint motion[41, 43, 45, 46, 290] may produce fractures of one or both of the two apposing joint surfaces. The resultant fracture fragments may consist[36, 37, 45] of cartilage[38] only (chondral fractures) or of cartilage and underlying bone (osteochondral fractures) (Fig. 4–18). The histologic zone of demarcation between calcified and uncalcified cartilage at the junction of uncalcified cartilage and subchondral bone in an articular surface is referred to as the *tidemark* (see Fig. 1–13).[35, 39, 46] The fracture line ordinarily runs parallel to the joint surface. The fracture may pass through uncalcified cartilage, the tidemark, or subchondral bone. This variation in the fracture line creates fragments that are more or less radiopaque, depending upon the quantity of calcified car-

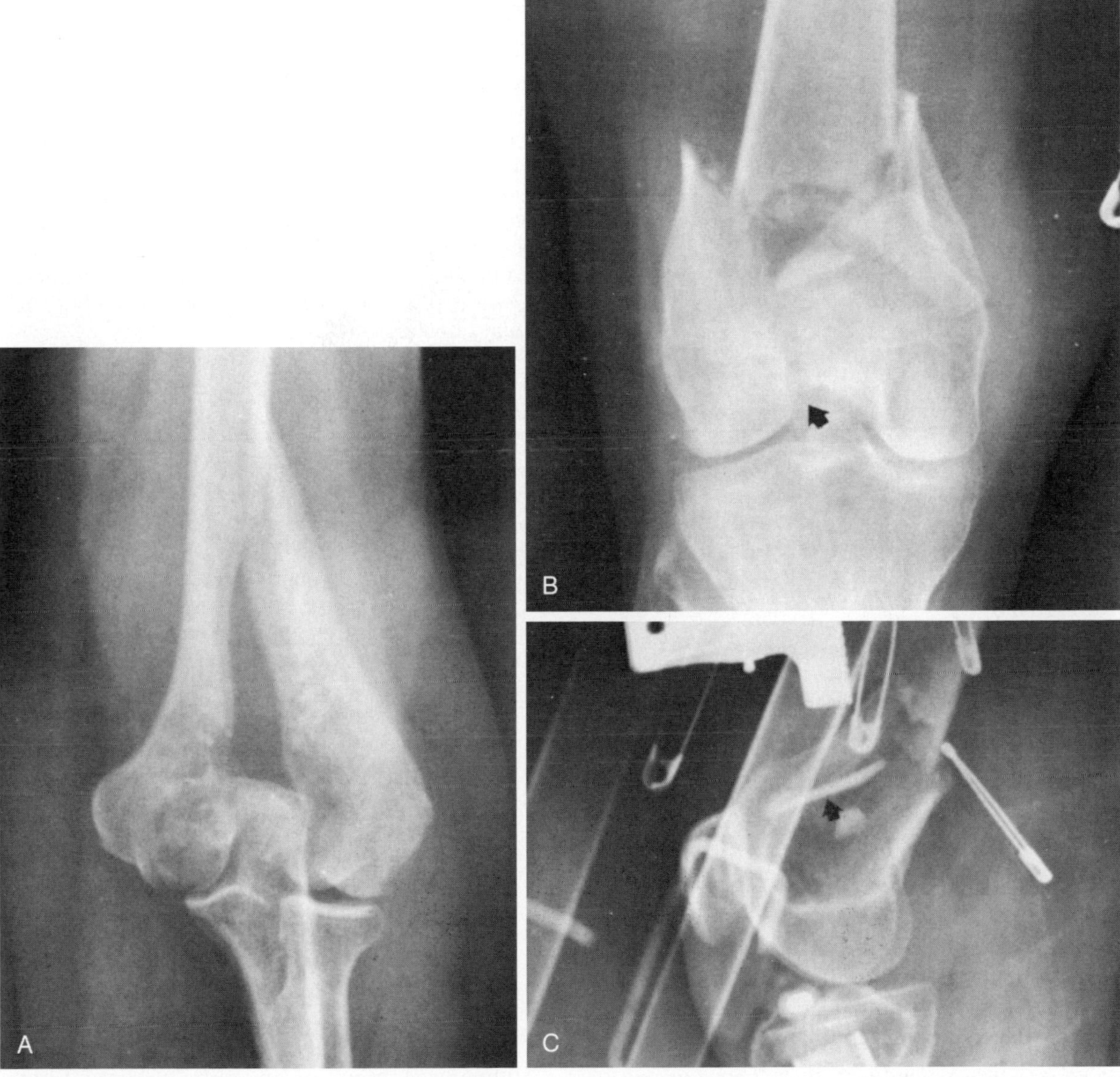

Figure 4–15. Intra-articular fractures of the condyles. *A*, Fracture involving a single condyle. In this vertical fracture in a 53-year-old woman, the fracture fragment is separated off the lateral condyle of the humerus. The fragment is rotated, and the joint is subluxated laterally. *B*, A Y-shaped intercondylar fracture of the distal femur with comminution in an 82-year-old woman. In addition to the V-shaped component extending above each condyle, note the vertical extension into the intercondylar notch (*arrow*) that identifies this as a Y-shaped intercondylar fracture. *C*, Lateral view demonstrates a characteristic posterior angulation of the distal fragment. This is caused by pull of the origins of the gastrocnemius muscles. Note the dense line of cortical bone (*arrow*). This depressed, anterior fragment is lying perpendicular to the x-ray beam, which accentuates the density of the fragment.

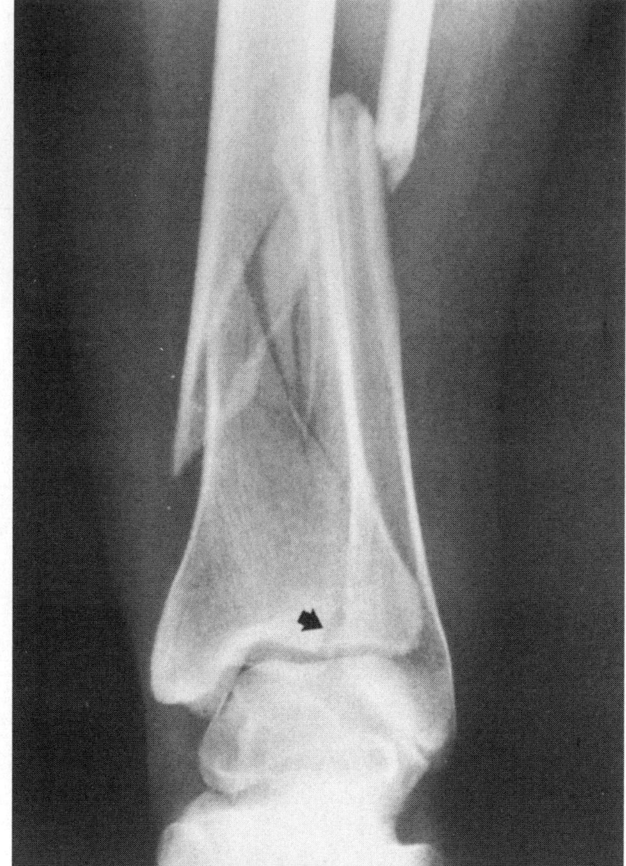

Figure 4–16. Comminuted fracture of the distal tibia with extension into the ankle mortise. The extension of the fracture (*arrow*) into the ankle joint is not as easily identified in this case as in Figure 4–2*B*. Every fracture of the distal shaft must be examined closely for evidence of extension into the adjacent joint.

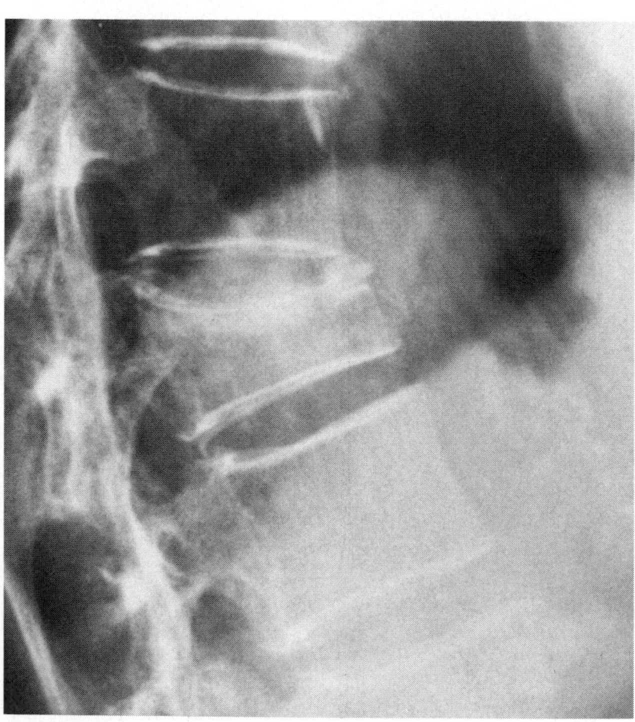

Figure 4–17. Compression fracture of T12 in a 73-year-old woman. The wedge-shaped deformity of the vertebral body is characteristic of a compression fracture of the vertebra. Note that this injury involves principally the superior end plate. There is increased density beneath the end plate because of impaction. The anterior superior cortex of the vertebra is disrupted.

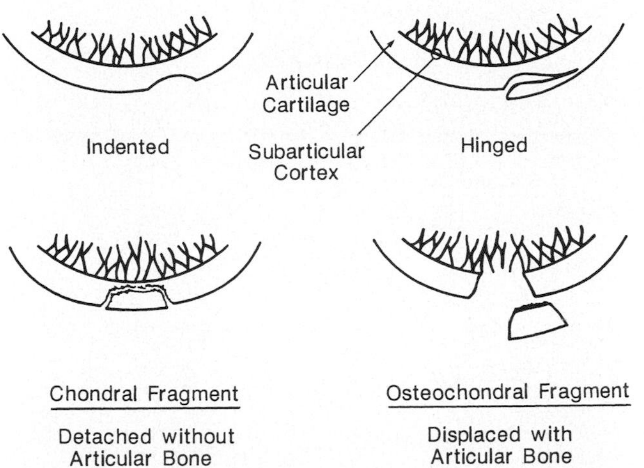

Figure 4–18. Types of osteochondral injury. Injuries of the joint surface include simple indentation; hinged tear of the cartilaginous surface; complete avulsion of a fragment limited to the joint cartilage, referred to as a chondral fragment; and complete avulsion of a fragment containing a piece of articular bone, more accurately referred to as an osteochondral fragment. The completely avulsed fragment may remain within the defect or be displaced and lie free within the joint.

tilage or subchondral bone present (Fig. 4–19). The cartilaginous joint surface and the adjacent subchondral bone are free of nerve endings; therefore, the initial fracture may not even be appreciated by the patient because of the insensitivity of the joint surface.[40]

Radiographic visualization of an osteochondral fracture will depend upon the amount of subchondral bone contained within the fragment (see Fig. 4–19). Obviously, if the fracture is a pure chondral fracture without subchondral bone, it will be impossible to visualize the fragment directly on radiographs. When a radiopaque fragment is visualized, the fragment will be much larger than the radiographic abnormality because of the attached radiolucent chondral articular surface.[40] In addition, it is quite likely that there will be more fragments than those visualized radiographically. Even when a fragment contains subchondral bone, it may be difficult to visualize on radiographs of an acute fracture because of the small size of the attached bone. Similarly, the site of origin usually is obscure and impossible to demonstrate.[42]

MRI is the best noninvasive method for demonstrating chondral and subchondral fractures (Fig. 4–20).[245, 315] Most patients are not referred for MRI until their injuries have failed to heal within the expected time frame. Fractures involving the articularing surfaces of bone are a common cause of chronic disability after joint injury. With the continuing development of new arthroscopic methods of treatment of acute traumatic osteochondral lesions,[253, 292] it is likely that earlier diagnosis of such lesions will gain further clinical importance.

Ultrasonography has been described in preliminary reports as an imaging modality capable of demonstrating osteochondral fractures and identifying resultant loose bodies at the knee[265] and elbow.[332] Progress in this area of research has been slow,[225, 283] and it seems unlikely that this modality will displace MRI from its preeminent position.

Bone Bruises

The concept of the bone bruise, or bone contusion, is one that came into currency with the advent of MRI.[237, 293, 345] Bone bruises involve medullary bone at joints and are characterized by a diffuse or localized pattern of low signal intensity on T_1-weighted or proton density images and of high signal intensity on T_2-weighted or inversion recovery images (Figs. 4–21 and 4–22). Technetium bone scans demonstrate increased activity in the same abnor-

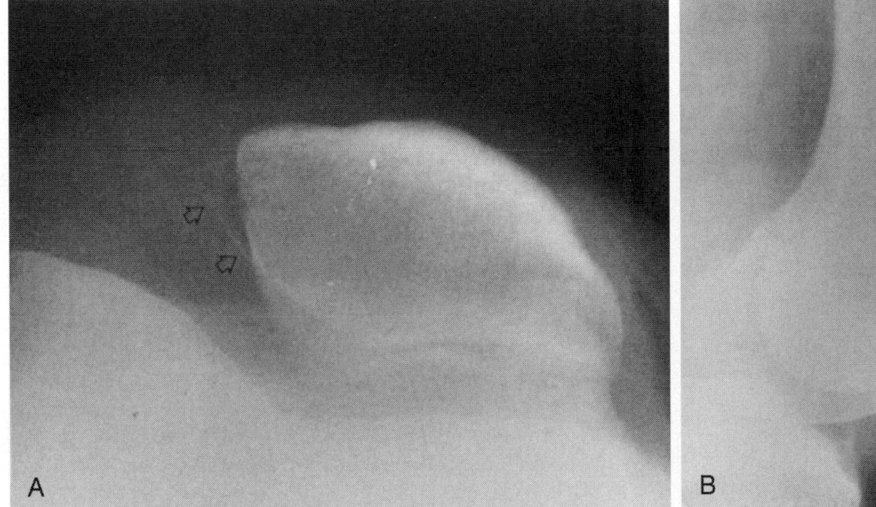

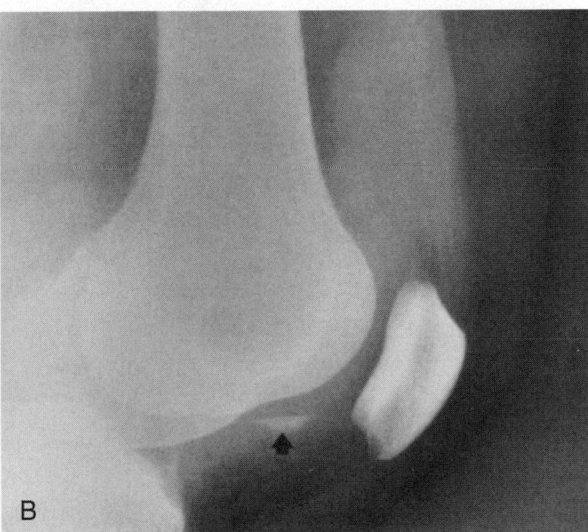

Figure 4–19. Osteochondral fractures of the knee. *A*, Sunrise view of the patella demonstrates a small osteochondral fracture (*arrows*) arising from the medial facet of the patella. *B*, A relatively large osteochondral fracture. The lateral view of the knee demonstrates a large osteochondral fragment (*arrow*). The fragment was found to arise from the lateral femoral condyle. The site of origin could not be identified on the radiograph. Note also the distention of the suprapatellar bursa, indicating the presence of a hemarthrosis.

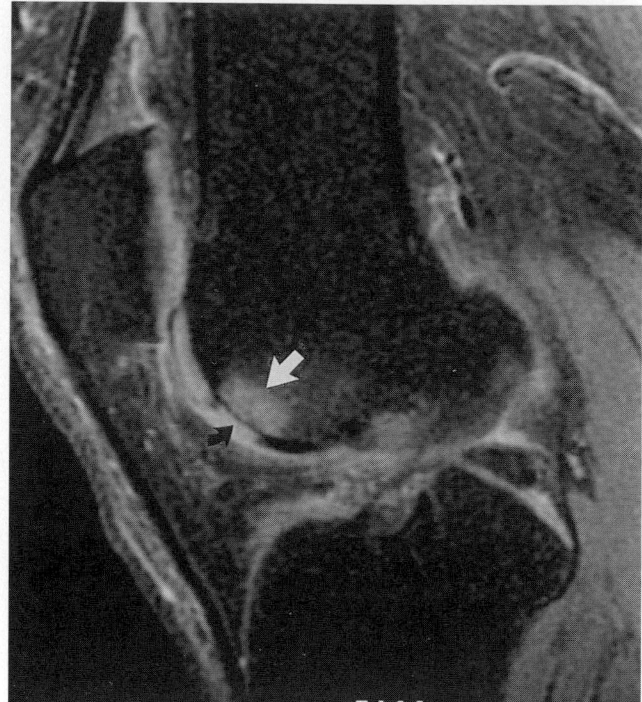

Figure 4–20. Osteochondral fracture of the femur with "bone bruise." Sagittal T_2-weighted fat-suppressed magnetic resonance image shows that a segment of articular cartilage (*arrow*) is missing from the knee at the lateral aspect of the patellofemoral groove. A bone bruise underlies the cartilage defect, indicating an impaction injury. (From Chew, F. S. [2000]. Skeletal Radiology Interactive 2.0, with permission.)

mal sites as on MRI.[201] Bone bruises often occur in association with collateral ligament or anterior cruciate ligament disruptions from compressive forces induced by the traumatic episode. They also can occur as a result of direct trauma (see Fig. 4–22) and twisting injuries.[201, 206] Radiologic-histologic correlation has confirmed that these lesions represent microfractures of cancellous bone and edema and bleeding in the fatty marrow.[311] Bone bruises appear to be sustained as the result of compression or impaction forces. These fractures may be associated with cartilaginous (see Fig. 4–20) or ligamentous injuries but may also occur as isolated findings. Most studies of bone bruises concern the knee,[289] but bone bruises also occur commonly at the ankle,[227] the femoral head,[279] the foot,[298, 327] and probably other sites that are less frequently examined by MRI following trauma. Bone bruises appear

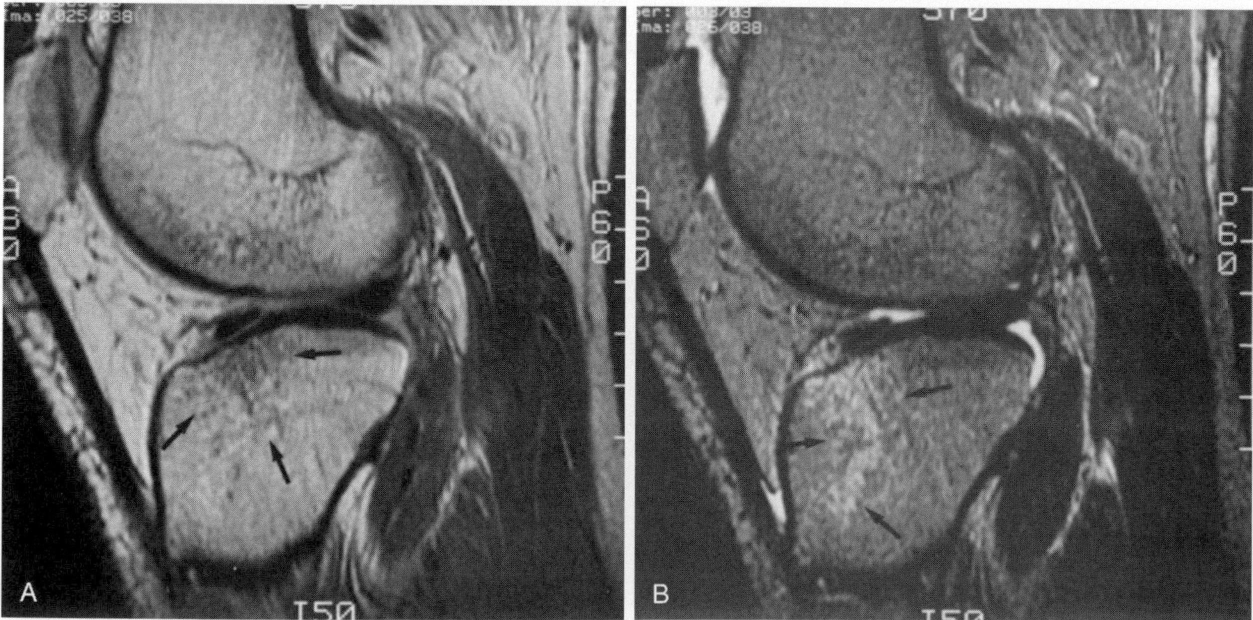

Figure 4–21. Occult intraosseous fracture, or bone bruise, in a 24-year-old man involved in a motorcycle accident 1 week before this magnetic resonance imaging examination. *A*, Sagittal proton density image (TR 2250 msec, TE 20 msec) shows speckled areas of decreased signal in the lateral tibial plateau (*arrows*). *B*, Corresponding T_2-weighted image (TR 2250 msec, TE 80 msec) reveals high signal intensity over a relatively more extensive area (*arrows*). (From Lee, J.K., & Yao, L. [1989]. Occult intraosseous fracture: Magnetic resonance appearance versus age of injury. Am. J. Sports Med., *17*:620, with permission.)

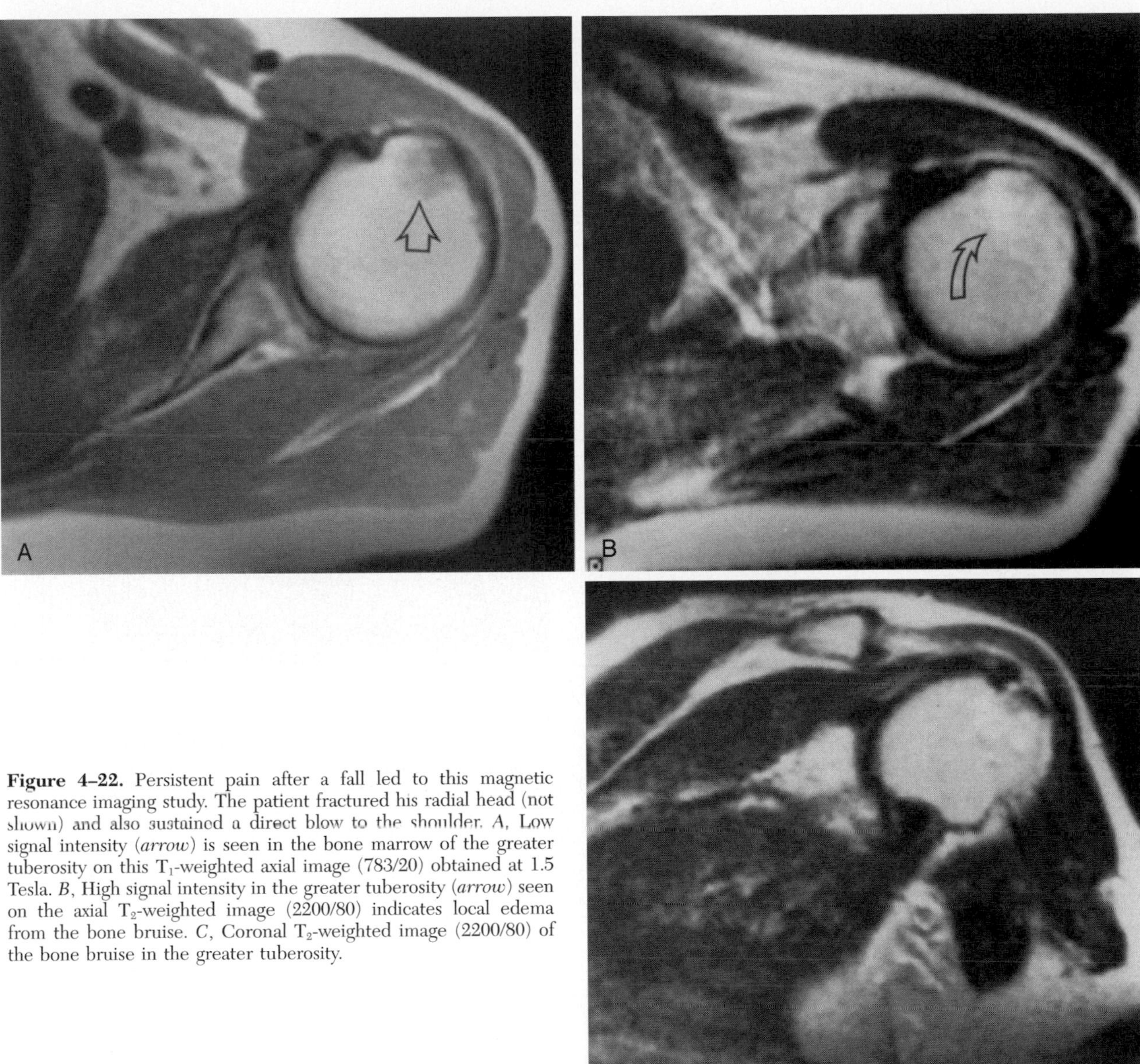

Figure 4–22. Persistent pain after a fall led to this magnetic resonance imaging study. The patient fractured his radial head (not shown) and also sustained a direct blow to the shoulder. *A*, Low signal intensity (*arrow*) is seen in the bone marrow of the greater tuberosity on this T_1-weighted axial image (783/20) obtained at 1.5 Tesla. *B*, High signal intensity in the greater tuberosity (*arrow*) seen on the axial T_2-weighted image (2200/80) indicates local edema from the bone bruise. *C*, Coronal T_2-weighted image (2200/80) of the bone bruise in the greater tuberosity.

to heal without specific treatment and the MRI findings gradually return to normal in 2 to 4 months.[291] The areas of high signal intensity on T_2-weighted images regress more rapidly than do those on the corresponding T_1-weighted or proton density images. Symptoms may resolve within a similar time frame. Late or continuing demonstration of marrow edema at a site of trauma may reflect a post-traumatic condition such as instability or altered joint biomechanics.[277, 320]

The impaction mechanism of bone bruising of subchondral bone implies that the traumatic forces are transmitted through the overlying articular cartilage. As would be expected, this cartilage also sustains traumatic injury, even if it remains in mechanical continuity with the subchondral bone and adjacent uninvolved portions of the joint. In fact, Johnson and coworkers[271] have demonstrated substantial damage to the homeostasis of articular cartilage overlying bone bruises. Their arthroscopic findings in such articular cartilage included softening (dimpling), fissuring, and overt chondral fracture. Histologic correlation revealed degeneration of the chondrocytes and loss of proteoglycan ground substance. In the contiguous subchondral bone, necrosis of osteocytes with empty lacuna was found.

Dislocations and Subluxations

An injury may involve the joint capsule and supportive tissues with or without displacement or fracture of the involved bone. Displacement of a bone in relation to the apposing bone at the joint is classified as a dislocation, subluxation, or diastasis.

A *dislocation* (Fig. 4–23) is a displacement of a bone

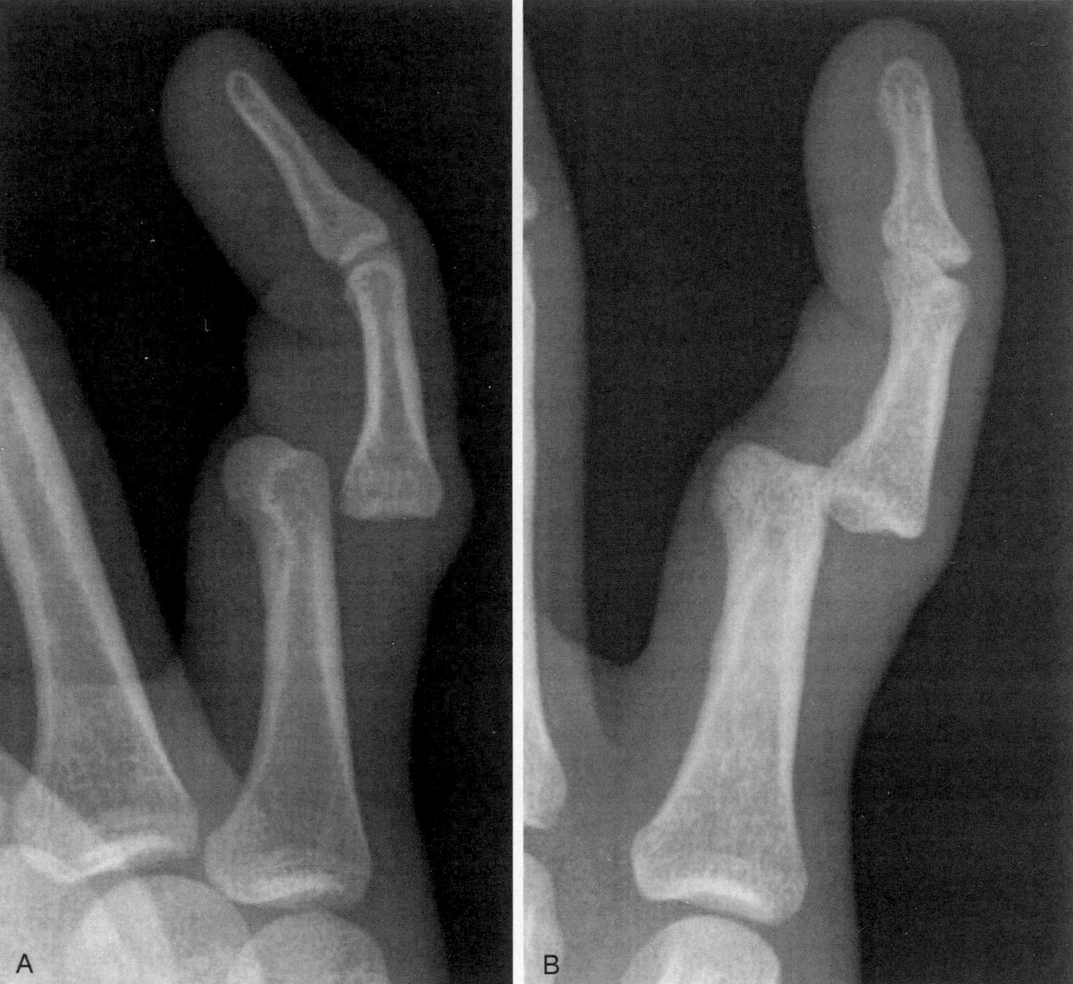

Figure 4–23. Dorsal (posterior) dislocation of the distal interphalangeal joint. *A*, Lateral radiograph shows dorsal dislocation of the distal phalanx relative to the middle phalanx. There is total loss of contact between the articular surfaces. *B*, Posteroanterior radiograph shows that dislocation is present but does not demonstrate the relationship of the bones as well as the lateral view does.

in relation to the apposing bone at the joint, resulting in a complete loss of continuity of the joint surfaces. When associated with a fracture of the involved bone, the injury is classified as a fracture-dislocation (Fig. 4–24*B*). Dislocations may be open or closed, depending upon the integrity of the skin. If the joint is exposed, an open dislocation is present. *Open* joint injuries[1] are particularly devastating. Immediate surgical closure is necessary to prevent subsequent joint destruction. The radiographic demonstration of air within the joint space (Fig. 4–25) establishes the presence of an open joint injury. If all of the major bones of the joint are involved, the dislocation is designated by the name of the joint involved (e.g., dislocation of the elbow). If a smaller bone or one of several bones of a joint is involved, the dislocation is designated by the name of the displaced bone; for example, patellar dislocation refers to dislocation of the patella, and lunate dislocation refers to dislocation of the lunate.

A *subluxation* (see Fig. 4–24*B*; see also Fig. 4–6*B*) is a displacement of a bone in relation to the apposing bone at the joint, resulting in partial loss of continuity of the joint surfaces. The joint surfaces are incongruous, but a significant portion remains apposed. The displacement is slight to moderate in degree. A subluxation may also be called a partial dislocation, and a joint in such a state is said to be *subluxated* (not "subluxed").

A *diastasis* (see Fig. 4–24*B*) is a displacement of a bone in relation to the apposing bone in a slightly movable or synarthrodial joint. It may be partial or complete. The separation involves either a fibrous (syndesmosis) or cartilaginous (symphysis) joint. It is named after the joint involved (e.g., tibiofibular diastasis at the ankle or diastasis of the symphysis pubis). Diastases are frequently associated with fractures of the involved bones or dislocations of adjacent joints. The associated fractures are usually remote from the diastasis and do not extend into the involved joint.

Stress, Insufficiency, and Pathologic Fractures

Terminology

Considerable imprecision and confusion surround the use of the terms stress fracture, fatigue fracture, insuffi-

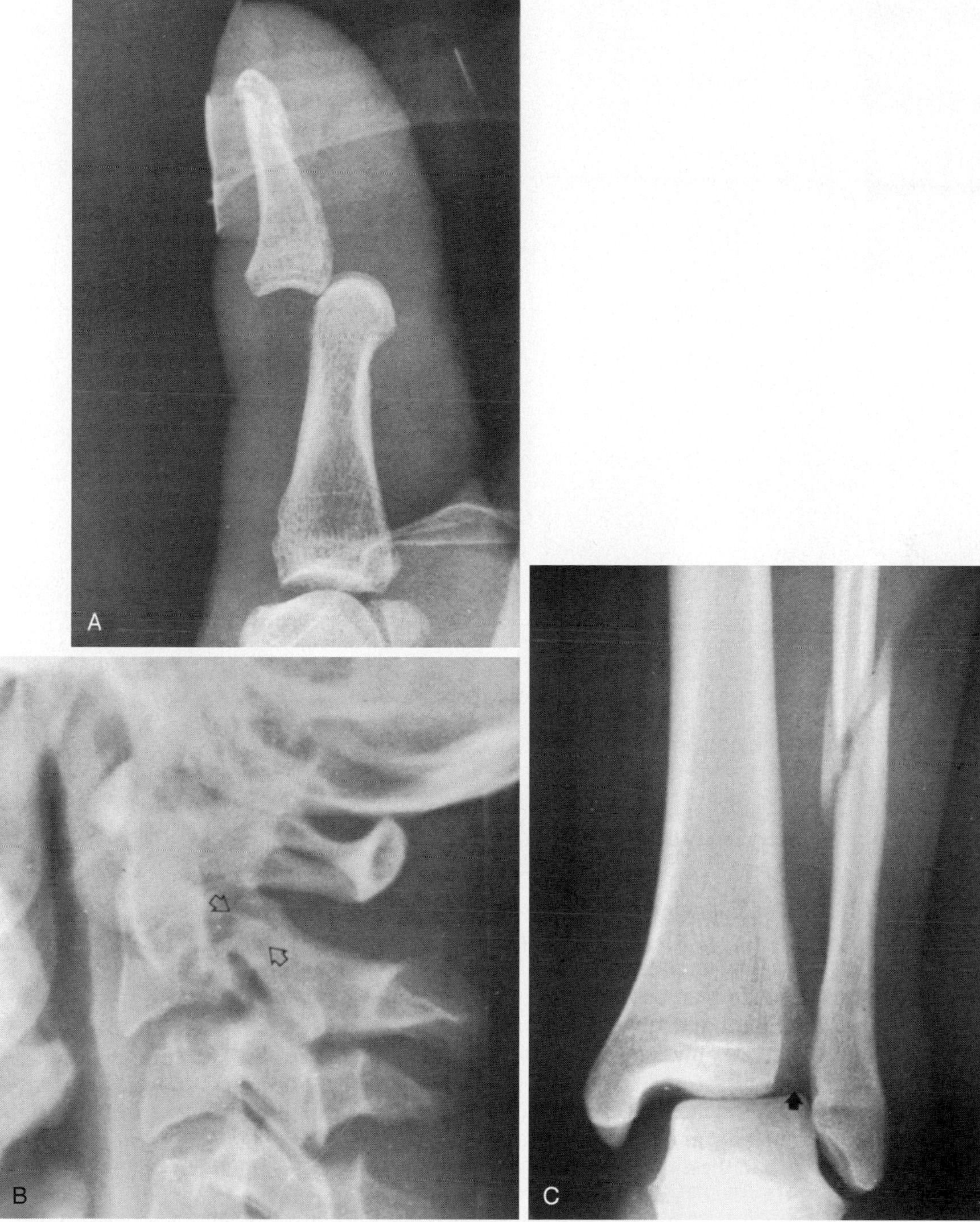

Figure 4–24. Joint injuries. *A*, Posterior dislocation of the interphalangeal joint of the thumb. There is complete disruption of the joint with no apposition of the articular surfaces. *B*, Subluxation of C2 upon C3, characteristic of a hangman's fracture. The body of C2 is anteriorly displaced relative to C3 by approximately 4 mm. This finding is associated with a bilateral fracture of the neural arch (*arrows*) of C2. These are the basic components of a hangman's fracture. This form of joint disruption is a subluxation, because some apposition of the joint surfaces remains. *C*, A diastasis of the tibiofibular syndesmosis is present (*arrow*). The normal width of the syndesmosis should not exceed 5 mm. The diastasis is associated with lateral dislocation or subluxation of the talus and an oblique fracture of the distal third of the shaft of the fibula.

ciency fracture, and pathologic fracture. For these specific types of fractures, definitions in common usage are not mutually exclusive; not all authors would completely agree with all aspects of the terminology used here.

A *stress fracture* is a fracture through normal bone that has been subjected to abnormal chronic repetitive stresses. The amount of biomechanical loading that constitutes the inciting abnormal chronic repetitive stress may vary from one patient to another. For example, a fracture of the metatarsal occurring in a highly trained, competitive marathon runner who recently increased her daily distance from 15 to 20 miles would be considered a stress fracture, but a similar fracture in an obese "couch potato" who begins a regimen of walking slowly on the treadmill while watching television would also be considered a stress fracture. As described subsequently, stress

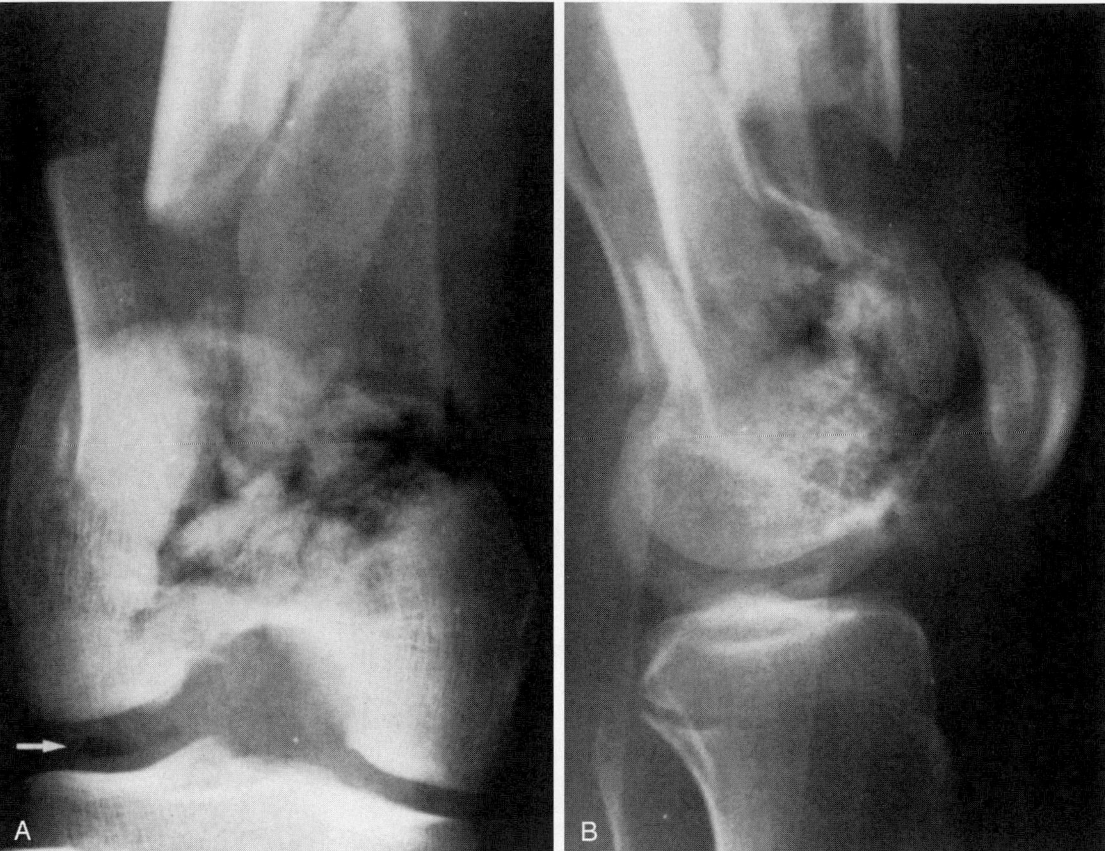

Figure 4–25. Open joint injury associated with a highly comminuted condylar and supracondylar fracture of the femur in a 33-year-old man. *A*, Anteroposterior view demonstrates air entrapped within the severely comminuted fracture. Note also the air within the lateral compartment of the knee *(arrow)*. *B*, Lateral view demonstrates air within the patellofemoral compartment of the joint. Air within the joint is radiographic evidence of an open joint injury; such evidence should be sought in every injury involving the end of a bone.

fractures occur under specific conditions of biomechanical loading. The term *fatigue fracture* may be used identically with stress fracture.

An *insufficiency fracture* is a fracture caused by stresses generated during normal activities through bone that has been weakened by disease such that the bone is abnormal in quantity, quality, or both. For example, fractures that result from normal activities in patients with osteoporosis, osteomalacia, osteopetrosis, or Paget's disease are considered insufficiency fractures. Many of the conditions in which insufficiency fractures typically occur are systemic, endocrine, or metabolic diseases. The bone in these conditions often has abnormal biomechanical characteristics.

A *pathologic fracture* is a fracture through bone that has been replaced by abnormal tissue. Examples of pathologic fractures are a fracture through a focal, lytic, metastatic bone lesion; a fracture through a bone diffusely involved by multiple myeloma or by a blastic osteosarcoma; a fracture through a bone with a focus of fibrous dysplasia; and a fracture through a bone with a unicameral bone cyst. Many of the conditions in which pathologic fractures typically occur are focal or neoplastic lesions. Any description of a pathologic fracture should include a description of the pathologic lesion through which the fracture extends.

Stress Fractures

Stress fractures occur in normal bones of healthy persons in response to the abnormal repetitive stress of activities such as unaccustomed exercise, athletics, or occupational work (Fig. 4–26).[54] There is no history of an episode of discrete trauma, and the typical presentation is one of pain during the activity that ceases when the activity stops. The type of stress fracture and the site in which it occurs vary with the activity. The likelihood of occurrence of a stress fracture is dependent upon the strength of the underlying bone structure, the magnitude of the repetitive stresses, and the time course during which such stresses are applied.[54, 58, 83] Excessive stresses may be generated even by people who are physically fit.[89]

The radiographic examination is within normal limits initially (Fig. 4–27), and usually no evidence of fracture is identified until 10 days to 3 weeks or more after the onset of symptoms. The presence or absence of radiographic findings is in large measure dependent upon the time elapsed since the onset of symptoms; the more time elapsed, the higher the percentage of positive radiographic findings. As many as 70% of initial radiographs can be normal and unrevealing, even when there has been a delay between onset of symptoms and presentation.[64] The radiographic findings[58, 73] vary with the site of involvement to some extent. The fracture may first be

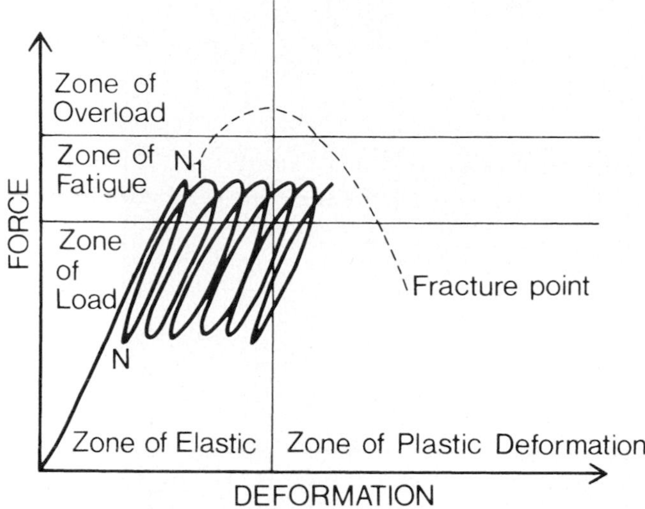

Figure 4–26. Modified stress-strain curve demonstrating the biomechanical effects of repeated strains, probably operative in the creation of stress fractures. Although the repeated stresses are below the limits of tolerance, their cumulative effect leads to crystalline failure and fracture, probably as a result of heat generated by hysteresis. (Adapted from Chamay, A. [1970]. Mechanical and morphological aspects of experimental overload and fatigue in bone. J. Biomed., 3:263, with permission.)

visualized as a thin line of transverse or occasionally oblique radiolucency (Fig. 4–28). Alternatively, a faint, fluffy periosteal callus (see Fig. 4–27*B*) may be visualized without evidence of a fracture line. A third form of radiographic manifestation identified particularly in the calcaneus[68] or the tibial plateau[61] (Fig. 4–29), and at times at the base of the first metatarsal,[58] is a line of endosteal sclerosis, indicating some degree of healing and possibly compression of medullary bone. A fourth form is evidence of periosteal reaction over a prolonged segment of the shaft of a long bone[96] without a discernible fracture of the cortex. This radiographic presentation is encountered

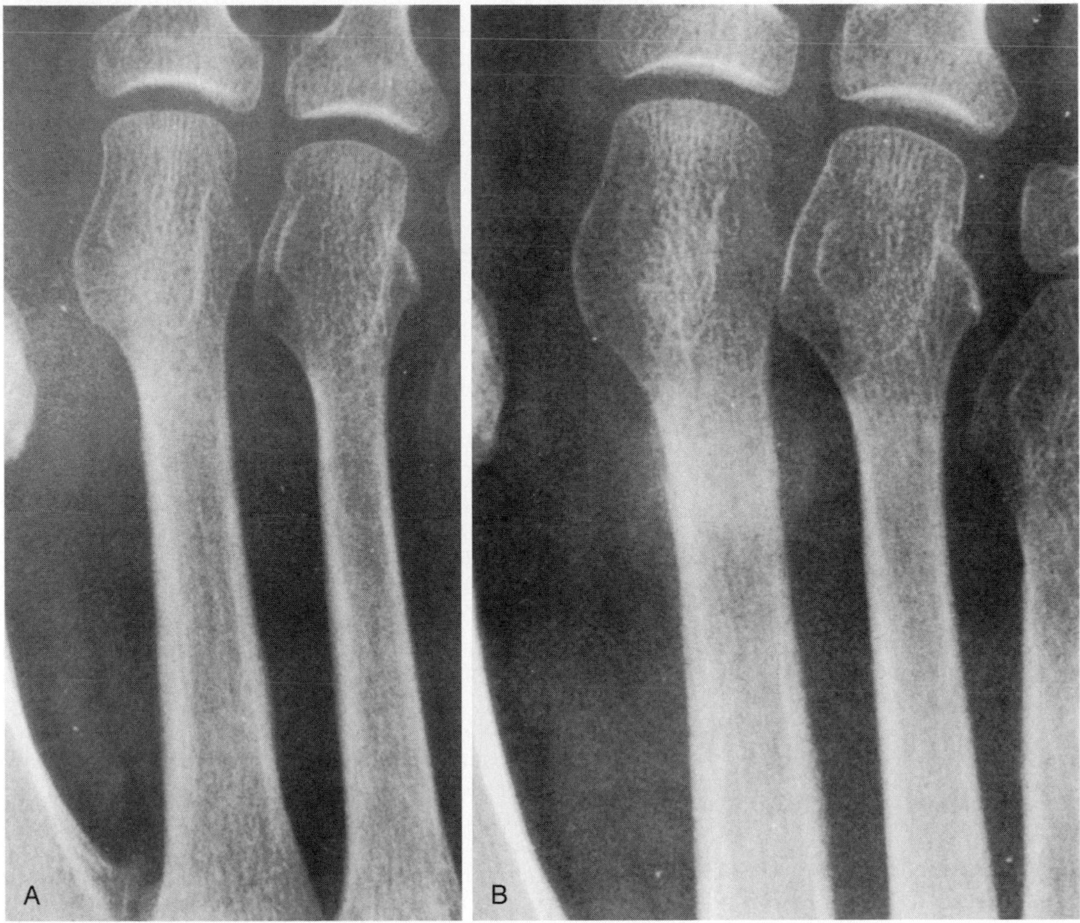

Figure 4–27. Stress fracture of the second metatarsal in a 61-year-old woman who had recently taken up jogging. *A*, The initial radiographic examination was normal. *B*, A second radiograph obtained 12 days later demonstrates fluffy periosteal callus formation about the neck of the second metatarsal. Close inspection demonstrates an underlying disruption of the cortex.

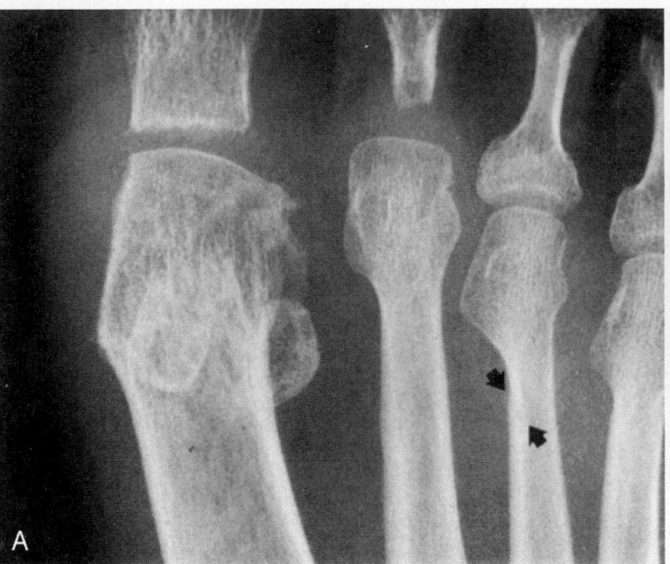

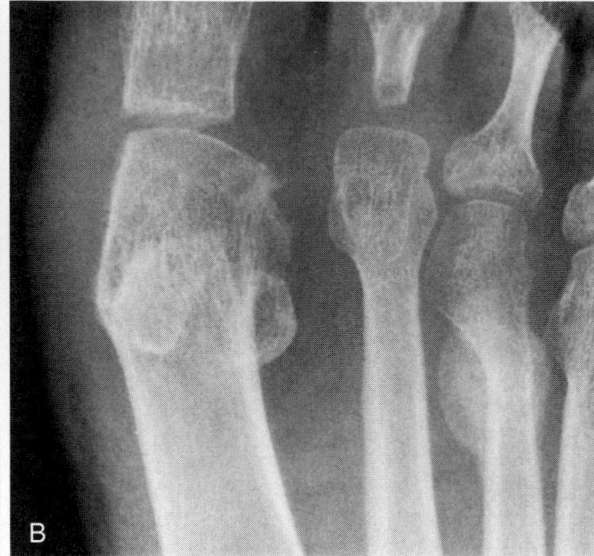

Figure 4–28. Stress fracture of the third metatarsal. *A*, Stress fractures manifested by a fracture line (*arrows*) in the neck of the third metatarsal. The patient had previously undergone surgical correction of a hallux valgus deformity. *B*, A radiograph obtained 3 weeks later demonstrates extensive callus formation. Note that there is also slight angulation at the fracture site.

in children or in the tibia as a manifestation of "shin splints."[69] More often in such cases, the radiographs are unrevealing but the bone scan reveals increased activity over an extended length of the diaphyseal cortex on both the frontal and lateral views (Fig. 4–30). With a linear cortical radiolucency, the differential diagnosis includes pseudofractures[65] associated with osteomalacia and Paget's disease. The possibility of pseudofracture, in the proper clinical setting, is particularly true of stress fractures of the anterior tibial cortex[56] and less commonly the anterior surface of the patella, which are wider and sometimes multiple and demonstrate little or no periosteal reaction at their margins (see Chapter 21 on the knee). Although they mimic such pseudofractures in appearance, they differ in location. Pseudofractures with this appearance occur in the medial cortex of the shaft of the femur and femoral neck, and in the lateral border of the scapula. Those stress fractures manifested by periosteal callus may be mistaken for a more sinister process (e.g., osteomyelitis or malignant disease)[91] if the examiner is unaware of a history of athletic activity or fails to recognize the characteristic location of the stress fracture. For instance, the posterior cortex of the proximal third of the tibia is such a common and typical location for a stress fracture (Figs. 4–31 through 4–33) that, irrespective of the patient's age, this possibility should be given first consideration when periosteal new bone formation is noted in this location.[57]

Stress fractures tend to occur in predictable locations, depending on the particular inciting activity. These are described in subsequent chapters. The most common sites of occurrence[58, 64, 65] are at the distal shaft of the

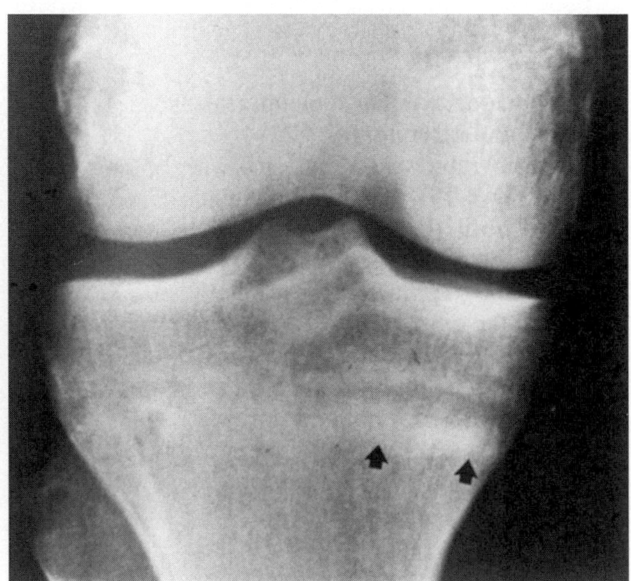

Figure 4–29. Stress fracture of the tibial plateau. The patient was a 26-year-old military recruit who complained of pain in the knee. Note the band of endosteal sclerosis (*arrows*). (Case courtesy of Jay Harold, MD, Oklahoma City, Okla.)

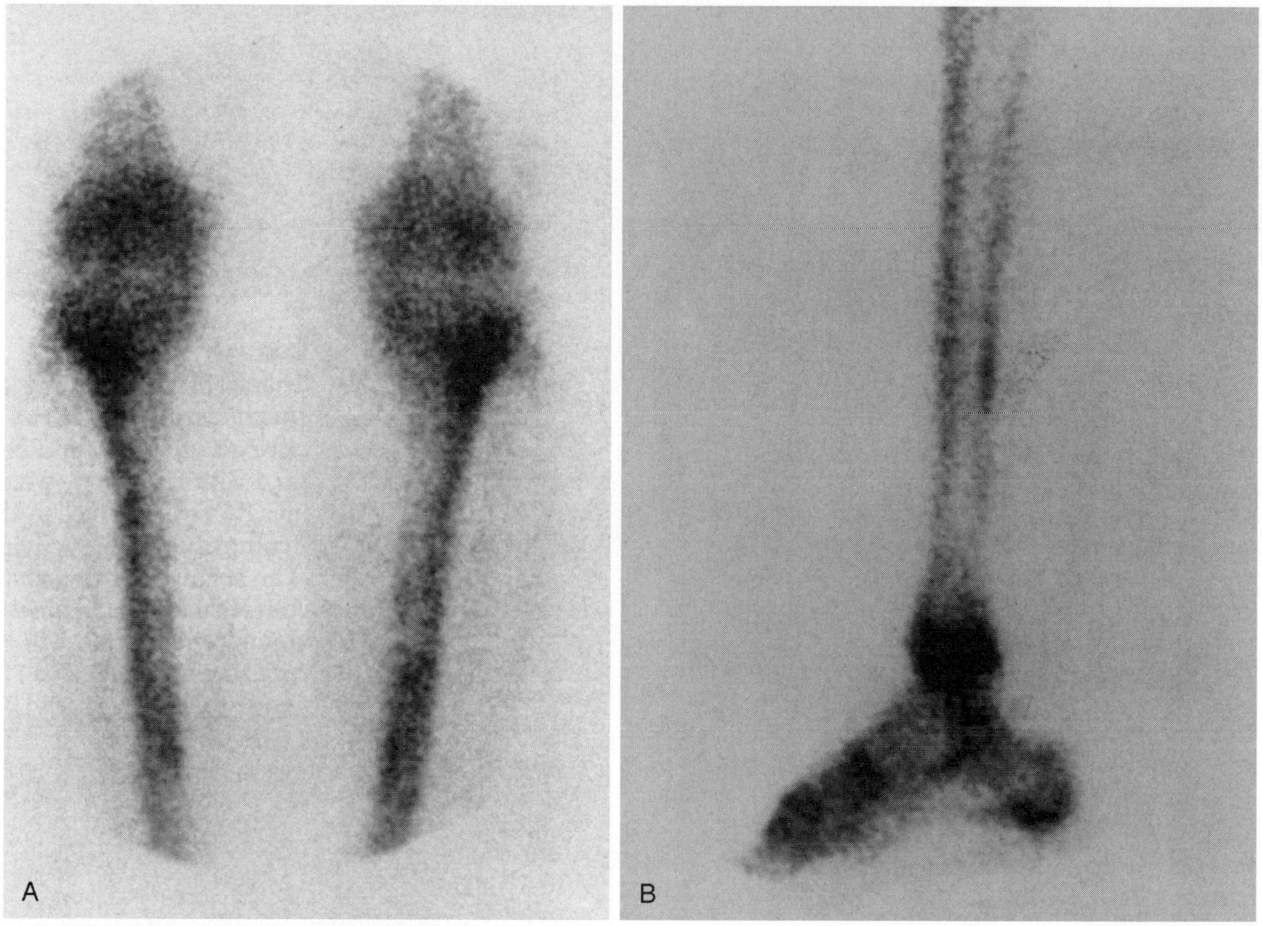

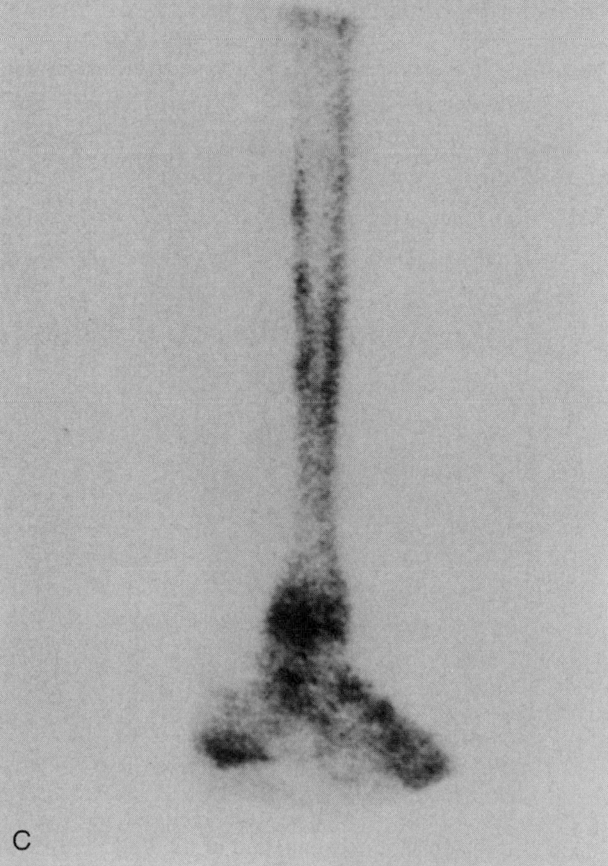

Figure 4–30. Radioisotopic technetium 99m bone scan demonstrating tibial shin splints in a 27-year-old physical fitness buff engaged in running and aerobic dancing. *A*, Anteroposterior view demonstrates increased radioactivity on both the lateral and medial cortices of both tibias. *B* and *C*, Medial views of the right and left tibias, respectively, demonstrate increased radioactivity on both the anterior and posterior cortices of the tibia. These findings are consistent with shin splints.

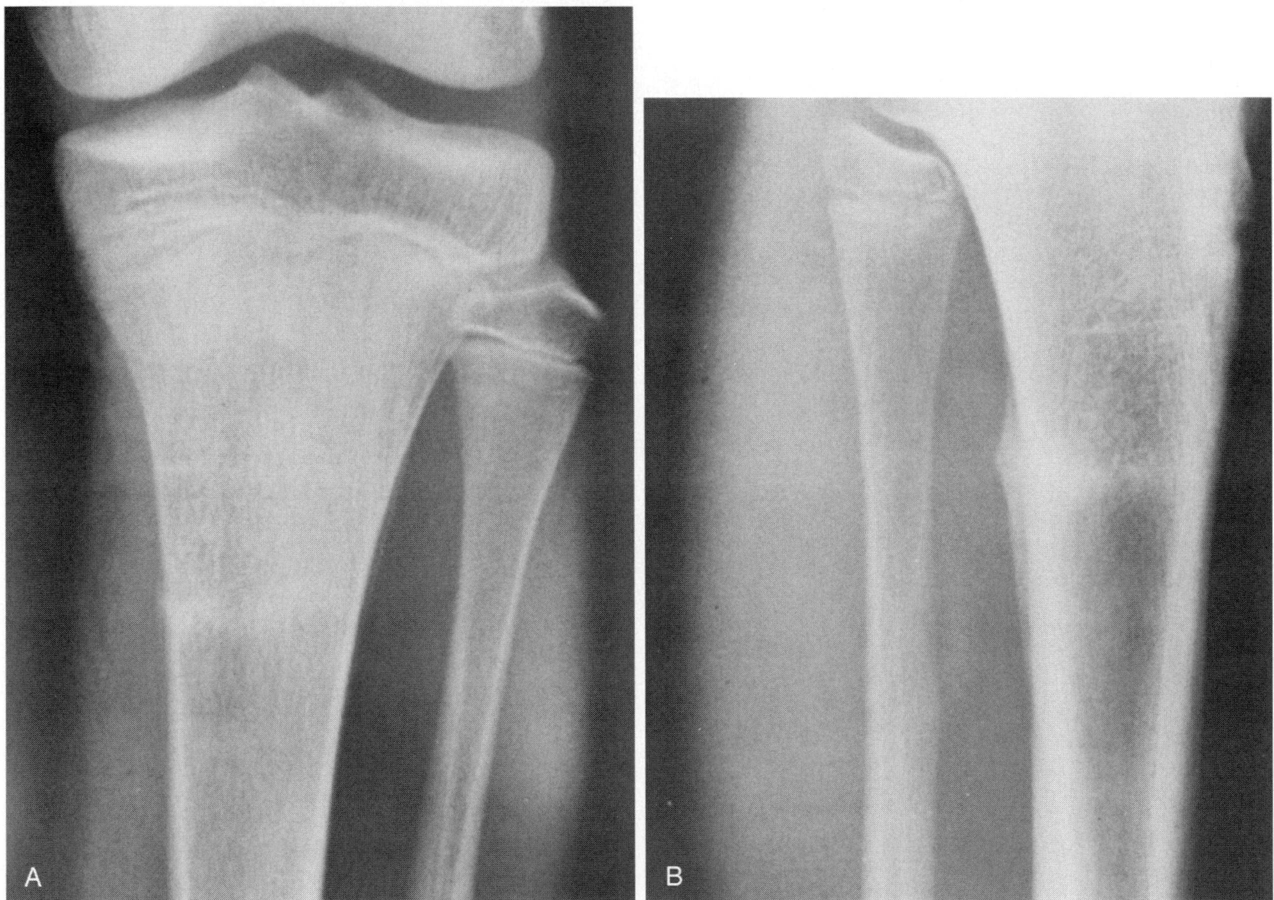

Figure 4–31. Stress fracture of the proximal tibia in a 13-year-old athlete. *A*, A band of increased density extends across the proximal shaft of the tibia, with overlying periosteal reaction. *B*, The fracture is much more clearly visualized on this lateral projection. Note the extensive periosteal reaction with callus formation on the posterior surface of the proximal end of the tibia. This location and appearance are typical for a stress fracture of the proximal third of the tibia.

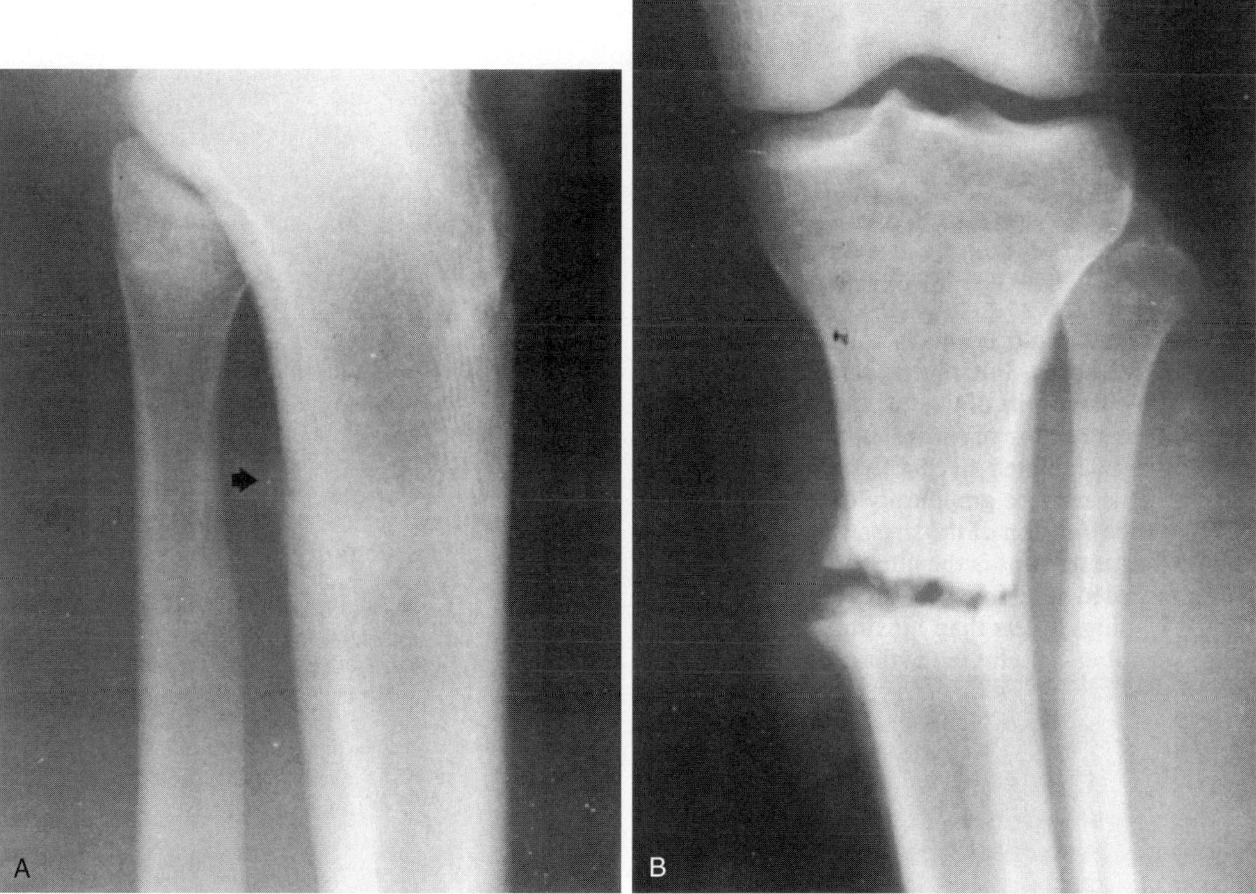

Figure 4–32. Stress fracture of the proximal tibia in a 20-year-old wrestler. *A*, The initial lateral radiograph demonstrates minimal periosteal callus formation (*arrow*) on the posterior surface. *B*, He persisted in his physical activities against medical advice and 5 weeks later sustained a complete fracture while wrestling. Note the callus formation at the medial margin of the fracture. This radiograph was obtained on the day of injury. The findings are typical of a stress fracture that went on to a complete fracture. (Case courtesy of Thomas Harle, MD, Houston, Tex.)

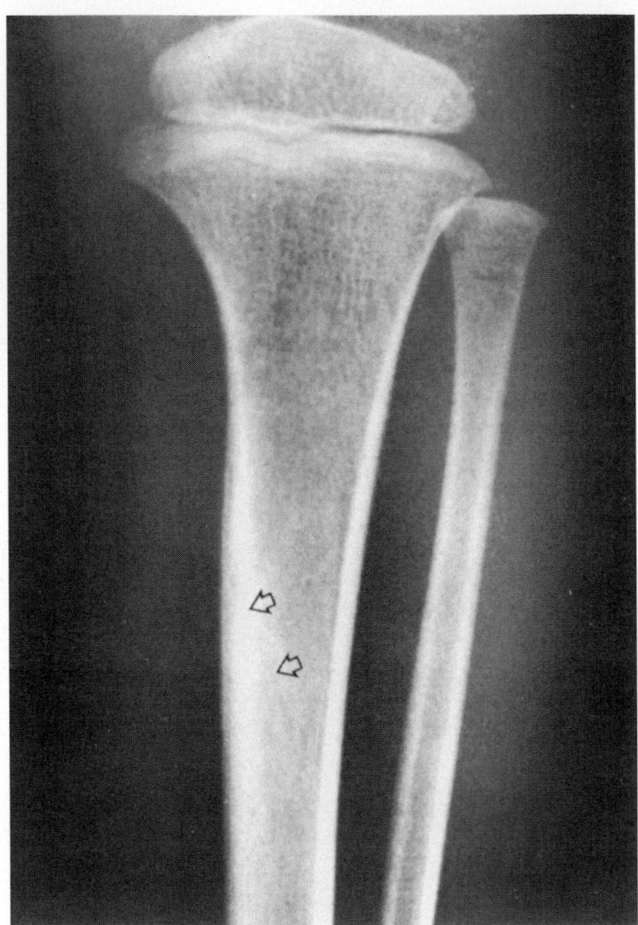

Figure 4–33. Stress fracture of the proximal tibia in a 4-year-old boy. Note the callus formation and the oblique lucency through the medial cortex (*arrows*). The patient had previously experienced a similar stress fracture of the opposite tibia. No predisposing factors could be identified. Presumably, this fracture resulted from the child's play activities.

second and third metatarsals, the tuberosity of the calcaneus, the proximal[52] (see Figs. 4–31 through 4–33) and distal shafts of the tibia and fibula, the shaft[49, 51] (Fig. 4–34) and neck[59, 62, 98] of the femur, and the ischial and pubic rami.[72, 77, 94] Rarer sites are the shaft[58] of the radius[82] and ulna,[71] the lateral margin[50] and the coracoid process[88] of the scapula, the first rib,[58, 74] other ribs,[67, 76] the clavicle,[55, 70] the tarsal navicular,[95] the scaphoid,[66] the humerus,[85] and the pedicles and laminae of the lumbar vertebrae.[47, 81]

MRI[53, 75, 77] is the preferred method for the detection and delineation of stress fractures when the diagnosis is in doubt for whatever reason—history, physical findings, or radiographic findings. In the acute stage, that is, at less than 1 month after onset, the T_1-weighted images demonstrate decreased signal within the marrow in a broad, extended band in the area of fracture, and the T_2-weighted images show signal intensity higher than that of fat in this same area (Fig. 4–35). Linear or broader arcs of increased signal are occasionally encountered in the cortex, and signals characteristic of edema are often identified in the juxtacortical and surrounding soft tissues. In later stages, a narrow, linear, at times undulant band of decreased signal intensity is identified within the intramedullary cavity contiguous with the cortex (Fig. 4–36). This linear band is seen on both T_1- and T_2-weighted images and is presumed to represent microfractures of the trabeculae. The increased signal on T_2-weighted images recedes and is not present as the lesion ages beyond 4 weeks. The linear band of decreased signal persists for some time thereafter.

Radionuclide bone scanning may also be useful in the diagnosis of stress fractures,[48, 63, 79, 80, 84, 86, 87, 97, 99] although its role has been greatly diminished by the use of MRI. The bone scan is positive in the presence of a stress fracture, revealing an area of increased activity. As with MRI, the bone scan will be positive before the radiographic findings are positive (see Fig. 4–34), with a sensitivity similar to that of MRI. If the appearance on bone scan is normal, the diagnosis of a stress fracture is most unlikely. The scan may also demonstrate or reveal occult, asymptomatic stress fractures on the opposite side of the bone. Such symmetrical stress fractures are not uncommon.[84, 86, 89] The bone scan remains positive during the entire healing process; therefore, the increased activity may persist for several months. If the patient refrains from activity immediately after a positive bone scan is obtained, the radiographic examination may never reveal any evidence of abnormality,[84, 86, 97] because the morphologic changes in the bone remain subliminal or microscopic. With an appropriate history of athletic or similar activity, a positive bone scan is sufficient to establish the diagnosis. It is not necessary to have abnormal radiographic findings.

Computed tomography (CT) plays a limited role in the diagnosis of stress fractures of the appendicular skeleton,[78, 92] but is of prime importance in the detection of stress fractures of the pars interarticularis and lamina

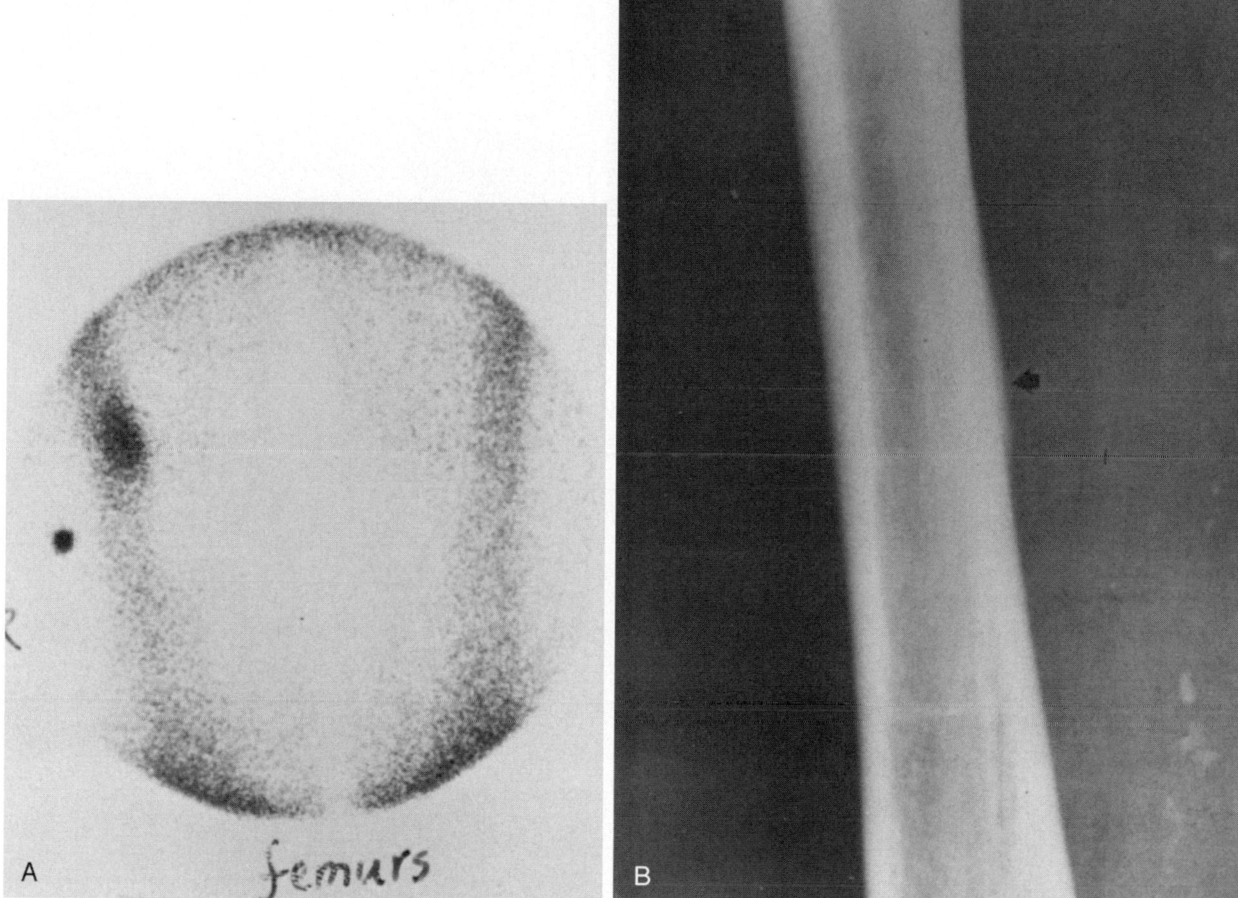

Figure 4–34. Stress fracture of the midshaft of the femur in a 53-year-old runner who had recently increased his training activities. *A*, A technetium 99m pyrophosphate bone scan demonstrates an area of increased radioactivity in the midshaft of the right femur. The radiographic examination at this time was normal. *B*, This anteroposterior radiograph of the femur was obtained 4 weeks after the initial examination and bone scan and demonstrates callus formation along the medial aspect of the femoral shaft (*arrow*), indicating the site of the stress fracture. (Case courtesy of Joseph Norfray, MD, Chicago, Ill.)

in the lower lumbar spine (see Chapter 13). In the long bones CT can demonstrate endosteal callus, which is much less apparent on radiographs. CT discloses edema of the overlying soft tissues and adjacent marrow. Marrow edema is evidenced by obliteration of the normal low signal of fat.[92] CT will also disclose linear, fissure-like lines of fracture in the cortex that may not be evident on radiographs. CT is especially helpful in identifying stress fractures with considerable periosteal reaction that may mimic other lesions such as osteoid osteoma.

Insufficiency Fractures

Insufficiency fractures occur in weakened bone and are caused by physiologic forces generated during normal activities. The involved bone is weakened by a disease process that results in a decrease in the amount of bone or in the quality and strength of bone, or both. Insufficiency fractures are to be differentiated from stress fractures, which occur through normal bone subjected to abnormal forces, and from pathologic fractures, which occur in bone that has been destroyed and replaced by abnormal tissue. Insufficiency fractures constitute one of the major causes of morbidity in a number of systemic diseases.

The most distinctive variety of insufficiency fracture occurs in the pelvic bones of elderly women with osteoporosis[102, 103] (Fig. 4–37) (see Chapter 19 for a full discussion). Similar fractures occur in patients with rheumatoid arthritis or renal osteodystrophy, in those taking steroids, and in patients who have received pelvic irradiation. In osteoporosis, the bone mass in the skeleton is decreased as the cortices and trabecula become thinner. In patients with renal osteodystrophy, the biomechanical quality of the bone is decreased as osteoid seams fail to mineralized normally and calcium is lost through the kidneys. Following irradiation, osteonecrotic bone may fail to remodel along lines of stress. Patients with pelvic insufficiency fractures present with a history of pain, and the radiographic findings are often obscure. Occasionally an ill-defined sclerosis can be seen in the sacral alae,[110, 115] or an obvious healing fracture of the pubic ramus may be visualized (Fig. 4–38). The body of the pubis may show patchy areas of lucency and sclerosis and, on occasion, an obvious loss of bone volume.[100] Bone scanning is helpful[106, 116] (Fig. 4–39). The diagnosis can be confirmed

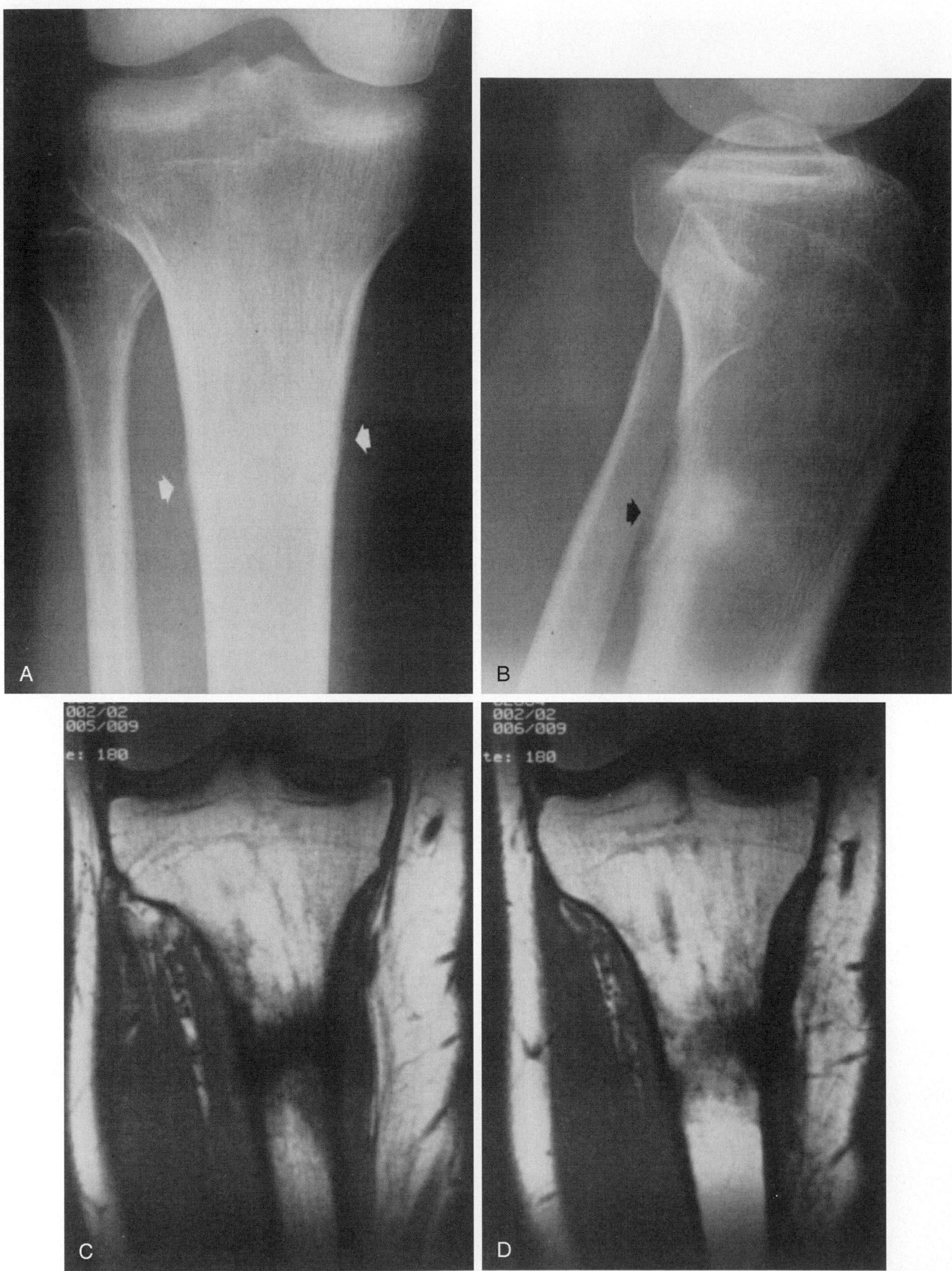

Figure 4–35. Magnetic resonance imaging examination of stress fracture of the proximal tibia in a 23-year-old man. *A* and *B*, Anteroposterior *(A)* and lateral *(B)* views demonstrate periosteal new bone formation on the medial, lateral, and posterior surfaces of the proximal tibia *(arrows)*. *C* and *D*, T_1-weighted coronal images of the posterior aspect of the shaft (*D* is 6 mm anterior to *C*) demonstrate the periosteal reaction but also reveal a zone of decreased signal intensity within the marrow adjacent to the cortex at the site of the stress fractures. (Case courtesy of Alan Schlesinger, MD, Ann Arbor, Mich.)

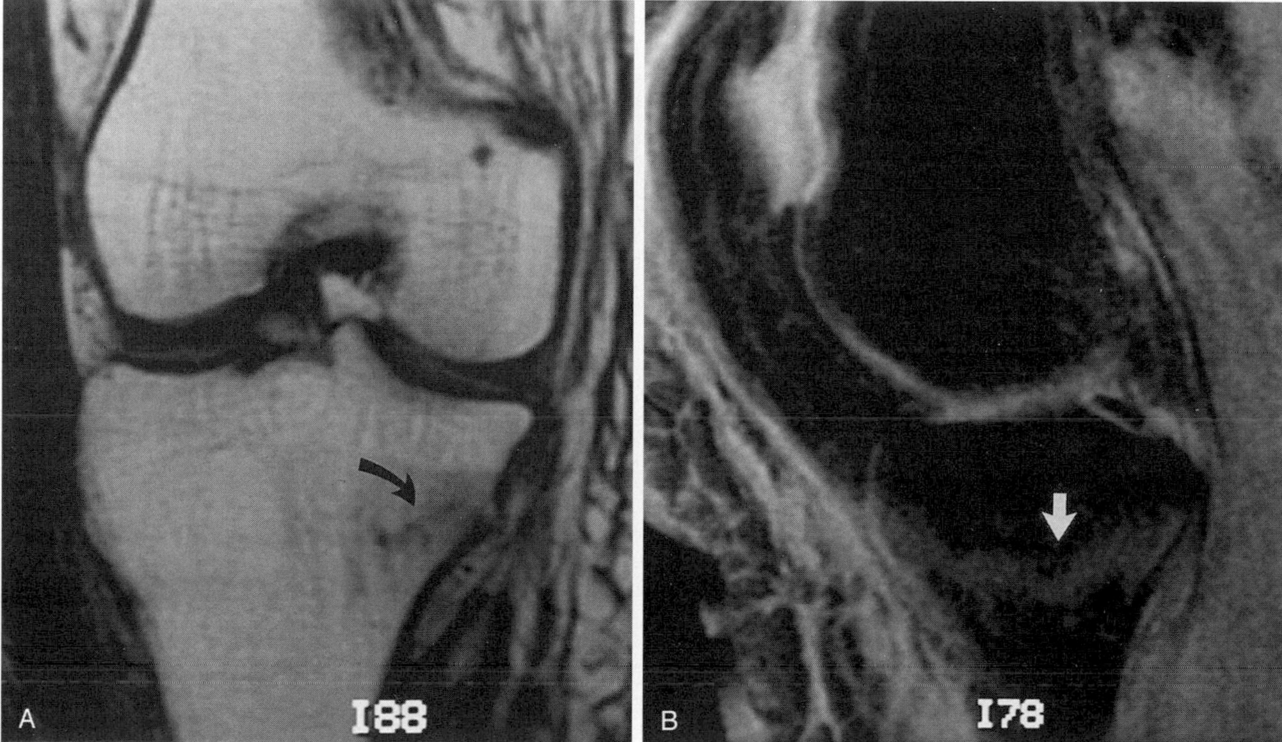

Figure 4–36. Stress fracture of the medial proximal tibial metaphysis demonstrated on magnetic resonance imaging examination. *A*, Coronal T_1-weighted image shows a horizontal fracture line (*arrow*) involving the medial cortex. *B*, Sagittal T_2-weighted fat-suppressed image through the medial aspect of the proximal tibia shows marrow edema (*arrow*) surrounding the fracture. (From Chew, F.S. [2000]. Skeletal Radiology Interactive 2.0, with permission.)

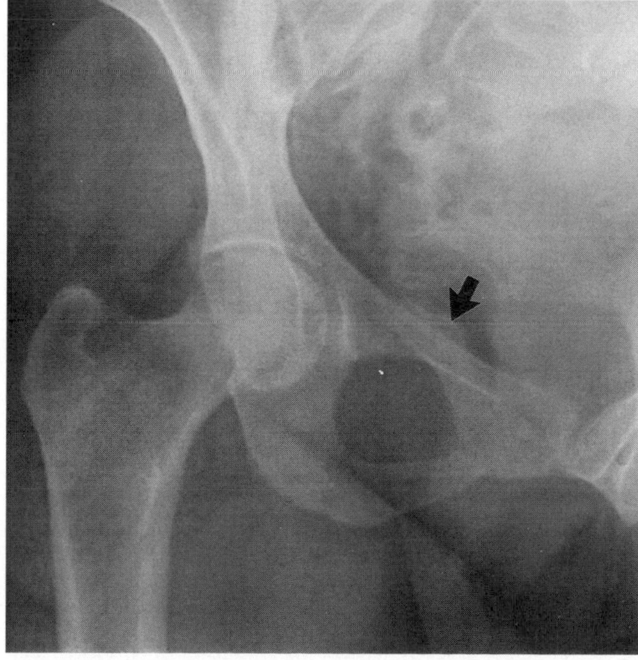

Figure 4–37. Insufficiency fracture. This radiograph, obtained in an elderly woman, demonstrates a healing insufficiency fracture of the superior pubic ramus, evident as fluffy periosteal callus (*arrow*).

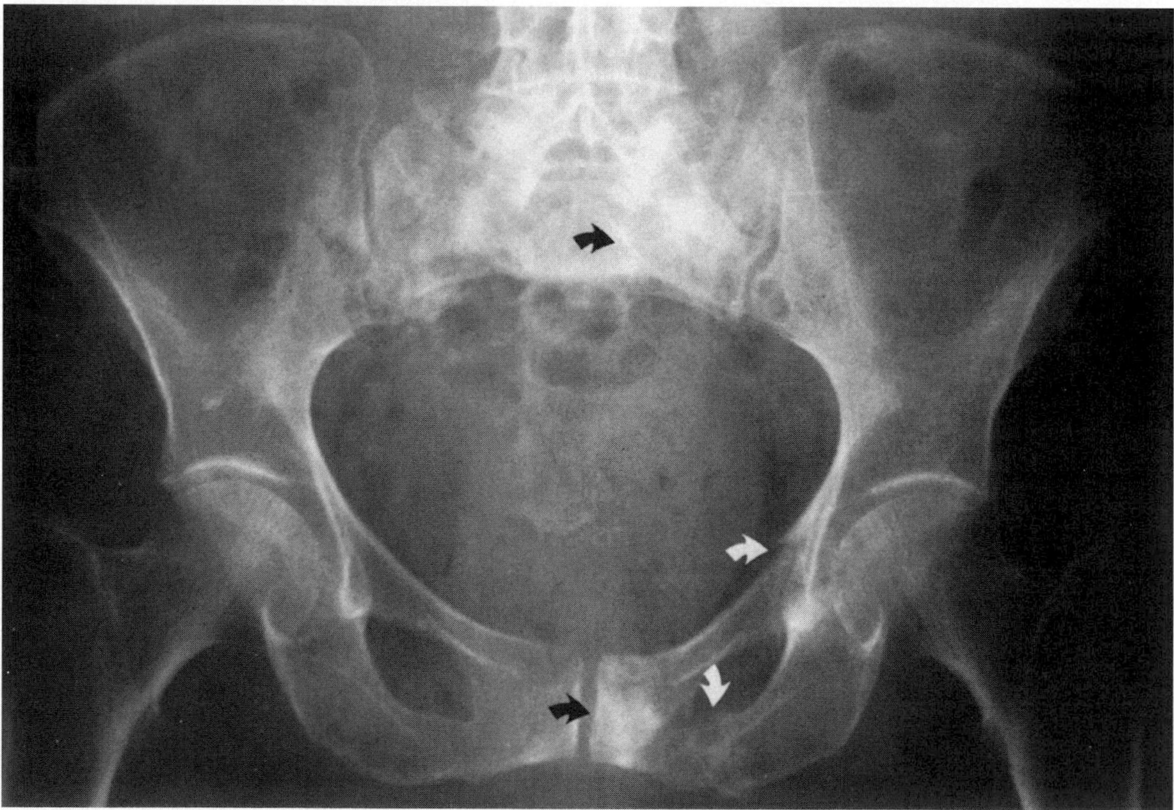

Figure 4–38. Insufficiency fractures of the pelvis in an 86-year-old woman with osteoporosis. The patient complained of pain in the left lower back and left anterior pelvis of approximately 1 month's duration. A history of trauma was denied. Note the obvious fractures of the left pubic ramus, both inferiorly and superiorly (*white arrows*), and areas of mottled sclerosis in the body of the left pubis and left sacral ala (*black arrows*). The latter finding could easily be misconstrued as sites of blastic metastases. The location and appearance of the findings in this case are typical of insufficiency fractures of the pelvis. The findings are often bilateral and symmetrical.

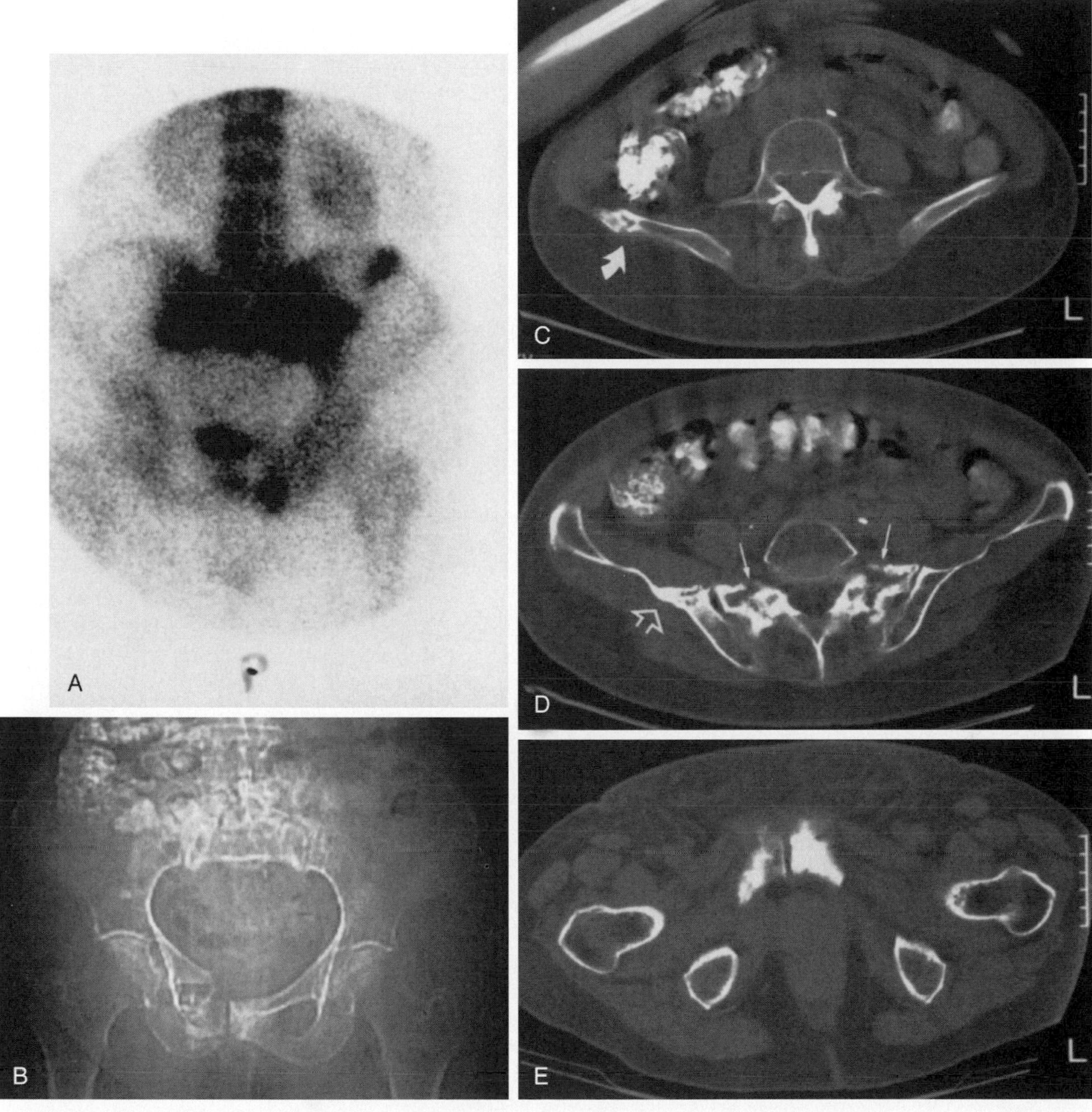

Figure 4–39. Insufficiency fractures of the pelvis in a 79-year-old woman with osteoporosis who presented with a 6-week history of increasing pelvic pain. *A*, Posterior view from a radioisotopic bone scan demonstrates increased radioactivity in both sacral alae and in a linear band extending from the sacroiliac joint through the left iliac bone. There is also increased activity in the body and inferior ramus of the right pubic bone. A small amount of activity is present within the bladder. *B*, Digital anteroposterior radiograph of the pelvis demonstrates a comminuted fracture of the right pubic bone and sclerosis within the body of the left pubic bone. The sacrum and iliac wings are obscured by residual contrast within the colon. *C*, CT through the iliac wings demonstrates a fracture of the right iliac wing (*arrow*) with sclerosis of the margins of the fracture but without a surrounding soft tissue mass. *D*, CT of the sacrum demonstrates sagittally oriented fractures through both sacral alae (*arrows*) surrounded by irregular sclerosis and lysis without associated soft tissue mass. There is also sclerosis in the iliac margin of the sacroiliac joint on the right (*open arrow*), which represents the medial extent of the iliac fracture. *E*, CT of the body of the pubic bones demonstrates irregular sclerosis that is more marked on the left. The absence of soft tissue mass and overt bone destruction and the distribution of findings in this case readily identify these lesions as insufficiency fractures and distinguishes them from foci of metastatic disease.

by CT,[103, 105] which demonstrates patchy sclerosis, often with fissure-like fractures and no associated soft tissue mass (see Fig. 4–39). The absence of soft tissue mass aids in distinguishing insufficiency fracture from metastatic disease, which is often a clinical consideration in these patients.[107] MRI also can establish the diagnosis of pelvic insufficiency fractures in the rami[268, 296] and around the acetabulum[263, 302] and sacrum.[243, 385]

Senile osteoporosis is associated with a high incidence of fracture, particularly in the femoral neck and subcapital area of the femur. Such fractures may occur after rather trivial trauma, and it has been suggested that they may better be termed insufficiency fractures rather than traumatic fracture.[60]

In certain conditions, particularly rheumatoid arthritis[90, 144, 160, 167] (whether or not steroids are used), peculiar forms of fractures may occur, principally in the lower extremity, with no more than normal activity. Such fractures often present as linear, bandlike densities in the metaphysis paralleling the joint surface (Fig. 4–40) and are similar in appearance to stress fractures in the same location.[104] The combination of osteoporosis due to rheumatoid arthritis and corticosteroid therapy, joint stiffness, contracture, angular deformity of the extremity, and the unaccustomed exercise after surgery for joint reconstruction predisposes to the occurrence of these fractures. At times the fracture may follow resumption of ambulation after periods of prolonged bed rest. The pain and disability caused by these fractures is often attributed to rheumatoid joint involvement. The fractures may not be visible on radiographs obtained shortly after the onset of symptoms, and serial examinations may be required for diagnosis. These fractures[90] are likely to occur in the distal or proximal tibia or fibula or in the femoral neck. Similar fractures have also been described after joint replacement for osteoarthritis in patients with osteoporosis,[109] as well as in persons with osteoporosis alone[111] or associated with pyrophosphate arthropathy.[114] Such fractures also occur in patients treated with fluorides for osteoporosis.[117] Insufficiency fractures of the sternum are known to occur in osteoporotic persons with severe dorsal kyphosis.[101, 108, 113]

Transversely oriented insufficiency fractures are common in bone affected by Paget's disease,[119, 157, 171] particularly the shafts of the weight-bearing bones (Fig. 4–41), the femur and tibia, and to a lesser extent the humerus and the vertebral bodies. Although the bone in the sclerotic phase of Paget's disease may appear enlarged, thickened, and extremely dense, it is not as strong as normal bone.

Congenital or developmental disease may result in numerous and repeated fractures of bone.[149] This feature is the hallmark of osteogenesis imperfecta. The congenita form of this disease is well known and easily recognized radiographically by the characteristic thin cortex, the numerous fractures in various stages of healing, and the overall deformity secondary to previously healed fractures (Fig. 4–42). The tarda form is less easily recognized because of the apparent delay in onset of the osseous fragility, the otherwise normal radiographic appearance of the involved bone, and the relative infrequency of fractures.

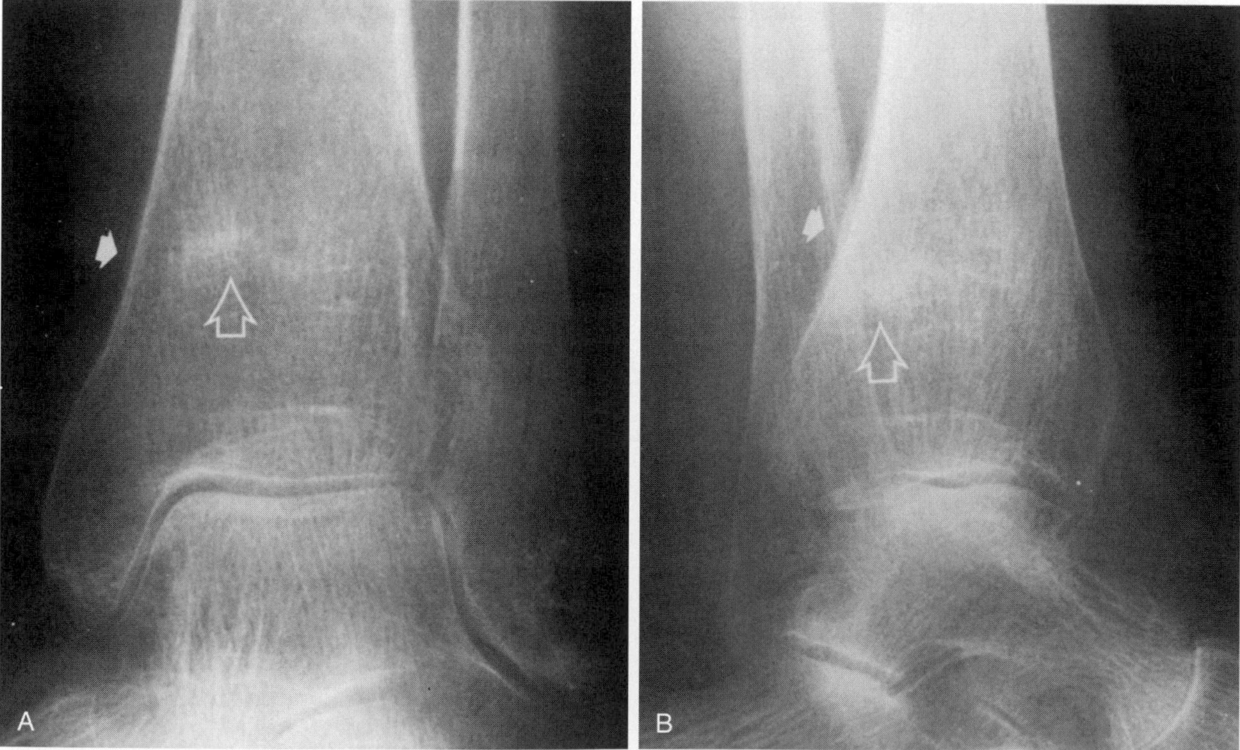

Figure 4–40. Insufficiency fracture of the distal tibia in a 65-year-old woman with rheumatoid arthritis who presented with ankle pain. *A*, Internal oblique view of the ankle demonstrates diffuse osteoporosis and a symmetrical narrowing of the joint space, findings consistent with rheumatoid arthritis. There is an irregular, poorly defined band of sclerosis (*open arrow*) in the tibial metaphysis with overlying compact periosteal new bone formation (*arrow*). *B*, Lateral view. The bandlike area of sclerosis (*open arrow*) extends to the posterior cortex. Evidence of overlying periosteal reaction is present (*arrow*). This appearance is typical of insufficiency fractures occurring in the proximal and distal tibia.

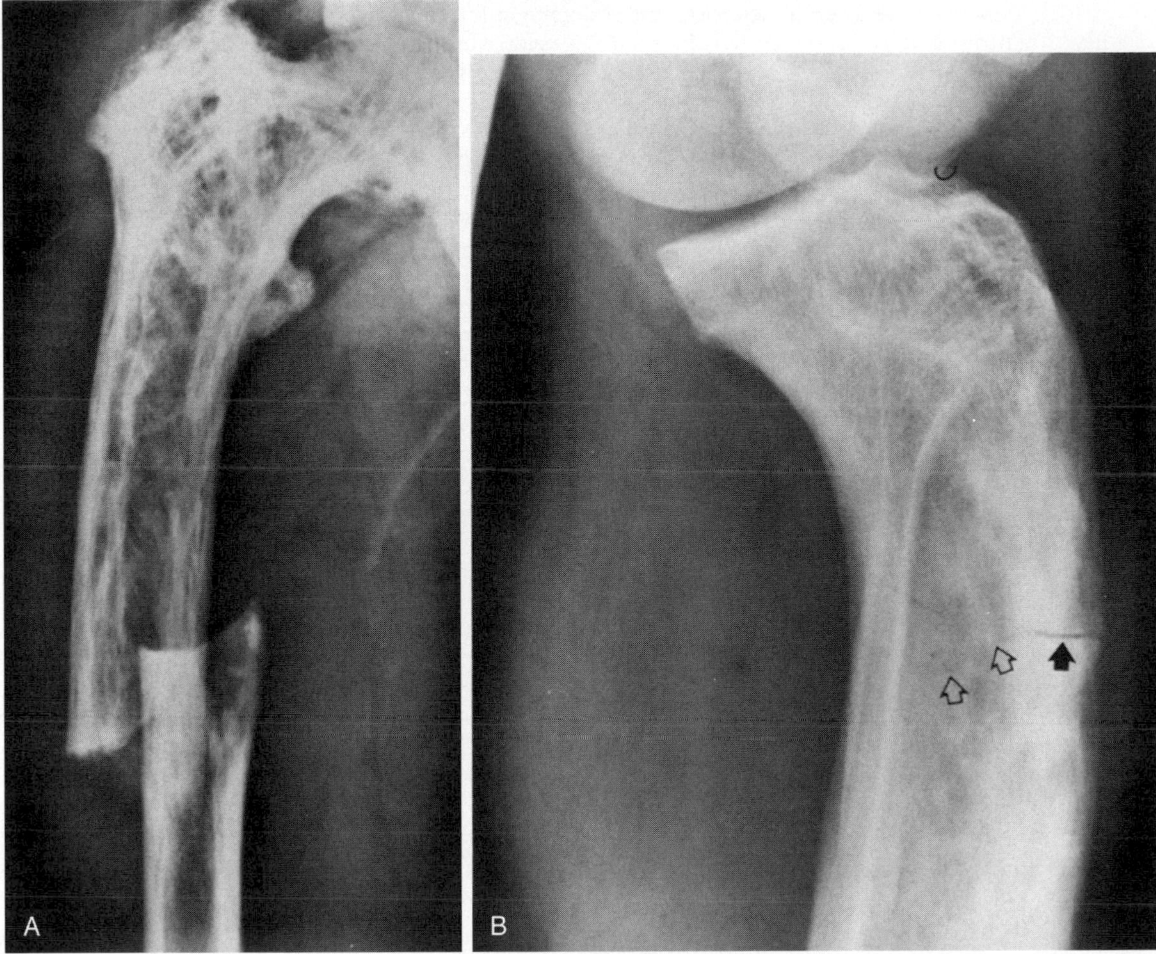

Figure 4–41. Insufficiency fracture in Paget's disease of bone. *A*, There is a slightly oblique fracture through the proximal shaft of the femur. The thickening of the cortex and coarsening of the trabecular pattern of the femur are the classic features of Paget's disease. *B*, Stress fracture through a pseudofracture in a 50-year-old man. He sustained the injury as he twisted his leg during a fall. Note the classic pseudofracture of the anterior cortex (*black arrow*). A fine fracture line extends from the posterior surface of the pseudofracture (*open arrows*).

When repeated fractures occur in response to minor trauma in what appears to be radiographically normal bone, the diagnosis of osteogenesis imperfecta of the tarda form should be considered, and other stigmata of this disease (e.g., blue sclera) should be sought.

Although the bones are denser than normal in osteopetrosis (Fig. 4–43) and pyknodysostosis (Fig. 4–44), they are reduced in strength because they fail to remodel along lines of stress, and are therefore subject to insufficiency fractures. When a transverse or any other form of fracture occurs in unusually dense bone, this possibility must be considered.

Certain metabolic disorders lead to a diffuse loss of bone substance (osteoporosis)[118, 138, 144, 159, 160, 167, 168] or bone mineral (osteomalacia),[146, 163, 172] making the skeleton more susceptible to injury. Chronic renal disease results in a specific disorder of bone, renal osteodystrophy. In this disorder, fractures may occur in bone weakened by osteomalacia[122, 132, 156, 165] (Fig. 4–45) or through deposits of amyloid, the latter usually in the femoral neck.[123, 124] Although fractures of bone are unusual,[155, 163, 172] epiphyseal separations occur in children and adolescents with this disorder, involving particularly the proximal femoral epiphysis. It is rare for an insufficiency fracture to occur in osteomalacia associated with even advanced hyperparathyroidism,[148] except for those cases involving cystic, expansile brown tumors (Fig. 4–46). Because brown tumors replace the bone, such fractures are more properly considered pathologic. Recurrent fractures of the metatarsals[137] and femoral shaft fractures through preexisting pseudofractures[128] have been reported in adult hypophosphatasia.

Fractures occur in previously irradiated bone, usually in the pectoral girdle, clavicle, ribs, and scapula in patients who have undergone treatment for carcinoma of the breast,[143, 154] or in the femoral neck[142] and pelvis, particularly the sacrum (Fig. 4–47) and pubis, in patients who have received treatment for gynecologic or urologic malignancy.[139] The affected bone characteristically contains patchy areas of sclerosis and lucency, indicative of radiation osteitis. One or more fractures of variable age may be present. It is important to distinguish such fractures from pathologic fractures associated with metastatic disease to avoid unnecessary and contraindicated irradiation of the lesion. The characteristic appearance of the surrounding bone, absence of lesions outside the irradiated field, and lack of an associated soft tissue mass (best determined by MRI or CT) are helpful in this regard.

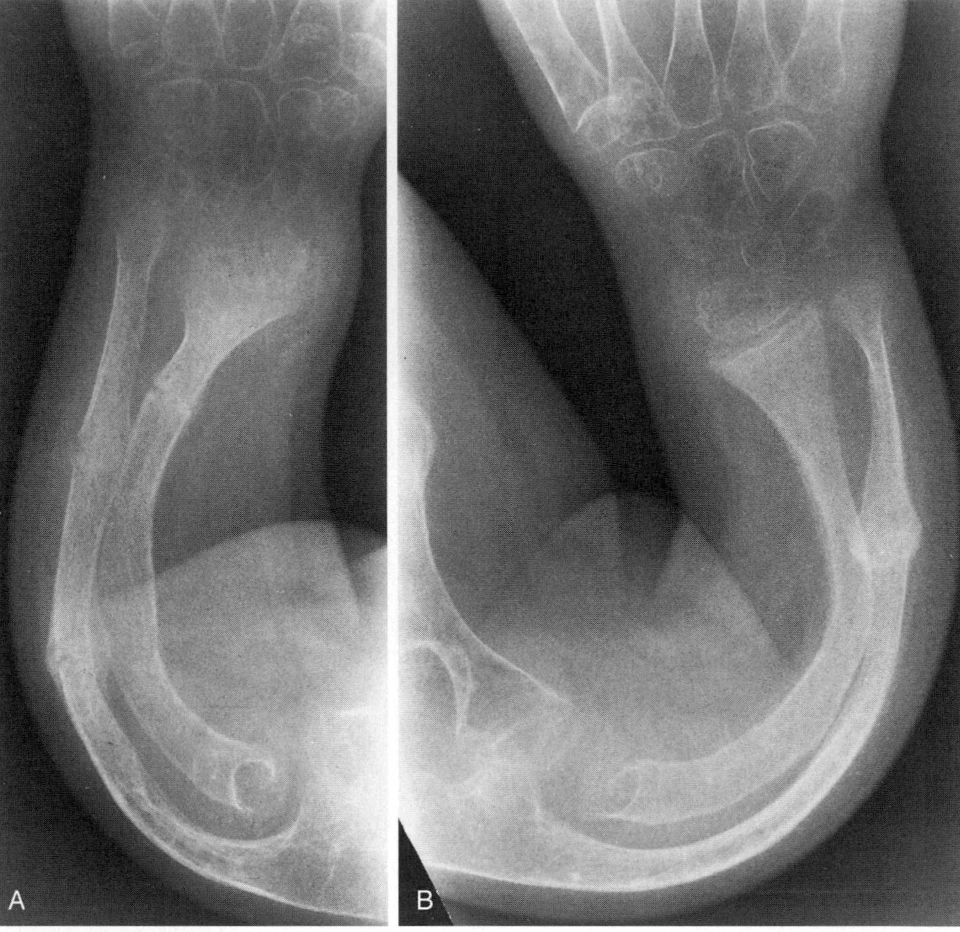

Figure 4–42. Insufficiency fractures in a child with osteogenesis imperfecta. *A* and *B*, Anteroposterior radiographs of both forearms show osteopenic bone with severe bowing deformities. Healing fractures of various ages are present. (From Chew, F.S., Maldjian, C., & Leffler, S.G. [1999]. Musculoskeletal Imaging: A Teaching File. p. 721. Lippincott Williams & Wilkins, Philadelphia, with permission.)

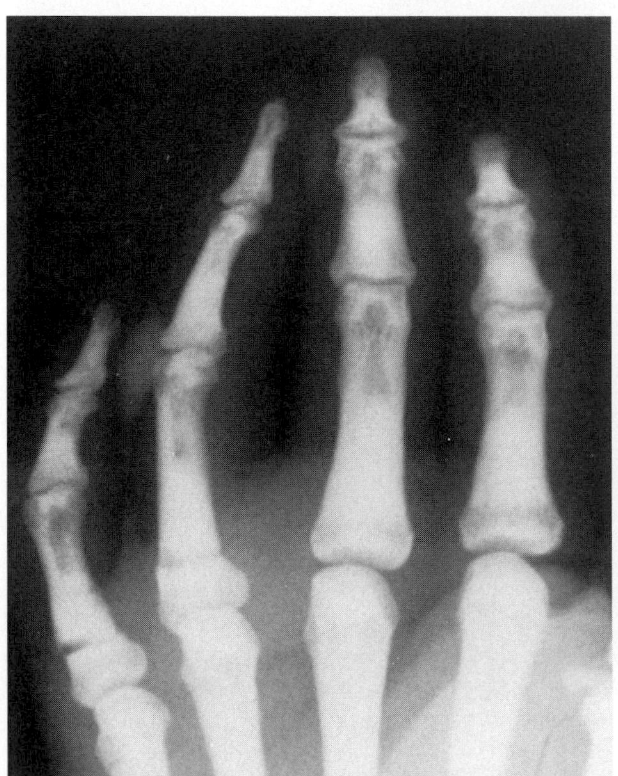

Figure 4–43. Insufficiency fractures at the base of the proximal phalanges of the fourth and fifth digits in a 26-year-old man with osteopetrosis. The fractures are transversely oriented through dense sclerotic bone. The distribution of sclerosis in the phalanges and metacarpals is characteristic of osteopetrosis. (Case courtesy of Jasmid Tehranzadah, MD, Irvine, Calif.)

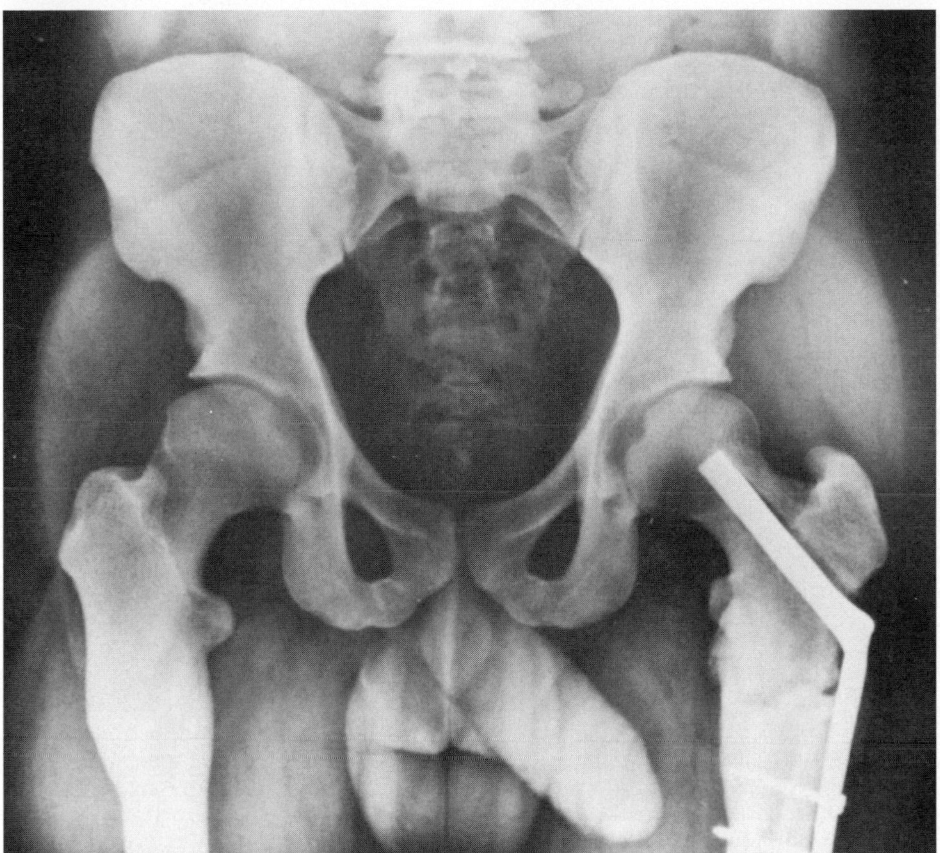

Figure 4–44. The patient was a 27-year-old man who had pyknodysostosis, characterized by an increase in the density and fragility of the skeletal system. Note the deformity of the right femur, indicating a healed subtrochanteric fracture. There has been a more recent subtrochanteric fracture on the left. A Jewett nail is in place.

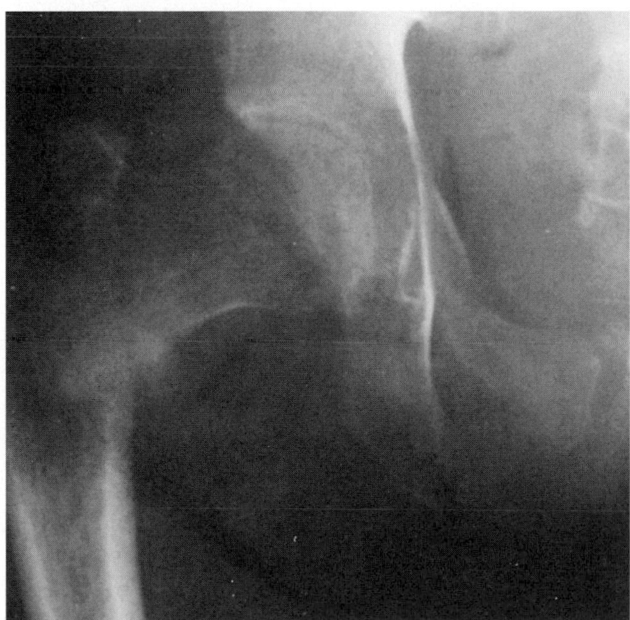

Figure 4–45. Insufficiency subtrochanteric fracture of the right femur in a 23-year-old woman with systemic lupus erythematosus and chronic renal failure, sustained while walking. Note diffuse osteopenia, representing a combination of osteomalacia and osteoporosis. The patient had experienced a similar fracture on the opposite side 15 months previously, as well as fractures of the superior and inferior portions of the pubic ramus before that.

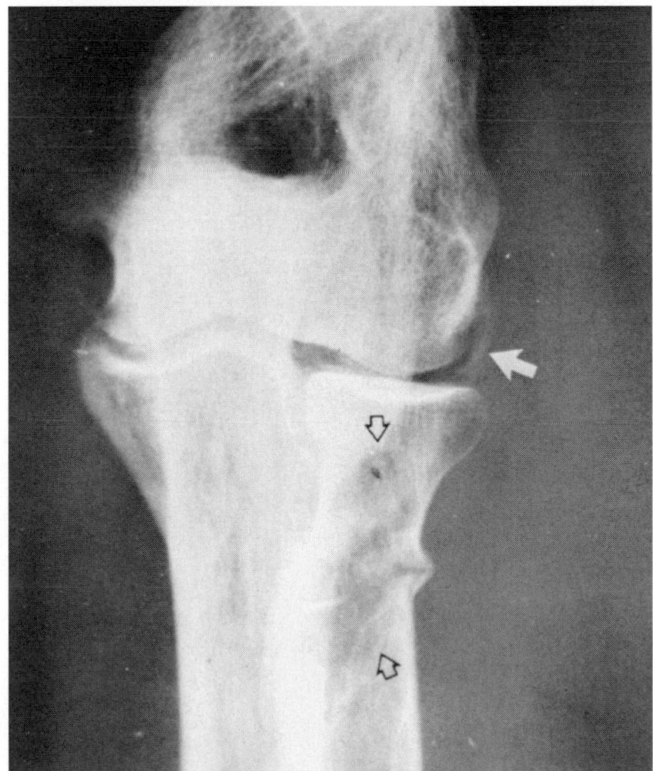

Figure 4–46. A 46-year-old man with primary hyperparathyroidism sustained an eggshell fracture through a brown tumor in the proximal third of the radius (*open arrows*). Note also the presence of chondrocalcinosis (*arrow*).

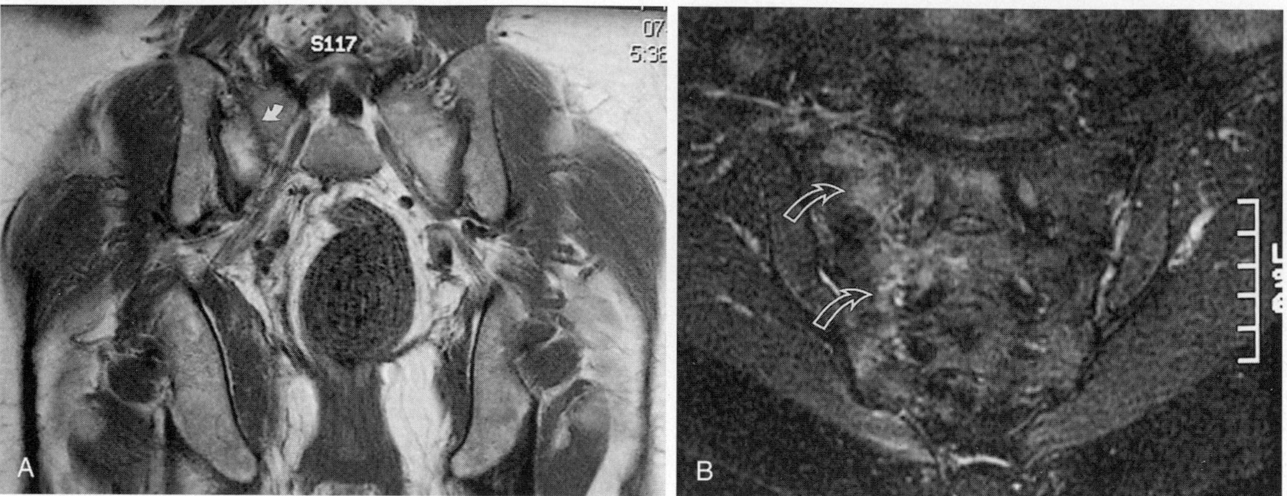

Figure 4–47. Insufficiency fractures of the sacrum after pelvic irradiation, demonstrated on magnetic resonance imaging examination. *A*, Coronal T_1-weighted image shows a low-signal-intensity nondisplaced insufficiency fracture (*arrow*) extending in the sagittal plane through the right sacral wing. *B*, Oblique coronal T_2-weighted fat-saturated image shows high signal intensity extending vertically through the right sacral wing (*arrows*). (From Chew, F. S. [2000]. Skeletal Radiology Interactive 2.0, with permission.)

Some evidence suggests that patients with homozygous β-thalassemia[129] have frequent and multiple insufficiency fractures, usually involving the lower extremity. Delayed healing and resultant deformities are common. Compression fractures of the spine occur.

Insufficiency fractures are frequently sustained by quadriplegic or paraplegic patients (Fig. 4–48) in the denervated limbs.[130, 140] Limbs affected by poliomyelitis are also easily fractured. With denervation the limb undergoes both soft tissue wasting and disuse osteoporosis, resulting in reduced bone strength. The limbs affected by spinal cord injury are also insensate to various degrees, and the patient is often unaware that a fracture has occurred.

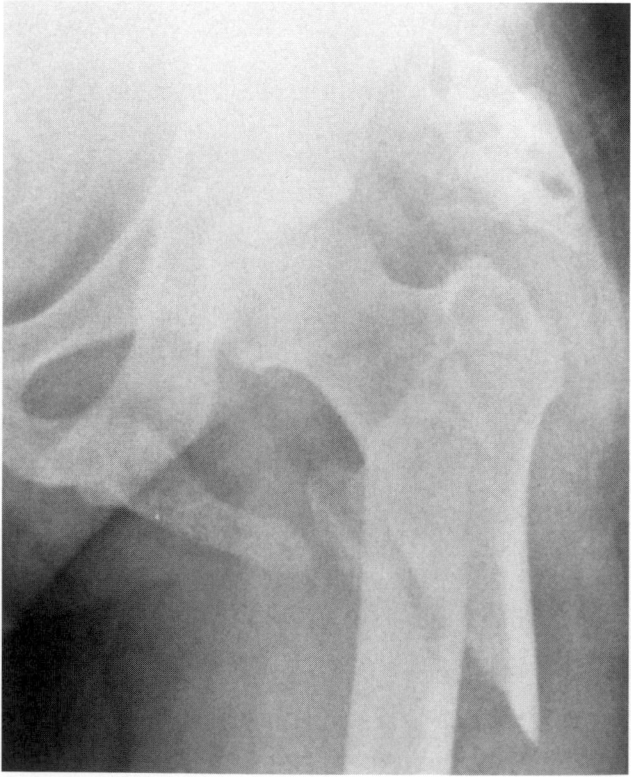

Figure 4–48. Oblique subtrochanteric fracture in a 26-year-old paraplegic man, sustained in a fall. He noted swelling 2 days later. Note the periarticular ossification typically found with paraplegia.

The hallmark of neurotrophic arthritis (Fig. 4–49) is repeated fractures leading to fragmentation of the joint surface. This condition is noted most commonly in the feet of diabetics and characteristically involves the tarsal joints, usually the tarsometatarsal joints, leading to a Lisfranc fracture-dislocation (see Fig. 4–49).[127, 169] When numerous fracture fragments are present the diagnosis is less challenging than when a single osteochondral fracture or a more subtle form of fracture, such as a depressed fracture of the tibial plateau, is encountered (Fig. 4–50). Under these circumstances, the patient's history and laboratory data and radiographic examination of additional joints are required to substantiate the diagnosis.

Pathologic Fractures

Pathologic fractures occur in bone that has been destroyed and replaced by diseased tissue.[90, 112, 158] The disease may be a focal process, a regional condition, or a generalized systemic disorder. The most common underlying focal pathologic process is a metastatic tumor (Fig. 4–51). The initial manifestation of focal benign lesions[152] or metastatic disease[126] is often pain accompanying the occurrence of a pathologic fracture.

There are both clinical and radiographic clues[164] to the pathologic nature of a fracture. Characteristically, the fracture arises from stresses of low magnitude that normal bone would easily withstand. There is frequently a history[9, 12, 126, 153] of preexisting pain or a mass or swelling in the area before the occurrence of the minimal or trivial traumatic episode[153] that resulted in the fracture. Radiographically, the fracture traverses an area of abnormal thinning, expansion, or bone destruction (Fig. 4–52). A

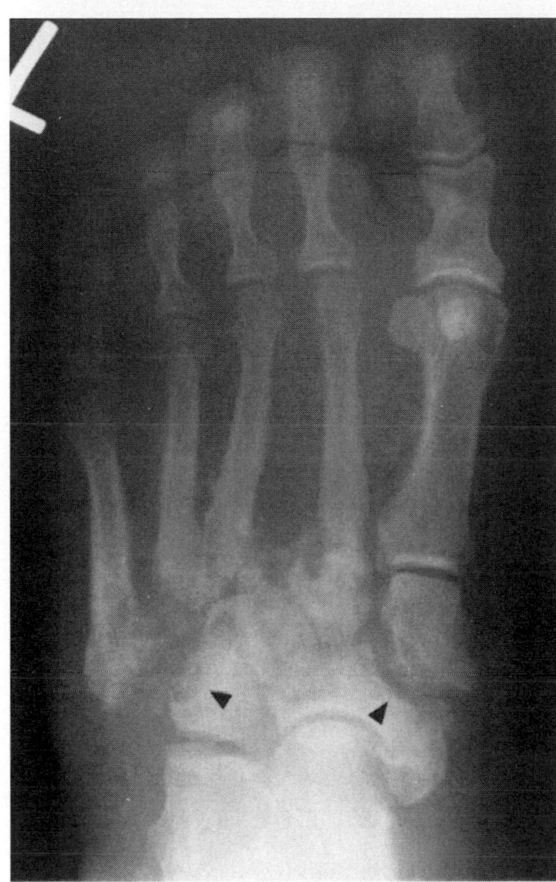

Figure 4–49. Neuropathic arthropathy in a 48-year-old diabetic man who presented with a severely swollen foot. The oblique radiograph of the foot demonstrates a fracture-dislocation of the metatarsal joints, a so-called Lisfranc's fracture-dislocation. Note the periosteal bone formation about the shaft of the metatarsals and the sclerosis and fragmentation of the bones, particularly of the cuboid and navicular bones (*arrowheads*). There is considerable soft tissue swelling. These findings are indicative of a neuropathic joint.

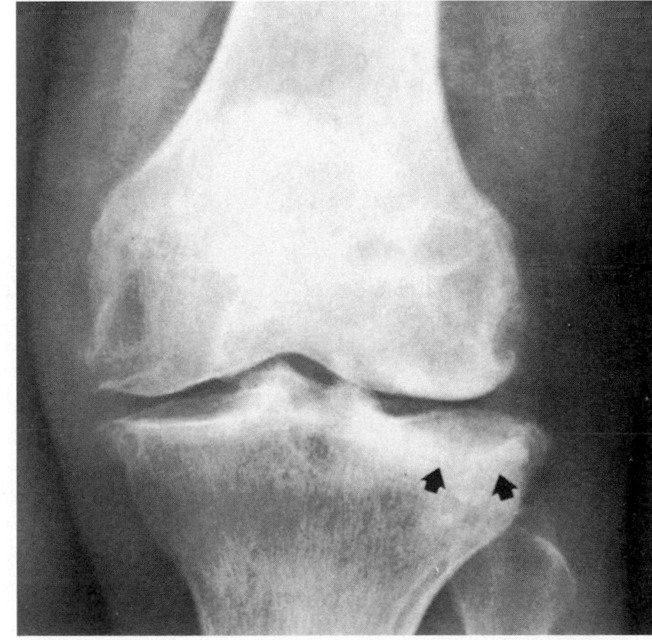

Figure 4–50. Neurotrophic arthritis in a 73-year-old man with tabes dorsalis. Note the depressed fracture of the lateral tibial plateau (*arrows*). Findings on the opposite side were similar. The patient denied pain or a history of trauma. Results on VDRL testing were positive in both blood and spinal fluid. The tibial plateau fracture is manifested by distortion of the cortical margin and an apparent increase in bone density due to impaction of fracture fragments. Similar changes may occur as the result of pyrophosphate arthropathy.

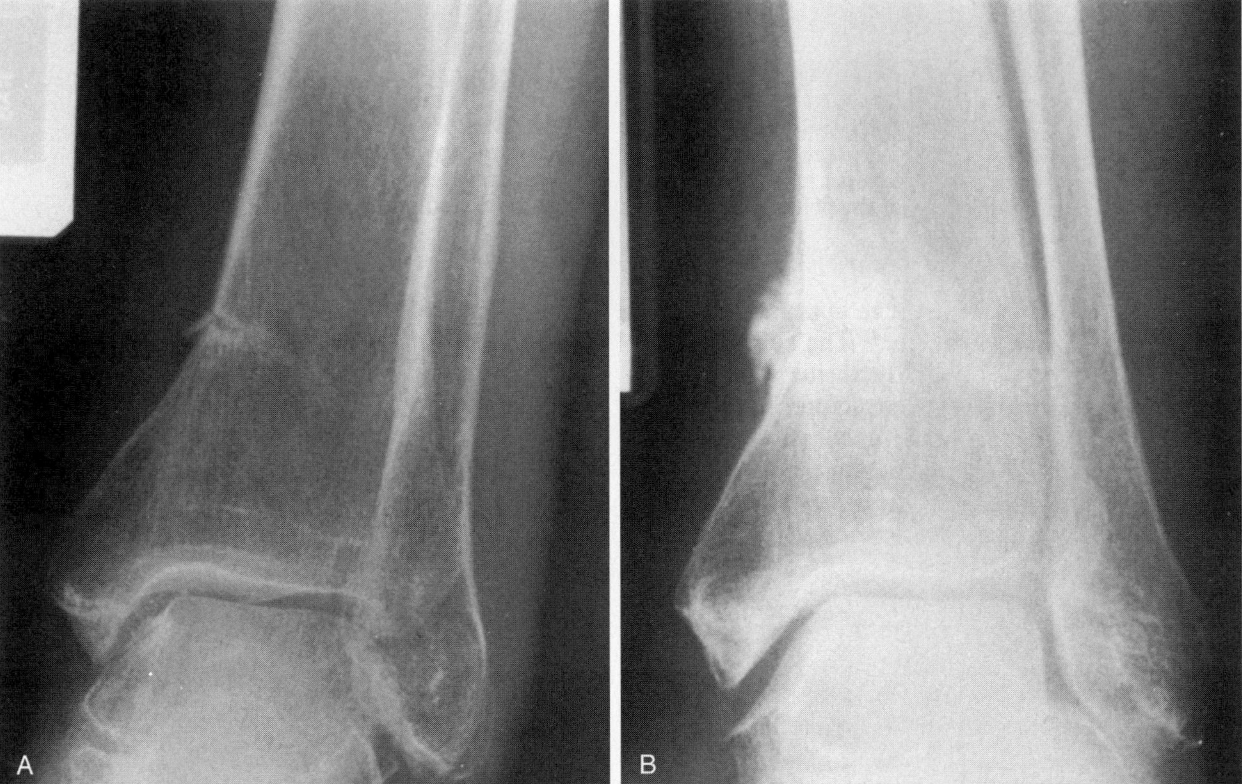

Figure 4–51. Insufficiency fracture of the distal tibia in a 72-year-old man who denied a history of trauma or increased physical activity. *A*, The initial radiographic examination demonstrates disruption of the medial cortex of the distal tibia. *B*, A second examination 6 weeks later demonstrates extensive callus formation and a linear fracture line with surrounding sclerosis extending across the width of the tibia.

characteristic orientation for a fracture involving diseased bone in the appendicular skeleton is transverse to the long axis (Fig. 4–53). (Transverse fractures are relatively uncommon in normal bone outside of the diaphysis, particularly in the metaphysis or metadiaphysis.) Therefore, when a transverse fracture is encountered, an underlying pathologic process must be considered. Incomplete linear fractures (Fig. 4–54*A*) involving areas of bone abnormality may occur. Expansile, ballooned lesions, such as giant cell tumor (see Fig. 4–54*A*), aneurysmal bone cyst, or enchondroma (see Fig. 4–54*B*) in short bones, with extreme thinning of all or a portion of surrounding cortex, are particularly associated with incomplete fracture from minor trauma. A fracture in such a lesion can result from the most trivial accident. A comminuted, depressed fracture, similar to a depressed fracture of the skull, can occur in a person with an expanded lesion as a result of bumping into a sharp object such as the edge of a chair. The fracture sustained in such lesions is similar to the cracking of an egg and may be described as an "egg-shell" fracture.

Most pathologic fractures in adults occur in an area of metastatic disease involving the spine, femur,[136, 157] or humerus,[121, 125, 126, 141, 145, 162] but any bone may be involved. Fractures occasionally occur through bone erosions and subchondral cysts in rheumatoid arthritis,[161] as well as through subchondral cysts in pyrophosphate arthropathy.[166] Fractures in areas of osteomyelitis[120, 131] (Fig. 4–55) or sarcoidosis[135, 170] (Fig. 4–56) are rare. If a fracture occurs in an area of chronic osteomyelitis, the possibility of a superimposed squamous cell carcinoma should be considered.

Pathologic fractures of the spine (Fig. 4–57) result in collapse or compression of the vertebral body.[134, 150, 151] Therefore, a compressed vertebra in individuals over 40 years of age should be viewed with suspicion, and evidence of associated bone destruction in the involved or adjacent vertebrae should be sought. This evidence is most easily obtained by viewing the pedicles to look for loss in their cortical margins, but any associated loss of cortex in the vertebral body is of equal diagnostic significance. The pedicles are frequently spared in multiple myeloma, although this disease is a common cause of pathologic fractures of the vertebrae. Therefore, the presence of intact pedicles does not exclude the possibility of a pathologic fracture in the spine.

In the long bones the most common site of pathologic fracture from metastatic disease is the femur,[121, 125, 133, 136, 147, 157] particularly the femoral shaft (see Fig. 4–52) and subtrochanteric regions.[171] In this region the course of fracture lines in normal bone is frequently transverse, and fracture lines in pathologic bone may be oblique. To avoid oversight, all fractures in these locations occurring in older persons must be viewed with suspicion[133] and the fragments examined closely for signs of bone destruction (Fig. 4–58). If there is any question, a biopsy should be performed. This procedure is easily done because most of the fractures are treated by open reduction and internal fixation.

Certain fractures should be considered pathologic until

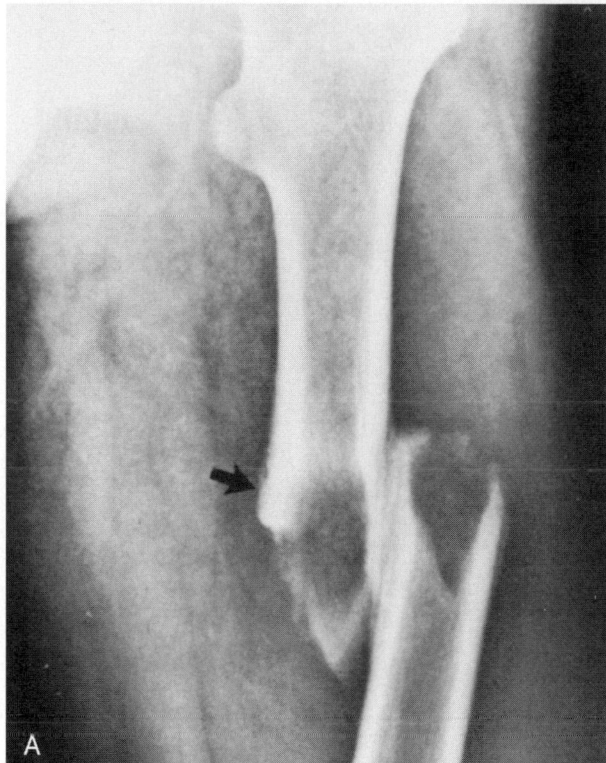

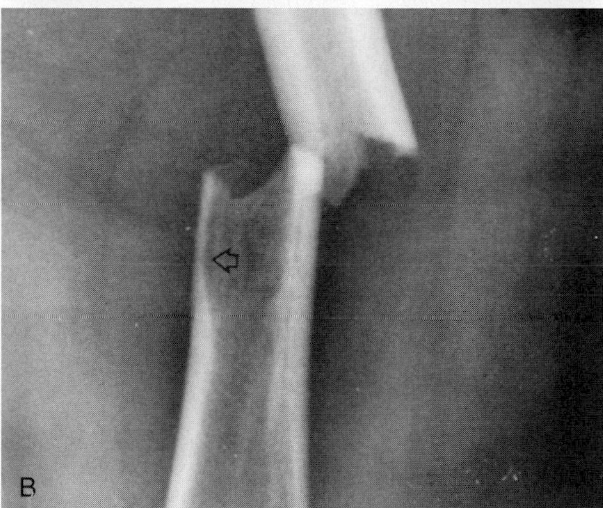

Figure 4–52. Pathologic fractures of the femoral shaft. *A*, The patient "felt something snap" in his leg as he stepped from a bar stool. He was subsequently found to have carcinoma of the lung. There is an oblique fracture through an obvious area of lucency with surrounding periosteal reaction (*arrow*). *B*, The patient sustained this fracture when she tripped and fell. She was subsequently found to have carcinoma of the colon. Note that the pathologic nature of the fracture is not as obvious as in *A*. There is a lytic focus located principally in the distal fragment, with erosion of the endosteal surface of the shaft (*arrow*).

proven otherwise. Isolated avulsion fractures of the lesser trochanter are not uncommon athletic injuries in adolescents, in whom the apophyseal plate is still open. Once the apophyseal plate closes, however, isolated lesser trochanter fractures are usually pathologic, with an underlying metastasis. Similarly, isolated avulsion fractures of the ischial tuberosity occur in adolescent athletes, but once the apophysis closes, such fractures are usually pathologic. Surgical neck fractures of the humerus are common in adults, particularly those over the age of 50 years, but in children, they are usually pathologic.

Indications for Radiography in Trauma

A radiograph is not a substitute for obtaining a medical history or for performing a physical examination. Selection of those patients requiring radiography should be made on the basis of history and physical examination. Unfortunately, this approach is not universally recognized or practiced, resulting in unnecessary examinations.

When does a patient require a radiograph following an injury? This question is not easily answered. The decision involves multiple, intermeshed considerations—the desire of the physician not to miss any injury, the patient's expectations of care and need for radiography, the physician's need to reassure the patient that no injury is present, and the latent fear of liability and other medicolegal considerations. These considerations, combined with the paucity of objective screening guidelines, exert great pressure on the physician to subject virtually every patient with a complaint or history of trauma, however trivial, to radiography.[18, 32]

Diagnostic imaging in the setting of known or suspected skeletal trauma may be used to detect and document the presence or absence of fracture or other injury, to provide information for clinical management and possibly surgical planning, and to monitor the subsequent clinical course for progress and possible complications. Imaging methods commonly applied in the setting of acute trauma include radiography, CT, and MRI. Special radiographic techniques, conventional tomography, radionuclide imaging, arthrography, and ultrasonography may be applicable occasionally. Specialized imaging methods may also be indicated for the evaluation of associated injuries of vascular, neurologic, or other soft tissue structures.

Most fractures can be identified on radiographs, although sometimes a second look following examination of the patient is required. When technically acceptable radiographs are normal and fractures are suspected nonetheless, cross-sectional imaging methods may be used when a management decision is critical (e.g., surgery versus no surgery). In some circumstances follow-up radiographs may be more appropriate than additional imaging, particularly when treatment such as a splint or cast would be instituted anyway. The onset of fracture healing typically makes nondisplaced fractures more evident.

Overall, the positive yield in radiography of the extremities for trauma is approximately 20%.[18] In Lee and Chew's study of emergency room radiography,[281] 75% of skeletal radiographs obtained in the emergency room after trauma were normal. The examinations with the greatest proportion of normal were the cervical spine (89% were normal), the thoracic spine (87% were normal), and the knee (86% were normal). The proportion of studies with abnormal findings can be increased by tightening the clinical criteria for ordering radiographs

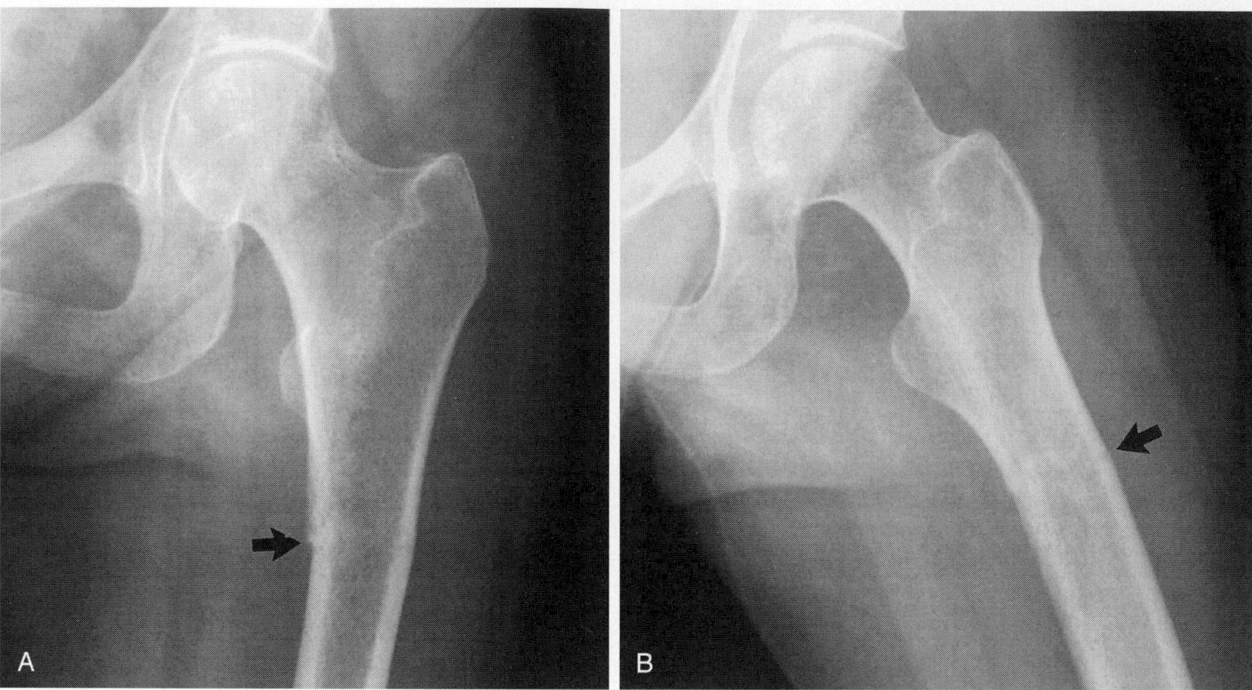

Figure 4–53. Pathologic fracture. Anteroposterior *(A)* and frog-leg lateral *(B)* radiographs of the left hip of a woman with metastases from breast carcinoma diffusely involving the femoral shaft. A minimally impacted transverse fracture is present *(arrow)*. There is no focal lesion. (From Chew, F.S. [2000]. Skeletal Radiology Interactive 2.0, with permission.)

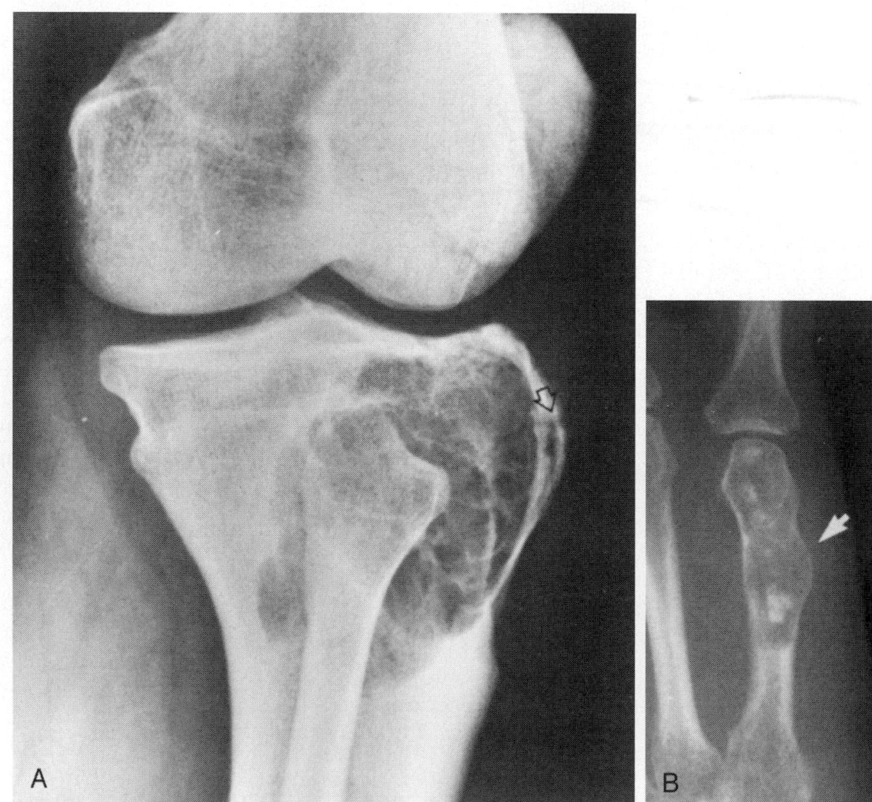

Figure 4–54. Pathologic fractures in patients with benign tumors. A, The patient was a 28-year-old man who sustained this fracture when he bumped his knee against a chair. The sharply defined, lobulated lucency that abuts on the cortical surface of the tibial plateau is typical of a giant cell tumor. Note the incomplete fracture through the cortex *(arrow)*, well visualized only in the oblique projection. *B*, Fracture *(arrow)* through an enchondroma of the distal shaft and head of the fifth metacarpal. The sharp definition of the lesion with expansion of the cortex and chondroid matrix is indicative of an enchondroma. These tumors are more commonly located in the phalanges.

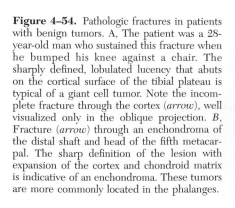

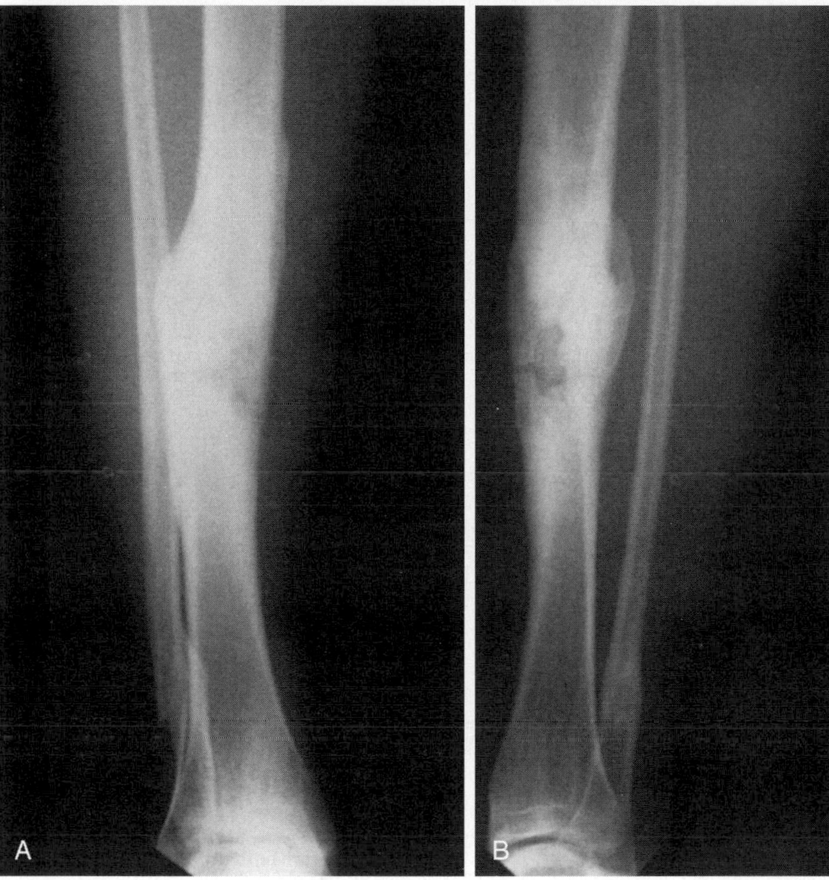

Figure 4–55. The patient stumbled and incurred a pathologic fracture through an area of chronic osteomyelitis. The initial injury, an open fracture-dislocation of the tibia and fibula, had occurred 6 years previously; at that time a pedicle graft was required to cover the soft tissue deficit. *A*, Anteroposterior view demonstrates considerable sclerosis about the well-healed fracture of the midshaft of the tibia. There is also a well-healed fracture of the distal shaft of the fibula. A new lucent transverse fracture courses through a vaguely defined radiolucency in the midportion of the lesion. *B*, The intramedullary lucent focus is well defined, as is the line of fracture. The lucency proved to be a chronic bone abscess.

and reducing the percentage of patients referred for radiography.[18, 33]

The Ottawa ankle and foot rules (Table 4–1)—a set of historical, clinical, and functional criteria developed for rational ordering of radiographs in the setting of ankle injury[329, 330]—have proved to be effective in determining which patients with blunt ankle trauma do not need radiographs.[286, 301, 335, 341] Similar sets of rules, the Ottawa knee rules[328] and the Pittsburgh knee rules,[232] have been validated for use in patients with blunt knee trauma[334, 338] (Table 4–2). The Pittsburgh knee rules in one retrospective study had better diagnostic performance than the Ottawa knee rules.[321] These clinical rules appear to be practicable in clinical settings and have gained acceptance by many physicians.[262] Some emergency rooms have been successful in implementation of these rules by triage nurses.[317] The American College of Radiology (ACR) has published several series of criteria for the appropriateness of diagnostic imaging in a variety of clinical circumstances, including suspected ankle injury, cervical spine trauma, acute shoulder trauma, acute trauma to the hand and wrist, and acute trauma to the knee.[223] These criteria are freely available on the ACR World Wide Web (www.acr.org).

Most radiographic examinations are requested either to confirm a clinically suspected abnormality or because of difficulty in excluding a significant bone injury on clinical grounds alone.[19] Most physicians err on the side of caution when deciding which patients to radiograph. When a decision not to obtain a radiograph is based on sound clinical grounds, fractures will be missed infrequently, and those missed will almost always be less severe and relatively inconsequential.[20, 23] Many requests for radiographs, however, are made simply to reassure the

Table 4–1. Clinical Decision Rules for Use of Radiography in Acute Ankle Injury

Ottawa Ankle Rules

Ankle radiographs are necessary only if
(1) there is pain near the malleoli, *and*
(2) either
  (a) there is inability to bear weight for four steps both immediately following injury and in the emergency department, *or*
  (b) there is bone tenderness at the posterior edge or tip of either malleolus.

Ottawa Foot Rules

Foot radiographs are necessary only if
(1) there is pain in the midfoot, *and*
(2) either
  (a) there is inability to bear weight for four steps both immediately following injury and in the emergency department, *or*
  (b) there is bone tenderness at the navicular or the base of the fifth metatarsal.

From Stiell, I.G., Greenberg G.H., McKnight, R.D. et al. (1993). Decision rules for the use of radiography in acute ankle injuries. Refinement and prospective validation. J.A.M.A., *269*:1127. Copyright © 1993 American Medical Association.

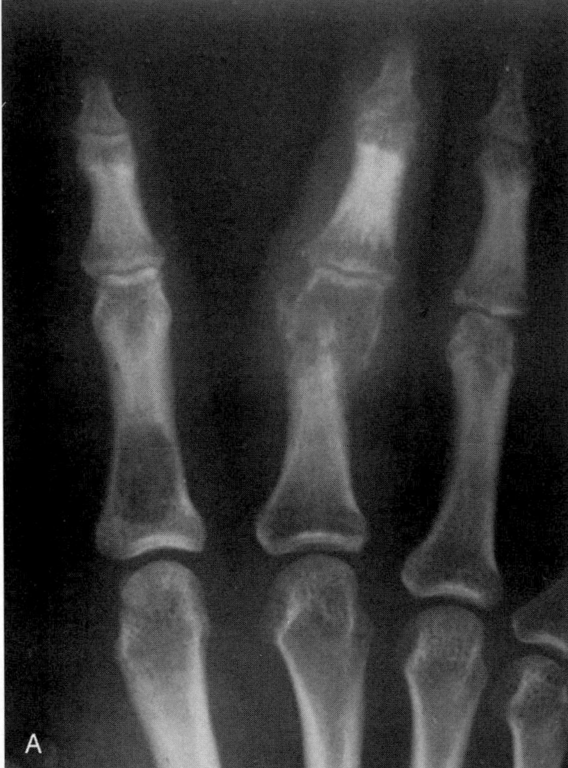

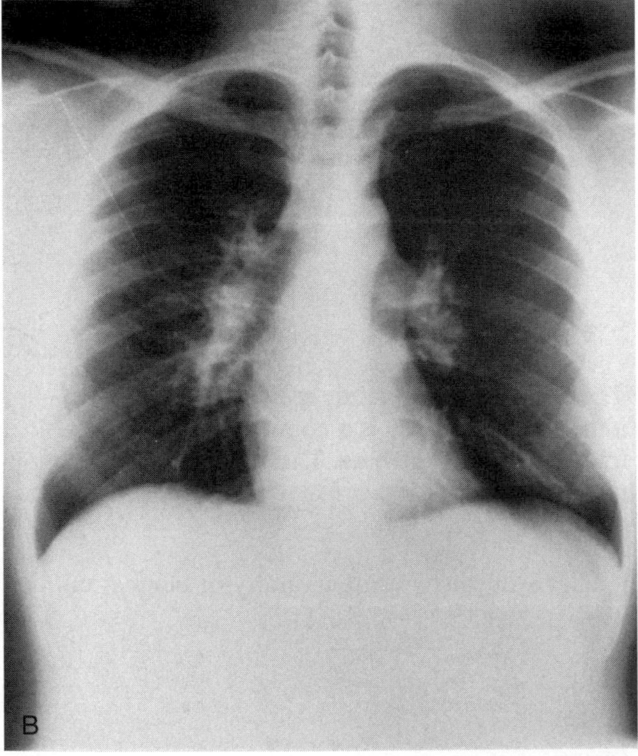

Figure 4–56. Pathologic fracture through a focus of sarcoidosis in the proximal phalanx of the long finger of a 32-year-old black man, who sustained the injury while playing deck tennis. *A*, There is an obvious angulated transverse fracture through a moderately well-defined, lytic process in the distal aspect of the proximal phalanx of the long finger. The lysis extends to the subarticular bone and appears to permeate portions of the cortex in the shaft. There is a well-defined lytic focus in the proximal phalanx of the index finger as well. *B*, The patient had no previous medical history, but this chest radiograph demonstrated bilateral and right peritracheal hilar adenopathy, consistent with sarcoidosis. A biopsy of the lesion in the phalanx confirmed this diagnosis.

Table 4–2. Clinical Decision Rules for Use of Radiography in Acute Knee Injury

Ottawa Knee Rules*

Knee radiographs are necessary only if there are one or more of the following findings related to age, tenderness, or function:
(1) age 55 years or greater, *or*
(2) tenderness at head of fibula, *or*
(3) isolated tenderness of patella, *or*
(4) inability to flex to 90 degrees, *or*
(5) inability to bear weight for four steps both immediately following injury and in the emergency department.

Pittsburgh Knee Rules†

Knee radiographs are necessary only if
(1) blunt trauma or a fall is mechanism of injury, *and*
(2) either
  (a) age younger than 12 years or older than 50 years, *or*
  (b) inability to walk four weight-bearing steps in the emergency department.

*From Stiell, I.G., Greenberg, G.H., Wells, G.A. et al. (1996). Prospective validation of a decision rule for the use of radiography in acute knee injuries. J.A.M.A., 275:611. Copyright © 1996 American Medical Association.

†From Bauer, S.J., Hollander, J.E., Fuchs, S.H., & Thode, H.C. Jr. (1995). A clinical decision rule in the evaluation of acute knee injuries. J. Emerg. Med., *13*:611, with permission from Elsevier Science.

patient. Medicolegal considerations lurk in the background in every case, but the fear of litigation rarely serves as the sole indication for radiography.

Obtaining the Radiograph

The patient must be positioned appropriately for standard radiographic studies, obtained in a minimum of two planes perpendicular to one another; additional unusual or nonstandard positions may be required occasionally and should be tailored to the occasion by the radiologist. A radiographic tube that can be positioned for cross-table lateral views is very useful, especially in an emergency department, for a lateral projection in patients who have multiple or severe injuries or who cannot turn for some other reason. Properly exposed films are necessary to prevent overlooking fractures (Fig. 4–59). Radiographs obtained using fixed equipment are better technically and yield more diagnostic information compared with radiographs obtained using portable equipment. Whenever it is medically prudent to do so, the patient should be brought to the x-ray equipment rather than vice versa. Body part thickness affects detail because of scattered radiation. A Bucky grid is necessary for radiographs of the pelvis, abdomen, and other thick body parts to absorb the unwanted scattered radiation. Decreasing the size of the exposed area also improves image detail by decreasing the amount of scattered radiation.

A radiograph may not demonstrate a subtle or even occasionally a not-so-subtle fracture for multiple reasons: patient motion, insufficient exposure or overexposure, patient body size, insufficient number of views of the area (Fig. 4–60), or use of a film-screen system that provides insufficient resolution of detail. Patient motion with resultant blurring of the radiographic image will defeat all other efforts at obtaining a satisfactory radiograph. This potential problem is not insignificant in patients with

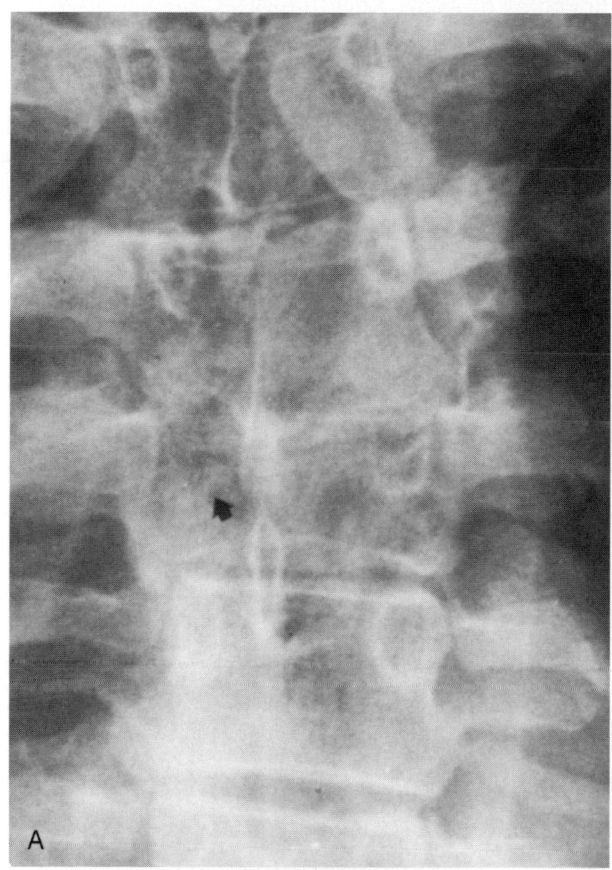

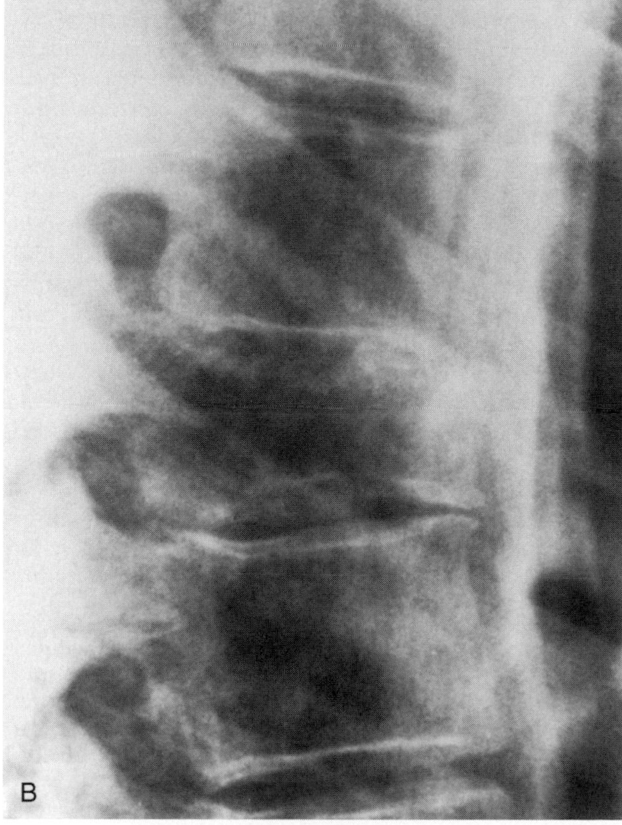

Figure 4–57. Pathologic fracture of the fifth thoracic vertebra in a 38-year-old woman with carcinoma of the breast. *A*, The anteroposterior projection demonstrates loss of the height of the fifth vertebra and absence of the right pedicle (*arrow*). *B*, The collapsed fifth vertebral body is wedge shaped. There is cortical destruction of the superior end plate.

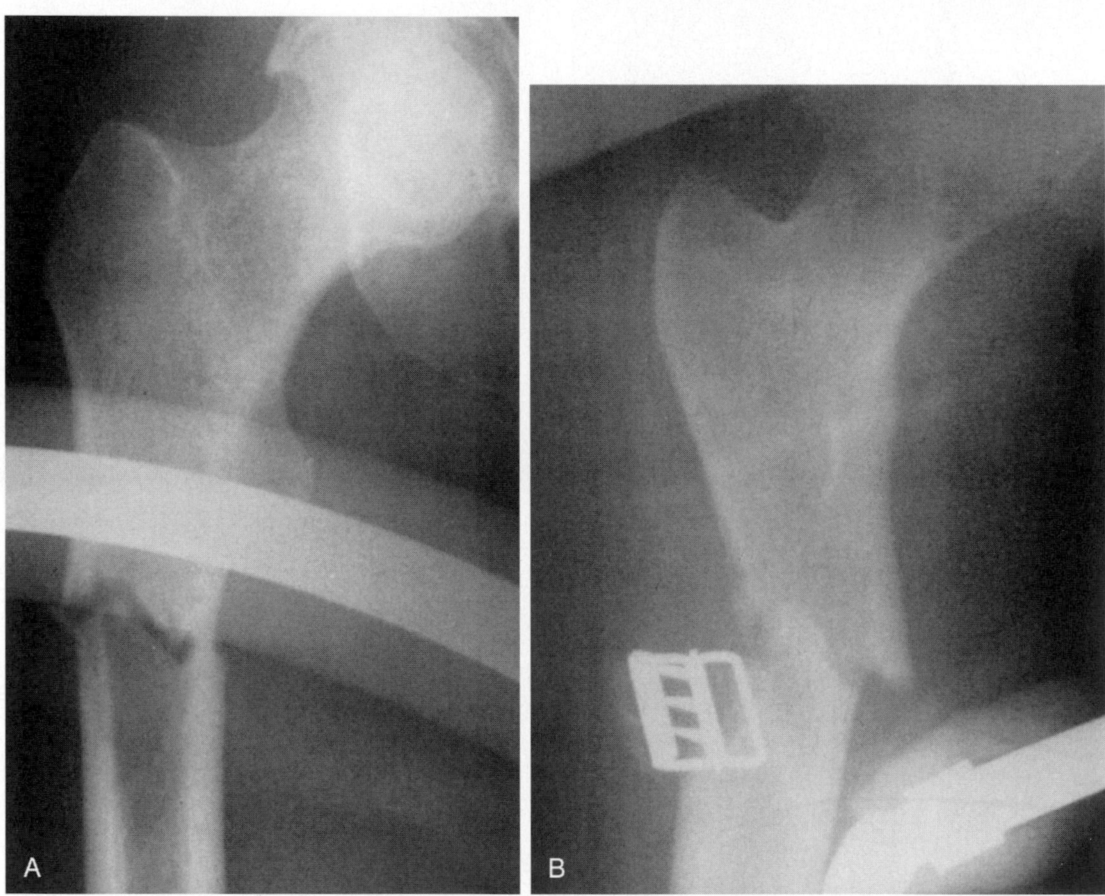

Figure 4–58. Pathologic fracture of the subtrochanteric region of the femur in a 38-year-old woman with carcinoma of the breast. The injury was sustained in a fall from a standing height, and represented the first manifestation of disease. *A*, Initial anteroposterior radiograph demonstrates the transverse fracture of the subtrochanteric region of the femur associated with a poorly defined lucency of medullary bone distal to the fracture line. *B*, Lateral radiograph again demonstrates the fracture, but there is no obvious abnormality within the intermedullary bone. However, close inspection of the area of the overlying strap reveals poorly defined destruction of the posterior cortex in this region. This finding probably represented an intracortical metastatic focus. Any transverse fracture in the subtrochanteric femur is highly likely to represent a pathologic fracture, and an underlying process must be excluded.

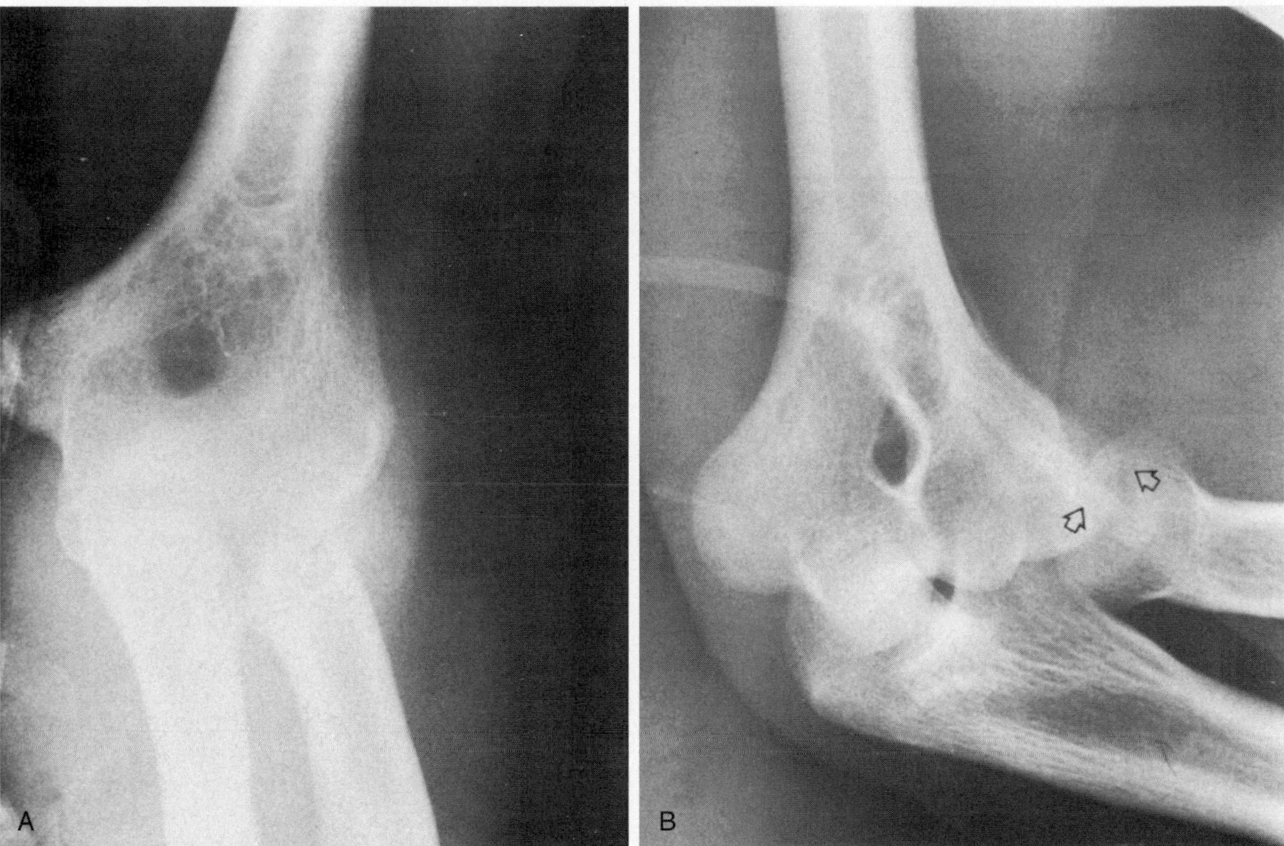

Figure 4–59. *A*, Limited extension of the elbow due to a large joint effusion and pain plus underexposure of the radiograph prevents detection of a radial head fracture. *B*, Improvement in the exposure technique allows visualization of the radial head fracture (*arrows*). The patient was unable to fully extend the elbow for routine views, and the fracture could not be seen on any other projection. Occasionally a less than optimal examination is all that is possible. A fracture is much more easily missed under such circumstances.

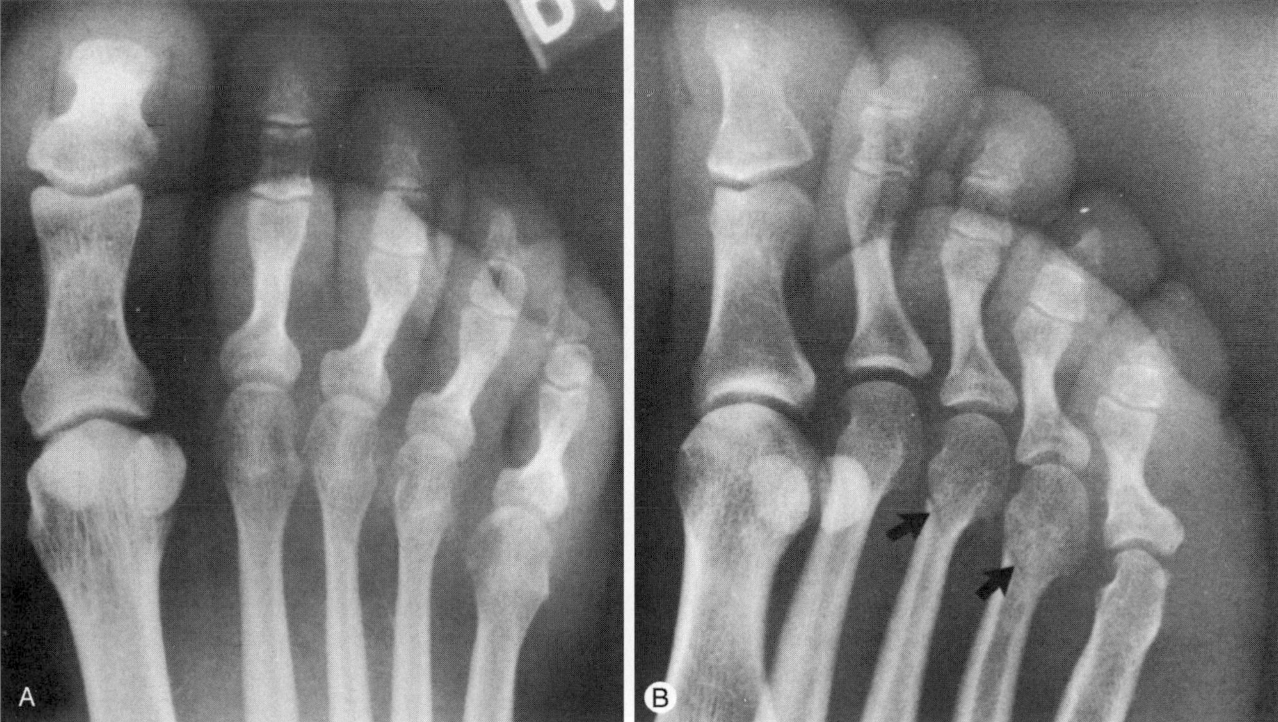

Figure 4–60. Failure of anteroposterior view to demonstrate fracture. *A*, No fracture could be identified on this anteroposterior view or on the lateral projection. Clinical findings included pain over the third and fourth metatarsophalangeal joints. *B*, Nondisplaced fractures (*arrows*) of the distal third and fourth metatarsal bones are clearly visualized only with the oblique view.

acute fractures, who may have multiple injuries, may be combative, or, because of pain or weakness, may have difficulty maintaining the necessary position for routine views of the fracture. A radiographic tube on an overhead crane that can be placed to permit an almost infinite number of projections, including cross-table lateral views, allows the patient to assume the most comfortable position with a minimum of turning during the examination. Immobilizing the part being radiographed with sandbags, sponges, and 2-inch-wide adhesive tape as needed also helps reduce motion in certain situations. Use of a fast film-screen combination will reduce the exposure time as well as the possibility of motion. Rare earth film-screen combinations have been useful in this respect. With computed radiography or digital radiography, high-resolution detectors and algorithms should be used. Image detail can also be improved by decreasing the focal spot size of the x-ray tube or by increasing the source-to-image distance (SID). Both of these changes improve the geometry and reduce geometric unsharpness in the image.

A minimum of two views of any fracture taken at 90 degrees to one another is necessary. Usually one view is taken in the anteroposterior or posteroanterior projection and the other in a lateral projection. Additional oblique projections or special-angle views (e.g., axillary view in the shoulder, frog-leg view of the hip, scaphoid view of the wrist, or internal oblique view of the ankle) are used frequently or even routinely (see Fig. 4–60). Some fractures, especially of the scaphoid, the radial head and neck, the acetabulum, the femoral neck, and the osteochondral structures of the knee, are often difficult to identify, even with a full set of routine views. In general, because of the possibility of overlooking an abnormality, an incomplete set of views should not be accepted as a complete examination. In certain circumstances—for example, as with an uncooperative patient or a multiply injured patient, or in an emergency medical situation—a complete examination cannot be performed. The study should be completed at a later time if at all possible.

Detection of Skeletal Injury by Imaging

The detection of a fracture or dislocation on a radiograph is significantly enhanced by knowledge of patient history and physical examination findings.[16, 17, 24] The provision of this information guides the radiologist to the area of interest and at the same time allows the practitioner to comfortably dismiss considerations remote from this site as likely to be of no consequence. For a variety of reasons, however, this information is frequently not provided on the radiographic request. If the radiologist has the opportunity to examine the patient or to discuss the case directly with the referring clinician, the problem can be circumvented, but such measures are frequently not possible for a number of reasons. One method used to circumvent this problem is to ask the x-ray technician to take a simple history and perform a basic physical examination and to record the information obtained for use by the radiologist. Alternatively, other authors have suggested that metal markers be placed on the radiograph pointing to areas of tenderness or other abnormalities.[28] Either method will improve the accuracy of detection and should receive serious consideration in any emergency room or other facility dealing with acute skeletal injuries.

Radiography

A *fracture* is a disruption in the continuity of a bone. This disruption is evidenced on a radiograph predominantly as an abnormal line of radiolucency, the width of which is dependent upon the degree of displacement of the fracture fragments. Obviously, the greater the displacement, the more evident the fracture line. In the absence of displacement, the line may be very thin and quite difficult to perceive. Furthermore, the clarity of the fracture line on the radiograph is dependent on how the fracture is aligned in relation to the x-ray exposure beam. If it is perfectly aligned, the fracture line is sharply defined. The clarity decreases with increasing angulation of the fracture line. As its obliquity approaches 45 degrees, the fracture line becomes more obscure and poorly defined, until finally it is completely obscured on the radiograph (Fig. 4–61). Although this obscuration may occur in one radiographic view or projection, it is unlikely to occur in another view obtained simultaneously at 90 degrees to the original projection. Thus, in practice, two radiographic views of the part in question obtained at 90 degrees to each other, usually an anteroposterior and a lateral projection, are considered the minimum necessary to establish or exclude the presence of a fracture. I estimate that the fracture is seen on both views 90% of the time; 5% of the time a fracture may be visualized on only one of the two views. In the remaining 5% an additional oblique or special projection may be necessary to identify a fracture (Fig. 4–62) that is otherwise obscure on both the standard anteroposterior and lateral projections. This is much more commonly the case at the end of a bone than in the shaft; thus, a minimum of three views—the anteroposterior, the lateral, and an appropriate oblique (see Fig. 4–62)—are needed to safely exclude fractures about the joints. As a practical matter, these three views are useful for the distal joints, but a lateral projection of the proximal major joints (hip and shoulder) lacks detail because of superimposition and is often not obtained. Fractures of the shaft are more likely to be angulated, which makes them more obvious.

Irregularity of the cortex (Fig. 4–63) is the second manifestation of a fracture. This is more easily identified in the long and short bones than in irregular bones. The shafts of long and short bones are cylindrical and gradually flared at both ends. Any digression from this pattern should be viewed with suspicion. The irregularity commonly takes the form of an angular projection or distortion in the flare of the metaphysis, particularly as seen in torus fractures in children. Abrupt offsets in the cortical margins of a bone or lines formed by the tangential projection of cortical bone, such as the ilioischial line of the pelvis, foraminal lines of the sacrum (Fig. 4–64), or innominate line of the orbit, indicate the presence of a fracture. Interruptions or changes in arcs formed by curved bones such as the ribs may be the only direct manifestation of a fracture.

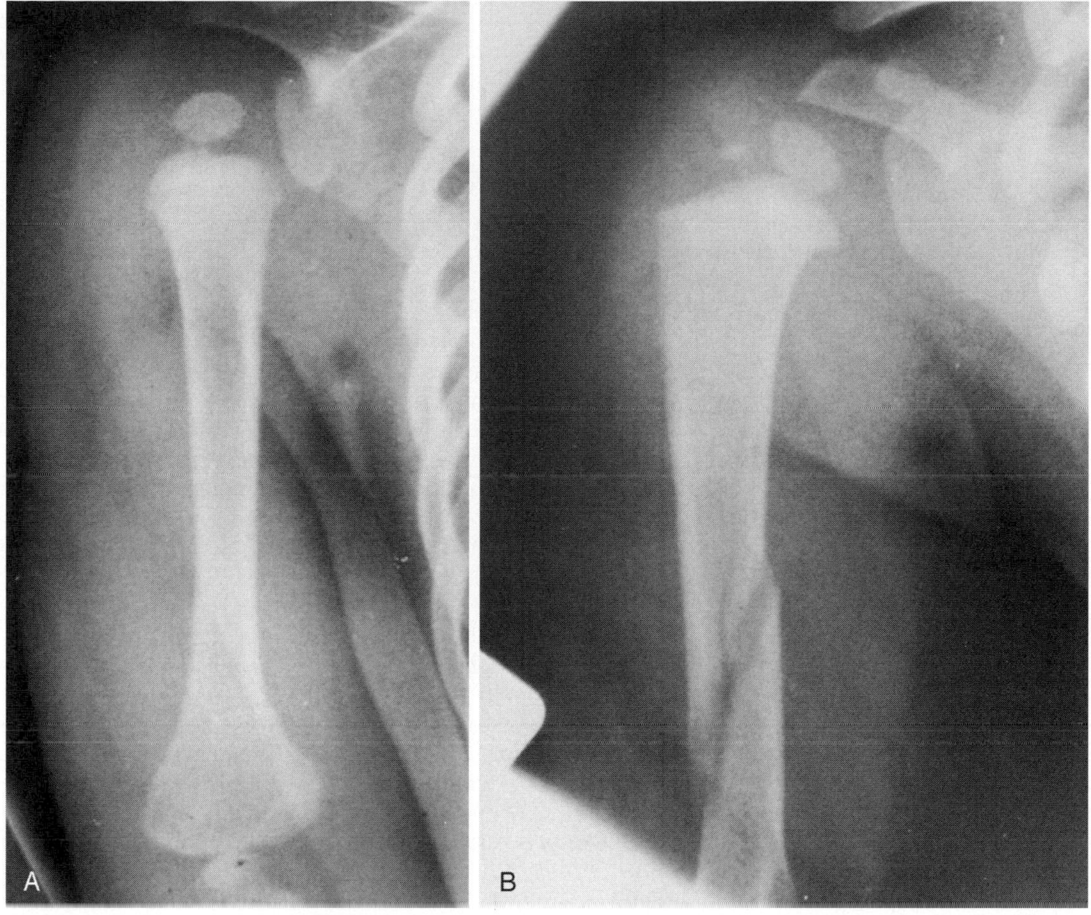

Figure 4–61. Fracture of humeral shaft in an 8-month-old boy. *A*, The anteroposterior view of the humerus reveals no evidence of fracture. There is soft tissue swelling surrounding the humeral shaft. *B*, Lateral view of the humerus clearly demonstrates a spiral fracture of the midshaft. This case is an excellent example of why the presence of a fracture should never be excluded on the basis of only one view of a bone.

Fractures can also be manifested by an increase in bone density. Compression forces may result in a poorly defined or blurred area of increased bone density due to the impaction of bone fragments (Figs. 4–65 and 4–66). This finding is common in compression fractures of the vertebrae. In comminuted fractures, fragments can be angulated toward the x-ray exposure beam, resulting in increased density. This cause for increased density is useful in recognition of depressed skull fractures. An overlap of fragments creates a sharply defined line of increased density (see Fig. 4–67*B*), the width of which is a measure of the amount of overlap.

There are radiographic changes in the soft tissues that give indirect evidence of an underlying fracture.[25] In some cases these changes may be the only manifestation of injury. They serve as an indication for closer scrutiny of the initial radiographs or point to the need for additional views to disclose an otherwise inapparent fracture. These soft tissue changes are swelling (see Fig. 4–62*A*), obliteration of fascial planes (see Fig. 4–63*B*), joint effusion (see Fig. 4–62*B*), and lipohemarthrosis, or fat in the joint (see Fig. 4–66*A*).

Although the swelling of soft tissues points to the area of injury, this finding is quite nonspecific because it is as likely to be the result of an injury limited to the soft tissues. Furthermore, it is quite possible that the soft tissue injury is remote from the fracture site.

Changes in certain fascial planes have been found to constitute a reliable indicator of associated bone injury, particularly those in the fascial plane overlying the pronator quadratus muscle (see Fig. 4–63*B*) on the volar aspect of the distal radius and ulna. The fascial plane is visualized as a fine line of radiolucency because of the presence of fat. Fractures of the radius frequently result in obliteration of the fascial plane because of hemorrhage within it, or the fascial plane becomes displaced forward because of hemorrhage and edema within the underlying muscle. Other diagnostically useful fascial planes are found about the hip and elbow.

The presence of a joint effusion (see Figs. 4–1, 4–62*B*, and 4–66) in an otherwise normal person with a history of trauma is a highly specific indicator of intra-articular soft tissue injury or intra-articular fracture. Under these circumstances the effusion is secondary to hemorrhage into the joint. The ease with which joint effusions can be identified varies from joint to joint. They are readily identifiable and are very useful signs in the elbow and knee.

An intra-articular fracture that extends into the marrow cavity allows egress of fatty marrow into the joint. If a

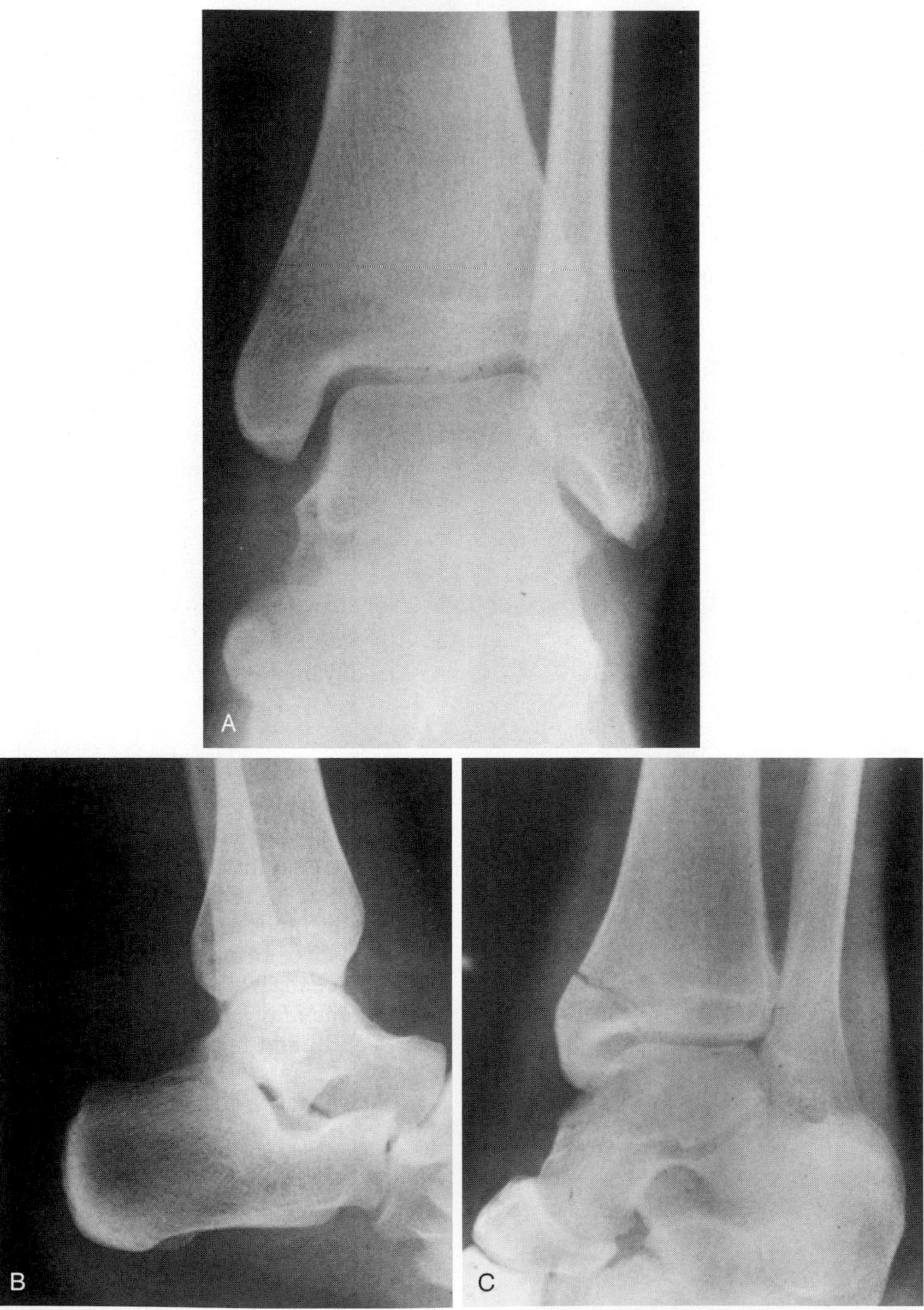

Figure 4–62. Fracture of the medial malleolus apparent only on oblique view. *A*, The anteroposterior view reveals soft tissue swelling about the medial malleolus but no evidence of fracture. *B*, Lateral view demonstrates the presence of a joint effusion, but the fracture is not identified. *C*, Internal oblique view clearly demonstrates a linear nondisplaced fracture of the medial malleolus.

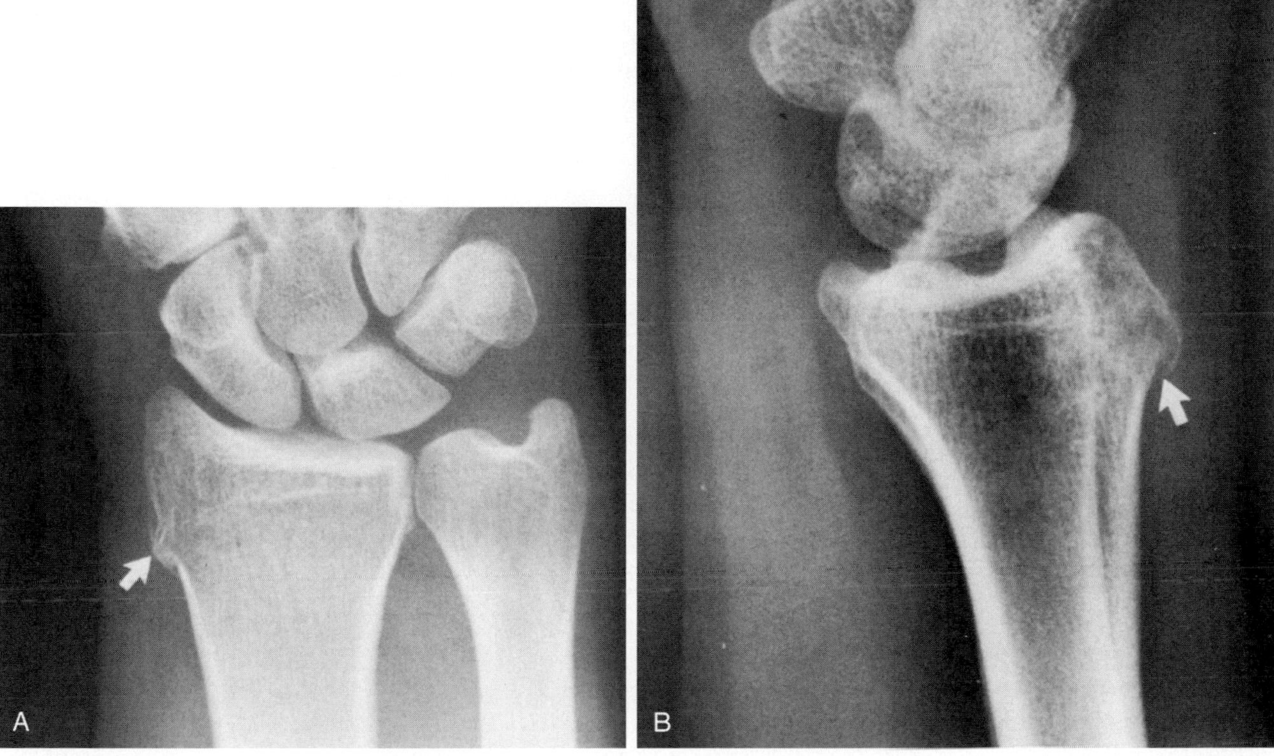

Figure 4–63. Incomplete fracture of the distal radius in a 33-year-old woman who fell while roller skating. *A*, A posteroanterior projection demonstrates distortion (buckling) of the cortex on the distal radius (*arrow*). *B*, The cortex on the dorsal surface of the radius is disrupted (*arrow*). There is partial obliteration of the pronator quadratus fascial plane over the volar surface of the distal radius in association with the fracture.

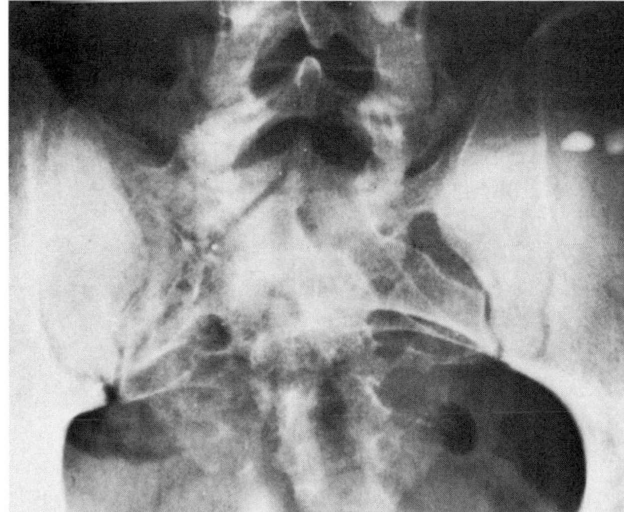

Figure 4–64. Traumatic fracture of the sacrum manifested by disruption of sacral foraminal lines. Note the intact superior cortical margins of the sacral foramina on the left and the disruption of the sacral foraminal lines on the right, indicating a line of fracture.

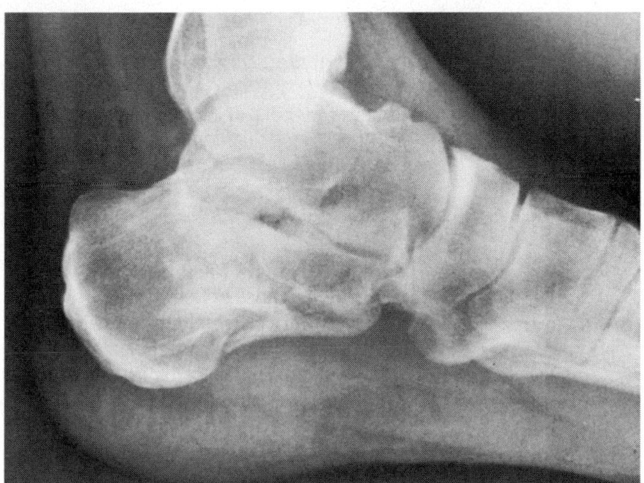

Figure 4–65. Compression fracture of the calcaneus. Impaction of fracture fragments is manifested as areas of increased density. The fracture is comminuted.

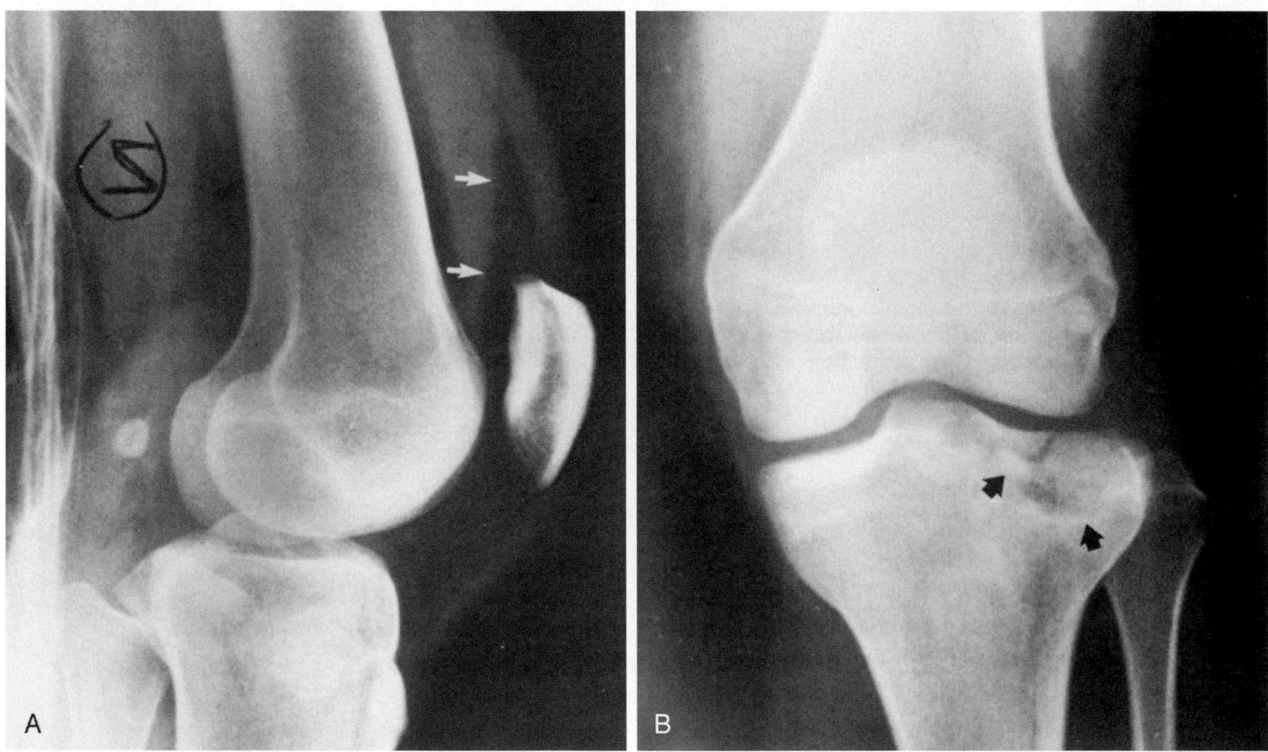

Figure 4–66. Depressed fracture of the lateral tibial plateau with lipohemarthrosis. *A*, Lateral view obtained with a horizontal beam demonstrates a fat-fluid level in the distended suprapatellar bursa (*arrows*). The depressed fracture of the lateral tibial plateau is also visualized. *B*, The anteroposterior view clearly demonstrates the depressed fracture of the lateral tibial plateau, manifested as disruption of the articular cortex and increased radiodensity of the impacted, depressed fragment (*arrows*).

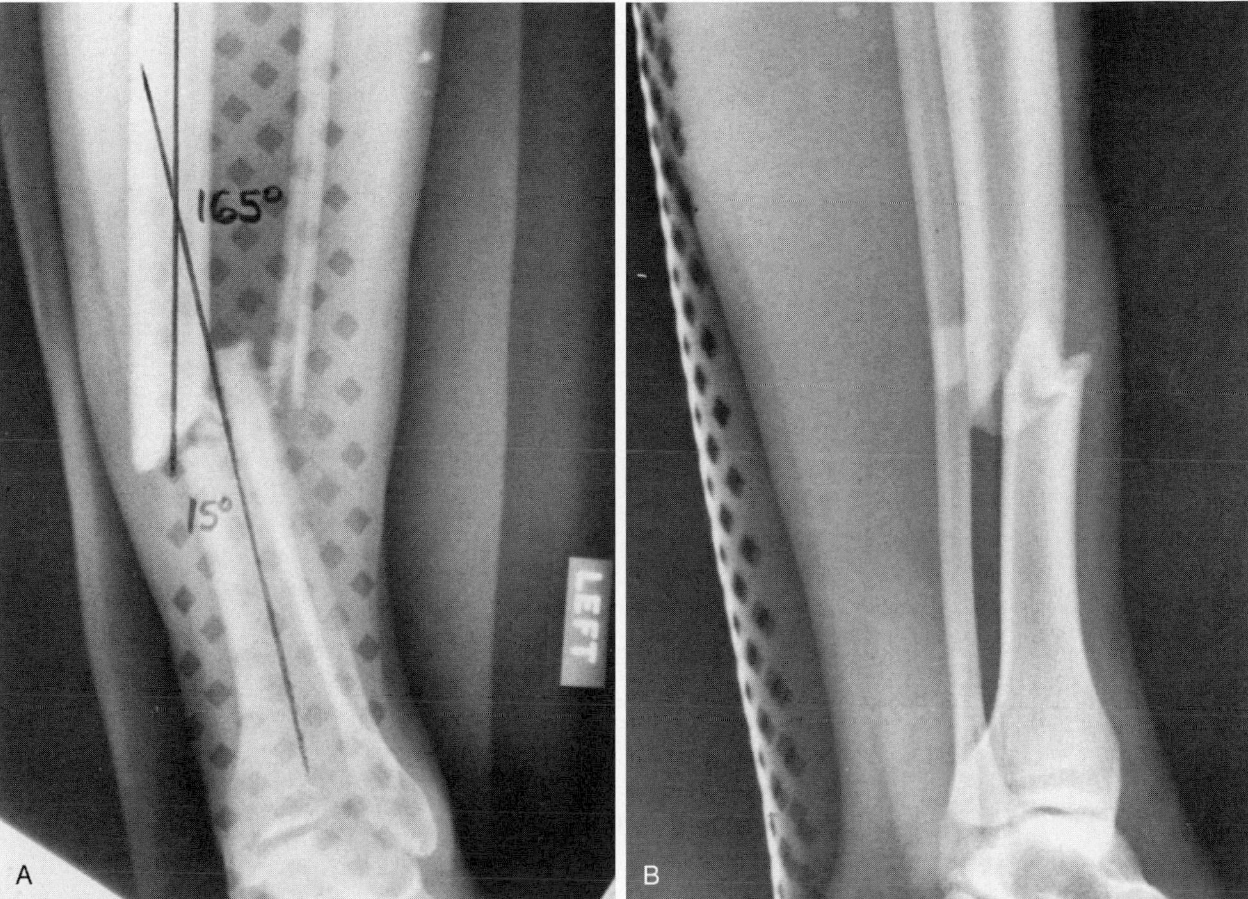

Figure 4–67. Oblique fractures at the junction of the middle and distal thirds of the tibia. *A*, A minimally comminuted oblique fracture can be seen at the junction of the middle and distal thirds of the tibial shaft. The distal fragment is angulated laterally at 15 degrees, resulting in a 165-degree medial angulation at the fracture site. The distal fragment is offset by approximately half the width of the shaft both anteriorly and laterally. There is an associated transverse fracture of the fibula with similar angulation of the distal fragments. The distal fragment lies medial to the proximal fragment with 1.5 cm of overriding. (The checkered pattern of lucencies is caused by the posteriorly placed aluminum splint in which the leg is held.) *B*, Lateral view demonstrates the anterior offset and minimal comminution of the tibial fracture as well as the overriding of the fracture fragments. The apparent density of bone is increased because of superimposition.

portion of the joint fluid is then removed, a layer of this fat forms on the surface of the bloody joint fluid. This condition is called *lipohemarthrosis* and is a highly specific indicator of intra-articular fracture. Joint aspiration is performed frequently in the knee, but less commonly in other joints, for the purpose of identifying lipohemarthrosis. Fat-fluid levels may also be identified radiographically by use of a horizontal exposure beam (see Fig. 4–66*A*). This maneuver is useful in disclosing fractures involving the knee. A horizontal-beam lateral projection demonstrates the fat-fluid level in the suprapatellar recess. Lipohemarthrosis has also been demonstrated in the shoulder by examining the patient in the upright position. This sign has not been used to any significant degree in other smaller joints. Fat-fluid levels are easily demonstrated on CT or MR images.

Indirect forces are unlikely to result in an isolated solitary fracture of one of the two paired bones, the radius and ulna and the tibia and fibula. Therefore, identification of a fracture in one should alert the examiner to the possibility of a fracture in the other (Fig. 4–68) or, alternatively, to an associated dislocation. Similarly, a solitary fracture in a ring or arch bone, as in the pelvis (Fig. 4–69) or mandible, respectively, should suggest the possibility of an associated second fracture or dislocation. Bone is sufficiently brittle, like a pretzel, to make this association a distinct possibility. In actual fact, there is sufficient resilience, as in a bagel, to make it possible for a solitary fracture to occur, but it is an excellent rule of thumb to search for the frequent, easily and often overlooked second fracture or dislocation.

Computed Tomography

CT is of major importance in the assessment of trauma of the axial skeleton (the skull, face, spine, pelvis, and hips) but plays a limited role in the initial detection of appendicular trauma. The axially oriented images allow visualization of the spinal canal, facial skeleton, and pelvis and hip free of overlap and thus demonstrate considerably more fractures than those seen on radiographs while improving the appreciation of the spatial relationship between fragments. A fracture is displayed on a CT scan much the same as on the radiograph and is manifested by linear disruption of the cortex, but CT also visualizes

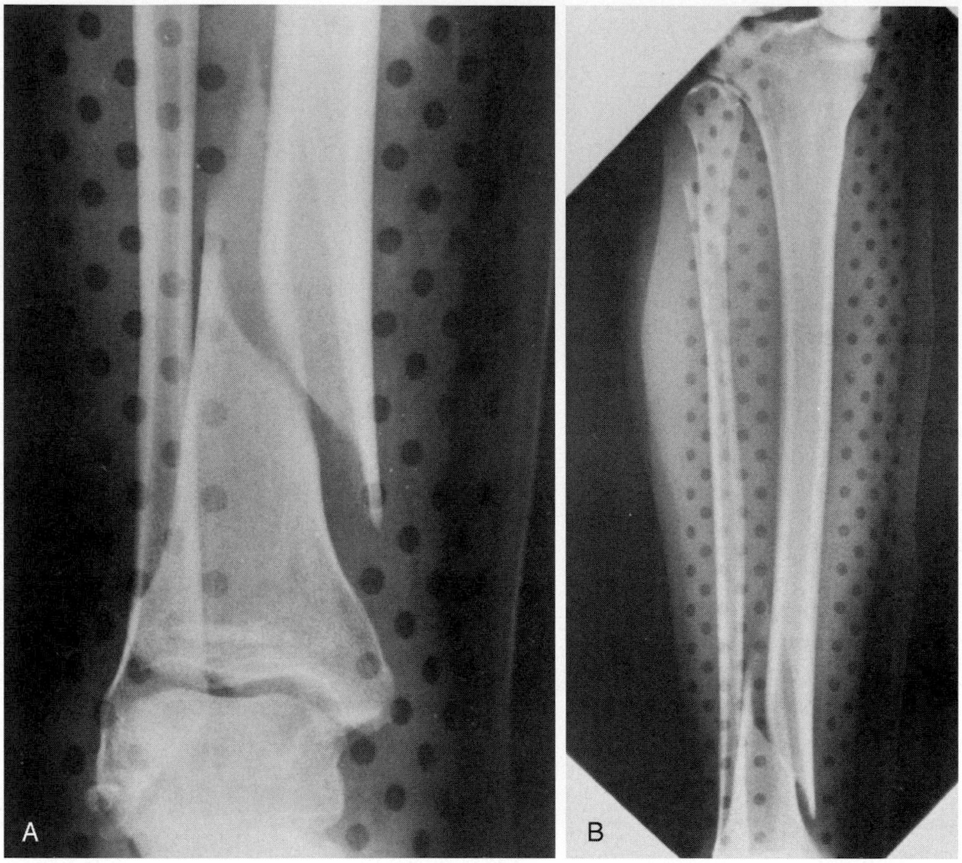

Figure 4–68. Fracture of the distal tibia and proximal fibula. *A*, A spiral fracture of the distal third of the tibia is evident. The distal fragment is offset by approximately 50% of the width of the shaft, associated with 2 cm of overriding. Radiographic examination of the entire length of the tibia and fibula is required to demonstrate an associated fracture of the fibula. *B*, An anteroposterior view of the entire tibia and fibula demonstrates the associated fracture of the proximal fibula.

fractures in medullary bone and associated soft tissue changes to much better advantage than is possible with plain radiography.

Acutely traumatized patients, especially those with severe injuries often have a limited ability to move in order to assume the necessary positions for radiographs. There tends to be an inverse relation between the quality of the radiograph study that can be obtained and the severity of the patient's injuries. CT has been particularly useful in this regard because it is unnecessary for the patient to change position during the study, but some fractures may be missed by CT.[198, 210]

The areas in which CT is most useful for fracture evaluation include the pelvis[189, 222] (Fig. 4–70), entire spine,[210] skull base,[192] facial bones,[188, 198] calcaneus,[187, 191] sternum,[218] and midfoot.[44] The cervical spine is a particular anatomic site in which CT in the acute setting is valuable,[267, 280] not only for evaluating fractures identified on radiographs[274] but also for screening levels not adequately demonstrated on radiographs, such as the craniocervical[242, 244] or cervicothoracic junctions,[333] or for screening of the entire cervical spine.[238, 241] Also, fractures that extend into a joint or dislocations with associated fracture can be characterized for the number and position of fracture fragments and the extent of articular surface disruption. CT scans of fractures of the hip (Fig. 4–71),[189] knee,[213] ankle,[202] midfoot and hindfoot,[186, 187, 191] sternoclavicular,[218] shoulder, wrist, and elbow joints are frequently used to determine whether operative intervention is needed or for preoperative planning. CT is useful for evaluating the quality of closed reduction or open reduction and internal fixation, especially of complicated fractures and when problems arise. In the setting of the multiply traumatized patient, CT is frequently performed for rapid evaluation of the chest and abdomen. Modern helical CT scanners have become so specialized in their operation that protocols that are optimal for acquiring and displaying images of the abdomen, for example, may be less suitable for displaying possible fractures of the lumbar spine or pelvis.[300] To obtain the best images of the skeleton using a helical CT scanner, the examiner should use a bone reconstruction algorithm, a slice thickness of 3 to 5 mm, a 1-to-1 pitch (slice thickness compared with rate of table feed), and bone windows and levels. If re-formations of images in other planes or in three dimensions are required, the helical image data may be reconstructed on the computer as 1-mm-thick slices, and those slices may be used to perform the re-formations. Once protocols have been established, these activities can be performed routinely by the technologist operating the CT scanner.

Acetabular fractures and fracture-dislocations of the hip are frequently complex.[216] Cartilaginous debris or small bone fragments present within the joint can prevent adequate reduction and can cause further damage to the joint.[217] Fractures of the pubic rami not infrequently are accompanied by fracture extension into the acetabulum that may not be evident on radiographs[211] but is obvious on a CT scan. CT demonstrates the configuration and extent of fractures, the position of loose bone fragments in the joint, and, occasionally, a fracture not detected with radiography. CT is definitely indicated when there is a

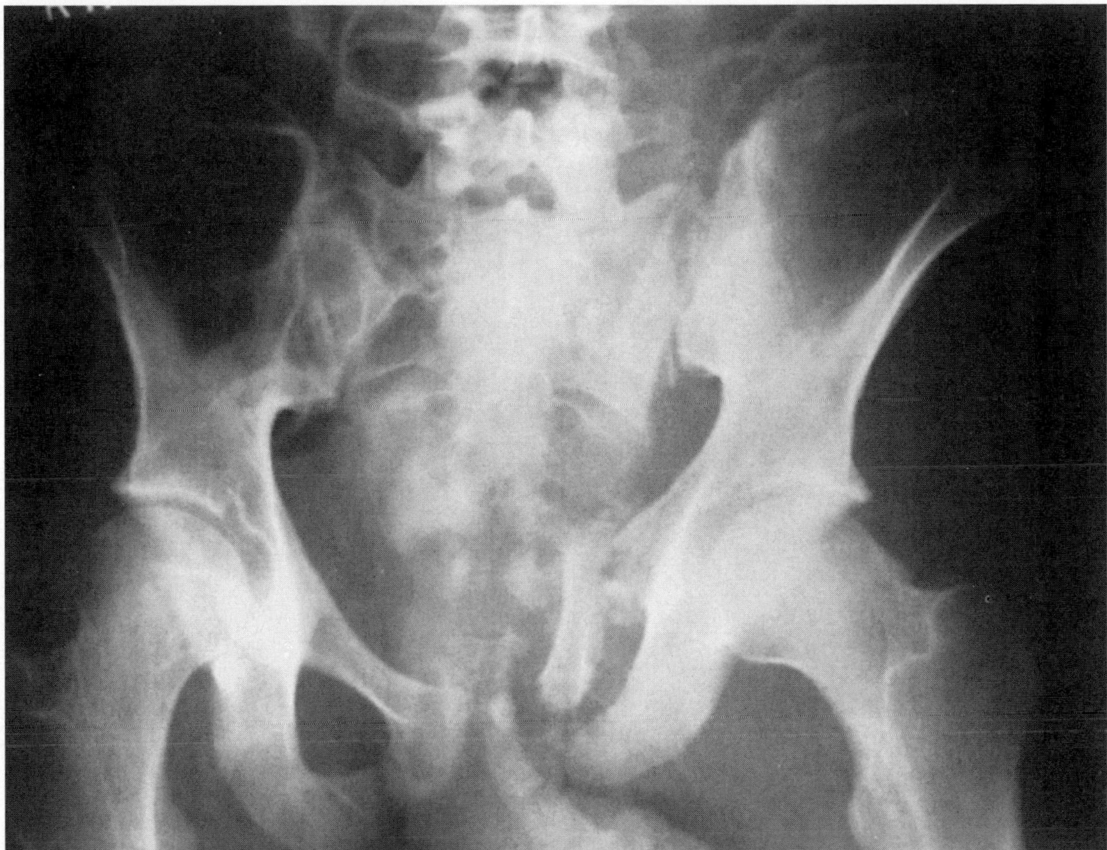

Figure 4–69. Malgaigne fracture of the pelvis in a 28-year-old man injured in an automobile accident. High-impact forces commonly result in fractures involving both the anterior and posterior portions of the pelvis. In this example there are obvious fractures of the superior and inferior portions of the pubic ramus on the left associated with disruption of the left sacroiliac joint posteriorly. Note the vertical displacement of the left innominate bone. In injuries involving rings or arcs of bone, such as the pelvis or mandible, fractures commonly occur at more than one site.

possibility of loose bodies trapped in the joint, as evidenced by widening of the joint space after reduction[199, 216] (Fig. 4–72). Because of the probability of severe degenerative sequelae following complex fractures of the medial acetabular wall, CT is indispensable for evaluation of fractures in this area and for planning surgical reduction.

CT clearly demonstrates the position of fracture fragments and their relation to one another in complex shoulder fractures and will clearly demonstrate dislocation of a sternoclavicular joint.[203] Radiography can demonstrate the presence of the same pathologic process, but usually with at least some difficulty, and not with the same certainty and clarity as for CT.

Helical CT (also called spiral CT) has a growing role in the evaluation of acute musculoskeletal trauma.[310] Some fractures, particularly nondisplaced fractures that are oriented in the axial plane, are better seen on volume-rendered images. Complex injuries can be better demonstrated with volume-rendered images, and complicated spatial information about the relative positions of fracture fragments can be easily demonstrated to the orthopedic surgeons. The use of intravenously administered contrast material allows simultaneous evaluation of osseous and vascular structures within the affected area.

Image reformatting is available currently with all commercial CT scanners.[204] This mode allows a structure to be imaged in at least three planes. Typically these images are slices showing a cut surface similar to that seen on routine axial images but merely in a different plane (e.g., sagittal or coronal). They are two-dimensional images and are referred to as such. Some CT scanners and free-standing units are capable of reformatting axial CT data into simulated three-dimensional images. These reformatting programs may allow subtraction of overlying bone, such as a femoral head, to permit better visualization of an underlying acetabular fracture. By means of shading and highlighting, an illusion of three dimensions is achieved even though the image is presented on a two-dimensional monitor screen or film. Usually a series of rotational images are generated that can be rotated around a preselected axis, permitting study of any part of the object by the viewer. These images are referred to as three-dimensional images.

Three-dimensional (3-D) medical images of computed tomographic data sets can be generated with a variety of computer algorithms.[248] The three most commonly used techniques are shaded surface display, maximum intensity projection, and, more recently, 3-D volume rendering. Implementation of 3-D volume rendering involves volume data management, which relates to operations including acquisition, resampling, and editing of the data set; rendering parameters including window width and level, opacity, brightness, and percentage classification;

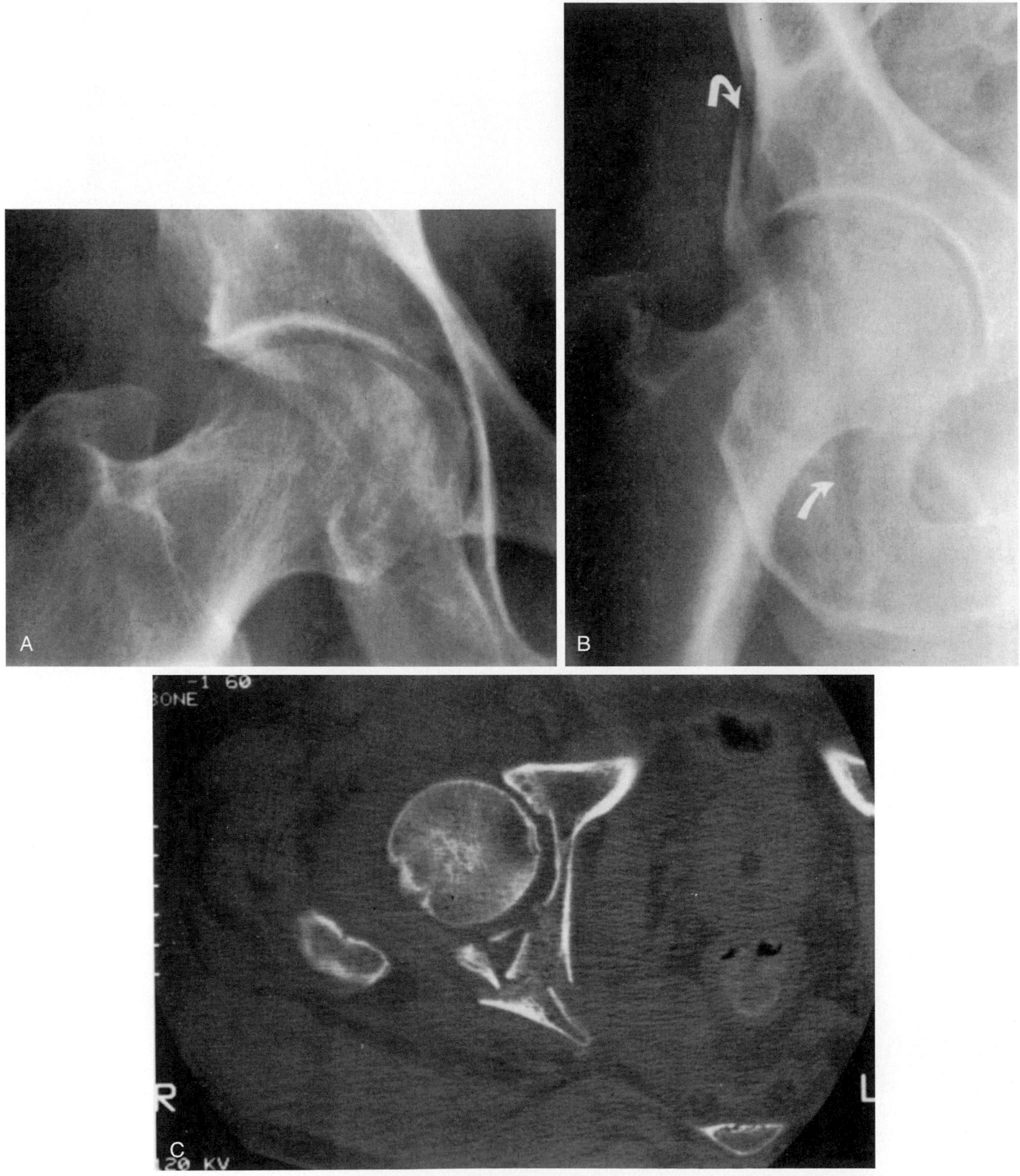

Figure 4–70. A posterior acetabular fracture in a 65-year-old man. *A*, The fracture was overlooked initially. *B*, After it was determined that the patient was unable to bear weight, additional Judet views were obtained, demonstrating the fracture more clearly (*arrows*). *C*, A computed tomography scan shows the comminution of the fracture and the lack of posterior restraint resulting in instability of the femoral head. The presence of instability can be suspected from the radiographs, but the severity can be demonstrated only with computed tomography.

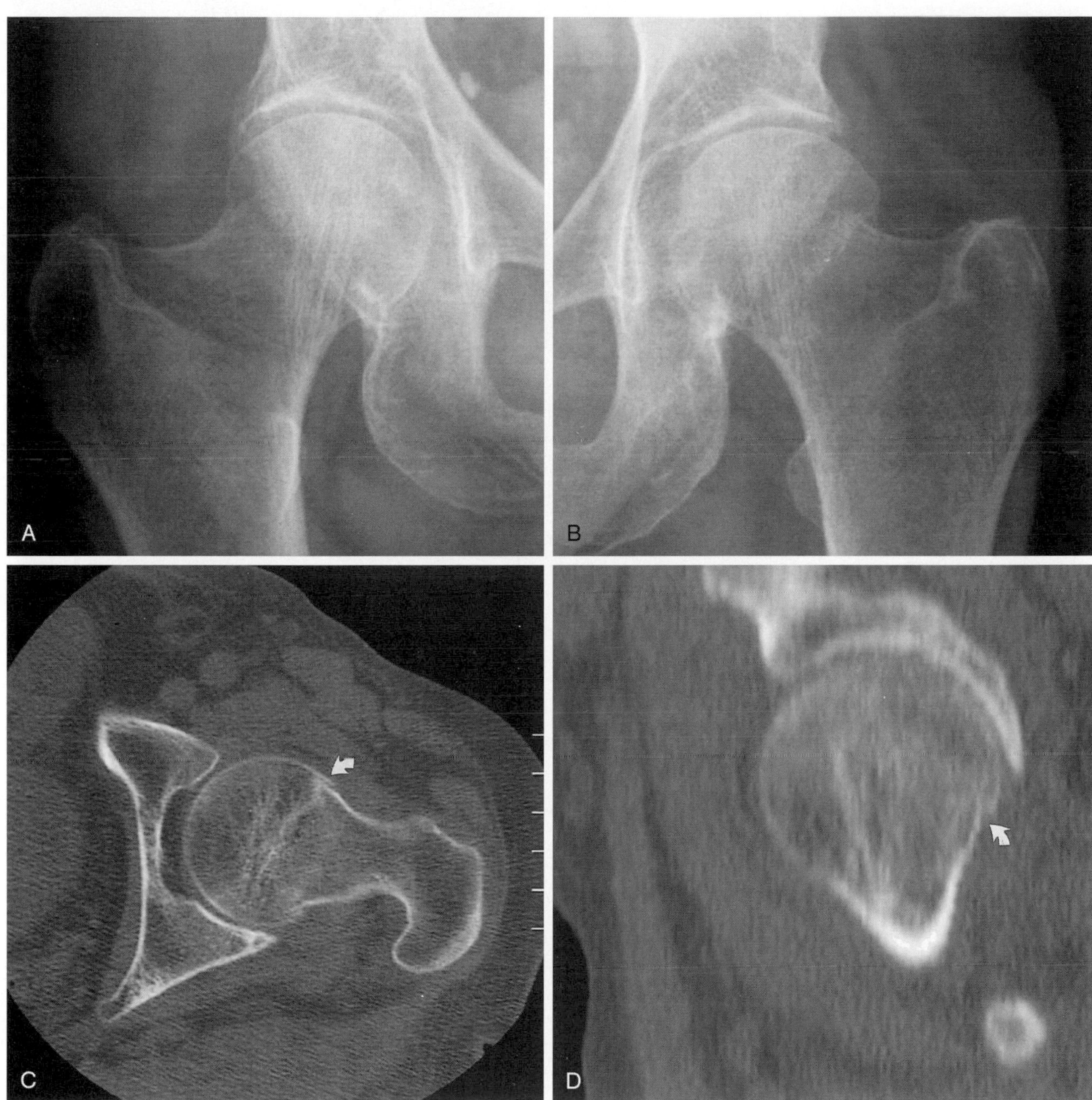

Figure 4–71. Radiographically equivocal subcapital hip fracture in a 79-year-old woman. Radiographs of the right and left hips (*A* and *B*) showed no displaced fracture; the findings were considered equivocal for the presence of an impacted or nondisplaced fracture. *C*, Axial computed tomography scan showed an impacted subcapital fracture on the left (*arrow*). *D*, Sagittal computed tomographic reformated image also showed the impaction (*arrow*). (From Chew, F.S. [2000]. Skeletal Radiology Interactive 2.0, with permission.)

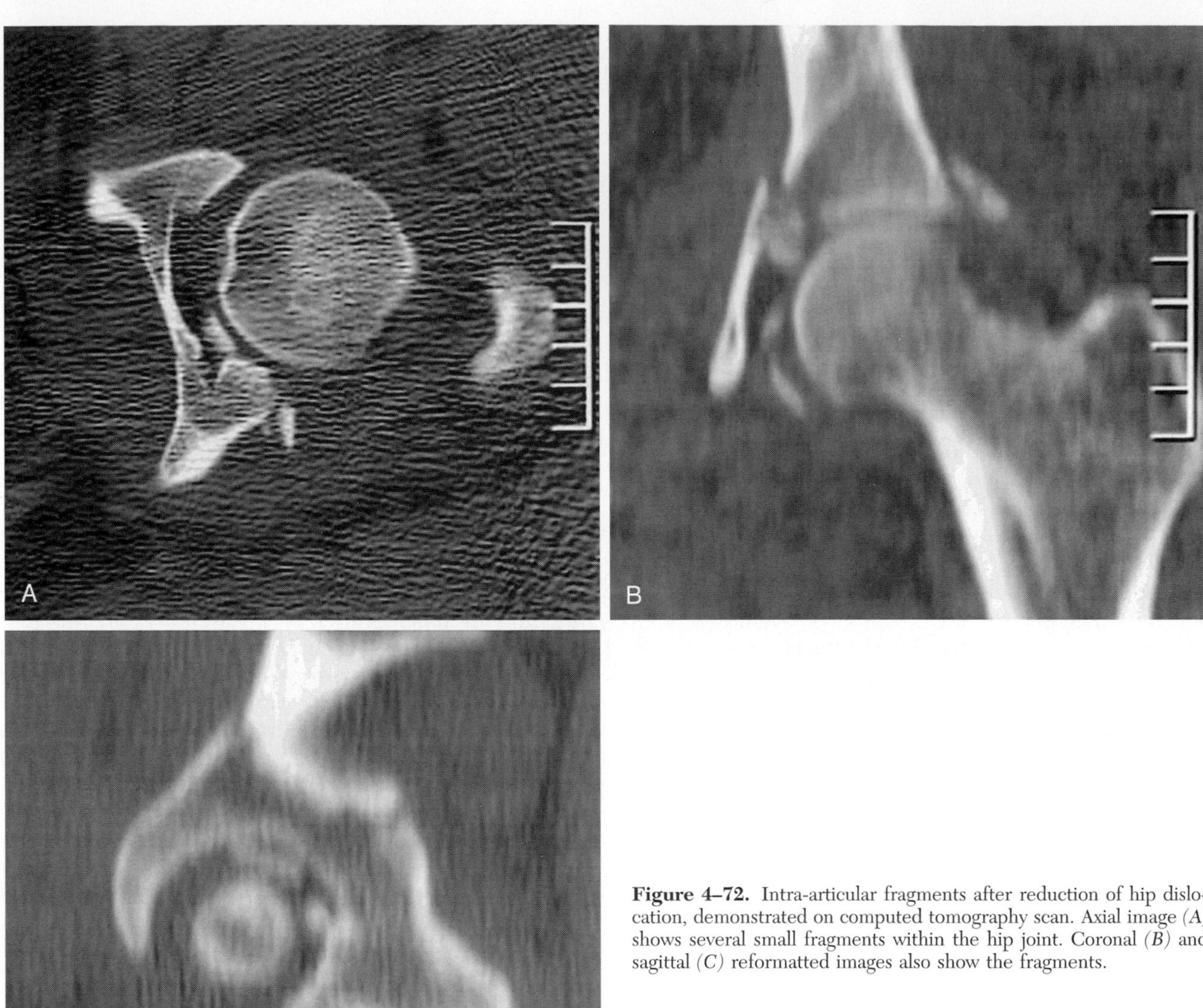

Figure 4–72. Intra-articular fragments after reduction of hip dislocation, demonstrated on computed tomography scan. Axial image *(A)* shows several small fragments within the hip joint. Coronal *(B)* and sagittal *(C)* reformatted images also show the fragments.

and image display, which comprises techniques such as "fly-through" and "fly-around," multiple-view display, obscured structure and shading depth cues, and kinetic and stereo depth cues. An understanding of both the theory and method of 3-D volume rendering is essential for accurate evaluation of the resulting images. 3-D volume rendering is useful in a wide variety of applications but is just now being incorporated into commercially available software packages for medical imaging.

Magnetic Resonance Imaging

The recent widespread availability of MRI has had a great impact on musculoskeletal radiology. MRI provides the best definition of soft tissues of any imaging technique currently available. Bone, muscle, fat, fluid, bone marrow, tendons, ligaments, cartilage, and vascular structures can be distinguished from one another. Multiplanar imaging is usual and is a distinct advantage of this method. Radiofrequencies introduced into a magnetic field induce radio signals within hydrogen nuclei in tissues, which in turn are detected and constructed into images by computer. In contrast, routine radiography and CT use x-ray sources and image differences of photon attenuation within tissues.[194] The relaxation times, T_1 and T_2, and proton density are the most common physical characteristics measured by MRI for diagnosis. T_1 reflects the interaction of excited nuclei with surrounding nuclei, and T_2 reflects the interaction of nuclear spin of excited nuclei with spins of surrounding nuclei. Proton density denotes the number of excited hydrogen nuclei or protons per unit area. Con-

traindications to the use of MRI include the presence of magnetically active cardiac pacemakers and intracranial aneurysm clips.[194] Most orthopedic appliances are not significantly ferromagnetic and cause artifacts in the MR image only in their immediate surrounding area. A broad range of ferromagnetic metal–containing materials have been shown to affect MRI, with variable implications for patient safety.[246, 309] Even body piercings, tattoos, and even facial cosmetics may be problematic.[255, 270, 272, 343] Each institution performing MRI should have policies and procedures in place for identifying patients at risk and preventing them from entering the scanner.[256, 273]

MRI is capable of detecting fractures but has a limited role in their diagnosis and management because other methods are much simpler and much less expensive.[196] Diagnosis of a fracture with MRI characteristically is preceded by a normal radiographic study. Typically, the MRI study is requested to evaluate for soft tissue injury to account for the patient's pain, and the fracture that is found is unexpected.[180, 206] Occult fractures, stress fractures, and osteochondral fractures have been identified under these circumstances.[179, 180, 201, 206, 221] Occult fractures on T_1-weighted and T_2-weighted MR images demonstrate linear low signal intensity crossing the bone marrow, with a configuration similar to that seen for a fracture on radiographs.[180, 194, 206] On T_2-weighted images there is increased signal intensity in the area surrounding the low-signal-intensity linear fracture line. Although the time duration after trauma before MRI demonstrates positive findings of an occult fracture has not been established, patients examined within 24 hours of symptom onset have had positive studies.[180] The tibial plateaus, proximal femur, and distal femur have been frequent sites of these fractures.[180, 206]

Stress fractures cause two patterns of abnormality on MR images. The most frequent is a linear zone of decreased signal intensity perpendicular to the cortex surrounded by a larger, poorly defined, less dark area on T_1-weighted images. On T_2-weighted images the linear zone remains dark but the surrounding area becomes brighter, presumably as a result of edema.[206] The second pattern seen is an amorphous area of decreased signal intensity on T_1-weighted images without any linear component. On T_2-weighted images the same area contains scattered areas of increased signal intensity. The findings with this pattern cannot be distinguished from a bone bruise except by history.[206]

Osteochondral fractures cause two different abnormal patterns on MR images.[206] When the fragment is displaced, it is best seen with T_2-weighted images, especially if an effusion is present. It will appear as a small area of decreased signal intensity within the surrounding sea of high signal intensity from the effusion. Impacted osteochondral fractures cause a low signal intensity on T_1-weighted and T_2-weighted images at the impaction site. The surrounding area of medullary abnormality usually has increased signal intensity on T_2-weighted images, presumably as a result of surrounding edema.

MRI may be used to detect and characterize osteonecrotic bone fragments, particularly in the femoral head, scaphoid proximal pole, and talar dome. MRI is the most specific and sensitive method available for detecting early stages of osteonecrosis.[177, 194, 207, 208, 219] Although MRI is able to detect changes of avascular necrosis before other imaging modalities, the pathologic condition exists at a cellular level even before it is detectable with MRI.[183] The specificity of MRI findings in osteonecrosis also allows differentiation from other disease entities with a high degree of diagnostic certainty.[185]

MRI examination of growth plate fractures was found by Jaramillo and associates to be superior to radiography.[195] MRI changed the radiographically assigned Salter-Harris classification of growth plate fractures in 6 of 12 patients examined within 6 months of the injury. The change in classification typically was to a more complex type of fracture (e.g., type 3 to type 4). MRI can also find additional occult fractures whose presence will change management.[249]

MRI is equal in sensitivity to bone scanning in the disclosure of skeletal injury and may do so in the presence of a normal radiograph.[21, 34] It is more often used in those cases in which radiography fails to demonstrate any abnormality (Fig. 4–73); more frequently, unsuspected fractures or bone bruises (see Fig. 4–21) are disclosed when the knee[26, 34] is evaluated with MRI for meniscal or ligamentous injury, or when the shoulder is examined for possible rotator cuff or labial abnormalities. MRI is frequently performed in the assessment of spinal trauma to evaluate the status of the spinal cord for intrinsic injury or compression by bony fragments, herniated intervertebral discs, or hematomas.

MRI demonstrates associated soft tissue swelling, hemorrhage, and joint effusions.[15] Tears and lacerations of ligaments and tendons are readily demonstrated by frank disruption of these low-signal-intensity structures with surrounding hematomas or by the appearance of high-signal-intensity areas within the substance of a tendon or ligament (Fig. 4–74).

MRI can be used to confirm a suspected stress or insufficiency fracture or an otherwise obscure fracture of the femoral neck (Fig. 4–75).[21, 304] The fracture is manifested on T_1-weighted or proton density images by a line or band of low signal intensity in the intramedullary space that is often contiguous with the cortex and surrounded by patchy areas of reduced signal, presumably representing edema within the marrow. On T_2-weighted images, the line of fracture remains of low signal intensity, but the surrounding edema now is of increased signal intensity, corresponding to hemorrhage and edema. The low-signal-intensity line of the fracture is presumed to represent a series of impacted microfractures of the trabeculae. Although MRI generally is a more costly procedure than radionuclide bone scanning, if a limited MRI study is performed, it represents a cost-effective alternative.[294, 316] MRI has the advantages of rapid imaging with immediate diagnosis, provision of anatomic detail for possible surgical planning, and specificity in identifying alternative diagnoses.

Patterns of abnormal signal on MR images have been correlated with fracture mechanisms (Table 4–3).[257, 303] With avulsion fractures, marrow edema tends to be minimal or absent. Whereas with fractures from impaction, shearing, or penetrating trauma, edema tends to be extensive.

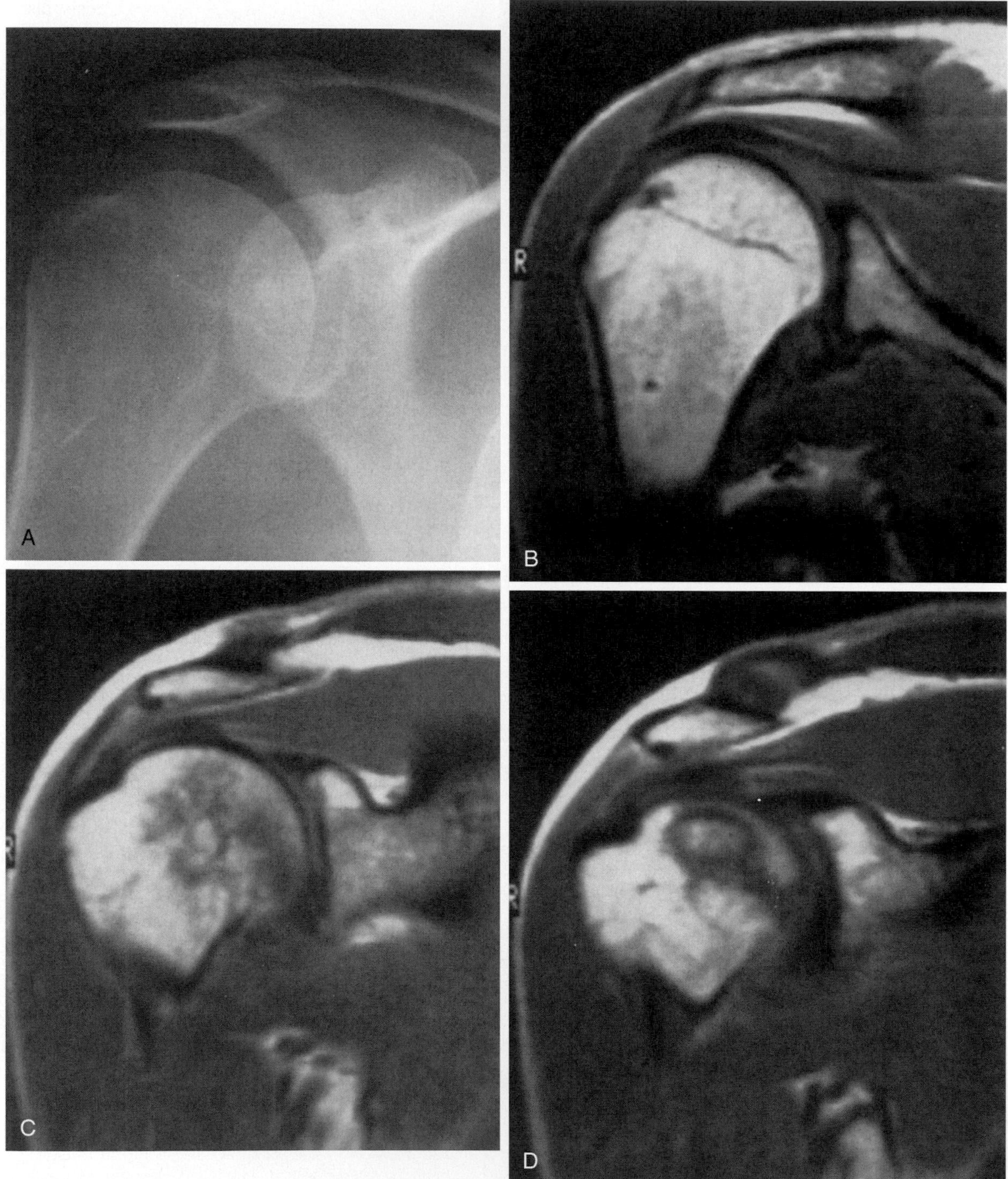

Figure 4–73. Magnetic resonance imaging of a bone bruise in a 41-year-old man who fell on his shoulder from a standing height. *A*, Anteroposterior view of the shoulder fails to demonstrate any evidence of abnormality. All radiographs in various projections were normal. *B–D*, T_1-weighted images of the shoulder. Posteriorly *(B)*, there is no evidence of abnormality. The midportion of the head *(C)* demonstrates a poorly defined, patchy area of decreased signal intensity within the humeral head. Anteriorly *(D)*, there is a circular area of low signal intensity, consistent with a fracture that appears to extend to the joint surface. The patchy areas of decreased signal intensity are indicative of a bone bruise, or occult interosseous fracture.

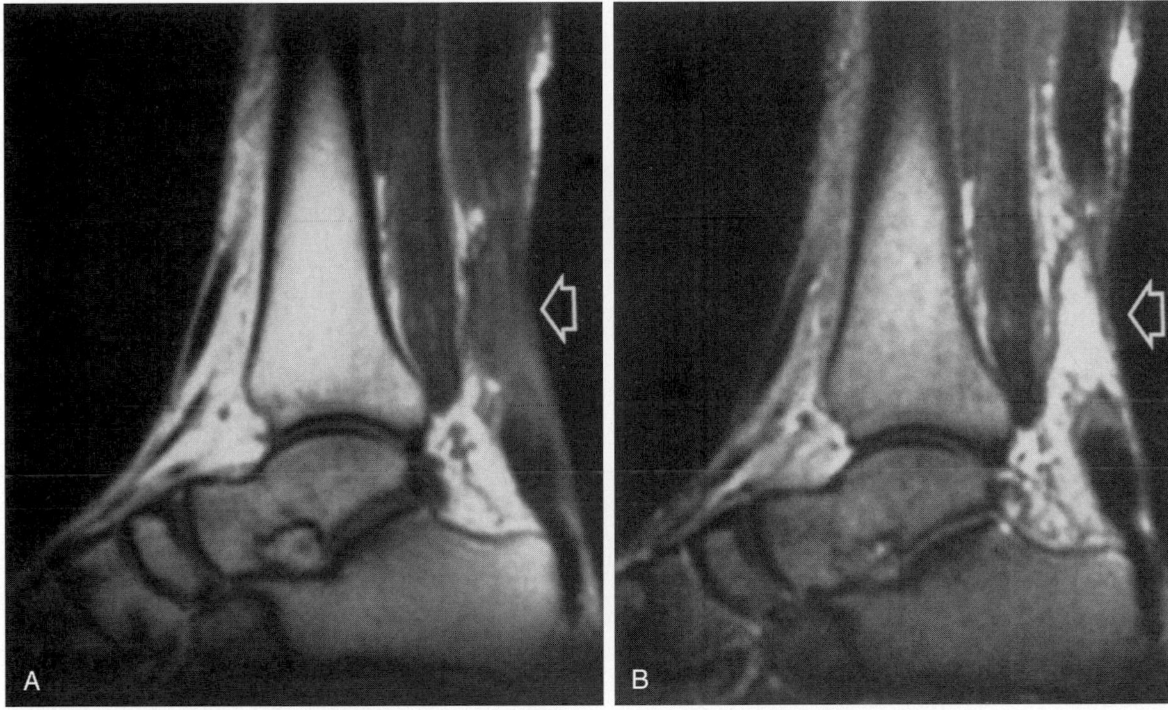

Figure 4–74. Magnetic resonance imaging examination of completely disrupted Achilles tendon in a 40-year-old man. He sustained the injury during a volleyball game when another player fell on the back of his lower leg. *A*, T_1-weighted image demonstrates an area of poorly defined signal encroaching upon the pre–Achilles tendon fat (*arrow*). *B*, T_2-weighted image demonstrates high signal intensity in the same area, consistent with recent hematoma (*arrow*).

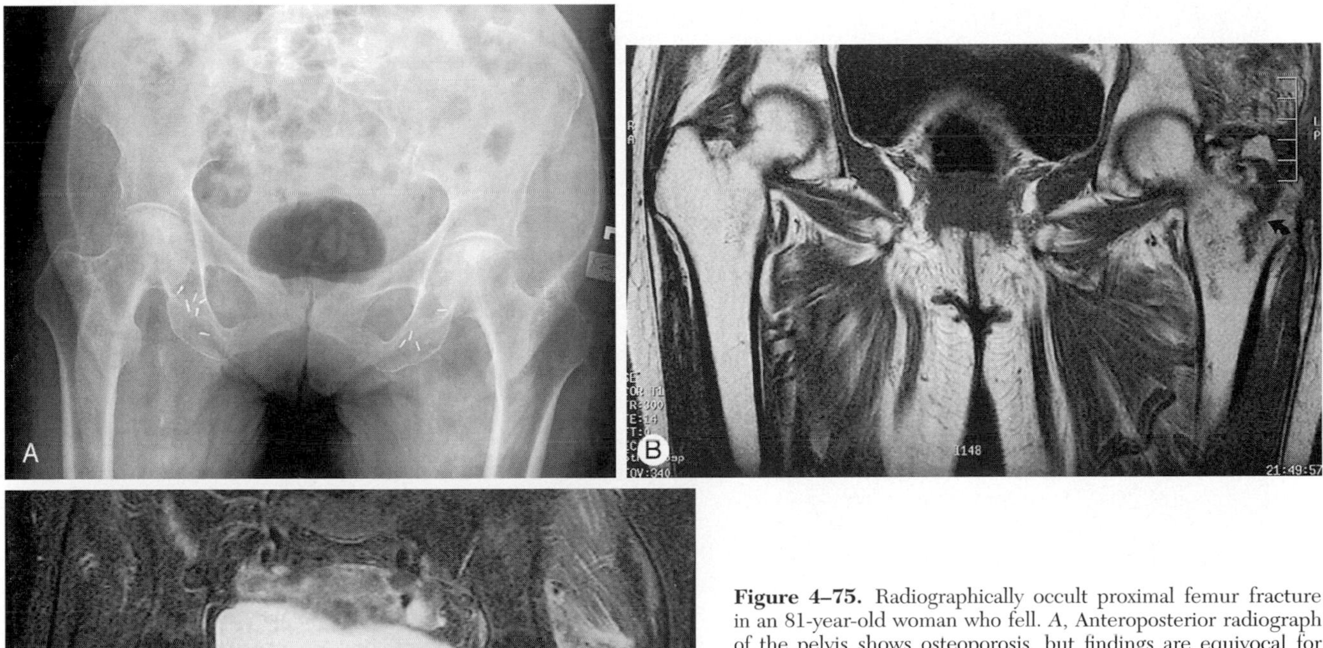

Figure 4–75. Radiographically occult proximal femur fracture in an 81-year-old woman who fell. *A*, Anteroposterior radiograph of the pelvis shows osteoporosis, but findings are equivocal for the presence of fracture. *B*, Coronal T_1-weighted magnetic resonance image shows an incomplete, nondisplaced intertrochanteric fracture on the left (*arrow*). The patient reported pain on the left side. *C*, Coronal T_2-weighted fat-suppressed magnetic resonance image shows the fracture line with surrounding marrow edema (*arrow*). The increased signal intensity in the surrounding musculature represents hematoma.

Table 4–3. Patterns of Injury on Magnetic Resonance Imaging (MRI) by Mechanism

Mechanism and Injury	Key MRI Features
Impaction	
Bone bruise	Diffuse marrow edema and hemorrhage
Nondisplaced fracture	Diffuse marrow edema and hemorrhage with cortical disruption
Wedge or compression fracture	Diffuse marrow edema and hemorrhage with altered anatomic fracture configuration
Distraction	
Nondisplaced avulsion fracture	Minimal marrow edema and hemorrhage at insertion of tendon or ligament
Displaced avulsion fracture	Minimal marrow edema and hemorrhage at insertion of tendon or ligament with displacement of osseous fragment
Chronic avulsion fracture	Minimal marrow edema at insertion of tendon or ligament often associated with local cystic change
Shearing or penetration	
Nondisplaced fracture	Bone bruising with linearity, often with a definite hypointense fracture line
Displaced fracture	Minimal bone brusing with linearity and displacement of bone fragment

From Eustace, S.J. (1999). Magnetic Resonance Imaging of Orthopedic Trauma. p. 64. Lippincott Williams & Wilkins, Philadelphia, with permission.

Radionuclide Bone Scanning

The diagnosis of a fracture using radionuclide bone scanning is made by demonstrating a focus of increased radioactivity in the area in question. Bone scanning is more sensitive than radiography; therefore, a bone scan may be positive despite a normal radiographic appearance. The principal use of bone scanning in trauma has been in the demonstration of otherwise occult fractures (Fig. 4–76).[14] Ninety-five percent of all patients with fractures have abnormal bone scans within 72 hours after injury, and 80% have abnormal scans within 24 hours.[27, 205] The rate and speed of positivity is age dependent, being delayed in the elderly.[31, 118] False-negative scans of fractures are therefore infrequent and occur primarily in older patients.[205, 214] Bone scanning plays a major role in the detection of stress and insufficiency fractures.

Radionuclide bone scanning is occasionally useful for fracture evaluation in situations in which cross-sectional imaging is not available. It is useful to detect subtle fractures when the radiographic examination is negative but there exists a strong clinical suspicion of a fracture.[205] In this respect, bone scanning has been proved most useful for hip, scaphoid, and stress fractures.[212, 214] The age of a vertebral compression fracture can also be estimated from serial bone scans,[209] and bone scanning can be used to determine the progress of fracture healing.[205] Avascular necrosis can be identified or predicted on the basis of a bone scan earlier than with radiographs. Early identification of necrosis is most useful in evaluating the femoral head because of the frequent occurrence of avascular necrosis after fracture of the femoral neck.

Technetium 99m–labeled phosphate or diphosphonate compounds are the radiopharmaceuticals of choice for bone scanning.[181] Whole-body bone scanning is performed with a gamma camera. Both anterior and posterior views are obtained. The scan is obtained from 2 to 6 hours after injection of the radiopharmaceutical, depending on the specific compound used. This time delay between injection and imaging is one of the major disadvantages of the bone scan in emergency room patients, and few if any alternative diagnoses can be offered in the event of a negative scan. Cross-sectional imaging modalities require a much shorter total examination time. Radiopharmaceuticals used in bone scanning are very sensitive to changes in bone metabolism such as those caused by fracture,[55] but the abnormal nuclide accumulation is nonspecific.[178, 197, 215] This nonspecificity is one of the greatest difficulties with the modality.[197]

Matin has described three phases of fracture healing as demonstrated by bone scanning.[205] In the first stage, diffuse increased activity surrounds the fracture site. The fracture line is sometimes visible. This stage lasts 3 to 4 weeks. The second stage lasts approximately 8 to 12 weeks; in this stage, well-defined linear distribution of intense nuclide activity is demonstrated at the fracture site. In the third stage, the activity gradually diminishes until the scan returns to normal. The bone scan reverts to normal sooner with rib fractures than with vertebral body or long bone fractures. The bone scan in approximately 90% of fractures of ribs, vertebrae, and distal extremities returns to normal by 2 years after injury, and in 95% of the fractures it is normal by 3 years. The bone scan remains positive longer in fractures treated with open reduction and internal fixation[205] and in fractures that heal with deformity[197] than in those treated with closed reduction that heal with normal anatomic alignment. The healing response as measured by radionuclide uptake intensity is often less striking in osteoporotic than in normal bone.[181] A bone scan may be positive more than 40 years after a long bone fracture has healed, even in the absence of persistent radiographic evidence of a fracture defect. As a general rule, bone scans return to normal in an uncomplicated healed fracture earlier in younger than in older patients.[205]

Because of the nonspecificity of bone scans, problems in interpretation arise. Traumatic synovitis accompanying a fracture adjacent to the joint may result in abnormal activity on the scan that can obscure the fracture. In such cases the scan must be repeated several days later. A fracture of the scaphoid is a likely site of this problem. Periosteal tears or ligament avulsions may also cause a transiently positive scan.[214] The increased nuclide activity caused by such an abnormality should return to normal or decrease in intensity within a few days, whereas a fracture will demonstrate increasing abnormal activity for several weeks and then persisting abnormal activity for several months.[205, 214] Lesions that were present before the traumatic episode, such as metastatic disease or previously healed fractures, can cause abnormal activity that may be confusing. Serial scans may be necessary in cer-

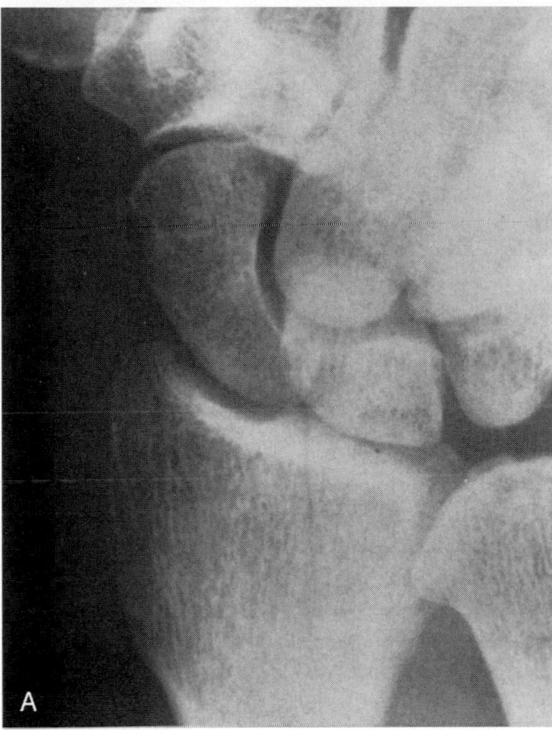

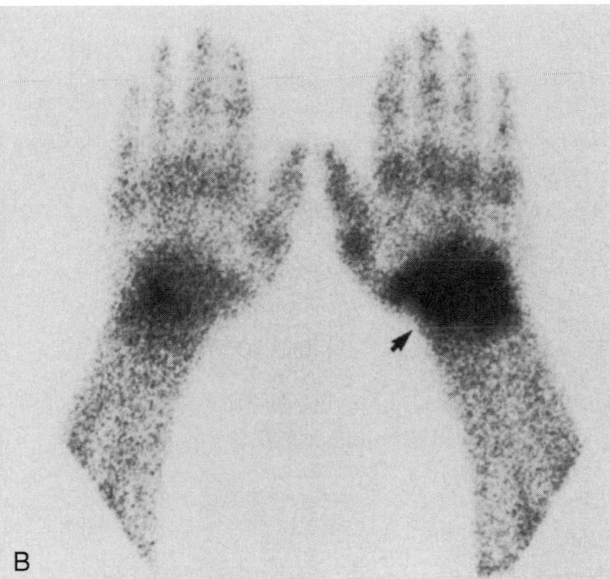

Figure 4–76. Detection of occult fracture of the scaphoid by technetium 99m radioisotopic bone scan in a 40-year-old radiologist injured in a fall while playing tennis. *A*, Posteroanterior radiograph of the scaphoid fails to reveal any evidence of fracture. *B*, Technetium 99m radioisotopic bone scan demonstrates diffuse increase in radioactivity throughout the carpus, with a focus of greater intensity in the scaphoid (*arrow*), identifying an otherwise occult fracture of the waist of the scaphoid.

tain cases to distinguish an old lesion from a new traumatic lesion. Synovitis from arthritis can cause abnormal activity. Increased nuclide activity on both sides of the joint, unchanged activity on serial scans, and multiple joint involvement are helpful to distinguish arthritis from a recent fracture.

Bone scanning can be used for grossly determining the age of a compression fracture in the spine.[182] This determination may be important in cases of litigation and worker's compensation but may also be useful in certain patients with metastatic disease and in patients receiving steroid therapy. Serial studies are necessary to demonstrate progression of the nuclide activity.[182, 205] Old fractures will demonstrate no change of activity on serial studies, whereas a recent fracture will show progressive increase in activity during healing followed by a decrease of activity.

Stress fractures and insufficiency fractures usually cannot be identified radiographically until 2 to 3 weeks after the onset of symptoms but are demonstrated by bone scanning as early as 1 to 3 days after occurrence.[184] The scan may remain positive for 16 to 18 weeks. If the patient refrains from activity, it is possible that the radiographs may remain normal, never revealing the stress fracture despite the positive nuclide scan. The injury remains submacroscopic and thus inapparent on the radiograph but would be visible on MR images. The normal response to increased stress is bone remodeling.[220] There is initial resorption of bone followed by accelerated osteoblastic replacement. If the accelerated physical activity is too great, bone resorption can outstrip the replacement capacity, resulting temporarily in a weak cortex and microfractures. If activity continues, the fractures may become complete and displaced.

Fluoroscopy

Fluoroscopy is most often used in relation to fractures during open reduction and internal fixation. A C-arm radiographic unit provides the surgeon with rapid visualization of the fracture alignment in two different perpendicular planes. Possible excessive patient radiation exposure is always of concern, as is accumulated excessive radiation exposure to the operating room personnel as well. The radiographic unit should have an image intensifier. A further way to reduce radiation exposure is with use of a digital x-ray unit that allows radiographic images to be captured and replayed on the monitor. This technique helps to avoid prolonged continuous fluoroscopy. Fluoroscopy should be used for visualization of the fracture position, and manipulation should be done with the fluoroscopic unit turned off.

Fluoroscopy may also be useful in cases of suspected nonunion of a long bone fracture. Under fluoroscopic control the fracture can be stressed to prove motion at the nonunion site.

Occasionally, fluoroscopy can be useful for positioning a difficult-to-see fracture for radiographic examination. Fluoroscopic guidance should not be used routinely for positioning. It is useful only rarely for those fractures that can only be seen on nonroutine views. It may actually decrease patient exposure by reducing the number of radiographs positioned blindly to optimally demonstrate a small area of interest.

Arthrography

Arthrography is performed by injecting contrast medium into a joint and then obtaining images. Radiographic and fluoroscopic arthrography are seldom performed, but CT and MR arthrography may sometimes demonstrate structures and abnormalities that would be obscure without the use of contrast. There are no indications for these procedures in the setting of acute trauma.

Radiography with Stress Views

Excessive stress to a joint may cause a fracture of an adjacent bone or rupture of a ligament. Radiographs obtained while stress is applied to the joint are used to evaluate a joint for ligamentous rupture. The acromioclavicular, the knee, and the ankle are the joints most likely to sustain ligamentous injury without accompanying fractures and to potentially need evaluation with stress radiographs. When a ligament is torn in one of these three joints, the bones making up the joint may return to normal or near-normal position and appear normal except for soft tissue swelling. Avulsion of a ligament from its bony attachment may or may not be accompanied by a small rim of bone that was avulsed as the ligament tore loose from the bone (Fig. 4–77). It is in the last case, in which there is no bony avulsion, that stress radiographs may be useful. They are indicated when there is a clinical question of instability or disruption of a joint or when there is radiographic uncertainty or a hint of abnormal separation of bones that make up a joint[200] (see Fig. 4–77). Ligamentous injuries are notoriously difficult to diagnose radiographically because the only finding is usually nonspecific soft tissue swelling adjacent to the joint. Improved soft tissue detail with computed radiography systems is making possible the diagnosis of lesions that would be occult on conventional film-screen systems. The importance of diagnosing a ligamentous injury cannot be overemphasized. The detachment of a ligament may be equivalent to a fracture insofar as the stability of a joint is concerned,[200] and failure to address the injury adequately may lead to early post-traumatic osteoarthritis.

Stress films of acutely injured joints are not particularly useful. The rapid onset of swelling and muscle spasm following injury may mask the presence of a torn ligament.[193] Pain and guarding may be so severe that stress films can be obtained only with the patient under anesthesia.

Conventional Tomography

Tomography is an analog x-ray technique used to image a structure or object obscured by overlapping shadows on the radiograph. Tomography blurs out objects above and below a given plane in the patient's body. Rather than improving image detail, tomograms actually degrade it.[190] The reason why pathologic processes may be seen better with tomography, or seen with tomography and not seen with radiographs, is that overlapping objects that may obscure a possible fracture line are blurred out.

In a tomographic x-ray unit, the x-ray tube and the film tray are connected by a rod that is attached to a fulcrum. During exposure, the tube and film tray move in reciprocal directions while the patient remains stationary. The portion of the patient at the level of the fulcrum is in focus, while the portions above and below are blurred. Sections at multiple levels through the area of interest are obtained by moving the radiographic tabletop up or down in small increments for successive exposures. With the ready availability of CT, a far superior technique, the role of conventional tomography is almost historical. Most tomographic x-ray units remaining in service were not designed for skeletal work.

Sonography

When applied to the musculoskeletal system, typically sonography is used to evaluate the soft tissues and not the bones.[20] Nevertheless, it is currently considered by some authorities to be the method of choice for examining infants during their first year for congenital hip dysplasia.[20, 33] A report of a femoral fracture and a clavicular fracture diagnosed in two infants using sonography is intriguing, especially because the radiographic findings were normal.[20] The rapidly performed study and the thin soft tissue that has to be penetrated make this modality attractive for use with infants. On sonographic studies performed on cadaveric bones, cortical discontinuities of 1 mm or more were detected using 7.5-MHz linear-array transducers and 3.5-MHz sector transducers,[264] suggesting possible applications in bones close to the skin surface. Limited clinical studies have shown that sonography can be more sensitive than radiography in the detection of acute rib fractures in adults.[266] It has been used to detect radiographically occult fractures of the foot and ankle[342] and nondisplaced fractures of the greater tuberosity of the humerus.[305] Sonography can provide important information about the soft tissues surrounding fracture sites in long bones and can indicate callus formation at an early stage. Sonography is more sensitive than conventional radiography in showing the early phases of organization of the callus, and its progression to bridging new bone formation. Sonography also clearly showed a disorganized echo pattern at the fracture site of the patients with nonunion.[284] Sonography can detect[275] and guide management of clavicular fractures in infants.[240] More investigation and perhaps better instrumentation are clearly needed to define the role of sonography in acute fracture detection.

Factors Affecting Detection of Fractures

Normal Structures and Anatomic Variants

Several normal structures or anatomic variants may be confused with or mistaken for a fracture.[173, 175, 176] Fortunately these structures are more or less predictable in appearance and location. In most cases this predictabil-

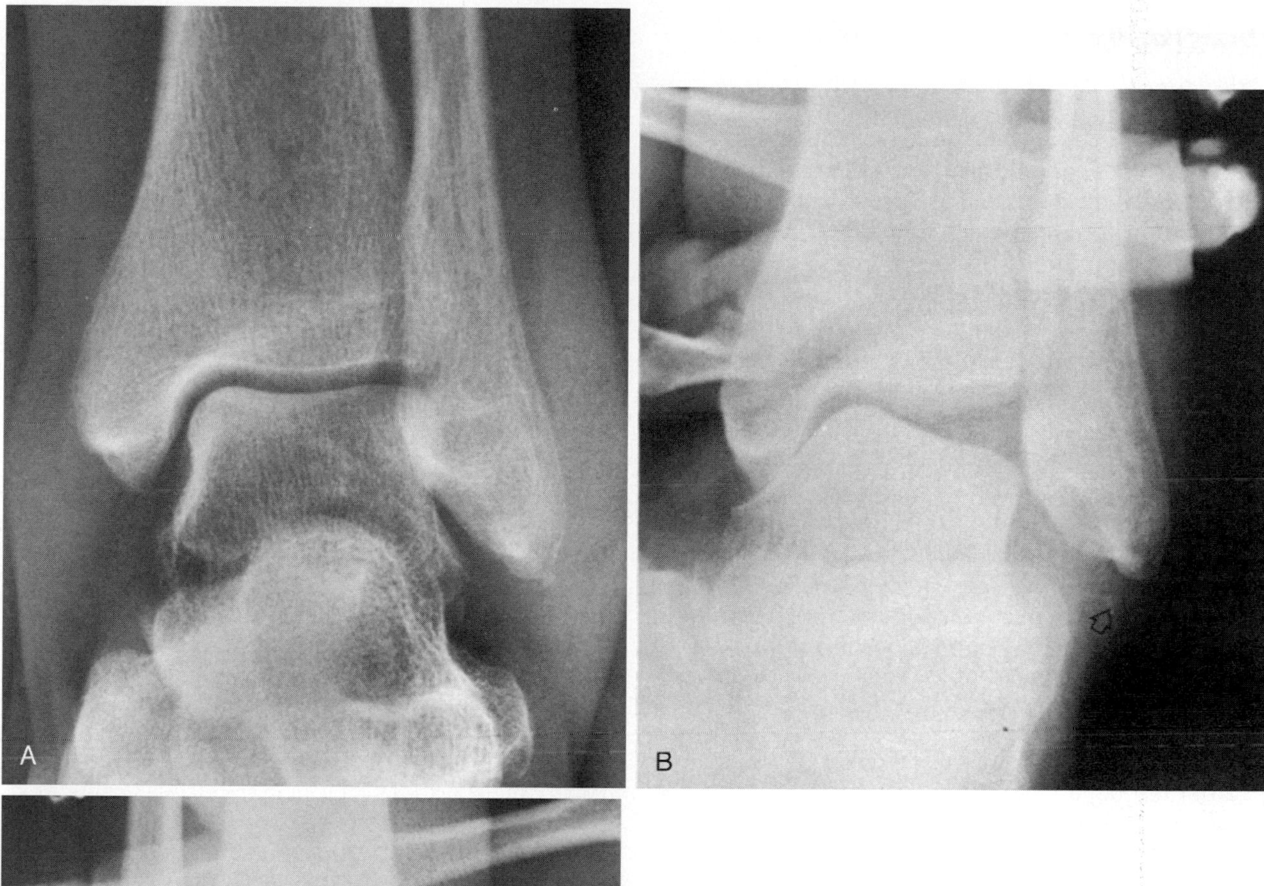

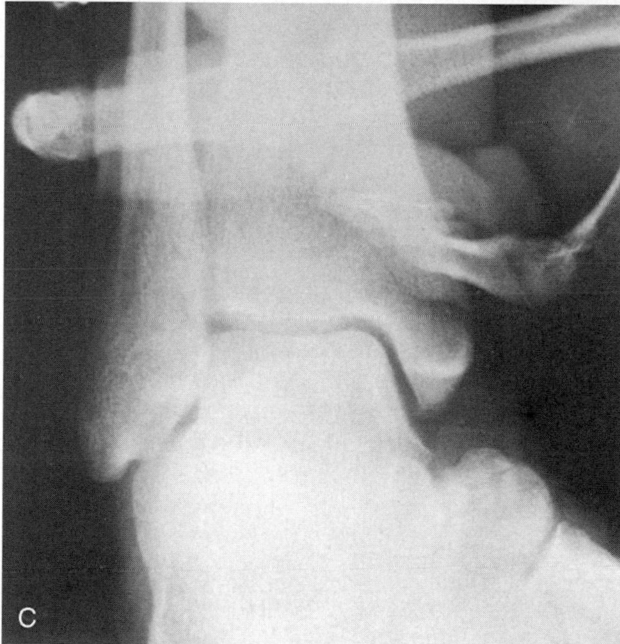

Figure 4–77. Use of stress views in radiographic evaluation of injury. *A*, On the anteroposterior view of the left ankle with lateral soft tissue swelling, no definite fracture is visible. *B*, Varus stress and internal rotation allow demonstration of a small bone fragment (*arrow*) that avulsed with the fibulocalcaneal ligament from its attachment to the tip of the lateral malleolus. The abnormal rotation of the talus is possible after loss of the lateral ligamentous support. *C*, Comparison stress view of the contralateral ankle. Regrettably, the hand of the examiner is included on the radiograph. A leaded protective glove and apron should be worn if there is a possibility of exposure to the x-ray beam during the performance of any examination.

ity allows for confident discrimination and accurate designation as to their true origin, thus minimizing a potential source of erroneous diagnosis. Reference atlases of anatomic variants are valuable to keep in the image interpretation area.[276, 319]

Vascular channels for nutrient arteries (Fig. 4–78*A*) in the long and short bones may mimic nondisplaced linear fractures. These channels are differentiated by their smooth course and slightly eburnated margins, in contrast with the irregular course and absence of eburnation on the margins of a fracture line. The vascular channels of long and short bones are reasonably predictable in location and direction. They generally course diagonally through the cortex in such a manner that the inner limit of the channel lies farther from the faster-growing end of the bone than the outer limit. Generally speaking, then, the channels point toward the knee, away from the elbow, and toward the distal ends of the digits. Frequently the cortex is slightly thickened at the point of entrance into the medullary canal. Because of their small size, vascular channels are visualized on a radiograph only when viewed in profile. Therefore, the lucency of the channel is con-

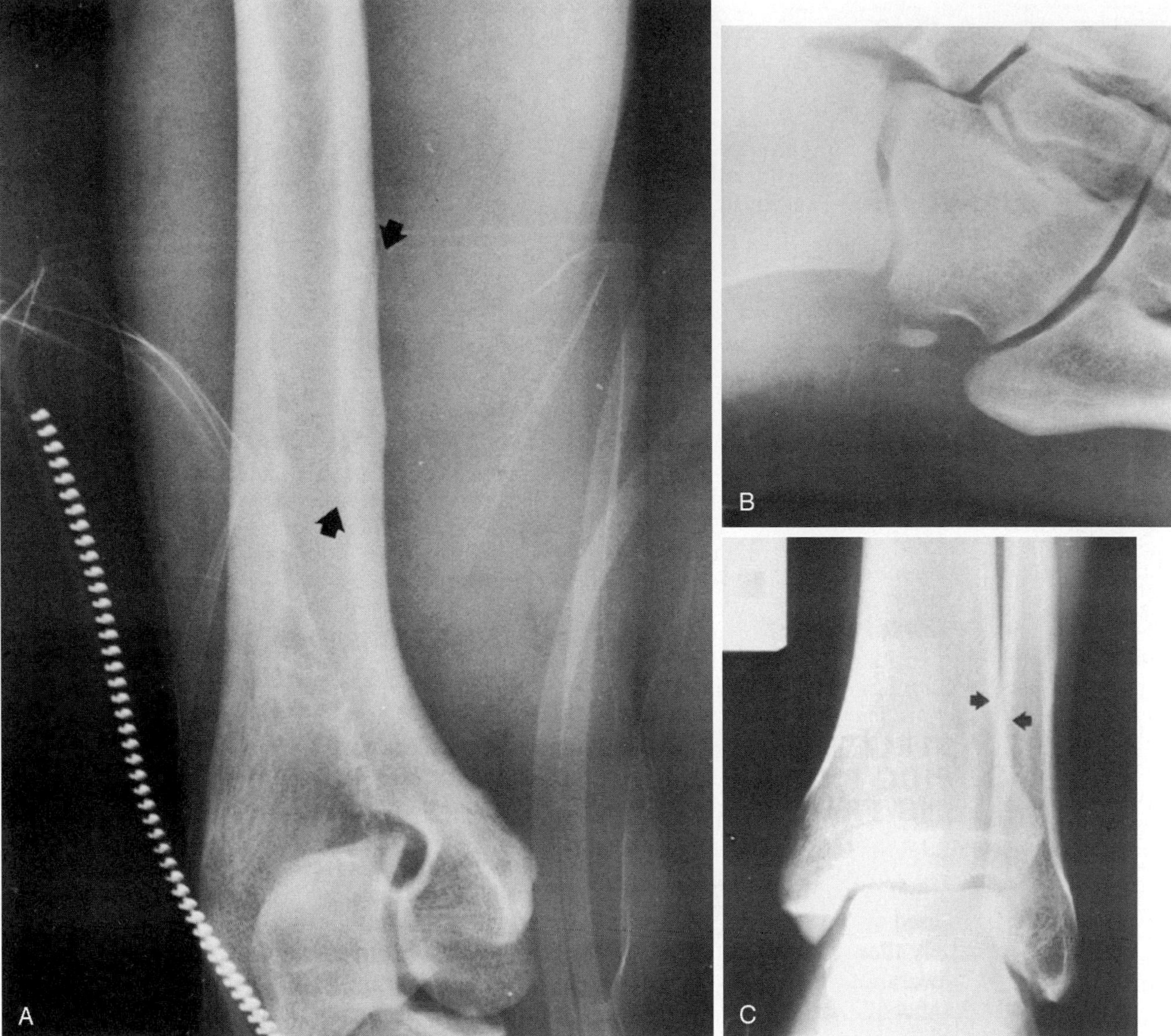

Figure 4–78. Normal radiographic findings that have the appearance of fractures. *A*, Vascular channel of the distal shaft of the humerus (*arrows*). The vascular canal in the medial cortex of the distal shaft of the humerus is clearly visualized. It is not as lucent as a fracture line. The margins of the canal are sharply defined and smooth. *B*, Accessory center of ossification. At the lateral margin of the cuboid on this oblique view of the foot, there is a small ossific radiodensity. It has a sharply defined cortical margin, and the apposing margin of the cuboid is intact. This feature clearly identifies it as an accessory center of ossification, in this case for the os peroneum. *C*, Mach effect simulating fracture. Note the lucent line (*arrows*) in the cortices of both the tibia and the fibula. This appearance, termed the Mach effect, is a visual artifact often present at the overlap of the two bones. There is no defect within the cortex of the bone. The Mach effect should not be mistaken for a fracture.

fined to the peripheral cortex of the bone and should neither extend into the medullary canal nor appear to involve any portion of the cortex not projected in profile.

Lines of junction between portions of growing bones may be confused with fractures. Their course is predictable, and junction lines should always be considered before diagnosis of a fracture in the region and direction they occupy. The age at appearance and closure of an epiphysis and apophysis should be generally known and should be considered before diagnosis of a fracture in children and adolescents. It should be quite unusual to mistake an apophysis and an epiphysis for a fracture in view of their sclerotic margins and predictable location and configuration. Rather, a more common problem is failure to recognize that they are displaced and that an apophyseal avulsion or epiphyseal separation is present. Certain epiphyses arise from multiple centers, such as in the proximal humerus, or have a tendency to be bifid, such as in the distal phalanx of the great toe, and these structures could be mistaken for fractures by the unaware. The apposing margins of such epiphyseal elements are sclerotic, smooth, and somewhat rounded and can be readily distinguished from fracture lines.

Small elements of bone, particularly *secondary centers of ossification* (see Fig. 4–78*B*) and, to a lesser extent, *sesamoids*, are at times difficult to distinguish from avulsion fractures. These are particularly troublesome about the foot and ankle and less so about the hand and wrist. The distinction lies in demonstration of the nature of the margin of the apposing bony surfaces. The apposing

borders of a sesamoid or secondary center of ossification and the adjacent bone are smooth, sharply defined, and sclerotic, whereas the apposing margins of an avulsion fracture are irregular and less well defined and lack sclerosis. The locations of secondary centers of ossification and sesamoids are well known and predictable. They do vary in frequency, however. Diagrams and radiographic demonstrations of these structures[173, 176] appear in Chapters 17 and 23.

Visual Perception

Mach bands are recognized under a variety of circumstances as lucent or dense lines due to overlap of radiographic shadows.[251] For example, when two bones overlap, a line of lucency may be encountered that parallels the periphery of the cortex of one of the two bones (see Fig. 4–78*C*). This optical illusion was described by Ernest Mach and is known as the Mach effect.[174] The Mach effect has been classically described as resulting from lateral inhibitory impulses in the retina of the eye, but it has been the subject of considerable research, and a number of alternative explanations have yet to be disproved.[306] Densitometric measurements at such boundaries have failed to demonstrate any actual change in density.[278] The eye tends to enhance the border between two adjacent or superimposed objects, thereby improving their visual discrimination—a form of edge enhancement. This phenomenon is commonly noted on radiographs of the ankle as the tibia overlaps the fibula. It may be encountered where clothing or skin folds overlie the bones, adjacent to hardware and metallic foreign bodies, adjacent to gas collections, along fat planes and fascial planes, and in other areas where sharp boundaries are present. Mach bands may be mistaken for nondisplaced fractures. Mach bands may also be seen on digital images.[252] The best place to observe these are on the gray scale step legends that are commonly included on CT images. Some computer algorithms for processing digital image data include edge enhancement, which may contribute to misinterpretation of digital images.

Digital Imaging

The expanding use of digital imaging in radiology has forced a growing number of physicians to become familiar with viewing images on the computer monitor (soft copy), as opposed to viewing images on film (hard copy). In transitional settings, hard copy images are simply printed from the digital data. Although the computer and network infrastructure necessary for so-called filmless radiology is very expensive, requiring a picture archiving and communication system (PACS), it confers undeniable advantages in terms of simultaneous availability, compact storage, and rapid retrieval (availability of any image at any time in any location). The integration of digital images into the computerized medical record is a laudable goal in medicine that is easily within reach. The radiologist may encounter three types of computerized radiographic images. Conventional analog film-screen radiographs that have been passed through a film digitizer are commonly used for teleradiology, the remote viewing of radiographs. The information content of such digitized images can be no better than the original film, and some data suggest these images are inferior in terms of diagnostic performance, even when high-resolution laser digitizers are used.[344] Computed radiography (CR) is a method of extracting a digital image from a special cassette that captures a latent radiologic image on a photostimulable storage phosphor plate. The plate is then scanned by a laser to produce digital data that are converted to an image. The theoretical spatial resolution of computed radiographs may be less than an analog film, but the contrast scale tends to be much better, and studies suggest diagnostic equivalence of computed radiographs to analog radiographs in both soft copy and hard copy formats.[282, 301] In clinical application, CR cassettes may be used by radiographic technologists in a manner similar to analog film-screen cassettes. One should be forewarned that images do not appear instantaneously because the plates have to be scanned by the laser to produce the image. Direct digital radiography uses an image detector array, of which there are several types, to capture a digital image without the necessity for laser scanning. Direct digital radiography produces images that are equivalent to and in some parameters better than conventional film-screen images.[307] The American College of Radiology has established standards covering various aspects of filmless radiology, including standards for display stations. These standards are available at their website (http://www.acr.org). Use of image interpretation tools such as window and level, magnification, rotation and flip, and annotation may affect interpretation. The luminance (brightness) of the monitor (and the level of ambient light) has an effect on perceived image quality, and a common major factor for better perception of digital images on radiologists' workstations compared with clinician workstations is the environment. Various image processing algorithms for edge enhancement, unsharp masking, and other techniques may have been applied to the digital data either in acquisition or post-processing, and if image compression has been used, some digital information may have been lost. The effects on diagnostic performance of digital radiologic imaging will require continuing study, but these technologies are proliferating rapidly and will soon replace conventional film-screen methods.

Description of Fractures and Joint Injuries

The maintenance of proper patient records requires an accurately written description of all fractures and dislocations. This approach is necessary in terms of sound medical practice and any future legal considerations. More important, however, the disciplined practice of the physician, whether radiologist or orthopedist, of writing a full description ensures that all aspects of the injury have been considered, reviewed, and noted and that the physician is fully aware of the problem at hand. Good judgment requires that as much information as possible be obtained before initiation of treatment. An accurate

diagnosis directs the physician to proper treatment and best assures a good result. No matter how apparently trivial the injury, a hastily taken history, perfunctory physical examination, and cursory glance at the radiographs reflect poor judgment and frequently lead to inaccurate diagnosis, inappropriate treatment, and poor results.

Many physicians expect that all abnormalities will be immediately apparent on simply looking at a radiograph. This is not true. Radiographs require interpretation and must not simply be "looked at." Unless findings are specifically sought, they will be overlooked. The eye is immediately taken and held by the obvious; therefore, it is important to specifically seek out related, less obvious findings that may have an impact on the treatment plan and prognosis. The "satisfaction of search" effect describes the adverse effect of finding an abnormality on continuation of the search for additional abnormalities; when one abnormality is found, the tendency is to stop looking for a second or a third.[234] The causes of this effect have been studied but remain elusive.[11, 235] This satisfaction of search effect may be a significant source of error in the interpretation of skeletal radiographs.[230] Perhaps this effect can be minimized by a disciplined intellectual effort to complete the search. Radiologists have not been found to have special or extraordinary perceptual abilities not found in laypersons[299]; rather, their skills are based on knowledge, experience, and discipline. The specifics of the clinical history,[236, 313] access to previous radiologic images or reports,[226, 233] and preconceptions[331] also have a significant effect on fracture detection.

Elements of Fracture Description

A full description of a fracture (see Fig. 4–67) includes a statement about the location, direction, and nature of the fracture line and whether the fracture is open or closed and simple or comminuted.[5, 6] This is followed by a description of the alignment and apposition of the fracture fragments.

Obviously, it is much easier and more dependable to determine that a fracture is open by visual inspection of the injury than by viewing radiographs of the injured part. It is often impossible to state that a fracture is open on the basis of its radiographic appearance. If a fragment of bone protrudes beyond the skin, it is certain that the fracture is open. However, it should be equally obvious that the reverse is not true: failure to visualize a bone fragment beyond the overlying skin cannot exclude the presence of an open fracture. It is possible that the radiographs obtained do not "view" the open wound in tangent, so that the protruding fragment overlies the fracture site, or the bone may be exposed but does not protrude through the skin. The presence of air within the soft tissues in proximity to bone fragments in an acute fracture is a reliable sign of an open fracture. In the main, however, this determination is clinical and not radiographic.

The presence of comminution is noted, as well as the degree of comminution—minimal, moderate, or severe. If there are a few small bone fragments adjacent to the fracture line, the comminution is minimal; if the fracture is composed of many relatively large fragments, the comminution is severe. Moderate comminution lies between these two extremes. The presence and position of characteristic butterfly fragments and segmental fractures are noted.

The direction and nature of the fracture line are described. The fracture is complete or incomplete and transverse, oblique, or spiral. In children the fracture may be described as a greenstick, torus, or bowing fracture.

The location of the fracture is stated in relation to its position in the shaft of long and short bones as proximal third, distal third, or midshaft; it is also described in relation to anatomic points or projections at the ends of long bones and in irregular bones, such as the lateral malleolus of the fibula, the medial tibial plateau, and waist of the scaphoid. It should always be noted whether or not the fracture at the end of a bone extends into the joint surface—that is, whether or not the fracture is intra-articular.

Generally speaking, in a radiographic report a fracture is presumed to be closed, complete, simple, and extra-articular unless the report specifically states otherwise (i.e., obviously open, incomplete, comminuted, and intra-articular). The designations closed, complete, simple, and extra-articular are utilized infrequently.

The position of a fracture refers to the relationship of the fractured ends of the bone at the fracture site. Alignment of a fracture refers to the relationship of the longitudinal axes of the fracture fragments one to another. With a nondisplaced fracture the bone is in normal position and alignment; the fragments are perfectly apposed without angulation. Displacement results in a change in either position or alignment or both of the fracture fragments.

Angulation of a fracture fragment results in malalignment. The description of this angulation is a source of considerable confusion. There are two methods of description. In the first—and preferred—method, the direction of the angulation of the long axis of the distal fragment is described relative to the long axis of the proximal fragment. In Figure 4–67*A*, there is "lateral angulation" of the distal fragment. The angle may be measured in degrees; the angle of displacement in the example shown is 15 degrees. In the second method of describing angulation, the direction of the apex of the angle formed by the displacement is described. Figure 4–67*A* also shows "apex medial angulation" at the fracture site. The resultant angle may be measured in degrees; in the example shown, the angle is 165 degrees. Angulation may be described as anterior or posterior, medial or lateral, or varus or valgus, or as a combination, such as posteromedial or anterolateral. Consistency is very important. One method or the other should be utilized, and one should not be confused with the other. Textbooks tend to favor the method of describing the angulation of the distal fragment, and we advocate specifying the particular method used in each communication. Because fracture angulation is measured from radiographs, which are two-dimensional representations of a three-dimensional situation, if the plane of angulation is not parallel to the plane in which the radiograph was obtained, the magnitude and perhaps even the direction of angulation may be in error. Note that in Figure 4–67*B*, the fracture appears to have no angulation

at all. Mathematical methods applied to two or more views have been devised to improve the accuracy of the radiographic analysis of angulation,[13, 30] but these methods are cumbersome and not generally utilized.

Fracture fragments that are not perfectly apposed are said to be displaced (see Fig. 4–67*B*). The direction of the displacement is stated in terms of the resting place of the distal fragment relative to the proximal fragment (e.g., displaced medially, anteriorly, or posterolaterally). The amount of displacement is measured in terms of the width of the shaft or width of the cortex or by actual measurement in millimeters (e.g., displaced half the width of the shaft medially, or displaced the width of the cortex laterally, or 8 mm of displacement anteromedially). If the displacement is such that the fracture fragments are not apposed, the fracture is said to be completely displaced. If, in addition, the limb is foreshortened in appearance and the distal fragment lies alongside the proximal fragment, the fragments are said to be overriding (see Fig. 4–67*B*). The extent of overriding is commonly measured in centimeters (e.g., 2 cm overriding of the fracture fragments).

If the fragments are separated by soft tissue and are not in direct apposition, they are said to be distracted. Distraction is measured in millimeters or centimeters (e.g., 8 mm of distraction of the fracture fragments). Distraction is often used in describing avulsion fractures of tendons in which muscular contraction has pulled the fragment away from its normal position.

Rotation about the longitudinal axis is much more easily determined by clinical evaluation than by radiographs. To be obvious on the radiograph, considerable rotational displacement is necessary (Fig. 4–79), and specific landmarks, such as the joints above and below the fracture, should be present on the same radiograph. Naimark and associates[29] have drawn attention to the fact that, in the absence of comminution, whenever there is a marked disparity between the diameters of the bones immediately proximal and distal to a fracture of the radius, a significant rotational deformity must be considered. This rule applies only when the cross-section of the bone at the fracture is ovoid, as is the case with the radius.

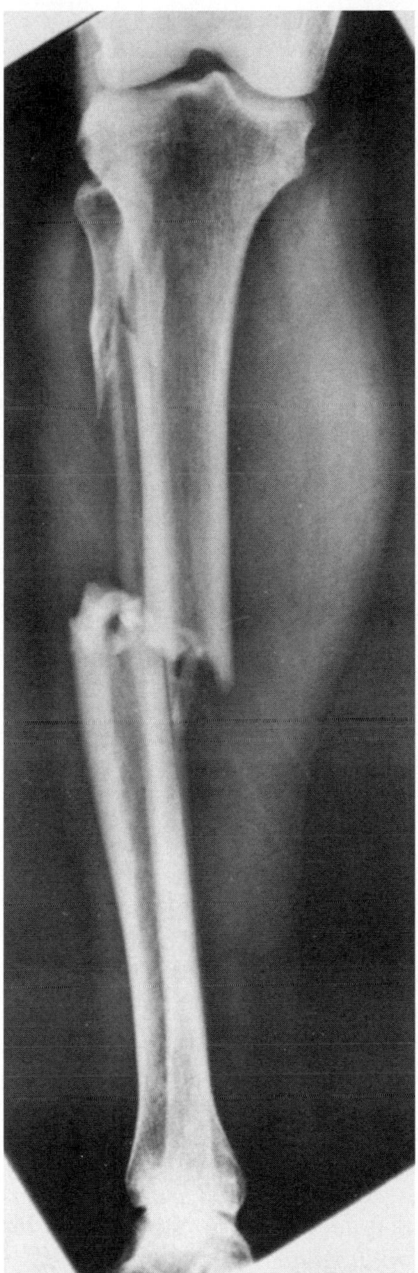

Figure 4–79. Midshaft fracture of tibia with 90-degree rotation of the distal fragment. There is a slightly oblique, minimally comminuted fracture of the midshaft of the tibia with a lateral offset of the distal fragment without apposition of the fracture fragments. A comminuted fracture of the proximal fibula is also present. The film was obtained diagonally on a 14 by 17-inch cassette, which allows demonstration of the 90-degree external rotation of the distal fragment. Note that the knee is seen in an anteroposterior projection, whereas the ankle is viewed as in a lateral projection.

The Radiology Report

The most important item in a radiology report of diagnostic images obtained in the setting of trauma is the presence or absence of fracture or dislocation. When such injury is absent, the report should state "no fracture or dislocation" or "negative for fracture," rather than "normal." When a fracture or dislocation is present, be certain to indicate specifically which bones and joints are involved before launching into a detailed description.

It should first be determined whether the fracture is complete or incomplete. Incomplete fractures are characteristically neither displaced nor angulated in adults but may show slight angulation in children. An incomplete fracture is reported as extending in a given direction from a designated portion of the cortex—for example, "an oblique, incomplete fracture extends from the medial cortex of the distal humerus." Unless the report states otherwise, a complete fracture is always implied.

Avulsion fractures are described as arising from an anatomic site (e.g., an avulsion fracture of the lateral malleolus), and by their size, either by specific measurements in millimeters and centimeters or, when quite small, in general terms such as minute or small. The direction of displacement and amount of measured distraction are also stated.

There are numerous classifications of various types of fractures in the literature. Fracture classification systems

are a means by which physicians communicate, make treatment decisions, estimate prognosis, and report and compare results. The ideal fracture classification is reliable, reproducible, all-inclusive, mutually exclusive, logical, and clinically useful.[287] Unfortunately, such classification systems, if they exist at all, have not gained general acceptance. As a general rule, fracture classifications should not be used in describing or reporting a fracture. With very few exceptions they are not universally known and utilized, and their use may therefore result in misunderstanding, or may communicate no information at all. It is quite likely that any orthopedic surgeon will be generally familiar with a given classification, but an emergency room physician, family practitioner, or generalist is not likely to appreciate its significance or to receive any useful information from its use. Radiologists should avoid such classifications and should choose a system they fully understand and use it correctly. Furthermore, a large body of literature indicates that interobserver variation in the application of fracture classifications is too great for these systems to be useful. Regions that have been studied in this way include the proximal humerus,[322, 323] the distal radius,[228, 269] the proximal femur,[229, 260, 261, 336] the tibia,[254, 288] and the ankle.[297, 337] Even if they could be applied precisely, some classifications may have no prognostic value.[259] Some classifications are ambiguous and difficult to apply; other classifications were not derived from imaging features and are difficult to apply using only imaging features.[339] In some classifications, even increasing the amount of imaging information with additional views, CT, or other means does not help reproducibility.[247, 325, 326] Many of the established morphologic classifications are being replaced by rapidly evolving treatment-oriented classifications and, as such, are beyond the purview of the radiologist.[258, 312]

The Salter-Harris classification of epiphyseal injuries is an exception to the general rule against the use of fracture classifications. It has broad application because it can be utilized to describe injuries in all portions of the appendicular skeleton and therefore is very convenient. Furthermore, it is well known and commonly utilized by most physicians who treat children's fractures (see Chapter 5 on children's fractures).

Eponyms—fractures or injuries that carry a person's name—bring color to what might otherwise be considered a sterile endeavor, the description of fractures. They hark back to an ancient lineage, the greats of yesteryear, and add a strand of continuity and professional heritage.[4] Unfortunately, they may also add confusion. They do not necessarily convey the same message to all users. Despite the aura of familiarity, they are probably best avoided. Various eponyms are defined in subsequent chapters, and it is often advantageous for the practitioner to be generally aware of what others may be referring to when these terms are used. Ravitch[7] has said of eponyms: "Given an eponym one may be sure (1) that the man so honored was not the first to describe the disease . . . or (2) that he misunderstood the situation, or (3) that he is generally misquoted, or (4) that (1), (2), and (3) are all simultaneously true." *Sic transit gloria.*

A dislocation is described by the joint involved and the direction of displacement of distal components (e.g., a posterolateral dislocation of the elbow joint). If a smaller bone or one of several bones of a joint is involved, the dislocation is designated by the name and direction of displacement of the involved bone (e.g., a lateral dislocation of the patella or volar dislocation of the lunate). It is good practice always to specify whether or not there is an associated fracture of the involved bones. Subluxations are similarly reported.

The recording of soft tissue changes relating to a fracture is dependent upon their importance to the presence or severity of the underlying injury. Joint effusions and lipohemarthroses are always reported because they imply an intra-articular injury when a history of trauma is given. There may be no obvious associated fracture, but the observation of an effusion is crucial to the care of the patient. Soft tissue swelling is recorded when associated with a relatively minor fracture or no obvious fracture at all, because it in some ways attests to the seriousness of the injury. In the presence of subtle fractures the description of surrounding soft tissue swelling or fascial plane obliteration lends support to the diagnosis; such information should therefore be recorded. However, if a fracture is obvious or gross, recording the expected soft tissue swelling only clutters the report.

Injuries resulting from firearms require a description of the retained fragments.[22] The course of a bullet can often be detected as a line of small metallic fragments.

References

General

1. Collins, D.N., & Temple S.D. (1988). Open joint injuries. Classification and treatment. Clin. Orthop., *244*:48.
2. Gustilo, R.B., Simpson, L., Nixon, R. et al. (1969). Analysis of 511 open fractures. Clin. Orthop., *66*:148.
3. Heppenstall, R.B. (1980). Fracture Treatment and Healing. W.B. Saunders Co., Philadelphia.
4. Peltier, L.F. (1983). Fractures of the distal end of the radius. An historical account. Clin. Orthop., *187*:18.
5. Pitt, M.J., & Speer, D.P. (1982). Radiologic reporting of orthopedic trauma. Med. Radiogr. Photogr., *58*:14.
6. Pitt, M.J., & Speer, D.P. (1990). Radiologic reporting of skeletal trauma. Radiol. Clin. North Am., *28*:247.
7. Raviteh, M.M. (1979). Dupuytren's invention of the Mikulicz enterotome with a note on eponyms. Perspect. Biol. Med., *22*:170.
8. Renner, R.R., Mauler, G.G., & Ambrose, J.L. (1978). The radiologist, the orthopedist, the lawyer and the fracture. Semin. Roentgenol., *13*:7.
9. Rockwood, C.A. Jr., Green, D.P., & Bucholz, R.W. (1996). Rockwood and Green's Fractures in Adults. 4th Ed. Lippincott Williams & Wilkins, Philadelphia.
10. Rogers, J.F., Bennett, J.B., & Tullos, H.S. (1984). Management of concomitant ipsilateral fractures of the humerus and forearm. J. Bone Joint Surg. [Am.], *66*:552.
11. Schultz, R.J. (1990). The Language of Fractures. 2nd Ed. Williams & Wilkins, Baltimore.
12. Wilson, J.N. Ed. (1976). Watson-Jones Fractures and Joint Injuries. 5th Ed. Churchill Livingstone, Edinburgh.

Radiographic Considerations

13. Bar, H.F., & Breitfuss, H. (1989). Analysis of angular deformities on radiographs. J. Bone Joint Surg. [Br.], *71*:710.
14. Batillas, J., Vasilas, A., Pizzi, W.F., & Gokcebay, T. (1981). Bone scanning in the detection of occult fractures. J. Trauma, *21*:564.
15. Beltran, J., Noto, A.M., Herman, L.J. et al. (1986). Joint effusions: MR imaging. Radiology, *158*:133.
16. Berbaum, K.S., El-Khoury, G.Y., Franken, E.A. et al. (1988). Impact of clinical history on fracture detection with radiography. Radiology, *168*:507.
17. Berbaum, K.S., Franken, E.A., & El-Khoury, G.Y. (1989). Impact of clinical history on radiographic detection of fractures: A comparison of radiologists and orthopedists. A.J.R. Am. J. Roentgenol., *153*:1221.
18. Brand, D.A., Frazier, W.H., Kohlhepp, W.C. et al. (1982). A protocol for

selecting patients with injured extremities who need x-rays. N. Engl. J. Med., *306*:333.
19. DeLacey, G., Barker, A., Wignall, B. et al. (1979). Reasons for requesting radiographs in an accident department. B.M.J., *1*:1595.
20. DeLacey, G., & Bradbrooke, S. (1979). Rationalising requests for x-ray examination of acute ankle injuries. B.M.J., *1*:1597.
21. Deutsch, A.L., Mink, J.H., & Waxman, A.D. (1989). Occult fractures of the proximal femur: MR imaging. Radiology, *170*:113.
22. Dodd, G.D., & Budzik, R.F. Jr. (1989). Identification of retained firearm projectiles on plain radiographs. A.J.R. Am. J. Roentgenol., *154*:471.
23. Guly, H.R. (1986). Fractures not x-rayed. Arch. Emerg. Med., *3*:159.
24. Hall, F.M. (1989). Clinical history, radiographic reporting, and defensive radiologic practice. Radiology, *170*:575.
25. Harris, J.H. Jr. (1981). The importance of soft tissues in certain skeletal traumatic lesions. Radiol. Clin. North Am., *19*:601.
26. Jackson, D.W., Jennings, L.D., Maywood, R.M., & Berger, P.E. (1988). Magnetic resonance imaging of the knee. Am. J. Sports Med., *16*:29.
27. Matin, P. (1979). The appearance of bone scans following fractures, including immediate and long-term studies. Clin. Sci., *20*:1227.
28. Miller, W.T. (1989). Impact of clinical history on fracture detection with radiography. Radiology, *170*:576.
29. Naimark, A., Kossoff, J., & Leach, R.E. (1983). The disparate diameter. A sign of rotational deformity in fractures. J. Assoc. Can. Radiol., *34*:8.
30. Sartoris, D.J. (1985). Quantitative assessment of distraction and angulation following long bone fracture. Invest. Radiol., *20*:222.
31. Slavin, J.D. Jr., Mathews, J., & Spencer, R.P. (1985). Bone imaging in the diagnosis of fractures of the femur and pelvis in the sixth to tenth decades. Clin. Nucl. Med., *11*:328.
32. Vandemark, R.M. (1990). Radiology of the cervical spine in trauma patients: Practice pitfalls and recommendations for improving efficiency and communication. A.J.R. Am. J. Roentgenol., *155*:465.
33. Vargis, T., Clarke, W.R., Young, R.A., & Jensen, A. (1983). The ankle injury—indications for the selective use of x-rays. Injury, *14*:507.
34. Yao, L., & Lee, J.K. (1988). Occult intraosseous fracture: Detection with MR imaging. Radiology, *167*:749.

Chondral and Osteochondral Fractures

35. Bullough, P.G., & Jagannath, A. (1983). The morphology of the calcification front in articular cartilage. Its significance in joint function. J. Bone Joint Surg. [Br.], *65*:72.
36. Clarke, I.C. (1972). The microevaluation of articular surface contours. Ann. Biomed. Eng., *1*:31.
37. Clarke, I.C. (1974). Articular cartilage: A review and scanning electron microscope study. II. The territorial fibrillar architecture. J. Anat., *118*:261.
38. Donohue, J.M., Buss, D., Oegema, T.R., & Thompson, R.C. Jr. (1983). The effects of indirect blunt trauma on adult canine articular cartilage. J. Bone Joint Surg. [Am.], *65*:948.
39. Landells, J.W. (1957). The reactions of injured human articular cartilage. J. Bone Joint Surg. [Br.], *39*:548.
40. Makin, M. (1951). Osteochondral fracture of the lateral femoral condyle. J. Bone Joint Surg. [Am.], *33*:262.
41. Mankin, H.J. (1983). The response of articular cartilage to mechanical injury. J. Bone Joint Surg. [Am.], *64*:460.
42. Matthewson, M.H., & Dandy, D.J. (1978). Osteochondral fractures of the lateral femoral condyle. J. Bone Joint Surg. [Br.], *60*:199.
43. Milgram, J.W. (1978). Radiological and pathological manifestations of osteochondritis dissecans of the distal femur. Radiology, *126*:305.
44. Milgram, J.W. (1986). Injury to articular cartilage joint surfaces: Displaced fractures of underlying bone. Clin. Orthop., *206*:236.
45. Milgram, J.W., Rogers, L.F., & Miller, J.W. (1978). Osteochondral fractures: Mechanisms of injury and fate of fragments. A.J.R. Am. J. Roentgenol., *130*:651.
46. Thompson, R.C., & Robinson, H.J. (1982). Articular cartilage matrix metabolism. J. Bone Joint Surg. [Am.], *63*:327.

Stress Fractures

47. Abel, M.S. (1985). Jogger's fracture and other stress fractures of the lumbosacral spine. Skeletal Radiol., *13*:221.
48. Ami, T.B., Treves, S.T., Tumeh, S. et al. (1987). Stress fractures after surgery for osteosarcoma: Scintigraphic assessment. Radiology, *163*:157.
49. Blatz, D.J. (1981). Bilateral femoral and tibial shaft stress fractures in a runner. Am. J. Sports Med., *9*:322.
50. Brower, A.C., Neff, J.R., & Tillema, D.A. (1977). An unusual scapular stress fracture. A.J.R. Am. J. Roentgenol., *129*:519.
51. Butler, J.E., Brown, S.L., & McConnell, B.G. (1982). Subtrochanteric stress fractures in runners. Am. J. Sports Med., *10*:228.
52. Cahill, B.R. (1977). Stress fracture of the proximal tibial epiphysis: A case report. Am. J. Sports Med., *5*:186.
53. Castillo, M., Tehranzadeh, J., & Morillo, G. (1988). Atypical healed stress fracture of the fibula masquerading as chronic osteomyelitis. Am. J. Sports Med., *16*:185.
54. Chamay, A. (1970). Mechanical and morphological aspects of experimental overload and fatigue in bone. J. Biomech., *3*:263.
55. Cummings, C.W., & First, R. (1975). Stress fracture of the clavicle after a radical neck dissection. Plast. Reconstr. Surg., *55*:366.
56. Daffner, R.H. (1984). Anterior tibial striations. A.J.R. Am. J. Roentgenol., *143*:651.
57. Daffner, R.H., Martinez, S., Gehweiler, J.A. Jr., & Harrelson, J.M. (1982). Stress fractures of the proximal tibia in runners. Radiology, *142*:63.
58. Devas, M. (1975). Stress Fractures. Churchill Livingstone, Edinburgh.
59. Dhoury, P., Metges, P.J., Pattin, S. et al. (1987). Fractures de fatigue: Maladie de pauzat du col femoral. Semin. Hop. Paris, *63*:1317.
60. Dorne, H.L., & Lander, P.H. (1984). Spontaneous stress fractures of the femoral neck. A.J.R. Am. J. Roentgenol., *144*:343.
61. Engber, W.D. (1977). Stress fractures of the medial tibial plateau. J. Bone Joint Surg. [Am.], *59*:767.
62. Erne, P., & Burchhardt, A. (1980). Femoral neck fatigue fracture. Arch. Orthop. Trauma Surg., *97*:312.
63. Geslien, G.E., Thrall, J.H., Espinosa, J.L., & Older, R.A. (1976). Early detection of stress fractures using 99mTc-polyphosphate. Radiology, *121*:683.
64. Greaney, R.B., Gerber, F.H., Laughlin, R.L. et al. (1983). Distribution and natural history of stress fractures in U.S. Marine recruits. Radiology, *146*:339.
65. Grusd, R. (1978). Pseudofractures and stress fractures. Semin. Roentengenol., *13*:81.
66. Hanks, G.A., Kalenak, A., Bowman, L.S. et al. (1989). Stress fractures of the carpal scaphoid. J. Bone Joint Surg. [Am.], *71*:938.
67. Holden, D.L., & Jackson, D.W. (1985). Stress fractures of the ribs in female rowers. Am. J. Sports Med., *12*:342.
68. Hopson, C.N., & Perry, D.R. (1977). Stress fractures of the calcaneus in women marine recruits. Clin. Orthop., *128*:159.
69. Johnell, O., Rausing, A., Wendeberg, B., & Westlin, N. (1982). Morphologic bone changes in shin splints. Clin. Orthop., *167*:180.
70. Kaye, J.J., Nance, E.P., & Green, N.E. (1982). Fatigue fracture of the medial aspect of the clavicle. Radiology, *144*:89.
71. Kendall, H.K. (1984). Stress fractures of the diaphysis of the ulna in a body builder. Am. J. Sports Med., *12*:405.
72. Kim, S.M., Park, C.H., & Gartland, J.J. (1987). Stress fracture of the pubic ramus in a swimmer. Clin. Nucl. Med., *12*:118.
73. Kittleson, A.C., & Whitehouse, W.M. (1966). Stress, greenstick and impaction fractures. Radiol. Clin. North Am., *4*:277.
74. Lankenner, P.A. Jr., & Micheli, L.J. (1985). Stress fracture of the first rib. J. Bone Joint Surg. [Am.], *67*:159.
75. Lee, J.K., & Yao, L. (1988). Stress fractures: MR imaging. Radiology, *169*:217.
76. McKenzie, D.C. (1989). Stress fracture of the rib in an elite oarsman. Int. J. Sports Med., *10*:220.
77. Moran, J.J.M. (1987). Stress fractures in pregnancy. Am. J. Obstet. Gynecol., *158*:1274.
78. Murcia, M., Brennan, R.E., & Edeiken, J. (1982). Computed tomography of stress fracture. Skeletal Radiol., *8*:193.
79. Nagle, C.E. (1986). Cost-appropriateness of whole body vs limited bone imaging for suspected focal sports injuries. Clin. Nucl. Med., *11*:469.
80. Norfray, J.F., Schlachter, L., Kernahan, W.T. Jr. et al. (1980). Early confirmation of stress fractures in joggers. J. A. M. A., *243*:1647.
81. Papanicolaou, N., Wilkinson, R.H., Emans, J.B. et al. (1985). Bone scintigraphy and radiography in young athletes with low back pain. A.J.R. Am. J. Roentgenol., *145*:1039.
82. Perry, C.R., Perry, H.M., & Burdge, R.E. (1984). Stress fracture of the radius following a fracture of the ulna diaphysis. Clin. Orthop., *187*:193.
83. Pilgaard, S., Poulsen, J.O., & Christensen J.H. (1976). Stress fractures. Acta Orthop. Scand., *47*:167.
84. Prather, J.I., Nusynowitz, M.L., Snowdy, H.A. et al. (1977). Scintigraphic findings in stress fractures. J. Bone Joint Surg. [Am.], *59*:869.
85. Rettig, A.C., & Beltz, H.F. (1985). Stress fracture in the humerus in an adolescent tennis tournament player. Am. J. Sports Med., *13*:55.
86. Roub, L.W., Gumerman, L.W., Hanley, E.N. et al. (1979). Bone stress: A radionuclide imaging perspective. Radiology. *132*:431.
87. Rupani, H.D., Holder, L.E., Espinola, D.A., & Engin, S.I. (1985). Three-phase radionuclide bone imaging in sports medicine. Radiology, *156*:187.
88. Sandrock, A.R. (1975). Another sports fatigue fracture. Radiology, *117*:274.
89. Schneider, H.J., King, A.Y., Bronson, J.L., & Miller, E.H. (1974). Stress injuries and developmental change of lower extremities in ballet dancers. Radiology, *113*:627.
90. Schneider, R., & Kaye, J.J. (1975). Insufficiency and stress fractures of the long bones occurring in patients with rheumatoid arthritis. Radiology, *116*:595.
91. Solomon, L. (1975). Stress fractures of the femur and tibia simulating malignant bone tumours. S. Afr. J. Surg., *12*:19.
92. Somer, K., & Meurman, K.O.A. (1982). Computed tomography of stress fractures. J. Comput. Assist. Tomogr., *6*:109.
93. Stafford, S.A., Rosenthal, D.I., Gebhardt, M.C. et al. (1986). MRI in stress fracture. A.J.R. Am. J. Roentgenol., *147*:553.
94. Tehranzadeh, J., Kurth, L.A., Elyaderani, M.K., & Bowers, K.D. (1982). Combined pelvic stress fracture and avulsion of the adductor longus in a middle-distance runner. Am. J. Sports Med., *10*:108.
95. Ting, A., King, W., Yocum, L. et al. (1988). Stress fractures of the tarsal navicular in long-distance runners. Clin. Sports Med., *7*:89.
96. Uhthoff, H.K., & Jaworski, Z.F.G. (1985). Periosteal stress-induced reactions resembling stress fractures. Clin. Orthop., *199*:284.

97. Wilcox, J.R., Moniot, A.L., & Green, J.P. (1977). Bone scanning in the evaluation of exercise-related stress injuries. Radiology, *123*:699.
98. Wolfgang, G.L. (1977). Stress fracture of the femoral neck in a patient with open capital femoral epiphyses. J. Bone Joint Surg. [Am.], *59*:680.
99. Zwas, S.T., Elkanovitch, R., & Frank, G. (1987). Interpretation and classification of bone scintigraphic findings in stress fractures. J. Nucl. Med., *28*:452.

Insufficiency Fractures

100. Casey, D., Mirra, J., & Staple, T.W. (1984). Parasymphyseal insufficiency fractures of the os pubis. A.J.R. Am. J. Roentgenol., *142*:581.
101. Chen, C., Chandnani, V., Kang, H.S. et al. (1990). Insufficiency fracture of the sternum caused by osteopenia: Plain film findings in seven patients. A.J.R. Am. J. Roentgenol., *154*:1025.
102. Cooper, K.L., Beabout, J.W., & Swee, R.G. (1985). Insufficiency fractures of the sacrum. Radiology, *156*:15.
103. De Smet, A.A., & Neff, J.R. (1985). Pubic and sacral insufficiency fractures: Clinical course and radiologic findings. A.J.R. Am. J. Roentgenol., *145*:601.
104. Fam, A.D., Shuckett, R., McGillivray, D.C., & Little A.H. (1983). Stress fractures in rheumatoid arthritis. J. Rheumatol. Arthritis, *10*:722.
105. Gacetta, D.J.& Yandow, D.R. (1984). Computed tomography of spontaneous osteoporotic sacral fractures. J. Comput. Assist. Tomogr., *8*:1190.
106. Gaucher, A., Pere, P., & Bannwarth, B. (1986). Insufficiency fractures of the pelvis. Clin. Nucl. Med., *11*:518.
107. Hall, F.M. (1984). Post-fracture pubic osteolysis simulating malignancy. J. Bone Joint Surg. [Am.], *66*:975.
108. Itani, M., Evans, G.A., & Park, W.M. (1982). Spontaneous sternal collapse. J. Bone Joint Surg. [Br.], *64*:432.
109. Lessniewski, P.J., & Testa, N.N. (1982). Stress fracture of the hip as a complication of total knee replacement. J. Bone Joint Surg. [Am.], *64*:304.
110. Lourie, H. (1982). Spontaneous osteoporotic fracture of the sacrum. J. A. M. A., *248*:715.
111. Manco, L.G., Schneider, R., & Pavlov, H. (1982). Insufficiency fractures of the tibial plateau. A.J.R. Am. J. Roentgenol., *140*:1211.
112. Pentecost, R.L., Murray, R.A., & Brindley, H.H. (1964). Fatigue, insufficiency, and pathologic fractures. J. A. M. A., *187*:1001.
113. Pere, P., Bannwarth, B., Gillet, P. et al. (1989). Les fractures par insuffisance osseuse du sternum. Rev. Rhum., *56*:843.
114. Ross, D.J., Dieppe, P.A., Watt, I., & Newman, J.H. (1983). Tibial stress fracture in pyrophosphate arthropathy. J. Bone Joint Surg. [Br.], *65*:474.
115. Scheib, J.S. (1989). Sacral insufficiency fracture. Orthopedics, *12*:1274.
116. Schneider, R., Yacovone, J., & Ghelman, B. (1985). Unsuspected sacral fractures: Detection by radionuclide bone scanning. A.J.R. Am. J. Roentgenol., *144*:337.
117. Schnitzler, C.M., & Solomon L. (1985). Trabecular stress fractures due to fluoride therapy for osteoporosis. Skeletal Radiol., *14*:276.

Pathologic Fractures

118. Arnold, J.S. (1973). Amount and quality of trabecular bone in osteoporotic vertebral fractures. Clin. Endocrinol. Metab., *2*:221.
119. Barry, H.C. (1967). Fractures of the femur in Paget's disease of bone in Australia. J. Bone Joint Surg. [Am.], *49*:1359.
120. Bohrer, S.P. (1971). Fracture complicating bone infarcts and/or osteomyelitis in sickle-cell disease. Clin. Radiol., *22*:83.
121. Bremner, R.A., & Jelliffe, A.M. (1958). The management of pathological fracture of the major long bones from metastatic cancer. J. Bone Joint Surg. [Br.], *40*:652.
122. Campeau, R.J., Bellah, R.D., & Varma, D.G.K. (1987). Pathologic fractures in a patient with renal osteodystrophy. Failure of early detection on bone scans. Clin. Nucl. Med., *12*:510.
123. Campistol, J.M., Gomez, J.M., Almirall, J. et al. (1988). Fracturas patologicas secundarias a la amiloidosis asociada a la hemodialisis. Nefrologia, *7*:357.
124. Campistol, J.M., Sole, M., Munoz-Gomez, J. et al. (1990). Pathological fractures in patients who have amyloidosis associated with dialysis. J. Bone Joint Surg. [Am.], *72*:568.
125. Carpenter, P.R., Ewing, J.W., Cook, A.J., & Kuster, A.H. (1977). Angiographic assessment and control of potential operative hemorrhage with pathologic fractures secondary to metastasis. Clin. Orthop., *123*:6.
126. Clain, A. (1965). Secondary malignant disease of bone. Br. J. Cancer, *19*:15.
127. Clohisy, D.R., & Thompson, R.C. (1988). Fractures associated with neuropathic arthropathy in adults who have juvenile-onset diabetes. J. Bone Joint Surg. [Am.], *70*:1192.
128. Coe, J.D., Murphy, W.A., & Whyte, M.P. (1986). Management of femoral fractures and pseudofractures in adult hypophosphatasia. J. Bone Joint Surg. [Am.], *68*:981.
129. Dines, D.M., Canale, V.C., & Arnold, W.D. (1976). Fractures in thalassemia. J. Bone Joint Surg. [Am.], *58*:662.
130. Drennan, J.C., & Freehafer, A.A. (1971). Fractures of the lower extremities in paraplegic children. Clin. Orthop., *77*:211.
131. Ed-Dars, M.S. (1987). Pathologische Frakturen als Komplikation von Osteomyelitis. Unfallchirurg, *90*:394.
132. Elmstedt, E. (1982). Spontaneous fractures in the renal graft recipient. Clin. Orthop., *162*:195.
133. Francis, K.C., Higinbotham, N.L., Carroll, R.E. et al. (1962). The treatment of pathological fractures of the femoral neck by resection. J. Trauma, *2*:465.
134. Gompels, B.M., Votaw, M.L., & Martel, W. (1972). Correlation of radiological manifestations of multiple myeloma with immunoglobulin abnormalities and prognosis. Radiology, *104*:509.
135. Guilford, W.B., Mentz, W.M., Kopelman, H.A., & Donohue, J.F. (1982). Sarcoidosis presenting as a rib fracture. A.J.R. Am. J. Roentgenol., *139*:608.
136. Habermann, E.T., Sachs, R., Stern R.E. et al. (1982). The pathology and treatment of metastatic disease of the femur. Clin. Orthop., *169*:70.
137. Harper, M.C. (1989). Metabolic bone disease presenting as multiple recurrent metatarsal fractures. Foot Ankle, *9*:207.
138. Jeffery, C.C. (1974). Spontaneous fractures of the femoral neck. Orthop. Clin. North Am., *5*:713.
139. Jones, A.R., & Lachiewicz, P.F. (1987). Pathologic Malgaigne fracture following pelvic irradiation. Clin. Orthop., *221*:226.
140. Korhonen, B.J. (1971). Fractures in myelodysplasia. Clin. Orthop., *79*:145.
141. Krishnamurthy, G.T., Tubis, M., Hiss, J., & Blahd, W.H. (1977). Distribution pattern of metastatic bone disease. A need for total body skeletal image. J. A. M. A., *237*:2504.
142. Leabhart, J.W., & Bonfiglio, M.(1961). The treatment of irradiation fracture of the femoral neck. J. Bone Joint Surg. [Am.], *43*:1056.
143. Lipshitz, H.I. (1979). Diagnostic Roentgenology of Radiotherapy Change. Williams & Wilkins Co., Baltimore.
144. Maddison, P.J., & Bacon, P.A. (1974). Vitamin D deficiency, spontaneous fractures, and osteopenia in rheumatoid arthritis. B.M.J., *4*:533.
145. Mall, J.C., Bekerman, C., Hoffer, P.B., & Gottschalk, A. (1976). A unified radiological approach to the detection of skeletal metastases. Radiology, *118*:323.
146. McGuire, M.H., Merenda, J.T., & Sundaram, M. (1989). Oncogenic osteomalacia. Clin. Orthop., *244*:305.
147. Menck, H., Schulze, S., & Larsen, E. (1988). Metastasis size in pathologic femoral fractures. Acta Orthop. Scand., *59*:151.
148. Mori, S., Shiraki, M., Fujimaki, H., & Ito, H. (1987). Bone fracture in elderly female with primary hyperparathyroidism: Relationship among renal function, vitamin D status and fracture risk. Horm. Metabol. Res., *19*:183.
149. Nerubay, J., Horoszowski, H., & Goodman, R. M. (1987). Fracture in progressive ossifying fibrodysplasia. Acta Orthop. Scand., *58*:289.
150. Newman, A.J., & Melhorn, D.K. (1973). Vertebral compression in childhood leukemia. Am. J. Dis. Child., *125*:863.
151. Nicholas, J.A., Wilson, P.D., & Freiberger, R. (1960). Pathological fractures of the spine: Etiology and diagnosis. J. Bone Joint Surg. [Am.], *42*:127.
152. Norman, A., & Schiffman, M. (1977). Simple bone cysts: Factors of age dependency. Radiology, *124*:779.
153. Onuigbo, W.I. (1975). Recognition and treatment of pathologic fractures in the nineteenth century. Surgery, *77*:553.
154. Overgaard, M. (1988). Spontaneous radiation-induced rib fractures in breast cancer patients treated with postmastectomy irradiation. Acta Oncol., *27*:117.
155. Parfitt, A.M., Massry, S.G., & Winfield, A.C. (1972). Osteopenia and fractures occurring during maintenance hemodialysis. A new form of renal osteodystrophy. Clin. Orthop., *87*:287.
156. Piraino, B., Chen, T., Cooperstein, L. et al. (1988). Fractures and vertebral bone mineral density in patients with renal osteodystrophy. Clin. Nephrol., *30*:57.
157. Poigenfurst, J., Marcove, R.C., & Miller, T.R. (1968). Surgical treatment of fractures through metastases in the proximal femur. J. Bone Joint Surg. [Br.], *50*:743.
158. Pugh, J., Sherry, H.S., Futterman, B., & Frankel, V.H. (1982). Biomechanics of pathologic fractures. Clin. Orthop., *169*:109.w444.
159. Ragab, A.H., Frech, R.S., & Vietti, T.J. (1970). Osteoporotic fractures secondary to methotrexate therapy of acute leukemia in remission. Cancer, *25*:580.
160. Rappoport, A.S., Sosman, J.L., & Weissman, B.N. (1976). Spontaneous fractures of the olecranon process in rheumatoid arthritis. Radiology, *119*:83.
161. Resnick, D., & Cone, R. (1984). Pathological fractures in rheumatoid arthritis: Sites and mechanisms. Radiographics, *4*:549.
162. Sim, F.H., & Pritchard, D.J. (1982). Metastatic disease in the upper extremity. Clin. Orthop., *169*:83.
163. Simpson, W., Kerr, D.S., Hill, A.V.L., & Siddiqui, J.Y. (1973). Skeletal changes in patients on regular hemodialysis. Radiology, *107*:313.
164. Slavin, J.D. Jr., Yoosufani, Z., & Spencer, R.P. (1987). Bone scan spot from separation of osseous fragments in pathologic fracture. Clin. Nucl. Med., *12*:659.
165. Skinner, H.B., Harris, J.R., Cook, S.D. et al. (1983). Bilateral sequential tibial and fibular fatigue fractures associated with aluminum intoxication osteomalacia. J. Bone Joint Surg. [Am.], *65*:843.
166. Stern, P.J., & Weinberg, S. (1981). Pathological fracture of the radius through a cyst caused by pyrophosphate arthropathy. J. Bone Joint Surg. [Am.], *63*:1487.
167. Taylor, R.T., Huskisson, E.C., Whitehouse, G.H., & Hart, F.D. (1971). Spontaneous fractures of pelvis in rheumatoid arthritis. B.M.J., *4*:663.
168. Taylor, S.D., & Kelly, T.M. (1989). Prolactinoma in a middle-aged man with an osteoporotic fracture. West. J. Med., *151*:80.
169. Varmarken, J.E., Olsen, C.A., & Kristiansen, B. (1988). Multiple fractures in a young diabetic patient. Injury, *19*:285.
170. Watson, R.C., & Cahen, I. (1973). Pathological fracture in long bone sarcoidosis. J. Bone Joint Surg. [Am.], *55*:613.
171. Zickel, R.E., & Mouradian, W.H. (1976). Intramedullary fixation of pathologi-

cal fractures and lesions of the subtrochanteric region of the femur. J. Bone Joint Surg. [Am.], *58*:1061.
172. Zingraff, J., Drueke, T., Roux, J.-P. et al. (1974). Bilateral fracture of the femoral neck complicating uremic bone disease prior to chronic hemodialysis. Clin. Nephrol., *2*:73.

Normal Structures and Radiographic Phenomena Mimicking Fractures

173. Caffey, J. (1972). Pediatric X-Ray Diagnosis. 6th Ed. Year Book Medical Publishers, Chicago.
174. Eaglesham, D.C. (1968). Visual illusions affecting radiographic interpretation. J. Can. Assoc. Radiol., *19*:96.
175. Keats, T.E. (1996). Atlas of normal roentgen variants that may simulate disease. Sixth edition. Mosby–Year Book.
176. Schmidt, H., & Freyschmidt, J. (1992). Koehler/Zimmer Borderlands of Normal and Early Pathologic Findings in Skeletal Radiology. 4th Ed., rev. and enl. Thieme Medical Publishers, Stuttgart.

CT and MR Imaging

177. Coleman, B.G., Kressel, H.Y., Dalinka, M.K. et al. (1988). Radiographically negative avascular necrosis: Detection with MR imaging. Radiology, *168*:525.
178. Corcoran, R.J., Thrall, J.H., Kyle, R.W. et al. (1976). Solitary abnormalities in bone scans of patients with extraosseous malignancies. Radiology, *121*:663.
179. Deutsch, A.L., & Mink, J.H. (1989). Magnetic resonance imaging of musculoskeletal injuries. Radiol. Clin. North Am., *27*:983.
180. Deutsch, A.L., Mink, J.H., & Waxman, A.D. (1989). Occult fractures of the proximal femur: MR imaging. Radiology, *170*:113.
181. Fordham, E.W., & Ramachandran, P.C. (1974). Radionuclide imaging of osseous trauma. Semin. Nucl. Med., *4*:411.
182. Freedman, G.S. (1973). Radionuclide imaging of the injured patient. Radiol. Clin. North Am., *11*:461.
183. Genez, B.M., Wilson, M.R., Houk, R.W. et al. (1988). Early osteonecrosis of the femoral head: Detection in high-risk patients with MR imaging. Radiology, *168*:521.
184. Geslien, G.E., Thrall, J.H., Espinosa, J.L., & Older, R.A. (1976). Early detection of stress fractures using 99mTc-polyphosphate. Radiology, *121*:683.
185. Glickstein, M.F., Burk, K.L., Schiebler, M.L. et al. (1988). Avascular necrosis versus other diseases of the hip: Sensitivity of MR imaging. Radiology, *169*:213.
186. Goiney, R.C., Connell, D.G., & Nichols, D.M. (1985). CT evaluation of tarsometatarsal fracture-dislocation injuries. A.J.R. Am. J. Roentgenol., *144*:985.
187. Guyer, B.H., Levinsohn, E.M., Fredrickson, B.E. et al. (1985). Computed tomography of calcaneal fractures: Anatomy, pathology, dosimetry, and clinical relevance. A.J.R. Am. J. Roentgenol., *145*:911.
188. Guyon, J.J., Brant-Zawadzki, M., & Seiff, S.T. (1984). CT demonstration of optic canal fractures. A.J.R. Am. J. Roentgenol., *143*:1031.
189. Harley, H.D., Mack, L.A., & Winquist, R.A. (1982). CT of acetabular fracture: Comparison with conventional radiography. A.J.R. Am. J. Roentgenol., *138*:413.
190. Haus, A.G., Collins, P.A., & Rossmann, K. (1973). A method of measuring image degradation in tomography. Radiology, *109*:219.
191. Heger, L., Wulff, K., & Seddiqi, M.S. A. (1985). Computed tomography of calcaneal fractures. A.J.R. Am. J. Roentgenol., *145*:131.
192. Holland, B.A., & Brant-Zawadzki, M. (1984). High-resolution CT of temporal bone trauma. A.J.R. Am. J. Roentgenol., *143*:391.
193. Hughston, J.C. (1962). Acute knee injuries in athletes. Clin. Orthop., *23*:114.
194. Jacobson, H.G. Ed. (1989). Musculoskeletal applications of magnetic resonance imaging. J. A. M. A., *262*:2420.
195. Jaramillo, D., Hoffer, F.A., Shapiro, F., & Rand, F. (1990). MR imaging of fractures of the growth plate. A.J.R. Am. J. Roentgenol., *155*:1261.
196. Kattapuram, S.V., Khurana, J.S., Rosenthal, D.I., & Ehara, S. (1989). Musculoskeletal applications of MRI. Radiat. Med., *7*:47.
197. Kim, H., Thrall, J.H., & Keyes, J.W. (1979). Skeletal scintigraphy following incidental trauma. Radiology, *130*:447.
198. Kreipke, D.L., Moss, J.J., & Franco, J.M. (1984). Computed tomography and thin-section tomography in facial trauma. A.J.R. Am. J. Roentgenol., *142*:1041.
199. Lasda, N., Levinsohn, E.M., Yuan, H., & Bunnell, W. (1978). Computerized tomography in disorders of the hip. J. Bone Joint Surg. [Am.], *60*:1099.
200. Lauge-Hansen, N. (1949). Ligamentous ankle fractures: Diagnosis and treatment. Acta Chir. Scand., *97*:544.
201. Lee, J.K., & Yao, L. (1989). Occult intraosseous fracture: Magnetic resonance appearance versus age of injury. Am. J. Sports Med., *17*:620.
202. Lindsjo, U., Hemmingsson, A., Sahlstedt, B. et al. (1979). Computed tomography of the ankle. Acta Orthop. Scand., *50*:797.
203. Levinsohn, E.M., Bunnell, W., & Yuan, H. (1979). Computed tomography in the diagnosis of dislocations of the sternoclavicular joint. Clin. Orthop., *140*:12.
204. Magid, D., & Frishman, E.K. (1989). Imaging of musculoskeletal trauma in three dimensions: An integrated two-dimensional/three-dimensional approach with computed tomography. Radiol. Clin. North Am., *27*:945.
205. Matin, P. (1979). The appearance of bone scans following fractures, including intermediate and long-term studies. J. Nucl. Med., *20*:1227.
206. Mink, J.H., & Deutsch, A.L. (1989). Occult cartilage and bone injuries of the knee: Detection, classification, and assessment with MR imaging. Radiology, *170*:823.
207. Mitchell, D.G., Rao, V.M., Dalinka, M.K. et al. (1987). Femoral head avascular necrosis: Correlation of MR imaging, radiographic staging, radionuclide imaging, and clinical findings. Radiology, *162*:709.
208. Mitchell, M.D., Kundel, H.L., Steinberg, M.E. et al. (1986). Avascular necrosis of the hip: Comparison of MR, CT, and scintigraphy. A.J.R. Am. J. Roentgenol., *147*:67.
209. Patton, D.D., & Woolfenden, J.M. (1977). Radionuclide bone scanning in diseases of the spine. Radiol. Clin. North Am., *15*:177.
210. Pech, P., Kilgore, D.P., Pojunas, K.W., & Haughton, V.M. (1985). Cervical spinal fractures: CT detection. Radiology, *157*:117.
211. Pearson, J., & Hargadon, E. (1962). Fractures of the pelvis involving the floor of the acetabulum. J. Bone Joint Surg. [Br.], *44*:550.
212. Prather, J.L., Nusynowitz, M.L., Sowdy, H.A. et al. (1977). Scintigraphic findings in stress fractures. J. Bone Joint Surg. [Am.], *59*:869.
213. Rafii, M., Firooznia, H., Golimbu, C., & Bonamo, J. (1984). Computed tomography of tibial plateau fractures. A.J.R. Am. J. Roentgenol., *142*:1181.
214. Rosenthall, L., Hill, R.O., & Chuang, S. (1976). Observation on the use of ^{99m}Tc-phosphate imaging in peripheral bone trauma. Radiology, *119*:637.
215. Shirazi, P.H., Rayudu, G.V.S., & Fordham, E.W. (1974). Review of solitary ^{18}F bone scan lesions. Radiology, *112*:369.
216. Shirkhoda, A., Brashear, H.R., & Staab, E. (1980). Computed tomography of acetabular fractures. Radiology, *134*:683.
217. Smith, G., & Loop, J. (1976). Radiologic classification of posterior dislocation of the hip: Refinements and pitfalls. Radiology, *119*:569.
218. Stark, P., & Jaramillo, D. (1986). CT of the sternum. A.J.R. Am. J. Roentgenol., *147*:72.
219. Totty, W.G., Murphy, W.A., Ganz, W.I. et al. (1984). Magnetic resonance imaging of the normal and ischemic femoral head. A.J.R. Am. J. Roentgenol., *143*:1273.
220. Wilcox, J.R., Moniot, A.L., & Green, J.P. (1977). Bone scanning in the evaluation of exercise-related stress injuries. Radiology, *123*:699.
221. Yao, L., & Lee, J.K. (1988). Occult intraosseous fracture detection with MR imaging. Radiology, *167*:749.
222. Young, J.W.R., & Resnik, C.S. (1990). Fracture of the pelvis: Current concepts of classification. A.J.R. Am. J. Roentgenol., *155*:1169.

Interpretation and Technique of Examination

223. ACR Appropriateness Criteria for Imaging and Treatment Decisions (1998). ACR Website Ed. American College of Radiology, Reston, Va.
224. Adamson, G.J., Wiss, D.A., Lowery, G.L., & Peters, C.L. (1992). Type II floating knee: Ipsilateral femoral and tibial fractures with intraarticular extension into the knee joint. J. Orthop. Trauma, *6*:333.
225. Adler, R.S. (1999). Future and new developments in musculoskeletal ultrasound. Radiol. Clin. North Am., *37*:623.
226. Aideyan, U.O., Berbaum, K., & Smith, W.L. (1995). Influence of prior radiologic information on the interpretation of radiographic examinations. Acad. Radiol., *2*:205.
227. Alanen, V., Taimela, S., Kinnunen, J. et al. (1998). Incidence and clinical significance of bone bruises after supination injury of the ankle. A double-blind, prospective study. J. Bone Joint Surg. [Br.], *80*:513.
228. Andersen, D.J., Blair, W.F., Steyers, C.M. Jr. et al. (1996). Classification of distal radius fractures: An analysis of interobserver reliability and intraobserver reproducibility.: J. Hand Surg. [Am.], *21*:574.
229. Andersen, E., Jorgensen, L.G., & Hededam, L.T. (1990). Evans' classification of trochanteric fractures: An assessment of the interobserver and intraobserver reliability. Injury, *21*:377.
230. Ashman C.J., Yu J.S., Wolfman, D. (2000). Satisfaction of search in osteoradiology. A.J.R. Am. J. Roentegenol., *175*:541.
231. Bansal, V.P., Singhal, V., Mam, M.K., & Gill, S.S. (1984). The floating knee. 40 cases of ipsilateral fractures of the femur and the tibia. Int. Orthop., *8*:183.
232. Bauer, S.J., Hollander, J.E., Fuchs, S.H., & Thode, H.C. Jr. (1995). A clinical decision rule in the evaluation of acute knee injuries. J. Emerg. Med., *13*:611.
233. Berbaum, K.S., Franken, E.A. Jr., & el-Khoury, G.Y. (1989). Impact of clinical history on radiographic detection of fractures: A comparison of radiologists and orthopedists. A.J.R. Am. J. Roentgenol., *153*:1221.
234. Berbaum, K.S., Franken, E.A. Jr., Dorfman, D.D. et al. (1990). Satisfaction of search in diagnostic radiology. Invest. Radiol., *25*:133.
235. Berbaum, K.S., Franken, E.A. Jr., Dorfman, D.D. et al. (1991). Time course of satisfaction of search. Invest. Radiol., *26*:640.
236. Berbaum, K.S., Franken, E.A. Jr., Anderson, K.L. et al. (1993). The influence of clinical history on visual search with single and multiple abnormalities. Invest. Radiol., *28*:191.
237. Berger, P.E., Ofstein, R.A., Jackson, D.W. et al. (1989). MRI demonstration of radiographically occult fractures. What have we been missing? Radiographics, 9:407.
238. Berne, J.D., Velmahos, G.C., El-Tawil, Q. et al. (1999). Value of complete cervical helical computed tomographic scanning in identifying cervical spine injury in the unevaluable blunt trauma patient with multiple injuries: A prospective study. J. Trauma, *47*:896.
239. Bernstein, J., Monaghan, B.A., Silber, J.S., & DeLong, W.G. (1997). Taxon-

omy and treatment—a classification of fracture classifications. J. Bone Joint Surg. [Br.], *79*:706.
240. Blab, E., Geissler, W., & Rokitansky, A. (1999). Sonographic management of infantile clavicular fractures. Pediatr. Surg. Int., *15*:251.
241. Blackmore, C.C., Ramsey, S.D., Mann, F.A., & Deyo, R.A. (1999). Cervical spine screening with CT in trauma patients: A cost-effectiveness analysis. Radiology, *212*:117.
242. Blacksin, M.F., & Lee, H.J. (1995). Frequency and significance of fractures of the upper cervical spine detected by CT in patients with severe neck trauma. A.J.R. Am. J. Roentgenol., *165*:1201.
243. Blomlie, V., Lien, H.H., Iversen, T. et al. (1993). Radiation-induced insufficiency fractures of the sacrum: Evaluation with MR imaging. Radiology, *188*:241.
244. Bloom, A.I., Neeman, Z., Slasky, B.S. et al. (1997). Fracture of the occipital condyles and associated craniocervical ligament injury: Incidence, CT imaging and implications. Clin. Radiol., *52*:198.
245. Bohndorf, K. (1999). Imaging of acute injuries of the articular surfaces (chondral, osteochondral and subchondral fractures). Skeletal Radiol., *28*:545.
246. Boutin, R.D., Briggs, J.E., & Williamson, M.R. (1994). Injuries associated with MR imaging: Survey of safety records and methods used to screen patients for metallic foreign bodies before imaging. A.J.R. Am. J. Roentgenol., *162*:189.
247. Brage, M.E., Rockett, M., Vraney, R. et al. (1998). Ankle fracture classification: A comparison of reliability of three X-ray views versus two. Foot Ankle Int., *19*:555.
248. Calhoun, P.S., Kuszyk, B.S., Heath, D.G. et al. (1999). Three-dimensional volume rendering of spiral CT data: Theory and method. Radiographics, *19*:745.
249. Carey, J., Spence, L., Blickman, H., & Eustace, S. (1998). MRI of pediatric growth plate injury: Correlation with plain film radiographs and clinical outcome. Skeletal Radiol., *27*:250.
250. Chen, C.E., & Wang, J.W. (1998). Floating knee with ipsilateral knee dislocation: Case report. J. Trauma, *44*:735.
251. Daffner, R.H. (1989). Visual illusions in the interpretation of the radiographic image. Curr. Probl. Diagn. Radiol., *18*:62.
252. Daffner, R.H. (1980). Visual illusions in computed tomography: Phenomena related to Mach effect. A.J.R. Am. J. Roentgenol., *134*:261.
253. Dhawan, A., & Hospodar, P.P. (1999). Suture fixation as a treatment for acute traumatic osteochondral lesions. Arthroscopy, *15*:307.
254. Dirschl, D.R., & Adams, G.L. (1997). A critical assessment of factors influencing reliability in the classification of fractures, using fractures of the tibial plafond as a model. J. Orthop. Trauma, *11*:471.
255. Elmquist, C., Shellock, F.G., & Stoller, D. (1995). Screening adolescents for metallic foreign bodies before MR procedures. J. Magn. Reson. Imaging, *5*:784.
256. Elster, A.D., Link, K.M., & Carr, J.J. (1994). Patient screening prior to MR imaging: A practical approach synthesized from protocols at 15 U.S. medical centers. A.J.R. Am. J. Roentgenol., *162*:195.
257. Eustace, S.J., (1999). Magnetic resonance imaging of orthopedic trauma. p. 57. Lippincott Williams & Wilkins, Philadelphia.
258. Evans, M.C., & Graham, H.K. (1999). Olecranon fractures in children: Part 1: A clinical review; Part 2: A new classification and management algorithm. J. Pediatr. Orthop., *19*:559.
259. Flinkkila, T., Raatikainen, T., & Hamalainen, M. (1998). AO and Frykman's classifications of Colles' fracture. No prognostic value in 652 patients evaluated after 5 years. Acta Orthop. Scand., *69*:77.
260. Gehrchen, P.M., Nielsen, J.O., Olesen, B., & Andresen, B.K. (1997). Seinsheimer's classification of subtrochanteric fractures. Poor reproducibility of 4 observers' evaluation of 50 cases. Acta Orthop. Scand., *68*:524.
261. Gehrchen, P.M., Nielsen, J.O., & Olesen, B. (1993). Poor reproducibility of Evans' classification of the trochanteric fracture. Assessment of 4 observers in 52 cases. Acta Orthop. Scand., *64*:71.
262. Graham, I.D., Stiell, I.G., Laupacis, A. et al. (1998). Emergency physicians' attitudes toward and use of clinical decision rules for radiography. Acad. Emerg. Med., *5*:134.
263. Grangier, C., Garcia, J., Howarth, N.R. et al. (1997). Role of MRI in the diagnosis of insufficiency fractures of the sacrum and acetabular roof. Skeletal Radiol., *26*:517.
264. Grechenig, W., Clement, H.G., Fellinger, M., & Seggl, W. (1998). Scope and limitations of ultrasonography in the documentation of fractures—An experimental study. Arch. Orthop. Trauma Surg., *117*:368.
265. Gregersen, H.E., & Rasmussen, O.S. (1989). Ultrasonography of osteochondritis dissecans of the knee: A preliminary report. Acta Radiol., *30*:552.
266. Griffith, J.F., Rainer, T.H., Ching, A.S. et al. (1999). Sonography compared with radiography in revealing acute rib fracture. A.J.R. Am. J. Roentgenol., *173*:1603.
267. Grossman, M.D., Reilly, P.M., Gillett, T., & Gillett, D. (1999). National survey of the incidence of cervical spine injury and approach to cervical spine clearance in U.S. trauma centers. J. Trauma, *47*:684.
268. Hosono, M., Kobayashi, H., Fujimoto, R. et al. (1997). MR appearance of parasymphyseal insufficiency fractures of the os pubis. Skeletal Radiol., *26*:525.
269. Illarramendi, A., Gonzalez Della Valle, A., Segal, E. et al. (1998). Evaluation of simplified Frykman and AO classifications of fractures of the distal radius. Assessment of interobserver and intraobserver agreement. Int. Orthop., *22*:111.
270. Jackson, J.G., & Acker, J.D. (1987). Permanent eyeliner and MR imaging. A.J.R. Am. J. Roentgenol., *149*:1080.
271. Johnson, D.L., Urban, W.P. Jr., Caborn, D.N. et al. (1998). Articular cartilage changes seen with magnetic resonance imaging–detected bone bruises associated with acute anterior cruciate ligament rupture. Am. J. Sports Med., *26*:409.
272. Kanal, E., & Shellock, F.G. (1998). MRI interaction with tattoo pigments. Plast. Reconstr. Surg., *101*:1150.
273. Kanal, E., & Shellock, F.G. (1992). Policies, guidelines, and recommendations for MR imaging safety and patient management. SMRI Safety Committee. J. Magn. Reson. Imaging., *2*:247.
274. Katz, M.A., Beredjiklian, P.K., Vresilovic, E.J. et al. (1999). Computed tomographic scanning of cervical spine fractures: Does it influence treatment? J. Orthop. Trauma, *13*:338.
275. Katz, R., Landman, J., Dulitzky, F., & Bar-Ziv, J. (1988). Fracture of the clavicle in the newborn. An ultrasound diagnosis. J. Ultrasound Med., *7*:21.
276. Keats, T.E. (1996). Atlas of Normal Roentgen Variants That May Simulate Disease. 6th Ed. Mosby–Year Book, St. Louis.
277. Labovitz, J.M., & Schweitzer, M.E. (1998). Occult osseous injuries after ankle sprains: Incidence, location, pattern, and age. Foot Ankle Int., *19*:661.
278. Lane, E.J., Proto, A.V., & Phillips, T.W. (1976). Mach bands and density perception. Radiology, *121*:9.
279. Laorr, A., Greenspan, A., Anderson, M.W. et al. (1995). Traumatic hip dislocation: Early MRI findings. Skeletal Radiol., *24*:239.
280. LeBlang, S.D., & Nunez, D.B. Jr. (1999). Helical CT of cervical spine and soft tissue injuries of the neck. Radiol. Clin. North Am., *37*:515.
281. Lee, S.I., & Chew, F.S. (1998). Radiology in the emergency department: Technique for quantitative description of use and results. A.J.R. Am. J. Roentgenol., *171*:559.
282. Lund, P.J., Krupinski, E.A., Pereles, S., & Mockbee, B. (1997). Comparison of conventional and computed radiography: Assessment of image quality and reader performance in skeletal extremity trauma. Acta Radiol., *4*:570.
283. Lund, P.J., Nisbet, J.K., Valencia, F.G., & Ruth, J.T. (1996). Current sonographic applications in orthopedics. A.J.R. Am. J. Roentgenol., *166*:889.
284. Maffulli, N., & Thornton, A. (1995). Ultrasonographic appearance of external callus in long-bone fractures. Injury, *26*:5.
285. Mammone, J.F., & Schweitzer, M.E. (1995). MRI of occult sacral insufficiency fractures following radiotherapy. Skeletal Radiol., *24*:101.
286. Markert, R.J., Walley, M.E., Guttman, T.G., & Mehta, R. (1998). A pooled analysis of the Ottawa ankle rules used on adults in the ED. Am. J. Emerg. Med., *16*:564.
287. Martin, J.S., & Marsh, J.L. (1997). Current classification of fractures. Rationale and utility. Radiol. Clin. North Am., *35*:491.
288. Martin, J.S., Marsh, J.L., Bonar, S.K. et al. (1997). Assessment of the AO/ASIF fracture classification for the distal tibia. J. Orthop. Trauma, *11*:477.
289. Mathis, C.E., Noonan, K., & Kayes, K. (1998). "Bone bruises" of the knee: A review. Iowa Orthop. J., *18*:112.
290. Milgram, J.W., Rogers, L.F., & Miller, J.W. (1978). Osteochondral fractures: Mechanisms of injury and fate of fragments. A.J.R. Am. J. Roentgenol., *130*:651.
291. Miller, M.D., Osborne, J.R., Gordon, W.T. et al. (1998). The natural history of bone bruises. A prospective study of magnetic resonance imaging–detected trabecular microfractures in patients with isolated medial collateral ligament injuries. Am. J. Sports Med., *26*:15.
292. Minas, T. (1999). The role of cartilage repair techniques, including chondrocyte transplantation, in focal chondral knee damage. Instr. Course Lect., *48*:629.
293. Mink, J.H., & Deutsch, A.L. (1989). Occult cartilage and bone injuries of the knee: Detection, classification, and assessment with MR imaging. Radiology, *170*:823.
294. Mlinek, E.J., Clark, K.C., & Walker, C.W. (1998). Limited magnetic resonance imaging in the diagnosis of occult hip fractures. Am. J. Emerg. Med., *16*:390.
295. Muller, E.J., Siebenrock, K., Ekkernkamp, A. et al. (1999). Ipsilateral fractures of the pelvis and the femur—floating hip? A retrospective analysis of 42 cases. Arch. Orthop. Trauma Surg., *119*:179.
296. Mumber, M.P., Greven, K.M., & Haygood, T.M. (1997). Pelvic insufficiency fractures associated with radiation atrophy: Clinical recognition and diagnostic evaluation. Skeletal Radiol., *26*:94.
297. Nielsen, J.O., Dons-Jensen, H., & Sorensen, H.T. (1990). Lauge-Hansen classification of malleolar fractures. An assessment of the reproducibility in 118 cases. Acta Orthop. Scand., *61*:385.
298. Nishimura, G., Yamato, M., & Togawa, M. (1996). Trabecular trauma of the talus and medial malleolus concurrent with lateral collateral ligamentous injuries of the ankle: Evaluation with MR imaging. Skeletal Radiol., 25:49.
299. Nodine, C.F., & Krupinski, E.A. (1998). Perceptual skill, radiology expertise, and visual test performance with NINA and WALDO. Acad. Radiol., *5*:603.
300. Novelline, R.A., Rhea, J.T., Rao, P.M., & Stuk, J.L. (1999). Helical CT in emergency radiology. Radiology, *213*:321.
301. O'Connor, P.J., Davies, A.G., Fowler, R.C. et al. (1998). Reporting requirements for skeletal digital radiography: Comparison of soft-copy and hard-copy presentation. Radiology, *207*:249.
302. Otte, M.T., Helms, C.A., & Fritz, R.C. (1997). MR imaging of supra-acetabular insufficiency fractures. Skeletal Radiol., *26*:279.

303. Palmer, W.E., Levine, S.M., & Dupuy, D.E. (1997). Knee and shoulder fractures: Association of fracture detection and marrow edema on MR images with mechanism of injury. Radiology, *204*:395.
304. Pandey, R., McNally, E., Ali, A., & Bulstrode, C. (1998). The role of MRI in the diagnosis of occult hip fractures. Injury, *29*:61.
305. Patten, R.M., Mack, L.A., Wang, K.Y., & Lingel, J. (1992). Nondisplaced fractures of the greater tuberosity of the humerus: Sonographic detection. Radiology, *182*:201.
306. Pessoa, L. (1996). Mach bands: How many models are possible? Recent experimental findings and modeling attempts. Vision Res., *36*:3205.
307. Piraino, D.W., Davros, W.J., Lieber, M. et al. (1999). Selenium-based digital radiography versus conventional film-screen radiography of the hands and feet: A subjective comparison. A.J.R. Am. J. Roentgenol., *172*:177.
308. Plint, A.C., Bulloch, B., Osmond, M.H. et al. (1999). Validation of the Ottawa Ankle Rules in children with ankle injuries. Acad. Emerg. Med., *6*:1005.
309. Pohost, G.M., Blackwell, G.G., & Shellock, F.G. (1992). Safety of patients with medical devices during application of magnetic resonance methods. Ann. N. Y. Acad. Sci., *649*:302.
310. Pretorius, E.S., & Fishman, E.K. (1999). Volume rendered three-dimensional spiral CT: Musculoskeletal applications. Radiographics, *19*:1143.
311. Rangger, C., Kathrein, A., Freund, M.C. et al. (1998). Bone bruise of the knee: Histology and cryosections in 5 cases. Acta Orthop. Scand., *69*:291.
312. Raskin, K.B. (1999). Management of fractures of the distal radius: Surgeon's perspective. J. Hand Ther., *12*:92.
313. Rickett, A.B., Finlay, D.B., & Jagger, C. (1992). The importance of clinical details when reporting accident and emergency radiographs. Injury, *23*:458.
314. Rosenthal, D.I., Christensen, S., & Emerson, R.H. (1994). "Handedness" of spiral fractures of the tibia. Skeletal Radiol., *11*:128.
315. Rubin, D.A. (1998). Magnetic resonance imaging of chondral and osteochondral injuries. Magn. Reson. Imaging, *9*:348.
316. Rubin, S.J., Marquardt, J.D., Gottlieb, R.H. et al. (1998). Magnetic resonance imaging: A cost-effective alternative to bone scintigraphy in the evaluation of patients with suspected hip fractures. Skeletal Radiol., *27*:199.
317. Salt, P., & Clancy, M. (1997). Implementation of the Ottawa Ankle Rules by nurses working in an accident and emergency department. J. Accid. Emerg. Med., *14*:363.
318. Sarup, S., & Bryant, P.A. (1997). Ipsilateral humeral shaft and Galeazzi fractures with a posterolateral dislocation of the elbow: A variant of the "floating dislocated elbow." J. Trauma, *43*:349.
319. Schmidt, H., & Freyschmidt, J. (1992). Koehler/Zimmer Borderlands of Normal and Early Pathologic Findings in Skeletal Radiology. 4th Ed., rev. and enl. Thieme Medical Publishers, Stuttgart.
320. Schweitzer, M.E., & White, L.M. (1996). Does altered biomechanics cause marrow edema? Radiology, *198*:851.
321. Seaberg, D.C., Yealy, D.M., Lukens, T. et al. (1998). Multicenter comparison of two clinical decision rules for the use of radiography in acute, high-risk knee injuries. Ann. Emerg. Med., *32*:8.
322. Sidor, M.L., Zuckerman, J.D., Lyon, T. et al. (1993). The Neer classification system for proximal humeral fractures. An assessment of interobserver reliability and intraobserver reproducibility. J. Bone Joint Surg. [Am.], *75*:1745.
323. Siebenrock, K.A., & Gerber, C. (1993). The reproducibility of classification of fractures of the proximal end of the humerus. J. Bone Joint Surg. [Am.], *75*:1751.
324. Simpson, N.S., & Jupiter, J.B. (1995). Complex fracture patterns of the upper extremity. Clin. Orthop., *Sept*:43.
325. Sjoden, G.O., Movin, T., Aspelin, P. et al. (1999). 3D-radiographic analysis does not improve the Neer and AO classifications of proximal humeral fractures. Acta Orthop. Scand., *70*:325.
326. Sjoden, G.O., Movin, T., Guntner, P. et al. (1997). Poor reproducibility of classification of proximal humeral fractures. Additional CT of minor value. Acta Orthop. Scand., *68*:239.
327. Soudry, G., & Mannting, F. (1995). Hot calcaneus on three-phase bone scan due to bone bruise. Clin. Nucl. Med., *20*:832.
328. Stiell, I.G., Greenberg, G.H., Wells, G.A. et al. (1996). Prospective validation of a decision rule for the use of radiography in acute knee injuries. J. A. M. A., *275*:611.
329. Stiell, I.G., Greenberg, G.H., McKnight, R.D. et al. (1993). Decision rules for the use of radiography in acute ankle injuries. Refinement and prospective validation. J. A. M. A., *269*:1127.
330. Stiell, I.G., Greenberg, G.H., McKnight, R.D. et al. (1992). A study to develop clinical decision rules for the use of radiography in acute ankle injuries. Ann. Emerg. Med., *21*:384.
331. Swensson, R.G., Hessel, S.J., & Herman, P.G. (1985). The value of searching films without specific preconceptions. Invest. Radiol., *20*:100.
332. Takahara, M., Ogino, T., Tsuchida, H. et al. (2000). Sonographic assessment of osteochondritis dissecans of the humeral capitellum. A.J.R. Am. J. Roentgenol., *174*:411.
333. Tan, E., Schweitzer, M.E., Vaccaro, L., & Spetell, A.C. (1999). Is computed tomography of nonvisualized C7–T1 cost-effective? J. Spinal Disord., *12*:472.
334. Tandeter, H.B., & Shvartzman, P. (1999). Acute knee injuries: Use of decision rules for selective radiograph ordering. Am. Fam. Physician, *60*:2599.
335. Tandeter, H.B., & Shvartzman, P. (1997). Acute ankle injuries: Clinical decision rules for radiographs. Am. Fam. Physician, *55*:2721.
336. Thomsen, N.O., Jensen, C.M., Skovgaard, N. et al. (1996). Observer variation in the radiographic classification of fractures of the neck of the femur using Garden's system. Int. Orthop., *20*:326.
337. Thomsen, N.O., Overgaard, S., Olsen, L.H. et al. (1991). Observer variation in the radiographic classification of ankle fractures. J. Bone Joint Surg. [Br.], *73*:676.
338. Tigges, S., Pitts, S., Mukundan, S. Jr. et al. (1999). External validation of the Ottawa knee rules in an urban trauma center in the United States. A.J.R. Am. J. Roentgenol., *172*:1069.
339. Van Raay, J.J., Raaymakers, E.L., & Dupree, H.W. (1991). Knee ligament injuries combined with ipsilateral tibial and femoral diaphyseal fractures: The "floating knee." Arch. Orthop. Trauma Surg., *110*:75.
340. Veith, R.G., Winquist, R.A., & Hansen, S.T. Jr. (1984). Ipsilateral fractures of the femur and tibia. A report of fifty-seven consecutive cases. J. Bone Joint Surg. [Am.], *66*:991.
341. Verma, S., Hamilton, K., Hawkins, H.H. et al. (1997). Clinical application of the Ottawa ankle rules for the use of radiography in acute ankle injuries: An independent site assessment. A.J.R. Am. J. Roentgenol., *169*:825.
342. Wang, C.L., Shieh, J.Y., Wang, T.G., & Hsieh, F.J. (1999). Sonographic detection of occult fractures in the foot and ankle. J. Clin. Ultrasound, *27*:421.
343. Weiss, R.A., Saint-Louis, L.A., Haik, B.G. et al. (1989). Mascara and eyelining tattoos: MRI artifacts. Ann. Ophthalmol., *21*:129.
344. Wilson, A.J., & Hodge, J.C. (1995). Digitized radiographs in skeletal trauma: A performance comparison between a digital workstation and the original film images. Radiology, *196*:565.
345. Yao, L., & Lee, J.K. (1988). Occult intraosseous fracture: Detection with MR imaging. Radiology, *167*:749.

Chapter 5

SPECIAL CONSIDERATIONS IN CHILDREN

with Sam T. Auringer, MD

There are appreciable differences among adults and infants, children, and adolescents in the manifestation of skeletal injury. The young are generally more agile and more able to avoid injury. The forces generated by falls and other accidents are not as great, because they weigh less and the leverage factor is reduced because of their shorter stature. Differences in bone structure and composition result in distinct biomechanical properties. The presence of growth centers not only modifies the skeletal response to traumatic forces but heightens the concern of parents and physicians because of the potential for growth disturbance.

The skeleton of the young is less brittle. It is more porous, the haversian canals are relatively larger, and the bones contain more water. The mineral content of growing bone is slightly less than that of the mature skeleton[45, 46, 49, 54] (Fig. 5–1). These factors result in the greater elasticity and plasticity of the growing skeleton. The differences are attributed more to the increased porosity and wetness than to the lesser mineral content[52] (Fig. 5–2). In addition, the periosteum is thicker, more elastic, and less firmly bound to bone. The periosteum is more likely to remain at least partially intact and attached to the fracture fragments, discouraging soft tissue interposition. This periosteum thus serves as a hinge between fragments, aiding materially in the reduction and stabilization of the fracture (see Fig. 5–13). Nonunion is quite rare.

Fractures constitute 10% to 25% of all pediatric injuries and are more common in boys than in girls. Playing accidents and sports-related activities are the cause of injury in the majority of fractures. The fracture rate is lower in late fall and winter and generally increases from May to October. Fractures most commonly occur in the late afternoon. The frequency of children's fractures has been clearly correlated with hours of available sunshine and play times.[56] Fractures of the distal forearm are the most frequent in childhood, accounting for nearly 25% of all fractures, followed by those of the phalanges (18.9%), the carpus and metacarpals (8.3%), and the clavicle (8.1%).[48]

An anteroposterior (AP) and a lateral radiograph will be sufficient except about joints, particularly the ankle, elbow, hand, and wrist, where oblique views are required.[55] Those physicians who practice outside pediatric centers may have limited experience with pediatric skeletal trauma, and the diagnosis can be more difficult.[13] Less experienced observers may require radiographs of the contralateral side for comparison. These films need not be obtained routinely, however.

As in adults, the presence of a joint effusion or hemarthrosis may point to an underlying, otherwise obscure injury. Joint effusions are most helpful in the elbow (Fig. 5–3), ankle, and knee. The reported incidence of fractures on follow-up examination in those patients who have a joint effusion on the initial examination varies widely.[14] Joint fluid without visible fracture is most likely to be identified in the elbow and ankle. The rate of initial detection varies with the experience of the observer and the use of oblique radiographs (see Fig. 5–3) and comparison views of the opposite extremity. The probability of detecting fractures on follow-up films is higher in those patients in whom comparison views were not taken or whose radiographs were not read by experienced observers. When a joint effusion is noted and no fracture is detected, a repeat examination in 7 to 10 days should be considered and performed in those children who have continued symptoms. In as many as half of the cases the symptoms will clear and additional radiographs are unwarranted. In more severe injuries and when symptoms persist, follow-up should be obtained. Thus, the presence of fluid in a joint or a joint effusion alerts the examiner to the possibility of an underlying bone injury; however, the probability of detecting fractures on follow-up films is relatively low, assuming that there has been a thorough examination initially.

Greenstick, Torus, and Bowing Fractures

The difference in biomechanical properties of bone gives rise to forms of incomplete fracture[26, 29, 35, 40] that are peculiar to children (Fig. 5–4). These are generally classified broadly as greenstick fractures,[44, 51, 52, 53] consisting of the classic greenstick, torus, and bowing varieties.

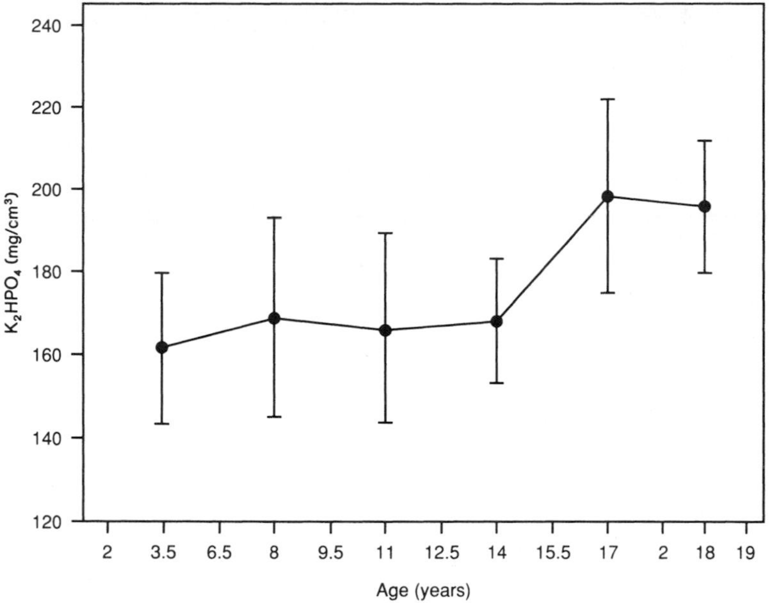

Figure 5–1. Vertebral bone density in children: The mean and standard deviation of trabecular bone density for children 2 to 19 years of age as determined by quantitative computed tomography (QCT). Bone mineral density is low during childhood but increases significantly at the time of puberty. (From Gilsanz, V., Gibbens, D. T., Roe, T. F., et al. [1988]. Vertebral bone density in children: Effect of puberty. Radiology, *166*:847, with permission.)

Classic Greenstick Fracture

The classic greenstick fracture (Figs. 5–4 and 5–5; see also Fig. 5–8) is the result of bending or angulation forces that place the convex side of the bone in tension and the opposite cortex or concave side in compression. These forces result in a fracture that is analogous to the break resulting from bending a green stick or twig. An incomplete transverse fracture is produced in the convex cortex by the tension forces and usually extends to the middle of the shaft, involving about one half the circumference of the bone. The fracture line may then turn at right angles to create a vertical or longitudinal split in either the proximal or distal component of the shaft, or in both. The concave cortex remains bent or bowed to a variable degree but is otherwise intact. These fractures are most common in the shafts of the radius and ulna and the clavicle.

Torus Fracture

The torus fracture (Fig. 5–6; see also Fig. 5–4) is a buckling of the cortex produced by compression forces.[50] A similar deformity may be produced in a green stick or twig by jamming its end into a hard surface. *Torus* is a Greek word meaning "round swelling." It is an architectural term used to designate the cap at the top or the

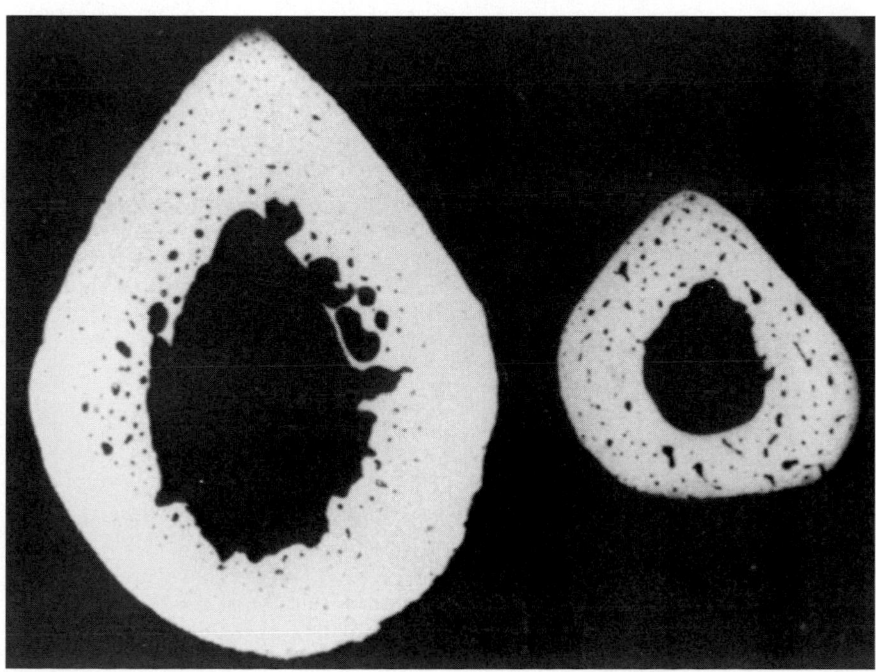

Figure 5–2. Microradiograph of the distal radial diaphysis of an adult and that of a child at 8 years of age. Children's bones are more porous than those of adults. Note the larger haversian canals in the child. (From Rang, M. [1983]. Children's Fractures. J. B. Lippincott, Philadelphia, with permission.)

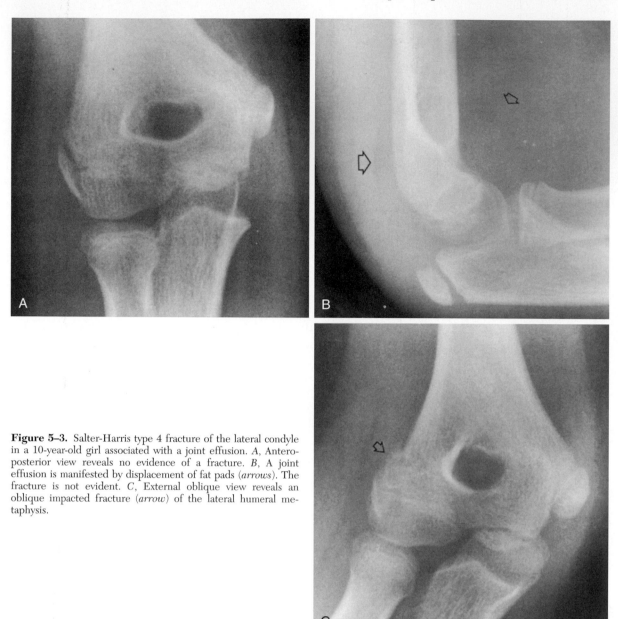

Figure 5–3. Salter-Harris type 4 fracture of the lateral condyle in a 10-year-old girl associated with a joint effusion. *A*, Anteroposterior view reveals no evidence of a fracture. *B*, A joint effusion is manifested by displacement of fat pads (*arrows*). The fracture is not evident. *C*, External oblique view reveals an oblique impacted fracture (*arrow*) of the lateral humeral metaphysis.

base of a Greek column. The degree of cortical buckling is variable, and at times the buckling may be quite subtle and easily overlooked. Such fractures almost always occur at the ends of long bones, in the metaphysis, and are best visualized in profile. It is important to keep in mind that the metaphysis of all long bones is gently flared or fluted, like the end of a musical horn. Torus fractures disrupt this smooth arc, and any irregularity in this flare must be viewed with suspicion. A series of microfractures in the crystalline structure of young bone allows cortical buckling to occur without the appearance of a lucent fracture line or obvious separation of fragments. In fact, impaction of fragments may give a slight, hazy increase in density to the fracture when viewed *en face*. These fractures are most frequently encountered in the distal radius and ulna and less commonly in the tibia and elsewhere.

A lead pipe fracture (Fig. 5–7; see also Fig. 5–4) is a combination of an incomplete transverse fracture of one cortex and a torus fracture of the contralateral side.[29] This injury is analogous to the deformity or fracture that occurs in a pipe made of lead when it is suddenly and forcefully bent. These fractures are relatively uncommon. They occur in the metaphysis in locations similar to those of torus fractures.

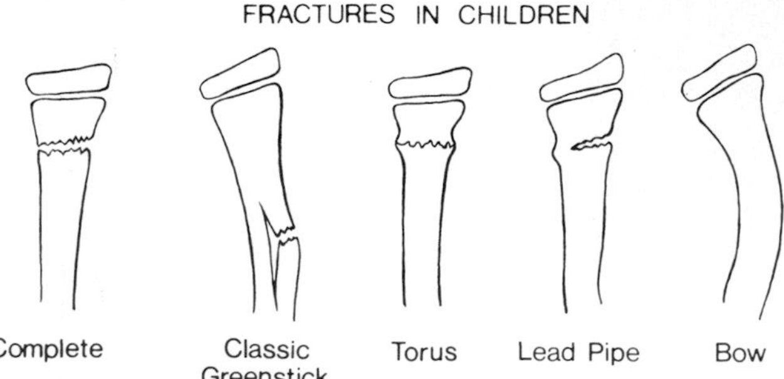

Figure 5–4. Types of fractures in children.

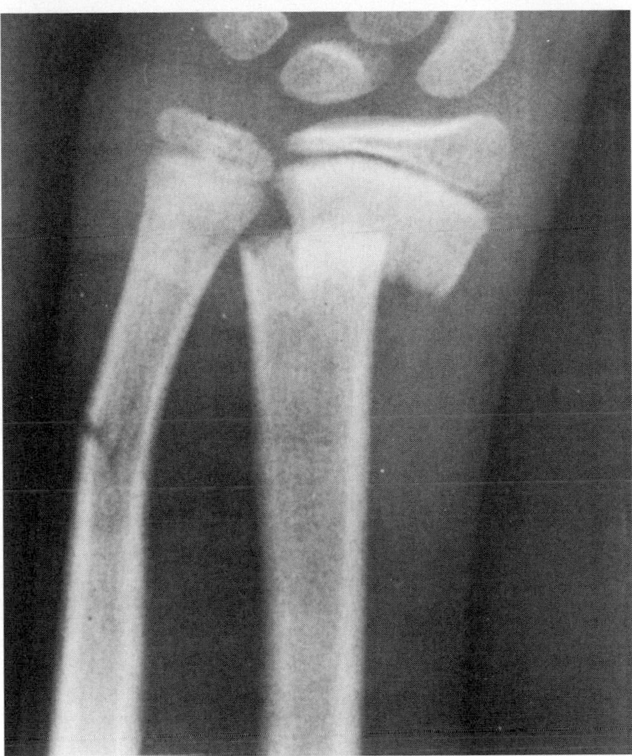

Figure 5–5. Greenstick fracture of the ulna and complete fracture of the distal radius in a 10-year-old boy. The convex cortex of the ulna is disrupted, and the fracture line extends across approximately 50% of the shaft and then turns at a right angle to create a longitudinal split. The concave cortex is bent but intact.

Bow Fracture

Young bones may be bent as a result of angulation and compressive forces without any of the generally expected radiographic evidence of fracture. The resultant bend or bow (see Fig. 5–4) usually affects the entire length of the bone in a broad curve, most commonly the radius, ulna (Fig. 5–8), and fibula (Fig. 5–9). These fractures are called bow or plastic bowing fractures.[5, 12, 26, 39, 57] They may easily be overlooked unless the observer is aware of this possibility or has comparison views of the contralateral side available. Scintigraphy[62] demonstrates diffuse increased activity in a major portion of the diaphysis over the length of bone.

Bow fractures are a manifestation of plastic deformation[5, 12, 52, 66] as visualized on a stress-strain curve (Fig. 5–10); the forces involved exceed the range of elastic strain that allows complete recovery of normal shape but are less than those required for the appearance of a frank complete or incomplete fracture. Histologically, in

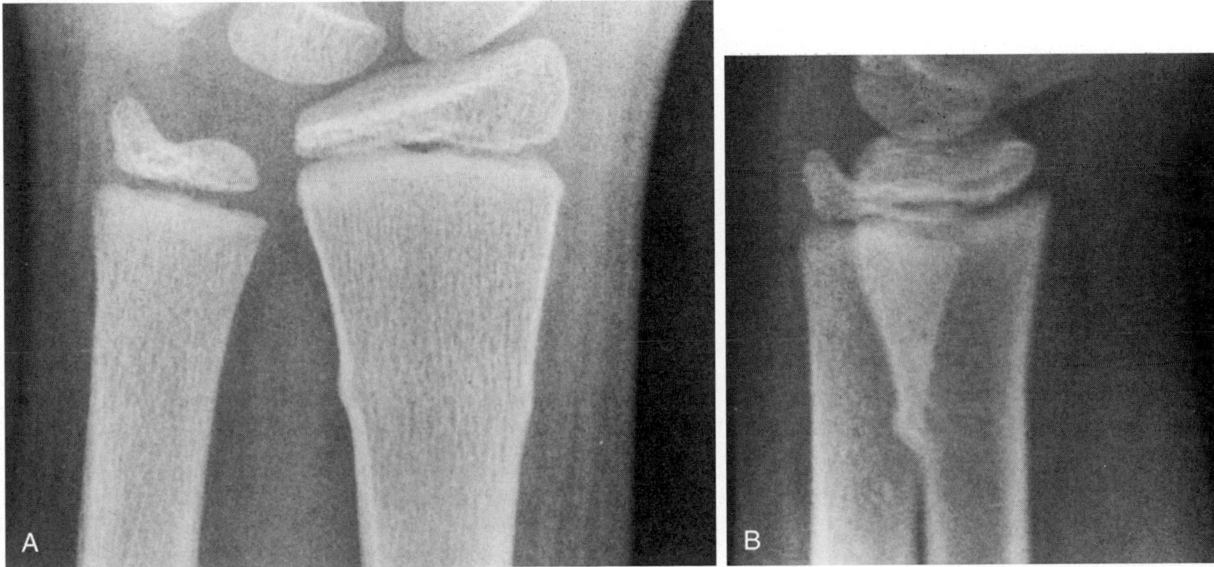

Figure 5–6. Torus fracture of the distal radius in a 10-year-old girl. *A*, Posteroanterior view demonstrates buckling of the medial and lateral cortices of the distal radial metaphysis. *B*, The lateral view demonstrates buckling on the dorsal cortex of the distal radial metaphysis. Buckle fractures of the dorsal cortex of the distal radius are very common but may be seen only on a true lateral view.

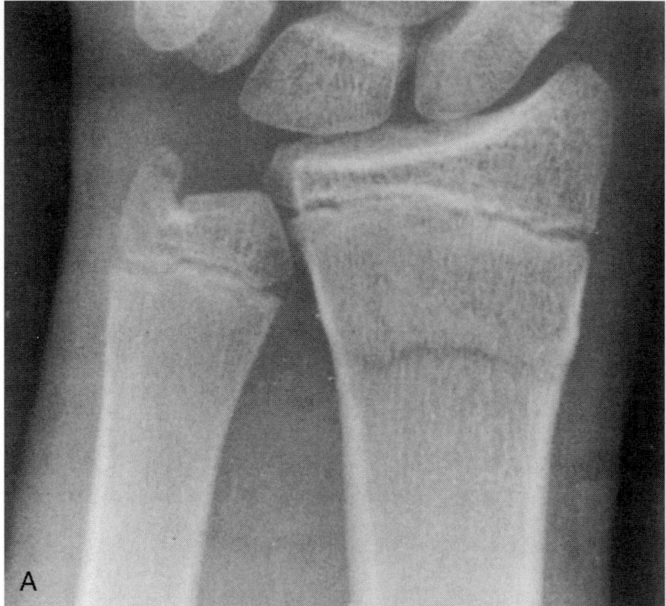

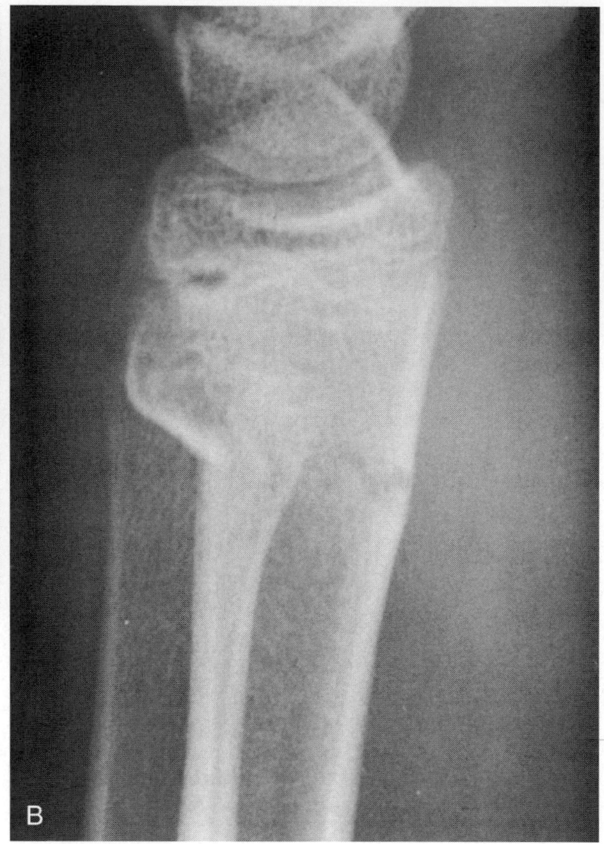

Figure 5–7. Lead pipe variety of fracture of the distal radius. *A*, Posteroanterior view demonstrates a transverse line of fracture across the distal radial metaphysis. There is an associated fracture of the tip of the ulnar styloid. *B*, Lateral view demonstrates marked buckling of the posterior cortex of the distal radius associated with an incomplete linear fracture involving the anterior cortex.

experimentally produced bow fractures a series of oblique microfractures[5] can be identified on the concave side of the bowing deformity. It is in this location that periosteal new bone formation may be seen subsequently in the very young as a manifestation of healing. This form of callus may be minimal or even absent in the older child or adolescent.[12] If the curvature is severe in the forearm, it may interfere with rotational movements.[5] If the fibula is severely curved, it may interfere with the proper alignment and apposition of bone fragments in an associated fracture of the tibia. It may be impossible to reduce the abnormal curvature, and therefore it may be necessary to create a complete fracture to eliminate the bow.

Toddler's Fracture

Infants and toddlers commonly present with limp of acute onset without a clear history of specific injury. Dunbar and associates[69] first reported a nondisplaced, oblique fracture of the distal shaft of the tibia as the source of the limp, which they termed *toddler's fracture* (Fig. 5–11). It has since been recognized that limp may also arise from occult fractures of the femur,[70] the metatarsals and tarsal bones (Fig. 5–12),[71, 75] pubic rami, or patella.[68] Such fractures occur during the usual activities of the toddler—the constant whirl with a tendency to trip, stumble, and fall.

Twenty percent of children who present with such a history have been found to have radiographic evidence of a fracture.[73] It is quite likely that additional fractures would be detected by bone scanning. The fractures are characteristically undisplaced and may be visualized only in one projection. Oblique views may be necessary.

Bone scans usually demonstrate a diffuse increase in activity over the entire length of the affected bone, even when a radiograph demonstrates a fracture of the metaphysis.[72, 74] Occasionally, with high-resolution techniques, the increased activity can be seen to be confined to an oblique band involving the diaphysis and metaphysis.

In a series of 100 cases,[73] 56% of toddler's fractures were located in the tibia and fibula, 30% in the femur, and 11% in the metatarsals; two occurred in the pubic rami and one in the calcaneus. In the tibia, 50% were located in the distal metaphysis, 32% in the proximal metaphysis, 10% in the diaphyses, and a single case within the physis. In the femur, just over half are located in the distal metaphysis, approximately one third in the diaphysis, and the remainder divided between the proximal metaphysis and physis.

Two thirds of children with toddler's fractures present between the ages of 1 and 3 years, 40% between the ages of 1 and 2, and 25% at age 1 or younger.[73] Over two thirds of those fractures in children younger than 1 year of age are fractures of the femur; less than 10% are of the femur in children over age 3, and none are of the femur in children older than the age of 5.

Toddler's fractures must be distinguished from those fractures resulting from child abuse. Toddler's fractures are commonly spiral or oblique in pattern and due to accidental trauma. Nonaccidental trauma or child abuse

is the most common cause of fractures in the first year of life, but not all fractures in the first year are due to abuse.[56]

Epiphyseal and Apophyseal Injury

The prevalence of epiphyseal injuries is variously reported from 6% to 30% of bone injuries in children younger than 16 years of age.[11, 21, 31, 51, 112] As the epiphyseal complex, consisting of the epiphysis, the physis or cartilaginous growth plate, and the metaphysis, is responsible for bone growth, the achievement of appropriate length of shaft, contour of bone ends, and proper axial relationships at the joints, the physician is rightfully concerned about the possibility of growth disturbance. However, deformities and significant shortening fortunately occur less often than might initially be anticipated following injuries of the epiphyseal complex.

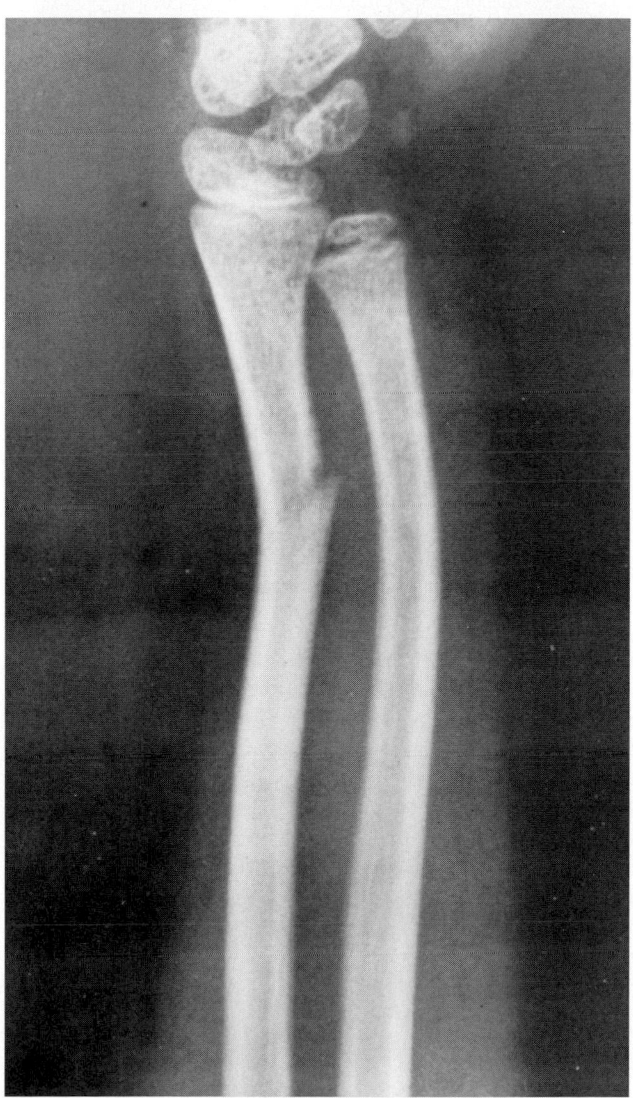

Figure 5–8. Bow fracture of the distal ulna associated with a greenstick fracture of the distal radius. Note that the ulna is bent, but there is no obvious break in the cortex. The apex of the bow within the ulna is at the level of the greenstick fracture of the radius. (Case courtesy of Leonard Swischuk, MD, Galveston, Tex.)

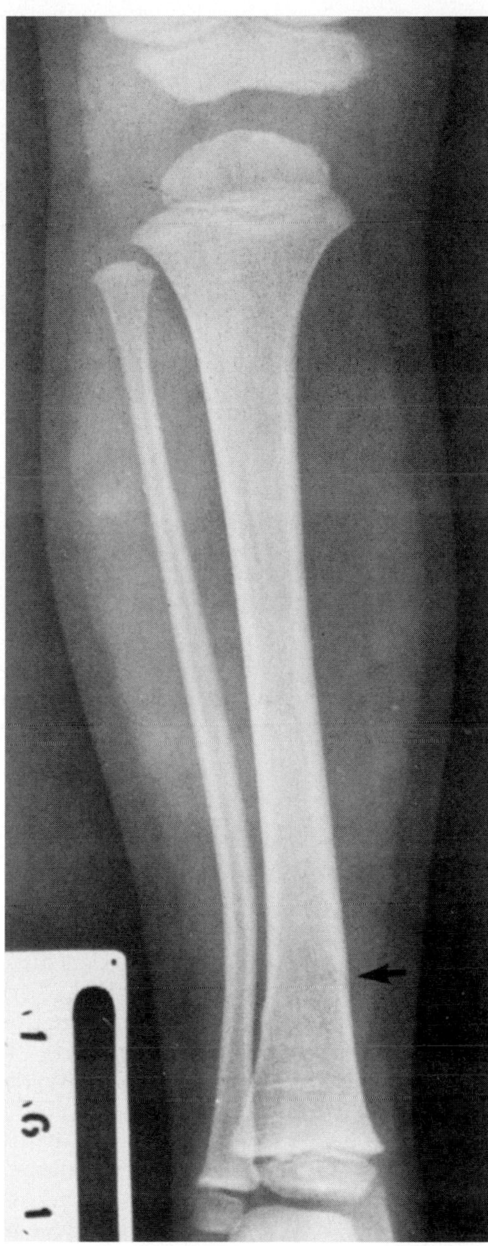

Figure 5–9. Bow fracture of distal fibula associated with greenstick fracture of distal tibia. The bowing of the fibula is obvious. There is no break within the cortex. A very faint incomplete fracture (*arrow*) is seen in the distal tibia with a break in the medial cortex.

In an amazing insight, the now noted Russian orthopedic surgeon G. A. Ilizarov recognized that longitudinal tension created by the growth plate in long bones was also responsible for morphogenesis of all soft tissues (i.e., muscles, nerves, and vasculature) as well as the longitudinal growth of bone.[97] This insight formed the premise for the tension external fixator treatment he devised for lengthening extremities.[101]

Poland,[28] in England, detailed the discovery, denial, and final acceptance of epiphyseal separation as an entity distinct from fracture. Epiphyseal separation was first described by Realdus Columbus in 1559 but was not generally accepted as an entity until the early 19th century. The investigations of European anatomists and sur-

geons confirmed the existence of this injury beyond all doubt by midcentury, and further clinical investigations by English and German surgeons resulted in its final acceptance. This work was culminated by publication of Poland's exhaustive, definitive treatise *Traumatic Separation of the Epiphyses*, in 1898.[28]

Epiphyseal separation in the young has been properly identified as the analogue[30] of dislocation[13] or ligamentous injury[25, 26] in the adult. It has been stated that the joint capsule and ligamentous structures are two to five times stronger[30] than the physis, or cartilaginous growth plate. Forces that would produce a ligamentous injury or dislocation of a major joint in an adult are more likely to result in epiphyseal separation or fracture in a child. Adolescence represents the transition period during which ligamentous and epiphyseal injuries may coexist, particularly for the adolescent athlete. Therefore, if clinical evaluation suggests either a dislocation[15] or ligamentous injury[36] in the young, the possibility of an underlying epiphyseal injury should be considered.

An apophysis is not responsible for bone growth in regard to length but is responsible for the development of a bony projection or protuberance to which a tendon is attached or from which muscles arise or insert. Muscles and tendons are stronger than the cartilaginous growth plate of the apophysis, and therefore a sudden, hard pull of the attached muscles or tendons may result in separation or fracture of the cartilaginous growth plate,[25] with displacement of the apophysis of variable degree. Thus, apophyseal separation or fracture in the young can be properly considered the analogue of muscle pull or strain in the mature.

Histologically the epiphyseal line or cartilaginous growth plate consists of four distinct zones[29, 30, 32, 84] in longitudinal section (Fig. 5–13*A*): (1) the germinal zone adjacent to the ossification center, composed of small resting or mother cells; next, (2) a zone of flattened cells arranged in columns, the proliferating zone; then, (3) the vesicular or hypertrophic zone, composed of swollen vacuolated cells maintaining the columnar arrangement; and finally, (4) the zone of provisional calcification at the metaphysis.

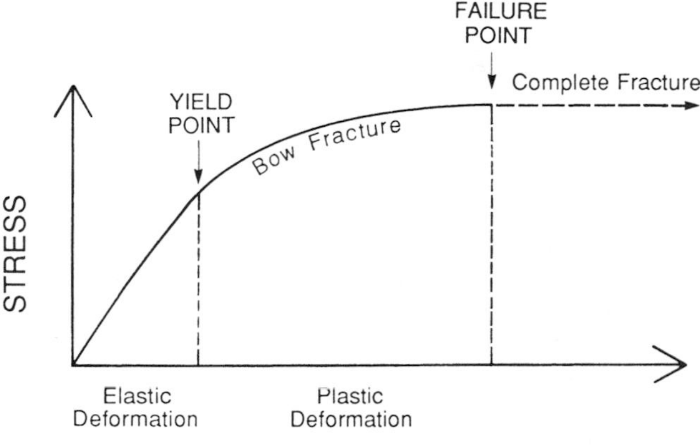

Figure 5–10. Stress-strain curve. Initially, strain is directly proportional to the force or stress applied. This is the zone of elastic deformation. In this zone, bone returns to normal after removal of the stress. Beyond the yield point, stress is no longer proportional to the resultant strain, and microfractures and deformities are created. This is the zone of plastic deformation. Stress beyond the yield point results in deformity of bone. Bow fractures of the diaphysis are the result of stresses in the plastic deformation range. At the failure point, the bone can no longer withstand the strain, and a frank fracture occurs.

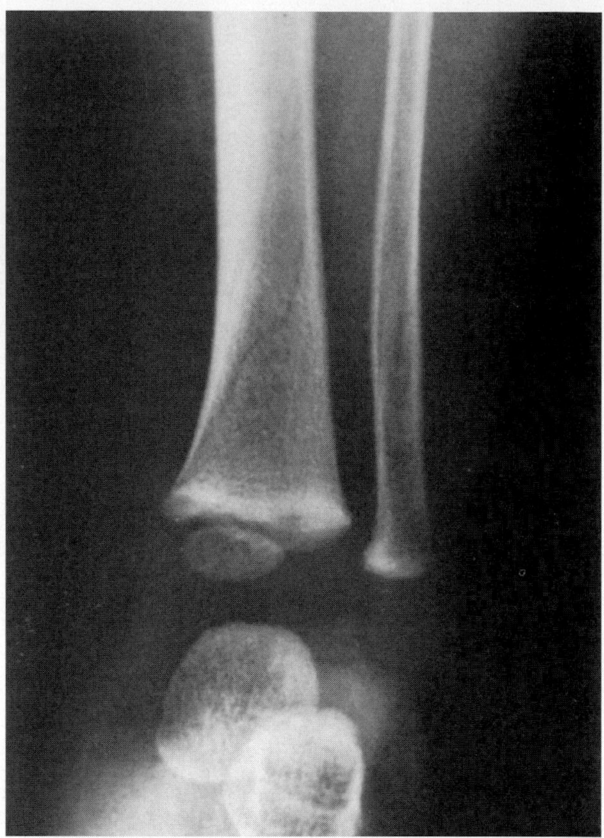

Figure 5–11. Toddler's fracture of the distal tibia in a 17-month-old boy who recently refused to bear weight on the left leg. Note the undisplaced oblique fracture of the distal tibial metaphysis. The fracture was not evident on the lateral view. Toddler's fractures are almost always undisplaced and often visualized in only one projection.

The cartilage cells lie in a matrix of chondroitin sulfate acid through which pass longitudinally arranged bundles of collagen fibers.[128] It is the matrix that provides resistance to shearing forces within the growth plate. The fibers have been compared to reinforcement rods within concrete. Abundant matrix exists in the first two zones, but matrix is considerably diminished in the third, or hypertrophic, zone by the enlargement of the cartilage cells. In the fourth zone the sparse matrix calcifies.[83, 103]

In general, the hypertrophic zone is the most vulnerable in the entire growth plate; it is through this layer that a fracture occurs as a result of a shearing force[82, 124, 125] (see Fig. 5–13*B*). Portions of the fracture line frequently involve the junction of the hypertrophic zone and zone of provisional calcification. The germinal cells are spared, and growth will continue, provided that there has been no interference with the blood supply.[32]

Fortunately the blood supply of the metaphysis and that of the epiphysis are separate; a line of fracture through the growth plate will not interfere with the arterial supply of the epiphysis or metaphysis (Fig. 5–14*A*). The metaphysis is centrally supplied by branches of the

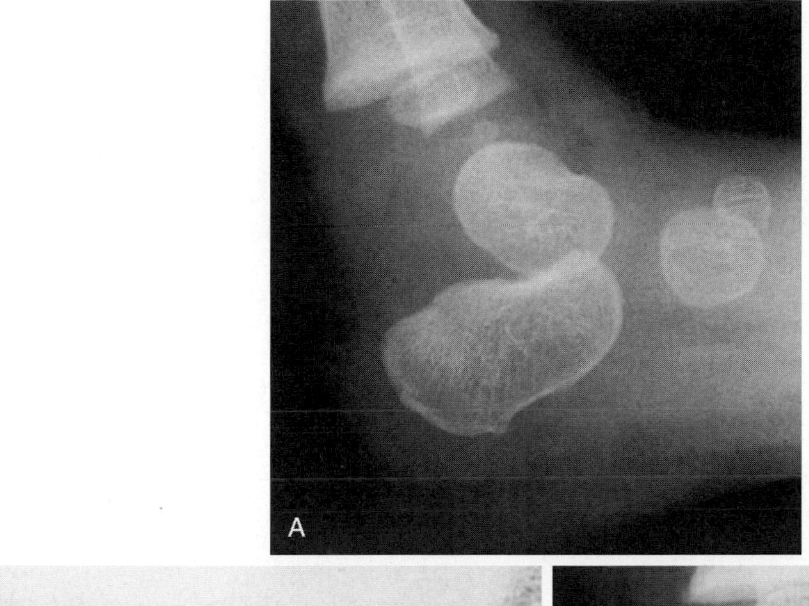

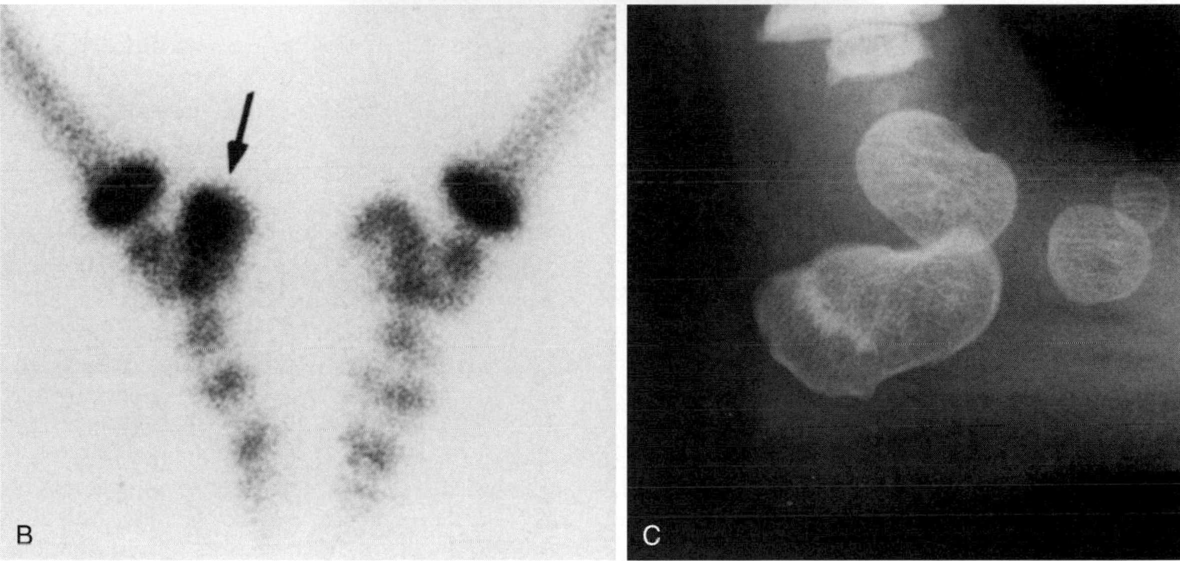

Figure 5–12. Toddler's fracture of the calcaneus in a 2-year-old child who presented with a limp and refused to bear weight on the left foot. *A*, Initial lateral radiograph of the foot demonstrates no evidence of abnormalities. *B*, Technetium 99m bone scan demonstrates focus of increased activity within the calcaneus (*arrow*). *C*, Follow-up radiograph demonstrates band of sclerosis, confirming toddler's fracture. (Case courtesy of James J. Conway, MD, Chicago, Ill.)

nutrient artery and numerous small branches of the periosteal arteries, originating from the diaphysis, at its periphery.[77] The vascular supply of the epiphysis consists of several periosteal vessels that arise from larger arteries about the joint. With this dual arrangement, the epiphyseal arteries supply nourishment for cartilaginous growth, whereas the metaphyseal arteries nourish ossification.[41, 42]

Following a separation, fibrin appears within the line of cleavage; the cartilage cells continue to grow, and the epiphyseal plate thickens as the cellular columns lengthen. In approximately 21 days[32] the fibrin is dissolved and the normal growth pattern restored. There is no resultant growth disturbance. Two exceptions to this arrangement exist, the proximal femur (see Fig. 5–14*B*) and proximal radial epiphyseal centers. As opposed to other epiphyseal centers, which are only partially intracapsular, these are located entirely within the joint and are covered entirely by articular cartilage. Because of this anatomy, at least a portion of the arterial supply must approach the epiphysis from the metaphysis. These arteries course in the perichondrium at the peripheral margins of the growth plate and are ruptured as the epiphysis is separated. Prognosis is dependent upon the degree of arterial disruption; the greater the vascular destruction, the more likely is a resultant growth disturbance.[41]

The pathway of injury, or vector of force, involved in epiphyseal injuries may serve as a prognostic indicator. A vertically oriented compressive or splitting force tends to involve all layers of the physis, whereas a horizontally oriented shearing force propagates along the zones of the growth plate. Fortunately for children, horizontally directed shearing forces are more common than vertically oriented forces that involve the germinal zone. Vertical fractures more often lead to growth arrest because they permit communication between epiphyseal and metaphyseal vessels, with the potential for subsequent formation

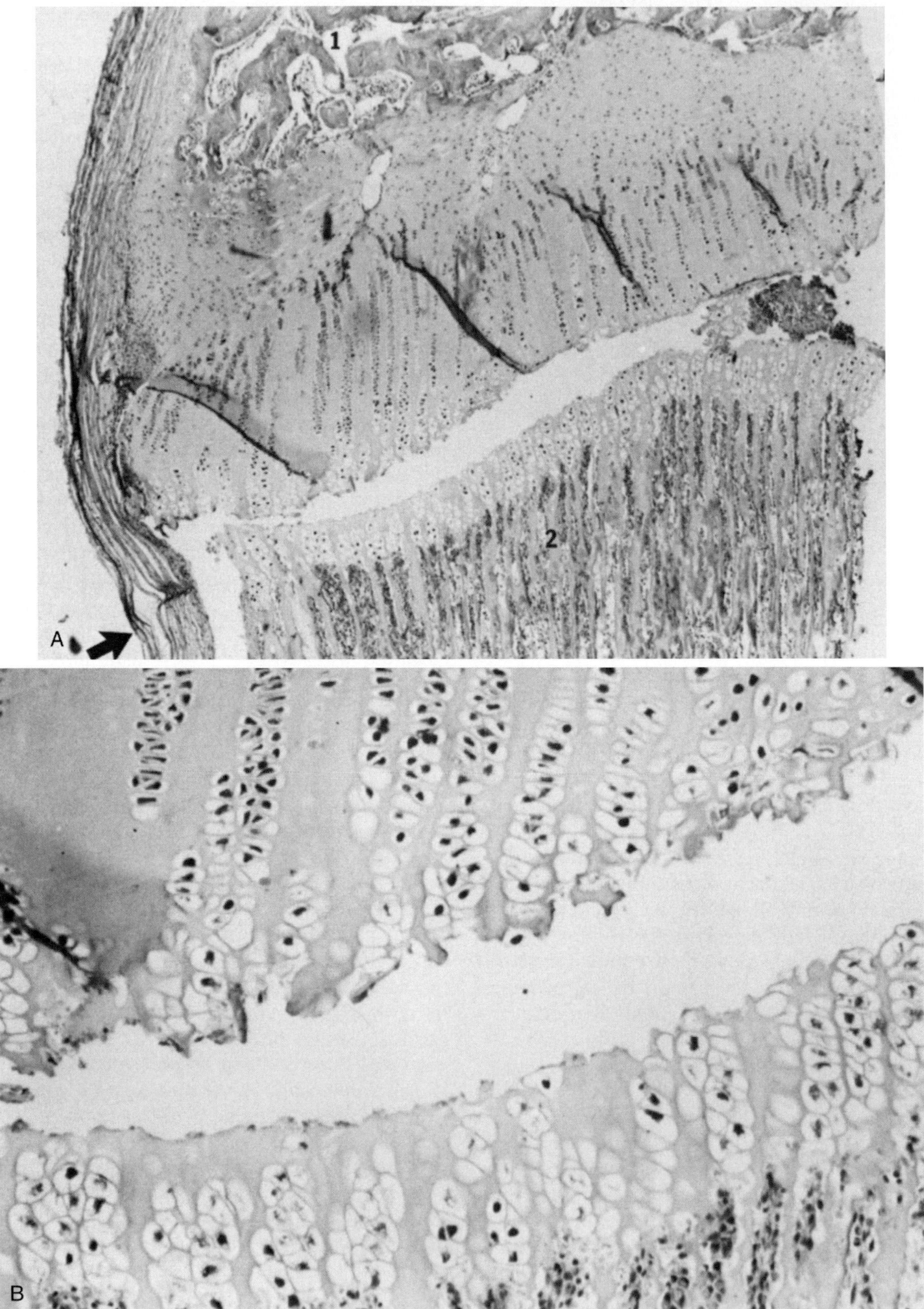

Figure 5–13. Experimentally produced fracture of the distal ulna of a rabbit. *A*, The line of fracture lies within the growth plate. Note that the periosteum (*arrow*) is intact but stripped from the metaphyseal fragment. 1, Epiphysis; 2, metaphysis. *B*, A higher power view demonstrates that the line of fracture lies within the hypertrophic zone.

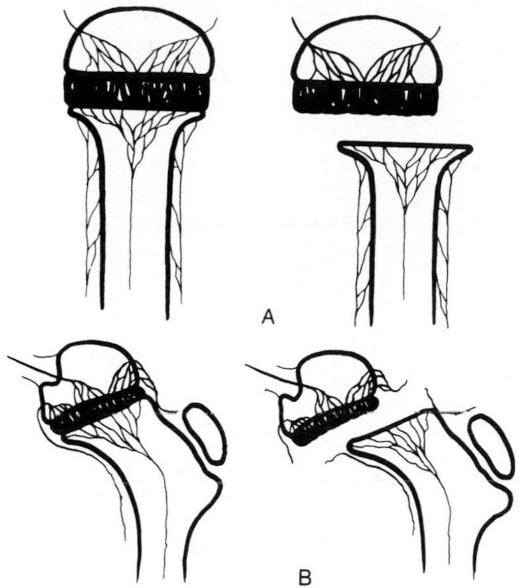

Figure 5–14. Blood supply to the growing end of bone. *A*, In most bones there is a separate blood supply to the epiphysis and metaphysis. Note that blood vessels about the joint supply the epiphysis, whereas the metaphysis receives its blood supply centrally from the branches of the nutrient artery and from vessels within the periosteum. A fracture across the growth plate does not disrupt the blood supply to either the epiphysis or the metaphysis. *B*, In the hip and in the proximal radius the growth plate is contained within the joint capsule, and the blood vessels entering the epiphysis must cross the growth plate. When a fracture occurs in the growth plate, these vessels are disrupted.

of a bone bridge (see Fig. 5–29).[30, 32, 82, 99, 100] Bone bridging results in cessation of growth at this point. The remainder of the epiphyseal complex continues to grow, creating an angular deformity.

Pure compression force crushes the cartilaginous growth plate, destroying a variable percentage of the resting cells without producing a clinically or radiographically apparent fracture. This injury is particularly devastating because it frequently results in growth arrest and deformity. It occurs most commonly in joints that move in only one plane (i.e., knee and ankle joints).

Approximately 80% of epiphyseal injuries[27, 30] occur between the ages of 10 and 16 years. The median age is 13 (Fig. 5–15). The exception to this general rule is injuries of the distal humerus, which usually occur before the age of 10. As would be expected, epiphyseal injuries occur much more frequently in males[30] than in females, and the age of maximal incidence is somewhat younger for girls (8 to 13 years) than for boys (11 to 14 years). Peterson's Olmstead County study reported a male-to-female ratio of 2:1 and incidence rates highest among 14-year-old boys and 11- to 12-year-old girls.[116] This male predilection is thought to be associated with the greater exposure of males to trauma and to the relative delay of epiphyseal closure in males rather than to any intrinsic difference in epiphyseal structure between the sexes.

The most common sites of epiphyseal injury (Fig. 5–16) are the distal radius,[23, 27, 30, 48, 109, 111, 112, 126] the distal tibia, and the phalanges of the hand, with rank ordering varying with reported series. In general, injuries of the distal epiphysis are more common than injuries of the proximal epiphysis in any given bone. Injuries of the proximal epiphyses of the femur, tibia, and radius are relatively rare.

Apophyseal separations occur predominantly in the pelvis[92] of the adolescent athlete. Typically, the patient reports an acute pop or snap occurring during a forceful muscular contraction, although chronic avulsive injury due to tight musculotendinous units may produce painful chronic traction apophysitis[79] (Fig. 5–17). Most frequently affected is the ischial apophysis, which serves as the insertion of the hamstrings.[25, 29] Avulsions of the anterior superior iliac spine and the medial epicondyle of the humerus are relatively common. Other pelvic apophyses, the trochanters of the femur, the olecranon and coronoid of the ulna, and the coracoid of the scapula are less commonly affected.

Classification

Salter-Harris Epiphyseal Injuries

The Salter-Harris classification of epiphyseal injuries[30, 32, 121] remains widely used, as it is a simple and practical

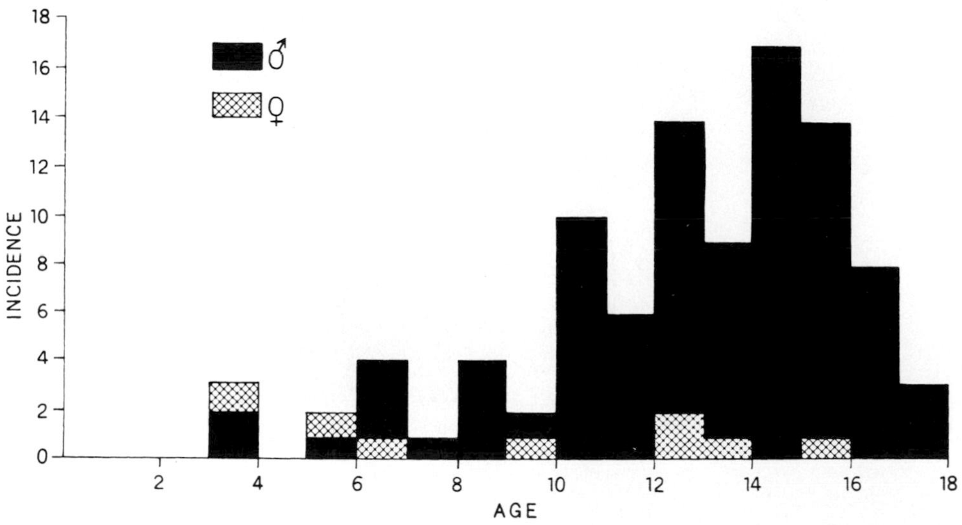

Figure 5–15. Age incidence in 107 epiphyseal injuries. (From Rogers, L. F. [1970]. The radiography of epiphyseal injuries. Radiology, *96*:289, with permission.)

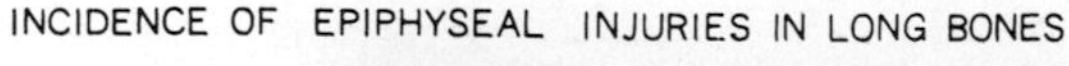

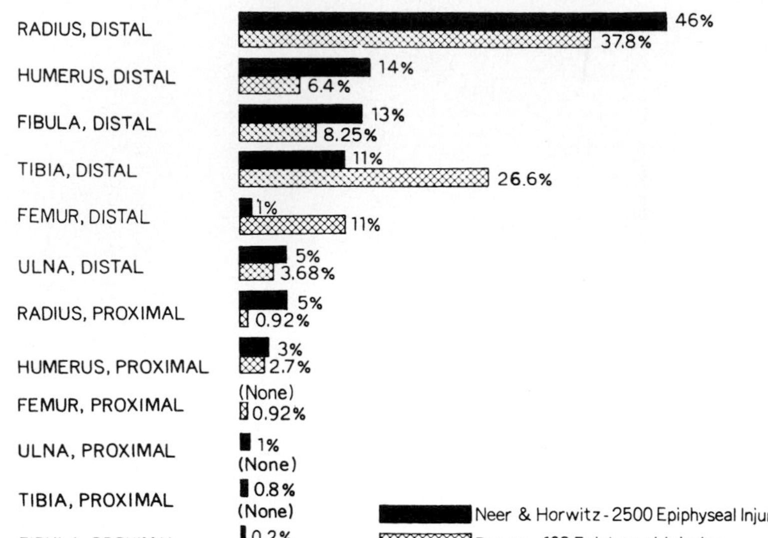

Figure 5–16. Comparison of the incidence of epiphyseal injuries in long bones in the series of Neer and Horwitz[23] and of Rogers.[30]

classification based on sound anatomic and clinical principles having prognostic significance. The classification is most appealing because a distinctive radiographic pattern emerges in each type[30, 111] (Fig. 5–18). Other, more complex classifications have been suggested by Ogden[51, 112] and Peterson.[117, 118] Peterson's classification provides quantification of the amount of physeal damage. Nevertheless, the Salter-Harris classification remains widely accepted throughout the world by all practitioners who deal with children, and it is reviewed in detail here.

Type 1

Type 1[30, 32] injuries are sometimes referred to as pure epiphyseal separations. Type 1 is characterized by a line of cleavage confined to the zone of hypertrophic cells without involvement of either the metaphysis or epiphyseal ossification center (Fig. 5–19*A*; see also Fig. 5–18). This type represents approximately 6% to 8.5% of all epiphyseal injuries and occurs most commonly in the phalanges.[121] The only radiographic evidence is a displacement of the epiphyseal ossification center. Generally this type is seen at a younger age than for other epiphyseal injuries, at a time when the physis is wide. It is most common under 5 years of age and particularly common as a result of birth injury.[15] It is often seen in the proximal end of the humerus and femur. The prognosis is generally favorable. Epiphyseal separations occurring in rickets (see Fig. 5–46), scurvy,[115] and slipped capital femoral epiphysis as seen in adolescents could be considered pathologic epiphyseal separations of this type.

Type 2

Type 2 injuries are by far the most common, comprising 75% of all epiphyseal injuries.[30, 32] Type 2 injuries of the distal radius (see Figs. 5–18 and 5–19*B*) account for one third to one half of all epiphyseal injuries in most

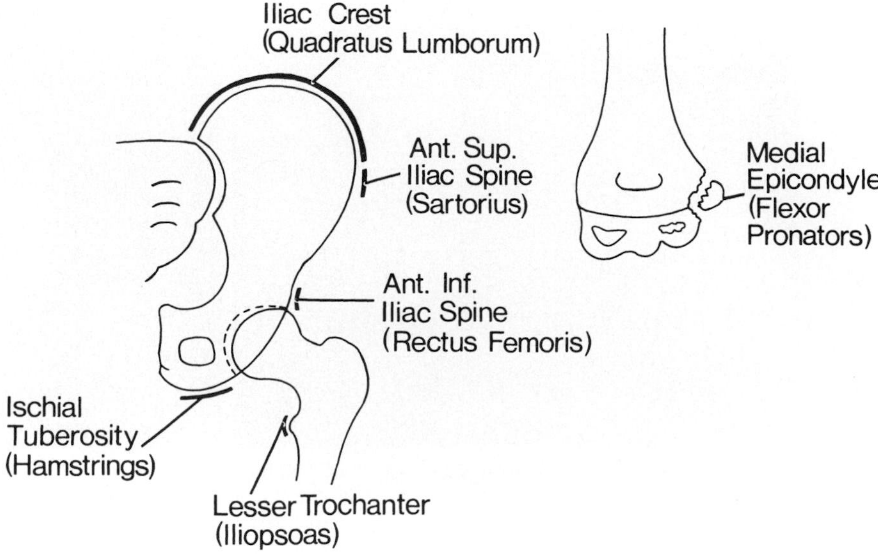

Figure 5–17. The common sites of apophyseal avulsion and muscle attachments that create the injury.

Type		Incidence
1	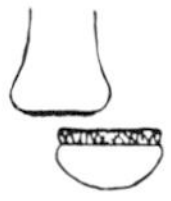	6%
2	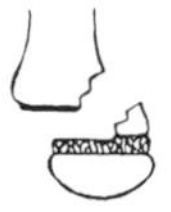	75%
3	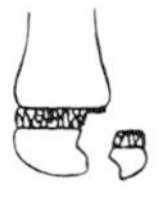	8%
4	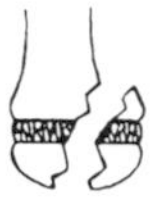	10%
5	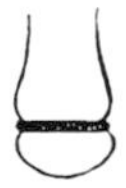	1%

Figure 5–18. Incidence of 118 injuries in 108 patients according to Salter-Harris classification. (From Rogers, L. F. [1970]. The radiography of epiphyseal injuries. Radiology, *96*:289, with permission.)

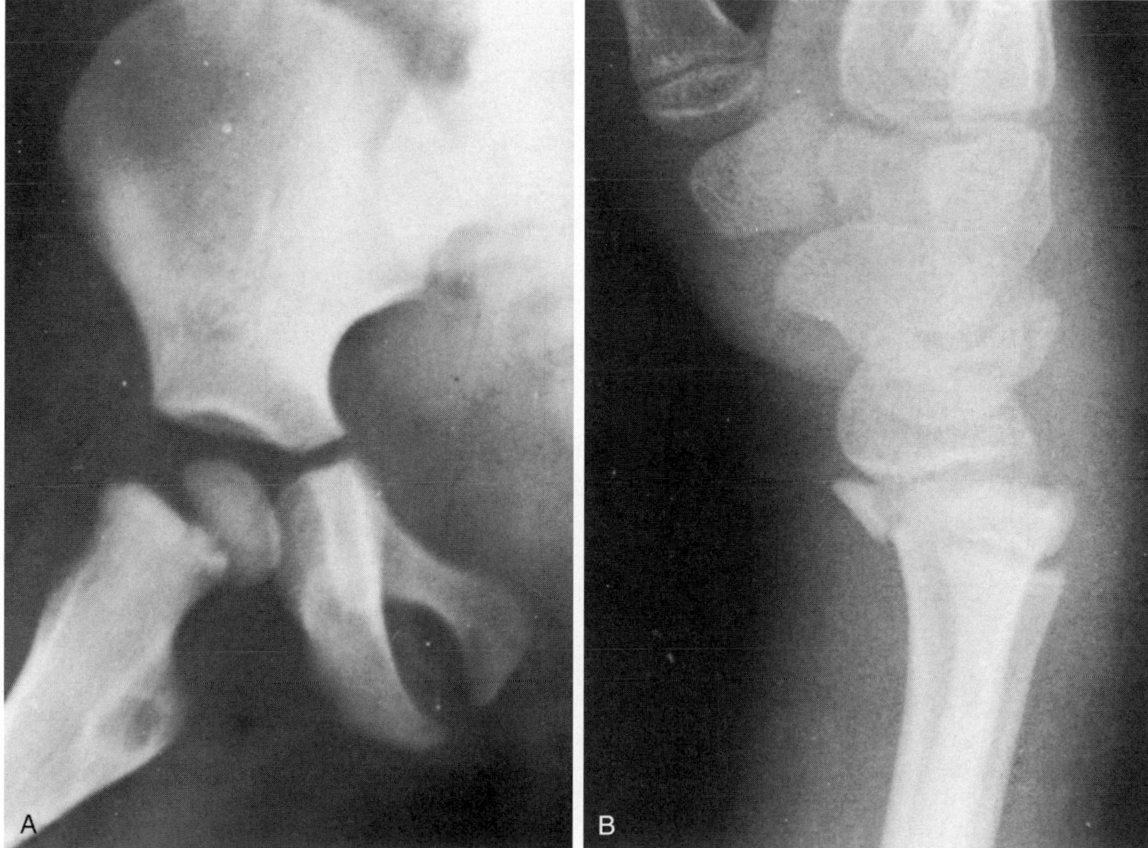

Figure 5–19. Salter-Harris epiphyseal injuries. *A*, Type 1. A 3-year-old girl fell from a second-story window and injured her hip. The line of fracture passes through the growth plate without involvement of either the metaphysis or the epiphysis. *B*, Type 2. A 12-year-old boy sustained injury to the distal radius in a fall. The distal radial epiphysis is displaced anteriorly in association with a fracture of the anterior corner of the metaphysis. (From Rogers, L. F. [1970]. The radiography of epiphyseal injuries. Radiology, *96*:289, with permission.)

series.[23, 30] The distal tibia, distal fibula, and phalanges account for most of the remainder. A fragment from the metaphysis accompanies the displaced epiphysis. Again, the line of cleavage is within the hypertrophic zone, but at some point it turns into the metaphysis, separating off a segment of bone. A type 2 injury is caused by shearing or avulsive forces that are converted to compressive forces on the side opposite the applied force by the apposing bone at the joint and the intact periosteum attached to the epiphysis. Although the hypertrophic zone is susceptible to a shear, it is resistant to compression.[32] The opposite applies to the fine new bone of the metaphysis; thus, the line of fracture extends into the metaphysis. The hallmark of this injury is the presence of the associated triangular metaphyseal fragment (Thurston-Holland fragment), referred to as the corner sign.[14] The prognosis is generally favorable.

Type 3

Type 3 injuries are the result of an intra-articular shearing force[30, 32] and account for approximately 8% of all epiphyseal injuries. The fracture runs vertically or obliquely through the epiphysis and growth plate into the hypertrophic layer and then horizontally to the periphery (Fig. 5–20*A*; see also Fig. 5–18), separating a portion of the epiphysis. Normally, displacement is minimal without an associated fracture of the metaphysis. This injury is seen most frequently at the distal tibia or distal phalanx and occasionally at the distal femur. The usual age at injury is early adolescence near the time of physeal closure. The prognosis is good; growth arrest and deformities are rare. However, the fragment must be replaced properly or an irregular joint surface can result.

Type 4

In type 4 injuries, a vertically oriented splitting force produces a fracture[30, 32] extending across the epiphysis growth plate, and metaphysis (see Fig. 5–18). A fragment consisting of a portion of both the metaphysis and the epiphysis is evident on radiographs (Fig. 5–21; see also Fig. 5–20*B*); 10% of epiphyseal injuries are of this type. The most common sites[30] are the lateral condyle of the humerus under age 10 years and the distal tibia over age 10 years. Growth arrest and limb shortening and physeal bars with angular deformities are distinct possibilities,[32] although the chances are decreased by proper open reduction and fixation.

Type 5

Fortunately the type 5 injury is rare,[89] comprising only 1% of epiphyseal injuries. This injury is presumably the result of a pure crushing injury (see Fig. 5–18). There is usually no immediate radiographic evidence (Fig. 5–22*A*), and the effects are apparent only later (Fig. 5–22*B*), manifested as bone shortening and joint deformities.[30, 32]

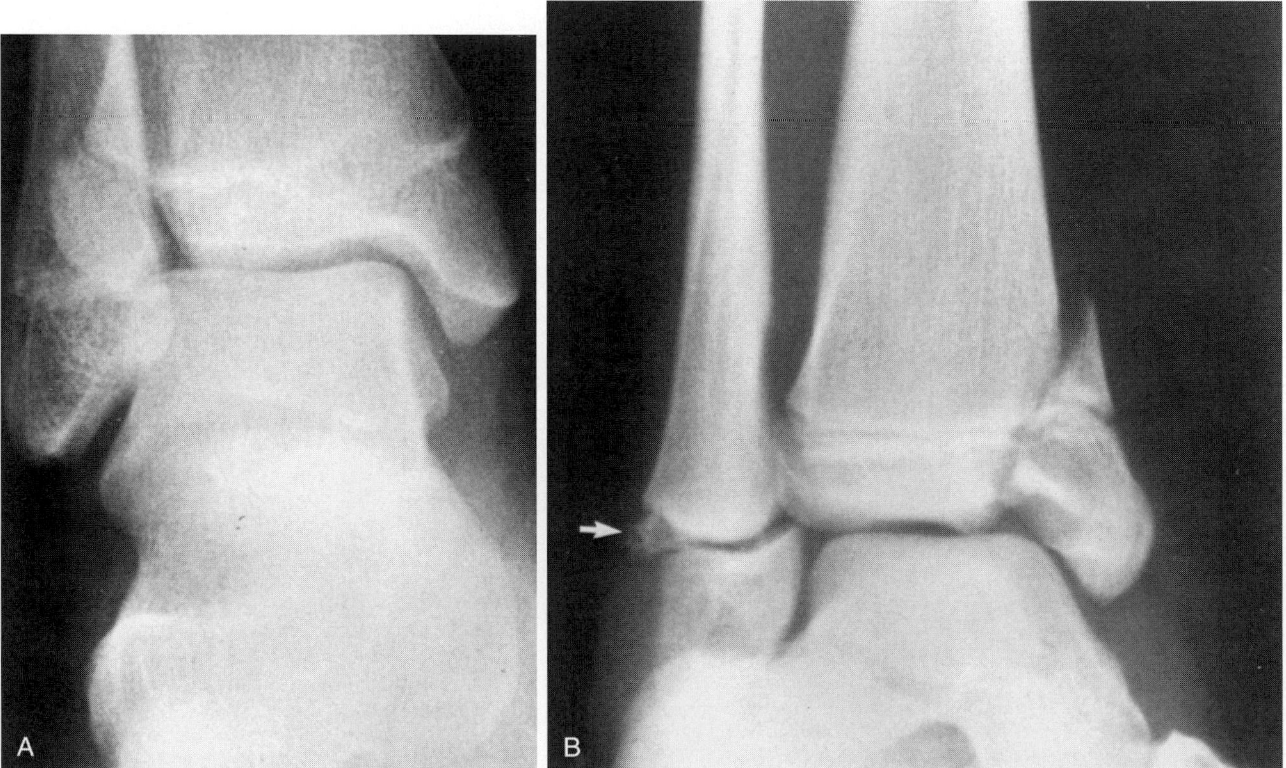

Figure 5–20. Salter-Harris epiphyseal injuries. *A*, Type 3. The foot of a 16-year-old boy was rotated externally in a fall, and the distal tibial epiphysis was fractured on its lateral margin. Note the minimal displacement and absence of metaphyseal involvement. (From Rogers, L. F. [1970]. The radiography of epiphyseal injuries. Radiology, *96*:289, with permission.) *B*, Type 4. A 15-year-old boy sustained this adduction injury of the ankle. There is a vertical fracture extending through the medial portion of the distal tibial epiphysis that also extends through the adjacent metaphysis, characterizing this as a type 4 injury. There is also a type 2 injury of the distal fibular epiphysis. Note the lamella or thin fragment of bone (*arrow*) that has been pulled from the adjacent fibular metaphysis.

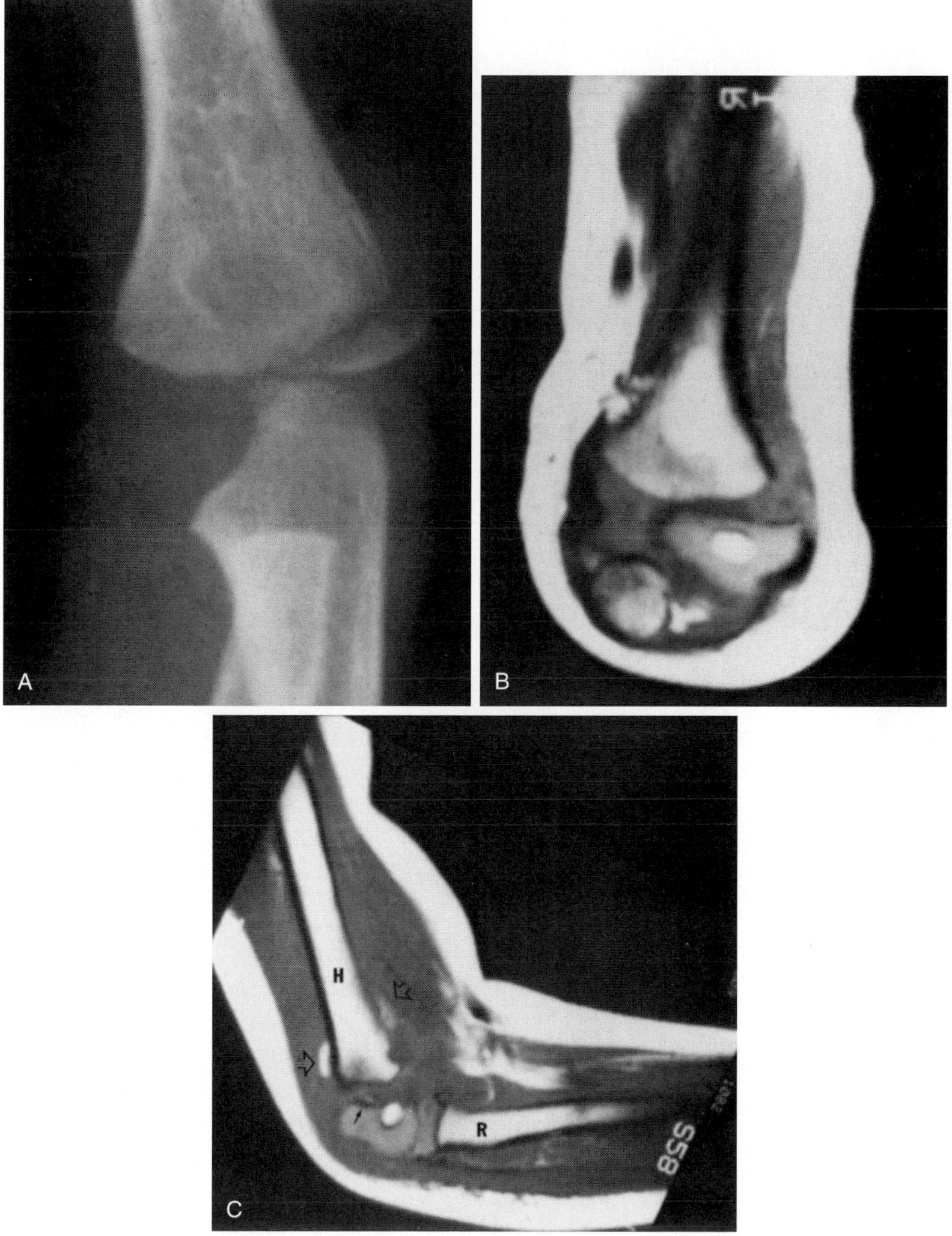

Figure 5–21. Salter-Harris type 4 fracture of the lateral condyle in a 21-month-old boy. *A*, Initial radiograph demonstrates fracture of the lateral distal metaphysis of the humerus. At this age, however, the majority of the distal humeral epiphysis is composed of cartilage, and the extension of the fracture into the epiphysis is not appreciated. This is particularly true in the absence of displacement of the ossification center. *B*, Magnetic resonance image in the coronal projection demonstrates the fracture through the distal humeral metaphyses and its vertical component through the midportion of the epiphysis. *C*, Sagittal magnetic resonance image demonstrates fracture through the physis. Note small flake of metaphyseal bone remaining attached to the epiphysis (*arrow*). The anterior and posterior fat pads (*open arrows*) are displaced by joint effusion. H, Humerus; R, radius.

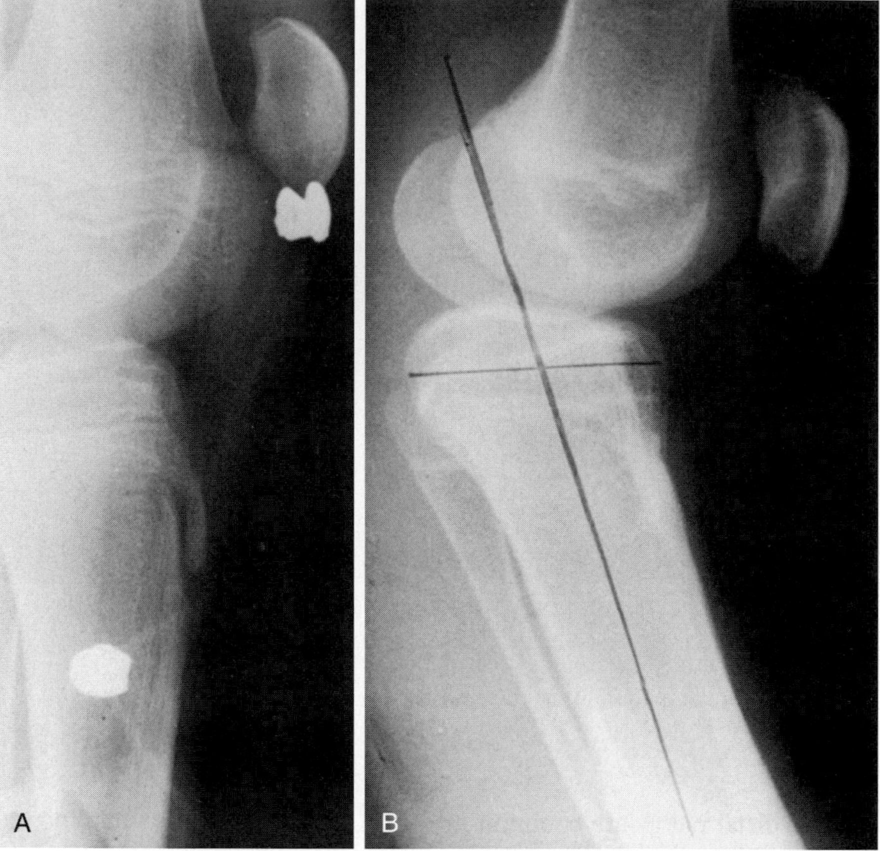

Figure 5–22. Salter-Harris epiphyseal injury, type 5. *A*, A 14-year-old boy sustained a fracture of the midshaft of the tibia in an automobile accident. No injury of the epiphyseal complex is apparent on the lateral or anteroposterior view obtained at the first examination. The shaft fracture healed normally. Angulation was first noted 1 year after injury. *B*, This lateral view was obtained 4 years after the injury and demonstrates closure of the growth plate anteriorly and resultant angulation. (From Rogers, L. F. [1970]. The radiography of epiphyseal injuries. Radiology, *96*:289, with permission.)

The distal femoral and proximal and distal tibial epiphyseal centers are most commonly affected, usually in association with fractures of the shaft of the femur or the tibia and fibula. Traumatic distal ulnar physeal arrest after distal radial fracture occurs and may also represent a type 5 injury.[119] Generally the age at injury is slightly higher (12 to 16 years) than is the average for other epiphyseal injuries. Sports and auto accidents account for the majority. The follow-up radiographic examination of shaft fractures of the lower extremity in adolescents should include the proximal and distal epiphyseal centers to detect any evidence of type 5 injury.

Birth Injuries

Separations of the epiphyses of the proximal[15] and distal humerus (Fig. 5–23) and proximal femur[107, 130] (see Fig. 20–69) may occur as a result of birth injuries[91] and have been properly termed *pseudodislocations*.[15] Similar cases have also been reported in the distal femur, distal tibia,[91] and fibula.[91]

These injuries typically occur in high-birth-weight babies of diabetic mothers who have a difficult delivery, often due to a breech presentation. They are often mistakenly diagnosed clinically as dislocations. The radiographic appearance may also be misinterpreted by the unwary as that of a dislocation, compounding the problem. At birth the primary ossification centers of the epiphyses at these sites are not ossified. Thus, the radiograph clearly demonstrates a displacement of the shaft but without ossification in the epiphysis to allow identification of its position. It is easily assumed that the epiphysis has been displaced with the shaft. However, traumatic dislocation of the joint probably never occurs at birth, and every instance of clinically suspected dislocation should be regarded as an epiphyseal fracture. The diagnosis may be established or confirmed by ultrasonography, magnetic resonance imaging (MRI), or arthrography if this is considered necessary.[100] In this setting, essentially all “dislocations” will ultimately be proved to be epiphyseal separations.

Following reduction these separations remain unstable, which may cause further diagnostic confusion for clinicians unfamiliar with these injuries. An unstable reduction is considered an indication for surgery and open reduction under most other circumstances; however, usually these separations do not require open reduction or pin fixation. Treatment by traction and closed casting is sufficient. In 6 to 10 days a repeat radiograph will demonstrate callus formation about the metaphysis and confirm the initial injury as an epiphyseal separation. If the lesion is identified promptly, the prognosis is satisfactory. Normal growth can be expected, particularly at the elbow and shoulder. The prognosis with hip injuries must be guarded.

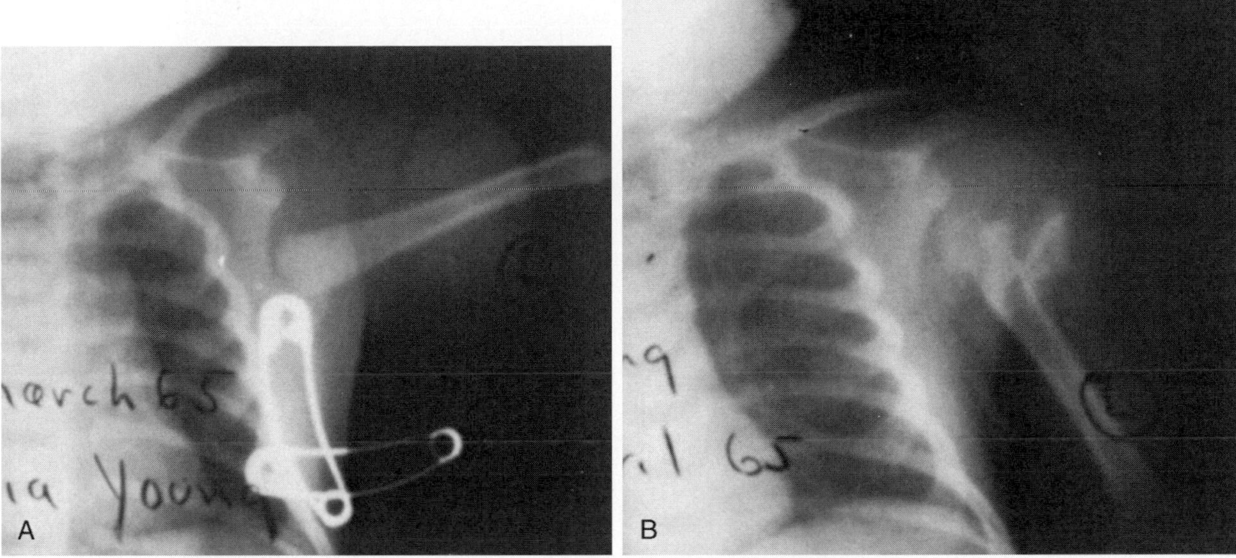

Figure 5–23. Separation of the proximal humeral epiphyses caused by birth injury. In the absence of an ossification center, this finding is easily mistaken for dislocation. *A*, Initial examination demonstrates medial and inferior displacement of the proximal humerus. No ossification center is present. *B*, Repeat examination at 2 weeks demonstrates callus formation at the margin of the metaphysis.

Stress Injuries of the Physis

Stress injuries occur in the physis of the distal radius and ulna,[87, 93, 122, 123] distal femur,[94] proximal tibia,[85] distal fibula,[121] and proximal humerus[95] of adolescent athletes. Radiographically they are evidenced by widening of the growth plate with slight irregularity and sclerosis of the metaphysis (Fig. 5–24). Those in the distal radius are common in gymnasts. Those involving the proximal humerus are usually confined to the lateral margin of the growth plate in baseball pitchers, and those in the distal femur usually involve only the lateral condylar portion of the physis. Stress injuries of the physis heal without growth disturbance if the athlete refrains from participation in the activity that caused the lesion, although so-called gymnast's wrist, or distal radial physeal dysfunction, has been associated with premature physeal arrest, with positive ulnar variance and tears of the triangular fibrocartilaginous complex.[76]

Radiographic Evaluation

The majority of epiphyseal injuries (Salter-Harris types 1 and 2) are manifested by displacement of the shaft relative to the ossification center and by widening of the growth plate. The greater the displacement, the more evident is the injury. At times, however, displacement or widening of the plate or both are minimal, necessitating comparative views of the contralateral extremity for verification and, occasionally, even discovery of the injury.[30] In the type 2 injury a triangular chip or fragment of the metaphysis accompanies the displaced epiphysis, aiding in demonstration of the injury (see Fig. 5–19*B*). Poland[28] published roentgenograms pointing out this fragment. Holland,[16] in 1929, stressed its importance, and it is now referred to as the Thurston-Holland fragment. The presence of this fragment is termed the *corner sign*. When the fragment is seen in profile, the corner sign is easily recognized. When the fragment is viewed *en face* or obliquely, the radiographic appearance may suggest cortical buckling or an incomplete metaphyseal fracture, or it may be entirely overlooked. The observer should then check for subtle widening of the growth plate. Oblique views with the central ray tangential to the metaphyseal area in question are helpful.

Werenskiold[43] and Bergenfeldt[3] emphasized the presence of a thin, fine flake or lamella of bone accompanying the epiphysis (see Fig. 5–20*B*). It is detached from the metaphysis and lies within or near the epiphyseal line. The *lamellar sign* differs from the corner sign in the size and position of the fragment. In the corner sign, the fragment is created by a compressive force and is found on the side of the fulcrum through which the forces were applied. The lamella formed by an avulsive force is found on the side opposite the fulcrum. In general, the greater the epiphyseal displacement, the larger the metaphyseal fragment will be. When the fragment is small, the displacement is minimal; when only widening of the growth plate is evident, a lamella may exist.

Poland[28] first considered that an immediate spontaneous reduction of epiphyseal separations could occur (Fig. 5–25). Clinically there is no deformity, only tenderness. The entity, now accepted, could not be proved until the advent of radiography. The radiographic proof is furnished by the presence of a corner sign, a lamellar sign, or widening of the growth plate with minimal or no epiphyseal displacement. Corner or lamellar fractures cannot occur without an associated fracture of the growth plate. Occasionally, only stress views will reveal the widening of the growth plate, but their use remains controversial, as stress may further disrupt the physis.[29, 30, 36]

With displacement and angulation of the metaphysis, the zone of provisional calcification becomes blurred or less sharply defined when viewed *en face*. Angulation is confirmed when the injury is viewed in profile.

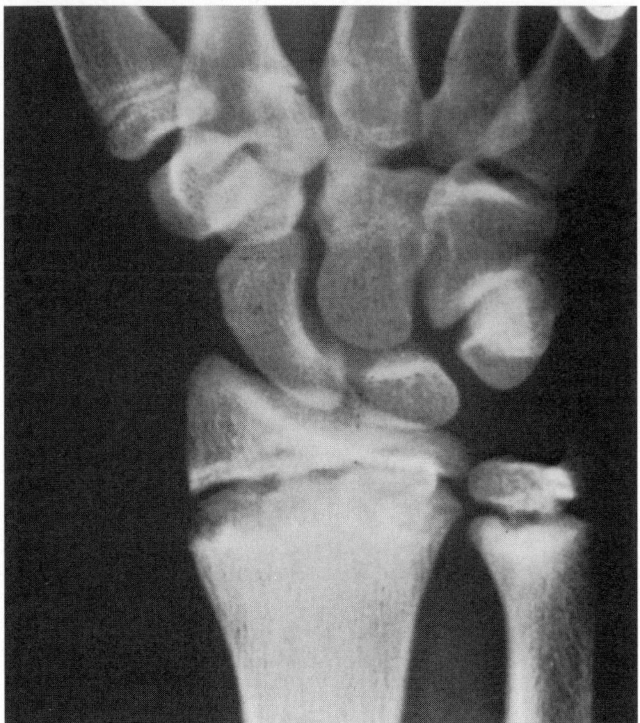

Figure 5–24. Stress injury of the distal radial and ulnar epiphyses in a 12-year-old gymnast who presented with intermittent pain in the wrist. There is an irregularity of the metaphysis and widening of the physes of both the distal radius and the ulna. The epiphyses are not displaced. The appearance of the only other visible physis, at the base of the first metacarpal, is within normal limits. Widening of the metaphyses and irregularity of the physes have been recognized as stress-induced changes in adolescent athletes, especially gymnasts.

Computed tomography (CT) with multiplanar reformatting capability is particularly useful for acute evaluation of complex fractures of the adolescent ankle including the triplane and Tillaux fractures.[127] MRI performed in the early post-traumatic period may detect occult physeal injuries, better characterize the path of injury and more accurately classify and determine the prognostic significance of an epiphyseal injury, and allow detection of concomitant soft tissue, ligamentous, and cartilaginous injuries. MRI is also useful for detecting injuries to unossified epiphyses, osteochondral injuries, occult scaphoid fractures, and bone marrow injuries such as bone bruises and stress fractures. MRI is the test of choice to evaluate for premature physeal arrest or physeal tethering by bone bridges, causing potential growth disturbances.[86, 98–100]

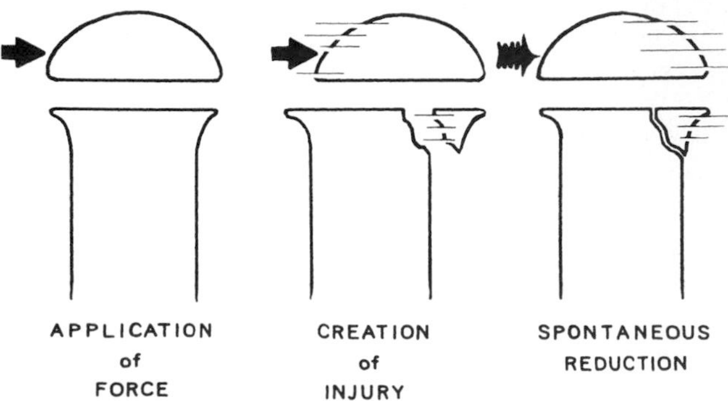

Figure 5–25. Spontaneous reduction of epiphyseal separation.

Apophyseal separations may be easily mistaken for avulsion fractures of bone (Fig. 5–26*A*) by those unfamiliar with this possibility. Although this is not a grievous error, it is certainly imprecise and reflects poorly on the radiologist's diagnostic capabilities. Views of the contralateral side will usually clarify the exact nature of the injury in question (see Fig. 5–26*B*); however, the ischial apophysis is located on the posterior inferior surface of the tuberosity and may be difficult to see when in its normal position. Similarly, the undisplaced anterior inferior iliac spine (see Fig. 5–26) is difficult to visualize.

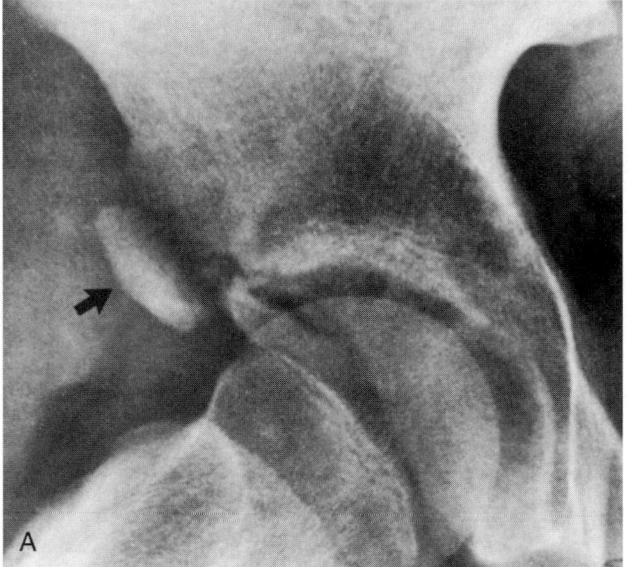

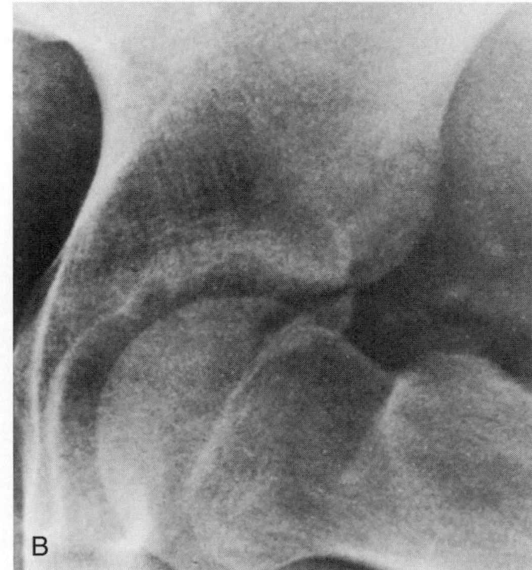

Figure 5–26. Avulsion of the anterior-inferior iliac spine in a 16-year-old boy that occurred while he was running. *A*, The apophyseal avulsion is readily identified *(arrow)*; it is separated 5 mm from the innominate bone. *B*, In this comparison view of the contralateral side, note that the outline of the apophyseal ossification center at the anterior inferior iliac spine is poorly visualized.

Treatment

One might assume that open reduction and fixation would be frequently required for all epiphyseal injuries. However, most type 1 and type 2 injuries usually require only closed reduction and casting.[4, 32, 40] It is the periosteum that lends stability to the reduced fracture.[1, 32, 47] The periosteum of the intact growing bone ensheathes the diaphysis and surrounds the epiphyseal line attaching to the margins of the epiphysis. A shearing force ruptures the periosteum on the side to which it is applied. On the opposite side the periosteum remains intact (see Fig. 5–13*A*), attached to the epiphysis and metaphyseal fragment, although stripped from a portion of the diaphysis. The intact periosteum has been compared to a hinge, allowing proper reduction and lending stability but preventing overcorrection.

It has been proved best not to attempt reduction of neglected type 1 and type 2 injuries. This is particularly true in children younger than 12 years of age, in whom considerable growth potential remains. Subsequent bone growth corrects the angulation and restores length (Figs. 5–27 and 5–28), frequently to such an extent that the examiner may be unable to determine which extremity was involved. For the same reason, repeated attempts to attain complete reduction are unnecessary and, in fact, may prove harmful by disrupting the blood supply, leading to growth arrest and deformity.[32]

Most type 3 and type 4 injuries require open reduction and fixation to prevent growth arrest and joint surface deformity. If the fracture is left displaced, a bar of bone may bridge the physis, joining the metaphysis to the epiphysis (Fig. 5–29) and preventing further growth in this region of the physis. Such bridging may ultimately result in an angular deformity of the joint surface or impair growth of the end of the affected bone.

Apophyseal separations or fractures usually do not require open reduction unless the apophyseal fragment is widely displaced. Following separation, an apophysis either may remain unattached to or develop a fibrous union with its site of origin. Alternatively, the entire area between the displaced apophysis and its site of origin may gradually fill in with bone, effectively, but at times excessively, enlarging the tuberosity from which it arose. Wide displacement of an apophysis results in shortening of the attached muscle, which in turn reduces the strength of the muscle by reducing the length of the lever arm. Overgrowth of a tuberosity may create mechanical problems because of size or give rise to symptoms because of the development of overlying bursae. These problems may be averted by open reduction and fixation of the displaced apophysis when necessary. The amount of displacement that necessitates open reduction varies from site to site; displacement of 1 cm or more is usually considered an indication for open reduction and pin fixation of the medial epicondyle of the humerus, whereas displacement of the ischial apophysis by 2 cm or more must be present before open reduction and pin or screw fixation is considered.

Prognosis

Of all epiphyseal injuries, 25% to 33% result in some shortening or deformity.[32, 37] Prognosis varies with patient

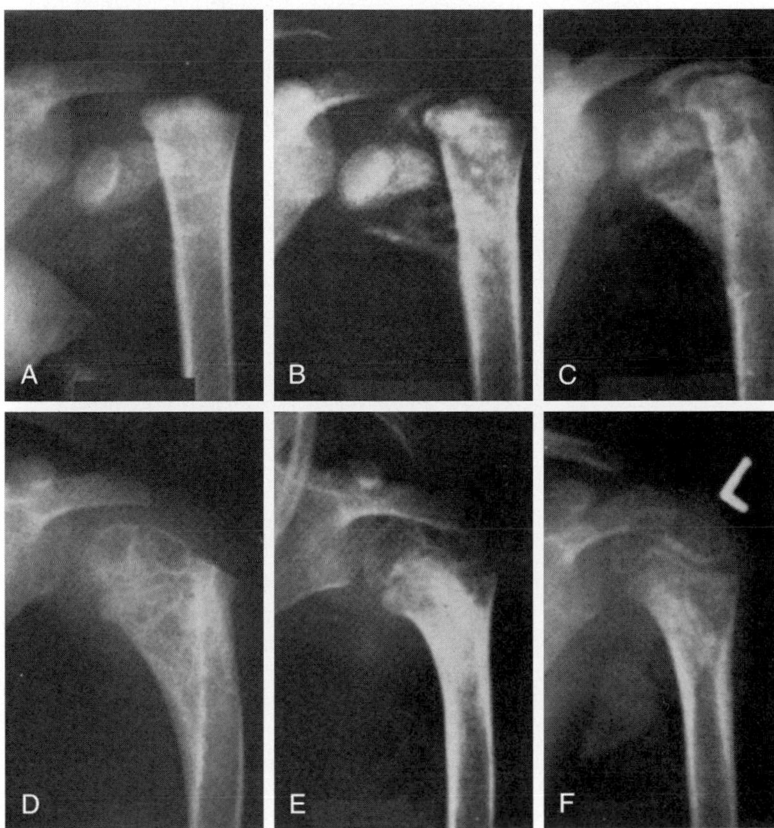

Figure 5–27. The patient was a 4-year-old girl who was struck by an automobile. The initial reduction of a severe fracture separation of the proximal humeral epiphysis was not maintained, and further attempts at remanipulation failed. Remarkable remodeling took place during the subsequent 30 months. Development of the humerus, however, was impaired by an associated incomplete brachial plexus injury. (From Sutton, D., & Grainger, R. G. [1975]. A Textbook of Radiology. Churchill Livingstone, Edinburgh, with permission.)

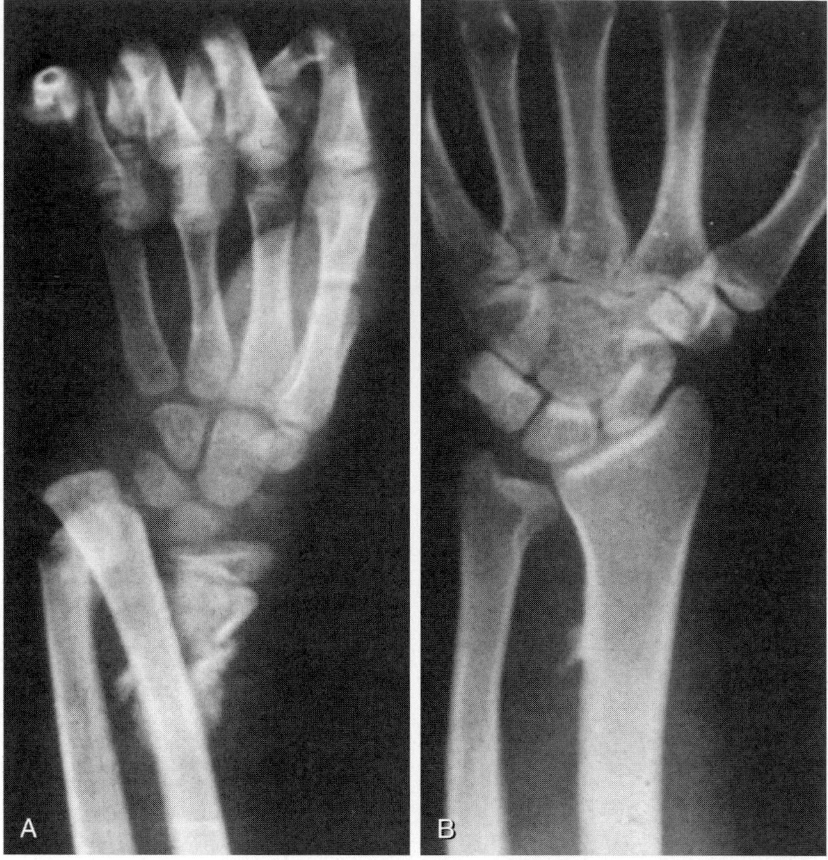

Figure 5–28. The patient was a 7-year-old girl who was struck by an automobile. She sustained multiple injuries, including this widely displaced epiphyseal separation of the left distal radius. *A*, Anteroposterior view of the left wrist on admission shows proximal fragment of the radius protruding through an open wound. Radial epiphyses, carpus, and hand are displaced proximally. *B*, Anteroposterior view of the left wrist 12 years after injury shows exostosis at the site of initial periosteal tear and remarkable regeneration of the distal radius. The open fracture was treated by excising the exposed bone at the level of the skin and packing the wound with petrolatum gauze. A plaster splint was applied with the hand in position of function. No attempt was made to reduce or change the position of the fracture. (From Wilson, J. C., Jr., & Aufranc, O. E. [1971]. Head injured child with fractures. J.A.M.A., *217*:1847, with permission. Copyright © 1971 American Medical Association.)

age, injury severity, anatomic site, fracture type, and the extent and manner of physeal disruption (Fig. 5–30).[32, 88, 117] Shortening or deformities are less well tolerated in the lower extremity because of weight bearing.[24]

In general, Salter-Harris type 1 injuries carry a favorable prognosis. In type 2 injuries minimal shortening is encountered but is rarely of a significant degree except at the knee and ankle. The prognosis with type 3 injuries is generally favorable, with rare deformity, and type 4 injuries frequently result in a joint deformity, either valgus (Figs. 5–31 and 5–32) or varus angulation. Type 5 injuries by definition carry an unfavorable prognosis, as shortening, angulation (see Fig. 5–22), or both[32] are present.

In truth, the prognosis based on the Salter-Harris classification is much more accurate in the upper than in the lower extremity. In the lower extremity, growth arrest and deformities are as likely to occur from type 2 as from type 4 injuries.[88, 107, 108, 120, 129] In any event, all proximal

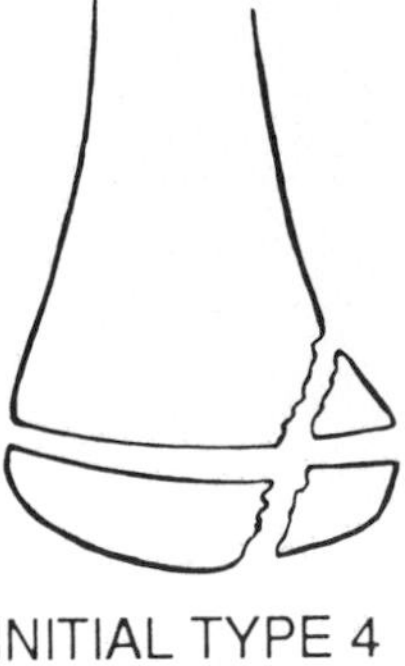

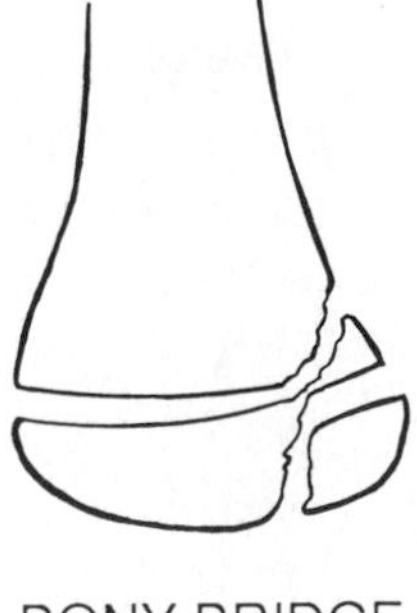

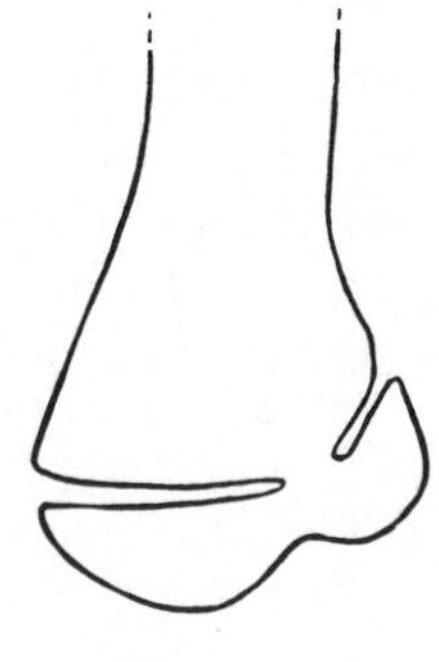

Figure 5–29. Growth disturbance in Salter-Harris type 4 injuries. The initial injury demonstrates a line of fracture across the metaphysis and contiguous epiphyses. If the fracture fragments are left undisturbed, a bone bridge may form between the epiphyses and metaphyses, essentially closing the physis in this area. As a result of premature closure, that portion of the bone is smaller and an angular deformity develops.

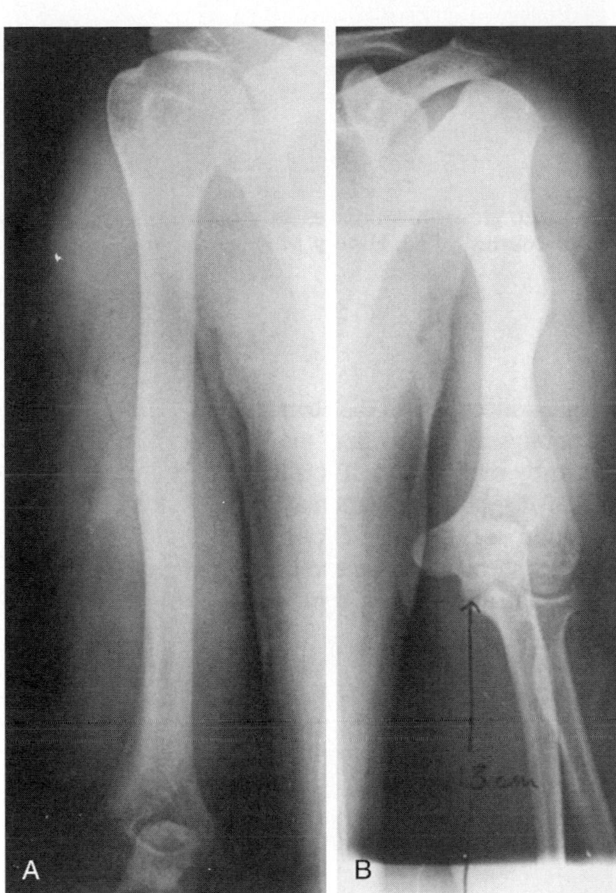

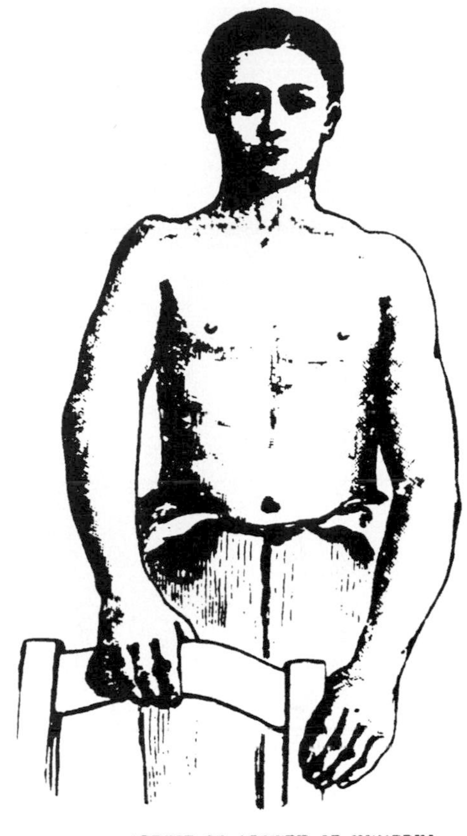

—ARREST OF GROWTH OF HUMERUS AFTER INJURY TO ITS UPPER EPIPHYSIS. (AFTER HELFERICH)

C

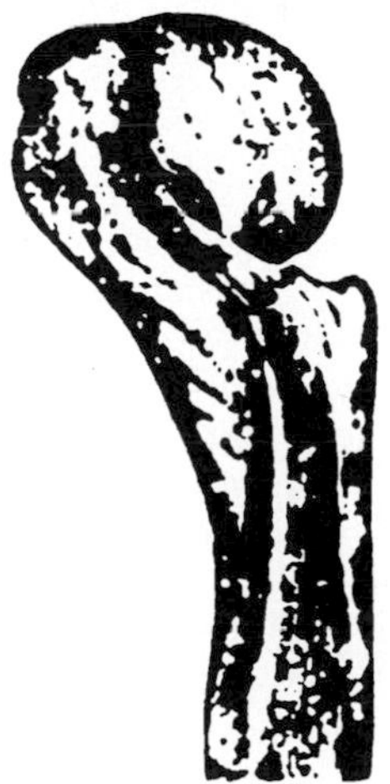

—OLD FRACTURE OF THE HUMERUS THROUGH THE LINE OF THE EPIPHYSIS UNITED BY BONE. DISPLACEMENT OF THE LOWER FRAGMENT INWARDS. (R. W. SMITH)

D

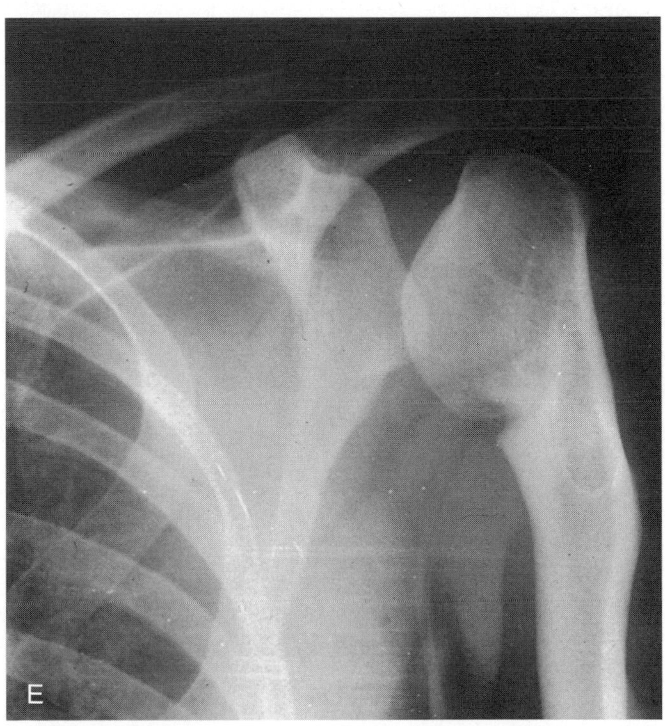

Figure 5–30. *A* and B, Residual shortening of the humerus from proximal epiphyseal injury. According to his history, at the age of 2 years the patient, now a 20-year-old man, had sustained an epiphyseal injury of the proximal left humerus, type unknown. The left humerus (*A*) is 13 cm shorter than the right (*B*). Despite severe shortening the handicap is minimal. (*A* and B, From Rogers, L. F. [1970]. The radiography of epiphyseal injuries. Radiology, 96:289, with permission.) *C,* Clinical appearance of a shortened humerus caused by previous injury of the proximal epiphysis at an early age. *D,* Drawing of deformity of the humerus caused by previous injury to the proximal epiphysis at an early age. *E,* Close-up view of the left shoulder of Figure 5–30*A* discloses a varus deformity of the humeral head that is strikingly similar to that diagrammed in Figure 5–30*D*. (*C* and D, From Poland, J. [1898]. Traumatic Separation of the Epiphyses. Smith, Elder, and Co., London.)

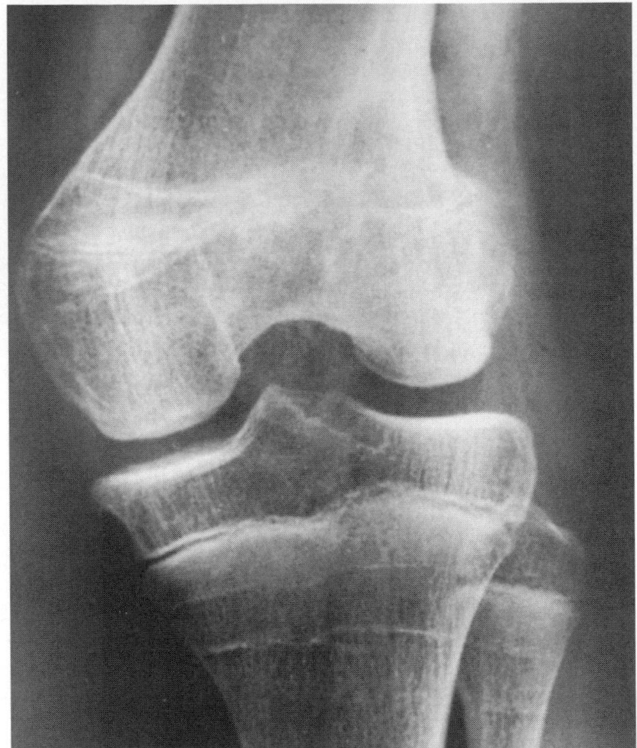

Figure 5–31. Valgus deformity of the knee in a 15-year-old boy who had sustained a Salter-Harris type 4 injury 4 years previously. Note that the distal lateral margin of the distal femoral growth plate has closed, and the lateral femoral condyle is underdeveloped, resulting in a valgus deformity of the knee.

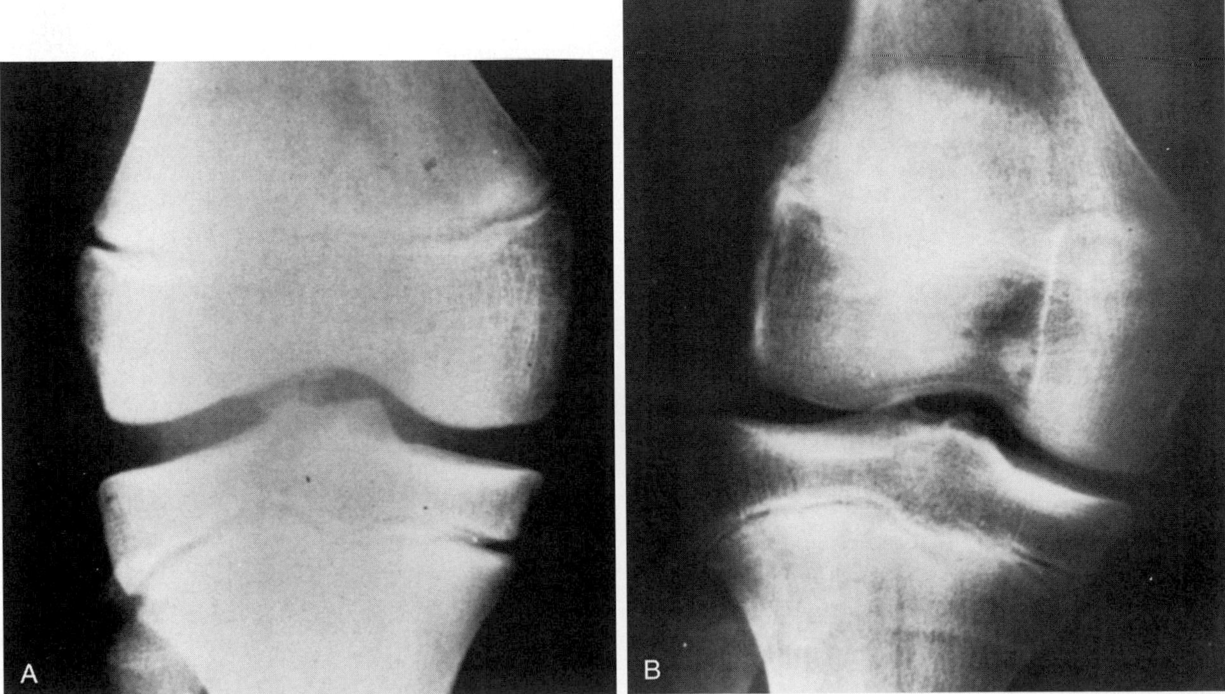

Figure 5–32. Salter-Harris type 5 injury of the distal femoral epiphysis in a 13-year-old boy who sustained an injury of the knee in an auto accident. *A*, Anteroposterior view demonstrates only a small avulsion fracture at the lateral margin of the epiphysis. *B*, Anteroposterior view 18 months after injury demonstrates closure of distal femoral epiphysis. Premature closure laterally resulted in a genu valgum deformity. There is no radiographic finding characteristic of type 5 injury. The compression forces generated by the initial injury led to growth disturbance, early closure of the growth plate, and subsequent angular deformity of the joint. (Case courtesy of J. J. Hinchey, MD, San Antonio, Tex.)

femoral epiphyseal injuries carry a poor prognosis irrespective of type, whereas the prognosis with all distal femoral, proximal tibial, and distal tibial injuries is guarded because of the potential for growth arrest.[126] In contrast, the prognosis with all distal fibular lesions is favorable.

Growth arrest is usually partial. Growth arrest as classified by Bright[80, 81, 131] may be type 1, purely peripheral; type 2, purely central; or type 3, combined peripheral and central. Partial growth arrest may be treated surgically[113] by resection of the bone bridge and interposition of a free fat graft or inert material.[80, 102, 105, 106, 110, 114] In general, at least 50% of the growth plate must remain and 2 or more years of growth must be anticipated before the procedure is undertaken.[81, 102, 104–106] It is therefore important to recognize bone bridging as early as possible to maximize the potential benefit of surgery.

MRI is a great aid in the evaluation of subsequent growth disturbance and is of particular value in the assessment of bone bridging the physis. Jaramillo and colleagues demonstrated that MRI can detect abnormalities in the physis associated with subsequent growth disturbances and provides accurate mapping of physeal bridging once growth disturbances occur.[98–100]

Age also is a factor in prognosis. Obviously, growth retardation or arrest results in greater deformity when it occurs at an early age (see Fig. 5–30). Prognosis with open injuries is less favorable than with closed injuries, regardless of type, because the danger of infection is introduced, and the blood supply to the epiphysis may be disrupted.

A variable time may elapse between the injury and cessation or retardation of growth. The epiphyseal line need not close to produce a deformity; only a decrease in the growth rate is required. In view of these considerations, a minimum of 2 years must elapse before the possibility of shortening or deformity can be excluded. During this period, radiographic re-evaluation should be performed at 3- to 6-month intervals, including comparison views of the contralateral extremity, to determine the comparative length and growth status of the affected extremity.[24] An early clue to the presence of a growth disturbance can be the development of growth arrest lines. If these lines are the result of constitutional causes, they parallel the adjacent growth plate. After trauma, if the line is tilted, curved, or focally depressed or absent, growth disturbance or arrest is likely.[96]

The Battered Child Syndrome

In the past 50 years a syndrome has emerged consisting of multiple, repeated traumatic injuries in young children.[137, 142] It was first described in 1946 by Caffey,[6] who reported the association of multiple fractures in the long bones of children suffering from chronic subdural hematomas, and who stated that these injuries "were either not observed or were denied when observed" by the parent or guardian. The designation of the syndrome as the "battered child syndrome" by Kempe and associates in 1962[17] led to a rash of publicity in the lay press, which was followed by an outpouring of articles in the medical literature fully describing the clinical, radiographic, psychological, and legal features of the syndrome. It has since been recognized that injuries in infants resulting from abuse had been described by Tardieu in the French literature in 1860.[151] The children are frequently younger than 2 and usually younger than 6 years of age when brought for medical attention. It is now accepted that these multiple injuries are inflicted by the parent or guardian.[8, 9, 34] Those who inflict such injuries are often ordinary in appearance and otherwise respectable citizens, who often seem incapable of doing such a thing. This fact made it hard for many to accept the traumatic origin of the syndrome.

The hallmark of the syndrome is clinical and radiographic evidence of repeated injury.[33, 34, 44] The clinical findings may consist of multiple bruises of variable age; body burns of variable age, commonly inflicted by scalding or cigarettes; a sullen demeanor; and findings inconsistent with the history given by the parent or guardian, such as for a 10-month-old who "fell out of the crib yesterday" or a 14-month-old who "pulled the teakettle off the stove"—activities exceeding the capabilities for the age of the child or injury exceeding that expected from the incident described. Often there is no history of trauma. The key to the radiographic diagnosis is the demonstration of characteristic patterns and distributions of fractures that have strong predictive values for abuse (Figs. 5–33 through 5–35).[2, 20, 44, 137] The radiographic hallmark of the syndrome is the classic metaphyseal lesions or corner and bucket handle fractures of the metaphysis, with (see Figs. 5–33*A* and *B* and 5–34*B*) or without (see Fig. 5–35*B*) associated epiphyseal displacement.[2, 32, 33, 44, 137, 139, 143] Fractures at other sites,[20, 134] such as posterior rib, scapular, spinous process, and sternal fractures, are highly suggestive.[38, 137, 140] These may be recognized on a radiograph obtained ostensibly for some other purpose, such as a chest examination (see Fig. 5–35*A*) for possible pneumonia. It is the radiologist's responsibility to alert the clinician to the possibility of the battered child syndrome when the findings suggest this diagnosis. Some of the radiographic features are practically diagnostic, whereas others are only suspicious, and in some instances of clinically unquestionable child abuse radiographic findings may be lacking altogether.[29, 30, 147]

The most common fractures in abused children involve the diaphyses of the long bones. However, in infancy the most common inflicted injuries involve the rib cage, metaphyses, and skull.[136, 137, 152] Epiphyseal separations are rare, and those that do occur are likely to involve either the distal or the proximal humerus.[143] Unsuspected fractures are uncommon beyond the age of 2,[148] and children over the age of 5 rarely sustain a fracture from abuse.[144] Eighty percent of fractures in abused children occur when the children are less than 18 months of age. This is in contrast to nonabused children, in whom 85% of fractures occur beyond the age of 5.[152]

Fractures of the ribs are very common in and quite characteristic of abuse.[148, 152] They are distinctly rare in the nonabused child, and those that do occur result from severe trauma in motor vehicle accidents and not the low-impact, "trip, stumble, and fall" injuries normally encountered in children. Rib fractures are easily over-

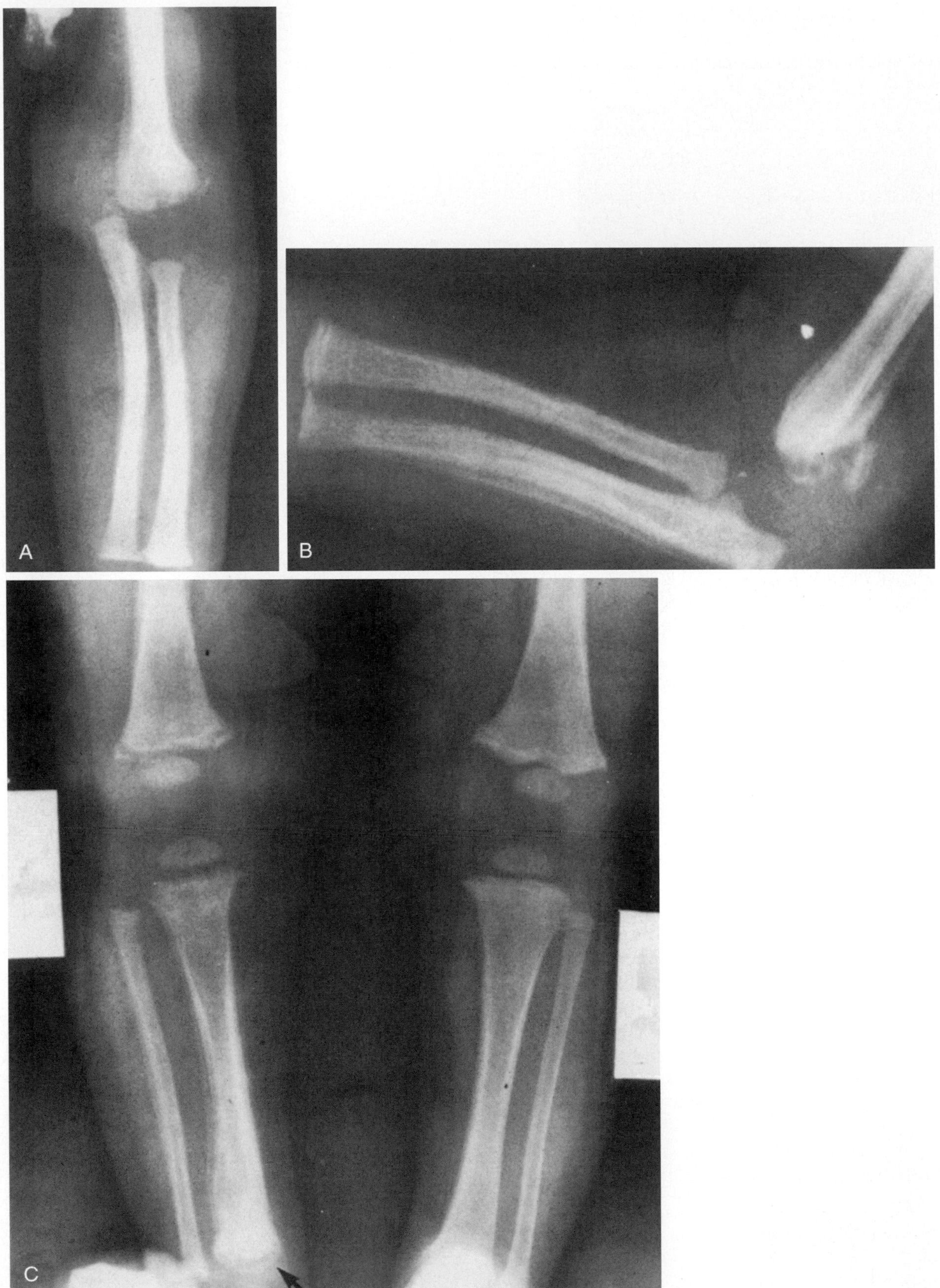

Figure 5–33. The patient was a battered child, age 8 months. *A*, Anteroposterior view of the arm reveals metaphyseal irregularities of the distal humerus. Both bones of the forearm are displaced medially, indicating separation of the distal humeral epiphysis; the ulna and, to a lesser extent, the radius are bowed. Note the periosteal new bone formation along the distal shaft of the humerus and the midshaft of the ulna. *B*, Lateral radiograph clearly demonstrates the extensive periosteal bone formation along the distal shaft of the humerus and the midshaft of the radius in addition to the metaphyseal irregularities of the humerus. *C*, Corner fractures are present at the distal femoral metaphysis on the right, with slight irregularity of the corner of the metaphysis on the left, probably indicating healed fractures. Periosteal new bone formation is present on the distal shaft of the right femur and along the entire shaft of the right tibia. Bucket handle fracture consisting of a large portion of the rim of the distal tibial metaphysis is present (*arrow*) on the right. The distal tibial metaphysis is broadened, suggesting a healed fracture in this area.

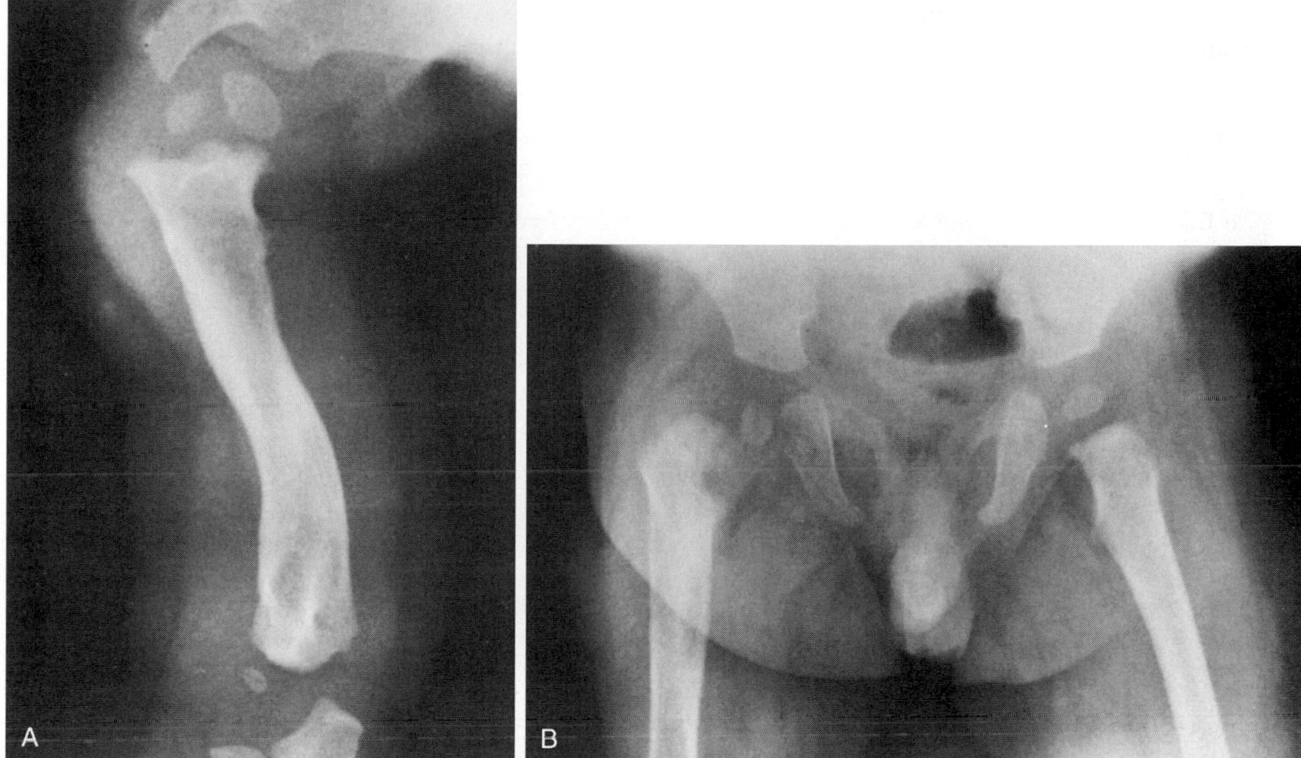

Figure 5–34. The patient was a battered child, age 10 months. *A*, In the humerus, there are irregularities at the corners of the metaphysis, both proximally and distally, in addition to abnormal contour of the shaft, indicating a healed fracture. *B*, Irregularities of the proximal femoral metaphysis are seen on the right, with displacement of the capital femoral epiphysis. The proximal femoral shaft on the right is abnormal in contour, being broadened with areas of sclerosis, which indicate a healed fracture. (Case courtesy of Andrew Poznanski, MD, Chicago, Ill.)

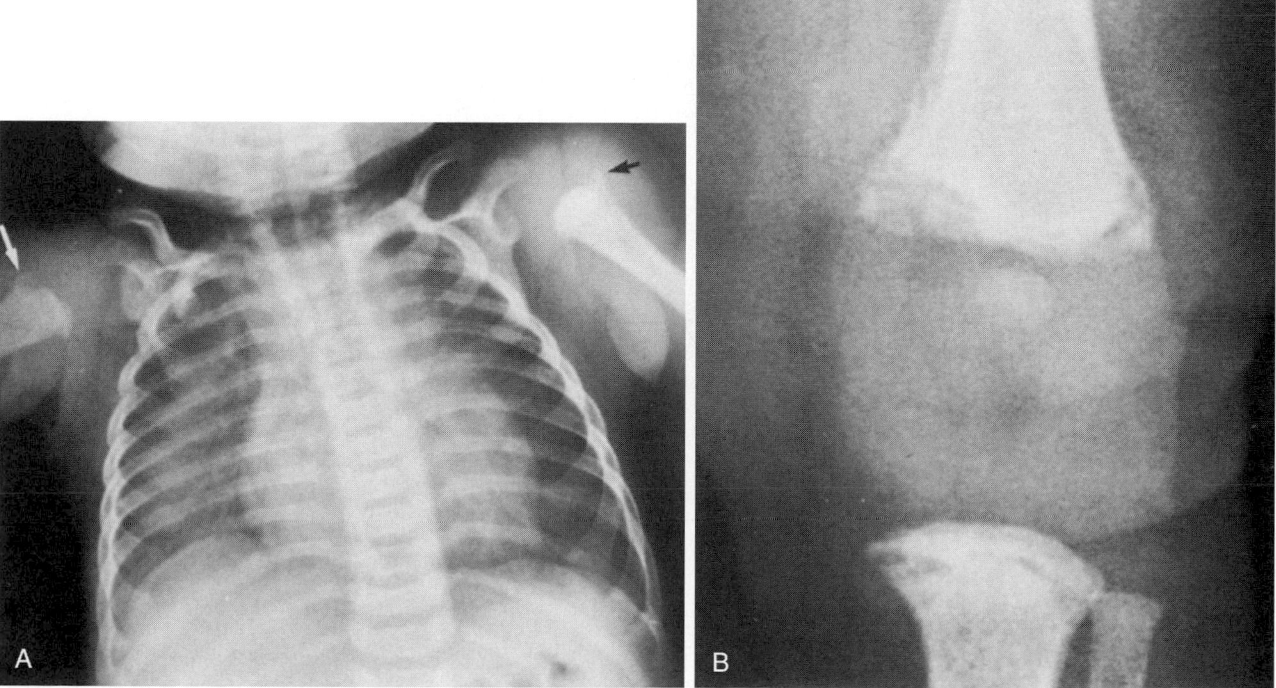

Figure 5–35. The patient was a battered child, 3 months of age. *A*, Chest radiograph was obtained because the patient had a fever. The irregularities of the proximal humeral metaphysis (*arrows*) were noted, and additional views of the extremities were obtained. *B*, Irregularities of the margins of the metaphyses of both the distal femur and the proximal tibia were identified. Note the periosteal new bone formation along the metaphysis of the distal femur. Similar though less extensive findings were present at other sites.

looked on radiographs. Although they can occur at any site, they are most common posteriorly and medially near the costal transverse process articulation and are usually multiple (Fig. 5–36). The characteristic rib fractures are due to thoracic compression or squeezing that flattens the chest and levers the posterior margin of the ribs over the transverse processes. Blows to the anterior chest may also cause fractures of the sternum and separation of the costochondral junctions. In any event, rib fractures or fractures of the sternum are very rare in infants and children from any cause other than abuse or high-impact motor vehicle accidents. Multiple rib fractures at any site would suggest child abuse in any circumstances other than high-impact motor vehicle or auto-pedestrian accidents. Posterior medial rib fractures are extremely difficult to visualize on the radiograph initially but may be identified subsequently as callus forms about the fracture on follow-up skeletal surveys.[141] However, they can be identified earlier by bone scanning (see Fig. 5–36).

Skull fractures are commonly encountered in abused children. However, linear skull fractures are of low specificity, whereas complex skull fractures are more suggestive (Fig. 5–37). Subdural hematomas and intracerebral hematomas frequently occur. Interhemispheric subdural hematomas are particularly common in the child who has been shaken and are quite suggestive of abuse (see Fig. 5–37*B*). In 80% of such infants, retinal hemorrhages will also be identified, and this combination is highly suggestive of abuse.[133, 142] Abused infants are at high risk for subsequent neurologic deficits. Skull films and noncontrast head CT are appropriate for acute evaluation, with MRI (and head ultrasound examination for infants) useful for full characterization of the nature and extent of intracranial injury. Abdominal injuries also occur, particularly pancreatic and bowel injuries, for which abdominal CT is indicated.[134, 137, 142, 149]

Many of the children are subjected to severe shaking[8] while held by the arms or legs, and this trauma presumably creates the classic metaphyseal lesions (see Fig. 5–33). Metaphyseal lesions in abused children are highly distinctive and have been termed *bucket handle* or *corner fractures*.[139] These lesions may form the basis for the diagnosis of abuse, particularly in infants younger than 2 years of age. Kleinman and associates[139] demonstrated that the basic histologic alteration is a series of microfractures through the primary spongiosa, the most immature portion of the distal metaphysis. This finding is in contradistinction to the plane of fracture of epiphyseal injuries of nonabused children, which occurs through the hypertrophic zone of the physis. The fracture results in the isolation of a mineralized disc of the distal metaphysis. The resultant radiographic appearance is dependent upon the radiographic projection and orientation of the plane of fracture (Fig. 5–38). When perpendicular it is seen as a linear lucency, and when tilted, as an arc of bone representing a typical bucket handle fracture (Fig. 5–39). The periosteum is tightly adherent to the metaphysis adjacent to the growth plate but relatively loosely attached to the remainder of the shaft. As the limb is shaken, the periosteum is pulled from the shaft, where it is loosely attached, and shears off portions of the metaphysis, where it is tightly attached.[7, 8, 47] As the periosteum is lifted, a subperiosteal hematoma forms, and subsequently new bone is laid down in the area. This form of injury is unlikely to occur under other circumstances, such as a fall. Repetitive injuries may cause periosteal new bone formation to become very exuberant and the metaphysis quite irregular. The peculiar and unusual nature of the radiographic findings initially made it difficult for many investigators to accept that they were of traumatic origin.

Not unexpectedly, many battered children have subsequently died of their injuries,[9, 34] and those who survive may be done severe psychological and physical harm. It is the radiologist's role and responsibility to alert the clinician to the possibility when this diagnosis is not expected and to confirm the diagnosis when suspected clini-

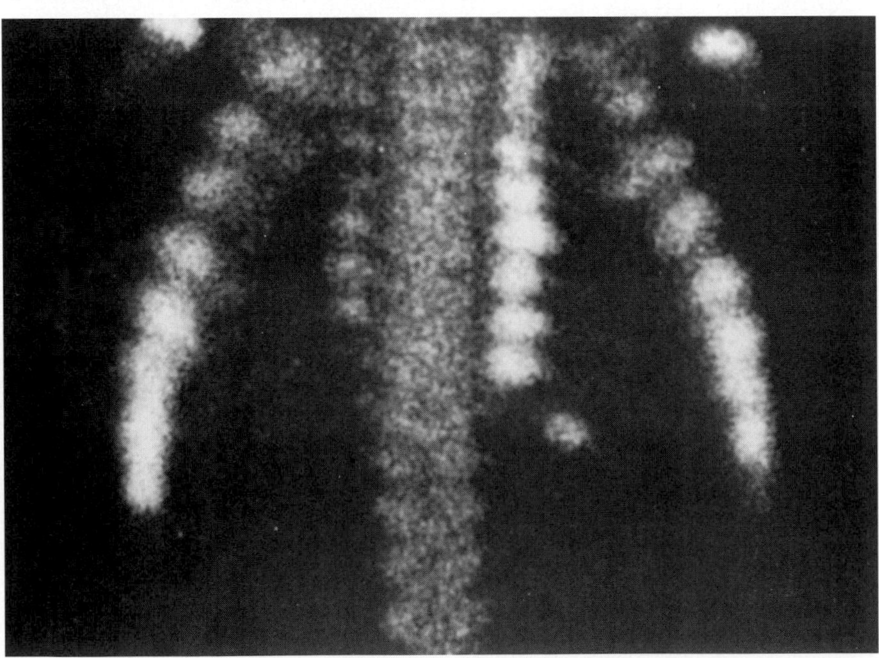

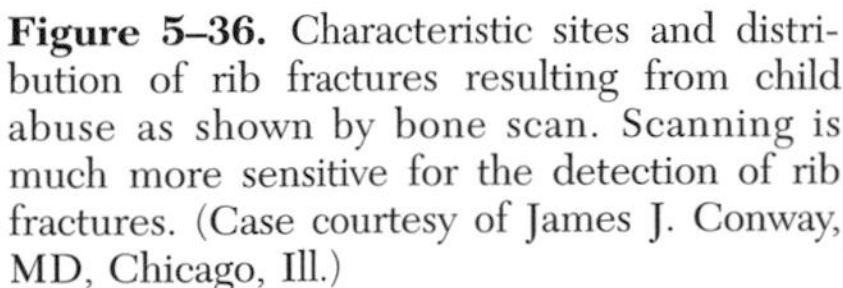

Figure 5–36. Characteristic sites and distribution of rib fractures resulting from child abuse as shown by bone scan. Scanning is much more sensitive for the detection of rib fractures. (Case courtesy of James J. Conway, MD, Chicago, Ill.)

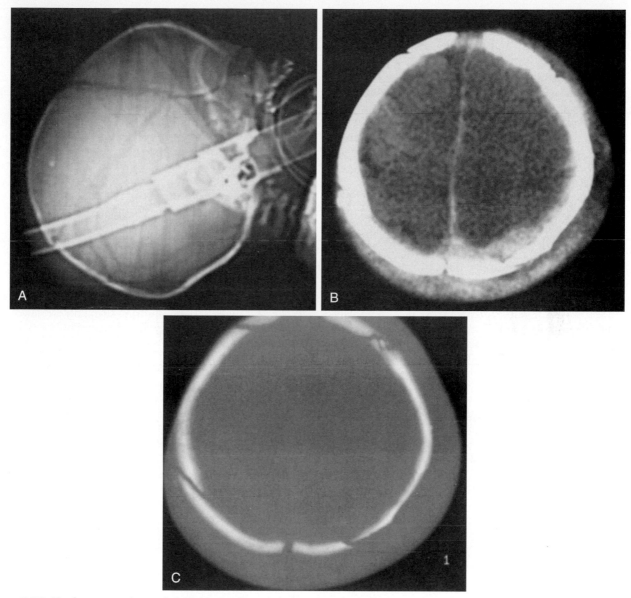

Figure 5–37. Head injury in a battered child. The mother struck the infant's head against the wall several times in an attempt to stop the child's crying. *A*, Lateral digital radiograph with overlying endotracheal tube in place demonstrates multiple complex fractures of the skull and diastasis of the coronal sutures. *B*, Computed tomography scan demonstrates subdural hematoma posteriorly with interhemispheric extension. There is also an intracerebral hematoma in the right hemisphere. *C*, Bone windows demonstrate multiple fractures and sutural diastasis. There is also a large subgaleal hematoma. (Case courtesy of Mary Ann Radkowski, MD, Chicago, Ill.)

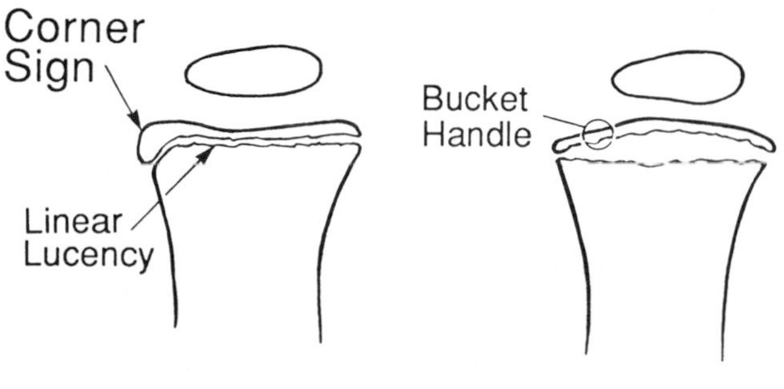

Figure 5–38. Characteristic metaphyseal fractures in child abuse. The appearance of fractures is dependent upon the alignment of the x-ray beam to the distal metaphyses and the presence or absence of displacement of the fracture fragments. If the beam is perpendicular and the fragment undisplaced, a fine linear fracture is seen in the distal metaphyses. If the metaphyseal fragment is displaced or tilted it has an arclike appearance, referred to as a "bucket handle." The fracture line is often obliquely oriented at the margin of the metaphyses, resulting in the characteristic "corner sign."

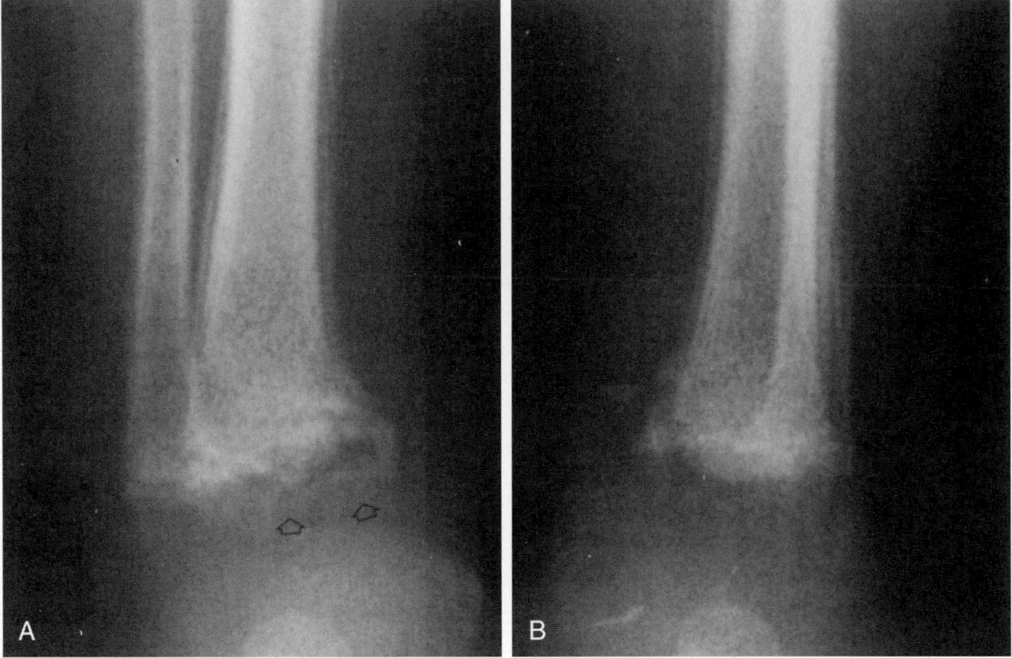

Figure 5–39. Bucket handle fractures of the distal tibia in a 13-month-boy. *A*, There is a characteristic bucket handle fracture on the right (*arrows*). *B*, On the left there is a corner fragment medially and a very thin bucket handle fragment distally. Periosteal elevation is present bilaterally. (Case courtesy of Mary Ann Radkowski, MD, Chicago, Ill.)

cally. The radiologic diagnosis of child abuse can be best accomplished by a well-performed skeletal survey that includes anteroposterior (AP) and lateral views of the skull and thorax, lateral cervical and lumbar spine views, oblique views of the hands, and AP views of the pelvis, humeri, forearms, femora, tibias, and feet, as recommended by the American College of Radiology (ACR).[137] Dedicated films should be obtained to confirm questionable findings.

Bone scanning has been advocated by some investigators as an initial screening procedure in suspected abuse.[150] However, it is nonspecific, and in fact the subtle metaphyseal fractures are difficult or impossible to detect because of the normally increased activity in this region.[144] Nonetheless, scanning is quite sensitive in detecting rib, spine, and subtle diaphyseal trauma, especially when the injury is acute and the radiographic appearance is normal.[135] Therefore, bone scanning plays a role in confirming evidence of abuse either when radiographic evidence of trauma is not present, nonspecific, or unifocal or when there is a strong clinical suspicion of abuse but the radiographic skeletal survey is negative.

It is well to keep in mind that similar skeletal manifestations are found in the condition of congenital indifference to pain and in other conditions associated with a neurosensory deficit, such as a myelomeningocele (see Fig. 5–47). However, the former condition is quite rare and the latter quite obvious to the clinician. Other diseases such as infantile cortical hyperostosis, congenital syphilis, scurvy, and osteogenesis imperfecta[132, 146] (see Fig. 5–43) may present as differential diagnostic possibilities.[147, 148] In general they are readily excluded by clinical and radiographic findings.

The radiologist and the clinician should transmit the possibility of the diagnosis of battered child syndrome verbally and not depend on the written request or report. The implications of this diagnosis are crucial for the child, and any delay in establishment of the diagnosis may jeopardize the child's well-being if not its very life.

Pathologic Fractures

Pathologic fractures are relatively infrequent in children. When encountered in a long bone they usually involve a simple bone cyst[44] or, less commonly, a nonossifying fibroma. A simple or unicameral bone cyst in children is commonly associated with a pathologic fracture (Fig. 5–40); indeed, pathologic fractures may even be considered characteristic of this lesion. A simple bone cyst is a purely osteolytic, well-defined, expansile lesion of the metaphysis, often found in the proximal humerus or femur. Incomplete fracture can occur through nonossifying fibromas (Fig. 5–41), which are eccentric, expansile, well-marginated lucent lesions commonly found in the distal end of the femur and proximal and distal ends of the tibia. Avulsion fractures from the thin peripheral cortex of these lesions have been reported.[159, 163] They have proved troubling because of the absence of a history of acute trauma and the presence of periosteal new bone formation. At first glance this constellation of findings suggests something sinister (e.g., malignant tumor or infection). It is likely that most such lesions represent avulsions by tendons inserting onto the surface of the involved bone as a result of repetitive activity such as running or other forms of exercise, and in this sense they represent stress or insufficiency fractures. The periosteal new bone formation is a healing response to injury similar to that

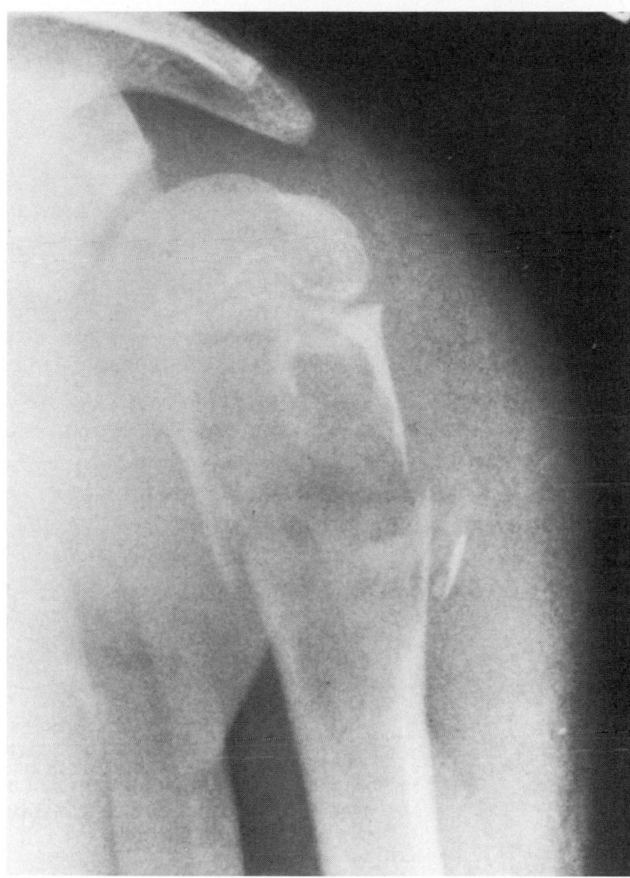

Figure 5–40. Pathologic fractures through a unicameral bone cyst of the proximal humerus in a 10-year-old boy. A transverse fracture with slight comminution at its lateral margin passes through a well-defined lucent, expansile lesion of the metaphysis. The lesion abuts the growth plate. Findings are characteristic of a unicameral bone cyst. The boy had injured his arm in a fall.

encountered in other, more orthodox stress fractures. The majority of patients with fractures through nonossifying fibromas can be managed nonoperatively.[156]

Compression fractures of the vertebral bodies are usually associated with osteoporosis secondary to the administration of steroids or due to infiltration in leukemia[166] or metastatic neuroblastoma (Fig. 5–42). Vertebra plana, or complete collapse of a vertebral body, is characteristic of histiocytosis X.

Multiple, recurring fractures are the hallmark of osteogenesis imperfecta.[26, 41] The congenita form (Fig. 5–43) is manifested at or shortly after birth. This form of the disease is readily diagnosed by the multiple thickened and deformed bones produced by repeated fractures with thin cortices. The tarda form (Fig. 5–44) may not manifest itself until adolescence or even until adult life, and the thin tubular bones and underlying osteoporosis may be difficult to appreciate. The associated clinical findings of wormian bones, blue sclerae, joint laxity, dentinogenesis imperfecta, and hearing loss are helpful and should be sought when repeated fractures occur in response to seemingly trivial trauma.[137]

Multiple fractures of the metaphyses of long bones constitute a hallmark of idiopathic juvenile osteoporosis.[154, 158, 160, 168, 169] This rare, nonhereditary condition of unknown etiology occurs in previously healthy 3- to 12-year-old children. They present with pain as a result of pathologic fractures, particularly about the feet, knees, and ankles. Diffuse osteoporosis is present, and vertebral fractures may occur. No specific biochemical abnormalities have been identified. Spontaneous remission occurs during puberty.

Multiple fractures of the ribs and long bones and rickets, also known as rickets of prematurity, characteristically occur in very-low-birth-weight infants, those weighing 1500 g or less.[162] With weight gain and appropriate nutrition, the fractures heal without subsequent deformity.

Osteoporotic bones in patients with β-thalassemia (Cooley's anemia) are prone to fracture from minor trauma[157] (see Fig. 5–45*B*). The red marrow hyperplasia results in cortical thinning, trabecular loss, and expansion of the medullary cavity. The fractures are most likely to occur in the metaphyses of long bones, which are severely affected by these changes. Deformities may result from recurrent and multiple fractures and from the accompanying partial closure of physes known to occur in association with this disease.

Pathologic epiphyseal separations occur in certain metabolic conditions, particularly renal osteodystrophy (Fig. 5–46), and less commonly in scurvy[115] and rickets. They are usually Salter-Harris type 1 injuries without involvement of the metaphysis. In renal osteodystrophy,[18, 26, 78] the proximal femoral, proximal humeral, and distal radial epiphyses are most frequently involved.

Patients with myelomeningocele[26, 44, 161, 165, 167] experience pathologic epiphyseal separations (Fig. 5–47) that characteristically involve the lower extremity. These separations are due to a combination of sensory deficiency, musculoligamentous laxity, and osteopenia. The injuries

RADIOLOGY OF SKELETAL TRAUMA

CHURCHILL LIVINGSTONE
A Harcourt Health Sciences Company

The Curtis Center
Independence Square West
Philadelphia, Pennsylvania 19106

Library of Congress Cataloging-in-Publication Data

Radiology of skeletal trauma / [edited by] Lee F. Rogers.—3rd ed.

p. ; cm.

Includes bibliographical references and index.

ISBN 0–443–06563–2 (set)—ISBN 9997634004 (v. 1)—ISBN 9997634012 (v. 2)

1. Fractures—Diagnosis. 2. Bones—Radiography. 3. Fractures—Tomography. I. Rogers, Lee F.
[DNLM: 1. Bone and Bones–injuries.
2. Fractures–radiography. WE 175 R727r 2002]

RD102.R64 2002 617.1′5—dc21

DNLM/DLC 2001–028375

Executive Editor: Lisette Bralow
Developmental Editor: Jennifer Shreiner
Manuscript Editor: Robin E. Davis
Production Manager: Mary Stermel
Illustration Specialist: Rita Martello

RADIOLOGY OF SKELETAL TRAUMA ISBN 0–443–06563–2

Printed in the United States of America.

Last digit is the print number: 9 8 7 6 5 4 3 2 1

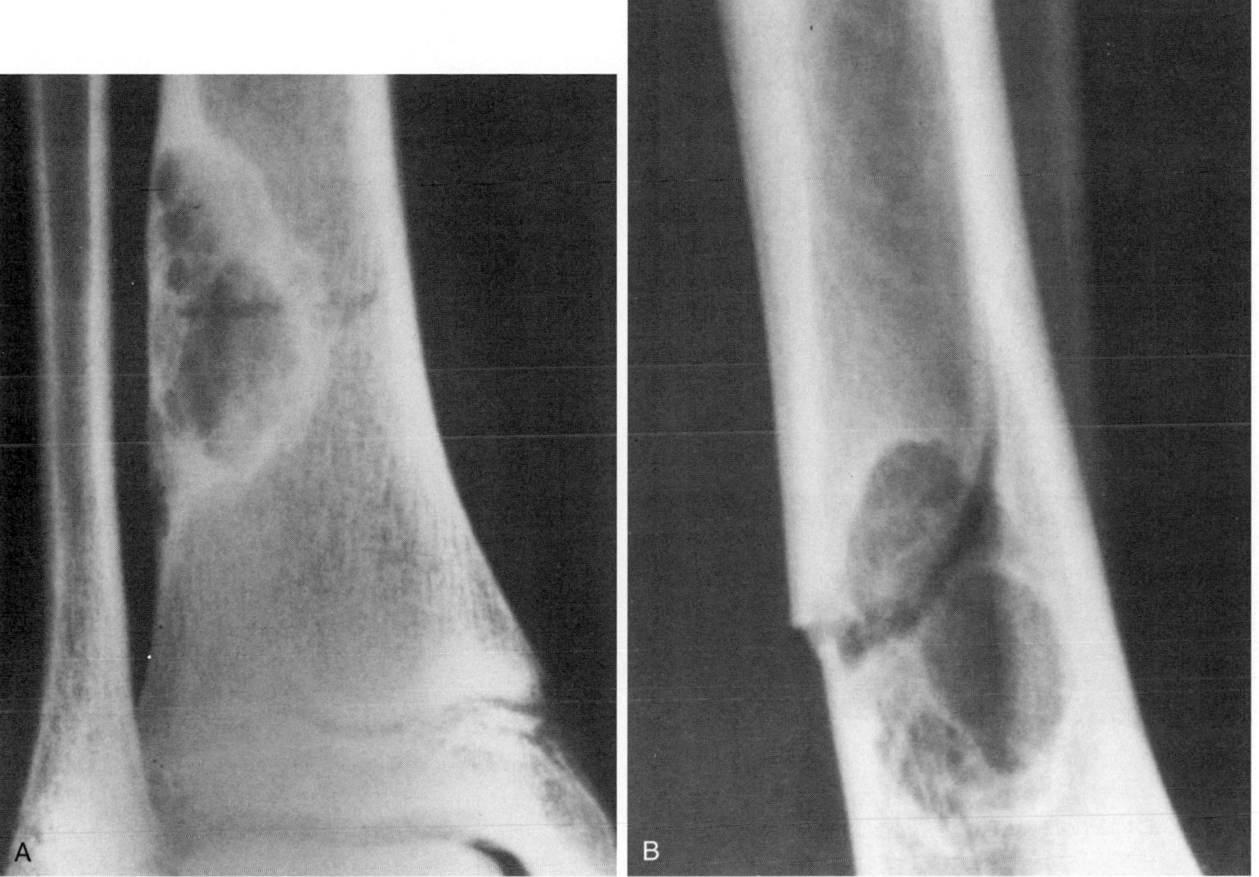

Figure 5–41. Pathologic incomplete fracture through a nonossifying fibroma of the distal end of the tibia in a 12-year-old boy. *A*, Anteroposterior view demonstrates a line of lucency extending through an eccentric, bubbly, well-marginated lesion of the distal tibial metaphysis. *B*, Lateral view demonstrates the incomplete greenstick fracture that extends through the lesion but does not involve the posterior cortex. The radiographic appearance of the lesion is typical of a nonossifying fibroma.

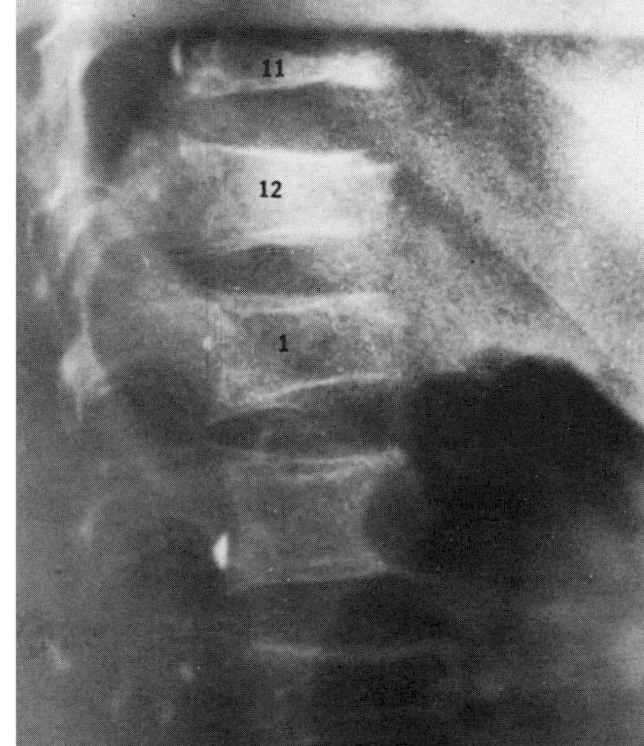

Figure 5–42. Pathologic fractures of multiple vertebrae in a 7-year-old girl with leukemia. Anterior wedging of variable degree is present in T11, T12, L1, and L3. Small droplets of residual contrast material (iophendylate [Pantopaque]) are also identified.

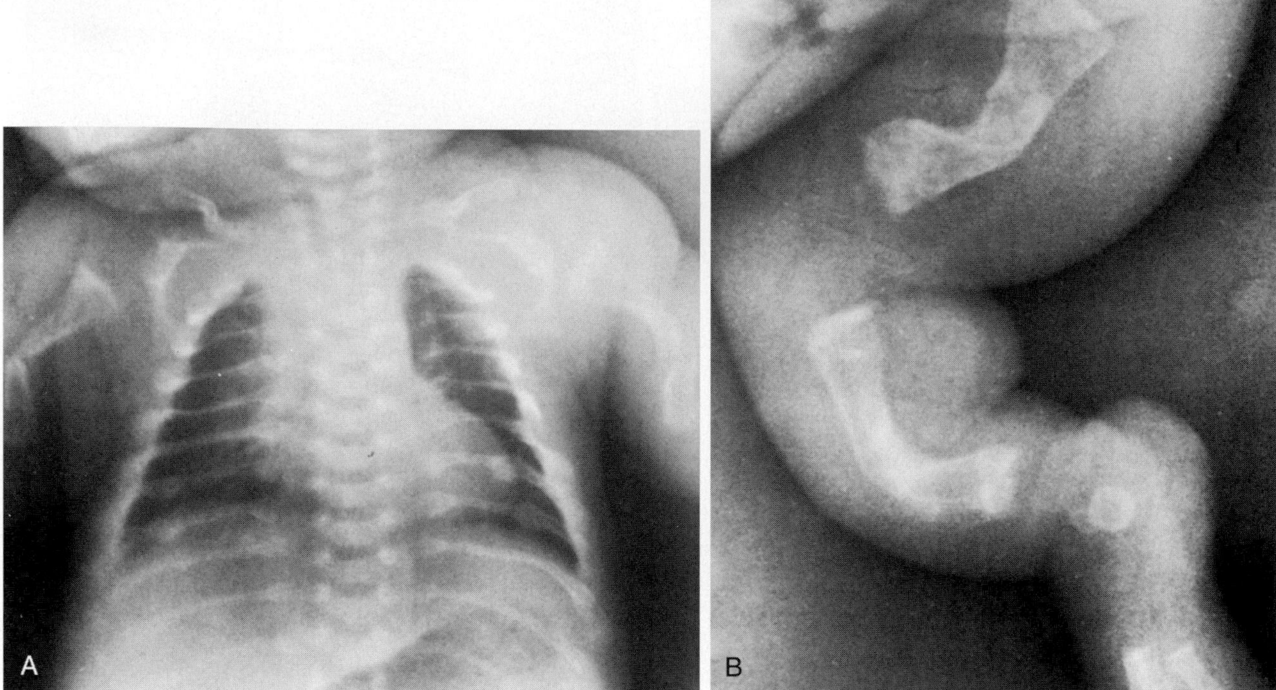

Figure 5–43. Osteogenesis imperfecta in a newborn. *A*, Note the bilateral fractures of the humerus and numerous fractures of the ribs with callus formation. The ribs are abnormally thin. *B*, In this view of the right lower extremity, the femur and tibia are greatly distorted by previous fractures. The cortices of the bones are thin.

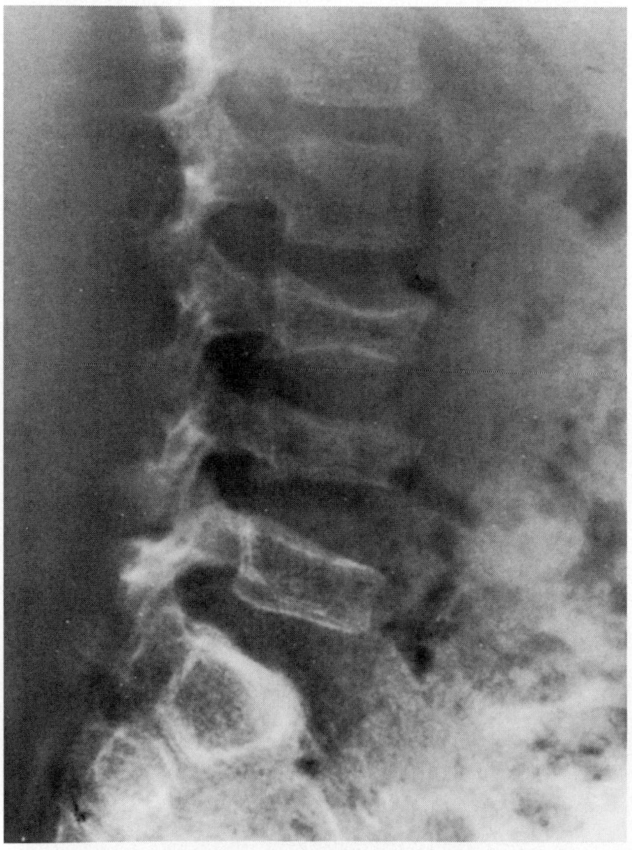

Figure 5–44. Appearance of the lumbar spine in a 5-year-old girl with osteogenesis imperfecta tarda who presented with back pain. She had had a previous femoral fracture; radiographs of the extremities were normal, however. Note the compression of the bodies of L3, L4, and L5. The bodies of L1 and L2 appear to be osteoporotic, having decreased density and thin cortices. The patient has blue sclerae.

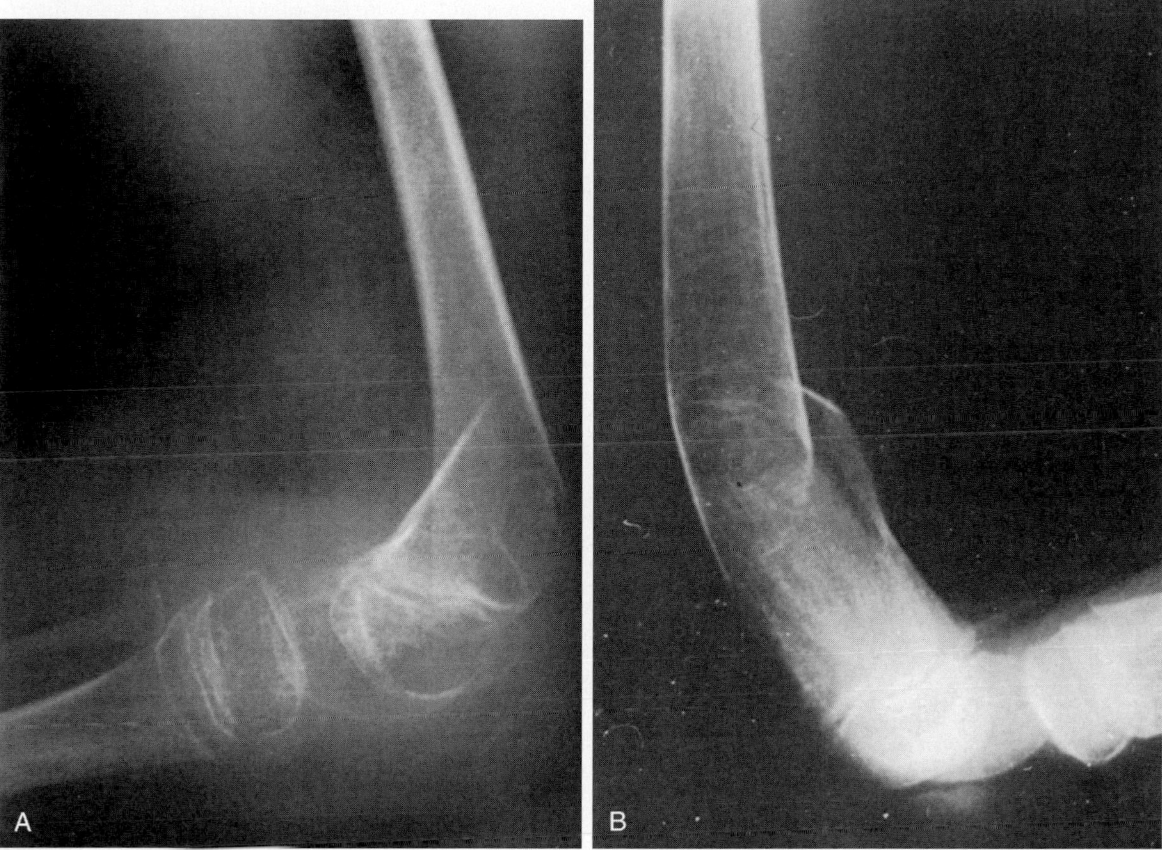

Figure 5–45. Pathologic fractures of the distal femoral metaphyses from two different causes. *A*, Supracondylar fracture in a 9-year-old girl who had a spinal cord deficit resulting in bone atrophy. The bones are markedly osteopenic and susceptible to fractures. *B*, Fracture in a young man with thalassemia. Note the profound thinning of the cortex caused by marrow hyperplasia. (Case courtesy of Jack Lawson, MD, New Haven, Conn.)

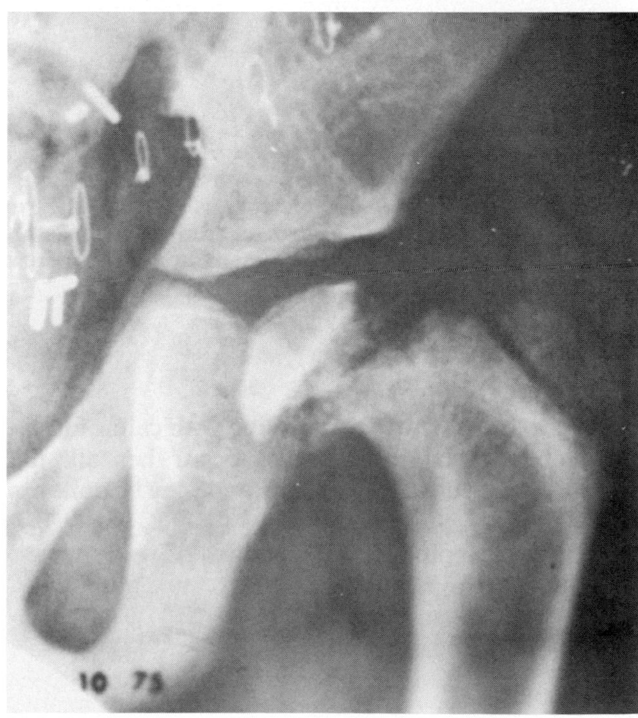

Figure 5–46. Pathologic separation of the proximal femoral epiphysis in a child with renal osteodystrophy. The femoral epiphysis is displaced medially and inferiorly. The growth plate is widened, and there are erosions and irregularities within the metaphysis. (Case courtesy of Andrew Poznanski, MD, Chicago, Ill.)

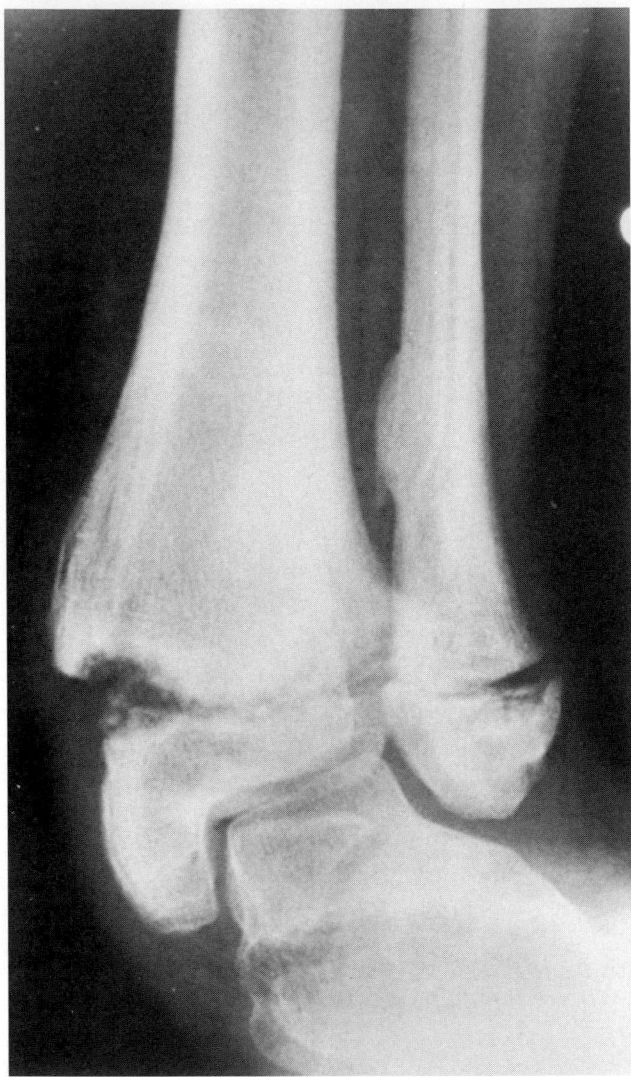

Figure 5–47. Pathologic fractures of the distal tibial epiphysis in a youngster with myelomeningocele. The epiphysis is tilted and displaced laterally with widening of the growth plate and marked irregularities of the medial metaphysis. There are similar changes in the distal fibular metaphysis. The findings are characteristic of the epiphyseal changes seen at the ankles in patients with myelomeningocele. (Case courtesy of Andrew Poznanski, MD, Chicago, Ill.)

are often not noted because of the lack of sensation. Repeated shearing fractures occur through the metaphysis, the epiphysis is displaced, and the growth plate is widened. The metaphysis becomes irregular because of the repeated fractures and healing with callus formation. Subperiosteal hemorrhages occur beneath the stripped periosteum. These areas calcify and may be quite extensive. Chronic stress or trauma to the poorly sensate limb produces micromotion at the zone of hypertrophy, yielding a widened, disorganized physis that predisposes to fracture, displacement, or delayed union.[167]

Pathologic fractures are also common in patients with cerebral palsy, whose osteoporotic long bones present long and fragile lever arms connected to stiff joints. Most fractures occur in the femoral shafts and supracondylar regions.[153]

Spontaneous epiphyseal separation of the proximal humerus and femur has been reported following radiotherapy for childhood malignancies.[90, 155, 164, 170] The radiation dose utilized is usually in excess of 4000 rads. Characteristically the separation is of the Salter-Harris type 1 variety and occurs 7 to 16 months after treatment.

References

General

1. Aitken, A. P. (1965). Fractures of the epiphyses. Clin. Orthop., *41*:19.
2. Baker, D. H., & Berdon, W. E. (1966). Special trauma problems in children. Radiol. Clin. North Am., *4*:289.
3. Bergenfeldt, E. (1933). Beiträge zur Kenntnis der traumatischen Epiphysenloösungun an den langen Röhrenknochen der Extremitaten. Eine klinischröntgenologische Studie. Acta Chir. Scand., *73*:1.
4. Blount, W. P. (1955). Fractures in Children. Williams & Wilkins, Baltimore.
5. Borden, S. IV. (1975). Roentgen recognition of acute plastic bowing of the forearm in children. A. J. R. Am. J. Roentgenol., *125*:524.
6. Caffey, J. (1946). Multiple fractures in the long bones of infants suffering from chronic subdural hematoma. A. J. R. Am. J. Roentgenol., *56*:163.
7. Caffey, J. (1957). Some traumatic lesions in growing bones other than fractures and dislocations: Clinical and radiological features. Br. J. Radiol., *30*:225.
8. Caffey, J. (1972). On the theory and practice of shaking infants. Am. J. Dis. Child., *124*:161.
9. Caffey, J. (1972). The parent-infant traumatic stress syndrome (Caffey-Kempe syndrome, battered babe syndrome). A. J. R. Am. J. Roentgenol., *114*:217.
10. Cail, W. S., Keats, T. E., & Sussman, M. D. (1978). Plastic bowing fracture of the femur in a child. A. J. R. Am. J. Roentgenol., *130*:780.
11. Compere, E. L. (1953). Growth arrest in long bones as result of fractures that include the epiphysis. J.A.M.A., *105*:2140.
12. Crowe, J. E., & Swischuk, L. E. (1977). Acute bowing fractures of the forearm in children: A frequently missed injury. Am. J. Roentgenol., *128*:981.
13. Dalzell, D. P., & Auringer, S. T. (1998). Problem children: Common fractures commonly missed. Postgrad. Radiol., *18*:170.
14. Donnelly, L. F., Klostermeier, T. T., & Klosterman, L. A. (1998). Traumatic elbow effusions in pediatric patients: Are occult fractures the rule? A. J. R. Am. J. Roentgenol., *171*:243.
15. Haliburton, R. A., Barber, J. R., & Fraser, R. L. (1967). Pseudodislocation: An unusual birth injury. Can. J. Surg., *10*:455.
16. Holland, C. T. (1929). A radiological note on injuries to distal epiphyses of the radius and ulna. Proc. R. Soc. Med., *22*:23.
17. Kempe, C. H., Silverman, F. N., Steele, B. F. et al. (1962). The battered-child syndrome. J.A.M.A., *181*:17.
18. Kirkwood, J. R., Ozonoff, M. B., & Steinbach, H. L. (1972). Epiphyseal displacement after metaphyseal fracture in renal osteodystrophy. A. J. R. Am. J. Roentgenol., *115*:547.
19. Kittleson, A. C., & Whitehouse, W. M. (1966). Stress, greenstick and impaction fractures. Radiol. Clin. North Am., *4*:277.
20. Kogutt, M. S., Swischuk, L. E., & Fagan, C. J. (1974). Patterns of injury and significance of uncommon fractures in the battered child syndrome. A. J. R. Am. J. Roentgenol., *121*:143.
21. Larson, R. L., & McMahan, R. O. (1966). The epiphyses and the childhood athlete. J.A.M.A., *196*:607.
22. Martin, W. III, & Riddervold, H. O. (1979). Acute plastic bowing fractures of the fibula. Radiology, *131*:639.
23. Neer, C. S. II, & Horwitz, B. S. (1965). Fractures of the proximal humeral epiphyseal plate. Clin. Orthop., *41*:24.
24. Nicholson, J. T., & Nixon, J. E. (1961). Epiphyseal fractures. J. Pediatr., *59*:939.
25. O'Donoghue, D. H. (1962). Treatment of Injuries to Athletes. W. B. Saunders Co., Philadelphia.
26. Ozonoff, M. B. (1992). Pediatric Orthopedic Radiology. 2nd Ed. W. B. Saunders Co., Philadelphia.
27. Peterson, C. A., & Peterson, H. A. (1972). Analysis of the incidence of injuries to the epiphyseal growth plate. J. Trauma, *12*:275.
28. Poland, J. (1898). Traumatic Separation of the Epiphyses. Smith, Elder and Co., London.
29. Rang, M. (1994). Children's Fractures. 2nd Ed. J. B. Lippincott Co., Philadelphia.
30. Rogers, L. F. (1970). The radiography of epiphyseal injuries. Radiology, *96*:289.
31. Sakakida, K. (1964). Clinical observations on the epiphyseal separation of long bones. Clin. Orthop., *34*:119.
32. Salter, R. B., & Harris, W. R. (1963). Injuries involving the epiphyseal plate. J. Bone Joint Surg. [Am.], *45*:587.
33. Silverman, F. N. (1953). The roentgen manifestations of unrecognized skeletal trauma in infants. J. Roentgenol., *69*:413.
34. Silverman, F. N. (1972). Unrecognized trauma in infants, the battered child syndrome, and the syndrome of Ambroise Tardieu. Radiology, *104*:337.

35. Silverman, F. N. (1978). Problems in pediatric fractures. Semin. Roentgenol., *13*:167.
36. Smith, L. (1962). A concealed injury to the knee. J. Bone Joint Surg. [Am.], *44*:1659.
37. Smith, M. K. (1924). The prognosis in epiphyseal line fractures. Ann. Surg., *79*:273.
38. Swischuk, L. E. (1969). Spine and spinal cord trauma in the battered child syndrome. Radiology, *92*:733.
39. Swischuk, L. E. (1994). Emergency Radiology of the Acutely Ill or Injured Child. 2nd Ed. Williams & Wilkins Co., Baltimore.
40. Tachdjian, M. O. (1990). Pediatric Orthopedics. 2nd Ed. W. B. Saunders Co., Philadelphia.
41. Trueta, J., & Amato, V. P. (1960). The vascular contribution to osteogenesis. III. Changes in the growth cartilage caused by experimentally induced ischaemia. J. Bone Joint Surg. [Br.], *42*:571.
42. Trueta, J., & Morgan, J. D. (1960). The vascular contribution to osteogenesis. I. Studies by the injection method. J. Bone Joint Surg. [Br.], *42*:97.
43. Werenskiold, B. (1927). A contribution to the röntgen diagnosis of epiphyseal separations. Acta Radiol., *8*:419.
44. Wilkinson, R. H., & Kirkpatrick, J. A. Jr. (1976). Pediatric skeletal trauma. Curr. Probl. Diagn. Radiol., *6*(2), March–April.
45. Cook, S. D., Harding, A. F., Morgan, E. L. et al. (1987). Association of bone mineral density and pediatric fractures. J. Pediatr. Orthop. 7:424.
46. Gilsanz, V., Gibbens, D. T., Roe, T. F. et al. (1988). Vertebral bone density in children: Effect of puberty. Radiology, *166*:847.
47. Jacobsen, F. S. (1997). Periosteum: Its relation to pediatric fractures. J. Pediatr. Orthop., *6*:84.
48. Lanoin, L. A. (1997). Epidemiology of children's fractures. J. Pediatr. Orthop., *6*:79.
49. Landin, L., & Nilsson, B. E. (1983). Bone mineral content in children with fractures. Clin. Orthop., *178*:292.
50. Light, T. R., Ogden, D. A., & Ogden, J. A. (1984). The anatomy of metaphyseal torus fractures. Clin. Orthop., *188*:103.
51. Ogden, J. A. (1982). Injury in the Child. Lea & Febiger, Philadelphia.
52. Rang, M. (1983). Children's Fractures. J. B. Lippincott Co., Philadelphia.
53. Rockwood, C. A. Jr., Wilkins, K. E., & King, R. E. (1996). Fractures in Children. 2nd Ed. J. B. Lippincott Co., Philadelphia.
54. Specker, B. L., Brazerol, W., Tsang, R. C. et al. (1987). Bone mineral content in children 1 to 6 years of age. Am. J. Dis. Child., *141*:343.
55. Swischuk, L. E. (1994). Emergency Radiology of the Acutely Ill or Injured Child. 2nd Ed. Williams & Wilkins, Baltimore.
56. Wilkins, K. E. (1996). The incidence of fractures in children. In Rockwood, C. A., Wilkins, K. E., & Beatty, J. H. Eds.: Fractures in Children. Vol. 3. 4th Ed. Lippincott-Raven Publishers, Philadelphia.

Plastic Bowing

57. Borden, S. (1974). Traumatic bowing of the forearm in children. J. Bone Joint Surg. [Am.], *56*:611.
58. Bowen, A. (1983). Plastic bowing of the clavicle in children. J. Bone Joint Surg. [Am.], *65*:403.
59. Cook, G. C., & Bjelland, J. C. (1979). Acute bowing fracture of the fibula in an adult. Radiology, *131*:637.
60. Demos, T. C. (1980). Traumatic (plastic) bowing of the ulna. Orthopedics, *3*:1112.
61. Manoli, A. (1978). Traumatic fibular bowing with tibial fracture: Report of two cases. Orthopedics, *1*:145.
62. Miller, J. H., & Osterkamp, J. A. (1982). Scintigraphy in acute plastic bowing of the forearm. Radiology, *142*:742.
63. Orenstein, E., Dvonch, V., & Demos, T. (1985). Acute traumatic bowing of the tibia without fracture. J. Bone Joint Surg. [Am.], *67*:965.
64. Rogers, L. F., Malave, S. Jr., White, H., & Tachdjian, M. O. (1978). Plastic bowing, torus and greenstick supracondylar fractures of the humerus: Radiographic clues to obscure fractures of the elbow in children. Radiology, *128*:145.
65. Rydholm, U., & Nilsson, J. E. (1979). Traumatic bowing of the forearm. Clin. Orthop., *139*:121.
66. Sanders, W. E., & Heckman, J. D. (1983). Traumatic plastic deformation of the radius and ulna. Clin. Orthop., *188*:58.
67. Steinstorm, R., Gripenberg, L., & Bergius, A. R. (1978). Traumatic bowing of forearm and lower leg in children. Acta Radiol., *19*:243.

Toddler's Fracture

68. Conway, J. J., & Poznanski, A. P. (1987). Acute compression injuries of bone: or, the toddler's fracture revised. Pediatr. Radiol., *17*:85.
69. Dunbar, J. S., Owen, H. F., Nogrady, M. B., & McLeese, R. (1964). Obscure tibial fracture of infants—the toddler's fracture. J. Can. Assoc. Radiol., *15*:136.
70. Gross, R. H. (1983). Causative factors responsible for femoral fractures in infants and young children. J. Can. Assoc. Radiol., *15*:136.
71. John, S. D., Moorthy, C. S., & Swischuk, L. E. (1997). Expanding the concept of the toddler's fracture. Radiographics, *17*:367.
72. Miller, J. H., & Sanderson, R. A. (1988). Scintigraphy of toddler's fracture. J. Nucl. Med., *29*:2001.
73. Oudjhane, K., Newman, B., Oh, K. S. et al. (1988). Occult fractures in preschool children. J. Trauma, *28*:858.
74. Park, H., Kernek, C. B., & Robb, J. A. (1988). Early scintigraphic findings of occult femoral and tibial fractures in infants. Clin. Nucl. Med., *13*:271.
75. Starshak, R. J., Simons, G. W., & Sty, J. R. (1984). Occult fracture of the calcaneus—another toddler's fracture. Pediatr. Radiol., *14*:37.

Epiphyseal Injuries

76. Albanese, S. A., Palmer, A. K., Kerr, D. R. et al. (1989). Wrist pain and distal growth plate closure of the radius in gymnasts. J. Pediatr. Orthop., *9*:23.
77. Arsenault, A. L. (1987). Microvascular organization at the epiphyseal-metaphyseal junction of growing rats. J. Bone Mineral Res., *2*:143.
78. Arvin, M., White, S. J. & Braunstein, E. M. (1990). Growth plate injury of the hand and wrist in renal osteodystrophy. Skeletal Radiol., *19*:515.
79. Aurinjen, S. T., & Anthony, E. Y. (1999). Common pediatric sports injuries. Semin. Musculoskeletal Radiol., *3*:247.
80. Bright, R. W. (1974). Operative correction of partial epiphyseal plate closure by osseous-bridge resection and silicone-rubber implant. J. Bone Joint Surg. [Am.], *56*:655.
81. Bright, R. W. (1982). Partial growth arrest: Identification, classification and results of treatment. Orthop. Trans., *6*:65.
82. Bright, R. W., & Elmore, S. M. (1968). Physical properties of epiphyseal plate cartilage. Surg. Forum, *19*:463.
83. Buckwalter, J. A. (1983). Proteoglycan structure in calcifying cartilage. Clin. Orthop., *172*:207.
84. Buckwalter, J. A., Mower, D., Schafer, J. et al. (1985). Growth-plate–chondrocyte profiles and their orientation. J. Bone Joint Surg. [Am.], *67*:942.
85. Cahill, B. R. (1977). Stress fracture of the proximal tibial epiphysis: A case report. Am. J. Sports Med., *5*:186.
86. Carey, J., Spence, L., Blickman, H. et al. (1998). MRI of pediatric growth plate injury: Correlation with plain film radiographs and clinical outcome. Skeletal Radiol., *27*:250.
87. Carter, S. R., & Aldridge, M. J. (1988). Stress injury of the distal radial growth plate. J. Bone Joint Surg. [Br.], *70*:834.
88. Chadwick, C. J., & Bentley, G. (1987). The classification and prognosis of epiphyseal injuries. Injury, *18*:157.
89. Du Boullay, T., & Gaubert, D. J. (1986). Etude experimentale des traumatismes du cartilage de croissance (type V de Salter). Chir. Pediatr., *27*:84.
90. Edeiken, B. S., Libshitz, H. I., & Cohen, M. A. (1982). Slipped proximal humeral epiphysis: A complication of radiotherapy to the shoulder in children. Skeletal Radiol., *19*:123.
91. Ekengren, K., Bergdahl, S., & Ekstrom, G. (1978). Birth injuries to the epiphyseal cartilage. Acta. Radiol. [Diagn.] (Stockh.), *19*:197.
92. Fernbach, S. K., & Wilkinson, R. H. (1981). Avulsion injuries of the pelvis and proximal femur. A. J. R. Am. J. Roentgenol., *137*:581.
93. Fliegel, C. P. (1985). Stress related widening of the radial growth plate in adolescents. Ann. Radiol., *29*:374.
94. Godshall, R. W., Hansen, C. A., & Rising, D. C. (1981). Stress fractures through the distal femoral epiphysis in athletes. Am. J. Sports Med., *9*:114.
95. Hansen, N. M. Jr. (1982). Epiphyseal changes in the proximal humerus of an adolescent baseball pitcher. Am. J. Sports Med., *10*:380.
96. Hynes, D., & O'Brien, T. (1988). Growth disturbance lines after injury of the distal tibial physis: Their significance in prognosis. J. Bone Joint Surg. [Br.], *70*:231.
97. Ilizarov, G. A., & Soibelman, L. M. (1969). Nekotorye klinikoeksperimental'-nye dannye beskrovnogo udlineniia nizhnikh konechnosttei. Exsp. Khir. Anaes., *4*:27.
98. Jaramillo, D., Hoffer, F. A., Shapiro, F., & Rand, F. (1990). MR imaging of fractures of the growth plate. A. J. R. Am. J. Roentgenol., *155*:1261.
99. Jaramillo, D., Kammen, B. F., & Shapiro, F. (in press). Evaluation of the cartilaginous path of physeal fracture-separations by MR imaging: An experimental study with histologic correlation in rabbits. Radiology.
100. Jaramillo, D., & Shapiro, F. (1998). Musculoskeletal trauma in children. Magn. Reson. Imaging Clin. N. Am., *6*:455.
101. Jones, C. B., Dewar, M. E., Aichroth, P. M. et al. (1989). Epiphyseal distraction monitored by strain gauges. J. Bone Joint Surg. [Br.], *71*:651.
102. Kasser, J. R. (1990). Physeal bar resections after growth arrest about the knee. Clin. Orthop., *255*:68.
103. Kawabe, N., Ehrlich, M. G., & Mankin, H. J. (1986). In vivo degradation systems of the epiphyseal cartilage. Clin. Orthop., *211*:244.
104. Langenskiold, A. (1975). An operation for partial closure of an epiphyseal plate in children, and its experimental basis. J. Bone Joint Surg. [Br.], *57*:325.
105. Langenskiold, A. (1981). Surgical treatment of partial closure of the growth plate. J. Pediatr. Orthop., *1*:3.
106. Langenskiold, A., Videman, T., & Nevalainen, T. (1986). The fate of fat transplants in operations for partial closure of the growth plate. J. Bone Joint Surg. [Br.], *68*:234.
107. Lindseth, R. E., & Rosene, H. A. Jr. (1971). Traumatic separation of the upper femoral epiphysis in a new born infant. J. Bone Joint Surg. [Am.], *53*:1641.
108. MacNealy, G. A., Rogers, L. F., Hernandez, R., & Poznanski, A. K. (1982). Injuries of the distal tibial epiphysis: Systematic radiographic evaluation. A. J. R. Am. J. Roentgenol., *138*:683.
109. Mann, D. C., & Rajmaira, S. (1990). Distribution of physeal and nonphyseal

fractures in 2650 long-bone fractures in children ages 0 to 16 years. J. Pediatr. Orthop., *10*:713.
110. Mayer, V., & Marchisello, P. J. (1984). Traumatic partial arrest of tibial physis. Clin. Orthop., *183*:99.
111. Mizuta, T., Benson, W. M., Foster, B. K. et al. (1987). Statistical analysis of the incidence of physeal injuries. J. Pediatr. Orthop., *7*:518.
112. Ogden, J. A. (1981). Injury to the growth mechanisms of the immature skeleton. Skeletal Radiol., *6*:237.
113. Olin, A. O., Creasman, C., & Shapiro, F. (1984). Free physeal transplantation in the rabbit. J. Bone Joint Surg. [Am.], *66*:7.
114. Osterman, K. (1972). Operative elimination of partial premature epiphyseal closure. Acta Orthop. Scand., *147*:17.
115. Quiles, M., & Sanz, T. A. (1988). Epiphyseal separation in scurvy. J. Pediatr. Orthop., *8*:223.
116. Peterson, H. A., Madhok, R., Berson, J. T. et al. (1994). Physeal fractures: Part 1. Epidemiology in Olmstead County, Minnesota, 1979–1988. J. Pediatr. Orthop., *14*:423.
117. Peterson, H. A. (1994). Physeal fractures: Part 3. Classification. J. Pediatr. Orthop., *14*:439.
118. Peterson, H. A. (1996). Physeal and apophyseal injuries. pp. 103–165. In Rockwood, C. A. Jr., Wilkins, K. E., & Beaty, J. H. Eds.: Fractures in children. 4th Ed. Lippincott-Raven Publishers, Philadelphia.
119. Ray, T. D., Tessler, R. H., & Dell, P. C. (1996). Traumatic ulnar physeal arrest after distal forearm fractures in children. J. Pediatr. Orthop., *16*:195.
120. Riseborough, E. J., Barrett, I. R., & Shapiro, F. (1983). Growth disturbances following distal femoral physeal fracture-separations. J. Bone Joint Surg. [Am.], *65*:885.
121. Rogers, L. F., & Pozwanski, A. F. (1994). Imaging of epiphyseal injuries. Radiology, *191*:287.
122. Rogers, L. F., Braunstein, E., DeSmet, A. A. et al. (1988). All-Star sports medicine film panel. Radiographics, *8*:235.
123. Roy, S., Caine, D., & Singer, K. M. (1985). Stress changes of the distal radial epiphysis in young gymnasts. Am. J. Sports Med., *13*:301.
124. Rudicel, S., Pelker, R. R., Lee, K. E. et al. (1985). Shear fractures through the capital femoral physis of the skeletally immature rabbit. J. Pediatr. Orthop., *5*:27.
125. Shapiro, F. (1982). Epiphyseal growth plate fracture-separations. A pathophysiologic approach. Orthopedics, *5*:720.
126. Shapiro, F. (1987). Epiphyseal disorders. N. Engl. J. Med., *317*:1702.
127. Siegal, M. J., & Luker, G. D. (1995). Pediatric applications of helical (spiral) CT. Radiol. Clin. North Am., *33*:997.
128. Speer, D. P. (1982). Collagenous architecture of the growth plate and perichondrial ossification groove. J. Bone Joint Surg. [Am.], *64*:399.
129. Spiegel, P. G., Cooperman, D. R., & Laros, G. S. (1978). Epiphyseal fractures of the distal ends of the tibia and fibula. J. Bone Joint Surg. [Am.], *60*:1046.
130. Weigl, K., & Conforty, B. (1974). Die traumatische epiphysenlosung am oberen femurende beim neugeborenene. Z. Orthop., *112*:1286.
131. Young, J. W. R., Bright, R. W., & Whitley, N. O. (1986). Computed tomography in the evaluation of partial growth plate arrest in children. Skeletal Radiol., *15*:530.

Child Abuse

132. Ablin, D. S., Greenspan, A., Reinhart, M., & Grix, A. (1990). Differentation of child abuse from osteogenesis imperfecta. A. J. R. Am. J. Roentgenol., *145*:1035.
133. Caffey, J. (1990). The whiplash shaken infant syndrome: Manual shaking by the extremities with whiplash-induced intracranial and intraocular bleedings, linked with residual permanent brain damage and mental retardation. Pediatrics, *54*:396.
134. Hilton, S. W., & Edwards, D. K. (1985). Radiographic diagnosis of nonaccidental trauma (child abuse). Appl. Radiol., *July/Aug.*:13.
135. Howard, J. L., Barron, B. J., & Smith, G. G. (1990). Bone scintigraphy in the evaluation of extraskeletal injuries from child abuse. Radiographics, *10*:67.
136. King, J., Diefendorf, D., Apthorp, J. et al. (1988). Analysis of 429 fractures in 189 battered children. J. Pediatr. Orthop., *8*:585.
137. Kleinman, P. K. (1998). Diagnostic Imaging of Child Abuse. 2nd Ed. Williams & Wilkins, Baltimore.
138. Kleinman, P. K. (1990). Diagnostic imaging in infant abuse. A. J. R. Am. J. Roentgenol., *155*:703.
139. Kleinman, P. K., Marks, S. C., & Blackbourne, B. (1986). The metaphyseal lesion in abused infants: A radiologic-histopathologic study. A. J. R. Am. J. Roentgenol., *146*:895.
140. Kleinman, P. K., & Zito, J. L. (1984). Avulsion of the spinous processes caused by infant abuse. Radiology, *151*:389.
141. Kleinman, P. K. (1996). Follow-up skeletal surveys in suspected child abuse. A. J. R. Am. J. Roentgenol., *167*:893.
142. McNeese, M. C., & Hebeler, J. R. (1977). The abused child. A clinical approach to identification and management. Clin. Symp., *29*:23.
143. Merten, D. F., Kirks, D. R., & Ruderman, R. J. (1981). Occult humeral epiphyseal fracture in battered infants. Pediatr. Radiol., *10*:151.
144. Merten, D. F., Radkowski, M. A., & Leonidas, J. C. (1983). The abused child: A radiological reappraisal. Radiology, *146*:377.
145. Nimkin, K., Kleinman, P. K., Teegas, S. et al. (1995). Distal humeral physeal injuries in child abuse: MR imaging and ultrasonography findings. Pediatr. Radiol., *25*:562.
146. Paterson, C. R. (1990). Osteogenesis imperfecta and other bone disorders in the differential diagnosis of unexplained fractures. J. R. Soc. Med., *83*:72.
147. Radkowski, M. A. (1983). The battered child syndrome: Pitfalls in radiological diagnosis. Pediatr. Ann., *12*:894.
148. Radkowski, M. A., Merten, D. F., & Leonidas, J. C. (1983). The abused child: Criteria for the radiologic diagnosis. Radiographics, *3*:262.
149. Sivit, C. J., Taylor, G. A., & Eichelberger, M. R. (1989). Visceral injury in battered children: A changing perspective. Radiology, *173*:659.
150. Sty, J. R., & Starshak, R. J. (1983). The role of bone scintigraphy in the evaluation of the suspected abused child. Radiology, *146*:369.
151. Tardieu, A. (1960). Etude medico-legale sur les services et mauvais traitments exerces sur des enfants. Ann. Hyg. Publ. Med. Leg., *13*:361.
152. Worlock, P., Stower, M., & Barbor, P. (1986). Patterns of fractures in accidental and non-accidental injury in children: A comparative study. Br. Med. J., *293*:100.

Pathologic Fractures

153. Brunner, R., & Doderlein, L. (1996). Pathologic fractures in patients with cerebral palsy. J. Pediatr. Orthop., *5*:232.
154. Dent, C. E., & Friedman, M. (1965). Idiopathic juvenile osteoporosis. Q. J. Med., *N.S.34*:177.
155. Dickerman, J. D., Newberg, A. H., & Moreland, M. D. (1979). Slipped capital femoral epiphysis (SCFE) following pelvic irradiation for rhabdomyosarcoma. Cancer, *44*:480.
156. Easley, M. E., & Kniesl, J. S. (1997). Pathologic fractures through nonossifying fibromas: Is prophylactic treatment warranted? J. Pediatr. Orthop., *17*:808.
157. Exarchou, E., Politou, C., Vretou, E. et al. (1984). Fractures and epiphyseal deformities in beta-thalassemia. Clin. Orthop., *189*:229.
158. Goodling, C. A., & Ball, J. H. (1969). Idiopathic juvenile osteoporosis. Radiology, *93*:1349.
159. Hoeffel, J. C., Voinchet, A., & Ligier, J. N. (1988). Avulsion fracture on benign cortical defect of the distal femur. Fortschr. Röntgenstr., *149*:336.
160. Houang, M. T. W., Brenton, D. P., Renton, P., & Shaw, D. G. (1978). Idiopathic juvenile osteoporosis. Skeletal Radiol., *3*:17.
161. Hyre, H. M., & Stelling, C. B. (1989). Radiographic appearance of healed extremity fractures in children with spinal cord lesions. Skeletal Radiol., *18*:189.
162. Koo, W. K. K., Sherman, R., Succop, P. et al. (1989). Fractures and rickets in very low birth weight infants: Conservative management and outcome. J. Pediatr. Orthop., *9*:326.
163. Kumar, R., Swischuk, L. E., & Madewell, J. E. (1986). Benign cortical defect: Site for an avulsion fracture. Skeletal Radiol., *15*:553.
164. Libshitz, H. I., & Edeiken, B. S. (1981). Radiotherapy changes of the pediatric hip. A. J. R. Am. J. Roentgenol., *137*:585.
165. Lock, T. R., & Aronson, D. D. (1989). Fractures in patients who have myelomeningocele. J. Bone Joint Surg. [Am.], *71*:1153.
166. Ribeiro, R. C., Pui, C., & Schell, M. J. (1988). Vertebral compression fracture as a presenting feature of acute lymphoblastic leukemia in children. Cancer, *61*:589.
167. Rodgers, W. B. Schwend, R. M., Janamillo, D. et al. (1997). Chronic physeal fractures in myelodysplasia: Magnetic resonance analysis, histologic description, treatment, and outcome. J. Pediatr. Orthop., *17*:615.
168. Smith, R. (1980). Idiopathic osteoporosis in the young. J. Bone Joint Surg. [Br.], *62*:417.
169. Towbin, R., & Dunbar, J. S. (1981). Generalized osteoporosis with multiple fractures in an adolescent. Invest. Radiol., *16*:171.
170. Wolf, E. L., Berdon, W. E., Cassady, J. R. et al. (1977). Slipped femoral capital epiphysis as a sequela to childhood irradiation for malignant tumors. Radiology, *125*:781.

Chapter 6

POLYTRAUMA: THE MULTIPLE-INJURY PATIENT

with Stuart E. Mirvis, MD

Trauma is the third most common cause of mortality in the United States. It is the leading cause of death in persons less than 40 years of age.[4] Over 400,000 people are permanently disabled by trauma each year.[55] They die and are maimed in large measure owing to multiple injuries, or polytrauma.

Polytrauma refers to multiple long bone fractures in association with other major visceral and soft tissue injuries (Fig. 6–1). The majority of polytrauma cases are the result of motor vehicle accidents[15] (54%), followed by motorcycle accidents (24%), auto-pedestrian accidents (17%), and falls or jumps from a height (5%).[7, 8, 19, 20, 24, 39, 42, 170, 172] Sports injuries, penetrating injuries, and assaults account for less than 5% each. Each victim sustains from 2.4[5, 9] to 5[17, 24] fractures in addition to major visceral injuries of the lung, spleen, liver, central nervous system (CNS), and genitourinary tract. The most common injuries are fractures of the long bones[33] (most often the femur, tibia, and fibula[34] (Fig. 6–2), pelvis, and spine associated with skull fracture or closed head injury; hemopneumothorax; lung contusion and rib fractures; and ruptures or lacerations of the spleen, liver, kidney, and bladder and urethra. In general, the incidence of thoracic injury approaches 60%, about two to three times that of intra-abdominal visceral injury. There is a tendency to regional concentration of injuries. Patients with fracture of the cervical spine tend to have a higher incidence of associated closed head injuries or skull fractures and facial fractures,[179] whereas patients with fractures of the thoracolumbar spine have a higher incidence of injuries of the spleen, liver, kidney, and bladder and associated pelvic fracture in addition to closed chest injuries.[20]

The average age of occurrence is just over 30 years,[20] most patients being between the ages of 10 and 50 years.[5, 7, 8, 9, 26, 39] The overall death rate is approximately 10% to 25%. Those over age 70 are more severely affected by accidents than any other age group.[34, 204] Trauma is the fifth leading cause of death in patients 65 years of age and older. Although they are less likely to be injured than persons in other age groups, older persons are more likely to experience fatal outcomes. The mortality due to accidents among the aged is five times higher than that of younger people.[34] Falls are more frequently a source of injury in the elderly than other causes, including motor vehicle accidents. In children, severe trauma ranks second to acute infections as the major cause of morbidity.[18] Motor vehicle–child pedestrian accidents are the leading source of multiple injuries in children, followed distantly by motor vehicle passenger accidents, bicycle–motor vehicle accidents,[41, 43] motorcycle accidents,[35] and falls from great heights.[29, 38] Children tend to survive multiple injuries better than adults.[18]

A motorcyclist is 13 times more likely to die in an accident than the driver of an automobile. It has been shown repeatedly that the use of helmets significantly decreases head injury, death, and disability in the motorcyclist.[5, 11, 22, 25, 30, 32, 44]

Injuries at multiple sites occur in varying combinations. Some combinations are predictable according to the cause of the injury and, to a lesser extent, the age of the patient. Others are less so. Some injuries are obvious on physical examination and others obscure because of the difficulties in performing a physical examination on the recumbent patient whose sensorium is often altered by CNS injury, shock, alcohol, or drugs. Diagnosis of multiple injuries can be further complicated by pressing needs for resuscitation, the treatment of immediately life-threatening shock, and abnormalities of the airway.

The cause of shock itself may not be immediately obvious. In the multiple trauma setting, shock is most frequently caused by intra-abdominal visceral injury.[27, 42] Severe shock may also be encountered from hemorrhage associated with pelvic fractures and, less commonly, femoral shaft fractures. In such cases the source of hemorrhage may not be immediately obvious. Cervical and high thoracic spinal cord injuries can produce "spinal shock," characterized by hypotension and bradycardia resulting from a loss of peripheral sympathetic vasomotor tone while cardiac vagal stimulation remains intact. In addition, patients in spinal shock suffer loss of abdominal wall muscle tone, skin sensation, and visceral pain perception, making the detection of intra-abdominal injury by physical examination quite difficult.[42] Under these circumstances, the need and requirement for radiography and other imaging procedures is superseded but should not ultimately be forgotten lest serious injuries be overlooked.

Systems of Trauma Care

It has been suggested that as many as a third of all deaths from trauma in the United States are medically

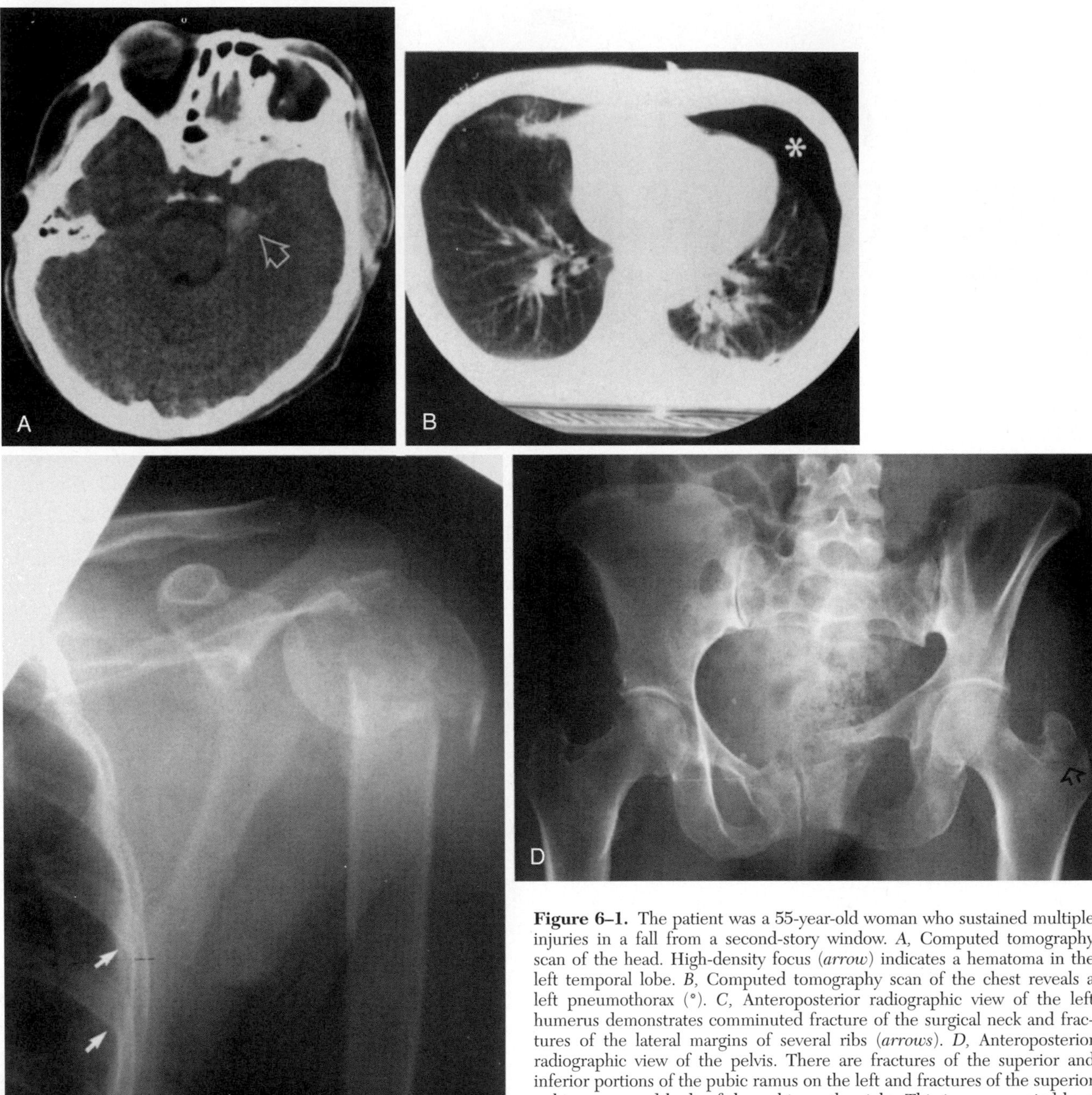

Figure 6–1. The patient was a 55-year-old woman who sustained multiple injuries in a fall from a second-story window. *A*, Computed tomography scan of the head. High-density focus (*arrow*) indicates a hematoma in the left temporal lobe. *B*, Computed tomography scan of the chest reveals a left pneumothorax (*). *C*, Anteroposterior radiographic view of the left humerus demonstrates comminuted fracture of the surgical neck and fractures of the lateral margins of several ribs (*arrows*). *D*, Anteroposterior radiographic view of the pelvis. There are fractures of the superior and inferior portions of the pubic ramus on the left and fractures of the superior pubic ramus and body of the pubis on the right. This is accompanied by a dislocation of the left sacroiliac joint and an avulsion fracture of the left greater trochanter (*arrow*). The patient was unconscious, and the fracture of the pelvis was not suspected on the basis of physical examination.

preventable.[15] Epidemiologic analyses of trauma care and outcomes comparing the experience in various medical facilities have demonstrated the wide variation in competence in caring for the multiply injured and the advantages afforded patients receiving care in adequately equipped centers with trained personnel.[47, 50, 51, 52, 54, 56] An organized system for care of the traumatized patient appears to be crucial to the success of care.[28, 46, 50] Management of the severely injured requires a team approach in trauma centers equipped and staffed around the clock.[48] Usually a general surgeon coordinates the care of a trauma team composed of emergency room physicians and anesthesiologists aided by radiologists and a host of surgical specialists: vascular, orthopedic, thoracic, urologic, and neurologic surgeons. Experience and efficiency of the staff are rewarded by greater survival and less ultimate morbidity of the patients. The recognition of this difference has led to the regionalization of trauma care.[48, 49, 55]

The designation of trauma facilities by the proper authorities is a political process[48] and requires the commitment of significant sums of money.[52] This is not easily

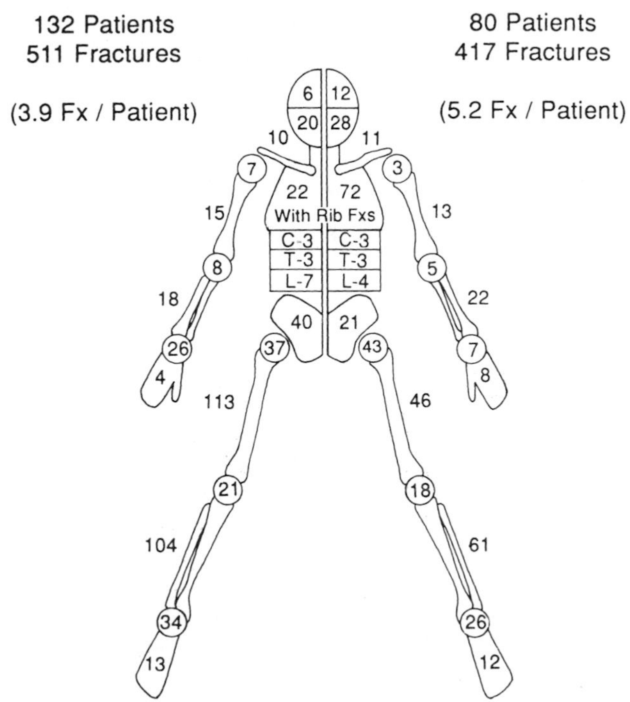

Figure 6–2. Distribution of fractures in two series of multiply injured patients. Those on the right represent 80 patients with 417 fractures (58 severely injured patients with 286 fractures) as reported by Goris and colleagues.[17] Those on the left represent 132 patients with 511 fractures as reported by Johnson and coworkers.[24] Note that the most common sites of fracture were in the femur and tibia and fibula in both series.

accomplished despite the clear demonstration of a significant decrease in morbidity and mortality[4, 51, 54, 57, 58] and a sharp reduction in preventable deaths when organized trauma care systems have been introduced (from an astonishing 73% to 9% in one study).

Imaging in the Multiple-Injury Patient

The initial evaluation of multiply injured patients is a challenge, and the risk of missing injuries in a patient population characterized by altered consciousness and life-threatening injury is high and real. During the initial examination and management, attention is drawn to the immediate need for resuscitative measures, establishment of an airway, and treatment of hemorrhage or shock. Although these concerns take precedence over the need for a radiographic examination,[3, 176, 177] it is necessary to assess the extent of obvious injuries and to determine the presence of abnormalities not apparent from physical examination. Both to assure patient safety and to enable an adequate radiographic examination, it is mandatory that life-threatening conditions be corrected and the patient's condition stabilized before a complete radiographic examination is undertaken.[173] A disciplined approach to the initial radiographic assessment will save lives and reduce morbidity.

The first requirement is an adequate radiographic facility.[159, 161, 164, 171] Some facilities utilize portable equipment[163]; however, a fixed radiographic installation—a dedicated trauma unit equipped with a floating-top pedestal table, and an upright Bucky apparatus paralleling the table top—is preferred. Such a unit minimizes the need to adjust or move the patient to obtain the required radiographs. A computed tomography (CT) scanner situated in the emergency room contributes substantially to meeting the immediate needs of patients. CT is required for the immediate evaluation of intracranial abnormalities and assessment of injuries of the liver, spleen, and kidney. CT also has a major role in the evaluation of certain skeletal injuries, particularly those of the spine and pelvis. Scintigraphy has been proved to be of little value in the assessment of the multiply injured patient.[166, 168]

"Hands-on" involvement of the radiologist adds immeasurably to the quality of the radiographic examination and diagnostic accuracy. Knowledge of the potential and limitations of various radiographic techniques enhances the care of the multiply injured patient.

Diagnostic imaging plays a crucial role in the initial work-up of hemodynamically stable or adequately resuscitated polytrauma patients in order to establish management and treatment priorities. Plain film radiography continues to serve as the major diagnostic screening study performed in the acute trauma setting. Other modalities including bedside sonography, CT, diagnostic and interventional angiography, and magnetic resonance imaging (MRI) have also become vital for the definitive diagnosis or exclusion of many injuries. Advances in diagnostic imaging technology have, in general, increased the accuracy and rapidity of identification of injuries, while improvements in interventional angiographic techniques have offered a definitive nonsurgical alternative for treatment of many types of vascular injury.

The ideal use or selection of diagnostic imaging studies should take into account several factors that may be unique to a given clinical setting. Such factors include the proximity and availability of the imaging technology to the patient resuscitation area and the quality and speed of the imaging equipment available. Other considerations include the experience and availability of radiology technologists to perform emergency imaging procedures in traumatized patients, the availability of expert interpretation of imaging studies, and the ability to communicate that interpretation in a timely fashion. In addition, the capacity to accurately monitor vital signs, maintain appropriate physiologic support, and respond therapeutically to sudden clinical deterioration both during transport to an imaging facility and during the diagnostic study is crucial.

Although the availability of sophisticated imaging studies offers the potential for improvements in speed and accuracy of diagnosis of acute traumatic injury, the smooth and appropriate integration of various diagnostic studies into the physical diagnosis, initial and ongoing resuscitation requirements, and management of the patient's injuries are not without controversy. The *physiologic* or *hemodynamic stability* of the patient is the single most important factor in determining whether the opportunity exists to perform diagnostic studies and, if so, the extent of such examination. For instance, a patient admitted in profound shock who fails to respond to initial resuscitation may not safely be subjected to any imaging studies at all or may undergo only a quick abdominal bedside sonogram for detection of gross hemoperitoneum. A patient who is admitted in hemodynamic shock but who responds well to aggressive and ongoing resuscitation may perhaps safely undergo rapid portable radiographic screening but would be at high risk with transport to a distant site for CT or MRI. A trauma patient who is initially hemodynamically stable and maintains stability in the resuscitation area may be an appropriate candidate for "off-site" imaging studies such as CT or MRI, depending on the level of clinical concern.

In some cases the priority of dealing with life-threatening injury to a single system may limit the potential for initial evaluation of other injuries, as when an initial cranial CT study demonstrates marked cerebral herniation requiring immediate craniotomy. The availability of extremely fast CT imaging performed using new multi–row detector spiral CT scanning should allow examination of other anatomic regions as needed, even in the clinical scenario just described.

The decision to perform a diagnostic imaging evaluation and the determination of the level of required imaging sophistication are the responsibility of the trauma team leader and may need to be revised according to changes in the patient's overall medical condition and the results of diagnostic studies already obtained. Close cooperation and clear communication among the trauma team physicians, nurses, imaging technologists, and radiologists are necessary to optimize any imaging assessment. The radiologist can and should be a valuable ally in selecting the type and order of diagnostic procedures to most efficiently answer particular clinical concerns.

Imaging Evaluation of Specific Anatomic Regions in the Polytrauma Patient

The purpose here is not to review specific imaging findings in various forms of traumatic injury. Rather, we offer a general diagnostic imaging approach to the work-up of various potential injuries in the setting of the multisystem–injured (polytrauma) patient. It should be noted, however, that a recommended imaging work-up may be well suited to some institutions but inappropriate or at least suboptimal for use in others.

Cervical Spine Assessment: Imaging Approach

In most trauma centers and emergency departments, a blunt trauma victim or patient with spinal penetrating trauma is presumed to have an unstable cervical spine injury until proven otherwise. The appropriate imaging evaluation of the cervical spine is controversial.[90] At the

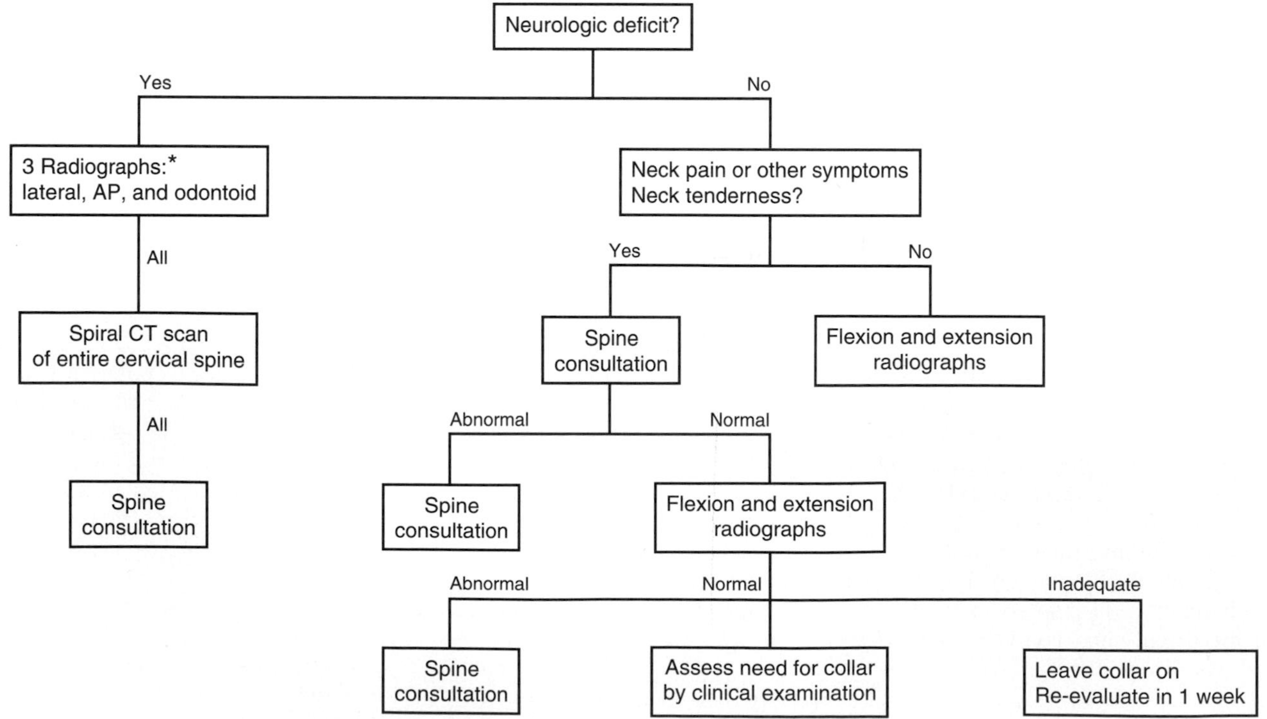

Figure 6–3. Guidelines for imaging the cervical spine at the Maryland Shock-Trauma Center determined by *reliability* of findings on physical examination of the patient. AP, Anteroposterior; CT, computed tomography; MRI, magnetic resonance imaging.

University of Maryland Shock-Trauma Center the application of diagnostic imaging studies performed is based substantially on the patient's clinical presentation (Fig. 6–3). Several studies have indicated that patients who are awake and alert and have no major distracting injuries can be reliably assessed clinically.[89, 95, 152] Those patients without cervical pain on palpation and full range of motion without discomfort are considered "cleared" and do not require imaging assessment.[89, 95, 152]

In patients who are alert and complain of neck pain, a three-view radiographic series consisting of cross-table lateral, anteroposterior, and open-mouth odontoid views and an orthopedic consultation are obtained. If the initial radiographic findings are normal, lateral view flexion-extension stress radiographs are obtained under physician supervision to exclude a significant ligament injury. Some clinicians prefer to obtain a lateral view of the spine with the patient in the upright position before removing the cervical collar or obtaining the flexion-extension stress views. Alternatively, a total cervical spine spiral CT study may be performed to assess for radiographically occult fractures. CT has been increasingly used as a screening study since the advent of commonly available spiral CT, which is more sensitive than radiography in the detection of subtle injury and can examine the entire cervical spine rapidly.[62, 63, 101] If findings on these studies are normal, the patient is immobilized in a soft cervical collar, and follow-up neutral lateral and flexion-extension stress views are obtained, if symptoms persist, in 7 to 10 days to exclude delayed manifestation of ligament injury.[74]

Patients with cervical pain in whom imaging studies yield positive results are maintained in rigid cervical immobilization and undergo further imaging work-up as directed by the orthopedic consultant. Patients who present with neurologic deficits referable to the cervical spinal cord remain immobilized, and neurosurgical consultation is obtained. In these patients, typically a three-view standard radiographic series is obtained, followed by spiral cervical spine CT. In most cases MRI is also performed to evaluate the extent of ligament injury and to assess for the presence of disc herniation, epidural hematoma, and other soft tissue injury. These findings may well have a bearing on the type of reduction and surgical fixation, if required, that is performed.

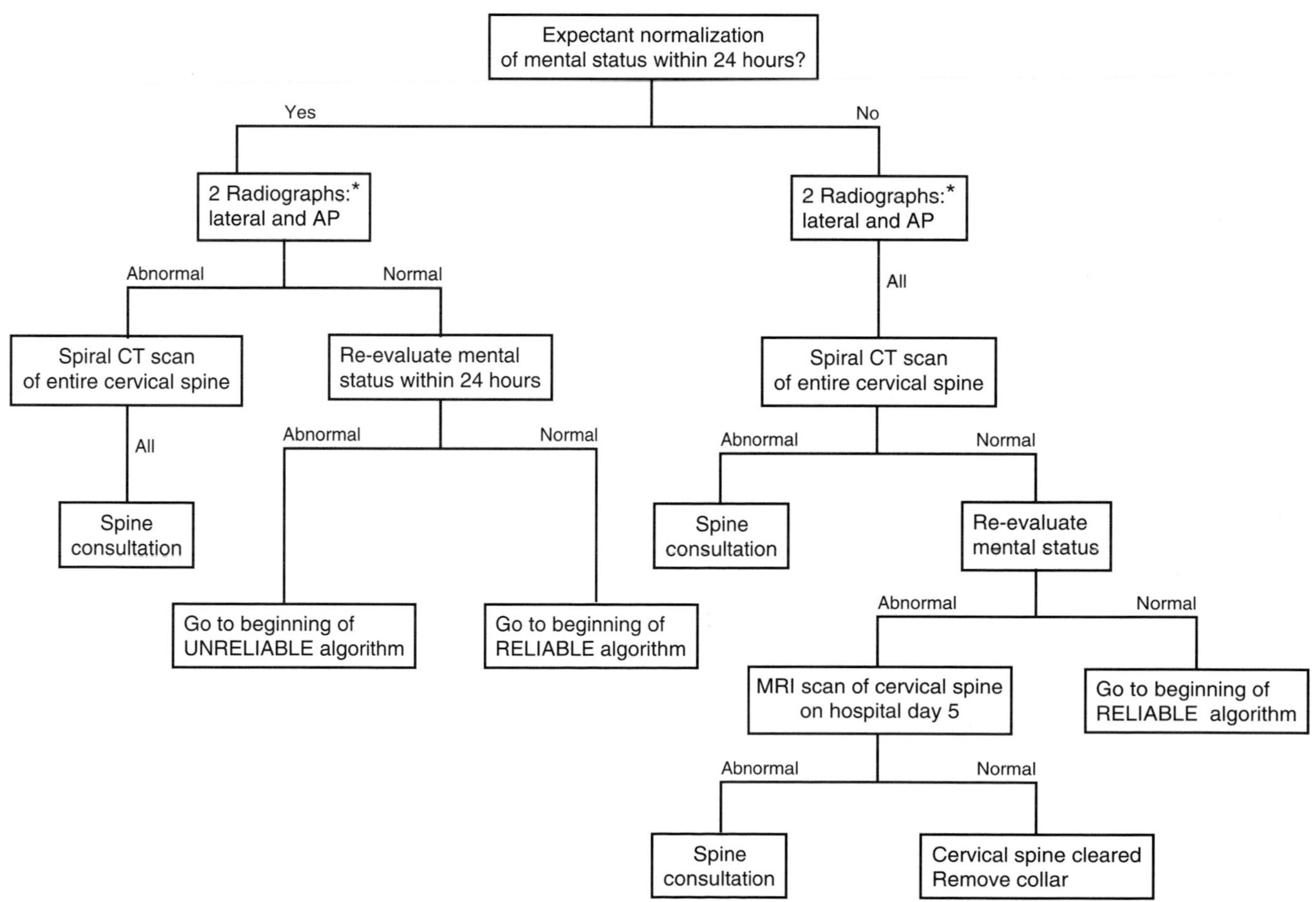

Figure 6–3 *Continued*

In patients who are unconscious or uncooperative or who have impaired mental status, or who, in the judgment of the admitting physician, are not reliable enough to respond appropriately to physical evaluation, the initial imaging study should be the three-view radiographic series (however, the open-mouth view is often difficult to obtain in this population). If this series yields normal results, a total cervical spiral CT study is performed to exclude osseous injury. The ability of the spiral CT examination to exclude all significant (potentially mechanically unstable) ligament injuries is, however, not established. If the spiral CT findings are normal and the patient is not expected to become alert and able to undergo a reliable physical examination within 5 days of injury, an MRI study of the cervical spine is performed. The MRI study is intended to reveal subtle ligament damage, disc herniation, epidural hematoma, and soft tissue edema that may not be detected by the cervical CT study.[72] If the MRI findings are normal, the cervical collar is removed. If, in the judgment of the clinical physician, the patient will, in a reasonably short time (1–3 days), become a candidate for a reliable physical examination of the cervical spine, rigid cervical immobilization is maintained until clinical assessment can be performed. Some common pitfalls leading to missed diagnoses in cervical spine image interpretation are listed in Table 6–1.

Thoracic Trauma Imaging

Increasing Utilization of Screening Computed Tomography

The chest radiograph serves as the best single screening study for diagnosis of thoracic injury. It is quickly obtained and provides a large amount of information regarding several potentially life-threatening thoracic injuries. Radiography is relatively accurate for the detection of pneumomediastinum, pulmonary contusion, moderate to large pleural effusions, and simple or tension pneumothorax, pneumopericardium, aspiration, and thoracic skeletal injury. Most chest radiographs obtained on hospital admission are acquired with the patient in the supine position, which makes identification of small pneumothoraces relatively more difficult because air ascends into the anterior inferior pleural space rather than outlining the visceral pleura at the lung apex.[158] Pleural effusions will potentially collect posteriorly, creating a hazy increase in hemithoracic density that may be difficult to perceive and may be impossible to detect when the effusions are bilateral and relatively equal in size. The quantity of pericardial fluid needed to create tamponade usually will not, in the acute setting, distort the cardiac contour enough to be appreciated radiographically (Fig. 6–4).

Recent studies have shown that the chest radiograph is relatively insensitive in the detection of several important thoracic injuries.[98, 115, 149] Chest CT detects much smaller pneumothoraces, hemothoraces, and pericardial effusions than can be visualized by radiography.[98, 115, 149] Although a small pneumothorax may not initially produce significant physiologic impairment, it may enlarge or develop a tension component, especially if the patient is receiving positive-pressure ventilation, leading to major cardiovascular and respiratory compromise. CT is far more accurate than radiography at identifying and quantifying pulmonary contusions and lacerations,[153] knowledge of which may explain difficulties in oxygenation and permit anticipation of complications such as pneumonia, infected traumatic pneumatoceles, or bronchopleural fistula.[117] Other trauma-related problems that are more readily diagnosed by CT are pericardial effusion, cardiac tamponade (see Fig. 6–4),[87] sternoclavicular dislocation,[148] transthoracic lung herniation,[131] and direct cardiac or pericardial injury.[100]

Table 6–1. Pitfalls in Cervical Spine Imaging Diagnosis

- Nondisplaced or minimally displaced fractures such as high odontoid (classic type 2) fractures[108]
- Failure to adequately assess the prevertebral soft tissues[107]
- Failure to observe alignment at C7–T1 level
- Failure to obtain *accurate clinical information* regarding symptoms
- Failure to search for multiple injuries when one obvious injury is detected
- Inappropriate determination of potential for mechanical instability of certain injuries
- Failure to review two-dimensional sagittal and other multiplanar reformatted images of the spine following axial computed tomography to better determine alignment
- Failure to communicate suspicions or diagnostic findings to clinical care team
- Failure to apply injury mechanism to guide search for other injuries associated with same mechanism

Focus on Selected Thoracic Injuries

Mediastinal Hemorrhage and Aorta and Great Vessel Injury

The presence of mediastinal hemorrhage is an important clue to the possibility of a major thoracic vascular injury, which most commonly involves the thoracic aorta. The chest radiograph provides the initial assessment of the mediastinal contour. Numerous articles have appeared in the literature describing the most reliable radiographic signs of hemomediastinum.[102, 108, 155] As larger series were reported, many of these signs were found to be less accurate than indicated by earlier, smaller series. Although it is true that most patients with hemomediastinum are found to have a "widened mediastinum" on chest radiograph, this finding is by no means accurate in indicating the presence or absence of vascular injury (Fig. 6–5). Indeed, patients in whom the mediastinum is seen to be very narrow or the mediastinum-to-chest width ratio is abnormal (<25%) may also have traumatic aortic injury. In patients with mediastinal hemorrhage, the probability of major thoracic vascular injury is no greater than 20%.[113] Analysis of the mediastinal contour offers the best chance of diagnosing mediastinal hemorrhage. Radiologic signs that serve as accurate markers for mediastinal hematoma include (1) obscuration of the aortic arch and descending aorta, (2) right paratracheal soft tissue density, (3) rightward displacement of the esophagus and trachea, and (4) widened left paraspinal stripe or extension of the stripe above the aortic arch.

Unfortunately, radiographic evaluation often gives a false-positive result for evidence of mediastinal blood and

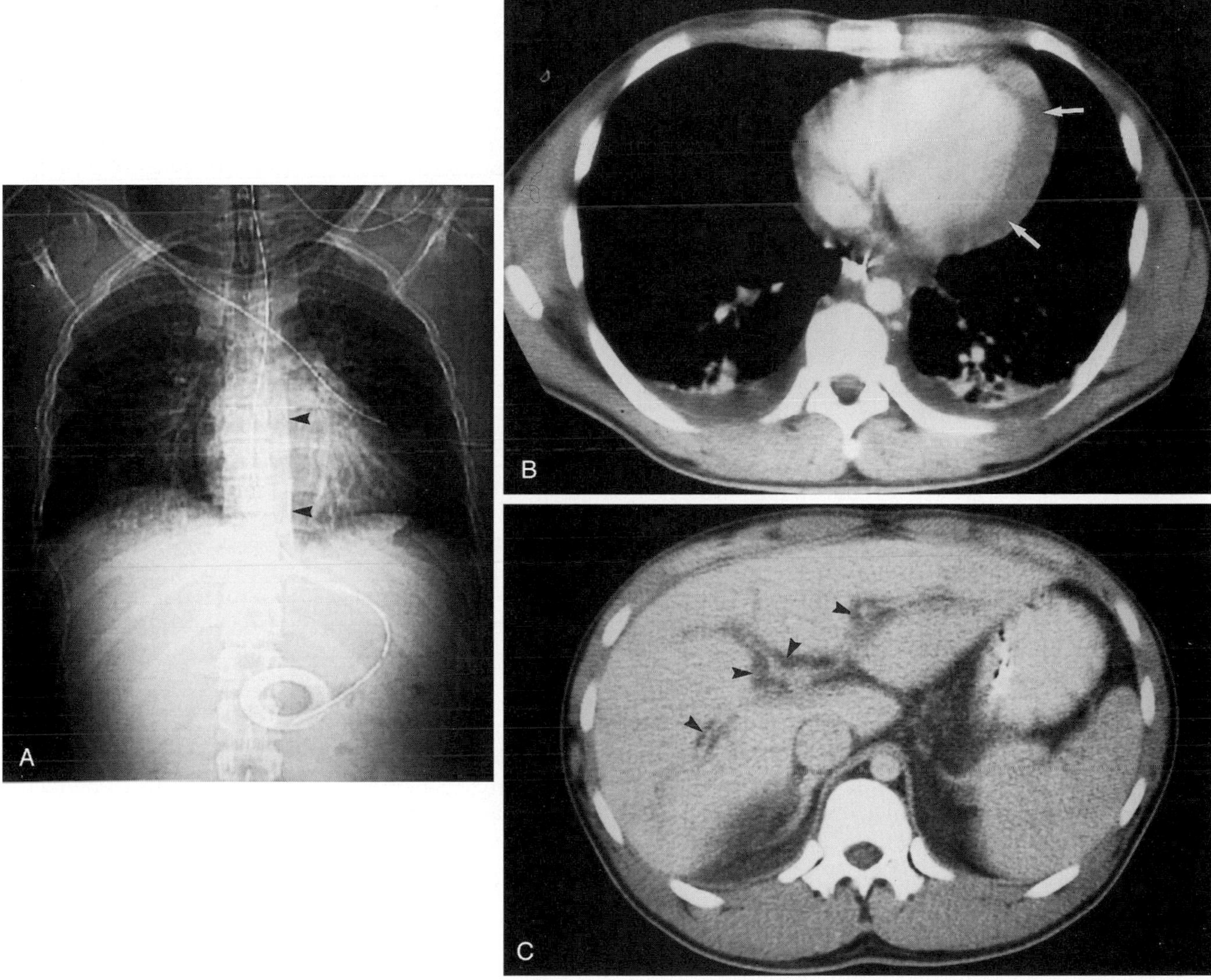

Figure 6–4. Post-traumatic pericardial tamponade. *A,* Scout anteroposterior chest film shows abnormal contour to the superior mediastinum and a wide left paraspinal stripe (*arrowheads*), suggesting hemorrhage, but a normal cardiac size and contour. *B* and *C,* CT study. The mid-cardiac level demonstrates a pericardial effusion (*arrows*) and small pleural effusions. *C,* Image obtained at the level of the upper abdomen shows distention of periportal lymphatics (*arrowheads*) and the inferior vena cava, indicating elevated venous return pressure. Note the small aorta due to decreased cardiac output. Tamponade was verified clinically and managed by pericardial window. (From Goldstein, L., Mirvis, S.E., Kostrubiak, I.S., & Turney, S.Z. [1989]. CT diagnosis of acute pericardial tamponade following blunt chest trauma. A.J.R. Am. J. Roentgenol. *152*:739.)

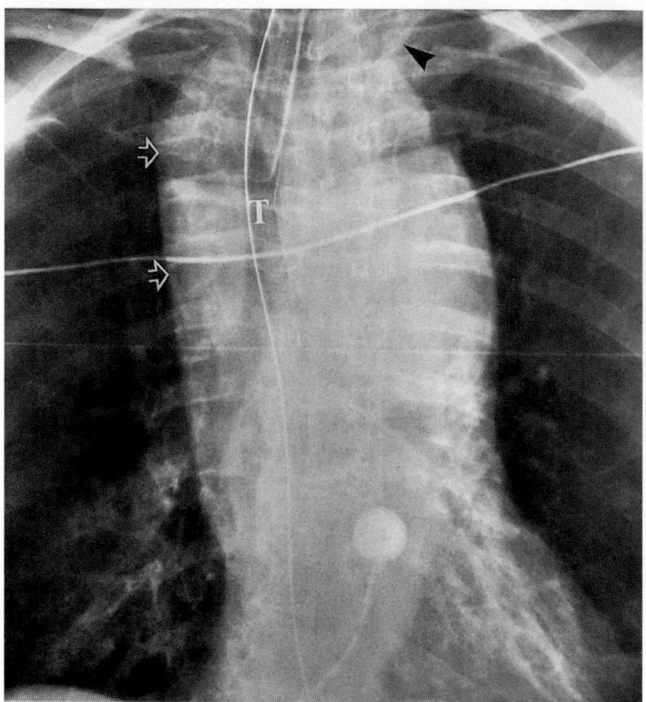

Figure 6–5. Radiograph demonstrating mediastinal hemorrhage. Supine view shows marked contour abnormalities of mediastinum including increased right paratracheal density (*open arrows*), displacement of the tracheal (T) and nasogastric tube to the right, and loss of the aortic arch and descending aortic lateral margins. The left paraspinal stripe is also widened and extends cephalad to form a small extrapleural apical hematoma (*arrowhead*). (From White, C.S., & Mirvis, S.E. [1995]. Pictorial review: Imaging of traumatic aortic injury. Clin. Radiology, *50*:281, with permission.)

therefore for potential great vessel injury. Some causes of false-positive diagnoses include (1) widening and distortion of the mediastinal contour due to supine positioning of the patient for the chest radiograph; (2) the presence of atelectasis, pleural effusion, lung contusions, or lung hematoma, which may obscure the mediastinal contours; (3) limited technical quality of studies, motion artifact, or the presence of overlying support tubes and lines; (4) mediastinal lipomatosis; (5) marked vascular ectasia or thoracic scoliosis of severe degree; and (6) mediastinal hemorrhage without vascular injury (a common cause).

Unless the mediastinal contours can be clearly and unequivocally defined, mediastinal hemorrhage cannot be excluded. Because aortic and other major thoracic arterial injuries are associated with a high incidence of vascular rupture and mortality within hours to days of admission,[61] such injury must be excluded quickly and definitively. Generally, arteriography has provided the diagnostic reference standard to exclude major arterial injury, but this study is costly, invasive, and time-consuming and may significantly delay other diagnostic or therapeutic procedures. Few centers provide immediate diagnostic arteriography on a 24-hour basis. In some cases the results of arteriography are atypical or nondiagnostic.[110]

If the appearance on the chest radiograph is either abnormal or equivocal in the depiction of the mediastinal contour, the next study, if readily available, should be CT with intravenous contrast enhancement. CT can assess the extent and location of any mediastinal hemorrhage and differentiate mediastinal blood from other causes of mediastinal contour abnormality.[111] In addition, CT, particularly spiral (helical) CT, has shown high accuracy in identifying or ruling out direct signs of aortic injury such as a pseudoaneurysm (Fig. 6–6), intimal flaps, intraluminal clot, contour irregularity, and aortic pseudocoarctation (sudden decrease in aortic luminal diameter distal to the injury).[111] In almost all cases the aortic vascular injury is associated with perivascular hemorrhage. In all studies reported to date, the absence of both mediastinal hematoma and direct signs of aortic injury has a 100% negative predictive value for aortic injury.[78, 82, 111] Also, the presence of a mediastinal hematoma localized to the anterior compartment or posterior mediastinum related to a fracture without direct signs of aortic injury also appears to exclude aortic injury.[111] Potential pitfalls in the use of CT to assess for aortic injury include atherosclerotic ulceration, ductus diverticulum, diverticular origin of the bronchial artery, atypical locations of aortic injury, such as in the arch or ascending aorta (Fig. 6–7*A*), and subtle aortic injuries. Very little information on CT accuracy for detection of proximal great vessel injury is available in the literature. Certainly CT can diagnose such injuries (Fig. 6–7*B*), but larger studies with arteriographic correlation are needed before the use of CT for detection of these injuries can be recommended. At present, the presence of hemorrhage around the aorta or great vessels remains an indication for thoracic angiography even if direct signs of vascular injury are absent. Before attributing mediastinal hematoma to a vascular injury, be certain to exclude the possibility of an underlying thoracic spinal fracture as the source (Fig. 6–8). The current Shock-Trauma Center protocol followed for CT assessment of the mediastinum of blunt trauma is presented in Figure 6–9.

Diagnosis of Acute Diaphragm Injury

Injury to the diaphragm occurs in 0.8% to 5.8% of major blunt abdominal trauma cases. Penetrating injury is far more common and is usually detected at surgical exploration. The imaging diagnosis is apparent at radiography in only about 50% (range 27–60%)[83] of blunt

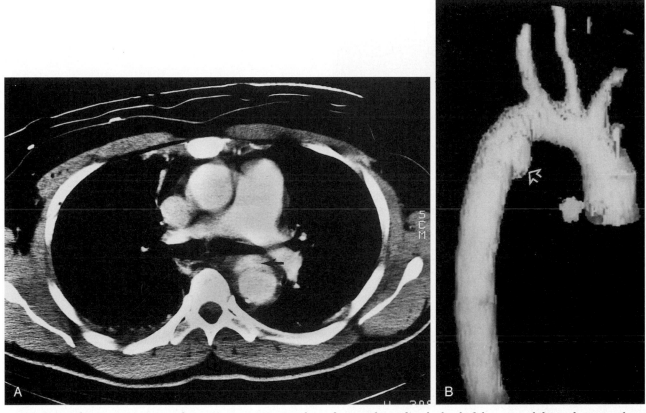

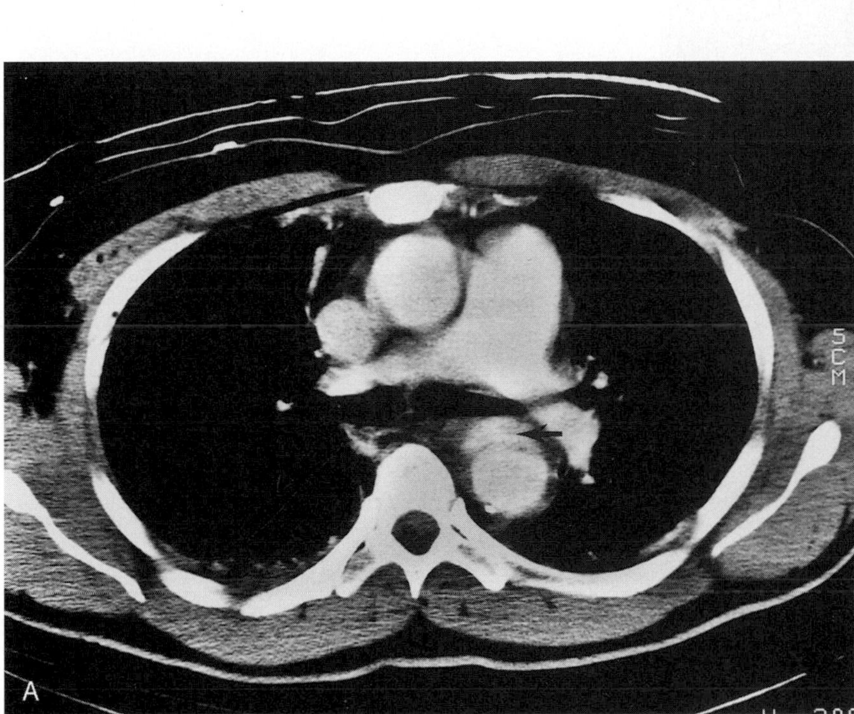

Figure 6–6. CT of traumatic aortic pseudoaneurysm. *A,* Contrast-enhanced image obtained at the level of the proximal descending aorta shows an anterior pseudoaneurysm arising from the aorta (*arrow*). There is a small amount of adjacent mediastinal blood within the mediastinal fat. *B,* Surface-contour 3-D reformatted image shows the pseudoaneurysm (*open arrow*) and its relationship to the major aortic branches. (From Mirvis, S.E., Shanmuganathan, K., Miller, B.H., et al. [1996]. Traumatic aortic injury: Diagnosis with contrast-enhanced CT. Five-year experience at a major trauma center. Radiology, *200*:413.)

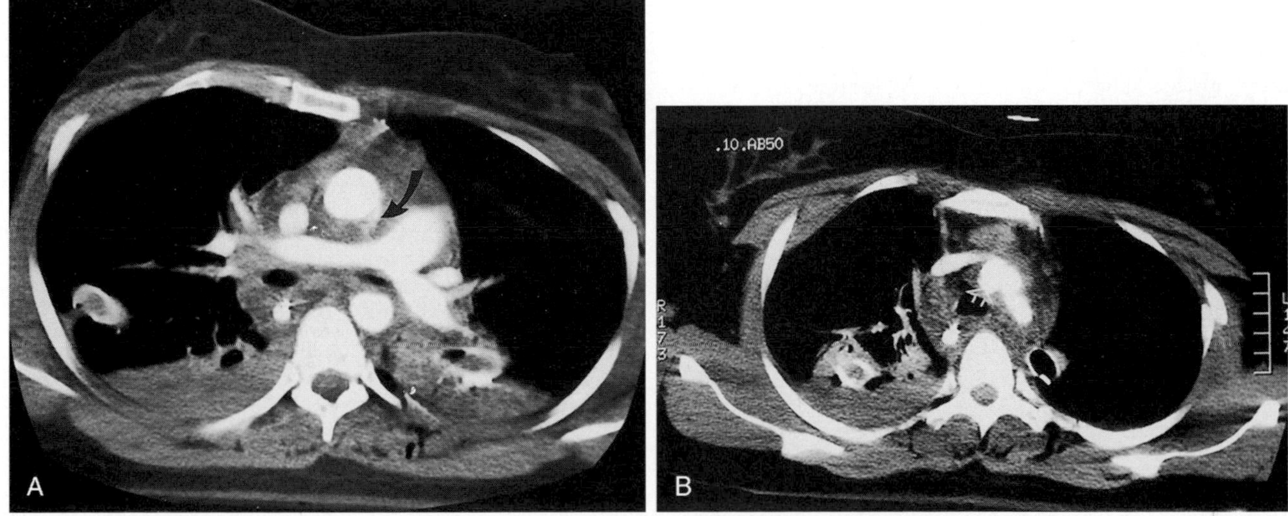

Figure 6–7. CT in evaluation of ascending aorta and right brachiocephalic arterial injuries in a fall victim. *A,* This image from a scan through the proximal ascending aorta, shows a leak of contrast from the left posterior aspect of the aorta (*curved arrow*). This finding proved to represent a focal pseudoaneurysm at surgery. Note the diffuse mediastinal hematoma. *B,* CT of right brachiocephalic arterial injury. This image shows irregular outpouching from the right brachiocephalic artery (*open arrow*) that also proved to be a pseudoaneurysm at surgery. There is also diffuse mediastinal hemorrhage in the superior mediastinum.

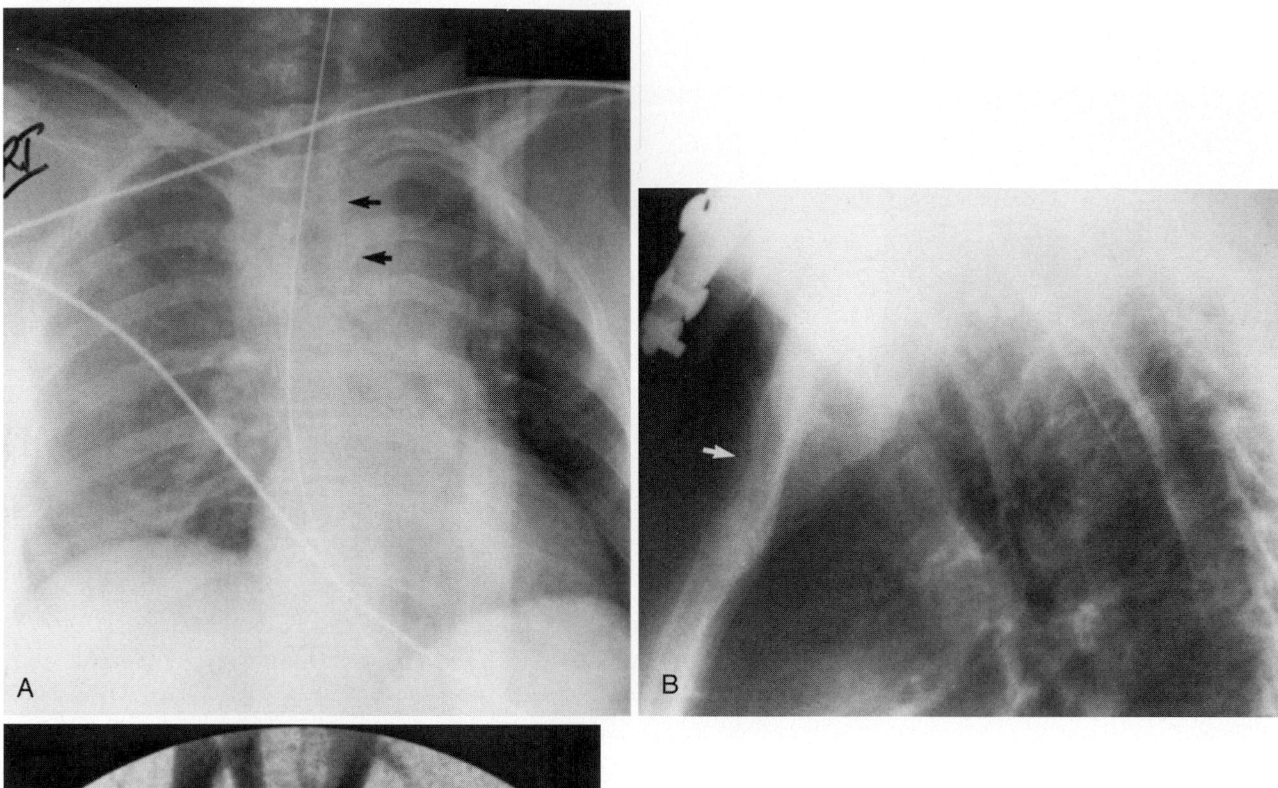

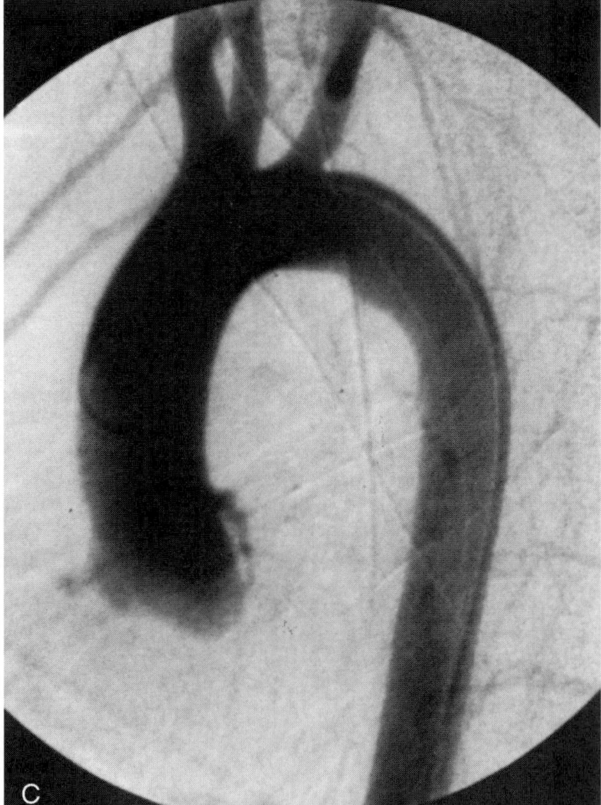

Figure 6–8. Fracture-dislocation of T3-T4 with mediastinal hematoma in a 38-year-old woman injured in a motor vehicle accident. *A,* Anteroposterior view of the chest demonstrates widening of the superior mediastinum with apical capping of both lungs. Note fractures of the first three ribs bilaterally. The trachea remains in the midline, and the nasogastric tube shows no displacement of the esophagus. Closer examination reveals lateral dislocation of C3 upon C3-C4 (*arrows*). *B,* Lateral radiograph of the chest. The fracture-dislocation of the upper spine is not demonstrated with certainty; however, there is a fracture of the manubrium (*arrows*). Such fractures are often associated with fractures or fracture-dislocations of the upper dorsal spine. *C,* Digital subtraction aortogram was performed in the left anterior oblique position and revealed that the aorta was intact. When a mediastinal hematoma is identified on a chest radiograph, every effort should be made to exclude the possibility of a fracture or fracture-dislocation of the thoracic spine before submitting the patient to aortography. The identification of a fracture or fracture-dislocation of the thoracic spine under these circumstances and in the absence of clinical signs of aortic rupture mitigates the need for aortography.

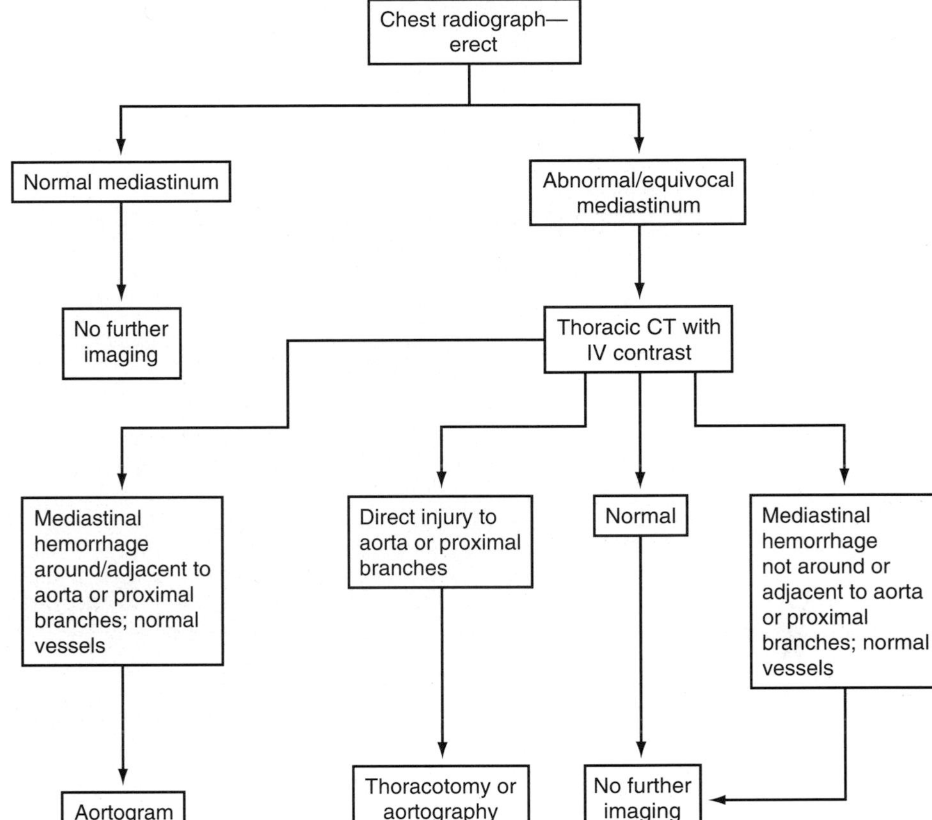

Figure 6–9. Algorithm for imaging assessment of potential traumatic aortic injury. CT, computed tomography, IV, intravenous.

trauma cases and depends on visualization of herniated abdominal structures, usually the stomach, above the level of the hemidiaphragm. Placement of nasogastric tube helps to localize the stomach and its relationship to the hemidiaphram. A constriction of the stomach or other herniated structure at the level of the diaphragm tear (the "collar sign") is pathognomonic for diaphragmatic injury (Fig. 6–10).[99] Injury to the left hemidiaphragm is more commonly diagnosed, because herniation of abdominal contents is more likely to occur than on the right side, where the liver blocks other abdominal tissues from reaching the tear. In about 18% of patients with diaphragm rupture, the diagnosis is suggested radiographically by a poorly defined or apparently elevated hemidiaphragm.[83] In such cases, follow-up radiography may be of value, because delayed presentation of herniation is not uncommon. The diaphragm may appear completely normal radiographically.[83] It is important to obtain chest radiographs in blunt trauma patients after they are removed from positive-pressure airway support, because positive intrathoracic pressure will delay or prevent transdiaphragmatic herniation, whereas typical negative intrathoracic pressure will promote it.

Causes of false-positive radiographic diagnosis of diaphragm tear include the presence of lacerations at the lung bases with air-fluid levels mimicking herniated bowel, phrenic nerve injury and diaphragm paralysis, and eventration of the hemidiaphragm[99] (Figs. 6–11 and 6–12). False-negative radiographic diagnosis is usually due to the presence of tears without associated herniation or mistaking the acute injury for a remote or congenital abnormality. Acute injuries are usually associated with mediastinal displacement away from the hernia contents and ipsilateral pleural effusion.

If the radiologic findings are suggestive but definitive diagnosis is required, CT scanning is an appropriate secondary study. CT can directly detect the point of diaphragm disruption and identify structures crossing the tear[99] (Fig. 6–13). Use of dedicated, thin-section CT technique with improved two-dimensional reformatted images optimizes diagnostic accuracy[99] (Fig. 6–14; see also Fig. 6–12). If CT remains nondiagnostic, then MRI can be used. MRI will show direct diaphragm discontinuity and herniation and typically requires only T_1-weighted sagittal and coronal imaging[140] (Fig. 6–15). MRI is very useful to confirm an intact diaphragm in blunt trauma patients with apparent elevation on plain radiographs[140] or to confirm a diaphragm rupture.

Usually, penetrating injury to the diaphragm is determined at surgical exploration performed for injury with proximity to the lower thorax or upper abdomen. CT can be useful in clarifying the course of a penetrating injury and in determining its relationship to the diaphragm. Obviously an object that crosses the plane between the chest and the abdomen has injured the diaphragm. Careful inspection of CT axial images in such cases may reveal the location and extent of such injuries (Fig. 6–16). Although most penetrating injuries to the left hemi-

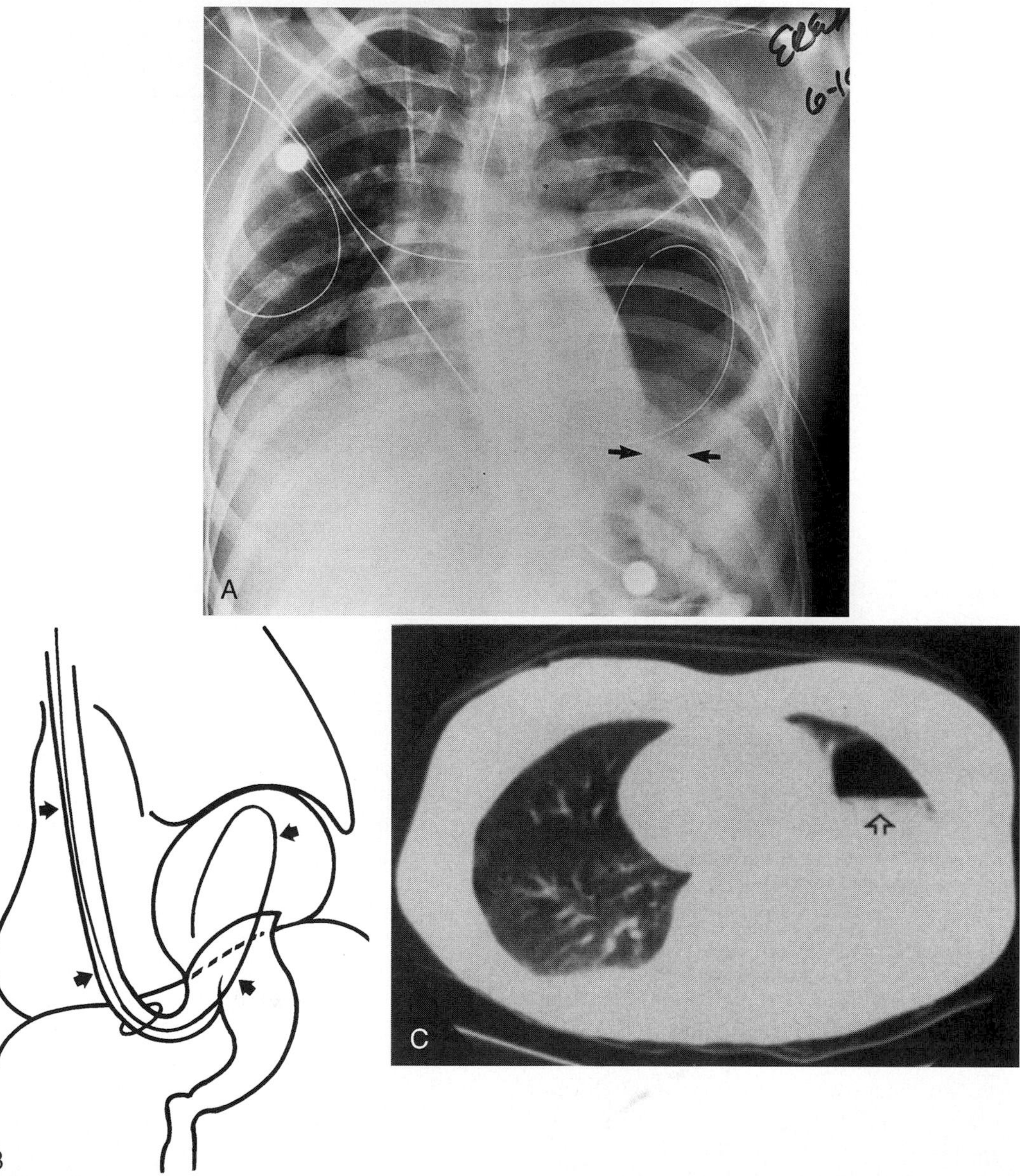

Figure 6–10. Traumatic left hemidiaphragm rupture. *A,* Semierect chest radiograph shows elevation of the stomach containing the nasogastric tube into the left thorax. Note that the gastric bubble tapers as it approaches the diaphragmatic tear (*arrows*), confirming a transdiaphragmatic course. Note that the nasogastric tube is coiled within the stomach (*arrows*). This confirms the presence of a ruptured diaphragm (as diagrammed in *B*). *B,* Diagram demonstrating rupture of left hemidiaphragm with herniation of stomach into the left chest. A nasogastric tube passes through the esophageal hiatus and then up into the displaced stomach (*arrows*), which confirms the diagnosis. *C,* Computed tomography scan confirms the diagnosis of diaphragmatic rupture. Note the gas within the stomach displaced into the left hemithorax. Note also the layered food contents (*arrow*), which identifies this structure with certainty as the stomach.

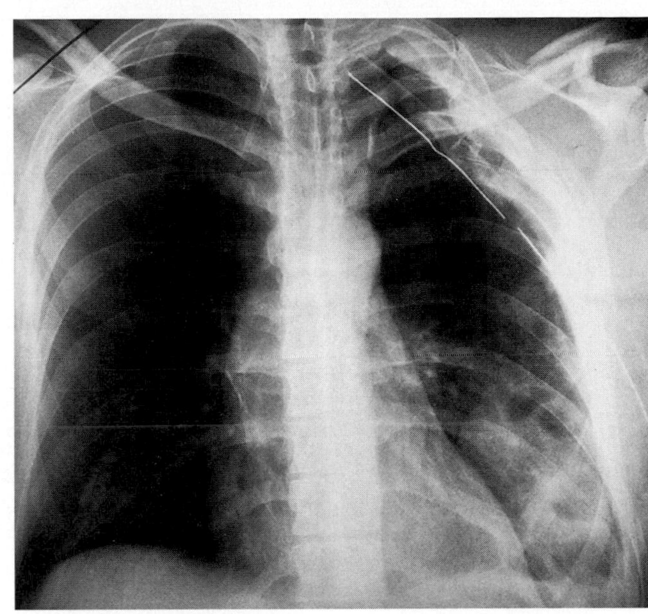

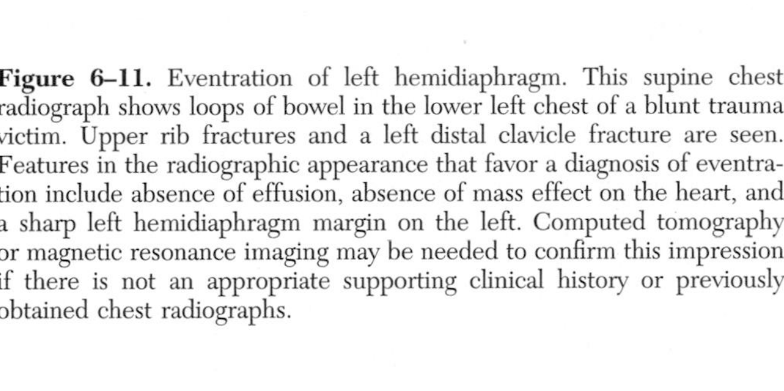

Figure 6–11. Eventration of left hemidiaphragm. This supine chest radiograph shows loops of bowel in the lower left chest of a blunt trauma victim. Upper rib fractures and a left distal clavicle fracture are seen. Features in the radiographic appearance that favor a diagnosis of eventration include absence of effusion, absence of mass effect on the heart, and a sharp left hemidiaphragm margin on the left. Computed tomography or magnetic resonance imaging may be needed to confirm this impression if there is not an appropriate supporting clinical history or previously obtained chest radiographs.

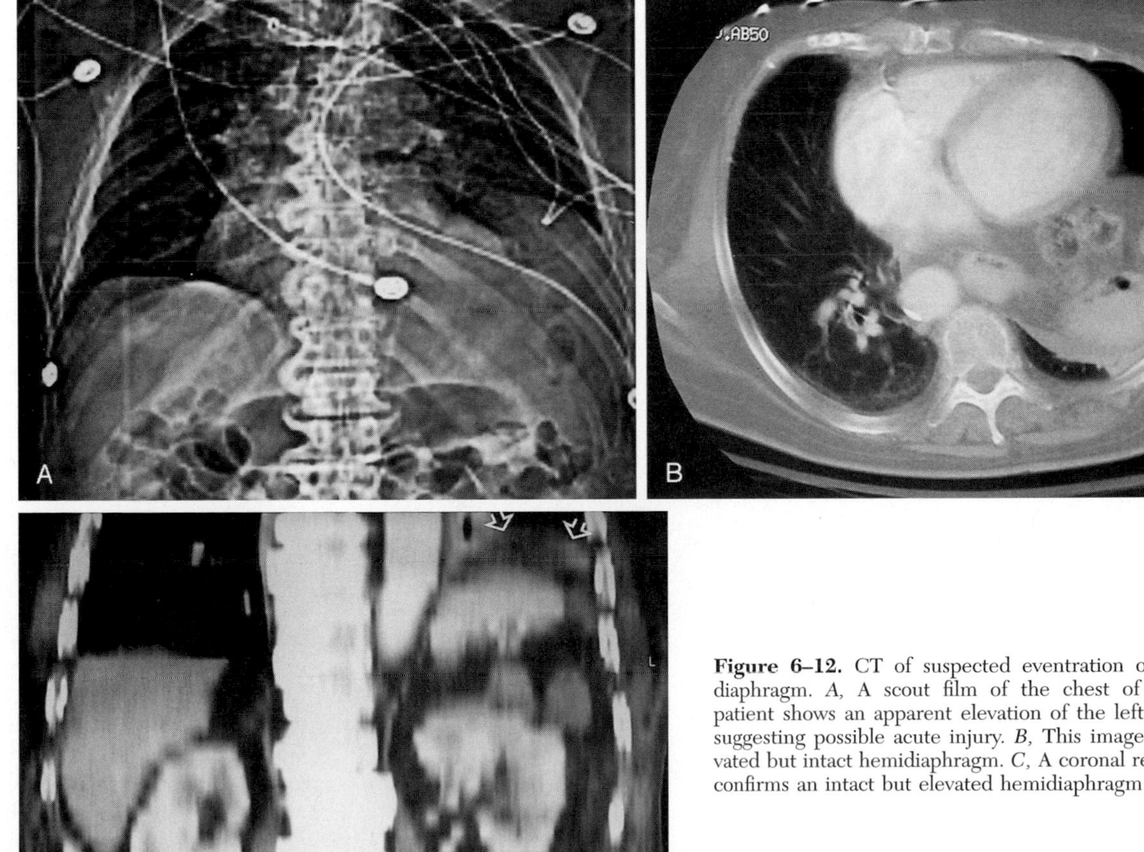

Figure 6–12. CT of suspected eventration of the left hemidiaphragm. *A,* A scout film of the chest of a blunt trauma patient shows an apparent elevation of the left hemidiaphragm, suggesting possible acute injury. *B,* This image suggests an elevated but intact hemidiaphragm. *C,* A coronal reformatted image confirms an intact but elevated hemidiaphragm (*arrows*).

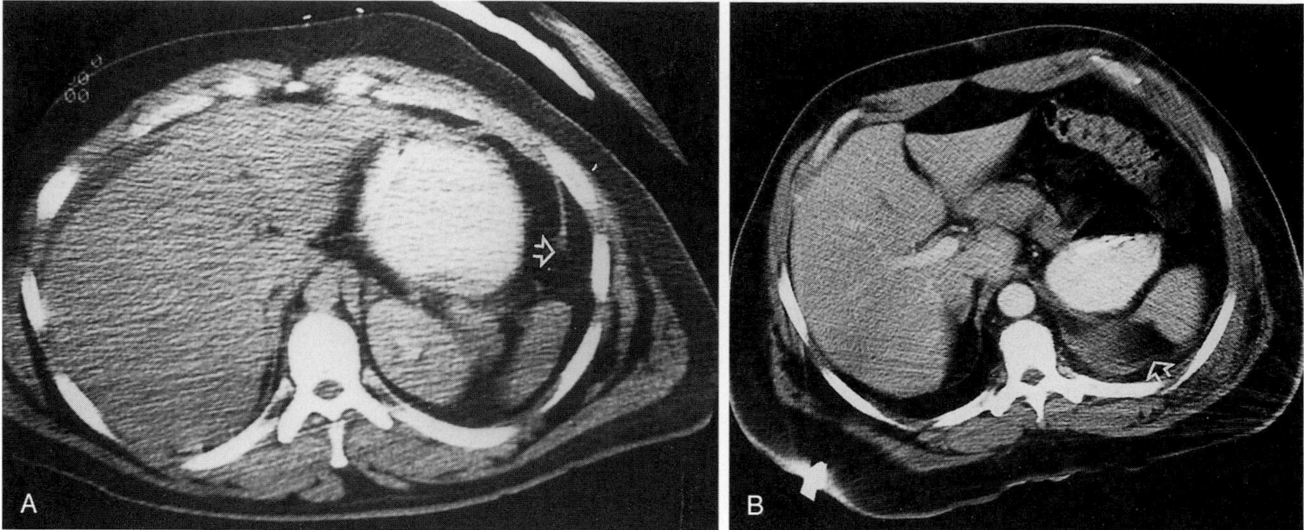

Figure 6–13. CT of direct diaphragm disruption. *A,* An image through the upper abdomen of a blunt trauma victim shows an interruption in the left hemidiaphragm (*arrow*) with fat and spleen herniating into the hemithorax. There is a small perihepatic fluid collection. *B,* An image from another patient also shows interruption of the left hemidiaphragm (*arrow*), with some hemorrhage at the injury site. (From Gelman, R., Mirvis, S.E., & Gens, D.R. [1991]. Diaphragmatic rupture due to blunt trauma: Sensitivity of plain chest radiographs. A.J.R. Am. J. Roentgenol., *156*:51.)

diaphragm are surgically or thorascopically repaired, minor tears on the right side may be observed, owing to the protective presence of the liver.

Trends in Diagnostic Imaging of Abdominal Trauma

Initial Screening Evaluation

The initial assessment of the trauma patient is clinical. Monitoring of vital signs and restoration of circulation, a patent airway, and respiration are the primary clinical goals. In most cases, if the patient's vital signs cannot be maintained adequately or necessitate ongoing high-level resuscitative measures, then operative management is required to identify and address sources of ongoing blood loss. In many cases the site(s) of hemorrhage are identified using bedside clinical assessment. Major sites of blood loss include the thoracic cavity, abdominal cavity, extraperitoneal space, and extremity wounds; previous blood loss occurring at the injury scene or on route to the medical facility is also an important consideration.

Diagnostic assessment for potential bleeding into the peritoneal cavity has undergone several changes since the early 1980s. Since the mid-1960s, diagnostic peritoneal lavage (DPL) has been commonly used in both hemodynamically stable and unstable patients to determine the presence or absence of intraperitoneal bleeding. The technique is relatively safe, simple to perform, and highly sensitive for detection of minimal hemoperitoneum.[104, 124] Some of the deficiencies of DPL are sensitivity for detection of minor parenchymal injuries that require no surgical treatment, inability to detect retroperitoneal bleeding sites, and "contamination" of the peritoneal cavity with hemorrhage from an extraperitoneal source such as the pelvis. Occasionally, false-negative results due to suboptimal technique or presence of adhesions or diaphragm injury may be obtained.[114] As the clinical trend toward nonoperative treatment of selected solid organ injuries has grown, the oversensitivity of DPL that led to many nontherapeutic celiotomies has become of major significance, especially as the complications and cost of such operations have become better appreciated.[128]

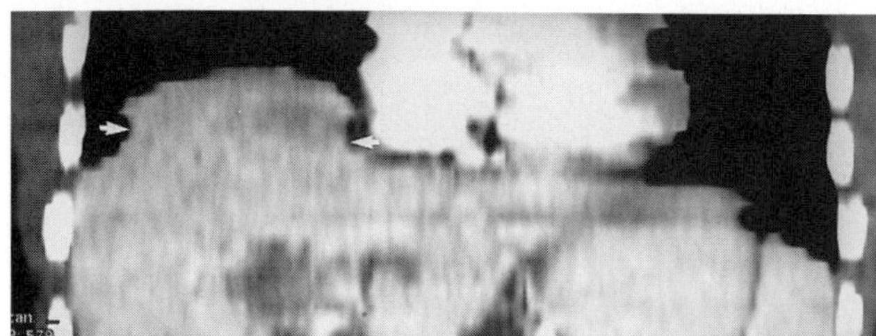

Figure 6–14. A 2-D reconstructed CT in suspected right diaphragm rupture. A reformatted image of the diaphragm demonstrates a collar sign (*arrows*) involving the liver indicating herniation through a tear. Appearance on the chest radiographs and axial images on the computed tomography scan (not shown) was equivocal.

Another diagnostic modality used in the assessment of abdominal trauma, particularly over the last past decade or so, in the United States has been sonography. Sonographic examination of the abdomen for blunt trauma has been performed in Europe since the 1970s.[60, 67, 85] Only relatively recently has the use of sonography in trauma been evaluated in the United States.[150] Because it is a rapidly performed, repeatable, noninvasive, and inexpensive study, sonographic evaluation has been advocated by many authorities as an effective triage tool to assess blunt abdominal trauma.[64, 65, 81] The use of screening sonography in the pediatric population is well established,[59, 85, 121] but its exact role in the adult blunt injury population is more controversial.[69, 106, 126] Different trends in the use of abdominal sonography in trauma have emerged. Some authors, mainly in Europe and Asia, advocate abdominal sonography performed by a radiologist (sonologist) as the primary screening tool in the trauma room.[64, 88, 157] In

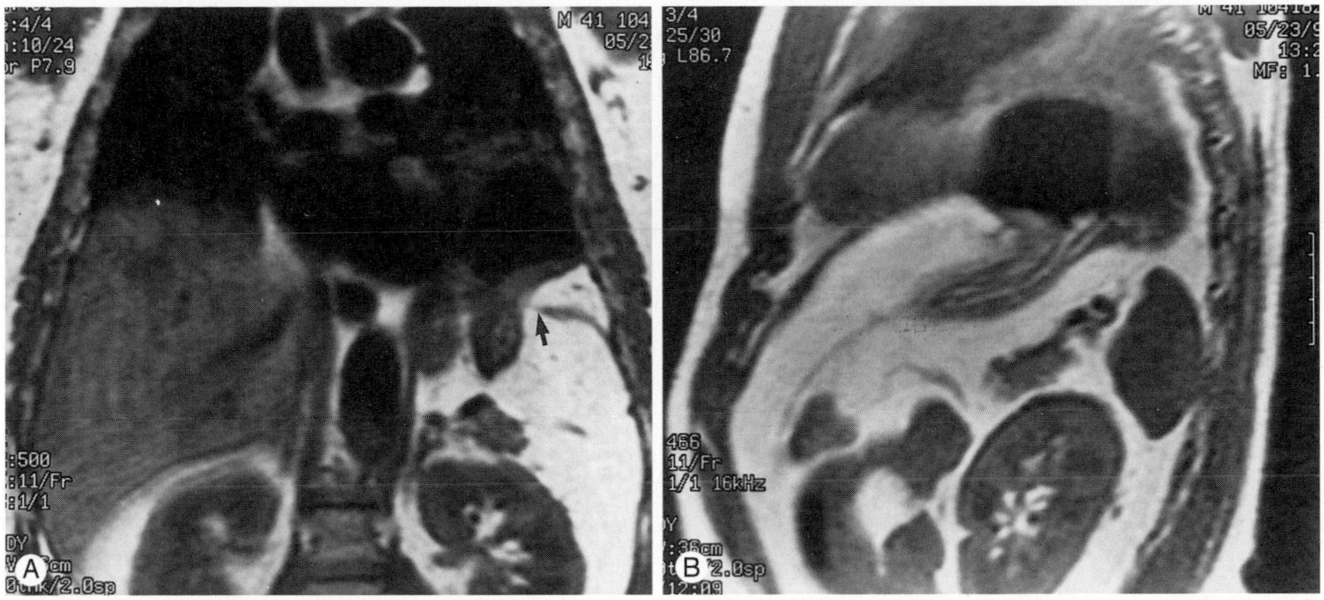

Figure 6–15. Suspected right hemidiaphragm injury. Coronal (*A*) and lateral (*B*), T_1-weighted MRI examination confirms left diaphragm rupture and gastric herniation (note the gastric "collar sign" at the diaphragm tear). Some retroperitoneal fat appears herniated on the sagittal view (*B*), and the torn edge of the diaphragm (*arrow*) is seen on the coronal view (*A*). There is atelectasis above the stomach. (From Shanmuganathan, K., Mirvis, S.E., White, C.S., & Pomerantz, S.M. [1996]. MR imaging evaluation of hemidiaphragms in acute blunt trauma. Experience in 16 patients. A.J.R. Am. J. Roentgenol. *167*:397.)

the United States and Canada, focused assessment with sonography for trauma (FAST) has generally been regarded as a rapid and reliable diagnostic test in blunt abdominal trauma victims, but only for the detection of free peritoneal fluid when performed by nonradiologists. FAST may therefore be useful as an initial imaging study and triage tool.[65, 105, 129] Some authors also advocate abdominal sonography as a cost-effective replacement for DPL and CT.[106]

The increasing use of abdominal sonography for evaluating patients with blunt abdominal trauma and the increasing number of associated clinical research studies

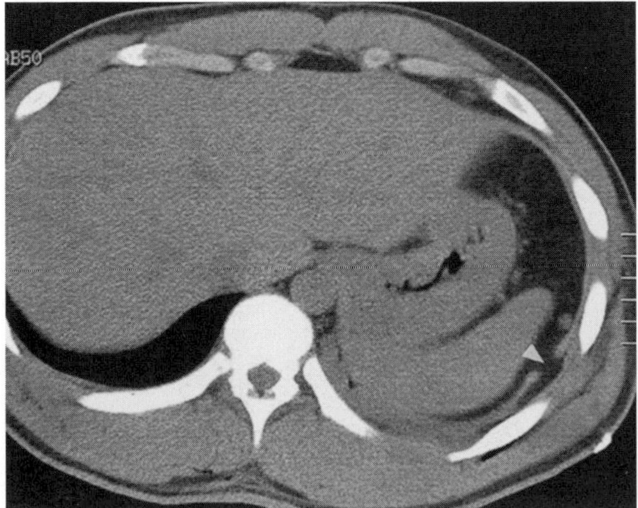

Figure 6–16. CT in evaluation of a knife wound to the diaphragm. This image shows a focal defect in the left hemidiaphragm (*arrowhead*) adjacent to the site of knife penetration (*radiodense marker* on skin). The injury was repaired by thoracoscopic surgery.

mandate standardization of methodology and terminology. The term *FAST* was first introduced in 1993[135] in an attempt to define and standardize the current role of sonography in the management of trauma victims. The following discussion reflects the findings of a 1997 international consensus conference on this diagnostic imaging approach.[132]

The FAST technique has been defined as real-time sonographic scanning of four regions: pericardial, perihepatic, perisplenic, and pelvic. This method of examination does *not* include direct visualization of parenchymal injuries. Indeed, it has been judged impracticable for surgeons to acquire and maintain the skill needed to identify parenchymal lesions by sonography when CT is readily available. In an unstable patient, a positive FAST result mandates exploratory laparotomy. A positive FAST result in a hemodynamically unstable patient is an indication for urgent laparotomy, and a negative FAST result should direct a search for extra-abdominal sources of hemorrhage. FAST may be useful as a general screening study to detect the presence of peritoneal free fluid in a hemodynamically stable blunt trauma patient. The amount and type of training needed for clinicians to achieve a high level of competence in performing the FAST study have not been clearly established.[132]

Although the use of FAST as an expedient tool for the identification of free fluid in the unstable blunt trauma patient seems prudent, its role in the stable trauma patient is perhaps more controversial. In this setting, there is typically more time for alternative diagnostic CT studies. The potential weaknesses of the FAST technique are listed in Table 6–2. The potential values and weaknesses of CT scanning in the setting of blunt abdominal trauma are listed in Table 6–3. The accuracy of FAST has been described in many studies, mainly from the surgical litera-

Table 6–2. Potential Limitations of Focused Assessment with Sonography for Trauma (FAST) in Hemodynamically Stable Blunt Trauma Victims

Patient-Related Factors
Open wounds over abdomen
Previous surgery and adhesions (potential)
Body habitus (obesity)
Lack of patient cooperation (movement)
Diagnostic Test Factors
Obscuration by bowel gas
Presence of clotted (nonliquid) blood
Nonhemorrhagic fluid collections (e.g., cysts, bowel loops, renal)
Operator-dependent/experience limited
Technical Factors
Limited transducer selection
Inappropriate gain setting for near and far field
Sonographic artifacts
Improper calibration of sonography machine

ture.* Studies performed at the University of Maryland Shock-Trauma Center have found some important limitations of FAST. A study by Sherbourne and colleagues[143] found that of 196 patients with intraabdominal injuries in whom FAST studies were performed, 50 (26%) had no evidence of hemoperitoneum by CT or sonography. Among these 50 patients, 10 required surgery for their intraperitoneal injuries. In a follow-up study conducted in 466 patients with 575 abdominal visceral injuries, Shanmuganathan and associates[138] used CT to assess for the presence of hemoperitoneum. No evidence of hemoperitoneum was seen in 157 (34%) of these 466 patients, including 57 (27%) of 210 splenic injuries, 71 (34%) of 206 hepatic injuries, 30 (48%) of 63 renal injuries, 4 (11%) of 35 mesenteric injuries, and 2 (29%) of 7 pancreatic injuries. Surgery or angiographic embolization was performed to treat injuries in 26 (17%) patients with no CT evidence of hemoperitoneum. This study suggests that the presence of hemoperitoneum alone as an indicator of abdominal visceral injury is insufficient.

A recent study reviewed results of FAST performed by nonradiologist physicians with variable levels of training and experience. In this study (P.A. Poletti, MD, personal communication, 2001), the FAST results were compared with results of abdominal CT performed subsequently. A total of 531 FAST examinations were performed. When CT results were used as the reference standard, the FAST technique was only 33% sensitive for the detection of abdominal injury. The positive predictive value was 45%, and the negative predictive value was 94%. Among the 531 patients, 23 required laparotomy or angiographic embolization. FAST yielded false-negative results in 8 (35%) of these 23 patients. Table 6–4 correlates the results of FAST and CT in this patient population. In this study, 24 patients with intra-abdominal injury had no evidence of hemoperitoneum as determined by either FAST or subsequent CT. CT demonstrated abdominal organ injury in 69 patients, with associated intraperitoneal free fluid in 45 of these patients.

At the Shock-Trauma Center, rapid availability of fast CT scanning and experienced interpretation has increased the use of CT for assessment of most stable trauma patients. According to individual physician preference, serial FAST studies combined with clinical assessment may be used as an alternative, but this approach typically requires at least a 6- to 12-hour observation period. Uniform guidelines for the performance of FAST by physicians without formal training in sonography need to be established to assure both quality interpretation and documentation of results. The potential for FAST to miss intra-abdominal organ injuries not accompanied by hemoperitoneum must also be emphasized.

*See references 59, 65, 67, 81, 88, 106, 121, 129, 132, 150, 157.

Identification of Hemorrhage by Computed Tomography: Implications for Management

The increasing use of fast conventional or spiral CT with timed-bolus intravenous contrast injection for assessment of abdominal trauma has led to improved recognition of active bleeding within the abdomen. Previous studies have shown that extravasated contrast material has a CT density higher than that of clotted blood or enhanced organ parenchyma, typically with a value within 10 Hounsfield units of that for an adjacent artery.[139] The contrast "blush" that is seen on CT (Fig. 6–17) may represent either contrast material that has extravasated into the surrounding parenchyma or a pseudoaneurysm of an injured artery. Vascular contrast may on occasion be seen leaking directly into the peritoneal cavity. The focus of contrast blush is usually surrounded by hematoma of lower CT attenuation.

The increasing recognition of active bleeding with use of CT has vital implications for patient management that have not yet been incorporated into organ injury classification systems (see later on). The demonstration of active bleeding has direct implications regarding the need for angiographic or surgical intervention.

Table 6–3. Use of Computed Tomography in the Hemodynamically Stable Blunt Trauma Victim

Potential Advantages	Potential Limitations
Can concurrently assess other body regions (spine, head, chest)	May not be available, or access difficult
Accurate in localizing site of bleeding	Monitoring may be more limited
Can quantify blood loss in gross fashion	Immediate access to patient more limited
Can distinguish intraperitoneal from extraperitoneal source of bleeding	Rapid, accurate interpretation needed
Can aid in determination of need for angiographic evaluation	?Accuracy for bowel/mesentery injury
Easy to document and store image data	Study slow with older technology
Easy to manipulate data in two-dimensional and three-dimensional formats	Expensive (professional charges and technical cost)
Very fast using spiral and multi-row detector technology	Requires x-ray exposure
Less operator-dependent results	
Can distinguish blood and clot from other fluids (urine, bile) in most cases	

Table 6–4. Correlation of Results with Focused Assessment with Sonography for Trauma (FAST) and Computed Tomography (CT)*

	Negative CT without FF n = 460	**Negative CT with FF** n = 2	**Positive CT** n = 69	**Positive CT with FF** n = 45	**Positive CT without FF** n = 24
Positive FAST n = 33	12 (36%)	2 (6%)	19 (58%)	15 (45%)	4 (12%)
Negative FAST n = 480	433 (90%)	0	47 (10%)	30 (6%)	17 (4%)
Indeterminate FAST n = 18	15 (83%)	0	3 (17%)	0	3 (17%)

*At the University of Maryland Shock-Trauma Center, August 1997–September 1998.

FF, intra-abdominal free fluid. Negative or positive CT refers to the presence of a traumatic injury only. Free fluid was found in one patient with negative CT findings and preexisting cirrhosis and was considered physiologic in another patient.

Unpublished data; From Pierre A. Poletti; MD, personal communication, 2001.

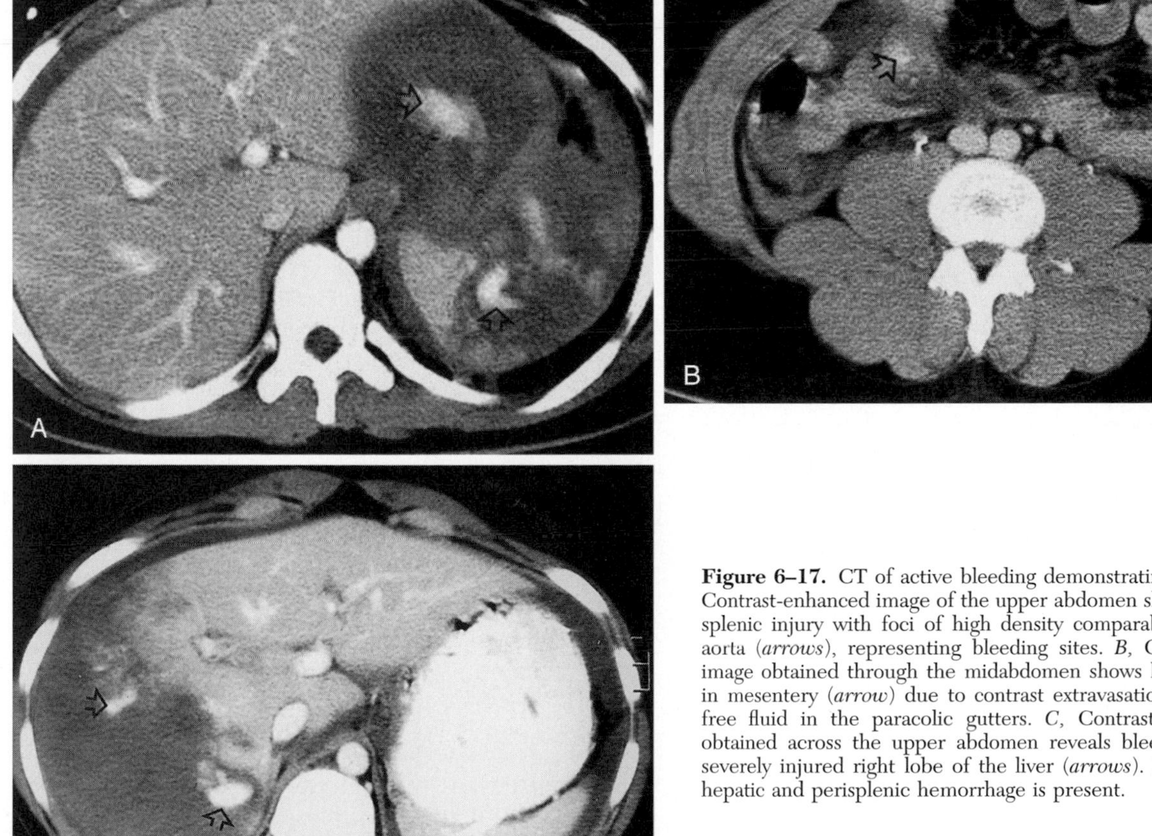

Figure 6–17. CT of active bleeding demonstrating CT "blush." *A,* Contrast-enhanced image of the upper abdomen shows a high-grade splenic injury with foci of high density comparable to that of the aorta (*arrows*), representing bleeding sites. *B,* Contrast-enhanced image obtained through the midabdomen shows high-density focus in mesentery (*arrow*) due to contrast extravasation. There is some free fluid in the paracolic gutters. *C,* Contrast-enhanced image obtained across the upper abdomen reveals bleeding sites in the severely injured right lobe of the liver (*arrows*). Evidence of perihepatic and perisplenic hemorrhage is present.

Trend Toward Nonoperative Management of Solid Organ Injury

Spleen Injury

Nonoperative management is the preferred treatment for splenic injury in children,[130] owing to the importance of preserving the immune functions of the spleen. The nonoperative management of splenic trauma in the adult has also gained popularity in recent years, but the selection criteria to identify patients for attempted nonoperative management are controversial.[68, 85, 118, 146] Many selection criteria are clinically based, including hemodynamic status, age, abdominal examination findings, and blood transfusion requirements, among others.[68, 85, 118, 146] Other criteria are imaging based and may include the presence of other abdominal injuries requiring surgery, magnitude of hemoperitoneum, grade of organ injury, and, more recently, evidence of ongoing bleeding by CT.[73, 79, 133, 142]

The surgical grading system for splenic injury is essentially quantitative, measuring extent of parenchymal laceration or hematoma and tissue viability (Table 6–5). A proposed CT splenic injury classification system is derived from the American Association for the Surgery of Trauma (AAST) version (Table 6–6). In general, CT classification systems have not been found to reliably predict the clinical outcome with attempted nonoperative management.[147] In part, this apparent failing may be related to the relatively small size of the series but may also reflect an important missing element in the proposed classification systems. Previous studies have shown that the presence of a CT contrast blush within the spleen is an extremely strong predictor for failure of nonoperative treatment[73, 79, 133] and that this failure rate can be significantly improved by use of splenic artery embolization.[73] Ideally, if CT scanning could reliably demonstrate the presence of vascular injuries, patients could be selected for splenic angiography on the basis of CT results. Shanmuganathan and associates[137] studied 78 patients with blunt splenic trauma who underwent both abdominal CT and splenic angiography. In this study, contrast-enhanced spiral CT was 81% sensitive, 84% specific, and 83% accurate in predicting the presence of a splenic vascular injury requiring angiography. Further prospective studies of this type are needed to verify and potentially improve upon these results.

In previous studies Sclafani[134] and Hagiwara[91] and their colleagues have shown that angiographic embolization is highly successful in the treatment of post-traumatic splenic vascular lesions, resulting in a 93% to 97% overall success rate for nonoperative treatment of hemodynamically stable patients with CT-diagnosed blunt splenic injury. Sclafani and coworkers[134] recommend the use of proximal coil embolization of the splenic artery to permit collateral blood flow to maintain viable splenic parenchyma and maximize splenic function. Boyd-Kranis and associates[66] describe the use of selective distal embolization of bleeding splenic artery branches. Regional splenic infarcts appeared more commonly in patients undergoing distal splenic embolization, but infections were quite rare in both the proximal and distal embolization groups.[66]

The optimal use of combined clinical and imaging criteria to select patients for attempted nonoperative management of splenic trauma, as well as the type of intravascular treatment of injured splenic vessels, awaits further study.

Table 6–5. AAST Spleen Injury Scale (1994 Revision)

Grade*	Type	Description of Injury
I	Hematoma	Subcapsular, <10% surface area
	Laceration	Capsular tear, <1 cm parenchymal depth
II	Hematoma	Subcapsular, 10–50% surface area; intraparenchymal, <5 cm in diameter
	Laceration	1–3 cm parenchymal depth that does not involve a trabecular vessel
III	Hematoma	Subcapsular, >50% surface area or expanding; ruptured subcapsular or parenchymal hematoma
	Laceration	>3 cm parenchymal depth or involving trabecular vessels
IV	Laceration	Laceration involving segmental or hilar vessels producing major devascularization (>25% of spleen)
V	Laceration	Completely shattered spleen
	Vascular	Hilar vascular injury that devascularized spleen

*Advance one grade for multiple injuries, up to grade III.
AAST, American Association for the Surgery of Trauma.
From Moore, E.E., Cogbill, T.H., Jurkovich, G.H., et al. (1995). Organ injury scaling: Spleen and liver (1994 revision). J. Trauma, 38:323.

Table 6–6. Computed Tomography Injury Severity Grades in Blunt Splenic Injury

Grade	Criteria
I	Capsular avulsion, superficial laceration(s), or subcapsular hematoma <1 cm
II	Parenchymal laceration(s) 1–3 cm deep, central/subcapsular hematoma(s) <3 cm
III	Lacerations >3 cm deep, central/subcapsular hematoma >3 cm
IV	Parenchymal fragmentation into two or more sections
V	Intraparenchymal contrast blush or extravasation beyond capsule; progression of injury by follow-up CT; devascularized (nonenhancing) spleen

Modified from Mirvis, S.E., Whitley, N.O., & Gens, D.R. (1989). Blunt splenic trauma in adults: CT-based classification and correlation with prognosis and treatment. Radiology, *171*:33.

Hepatic Injury

Increasingly, blunt hepatic trauma is being managed nonoperatively. Many hepatic injuries are limited and are not bleeding at the time of surgery; in these cases, nontherapeutic celiotomy with its costs and potential complications was the undesired result.[141] CT has fostered the trend toward nonoperative management by demonstrating the extent of the injury, the presence or absence of concurrent intraperitoneal injuries, progression or resolution of the injury, and the development of complications such as infection or biloma.[141] The surgical hepatic injury grading system developed through the AAST (Table 6–7) can estimate the extent of injury, as can a CT-based grading system derived from the surgical system (Table

Table 6–7. AAST Liver Injury Scale (1994 Revision)

Grade*		Injury Description
I	Hematoma	Subcapsular, nonexpanding, <10 cm surface area
	Laceration	Capsular tear, nonbleeding, <1 cm parenchymal depth
II	Hematoma	Subcapsular, nonexpanding, 10–50% surface area; intraparenchymal, nonexpanding <10 cm diameter
	Laceration	Capsular tear, active bleeding: 1–3 cm parenchymal depth, 10 cm in length
III	Hematoma	Subcapsular, >50% surface area or expanding; ruptured subcapsular hematoma with active bleeding; intraparenchymal hematoma >10 cm in depth or expanding
IV	Hematoma	Ruptured intraparenchymal hematoma with active bleeding
	Laceration	Parenchymal disruption involving 25–75% of hepatic lobe, or 1–3 Couinaud segments within a single lobe
V	Laceration	Parenchymal disruption involving >75% of hepatic lobe, or >3 Couinaud segments within a single lobe
	Vascular	Juxtavenous injuries (e.g., in retrohepatic vena cava/central major hepatic veins)
VI	Vascular	Hepatic avulsion

*Advance one grade for multiple injuries, up to grade III.
AAST, American Association for the Surgery of Trauma.
From Moore, E.E., Cogbill, T.H., Jurkovich, G.H., et al. (1995). Organ injury scaling: Spleen and liver (1994 revision). J. Trauma, *38*:323.

6–8). Most studies indicate that all grades of hepatic injury can be successfully managed without surgery if the patient maintains hemodynamic stability; therefore, the grading of these injuries has no value in selecting patients for surgery or nonoperative management.[144]

A recent prospective study of 63 patients with blunt hepatic injury conducted at the University of Maryland Shock-Trauma Center assessed clinical outcome with injury location. All patients with CT findings indicating injury severity grade of II or higher (see Table 6–6) underwent hepatic angiography after CT. The proximity of hepatic parenchymal injuries to the gallbladder fossa, porta hepatis, inferior vena cava, and major hepatic veins was analyzed.[123] Injuries involving at least one major hepatic vein had a statistically increased association with failed nonoperative management and delayed hepatic-related complications (Fig. 6–18). No other statistically significant correlation between site of injury and outcome of initial nonoperative treatment was found. In this study the presence of an arterial-phase contrast blush was 65% sensitive and 85% specific for an arteriographically confirmed hepatic artery injury. These results increased to 100% sensitive and 94% specific if only patients with CT grade II and grade III injurity severity were considered. It was determined that patients with injuries of CT grade I to III severity who did not have evidence of major hepatic vein involvement did not require hepatic angiography, whereas patients with injuries of CT grade IV and grade V severity without an arterial blush but with hepatic vein involvement did require angiography.[123] In this study, the need for operative or angiographic treatment of the liver increased with injury grade from II to V.

Table 6–8. Computed Tomography Scan-Based Injury: Severity Grades for Blunt Hepatic Trauma

Grade	Criteria
I	Capsular avulsion, superficial laceration(s) <1 cm deep, subcapsular hematoma <1 cm maximal thickness
II	Laceration(s) 1–3 cm deep, central/subcapsular hematoma(s) 1–3 cm in diameter
III	Laceration(s) >3 cm deep, central/subcapsular hematoma(s) >3 cm in diameter
IV	Laceration >10 cm deep; central/subcapsular hematoma >10 cm; lobar maceration or devascularization; injury extending into major hepatic vein
V	Bilobar tissue maceration; parenchymal contrast "blush"; arterial contrast extravasation beyond capsule

*Modified from Mirvis, S.E., Whitley, N.O., Vainwright, J.R., & Gens, D.R. (1989). Blunt hepatic trauma in adults. CT-based classification and correlation with prognosis and treatment. Radiology, *171*:27.

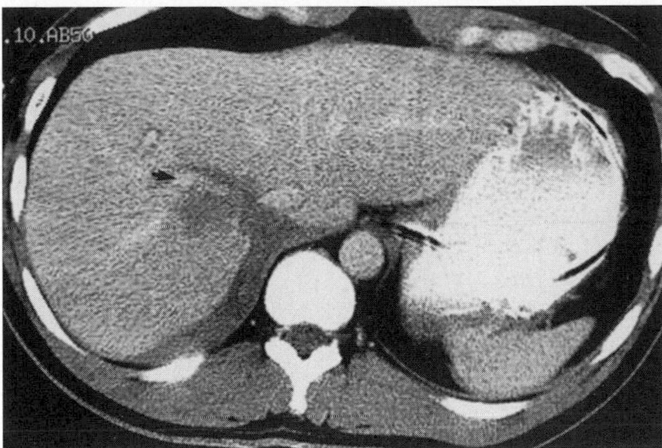

Figure 6–18. CT of a laceration involving the middle hepatic vein (*arrow*) and the region of the inferior vena cava. Hemorrhage extends along the bare area of the liver.

Bowel and Mesenteric Injury: Improving Diagnostic Accuracy

Bowel and mesenteric injuries are found in about 5% of patients who undergo laparotomy for blunt abdominal trauma.[77, 109] Clinical signs and symptoms of bowel injury such as abdominal tenderness, rigidity, and diminished bowel sounds are present in only 31% of patients.[77, 109] DPL has been used traditionally to detect free hemorrhage or intestinal contents as evidence of possible bowel or mesenteric injury and is considered by some authors to be superior to CT.[107] Again, limitations of DPL include its overly high sensitivity for detection of even minor injuries, its lack of sensitivity for detection of retroperitoneal injuries that may involve the duodenum or parts of the colon, and its nonspecificity regarding both site and extent of intraperitoneal injury. More recently, CT has been found in both surgical and imaging studies to have reasonably high accuracy for the detection and characterization of both bowel and mesenteric injuries.[77, 96, 109, 145]

It is helpful to administer oral contrast before the performance of CT in blunt trauma cases. Contrast may

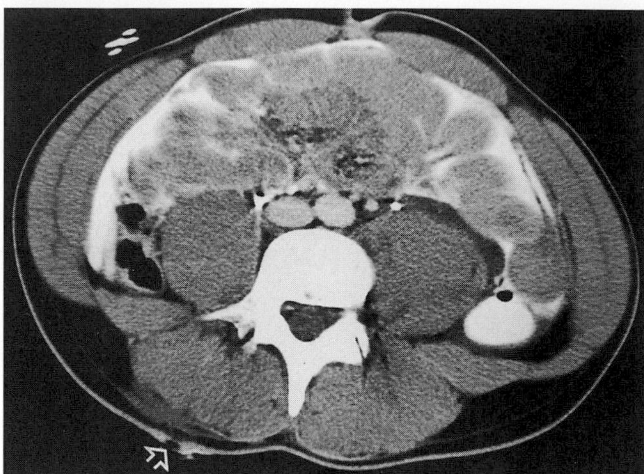

Figure 6–19. Contrast-enhanced CT image shows marked leak of oral contrast material into the peritoneal cavity, indicating full-thickness bowel disruption due to penetrating trauma. The wound site is marked by an *open arrow*.

be given orally or via nasogastric tube as soon as the patient is scheduled for abdominal CT scanning. An additional oral contrast load can be given in the CT scanning room. The oral contrast usually fills the stomach and at least the proximal small bowel. Although there are rare reports of aspiration related to oral contrast administration, in general its administration appears safe and without complications.[80] Opacification of the upper gastrointestinal tract can help assess for small bowel contusion, hematoma, and full-thickness tears (Fig. 6–19). In addition, this technique helps to delineate the pancreas and can be useful to diagnose pancreatic injury.

CT signs of bowel injury can be defined as diagnostic or suspicious and are shown in Table 6–9. In a retrospective study conducted at the Maryland Shock-Trauma Center, CT was 96% sensitive for detection of bowel injury and 88% accurate. CT was able to delineate a full-thickness injury with 92% sensitivity and 88% accuracy (K. Killeen, MD, personal communication, 2001). Other studies have reported similar results.[96, 145] The most sensitive findings for full-thickness bowel wall injury were pneumoperitoneum and free intraperitoneal fluid. It is important to review abdominal images in windows centered for lung or preferably bone, as small amounts of extraluminal air may be difficult to see in normal soft tissue window/level settings (Fig. 6–20). Mesenteric injuries appear as areas of streaky infiltration, hematomas, or active bleeding within the mesentery (see Fig. 6–16). The study by Dowe and colleagues showed that CT was 89% accurate in detection of mesenteric injury.[77] The presence of active bleeding or hematoma enveloping the adjacent bowel constitutes a definite indication for surgery. CT is only 75% accurate in differentiating surgical from nonsurgical injury (K. Killeen, MD, personal communication, 2001). Two entities that can obscure or mimic bowel injury include increased central venous pressure (CVP) and "shock bowel."[112, 136] Increased CVP may result from overresuscitation, cardiac tamponade, tension pneumothorax, or obstruction of the inferior vena cava by adjacent hematoma. It causes distention of the inferior vena cava and renal veins, periportal lymphedema, and bowel wall, mesenteric, and retroperitoneal edema (Fig. 6–21).[136] Shock bowel occurs after prolonged hypotension or cardiac arrest "in the field." The bowel appears thickened, dilated, and fluid-filled, and the wall enhances in a patchy pattern (Fig. 6–22). Usually, the inferior vena cava is collapsed, and there is no evidence of periportal lymphedema. In most cases the small bowel is primarily affected with both increased CVP and shock bowel, but the colon may rarely also be involved.[112]

Table 6–9. Computed Tomography Signs of Bowel Injury

Diagnostic	Suspicious
Pneumoperitoneum without known source	Bowel wall thickening >4 mm
Oral contrast extravasation	Free intraperitoneal fluid
Intramural, intramesenteric, retroperitoneal air without known source	Retroperitoneal fluid, especially anterior pararenal
Direct bowel wall discontinuity	Fluid between folds of mesentery ("triangles")
Extraluminal feces	Irregular bowel wall enhancement

Penetrating trauma to the flank and back in hemodynamically stable patients can be assessed by CT. The examination involves administration of oral, intravenous, and rectal contrast. The colonic contrast opacification is crucial to detect perforations in posterior retroperitoneal aspects of the bowel (Fig. 6–23). Any evidence of bowel perforation or intraperitoneal intrusion of the penetrating object necessities surgical exploration.

Potential Cervical Vascular Injury: Which Patients Need Imaging Assessment?

Injury to the carotid artery after blunt trauma appears to be rare.[127] The diagnosis certainly needs to be considered in patients with a central neurologic deficit unexplained on the basis of CT findings, or with evidence of post-traumatic cerebral infarction unaccounted for by sequelae of cerebral trauma. Unfortunately, many patients with traumatic carotid artery injury progress rapidly from an intact neurologic status to a profound and permanent neurologic deficit without the diagnosis being considered. It is unclear which blunt trauma patients are at significant increased risk for blunt carotid injury and should therefore undergo a screening study. Patients who have sustained direct injury to the neck or who have cervical hematoma are at higher risk, as are patients with clinical signs of carotid injury such as a thrill or diminished carotid pulse. Trauma patients with skull base fractures that cross the course of the petrous carotid artery appear to be at significantly increased risk for carotid artery injury that may result in infarction or carotid artery–cavernous sinus fistula formation.[125] Factors predisposing to carotid dissection such as hypertension, fibromuscular dysplasia, Marfan's syndrome, and cystic medial necrosis also carry an increased injury risk. Patients who sustain injury to the head, neck, and face all are *potentially*

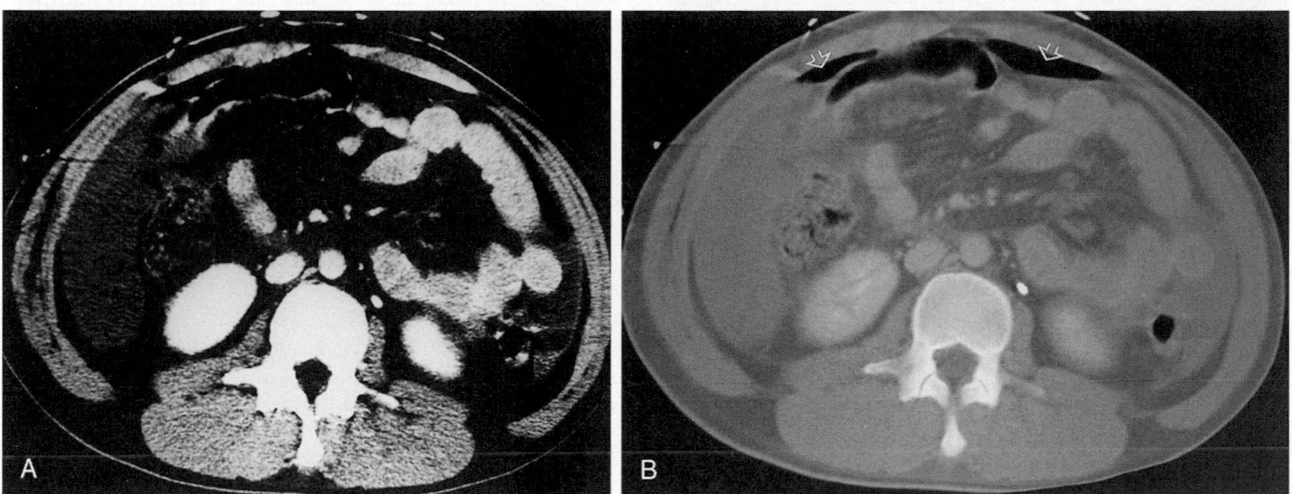

Figure 6–20. Review of abdominal CT for evaluation of blunt trauma with "extended" windows to detect pneumoperitoneum. *A,* Image obtained at midabdominal level using narrow windows (window 150 HU, center 50 HU) limits differentiation of air and fat and of intraluminal from extraluminal gas. *B,* Evaluation using wider windows and a lower center (window 1980 HU, center − 300) improves detection of pneumoperitoneum versus intraluminal gas (*arrows*).

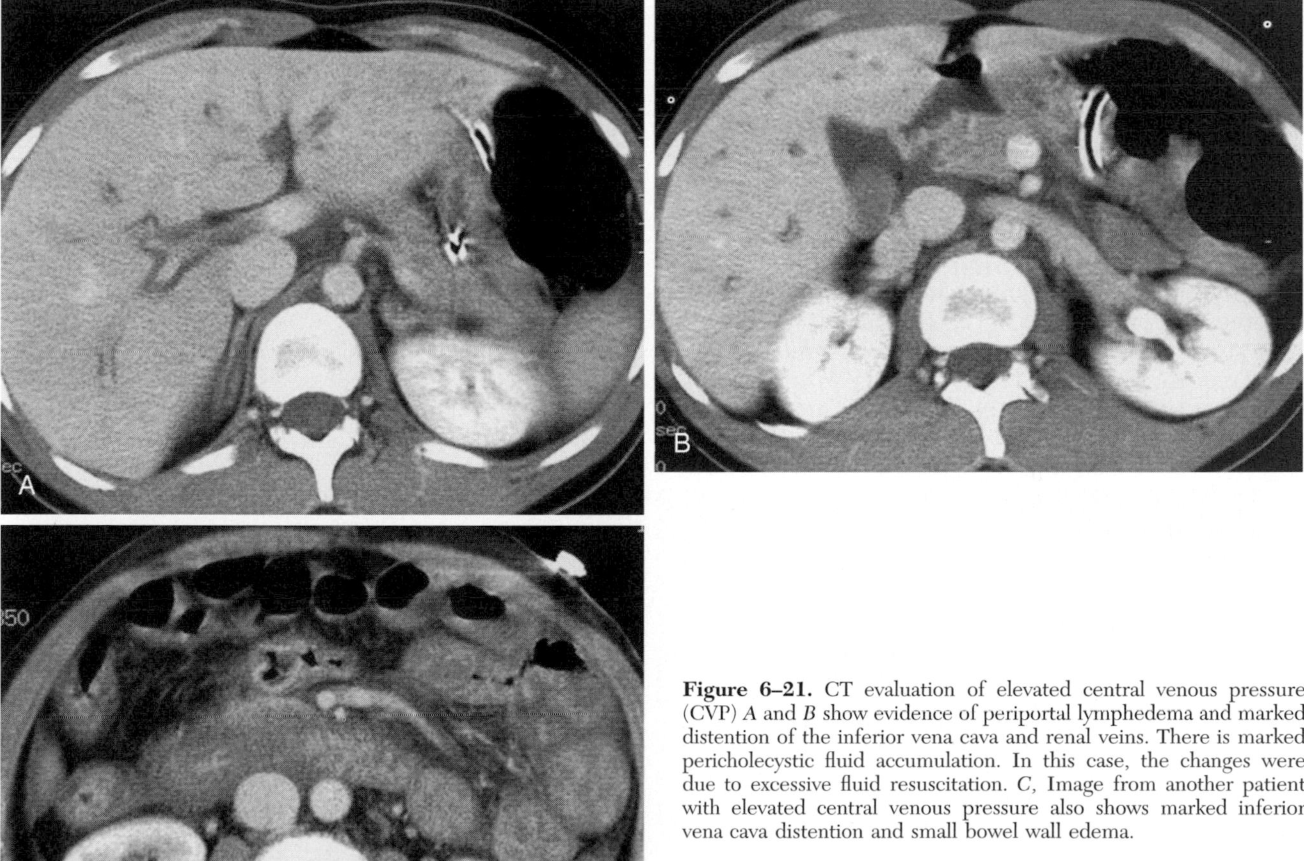

Figure 6–21. CT evaluation of elevated central venous pressure (CVP) *A* and *B* show evidence of periportal lymphedema and marked distention of the inferior vena cava and renal veins. There is marked pericholecystic fluid accumulation. In this case, the changes were due to excessive fluid resuscitation. *C,* Image from another patient with elevated central venous pressure also shows marked inferior vena cava distention and small bowel wall edema.

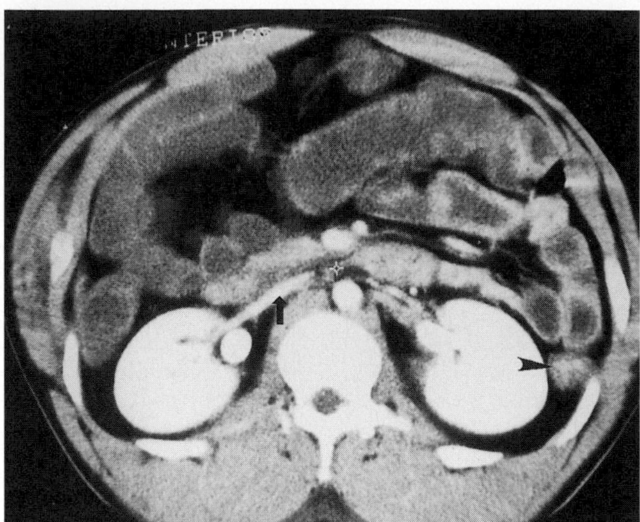

Figure 6–22. CT of "shock bowel." Contrast-enhanced image through the midrenal level shows a collapsed inferior vena cava (*arrow*) and renal veins. There is mild bowel wall thickening (in the small bowel) with diffuse but patchy enhancement of the small bowel wall. The small bowel is fluid filled and moderately distended. Enhancement of the kidneys is very bright, probably owing to slowed perfusion and contrast retention. The left colon (*arrowhead*) appears normal. (From Mirvis, S.E., Shanmuganathan, K., & Erb, R. [1994]. Diffuse small-bowel ischemia in hypotensive adults after blunt trauma (shock-bowel): CT findings and clinical significance. A.J.R. Am. J. Roentgenol., *163*:1375.)

at increased risk for carotid injury, but this population represents a considerable proportion of all blunt trauma cases, and the injury appears very uncommon.

An appropriate, cost-effective screening test is needed to evaluate the carotid artery both quickly and reliably. Rogers and coworkers[127] used computed tomographic angiography (CTA) as a screening study. They reported an improved time to diagnosis of carotid injury from a historical norm of 156 hours to an average of 5.9 hours when CTA screening was utilized in all patients. Magnetic resonance angiography (MRA) is an appropriate screening study but is more costly and more difficult to perform in the major trauma patient and requires patient transport. Although cervical angiography is the gold standard imaging test, it is expensive and invasive and also typically requires transport of the patient to another area of the radiology department. Further prospective studies comparing cervical CTA and sonography with cervical angiography are needed to determine the best screening study. Also, a clearer definition of the population at increased risk for the injury is needed. Once diagnosed, carotid injuries can be treated by surgery when the vessel is accessible or by anticoagulation or endovascular techniques[75, 76, 103] often depending on the exact clinical circumstances and available institutional resources.

Vertebral artery (VA) injury appears to occur more commonly than was suspected before the common use of MRA in assessing cervical spine trauma.[84, 156] Injury to the vertebral artery occurs in from 20%[84] to 46%[156] of patients who sustain cervical spine injuries with significant vertebral subluxation or dislocation. Fractures of the cervical spine that traverse the foramen transversarium also can cause VA injury.[154] In most cases it appears that VA injuries are not of clinical consequence, particularly if unilateral and involving the nondominant side. In a study by Demetriades and coworkers[84] of 22 patients with VA injury from blunt trauma, 18 were managed by observation alone, and 4 required intervention for bleeding or failed angiographic management.[84] Most VA injuries produce complete occlusion of the involved artery. An intimal injury with flow maintained through the injured region is associated with increased risk for embolization. In most patients with traumatic VA occlusion, reconstitution of flow is not seen at 2-year follow-up evaluation,[151] and this potentiality should be considered if future cervical vascular surgery is contemplated. At the Maryland Shock-Trauma Center, patients with cervical fractures that involve the VA foramen or with major cervical spine injuries, such as unilateral or bilateral facet dislocations, hyperflexion "teardrop," or hyperextension subluxation or dislocation, undergo MRA screening for VA injury.

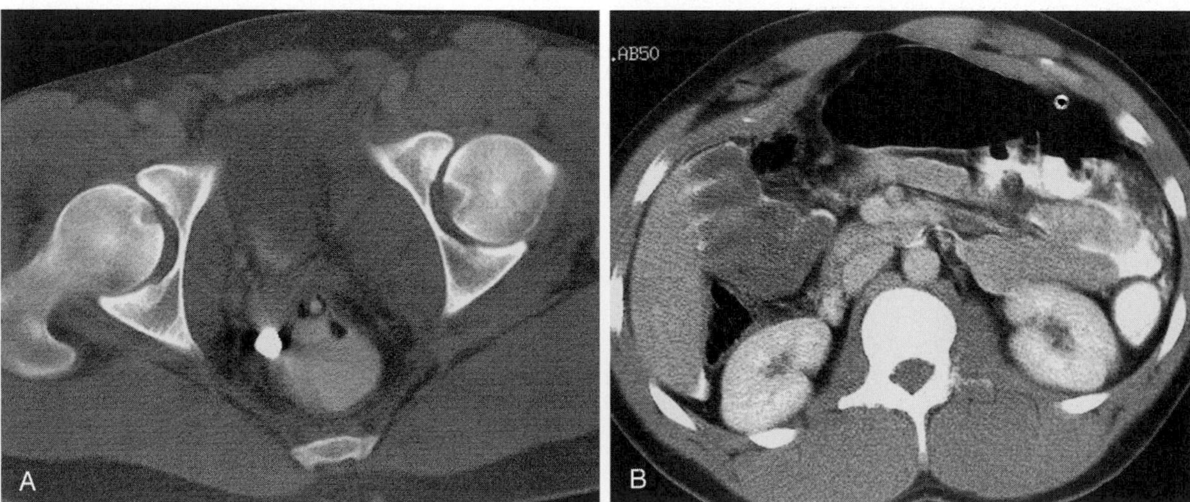

Figure 6–23. CT of penetrating trauma. *A,* This image shows a bullet adjacent to the rectum after a gunshot wound to the right gluteal region. *B,* This image was obtained after administration of colonic contrast and shows leakage of contrast into peritoneal cavity between bowel loops, indicating full-thickness disruption of the distal colon and peritoneal contamination.

Patients who sustain penetrating trauma to the cervical region are always considered at risk for vascular injury. Injuries to zone 1 (between the clavicles and the cricoid cartilage) and zone 3 (from the angle of the mandible to the skull base) are not easily accessible for clinical assessment and often require arteriographic evaluation.[184a] Zone 2 (from the cricoid cartilage to the angle of the mandible) injuries can be assessed clinically for evidence of major vascular injury and can be surgically explored if this intervention is indicated by signs such as bleeding, expanding hematoma, or palpable abnormality of the carotid pulse. Angiographic assessment may also be needed, perhaps less urgently, in patients with benign physical findings to rule out a subtle vascular injury. Montalvo and associates[116] have reported that color flow Doppler sonography can detect all "serious" zone 2 and zone 3 carotid and vertebral injuries and recommend it as the most appropriate screening test.[116]

The role of CTA in this clinical context is not well established but is expected to emerge as multi-row detector CT scanning becomes more widely available. CT can certainly assist in defining the course of a penetrating object in the neck. Proximity of a bullet or fragment to a major vessel or prevertebral soft tissue hematoma is an indication for angiography.[118]

Imaging of Trauma Patients: The Horizon

The application of current imaging technology has had a major impact on the management of polytrauma patients in assisting clinical triage, in guiding management decisions, and in enhancing therapeutic options. Many of the benefits of this technology are still filtering into common clinical practice. Cooperation between imaging specialists and trauma care physicians will permit the appropriate adaptation or integration of this modality into management strategies. The increased use of digital imaging, storage, and communication of data should foster the use of advanced imaging technology by providing secure and timely access to images.[71, 97, 122] The availability of multi-row CT detectors should allow faster scanning with improved image quality, particularly for multiplanar re-formatting and volumetric data. This capacity will expand the use of CTA for diagnosing vascular trauma and will provide the surgeon with preoperative images based on transparent color-coded volumetric data that reliably duplicate the intraoperative appearance of injuries from the surgical viewpoint. Further experience with endovascular treatment will extend options for injury management, increasing opportunities for potential avoidance of major surgical interventions.[70, 94, 120]

Diagnostic Oversights

Radiographic failures in the diagnosis of injuries are of various types, both of omission and of commission.[9, 175] Born and colleagues[162] reported that 55% of missed diagnoses were due to failure to obtain an x-ray film of the injured part at the time of hospital admission, and 23% were clearly visible on the admission film but overlooked. Ten percent were missed because of technically inadequate admission films (e.g., the fracture was obscured by the nameplate), inadequate or incomplete visualization of the involved bone, or inappropriate technique (i.e., either overexposure or underexposure). More than half (54%) occurred in patients with altered consciousness, and slightly more than a third (35%) occurred in patients who were intoxicated.

The physical examination of the multiply injured patient is difficult and, at best, unreliable in the diagnosis of injuries of the chest, abdomen, pelvis, or thoracolumbar spine.[1, 37, 165, 174, 175, 181] The difficulty is compounded if the patient is unconscious. Injuries of the heart, great vessels,[10] liver, and diaphragm[165] are often overlooked.[14] Most oversights related to injuries of the skeletal system involve the major joints or the thoracolumbar spine. Injuries are most commonly missed in unconscious patients with severe head injury[23] and in patients who have sustained blunt trauma to the chest.[3] The majority of such injuries occur in motor vehicle accidents.[169]

Most oversights are due not to lack of knowledge but to failure to consider certain common diagnostic possibilities, and many injuries are overlooked despite their well-recognized association with other, more readily apparent injuries.[177] Pelvic and thoracic injuries are especially difficult to identify in an unconscious patient (Fig. 6–24), and the routine radiographic examination of the pelvis[167] and chest may disclose otherwise obscure injuries.

Difficulties in the diagnosis of skeletal injuries by physical examination are well recognized. In the presence of a fracture of the shaft of a long bone, an injury of a proximal joint is likely to be overlooked[10, 176, 177] (Fig. 6–25). The proximal injury is masked by the deformity associated with the distal fracture. The importance of examining the shaft of an injured long bone along its length—from the joint above to the joint below—is well recognized, yet this advice is often unheeded.[27] The advice is less applicable to fractures at the ends of bones—for example, a Colle's fracture or a common fracture of the ankle. It is uncommon to examine the entire length of the bone with such fractures and, indeed, proximal injury is rare. However, with diaphyseal fractures, the radiographic examination must include the entire length of the bone and both of the joints proximal and distal to (above and below) the fractured shaft. This is particularly true for fractures of the femoral shaft, in which an associated fracture or fracture-dislocation about the hip is common[26, 40, 45] and radiography of the entire length of the femur and preferably the entire hemipelvis is necessary.

The association of femoral fracture with fracture or fracture-dislocation about the hip is ascribable to longitudinal compression force exerted along the length of the shaft (Fig. 6–26). In addition to the shaft fracture, the force may result in fractures about the knee.[2, 45] Therefore, on occasion, fracture of the femoral shaft is associated with fracture of the patella or proximal tibia as well as fracture-dislocation about the hip. Less commonly, with the knee held in extension, longitudinal compression force exerted along the length of the extremity may result in fracture of the tibia and fracture-dislocation of the hip (see Fig. 6–25). These associations reinforce the impor-

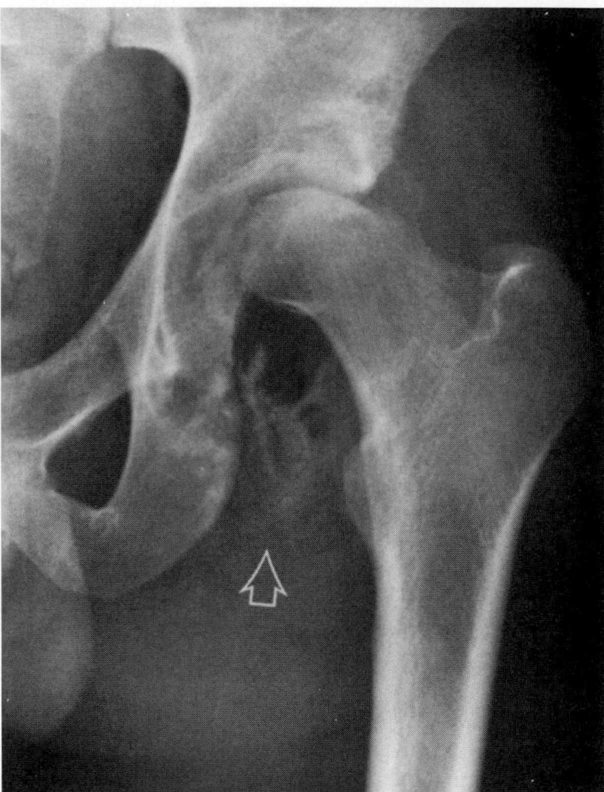

Figure 6–24. Delayed recognition of posterior fracture-dislocation of the left hip in a 22-year-old man who sustained a head injury in a motor vehicle accident. He was comatose for 10 days and complained of pain on initial ambulation. This radiograph was obtained 5 weeks after injury and demonstrates fracture-dislocation and periarticular ossification (*arrow*). The latter occurs in patients who are comatose or have sustained spinal cord injury. (From Rogers, L.F. [1985]. Problems in radiologic examination of patients with multiple injuries. Skeletal Radiol., *12*:103.)

tance of examining the entire length of the shaft. Therefore, radiographic examination of the pelvis is indicated in every patient who has a severe injury of the femur or tibia.[13, 36]

It has been noted that detection of one radiographic abnormality tends to interfere with the detection of additional abnormalities. This phenomenon is known as *satisfaction of search.*[160] In the evaluation of skeletal trauma, satisfaction of search leads to the failure to recognize second and third injuries that may be present. The examiner should be wary of this tendency. A familiarity with common associations of injuries is invaluable. For instance, fractures of the femoral shaft are often associated with fractures of the femoral neck and posterior dislocations of the hip; in the Monteggia fracture-dislocation of the forearm, a fracture of the proximal ulna is associated with a dislocation of the radial head. The second component of these injuries is often overlooked. The clinician can avoid such oversights by making it a point to specifically look for such associated injuries upon identification of the first injury.

Limited examinations may lead to oversights. At times, a single view of a part is obtained even though it is well known that a minimum of two views, usually projected at 90 degrees to each other, is necessary for the diagnosis of fractures and dislocations. A single radiographic view of a part should not be accepted as sufficient to rule out the presence of injury; the only possible exceptions are single radiographs of the chest or pelvis if these films show no abnormalities and if injury is not clinically evident. Oblique views may be obtained subsequently to either exclude or substantiate the presence of otherwise obscure injury suspected on the basis of persistent symptoms or physical signs.

Radiographs of the cervical spine must include all seven vertebrae; failure in this regard is the most common error in the radiographic evaluation of cervical spine injuries (Fig. 6–27). Fractures at the craniovertebral junction are at times associated with fractures lower in the cervical spine, in the area of the cervicothoracic junction. It is therefore important to make sure that the cervical spine is examined over its entire length despite the identification of an injury of the axis or atlas.

In 5% of patients who sustain spinal cord injury, a second spinal injury is present at a site remote from the primary injury[6, 180] (the one associated with neurologic deficit) (Figs. 6–28 and 6–29). If the primary injury is in the cervical spine, the second-level injury often is in the thoracolumbar spine. Other combinations are injuries in the upper part of the dorsal spine (primary) and the cervical spine (second-level) (see Fig. 6–28), the middorsal spine and either the cervical spine or the thoracolumbar junction, and the thoracolumbar junction and the lumbosacral junction (see Fig. 6–29). If a fracture is identified in C1 or C2, a second-level injury frequently occurs at the cervicothoracic junction. In any case of severe spinal or spinal cord injury, anteroposterior and lateral radiographs of the spine along its entire length should be obtained as soon as possible.

In the press of more important matters, undisplaced and minimally displaced fractures of the extremities may be overlooked in the initial evaluation and are frequently noted or suspected a few days after admission on the basis of findings on a subsequent physical examination, or a complaint noted by the patient, and confirmed by radiographic examination. These injuries include fractures of the radial head, scaphoid, tibial plateau, ankle, tarsals, metatarsals, metacarpals, and phalanges and dislocations of the carpus, tarsus, and tarsometatarsal and carpometacarpal joints. These injuries are associated with limited morbidity, and short delays in diagnosis are of little consequence. Longer delays may pose greater problems.

It is not enough to obtain appropriate radiographs of a patient with multiple injuries and interpret them correctly. The final responsibility is to make sure that the information is communicated to those involved in the patient's care. Unfortunately, at times a correct report is ignored or goes unread by the referring physician. When injuries are identified in this setting, it is best to communicate this information verbally to ensure that the patient receives full benefit of the radiographic examination.

Coding Systems for Severity of Injury

Methods have been devised for numerically describing the overall severity of injury.* These methods are of

*See references 182, 183, 185, 186, 189, 192, 194–198, 202, 203.

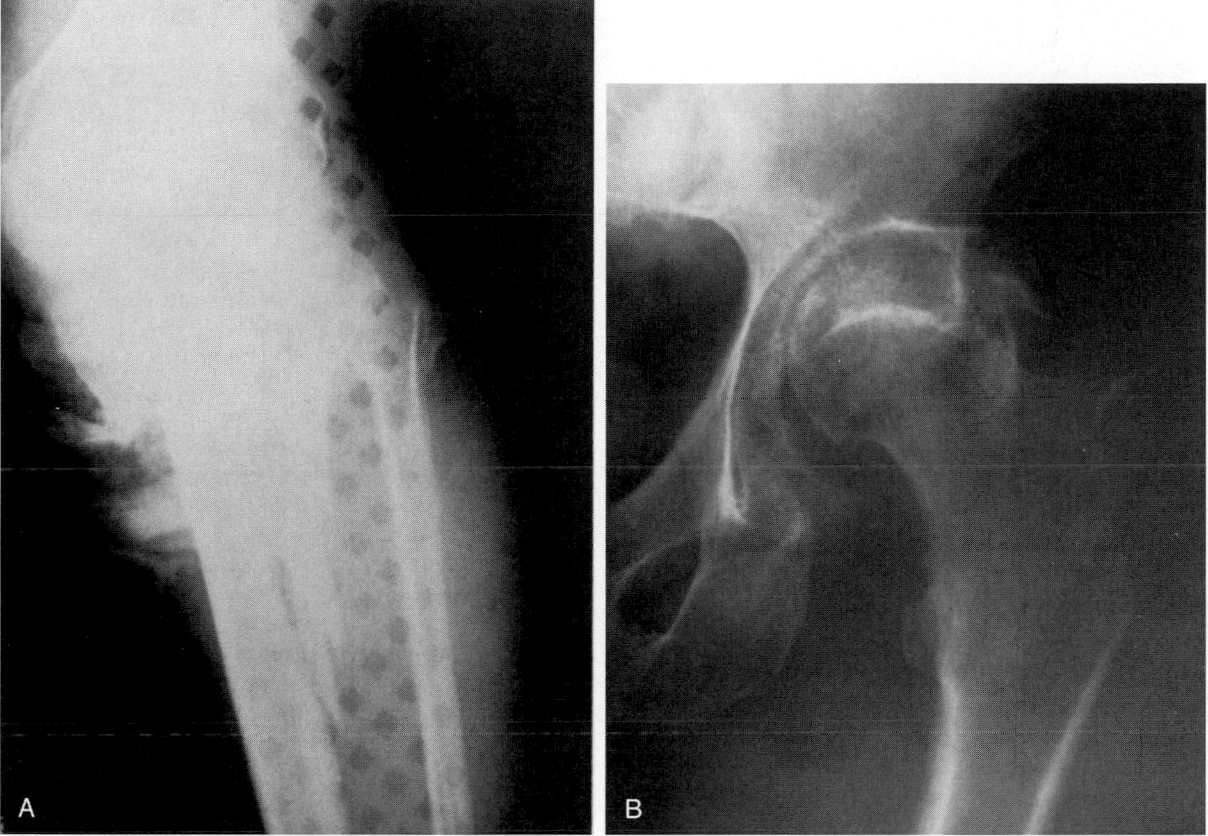

Figure 6–25. The patient was a 58-year-old man who sustained an open fracture of the proximal tibia with transection of the popliteal artery. *A*, Underexposed anteroposterior view of the left knee and proximal tibia demonstrates comminuted fracture. The presence of air, medial to the fracture, suggests this is an open injury. The patient underwent an open reduction and fixation of the fracture and the arterial injury was repaired. There were no complications. Twelve weeks after the injury the patient began ambulation and noted pain in the left hip. *B*, Anteroposterior view of the left hip demonstrates a previously unrecognized posterior fracture-dislocation of the hip. An anteroposterior view of the pelvis should be obtained in every patient who has sustained a fracture of the femur or tibia and fibula and in every unconscious patient who has a history of traumatic injury to exclude otherwise obscure injuries of the hip and pelvis.

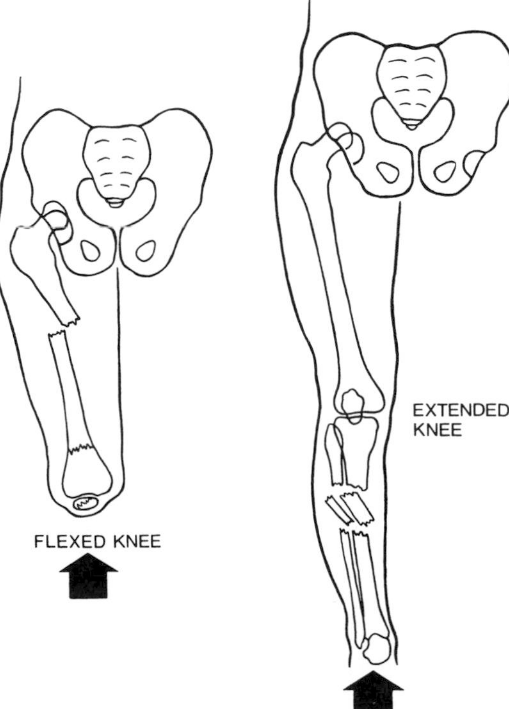

Figure 6–26. Posterior dislocation of the hip resulting from longitudinal compression forces may occur in association with fracture of the femoral shaft or other fractures about the knee when the knee is flexed. When the knee is extended, fracture of the tibia and fibula or other severe injury of the leg may also be associated with posterior dislocation of the hip. (From Rogers, L.F. [1985]. Problems in radiologic examination of patients with multiple injuries. Skeletal Radiol., *12*:103.)

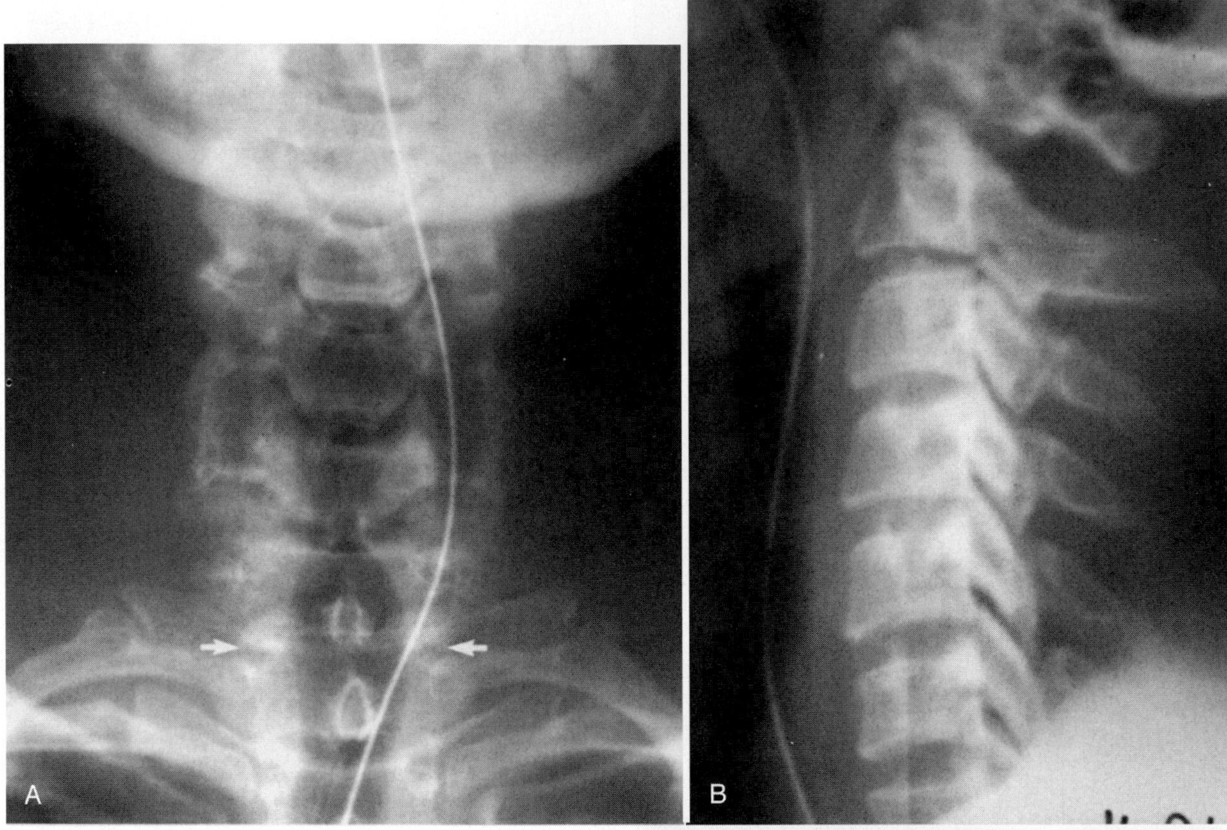

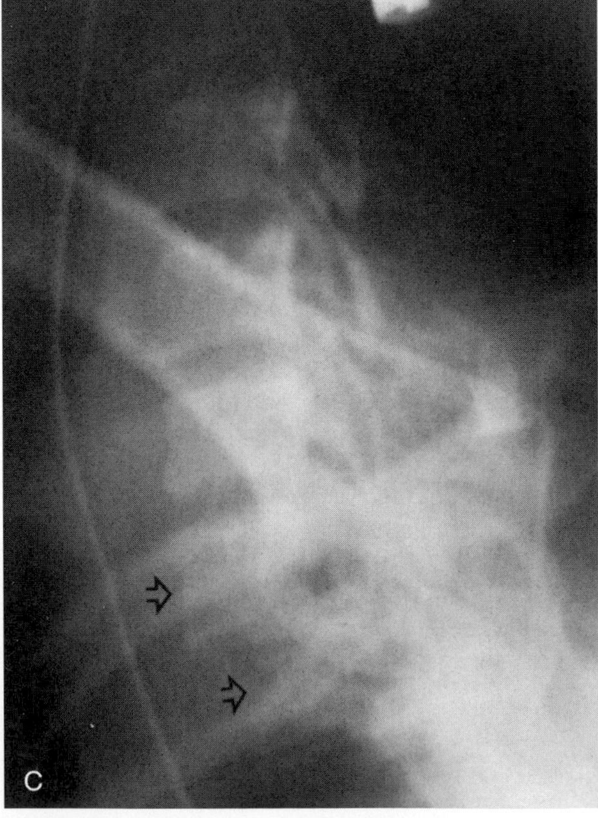

Figure 6–27. Fracture dislocation of C7–T1 in a 33-year-old man injured in a motor vehicle accident. *A,* Anteroposterior view of the cervical spine demonstrates loss of the disc space at C7–T1 (*arrows*), which should serve as a clue to the possibility of dislocation. There are no other significant findings. *B,* Lateral radiograph includes the superior half of the cervicothoracic junction and discloses no abnormality. *C,* Swimmer's view demonstrates anterior dislocation of C7 on T1 (*arrows*). All seven cervical vertebrae must be visualized to exclude injuries.

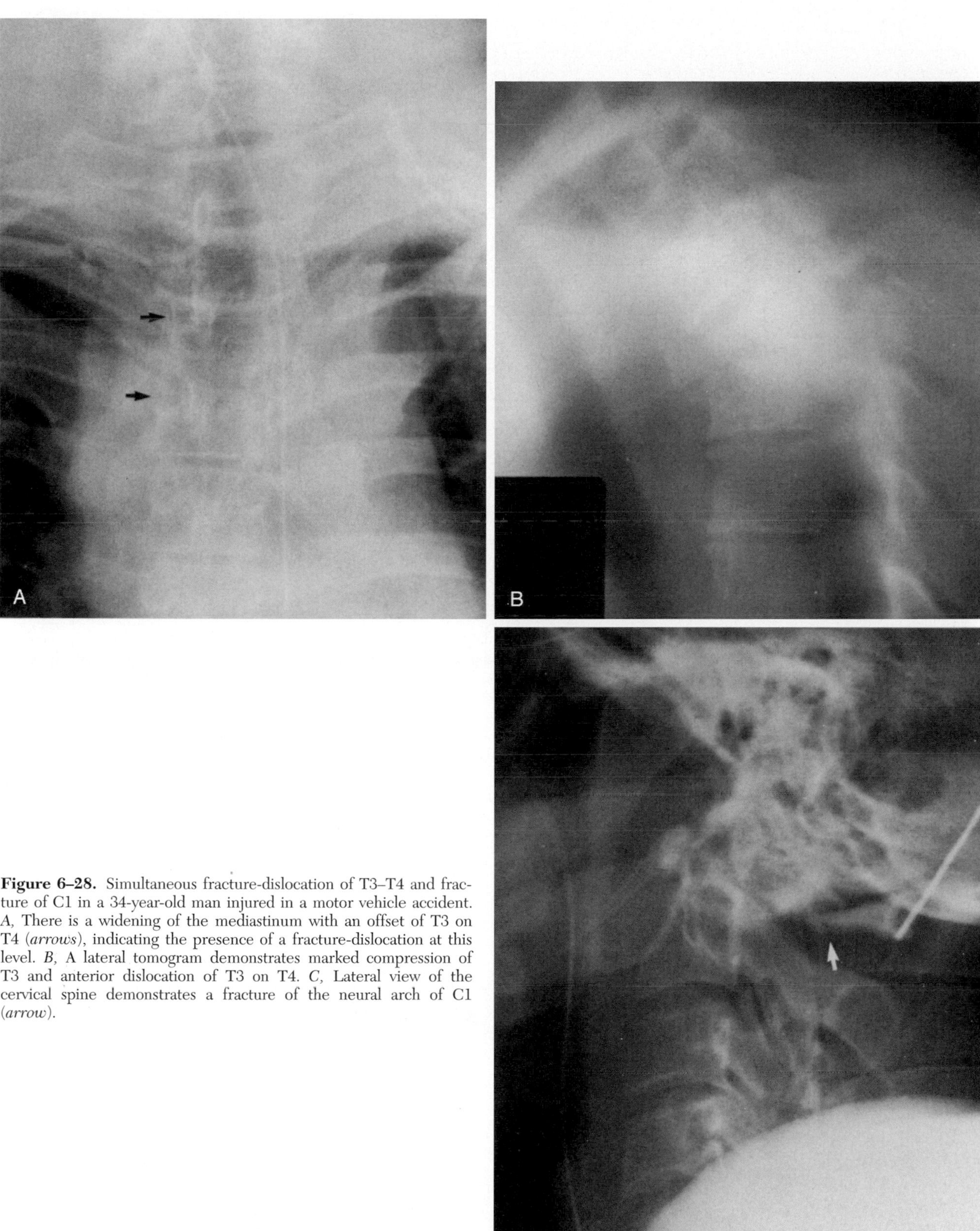

Figure 6–28. Simultaneous fracture-dislocation of T3–T4 and fracture of C1 in a 34-year-old man injured in a motor vehicle accident. *A,* There is a widening of the mediastinum with an offset of T3 on T4 (*arrows*), indicating the presence of a fracture-dislocation at this level. *B,* A lateral tomogram demonstrates marked compression of T3 and anterior dislocation of T3 on T4. *C,* Lateral view of the cervical spine demonstrates a fracture of the neural arch of C1 (*arrow*).

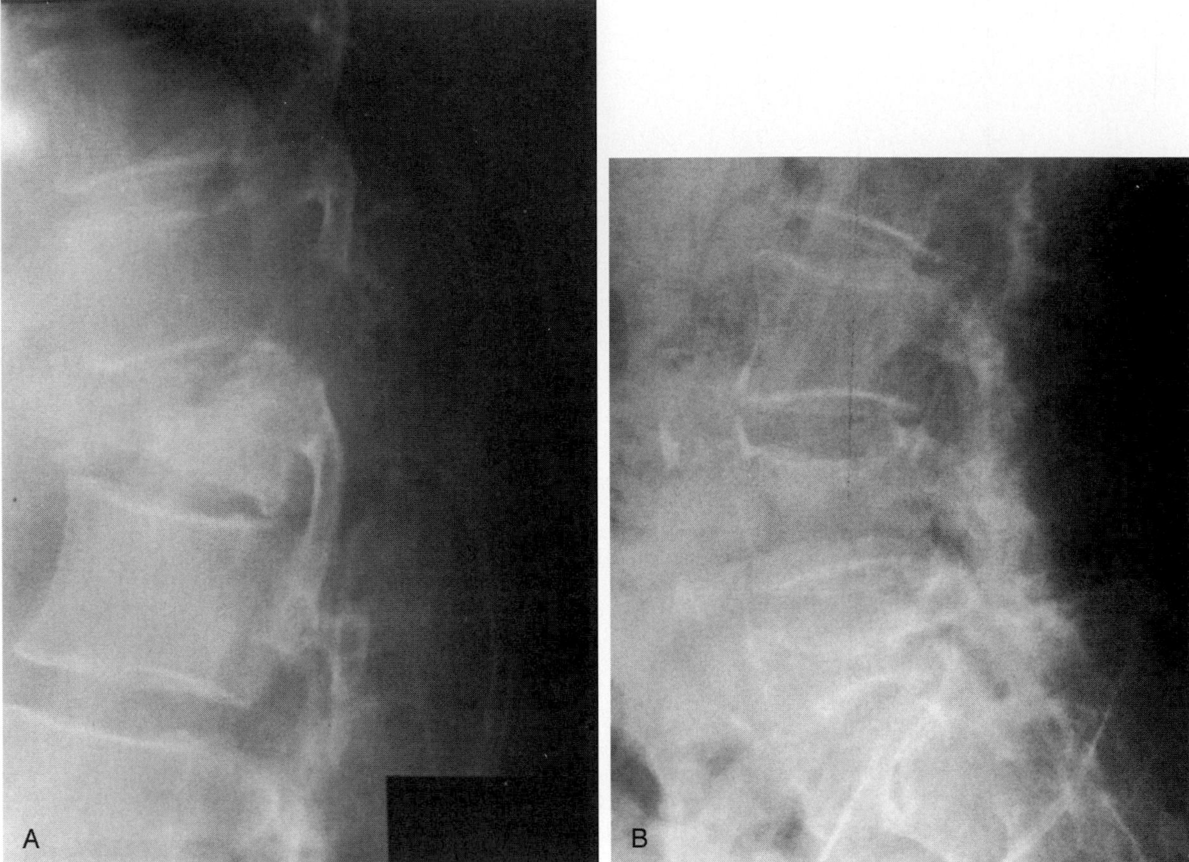

Figure 6–29. Fracture-dislocation of T12–L1 and compression fractures of L4 and L5 in a 58-year-old woman injured in a fall from a third-story window. *A,* Lateral view demonstrates marked wedging of T12 with slight posterior displacement of the spine above the level of vertebral compression. *B,* Lateral view of the lower lumbar spine demonstrates severe compression of L5 and moderate compression of the superior end plate of L4.

particular value in the study of populations and in comparing the intensity and outcome of injury sustained from various causes in varying age groups. Although coding systems are useful in the analysis of morbidity and mortality for groups of injured patients, their predictive utility in individual cases is questionable.[183, 190] The principal systems are the Abbreviated Injury Scale (AIS),[183, 188] the Modified Injury Severity Scale (ISS),[183, 196, 199, 200] the Glasgow Coma Scale (GCS),[201] the Hospital Trauma Index (HTI),[182] and the Hospital Trauma Index—Injury Severity Scale (HTI-ISS).[21]

The AIS[183, 187, 191, 193] (Table 6–10) was developed by the American Medical Association[188] and categorizes injuries in five body areas: general, face and neck, chest, abdominal and pelvic viscera, and extremities and pelvic girdle. The severity of each injury is graded on a 5-point scale: 1 point indicates a minor injury; 2, a moderate injury; 3, a severe but not life-threatening injury; 4, a severe injury with survival probable; and 5, a critical injury with survival uncertain. Each body area is graded separately.

The ISS,[21, 184, 191, 196, 199, 200] a modification of the AIS, was developed to deal specifically with the multiply injured patient. To determine the score, each body area is categorized according to the most severe injury to that area. The sum of the squares of the highest AIS score from each of three most severely injured body areas equals the ISS score. Table 6–11 presents an example of the calculation of an ISS score for a patient with multiple injuries consisting of a ruptured spleen, pulmonary contusion, sternal fracture, fracture of the femur, and fractured teeth. An ISS score of 25 points or more is associated with an increased risk of permanent impairment. A score of more than 40 points is predictive of death in 50% or more of cases.[184, 191, 196, 199]

The GCS[31, 190, 201] (Table 6–12) for neural injury consists of a graded scoring of the patient's physical examination for three different responses: eye opening, the level of verbal response, and the level of motor response. The total score is the sum of each of the three responses. The lower the score, the worse the injury.

The HTI[24, 182] (Fig. 6–30) was developed by the American College of Surgeons and utilizes objective diagnoses in rating injury severity rather than the subjective impressions[191] of the AIS. It also includes the presence and level of shock and an assessment of the cardiovascular status, which are not included in the AIS. The HTI is based on scoring the level of injury to six body systems; cardiovascular; nervous; abdominal; respiratory; extremities; and skin and subcutaneous tissues. The severity of injury is graded from 0 (no injury) to 5 (critical) in each system. The HTI-ISS is calculated in a manner similar to that for the ISS by summing the squares of the three highest HTI values.[24] A value of 18 or more is indicative of a significant multiple injury. The morbidity and mortality rates gener-

Table 6–10. Abbreviated Injury Scale

Score	Type
1	**MINOR**
	GENERAL
	Aches all over
	Minor lacerations, contusions, and abrasions (first aid—simple closure)
	All first-degree or small second- or third-degree burns
	HEAD AND NECK
	Cerebral injury with headache; dizziness; no loss of consciousness
	"Whiplash" complaint with no anatomic or radiologic evidence
	Abrasions and contusions of ocular apparatus (lids, conjunctiva, cornea, uveal injuries); vitreous or retinal hemorrhage
	Fracture and/or dislocations of teeth
	CHEST
	Muscle ache or chest wall stiffness
	ABDOMINAL
	Muscle ache, seat belt abrasion, etc.
	EXTREMITIES
	Minor sprains and fractures and/or dislocation of digits
2	**MODERATE**
	GENERAL
	Extensive contusions; abrasions; large lacerations; avulsions (less than 3 in. wide)
	HEAD AND NECK
	Cerebral injury with or without skull fracture, less than 15 min unconsciousness; no post-traumatic amnesia.
	Undisplaced skull or facial bone fractures or compound fracture of nose
	Lacerations of the eye and appendages; retinal detachment
	Disfiguring lacerations
	"Whiplash"—severe complaints with anatomic or radiologic evidence
	CHEST
	Simple rib or sternal fractures
	Major contusion of chest wall without hemothorax or pneumothorax or respiratory embarrassment
	ABDOMINAL
	Major contusion of abdominal wall
	EXTREMITIES AND/OR PELVIC GIRDLE
	Compound fractures of digits
	Undisplaced long bone or pelvic fractures
	Major sprains of major joints
3	**SEVERE: Not Life-Threatening**
	GENERAL
	Extensive contusions; abrasions; large lacerations involving more than two extremities, or large avulsions (greater than 3 in. wide)
	20–30% body surface—second- or third-degree burns
	HEAD AND NECK
	Cerebral injury with or without skull fracture, with unconsciousness lasting more than 15 min; without severe neurological signs; brief post-traumatic amnesia (less than 3 hrs)
	Displaced closed skull fractures without unconsciousness or other signs of intracranial injury
	Loss of eye or avulsion of optic nerve
	Displaced facial bone fractures or those with antral or orbital involvement
	Cervical spine fractures without cord damage
	CHEST
	Multiple rib fractures without respiratory embarrassment
	Hemothorax or pneumothorax
	Rupture of diaphragm
	Lung contusion
	ABDOMINAL
	Contusion of abdominal organs
	Extraperitoneal bladder rupture
	Retroperitoneal hemorrhage
	Avulsion of ureter
	Laceration of urethra
	Thoracic or lumbar spine fractures without neurologic involvement
	EXTREMITIES AND/OR PELVIC GIRDLE
	Displaced simple long bone fractures, and/or multiple hand and foot fractures
	Single open long bone fractures
	Pelvic fracture with displacement
	Dislocation of major joints
	Multiple amputations of digits
	Lacerations of the major nerves or vessels of extremities

Table continued on following page

Table 6–10. Abbreviated Injury Scale *Continued*

Score	Type
4	**SEVERE: Life-Threatening, Survival Probable**
	GENERAL
	Severe lacerations and/or avulsions with dangerous hemorrhage
	30–50% body surface—second- or third-degree burns
	HEAD AND NECK
	Cerebral injury with or without skull fracture, with unconsciousness lasting more than 15 min, with definite abnormal neurologic signs; post-traumatic amnesia 3–12 hr
	Compound skull fracture
	CHEST
	Open chest wounds; flail chest; pneumomediastinum; myocardial contusion without circulatory embarrassment; pericardial injuries
	ABDOMINAL
	Minor laceration of intra-abdominal contents (to include ruptured spleen, kidney, and injuries to tail of pancreas)
	Intraperitoneal bladder rupture
	Avulsion of the genitals
	Thoracic and/or lumbar spine fractures with paraplegia
	EXTREMITIES
	Multiple closed long bone fractures
	Amputation of limbs
5	**CRITICAL: Survival Uncertain**
	GENERAL
	Over 50% body surface—second- or third-degree burns
	HEAD AND NECK
	Cerebral injury with or without skull fracture with unconsciousness lasting more than 24 hr; post-traumatic amnesia more than 12 hr; intracranial hemorrhage; signs of increased intracranial pressure (decreasing state of consciousness, bradycardia under 60, progressive rise in blood pressure or progressive pupil inequality)
	Cervical spine injury with quadriplegia
	Major airway obstruction
	CHEST
	Chest injuries with major respiratory embarrassment (laceration of trachea, hemomediastinum, etc.)
	Aortic laceration
	Myocardial rupture or contusion with circulatory embarrassment
	ABDOMINAL
	Rupture, avulsion or severe laceration of intra-abdominal vessels or organs, except kidney, spleen, or ureter
	EXTREMITIES
	Multiple open limb fractures

From Committee on Injury Scaling (1985). The Abbreviated Injury Scale, 1985 Revision. American Association for Automotive Medicine, Des Plains, Ill., with permission.

Table 6–11. Modified Injury Severity Scale (ISS): Calculations

Regional AIS scores		
Abdomen	Ruptured spleen	5*
Chest	Pulmonary contusion	3*
	Fractured sternum	2
Limbs	Fractured femur	3*
Head and neck	Fractured teeth	1

ISS score

$$\begin{aligned} ISS &= 5^2 + 3^2 + 3^2 \\ &= 25 + 9 + 9 \\ &= 43 \end{aligned}$$

*The highest AIS score from each of the three most severely injured body areas.

Table 6–12. Glasgow Coma Scale

Eye opening
4. Spontaneous
3. To speech
2. To pain
1. None

Best verbal response
5. Oriented
4. Confused
3. Inappropriate
2. Incomprehensible
1. None

Best motor response
6. Obeys commands
5. Localizes pain
4. Withdraws
3. Flexes to pain
2. Extends to pain
1. None

From Teasdale, G., & Jennett, B. (1974). Assessment of coma and impaired consciousness. A practical scale. Lancet, 2:81, with permission.

System	Injury	Class	Index
Respiratory	No Injury	No injury	0
	Chest discomfort—minimal findings	Minor	1
	Simple rib or sternal fx, chest wall contusion with pleuritic pain	Moderate	2
	1st or multi-rib fx, hemothorax, pneumothorax	Major	3
	Open chest wounds, flail chest, tension pneumothorax, nl bp, simple lac diaphragm	Severe	4
	Acute resp failure (cyanosis), aspiration, tension pneumothorax, c̄ ↓ bp, bilateral flail, lac(s) diaphragm	Critical	5
Cardiovascular	No Injury	No injury	0
	< 10% (< 500 cc) bv loss; no change in skin perfusion	Minor	1
	10–20% bv loss (500–1000 cc); ↓ skin perfusion, urine normal (+30 cc/hr; myocard. cont. bp normal	Moderate	2
	20–30% bv loss (100–1,500 cc); ↓ skin perfusion, urine (<30 cc); tamponade, bp 80	Major	3
	30–40% bv loss (1,500–2,000 cc); ↓ skin perfusion, urine (<10 cc); tamponade, conscious, bp < 80	Severe	4
	40–50% bv loss; restless, agitated, coma, cardiac contusion or arrhythmia; bp not obtainable	Critical	5
	50% + bv loss; coma; cardiac arrest; no vital signs	Fatal	6
Nervous System	No Injury	No injury	0
	Head trauma c̄ or s̄ scalp lactns, no loss consciousness (coma); no fracture (fx)	Minor	1
	Head trauma c̄ brief coma (<15'), skull fx, cervical pain c̄ minimal fndgs, one facial fx	Moderate	2
	Cerebral injury c̄ coma (+15'); depressed skull fx; cervical fx c̄ neuro fndgs; multi facial fxs	Major	3
	Cerebral injury c̄ coma (+60') or neuro findings; cervical fx c̄ major neuro findings, i.e., paraplegia	Severe	4
	Cerebral injury c̄ coma c̄ no response to stimuli up to 24 h; cervical fx c̄ *quadriplegia*	Critical	5
	Cerebral injury c̄ no response to stimuli & c̄ dilated fixed pupil(s)	Fatal	6
Abdominal	No injury	No injury	0
	Mild abdominal wall, flank or back pain & tenderness s̄ peritoneal signs	Minor	1
	Acute flank, back or abdominal discomfort and tenderness; fx of a rib 7–12	Moderate	2
	One of: minor liver, sm bowel, spleen, kidney, body pancr, mesentery, ureter, urethra; fxs 7–12 rib	Major	3
	2 major: rupture liver, bladder, head pancr, duodenum, colon, mesentery (large)	Severe	4
	2 severe: crush liver; major vascular including: thor & abdom aorta, cavae, iliacs, hepatic veins	Critical	5
Extremities	No Injury	No injury	0
	Minor sprains & fx(s) — no long bones	Minor	1
	Simple fx(s): humerus, clavicle, radius, ulna, tibia, fibula, single nerve	Moderate	2
	Fx(s) multiple moderate, open moderate, femur (simple), pelvic (stable), dislocation major, major nerve	Major	3
	Fx(s) two major, open femur, limb crush or amputation, unstable pelvic fx	Severe	4
	Fx(s) two severe, multiple major	Critical	5
Skin & Subcutaneous	No Injury	No injury	0
	< 5% burn. abrasions, contusions, lacerations	Minor	1
	5–15% burn. extensive contusions, avulsions 3–6″ extensive lacerations (total 12″)	Moderate	2
	15–30% burn. avulsions 12″	Major	3
	30–45% burn. avulsions entire leg, thigh or arm	Severe	4
	45–60% burn (3rd degree)	Critical	5
	60% + burn (3rd degree)	Fatal	6

Definitions:

minor = trivial injury
moderate = minimal injury, short hospitalization anticipated
major = major injury, not immediately life-threatening
severe = life-threatening but survival probable
critical = survival uncertain
fatal = survival unlikely

Abbreviations:

bp — blood pressure
bv — blood volume
cpd — compound
c̄ — with
d — days
fndgs — findings
fx — fracture
i.p. — intraperitoneal
lac-lactns — lacerations
mult — multiple
nl — normal
rds — respiratory distress syndrome
s̄ — without
u — units
vent — ventilator
wnd — wound
↑ — increased
↓ — decreased
> — greater than
< — less than

Figure 6–30. Hospital Trauma Index. (From American College of Surgeons. [1980]. Committee on Trauma: Field categorization of trauma patients and Hospital Trauma Index. Bull. Am. Coll. Surg., *65*:28, with permission.)

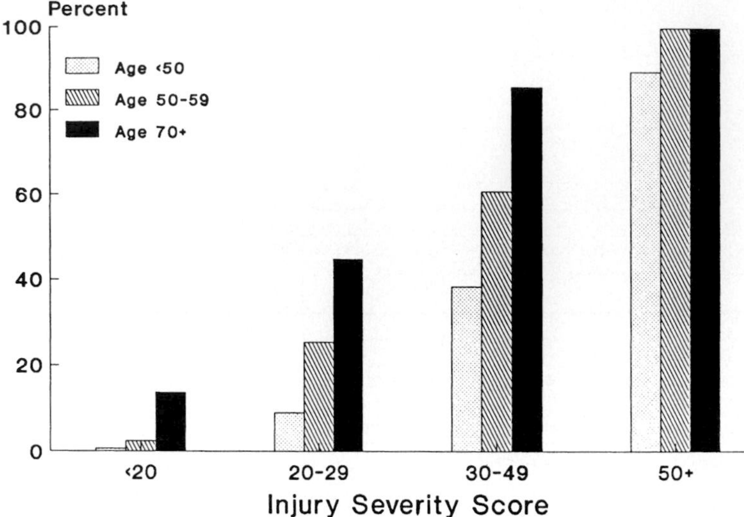

Figure 6–31. Mortality by Injury Severity Score for three age groups. Patients were hospitalized for motor vehicle crash injuries; those who were dead on arrival are excluded from calculations. (Adapted from Baker, S.P., O'Neill, B., Naddon, W., Jr., & Long, W.B. [1974]. The Injury Severity Score: A method for describing patients with multiple injuries and evaluating emergency care. J. Trauma, *14*:187, with permission.)

ally parallel the ISS or HTI-ISS scores.[16, 184, 200] (Fig. 6–31).

References

General

1. Anderson, S., Biros, M.H., & Reardon, R.F. (1996). Delayed diagnosis of thoracolumbar fractures in multiple-trauma patients. Acad. Emerg. Med., 3:832.
2. Bennett, F.S., Zinar, D.M., & Kilgus, D.J. (1993). Ipsilateral hip and femoral shaft fractures. Clin. Orthop. Rel. Res., *296*:168.
3. Blair, E., Topuzlu, C., & Davis, J.H. (1971). Delayed or missed diagnosis in blunt chest trauma. J. Trauma, *11*:129.
4. Bone, L. & Bucholz, R. (1986). The management of fractures in the patient with multiple trauma. J. Bone Joint Surg. [Am.], *68*:945.
5. Bried, J.M., Cordasco, F.A., & Volz, R.G. (1987). Medical and economic parameters of motorcycle-induced trauma. Clin. Orthop., *223*:252.
6. Calenoff, L., Chessare, J.W., & Rogers, L.F. (1978). Multiple level spinal injuries. Importance of early recognition. A.J.R. Am. J. Roentgenol., *130*:665.
7. Cass, A.S. (1984). The multiple injured patient with bladder trauma. J. Trauma, *24*:731.
8. Cass, A.S. (1984). Urethral injury in the multiple-injured patient. J. Trauma, *24*:901.
9. Chan, D., Kraus, J.F., & Riggins, R.S. (1973). Patterns of multiple fracture in accidental injury. J. Trauma, *18*:1075.
10. Chan, R.N.W., Ainscow, D., & Sikorski, J.M. (1980). Diagnostic failures in the multiple injured. J. Trauma, *20*:684.
11. Cookro, D.V. (1979). Motorcycle safety: An epidemiologic view. Arizona Med., *36*:605.
12. Council on Scientific Affairs, American Medical Association (1994). Helmets and preventing motorcycle- and bicycle-related injuries. J.A.M.A., *272*:1535.
13. Daffner, R.H., Riemer, B.L., & Butterfield, S.L. (1991). Ipsilateral femoral neck and shaft fractures: An overlooked association. Skeletal Radiol., *20*:252.
14. Garland, D.E., & Bailey S. (1981). Undetected injuries in head-injured adults. Clin. Orthop., *155*:162.
15. Gertner, H.R. Jr., Baker, S.P., Rutherford, R.B., & Spitz, W.U. (1972). Evaluation of the management of vehicular fatalities secondary to abdominal injury. J. Trauma, *12*:425.
16. Goris, R.J.A., & Draaisma, J. (1982). Causes of death after blunt trauma. J. Trauma, *22*:141.
17. Goris, R.J.A., Gimbrere, J.S.F., van Niekerk, J.L.M. et al. (1982). Early osteosynthesis and prophylactic mechanical ventilation in the multitrauma patient. J. Trauma, *22*:895.
18. Gratz, R.R. (1979). Accidental injury in childhood: A literature review on pediatric trauma. J. Trauma, *19*:551.
19. Gustilo, R.B., Corpuz, V., & Sherman, R.E. (1985). Epidemiology, mortality and morbidity in multiple trauma patients. Orthopedics, *8*:1523.
20. Harrington, T., & Barker, B. (1986). Multiple trauma associated with vertebral injury. Surg. Neurol., *26*:149.
21. Hebert, J.S., & Burnham, R.S. (2000). The effect of polytrauma in persons with traumatic spine injury. Spine, *24*:55.
22. Heilman, D.R., Weisbach, J.B., Blair, R.W., & Graf, L.L. (1982). Motorcycle-related trauma and helmet usage in North Dakota. Ann. Emerg. Med., *11*:25.
23. Irving, M.H., & Irving, P.M. (1967). Associated injuries in head injured patients. J. Trauma, *7*:500.
24. Johnson, K.D., Cadambi, A., & Seibert, B. (1985). Incidence of adult respiratory distress syndrome in patients with multiple musculoskeletal injuries: Effect of early operative stabilization of fractures. J. Trauma, *25*:375.
25. Kraus, J.F., Peek, C., McArthur, D.L., & Williams, A. (1994). The effect of the 1992 California motorcycle helmet use law on motorcycle crash fatalities and injuries. J.A.M.A., *272*:1506.
26. Laasonen, E.M., Penttila, A., & Sumuvuori, H. (1980). Acute lethal trauma of the trunk: Clinical, radiologic and pathologic findings. J. Trauma, *20*:657.
27. Light, T.R., Wu, J.C., & Ogden, J.A. (1980). Diagnosis and management of fractures in the multiply injured patient. Surg. Clin. North Am., *60*:1121.
28. Malisano, L.P., Stevens, D., & Hunter, G.A. (1994). The management of long bone fractures in the head-injured polytrauma patient. J. Orthop. Trauma, *8*:1.
29. Marcus, R.E., Mills, M.F., & Thompson, G.H. (1983). Multiple injury in children. J. Bone Joint Surg. [Am.], *65*:1290.
30. Martinez, R. (1994). Injury prevention: A new perspective. J.A.M.A., *272*:1541.
31. McCarroll, J.R., Braunstein, P.W., Weinberg, S.B. et al. (1965). The pathology of pedestrian automotive accident victims. J. Trauma, *5*:421.
32. McSwain, N.E. Jr., & Petrucelli, E. (1984). Medical consequences of motorcycle helmet nonusage. J. Trauma, *24*:233.
33. Meyers, M.H. (1984). The Multiply Injured Patient with Complex Fractures. Lea & Febiger, Philadelphia.
34. Oreskovich, M.R., Howard, J.D., Copass, M.K., & Carrico, C.J. (1984). Geriatric trauma: Injury patterns and outcome. J. Trauma, *24*:565.
35. Peek, C., Braver, E.R., Shen, H., & Kraus, J.F. (1994). Lower extremity injuries from motorcycle crashes: A common cause of preventable injury. J. Trauma, *37*:358.
36. Riemer, B.L., Butterfield, S.L., Ray, R.L., & Daffner, R.H. (1993). Clandestine femoral neck fractures with ipsilateral diaphyseal fractures. J. Orthop. Trauma, *7*:443.
37. Rupp, R.E., Ebraheim, N.A., Chrissos, M.G., & Jackson, W.T. (1994). Thoracic and lumbar fractures associated with femoral shaft fractures in the multiple trauma patient. Spine, *19*:556.
38. Scalea, T., Goldstein, A., Phillips, T. et al. (1986). An analysis of 161 falls from a height: The "jumper syndrome." J. Trauma, *26*:706.
39. Silva, J.F. (1984). Review of patients with multiple injuries treated at University Hospital, Kuala Lumpur. J. Trauma, *24*:526.
40. Shuler, T.E., Gruen, G.S., DiTano, O., & Riemer, B.L. (1997). Ipsilateral proximal and shaft femoral fractures: Spectrum of injury involving the femoral neck. Injury, *28*:293.
41. Siegel, J.H., Mason-Gonzalez, S., Dischinger, P. et al. (1993). Safety belt restraints and compartment intrusions in frontal and lateral motor vehicle crashes: Mechanisms of injuries, complications, and acute care costs. J. Trauma, *5*:736.
42. Soderstrom, C.A., McArdle, D.Q., Ducker, T.B., & Militello, P.R. (1983). The diagnosis of intra-abdominal injury in patients with cervical cord trauma. J. Trauma, *23*:1061.
43. Swierzewski, M.J., Feliciano, D.V., Lillis, R.P. et al. Deaths from motor vehicle crashes: Patterns of injury in restrained and unrestrained victims. J. Trauma, *37*:404.
44. Watson, G.S., Zador, P.L., & Wilks, A. (1980). The repeal of helmet use laws and increased motorcyclist mortality in the United States, 1975–1978. Am. J. Public Health, *70*:579.
45. Wolinsky, P.R., & Johnson, K.D. (1995). Ipsilateral femoral neck and shaft fractures. Clin. Orthop. Rel. Res., *318*:81.

Trauma Care Systems

46. Accidental Death and Disability. (1966). The Neglected Disease of Modern Society. National Academy of Sciences of the National Research Council, Committee on Trauma and Committee on Shock, Washington, D.C.
47. Breaux, C.W. Jr., Smith, G., & Georgeson, K.E. (1990). The first two years' experience with major trauma at a pediatric trauma center. J. Trauma, *30*:37.
48. Committee on Trauma of the American College of Surgeons. (1983). Hospital and prehospital resources for optimal care of the injured patient. A.C.S. Bull., *68*:11.
49. Detmer, D.E., Moylan, J.A., Rose, J. et al. (1977). Regional categorization and quality of care in major trauma. J. Trauma, *17*:592.
50. Gill, W., Champion, H.R., Long, W.B. et al. (1976). A clinical experience of major multiple trauma in Maryland. Md. State Med. J., *25*:55.
51. Kane, G., Wheeler, N.C., Cook, S. et al. (1992). Impact of Los Angeles County trauma system on the survival of seriously injured patients. J. Trauma, *32*:576.
52. McKenzie, E.J., Morris, J.A., Smith, G.S., & Fahey, M. (1990). Acute hospital costs of trauma in the United States: Implications for regionalized systems of care. J. Trauma, *30*:1096.
53. Moylan, J.A., Detmer, D.E., Rose, J., & Schulz, R. (1976). Evaluation of the quality of hospital care for major trauma. J. Trauma, *16*:517.
54. Mullins, R.J., Veum-Stone, J., Helfand, M. et al. (1994). Outcome of hospitalized patients after institution of a trauma system in an urban area. J.A.M.A., *271*:1919.
55. Tortella, B.J., & Trunkey, D.D. (1984). Trauma care systems. Trauma Q., *1*:17.
56. Waters, J.M. Jr., & Wells, C.H. (1973). The effects of a modern emergency medical care system in reducing automobile crash deaths. J. Trauma, *13*:645.
57. West, J.G., Cales, R.H., & Gazzaniga, A.B. (1983). Impact of regionalization. Arch. Surg., *118*:740.
58. West, J.G., Trunkey, D.D., & Lim, R.C. (1979). Systems of trauma care. Arch. Surg., *114*:455.

Imaging of Visceral Injury

59. Akgur, F.M., Aktug, T., Olguner, M. et al. (1997). Prospective study investigating routine usage of ultrasonography as the initial diagnostic modality for the evaluation of children sustaining blunt abdominal trauma. J. Trauma, *42*:626.
60. Asher, W.M., Parvin, S., Virgilio, R.W. et al. (1976). Echographic evaluation of splenic injury after blunt trauma. Radiology, *118*:411.
61. Ayella, R.J., Hankins, J.R., Turney, S.Z., & Cowley, R.A. (1977) Ruptures of the thoracic aorta due to blunt trauma. J. Trauma, *17*:199.
62. Berne, J.D., Velmahos, G.C., El-Tawail, Q. et al. (1999). Value of complete cervical helical computed tomographic scanning in identifying cervical spine injury in the unevaluable blunt trauma patient with multiple injuries: A prospective study. J. Trauma, *47*:896.
63. Blackmore, C.C., Ramsey, S.D., Mann, F.A., & Deyo, R.A. (1999). Cervical spine screening with CT in trauma patients: A cost-effectiveness analysis. Radiology, *21*:117.
64. Bode, P.J., Edwards, M.J., Kruit, M.C., & van Vugt, A.B. (1999). Sonography in a clinical algorithm for early evaluation of 1671 patients with blunt abdominal trauma. A.J.R. Am. J. Roentgenol, *172*:905.
65. Boulanger, B.R., Brenneman, F.D., McLellan, B.A. et al. (1995). A prospective study of emergent abdominal sonography after blunt trauma. J. Trauma, *39*:325.
66. Shanmuganathan, K., Mirvis, S.E., Boyd-Kranis, R. et al. (2000). Nonsurgical management of blunt splenic injury: Use of CT criteria to select patients for splenic angiography and potential endovascular therapy. Radiology, 217:75.
67. Branney, S.W., Wolfe, R.E., Moore, E.E. et al. (1995). Quantitative sensitivity of ultrasound in detecting free intraperitoneal fluid. J. Trauma, *39*:375.
68. Brasel, K.J., DeLisle, C.M., Olson, C.J., & Borgstrom, D.C. (1998). Splenic injury: Trends in evaluation and management. J. Trauma, *44*:283.
69. Chiu, W.C., Cushing, B.M., Rodriguez, A. et al. (1997). Abdominal injuries without hemoperitoneum: a potential limitation of focused abdominal sonography for trauma (FAST). J. Trauma, *42*:617.
70. Coldwell, D.M., Novak, Z., Ryu, R.K. et al. (2000). Treatment of posttraumatic internal carotid arterial pseudoaneurysms with endovascular stents. J. Trauma, *48*:470.
71. Cook, J.F., Hansen, M., & Brietweser, J. (1997). Optimizing radiology in the new picture archiving and communication system environment. J. Digit. Imaging, *10*:165.
72. D'Alise, M.D., Benzel, E.C., & Hart, B.L. (1999). Magnetic resonance imaging evaluation of the cervical spine in the comatose or obtunded trauma patient. J. Neurosurg., *91*:54.
73. Davis, K.A., Fabian, T.C., & Croce, M.A. et al. (1998). Improved success in nonoperative management of blunt splenic injuries: Embolization of splenic artery pseudoaneurysms. J. Trauma, *44*:1008.
74. Delfini, R., Dorizzi, A., Facchinetti, G. et al. (1999). Delayed post-traumatic cervical instability. Surg. Neurol., *51*:588.
75. Della Corte, F., Caricato, A., Pennisi, M.A. et al. (1999). Injury of the vertebral artery after closed head injury. Eur. J. Emerg. Radiol, *6*:255.
76. Demetriades, D., Theodorou, D., Asensio, J. et al. (1996). Management options in vertebral artery injuries. Br. J. Surg., *83*:83.
77. Dowe, M.F., Mirvis, S.E., Shanmuganathan, K. et al. (1997). CT findings of mesenteric injury after blunt trauma: Implications for surgical intervention. A.J.R. Am. J. Roentgenol., *168*:425.
78. Dyer, D.S., Moore, E.E., Mestek, M.F. et al. (1999). Can chest CT be used to exclude aortic injury? Radiology, *213*:195.
79. Federle, M.P., Courcoulas, A.P., Powell, M. et al. (1998). Blunt splenic injury in adults. Clinical and CT criteria for management with emphasis on active extravasation. Radiology, *206*:137.
80. Federle, M.P., Peitzman, A.B., & Krugh, J. (1997). Abdominal trauma: Use of oral contrast material for CT is safe. Radiology, *205*:91.
81. Fernandez, L., McKenney, M.G., McKenney, K.L. et al. (1998). Ultrasound in blunt abdominal trauma. J. Trauma, *45*:841.
82. Gavant, M.L., Menke, P.G., Fabian, T. et al. (1995). Blunt traumatic aortic rupture: Detection with helical CT of the chest. Radiology, *197*:125.
83. Gelman, R., Mirvis, S.E., & Gens, D. (1991). Diaphragmatic rupture due to blunt trauma. Sensitivity of plain chest radiographs. A.J.R. Am. J. Roentgenol., *158*:51.
84. Giacobetti, F.B., Vaccaro, A.R., Bos-Giacobetti, M.A. et al. (1997) Vertebral artery occlusion with cervical spine trauma: A prospective analysis. Spine, *22*:188.
85. Goan, Y.G., Huang, M.S., & Lin, J.M. (1998). Nonoperative management for extensive hepatic and splenic injuries with significant hemoperitoneum in adults. J. Trauma, *45*:360.
86. Goldberg, B.B., Clearfield, H.R., Goodman, G.A., & Morales, J.O. (1973). Ultrasonographic determination of ascites. Arch. Intern. Med., *131*:217.
87. Goldstein, L., Mirvis, S.E., Kostrubiak, I.S. & Turney, S.Z. (1989). CT diagnosis of acute pericardial tamponade following blunt chest trauma. A.J.R. Am. J. Roentgenol., *152*:739.
88. Goletti, O., Ghiselli, G., Lippolis, P.V. et al. (1994). The role of ultrasonography in blunt abdominal trauma: Results in 250 consecutive patients. J. Trauma, *36*:178.
89. Gonzales, R.P., Fried, P.O., Bukhalo, M. et al. (1999). Role of clinical examination in screening for blunt cervical spine injury. J. Am. Coll. Surg., *189*:152.
90. Grossman, M.D., Reilly, P.M., Gillett, T., & Gillett, D. (1999). National survey of the incidence of cervical spine injury and approach to cervical spine clearance in U.S. trauma centers. J. Trauma, *47*:684.
91. Hagiwara, A., Yukioka, T., Ohta, S. et al. (1997). Nonsurgical management of patients with blunt hepatic injury: Efficacy of transcatheter arterial embolization. A.J.R. Am. J. Roentgenol., *169*:1151.
92. Harris, J.H. Jr. (1994). Abnormal cervicocranial soft-tissues as a harbinger of subtle acute cervicocranial injury. Emerg. Radiol., *1*:42.
93. Harris, J.H. Jr. (1996). Injuries of diverse and poorly understood mechanisms. In Harris, J.H. Jr., & Mirvis, S.E. Eds.: The Radiology of Acute Cervical Spine Trauma. pp. 421–474. Williams & Wilkins, Baltimore.
94. Hemphill, J.C. 3rd, Gress, D.R., & Halbach, V.V. (1999). Endovascular therapy of traumatic injuries of the intracranial cerebral arteries. Crit. Care Clin., *15*:811.
95. Hoffman, J.R., Schriger, D.L., Mower, W. et al. (1992). Low-risk criteria for cervical spine radiography in blunt trauma. A prospective study. Ann. Emerg. Med., *21*:1454.
96. Janzen, D.L., Zweirewich, C.V., Breen, D.J., & Nagy, A. (1998). Diagnostic accuracy of helical CT for detection of blunt bowel and mesenteric injuries. Clin. Radiol., *53*:193.
97. Junck, K.L., Berland, L.L., Bernreuter, W.K. et al. (1998). PACS and CR implementation in a level I trauma center emergency department. J. Digit. Imaging, *11*:159.
98. Karaasian, T., Meuli, R., Androux, R. et al. (1995). Traumatic chest lesions in patients with severe head trauma: A comparative study with computed tomography and conventional radiograms. J. Trauma, 39:1081.
99. Killeen, K.L., Mirvis, S.E., & Shanmuganathan K. (1999). Helical CT of diaphragmatic rupture caused by blunt trauma. A.J.R. Am. J. Roentgenol., *173*:1611.
100. Killeen, K.L., Poletti, P.A., Shanmuganathan, K., & Mirvis, S.E. (1999). CT diagnosis of cardiac and pericardial injuries. Emerg. Radiol., *6*:339.
101. LeBlang, S.D., & Nunez, D.B. Jr. (1999). Helical CT of cervical spine and soft tissue injuries of the neck. Radiol. Clin. North Am., *37*:515.
102. Marnocha, K.E., Maglinte, D.D., Woods, J. et al. (1984). Mediastinal-width/chest-width ratio in blunt chest trauma: A reappraisal. A.J.R. Am. J. Roentgenol., *142*:275.
103. Marotta, T.R., Buller, C., Taylor, D. et al. (1998). Autologous vein–covered stent repair of a cervical internal carotid artery pseudoaneurysm: Technical case report. Neurosurgery, *42*:412.
104. McClellan, B.A., Hanna, S.S., Montoya, D.R. et al. (1985). Analysis of peritoneal lavage parameters in blunt abdominal trauma. J. Trauma, *25*:393.
105. McGahan, J.P., & Richards, J.R. (1999). Blunt abdominal trauma: The role of emergent sonography and a review of the literature. A.J.R. Am. J. Roentgenol., *172*:897.
106. McKenney, M., Lentz, K., Nunez, D. et al. (1994). Can ultrasound replace diagnostic peritoneal lavage in the assessment of blunt trauma? J. Trauma, *37*:439.
107. Meyer, D.M., Thal, E.R., Weigert, J.A., & Redman, H.C. (1989). Evaluation of computed tomography and diagnostic peritoneal lavage in blunt abdominal trauma. J. Trauma, *29*:1168.
108. Mirvis, S.E., Bidwell, J.K., Buddemeyer, E.U. et al. (1987). Value of chest radiography in excluding traumatic aortic rupture. Radiology, *163*:487.

109. Mirvis, S.E., Gens, D.R., & Shanmuganathan, K. (1992). Rupture of the bowel after blunt abdominal trauma: Diagnosis with CT. A.J.R. Am. J. Roentgenol., *159*:1217.
110. Mirvis, S.E., Pais, S.O., & Shanmuganathan, K. (1994). Atypical results of thoracic aortograms performed to exclude aortic rupture. Emerg. Radiol., *1*:24.
111. Mirvis, S.E., Shanmuganathan, K., Buell, J., & Rodriguez, A. (1998). Use of spiral computed tomography for the assessment of blunt trauma patients with potential aortic injury. J. Trauma, *45*:922.
112. Mirvis, S.E., Shanmuganathan, K., & Erh, R. (1994). Diffuse small-bowel ischemia in hypotensive adults after blunt trauma (shock-bowel): CT findings and clinical significance. A.J.R. Am. J. Roentgenol., *163*:1375.
113. Mirvis, S.E., Shanmuganathan, K., Miller, B.H. et al. (1996). Use of contrast-enhanced CT for the diagnosis of traumatic aortic injury. Five-year experience at a major trauma center. Radiology, *200*:413.
114. Mirvis, S.E., & Shanmuganathan, K. (1994). Trauma radiology: Part 1. Computerized tomographic imaging of abdominal trauma. J. Intensive Care Med., *9*:151.
115. Mirvis, S.E., & Shanmuganathan, K. (1994). Trauma radiology: Part II. Diagnostic imaging of thoracic trauma. A review and update. J. Intensive Care Med., *9*:179.
116. Montalvo, B.M., LeBlang, S.D., Nunez, D.B. Jr. et al. (1996). Color Doppler sonography in penetrating injuries of the neck. A.J.N.R. Am. J. Neuroradiol., *17*:943.
117. Moore, F.A., Moore, E.E., Haenel, J.B. et al. (1989). Post-traumatic pseudocyst in the adult: Pathophysiology, recognition, and selective management. J. Trauma, *29*:1380.
118. Nemzek, W.R., Hecht, S.T., Donald, P.J. et al. (1996). Prediction of major vascular injury in patients with gunshot wounds of the neck. A.J.N.R. Am. J. Neuroradiol., *17*:161.
119. Pachter, H.L., Guth, A.A., Hofstatter, S.R., & Spencer, P.C. (1998). Changing patterns in management of splenic trauma: The impact of nonoperative management. Ann. Surg., *5*:708.
120. Parodi, J.C., Schonholz, C., Ferreira, L.M., & Bergan, J. (1999). Endovascular stent-graft of traumatic arterial lesions. Ann. Vasc. Surg., *13*:121.
121. Patrick, D.A., Bensard, D.D., Moore, E.E. et al. (1998). Ultrasound is an effective triage tool to evaluate blunt abdominal trauma in the pediatric population. J. Trauma, *45*:57.
122. Peer, S., Vogl, R., & Jaschke, W. (1999). Sophisticated hospital information system/radiology information system/picture archiving and communication system (PACS) integration in a large-scale traumatology PACS. J. Digit. Imaging, *12*:99.
123. Poletti, P.A., Mirvis, S.E., Shanmuganathan, K. et al. (2000). CT criteria for management of blunt liver trauma: Correlation with angiographic and surgical findings. Radiology, *216*:418.
124. Powell, D.C., Bivins, B.A., & Bell, R.M. (1982). Diagnostic peritoneal lavage. Surg. Gynecol. Obstet., *155*:257.
125. Resnick, D.K., Subach, B.R., & Marion, D.W. (1997). The significance of carotid canal involvement in basilar skull fracture. Neurosurgery, *40*:1177.
126. Richards, J.R., McGahan, J.P., Simpson, J.L., & Tabar, P. (1999). Bowel and mesenteric injury: Evaluation with emergency abdominal US. Radiology, *211*:399.
127. Rogers, F.B., Baker, E.F., Osler, T.M. et al. (1999). Computed tomographic angiography for blunt cervical arterial injuries: Preliminary results. J. Trauma, *47*:438.
128. Ross, S.E., Dragon, G.M., O'Malley, K.F., & Rehm, C.G. (1995). Morbidity of negative coeliotomy in trauma. Injury, *26*:393.
129. Rozycki, G.S., Ochsner, M.G., Feliciano, D.V. et al. (1998). Early detection of hemoperitoneum by ultrasound. Examination of the right upper quadrant: A multicenter study. J. Trauma, *45*:878.
130. Ruess, L., Sivit, C.J., Eichelberger, M.R. et al. (1997). Blunt abdominal trauma in children: Impact of CT on operative and non-operative management. A.J.R. Am. J. Roentgenol., *169*:1011.
131. Sadler, M.A., Shapiro, R.S., Wagreich, J. et al. (1997). CT diagnosis of acquired intercostal lung herniation. Clin. Imaging, *21*:104.
132. Scalea, T.M., Rodriguez, A., Chiu, W.C. et al. (1999). Focused assessment with sonography for trauma (FAST): Results from an international consensus conference. J. Trauma, *46*:466.
133. Schurr, M.J., Fabian, T.C., Gavant, M.L. et al. (1995). Management of blunt splenic trauma. Computed tomographic contrast blush predicts failure of nonoperative management. J. Trauma, *39*:507.
134. Sclafani, S.J.A., Shaftan, G.W., Scalea, T.M. et al. (1995). Nonoperative salvage of computed tomography–diagnosed splenic injuries: Utilization of angiography for triage and embolization to hemostasis. J. Trauma, *39*:818.
135. Shackford, S.R. (1993). Focused ultrasound examination by surgeons: The time is now. J. Trauma, *35*:181.
136. Shanmuganathan, K., Mirvis, S.E., & Amerosa, M (1993). Periportal low density on CT with blunt trauma: Association with elevated central venous pressure. A.J.R. Am. J. Roentgenol., *160*:279.
137. Shanmuganathan, K., Mirvis, S.E., Boyd-Kranis, R. et al. (2000). Nonsurgical management of blunt splenic injury: Use of CT criteria to select patients for splenic arteriography and potential endovascular therapy. Radiology, *217*:75.
138. Shanmuganathan, K., Mirvis, S.E., Sherbourne, C.D. et al. (1999). Hemoperitoneum as the sole indicator of abdominal visceral injuries: A potential limitation of screening abdominal US for trauma. Radiology, *212*:423.
139. Shanmuganathan, K., Mirvis, S.E., Sherbourne, C.D. et al. (1993). Value of contrast-enhanced CT in detecting active hemorrhage in patients with blunt abdominal or pelvic trauma. A.J.R. Am. J. Roentgenol., *161*:65.
140. Shanmuganathan, K., Mirvis, S.E., White, C.S., & Pomerantz, S.M. (1996). MR imaging evaluation of hemidiaphragms in acute blunt trauma: Experience with 16 patients. A.J.R. Am. J. Roentgenol., *167*:397.
141. Shanmuganathan, K., & Mirvis, S.E. (1998). Evaluation of liver and pancreas after blunt trauma. In Gazelle, G.S., Saini, S., & Mueller, P.R. Eds.: Hepatobiliary and Pancreatic Radiology. pp. 171–204. Thieme, New York.
142. Shapiro, M.J., Krausz, C., Durham, R.M., & Mazuski, J.E. (1999). Overuse of splenic scoring and computed tomographic scans. J. Trauma, *47*:651.
143. Sherbourne, C.D., Shanmuganathan, K., Mirvis, S.E. et al. (1997). Visceral injury without hemoperitoneum: A limitation of screening abdominal sonography for trauma. Emerg. Radiol. *4*:301.
144. Sherman, H.F., Savage, B.A., Jones, L.M. et al. (1994). Nonoperative management of blunt hepatic injuries. Safe at any grade? J. Trauma, *37*:616.
145. Sivit, C.J., Eichelberger, M.R., & Taylor, G.A. (1994). CT in children with rupture of the bowel caused by blunt trauma: Diagnostic efficacy and comparison with hypoperfusion complex. A.J.R. Am. J. Roentgenol., *163*:1195.
146. Smith, J.S., Cooney, R.N., & Mucha, P. (1996). Nonoperative management of the ruptured spleen: A revalidation of criteria. Surgery, *120*:745.
147. Sutyak, J.P., Chiu, W.C., D'Amelio, L.F. et al. (1995). Computed tomography is inaccurate in estimating the severity of adult splenic injury. J. Trauma, *39*:514.
148. Thomas, D.P., Davies, A., & Hoddinott, H.C. (1999). Posterior sternoclavicular dislocation—A diagnosis easily missed. Ann. R. Coll. Surg. Engl. *81*:201.
149. Trupka, A., Waydhas, C., Hallfeldt, K.K. et al. (1997). Value of thoracic computed tomography in the first assessment of severely injured patients with blunt chest trauma: Results of a prospective study. J. Trauma, *43*:405.
150. Tso, P., Rodriguez, A., Cooper, C. et al. (1992). Sonography in blunt abdominal trauma. A preliminary progress report. J. Trauma, *33*:39.
151. Vaccaro, A.R., Klein, G.R., Flanders, A.E. et al. (1998). Long-term evaluation of vertebral injuries following cervical spine trauma using magnetic resonance angiography. Spine, *23*:789.
152. Velmahos, G.C., Theodore, D., Tatevossian, R. et al. (1996). Radiologic cervical spine evaluation in the alert asymptomatic blunt trauma victim. Much ado about nothing? J. Trauma, *40*:768.
153. Wagner, R.B., Crawford, W.O., & Schimpf P.P. (1988). Classification of parenchymal injuries of the lung. Radiology, *167*:77.
154. Weller, S.J., Rossitch, E., & Malek, A.M. (1999). Detection of vertebral artery injury after cervical spine trauma using magnetic resonance angiography. J. Trauma, *46*:660.
155. White, C.S., Mirvis, S.E., & Templeton, P.A. (1994). Subtle chest radiographic abnormalities in patients with traumatic aortic rupture. Emerg Radiol, *1*:72.
156. Willis, B.K., Greiner, F., Orrison, W.W., & Benzel, E.C. (1994). The incidence of vertebral artery injury after midcervical spine fracture or subluxation. Neurosurgery, *34*:435.
157. Yoshii, H., Sato, M., Yamamoto, S. et al. (1998). Usefulness and limitations of ultrasonography in the initial evaluation of blunt abdominal trauma. J. Trauma, *39*:45.
158. Ziter, F.M.H., & Westcott, J.L. (1981). Supine subpulmonary pneumothorax. A.J.R. Am. J. Roentgenol., *137*:699.

Diagnostic Oversights

159. Alzen, G., & Stargardt, A. (1995). New concept to optimize emergency diagnoses in patients with multiple injuries. Radiologe, *35*:406.
160. Ashman, C.J., Yu, J.S., & Wolfman, D. (2000). Satisfaction of search in osteoradiology A.J.R. Am. J. Roentgenol., *175*:541.
161. Ben-Menachem, Y., & Fisher, R.G. (1988). Diagnostic and interventional radiology in trauma. p. 187. In Mattox, K.L., Moore, E.E., & Feliciano, D.V. Eds. Trauma. Appleton & Lange, Norwalk, Conn.
162. Born, C.T., Ross, S.E., Iannacone, W. et al. (1989). Delayed identification of skeletal injury in multisystem trauma: The "missed" fracture. Trauma, *29*:1643.
163. Dunham, C.M., & Cowley, R.A. (comps). (1986). Shock Trauma/Critical Care Handbook. Aspen Publishers, Inc., Rockville, Md.
164. Eldar, R., & Inbar, A. (1987). Diagnostic radiology in disaster medicine: Implications for design, planning and organization of x-ray departments. Injury, *18*:247.
165. Feliciano, D.V., Bitondo, C.G., Mattox, K.L. et al. (1984). The missed injury: Sins in trauma care. A.A.S.T. Abstracts. J. Trauma, *24*:657.
166. Frawley, P.A., Mills, J.A., Murton, F., & Ware, R. (1995). Bone scanning in the multiply injured patient. Aust. N. Z. J. Surg., *65*:390.
167. Gillott, A., Rhodes, M., & Lucke, J. (1988). Utility of routine pelvic x-ray during blunt trauma resuscitation. J. Trauma, *28*:1570.
168. Hildingsson, C., Hietala, S.O., Toolanen, G., & Bjornebrink, J. (1993). Negative scintigraphy despite spinal fractures in the multiply injured. Injury, *24*:467.
169. Kingma, L.M. (1982). Radiological management of the patient with multiple injuries. Injury, *14*:17.
170. Mackersie, R.C., Shackford, S.R., Garfin, S.R., & Hoyt, D.B. (1988). Major skeletal injuries in the obtunded blunt trauma patient: A case for routine radiologic surgery. J. Trauma, *28*:1450.

171. Mulligan, M.E., McCarthy, M.J., Wippold, F.J. et al. (1988). Radiologic evaluation of mass casualty victims: Lessons from the Gander, Newfoundland, accident. Radiology, *168*:229.
172. Pal, J.M., Mulder, D.S., Brown, R.A., & Fleiszer, D.M. (1988). Assessing multiple trauma: Is the cervical spine enough? J. Trauma, *28*:1282.
173. Pilcher, D.B. (1981). Don't put the unstable on the x-ray table. J. Trauma, *21*:661.
174. Ravichandran, G., & Silver, J.R. (1982). Missed injuries of the spinal cord. Br. Med. J., *284*:953.
175. Reid, D.C., Henderson, R., Saboe, L., & Miller, J.D.R. (1987). Etiology and clinical course of missed spine fractures. J. Trauma, *27*:980.
176. Rogers, L.F. (1984). Common oversights in the evaluation of the patient with multiple injuries. Skeletal Radiol., *12*:103.
177. Rogers, L.F. (1985). Problems in radiologic examination of patients with multiple injuries. Appl. Radiol., *14*:59.
178. Roshkow, J.E., Haller, J.O., Hotson, G.C. et al. (1990). Imaging evaluation of children after falls from a height: Review of 45 cases. Radiology, *175*:359.
179. Scher, A.T. (1977). A plea for routine radiographic examination of the cervical spine after head injury. South Am. Med. J. *51*:885.
180. Teasdale, G., & Jennett, B. (1974). Assessment of coma and impaired consciousness: A practical scale. Lancet, 2:81.
181. Williams, D.R., Gaggoley, C., & Wortzman, D. (1988). Recognition of thoracic/lumbar spinal fractures in the multiple trauma patient. J. Trauma, *28*:1508.

Injury Scoring Systems

182. American College of Surgeons. (1980). Committee on Trauma: Field categorization of trauma patients and Hospital Trauma Index. Bull. Am. Coll. Surg., *65*:28.
183. Baker, S.P., & O'Neill, B. (1976). The injury severity score: An update. J. Trauma, *16*:882.
184. Baker, S.P., O'Neill, B., Haddon, W. Jr., & Long, W.B. (1974). The injury severity score: A method for describing patients with multiple injuries and evaluating emergency care. J. Trauma, *14*:187.
184a. Britt, L.D., Peyser, M.B. (2000). Penetrating and blunt neck trauma. p. 438. In Mattox, K.L., Feliciano, D.V., & Moore, E.E. Eds. Trauma. 4th ed. McGraw-Hill, New York.
185. Champion, H.R., & Sacco, W.L. (1988). Trauma scoring. p. 63. In Mattox, K.L., Moore, E.E., Feliciano, D.V. Eds.: Trauma. Appleton & Lange, Norwalk, Conn.
186. Champion, H.R., Sacco, W.J., Carnazzo, A.J. et al. (1981). Trauma score. Crit. Care Med., 9:672.
187. Committee on Injury Scaling. (1985). The Abbreviated Injury Scale, 1985 Revision. American Association for Automotive Medicine, Des Plains, Ill.
188. Committee on Medical Aspects of Automotive Safety. (1971). Rating the severity of tissue damage. I. The abbreviated scale. J.A.M.A., *215*:277.
189. Copes, W.S., Champion, H.R., Sacco, W.J. et al. (1990). Progress in characterizing anatomic injury. J. Trauma, *30*:1200.
190. Cottington, E.M., Young, J.C., Shufflebarger, C.M. et al. (1988). The utility of physiological status, injury site, and injury mechanism in identifying patients with major trauma. J. Trauma, *28*:305.
191. Goris, R.J.A. (1983). The injury severity score. World J. Surg., *7*:12.
192. Gormican, S.P. (1982). CRAMS scale: Field triage of trauma victims. Ann. Emerg. Med., *11*:132.
193. Joint Committee on Injury Scaling. (1976). The Abbreviated Injury Scale (AIS), 1976 Revision. American Association for Automotive Medicine, Morton Grove, Ill.
194. Lee, R.B., Bass, S.M., Morris, J.A. Jr., & MacKenzie, E.J. (1990). Three or more rib fractures as an indicator for transfer to a level I trauma center: A population-based study. J. Trauma, *30*:689.
195. Long, W.B., Sacco, W.J., Copes, W.S. et al. (1994). An evaluation of expert human and automated abbreviated injury scale and ICD-9 injury coding. J. Trauma, *36*:1.
196. Mayer, T., Matlak, M.E., Johnson, D.G., & Walker, M.L. (1980). The modified injury severity scale in pediatric multiple trauma patients. J. Pediatr. Surg., *15*:719.
197. McConigal, M.D., Cole, J., Schwab, W. et al. (1993). A new approach to probability of survival scoring for trauma quality assurance. J. Trauma, *34*:863.
198. Rutledge, R., Fakhry, S., Baker, C., & Oller D. (1993). Injury severity grading in trauma patients: A simplified technique based upon ICD-9 coding. J. Trauma, *35*:497.
199. Semmlow, J.L., & Cone, R. (1976). Utility of the injury severity score: A confirmation. Health Serv. Res., *Spring*:45.
200. Tandias, J., Ruiz, E., & Gustilo, R. (1975). Analysis of 200 multiple trauma patients at Hennepin County Medical Center. Minn. Med., *58*:514.
201. Teasdale, G., & Jennett, B. (1974). Assessment of coma and impaired consciousness. A practical scale. Lancet, 2:81.
202. van der Sluis, C.K., ten Duis, H.J., & Geertzen, J.H.B. (1995). Multiple injuries: An overview of the outcome. J. Trauma, *38*:681.
203. Young, J.C., Macioce, D.P., & Young, W.W. (1990). Identifying injuries and trauma severity in large databases. J. Trauma, *30*:1220.
204. Zietlow, S.P., Capizzi, P.J., Bannon, M.P., & Farnell, M.B. (1994). Multisystem geriatric trauma. J. Trauma, *37*:985.

Chapter 7

FRACTURE TREATMENT

with Ronald W. Hendrix, MD

The general aim of fracture treatment is to restore function and stability with an acceptable cosmetic result and minimum residual deformity. These goals are accomplished by means of manipulation, usually referred to as *reduction*, of the fracture fragments and their *fixation* by either external or internal means. *External* or *closed reduction* is accomplished without surgical incision by manipulation of the affected body part. *Open reduction* uses a surgical incision, direct or indirect manipulation of the fracture fragments, and usually the application or insertion of a surgical appliance or device to achieve and maintain the reduction. *External fixation* is accomplished by use of external fixators and pins, splints, or casts. *Internal fixation* uses metal plates and screws, wires, rods, or nails, either alone or in combination, to maintain the reduction.

Until plaster casting techniques became generally accepted, immobilization by the application of external wood and metal splints[61, 71] was the accepted, time-honored standard of fracture treatment in Western medicine. It is difficult to imagine treatment of fractures without the use of plaster casts. It is often assumed that they have been in general use for several centuries; in fact, they were not used until the mid-nineteenth century when Antonius Mathysen,[51, 61] a Flemish military surgeon, reported his invention of plaster of Paris–impregnated bandages and their use in the formation of circular plaster casts in the treatment of fractures. He published a short paper in 1852 and a monograph entitled *Du Bandage Platre et de son application dous le traitment des fractures* in 1854. This technique was popularized by its extensive use in the Crimean War from 1853 to 1856, but similar casting material had been used earlier by Arabian physicians.[51] There is evidence that limb molds made of clay were used as casting material in India. Bandages impregnated with wax, resins, or egg white had been used in antiquity in Western medicine, particularly in the treatment of nasal fractures, but they apparently were not used for immobilization at other fracture sites.

The plaster-of-Paris cast is made from a bandage of muslin stiffened by dextrose or starch and impregnated with hydrated calcium sulfate.[71] When water is added, an exothermic reaction takes place, the calcium sulfate crystallizes into a rock-hard, uniform mass, and heat is released ($CaSO_4 \cdot H_2O + H_2O \rightleftharpoons CaSO_4 \cdot 2H_2O$ + heat). The setting time is a few minutes, but the rate of drying may be varied by the addition of substances that accelerate (e.g., alum or hot water) or retard (e.g., sodium chloride) drying.

The cast can be applied directly to the skin (the skin-tight technique advocated by Böhler of Austria), or cotton wadding may be placed on the limb before the cast is applied. The Bologna cast technique uses cotton wadding and some degree of tension or compression by the plaster bandage. The most common method is the so-called third way, in which a padded cast is applied without significant tension.[67, 71] In America there are usually three layers of materials: the first, a tubular knitted stocking directly against the skin; the second, a layer of sheet wadding rolled around the part; and the third, the plaster bandage applied by rolling and shaping it over the sheet wadding. Plaster of Paris can also be used as a splint by fashioning a posterior trough (Fig. 7–1) instead of a full circular cast.

A plaster-of-Paris cast is, of course, radiopaque (Fig. 7–2). The degree of radiopacity is dependent not only on the thickness of the cast but on the wetness of the plaster. As a general rule, 8 to 16 kV is added during radiography to allow for the increased absorption of a wet cast. With a very thick cast or with severely osteopenic bone, it may be difficult to visualize the fracture site. Finer bony details are obscured under all conditions when a cast is present; therefore, if there is a question of healing that requires visualization of early callus formation or if there is a possibility of osteomyelitis, it is mandatory that the cast be removed prior to radiography to allow the recording of sufficient bone detail for the resolution of these questions.

The plaster-of-Paris cast can be cut by knife, shears, or mechanical saw. The cast may be split by a longitudinal cut (see Fig. 7–2) or bivalved by two longitudinal cuts on opposite sides to allow space for swelling and in turn prevent vascular compromise. Holes or windows can be cut into the cast (see Fig. 7–1*B*) to enable visualization of the underlying part. The holes may be round or oval. Rectangular or square windows weaken the cast by the concentration of forces at their angles and theoretically should be avoided. A cast may be wedged (Fig. 7–3) to improve the angulation at a fracture site. Wedging is most commonly performed in the treatment of tibial fractures. To wedge a cast, a transverse cut is made along approximately two thirds of the circumference of the cast. This cut is then opened by applying pressure to the distal portion of the limb. This opening is enlarged sufficiently to obtain the desired improvement in the angulation at the fracture site, which is then maintained by wedging a piece of sheet wadding, cork, or wood into the cut and applying plaster about the defect in the cast.

Fractures of the knee may be treated in a cast brace (Fig. 7–4*C* and *D*), a special modification of a long-leg cast in which separate casts above and below the knee

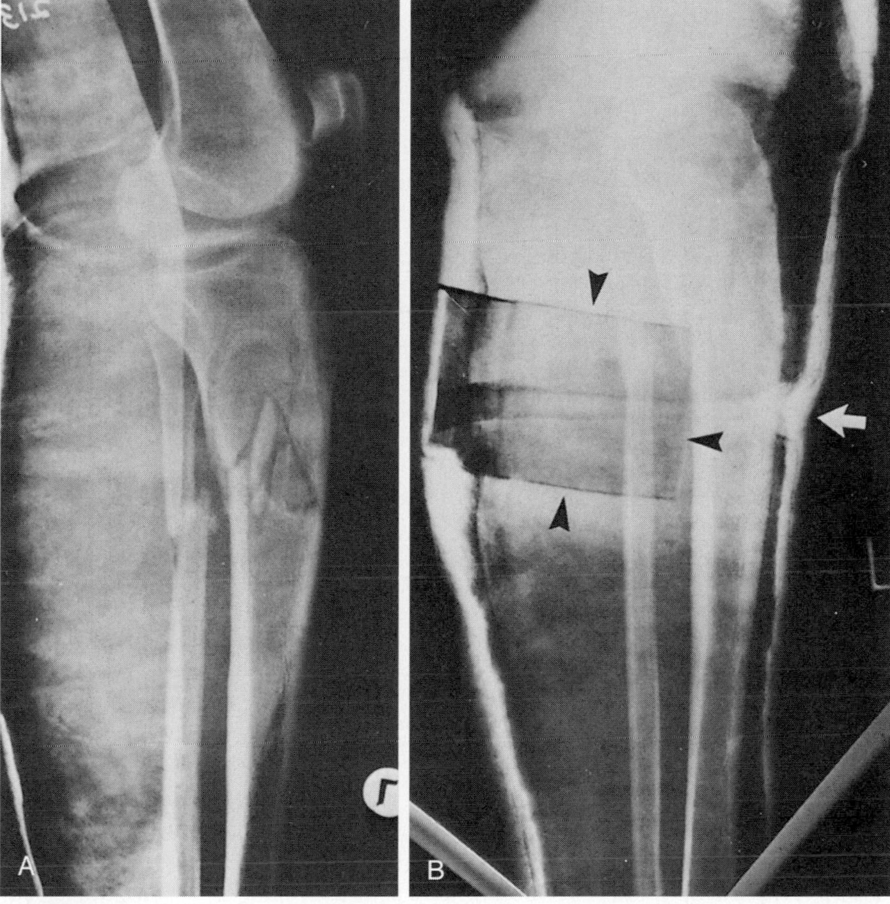

Figure 7–1. Casts used in the treatment of an open comminuted fracture of the proximal tibia and fibula. *A,* Initially, a molded posterior plaster splint was used so that the open anterior wound could be visualized and treated. Note that plaster overlies only the posterior aspect of the leg. *B,* A long leg cast was then used. The cast was wedged (*arrow*). A rectangular window was incised into the cast (*arrowheads*) so that the wound could be inspected.

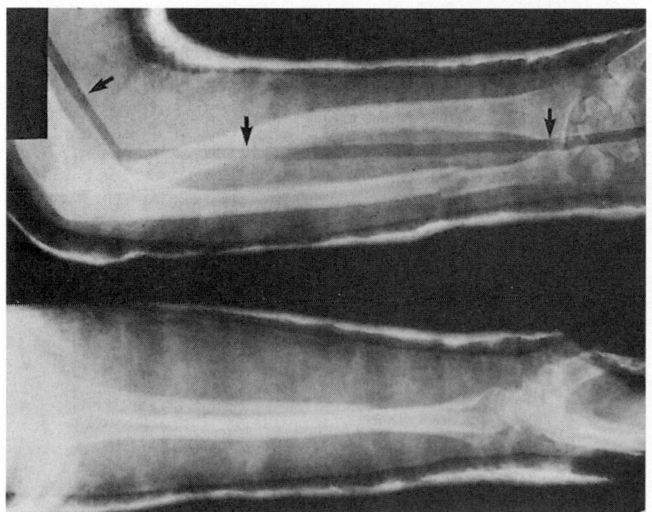

Figure 7–2. Long arm cast for treatment of fracture of both bones of the forearm. The forearm is held in the neutral position. A linear cut is made along the longitudinal axis of the cast and the cast spread to allow space for swelling. The cut causes a lucent band along the long axis of the cast (*arrows*). The cut is not visualized when viewed at a 90-degree angle.

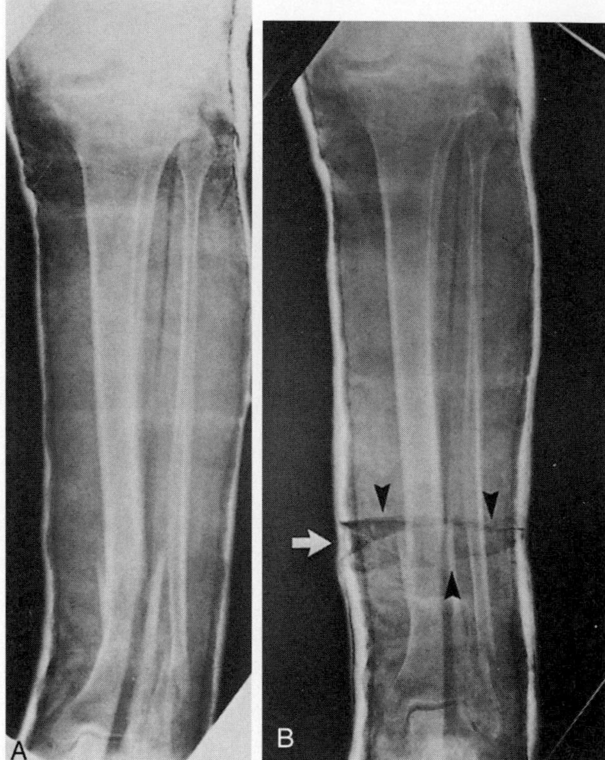

Figure 7–3. Wedging of cast to correct angulation. *A,* A comminuted fracture of the distal third of the tibia and fibula is enclosed in a long leg cast. There is a 20-degree medial angulation of the distal fragment. *B,* A transverse cut (*arrowheads*) was made in the cast at the level of the tibial fracture, and the cast was wedged open medially (*arrow*), which corrected the angulation of the tibial fracture.

are joined by two hinged braces incorporated into the plaster. This technique allows motion and prevents joint stiffness.

In the past two decades, Fiberglas or plastic materials have been used for casting. These materials are lightweight, waterproof, and radiolucent, and they are cured by light. Some materials may require that the entire casted limb be placed within a special circular apparatus for curing, which many surgeons have found to be time consuming and cumbersome. These casts are not used routinely in the initial treatment of fractures, but they have been useful in some situations after the first cast change.

Traction has been used routinely for centuries in the initial reduction of fractures and dislocations.[58, 62, 71] Only relatively recently, however, has continuous traction been used in the treatment of fractures. The traction may be applied to either the skin or the skeleton (see Fig. 7–4*A* and *B*). In skin traction, an adherent bandage or tape is applied directly to the skin, and traction is applied to the limb by attaching weights to the tape. Because the skin is irritated by the combination of the forces and tape, skin traction is usually used only temporarily before some form of definitive therapy. Skeletal traction was initially achieved by the use of tongs, but today application of tongs is limited to the production of cervical traction by attachment to the skull. Steinmann introduced a method of skeletal traction using thin metal rods measuring 2 to 6 mm in diameter,[62, 71] which he called *pins* (see Fig. 7–4*A* and *B*). These pins are placed transversely through the bone, and weights are attached by a system of rope or wire and pulleys. Steinmann pins are used frequently in the treatment of femoral fractures by placement of the pin in the proximal tibia or distal femur.

In severely comminuted or unstable fractures of the tibia, Steinmann pins may be placed proximal and distal to the fracture sites and their ends incorporated in a plaster cast—the pins-and-plaster technique (Figs. 7–5 and 7–6). The pins-and-plaster technique maintains length and alignment and prevents rotation of the fracture components. There are externally placed metallic devices (Fig. 7–7) designed to hold similarly placed pins above and below fractures. These external fixators are believed to have an advantage over the pins-and-plaster technique and have replaced it (see "External Fixation" for further discussion).

Open Fractures

Open fractures of long bones present special problems in fracture management. The possibility of significant complications, such as osteomyelitis, delayed union, nonunion, residual disability, or amputation, is quite high.[23] Open fractures have been classified by Gustilo, with greatest predictive weight given to soft tissue involvement,[23, 25] as indicated in Table 7–1. Care of an open fracture in sequence is as follows[26]:

1. Treat all open fractures as an emergency.
2. Care for life-threatening injuries first.
3. Start antibiotics immediately.
4. Débride immediately, with repeated débridement in 1 to 3 days.
5. Stabilize the fracture.
6. Close the wound within 7 to 10 days, if possible.
7. Perform early bone grafting of the fracture.
8. Rehabilitate the affected extremity.

Aggressive early treatment is important, with appropriate débridement and copious intermittent lavage being the most important steps in management.[26] Fracture sta-

Table 7–1. Gustilo's Classification of Open Fractures

Type I	Laceration less than 1 cm long and clean
Type II	Laceration greater than 1 cm long without extensive soft tissue damage
Type IIIA	Severely comminuted or segmental fractures regardless of wound size; Soft tissue coverage of the fractured bone is adequate; Extensive soft tissue damage
Type IIIB	Extensive soft tissue injury or loss of soft tissue with periosteal stripping and bone exposure, massive contamination, and severe comminution of the fracture
Type IIIC	Any open fracture with an associated arterial injury that must be repaired irrespective of soft tissue injury

Data from Gustilo and Anderson[23] and Gustilo and colleagues.[24, 25]

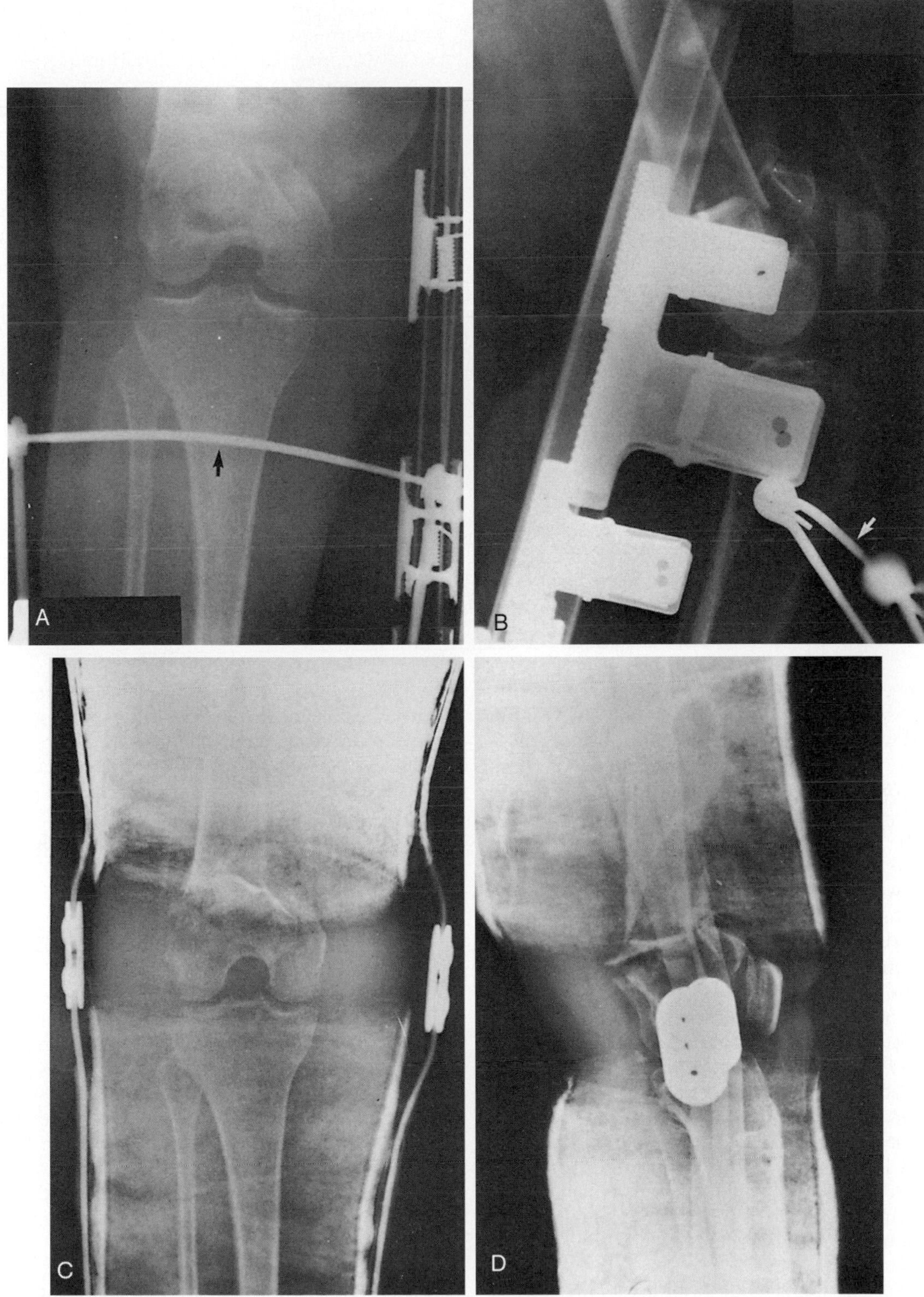

Figure 7–4. Comminuted supracondylar fracture of the femur, treated in balanced traction and cast brace. *A* and *B,* Anteroposterior (AP) and lateral views of the knee in a balanced traction device with a Steinmann pin (*arrow*) placed in the proximal tibia and attached to weights through a pulley system. *C* and *D,* AP and lateral views of the leg in a cast brace. Note the cast consists of two separate pieces, one above the knee and one below the knee, connected by a hinge on the medial and lateral surface. This setup allows motion of the knee joint.

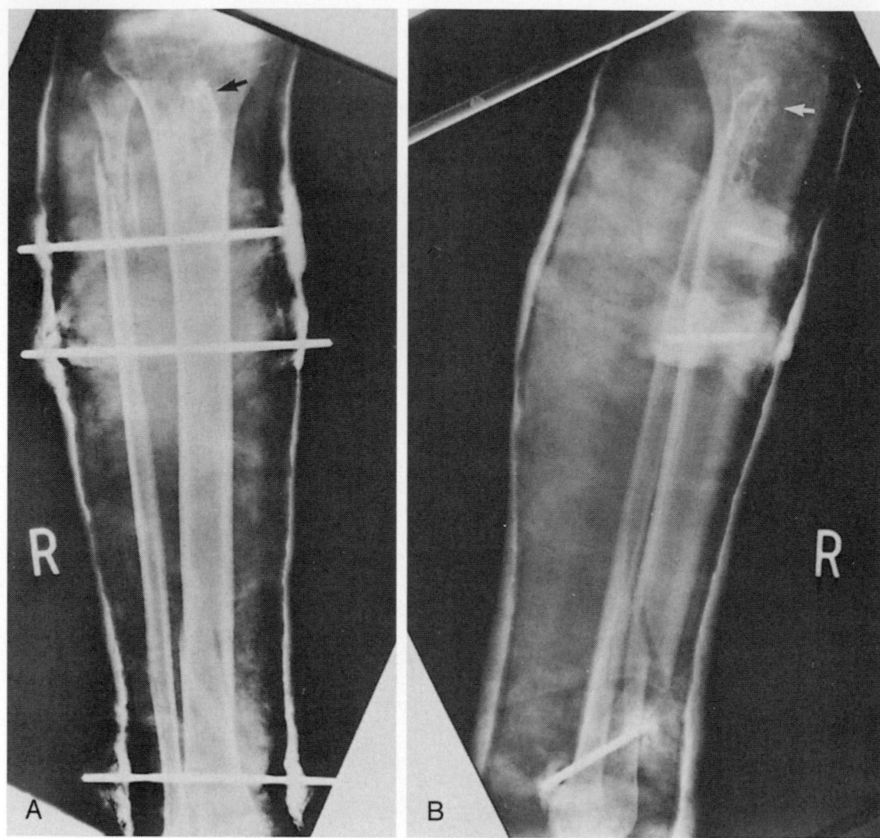

Figure 7–5. Pins-and-plaster technique used in the treatment of a spiral fracture of the distal third of the tibia and comminuted fracture of the proximal third of the fibula. *A* and *B,* Two pins are placed across the tibia proximal and one distal to the tibial fracture. The ends of the pin are incorporated into the cast, which controls both the length and rotation at the fracture site. Note the calcified bone infarct in the proximal tibia (*arrow*). The patient is an alcoholic with a previous history of pancreatitis.

bilization reduces the rate of infection and prevents further injury to adjacent soft tissues. Reduction and fixation are performed at the same time as initial débridement if the fracture is intra-articular. Intra-articular fractures must have anatomic reduction to expect reasonable future use of the joint.

Stabilization of fractures can be performed during the initial operative débridement. Either internal fixation or external fixation can be used. An external fixator is easy to apply with minimum operative trauma, and it allows easy access to the open wound later. Immediate fixation of type III fractures with intramedullary nailing or plate fixation carries a high infection rate and is discouraged.[14, 25] Fixation with a compression plate and screws is used for displaced intra-articular and metaphyseal fractures of the lower extremity and for upper extremity open fractures.[14, 26] Contraindications include severe contamination or extensive comminution; an external fixator is necessary in these cases. Types I and II open fractures can be treated immediately with an intramedullary nail, but infection is less likely if this treatment is used 10 to 14 days following wound closure.[14, 25] Skeletal traction may be used to maintain stability until the internal fixation is performed.

As soon as a clean, stable wound can be achieved, type III fractures can be treated with soft tissue reconstruction with coverage of exposed bone by a transported muscle pedicle or a free muscle transfer. These procedures prevent further contamination and infection, obliterate dead space, and provide coverage to allow later reconstruction.[26] Bone grafting of types I and II open fractures may be performed if severe comminution or bone loss is present. Local blood supply around these fractures should be minimally impaired, permitting bone grafting 2 to 3 weeks after the wound has healed. With type III open fractures there is significant soft tissue compromise, so autogenous bone grafting must be delayed for 6 weeks or more after wound healing. Type IIIC fractures with associated vascular injury carry a very high amputation rate of 42% to 70%.[25, 47]

Open Reduction and Internal Fixation

There are several acceptable indications for open reduction and internal fixation of fractures, which are chiefly related to the nature of the fracture and to a lesser extent are related to the skill and training of the surgeon. Although closed methods are generally preferred, certain fractures and certain situations do not lend themselves to a successful outcome without open reduction and fixation. The prime indication is the failure of closed manipulation. The instability of certain fractures is predictable from the outset on the basis of previous experience. A leading example of a situation in which healing is unlikely if closed methods are used is fractures of both bones of the forearm. Intertrochanteric or cervical fractures of the femur, although capable of healing without intervention, are fraught with frequent complications when treated by closed methods. Open reduction is also preferred because it substantially reduces the required length of hospital stay and the total expense incurred. Widely displaced avulsion fractures or transverse fractures of the patella

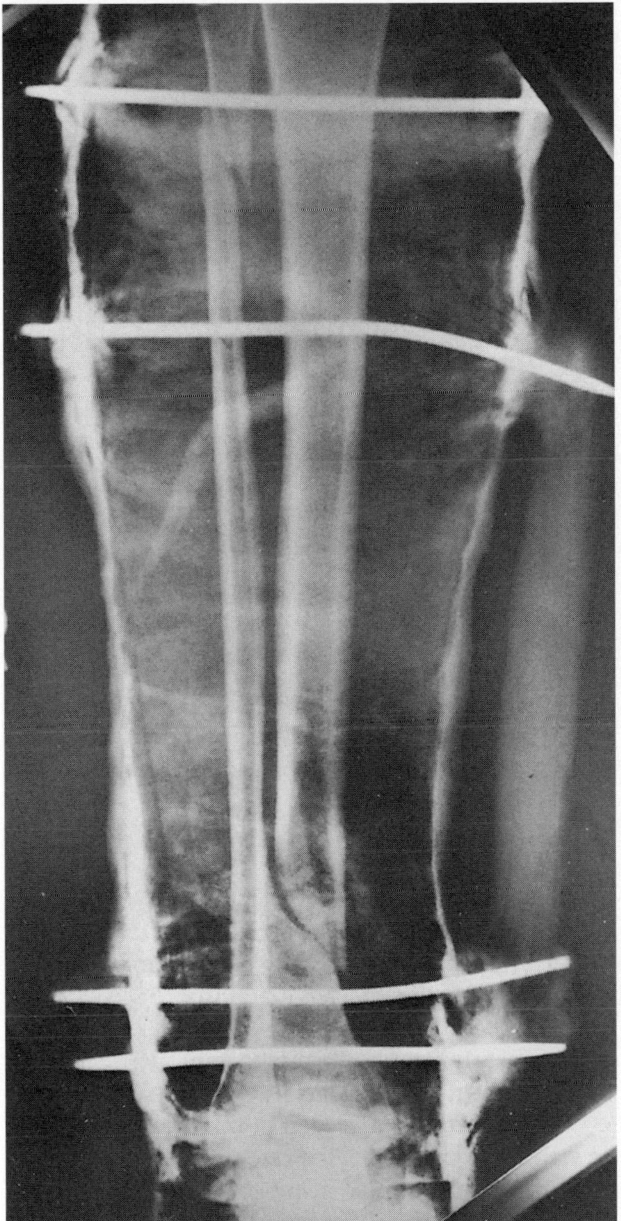

Figure 7–6. Pins-and-plaster technique using threaded Steinmann pins. Pins may be smooth (as in Figure 7–5A) or threaded (as demonstrated here). There are two pins distal and two pins proximal to the spiral fracture of the distal third of the tibia. There is also a spiral fracture of the proximal third of the fibula.

are unlikely to heal because of retraction of the attached muscles. In other cases, manipulation may have been attempted, but because of interposition of muscle or other soft tissue at the fracture site, apposition of the fracture fragments cannot be established. Reduction may be unsuccessful because one fragment has impaled surrounding muscle and is held by it; this is likely to occur in femoral shaft fractures.

Fractures involving the joint surface require accurate fixation of the fracture fragments. When a fragment of the joint surface—an osteochondral fracture—is avulsed free into the joint, usually it must be surgically removed to prevent further injury to the joint surface. Open reduction and fixation may also be indicated if there is significant associated arterial injury.

Open reduction and fixation of fractures imply the use of metal in some form. Metal may be used simply to place and hold the fragments in apposition or it may provide rigid fixation of the fracture. These two situations are not necessarily synonymous, and they should not be confused. Providing rigid fixation implies that the fracture has been stabilized and that external fixation may not be required, whereas placing and holding the fragments in apposition does not imply stabilization.

Sir Arbuthnot Lane[30, 46] of England championed the internal fixation of fractures, first using wire transfixion sutures and steel screws in the mid-1890s and then using German silver or steel plates in 1907. The development and acceptance of internal fixation were retarded by the problem of metal corrosion.[10, 11, 13, 68] When metal is placed in an electrolyte solution, an electric current is produced by its dissociation into metallic ions—the battery effect or galvanic corrosion. When two different metals are used and are in contact while in an electrolyte solution, one of the metals becomes positive and the other negative; in effect, one is an anode and the other a cathode because of the resultant electrolysis. These processes lead to corrosion and implant failure. There has been appreciable improvement with the introduction of more corrosive-resistant stainless steels, steel alloys, Vitallium, and titanium.

Wires are used as sutures or to encircle the shaft (i.e., cerclage) (Fig. 7–8) to hold bone fragments in apposition. Narrow metal bands—Parham bands (Fig. 7–9)—have been used circumferentially for the same purpose.

Screws are of two principal types. A *machine* or *cortical screw* is fully threaded from head to tip and is commonly used to transfix two fragments of cortical bone (Fig. 7–10). The *lag* or *cancellous screw* (Fig. 7–11) is not threaded beneath the head, in that portion referred to as the neck of the screw, and generally is not used in cortical bone, but it is thought by many to hold well in cancellous bone. Lag screws are used when it is inadvisable for the fixing screw to protrude beyond or through the opposite cortex.

Plates are strips of metal of varying width, thickness, and length that are secured to bone by screws inserted through circular holes or slots in the metal plate (see Figs. 7–10 and 7–22). One or two plates are used. They are placed longitudinally across the fracture with the fracture more or less at the midpoint of the plate. A minimum of four screws, usually an equal number proximal and distal to the fracture line, is used to transfix the plate.

A *compression plate* (see Fig. 7–10) is specially designed to allow or create axial compression forces to draw the fracture fragments into tight apposition during its application.[3, 59] This can be accomplished by fixing the plate to one side of a fracture and then applying a tension device to the other fracture fragment,[59] which pulls the plate toward it and thus draws the fragments into apposition. The other end of the plate is then transfixed with screws and the tension device is removed. This technique was popularized by Müller and associates[54] in the Arbeitsgemeinschaft für Osteosynthesfragen (AO), or its English

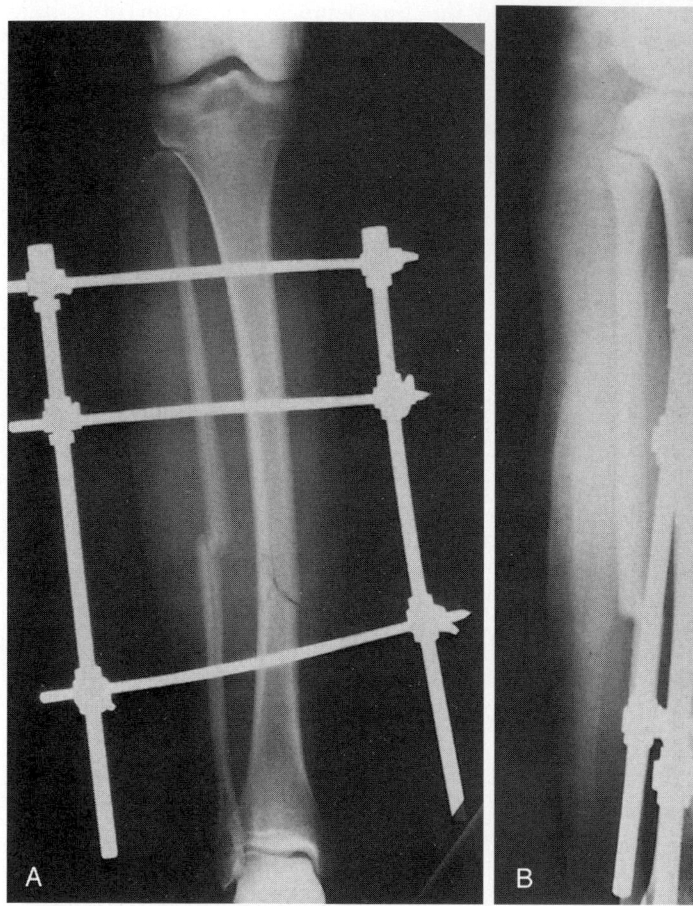

Figure 7–7. *A* and *B,* AP and lateral views of an external fixator used in the treatment of a fracture at the junction of the mid and distal thirds of the tibia with associated fracture of the fibula. Two pins are placed through the tibia proximal and one distal to the tibial fracture. These pins are then connected to threaded rods medially and laterally. The positions of the pins are then adjusted so that the fracture is in apposition with some degree of compression. This is a relatively simple external fixator device; others are more complicated, but the principle is the same.

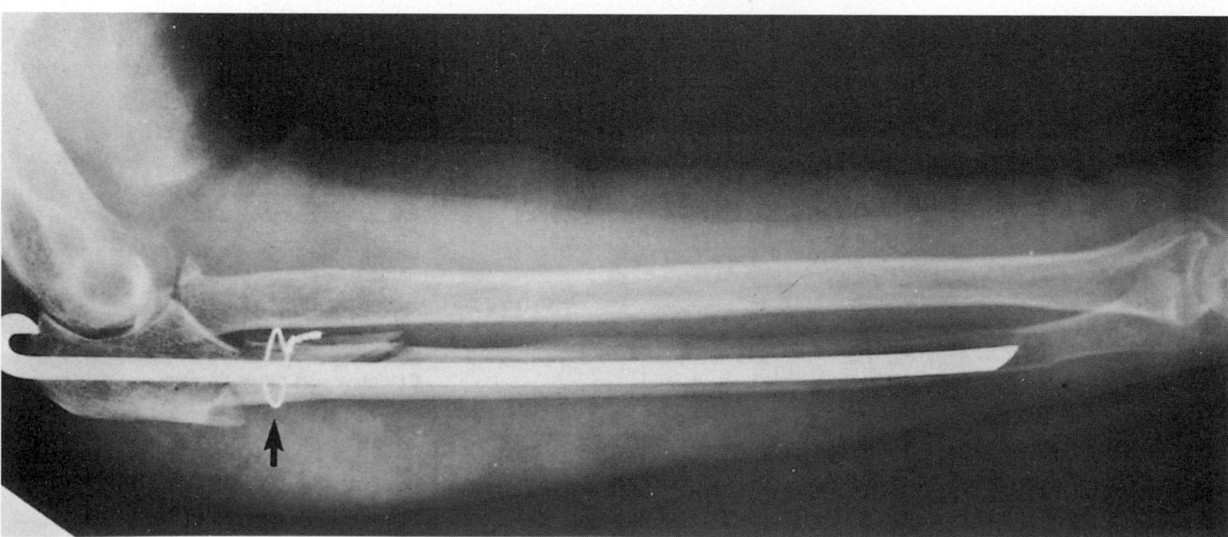

Figure 7–8. Rush rod and wire for cerclage used in treatment of a fracture-dislocation of the elbow. A Rush rod was inserted through the olecranon. Comminution at the fracture site required placement of a wire for cerclage (*arrow*). The radial head was excised.

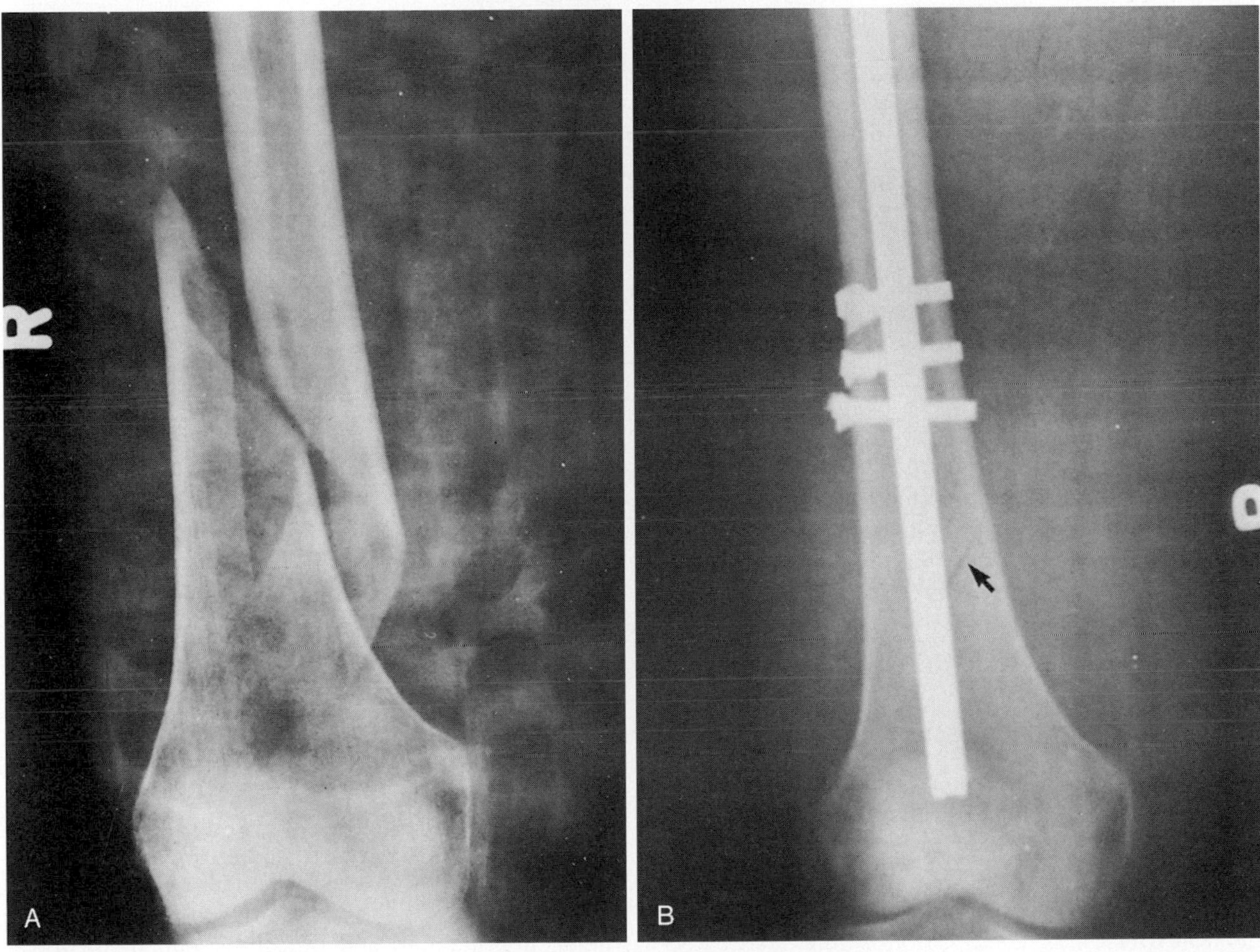

Figure 7–9. Spiral fracture of the distal third of the femur treated with Küntscher nail and three Parham bands. *A*, Anteroposterior view of the initial injury demonstrates a classic spiral fracture of the distal third of the shaft. The distal fragment is offset the width of the shaft, and there is approximately 2 cm of overriding of the fracture fragments. *B*, An immediate postoperative radiograph demonstrates the presence of the Küntscher nail and the three Parham bands. The reduction is so precise that it is difficult to identify the fracture line. Only the distal margin (*arrow*) is visualized. The obliteration of the fracture line is due to the accuracy of the reduction; it is not evidence of healing.

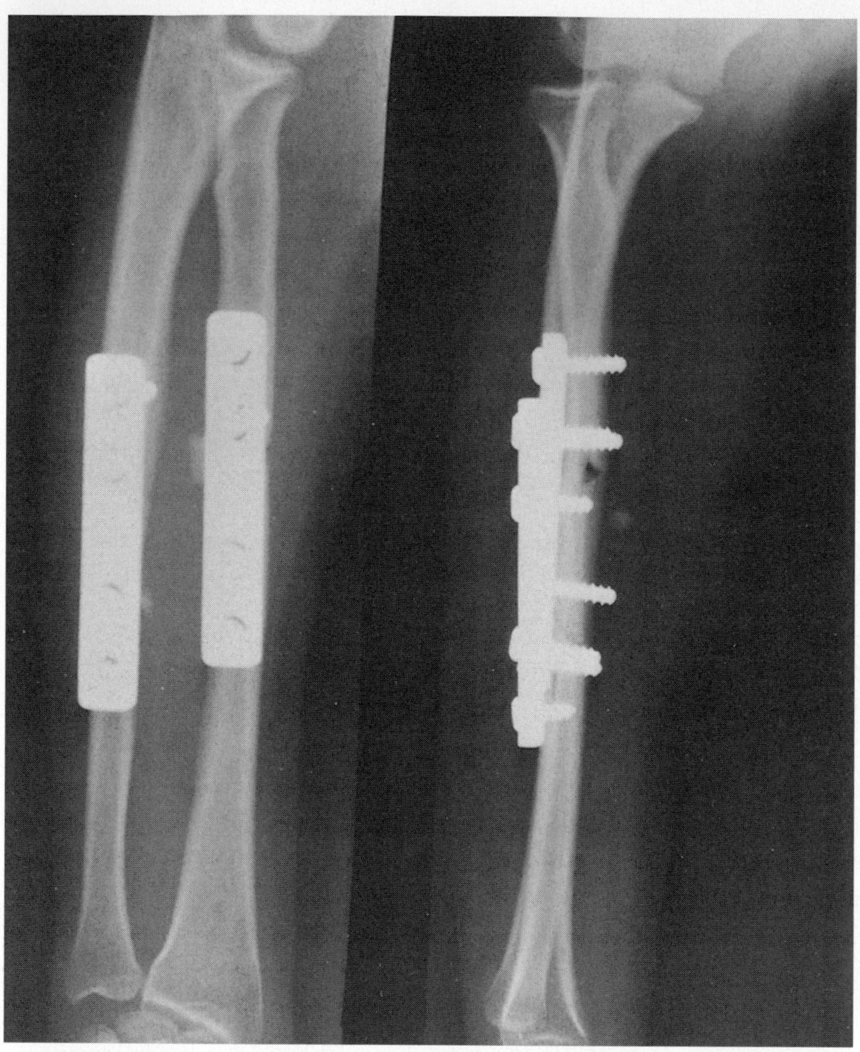

Figure 7–10. Compression plates and cortical screws used in the treatment of fractures of the middle third of both bones of the left forearm. There are two screws proximal to and two screws distal to the fracture in each plate. The holes within the plate are oval. The screws are threaded their entire length, identifying them as cortical screws.

designation, Swiss Association for the Study of Internal Fixation (ASIF). The ASIF has developed a whole system of plates, screws, and intramedullary nails to provide rigid internal fixation of fractures; thus, the term *AO compression plate* designates a compression plate of the organization's design. Compression plates have also been designed in which axial compression is generated by eccentric insertion of screws into oval or slotted holes.

For 40 years, the ASIF has directed the development and promulgation of correct surgical principles, instruments, and implants used for internal fixation.[49] Their work has been universally embraced by the orthopedic community. The group's tenets initially were anatomic reduction with rigid fixation to produce primary bone healing without callus. This goal was achieved using a wide subperiosteal exposure with reduction under direct vision. The entire circumference of the bone was exposed. Plates and screws were used for fixation. In the past decade, there has been a shift of emphasis from direct reduction and rigid fixation to techniques that emphasize preserving soft tissue and bone fragment vascularity while maintaining anatomic alignment and relative stability.[16, 49] Formation of callus is no longer deemed undesirable, and not all bone fragments must be returned to exact anatomic position unless they involve an articular surface. Soft tissue traction and fluoroscopic visualization are used during fracture manipulation. Longer plates with fewer screws are employed, and much less exposure of the fracture site is performed. The entire circumference of the bone is not exposed as was formerly.[49]

Certain plates are bent at one end for the purpose of being inserted into and transfixing one of the fracture fragments. These plates are referred to as *blade plates* (see Fig. 7–11), and they are most commonly used in the treatment of supracondylar fractures of the femur.

Intramedullary rods (see Fig. 7–8) and *nails* (Fig. 7–12; see Fig. 7–9) are metal devices of varying width and length inserted directly into the medullary cavity of a long bone to align and fix a shaft fracture. They are frequently used alone and do not require other forms of fixation. They serve as intramedullary splints of the fracture. Groves[22] of England introduced this method of treatment for femoral shaft fractures in 1918. Küntscher[41–45] of Germany perfected the method during World War II. There are many types of nails (see Figs. 7–9 and 7–12) in use that vary in design, particularly in their cross-sectional configuration. The Küntscher nail is a cloverleaf in cross section; others are diamond, oval, or square. This mismatch of shape with that of the intramedullary canal allows three-point frictional fixation between

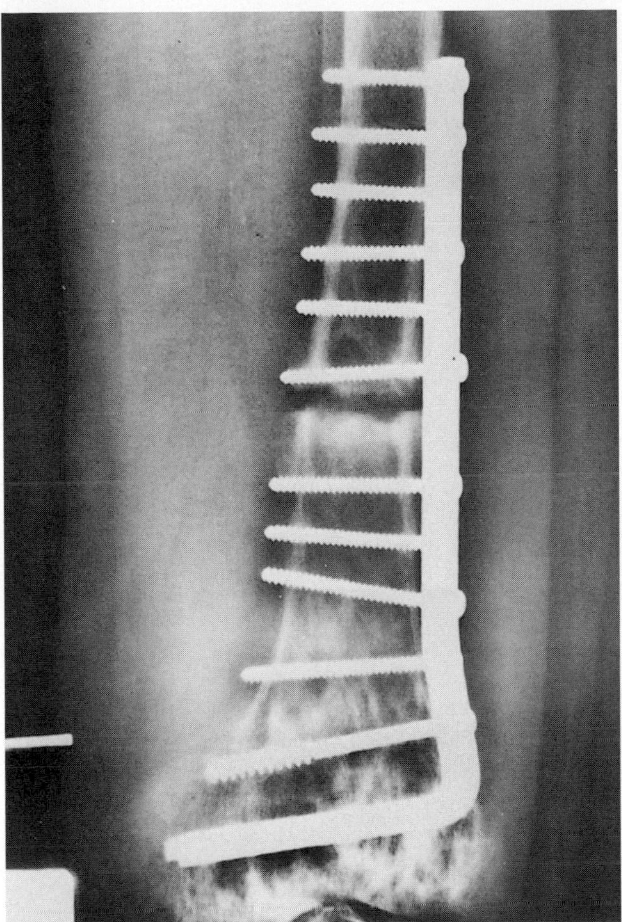

Figure 7–11. Blade plate used in the treatment of a transverse fracture of the distal shaft of the femur affected by Paget's disease. The plate is bent and inserted into the femoral condyles. A single lag or cancellous screw is used above the base of the plate. The remaining screws are machine or cortical screws. The cancellous screw has coarse threads, and its neck is not threaded.

the nail and the cortex for stability but allows room for revascularization of the cortex.[15] The nails measure 8 to 17 mm in diameter. The trend is to insert nails and rods blindly from the end of a bone (through the greater trochanter, tibial tubercle, or greater tuberosity) with radiographic control. The preference is to do this without opening the fracture site, although it cannot always be achieved. Not opening the fracture site preserves the soft tissue vasculature surrounding the fracture. Nails are primarily used in the treatment of femoral, tibial, humeral, ulnar, and radial fractures.

Intramedullary nails allow fixation of a fracture without surgically opening the fracture site, which is necessary if compression plating is used. As a result, fewer infections and nonunions occur than do in fractures treated with plate fixation.[9, 67] The intramedullary nails are of two types: reamed or unreamed. The unreamed nails may be small and flexible or large in diameter and very stiff.[14, 28] Several small flexible unreamed nails (e.g., Ender rods) are used simultaneously to completely fill the medullary cavity (Figs. 7–13 and 7–14) in order to provide stability, whereas a single large unreamed nail is used alone. Unreamed nails have the advantage of having an uncomplicated and quick insertion. They are thought to cause less damage to the medullary blood supply than reamed nails.[14] Disadvantages of intramedullary nail fixation, especially in the tibia and femur, include development of rotational deformity of the distal fracture fragment, particularly with distal fractures; shortening if the fracture is comminuted[2, 28]; and the possibility of a nail with too large a diameter getting stuck in the medullary cavity and, if forced, causing an additional fracture. Therefore, additional external support may also be needed to prevent shortening or torsion.

Reaming allows use of larger and therefore stiffer intramedullary nails that are less susceptible to fatigue fracture and increases contact area between the nail and the bone. Reaming also causes fat and other marrow elements to embolize into the general circulation.[15] Reamed nails fit tightly within the medullary cavity and

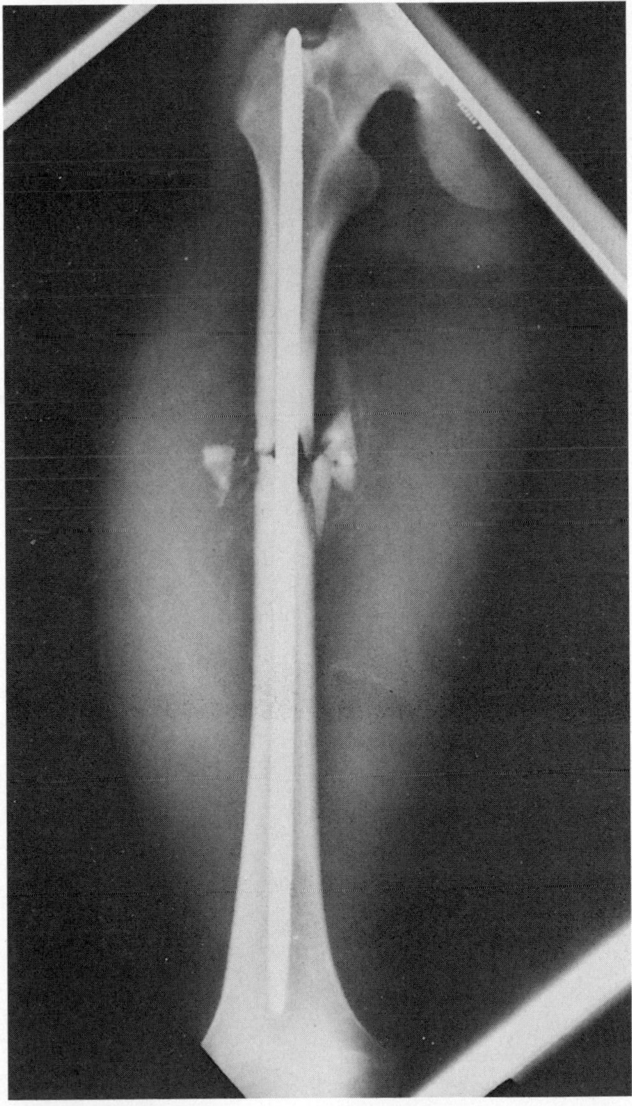

Figure 7–12. A Schneider nail used in the treatment of a midshaft fracture of the femur. The nail fits snugly within the medullary cavity. It protrudes through the greater trochanter, and its distal tip is located immediately proximal to the femoral condyles. The examination was performed 3 weeks after the insertion, and early callus formation is present at the fracture site.

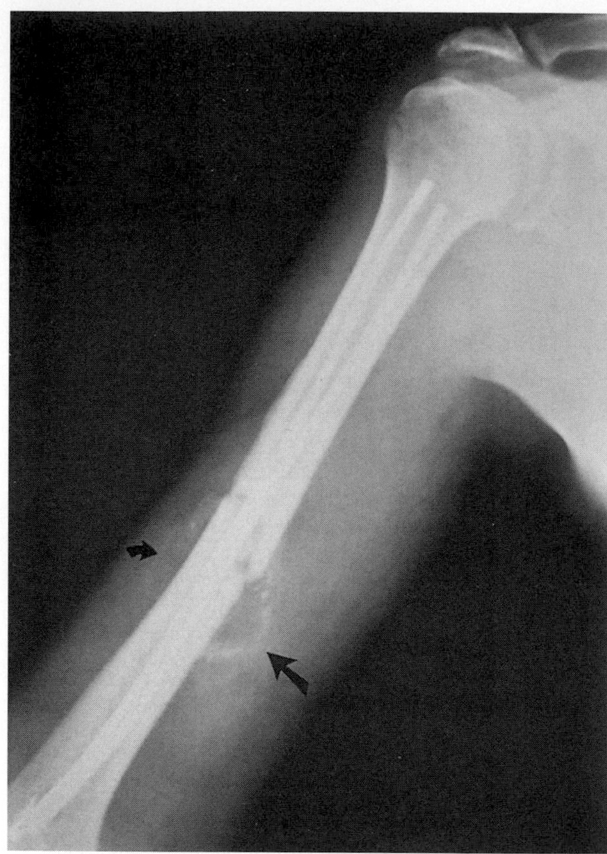

Figure 7–13. Midshaft humeral fracture with internal fixation with two Ender rods. The flexibility of the Ender rods allows a small amount of motion of the fractured bone ends with resulting exuberant calcified callus formation seen surrounding the fracture site (*arrows*).

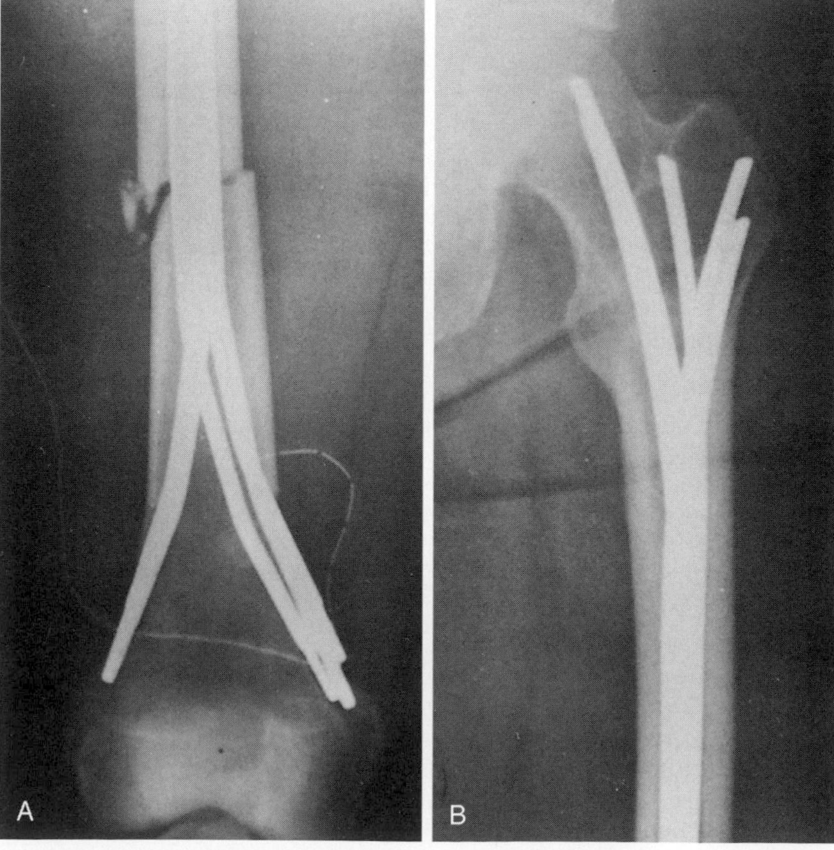

Figure 7–14. Ender rods used in the treatment of a fracture of the distal third of the shaft of the femur. *A,* This initial postoperative radiograph demonstrates five Ender rods inserted through holes cut in the medial and lateral cortex of the supracondylar portion of the femur. The rods are then passed up the shaft under fluoroscopic control. *Dashed line* represents a radiopaque marker in a drain within the surgical wound. *B,* To visualize the entire length of the rod, it is often necessary to obtain two radiographs. This separate examination of the proximal femur demonstrates the position of the proximal end of the five Ender rods.

impinge on the endosteal cortex of the bone to maintain rigid splinting.[28] They may be either locking or nonlocking nails. The locking variety has cross screws or bolts that are passed through the metaphyseal cortex of the long bone and through holes near the end of the nail and then through the opposite bony cortex, which locks the nail in place, preventing twisting or shortening of the bone by fracture fragments telescoping or sliding over one another (Fig. 7–15).[38] Screws can be inserted through both ends of the nail, usually two at each end, forming a very stable and stiff fracture fixation. Such fixation is called *static nailing* when interlocking screws are used at both ends of the nail and *dynamic nailing* when interlocking screws are used at only one end.[38] Rotational deformity and shortening are prevented by this very rigid fixation, and smaller diameter nails can be used that do not get stuck during insertion. They provide much more stable fixation than nonlocking nails and solve most of the problems of nonlocking nails. Even severely comminuted or segmental fractures (see Fig. 7–15) can be immobilized with interlocking nails without losing bone length during healing.[40] For the interlocking nails to work, it is necessary that the fracture occur far enough from the bone end to allow room to place the interlocking screws through unfractured bone. *Retrograde nailing* through the intercondylar notch into the femur allows nailing of the most distal metaphyseal fractures (Fig. 7–16).[29] No external support is needed with interlocking nails, and earlier weight bearing with joint use is possible, unlike with nonlocking nails. By 6 to 8 weeks, full weight bearing is possible with stable fractures.[2, 28] When healing is not evident on radiographs at 4 months, the distal screws may be removed to increase stress and stimulate bone production at the fracture site.[28, 55] Intramedullary rods are used mostly to treat tibial and femoral fractures. Fractures in the upper extremity are more often internally fixed with plates and screws than rods because of the difficulty of inserting the rods.[14]

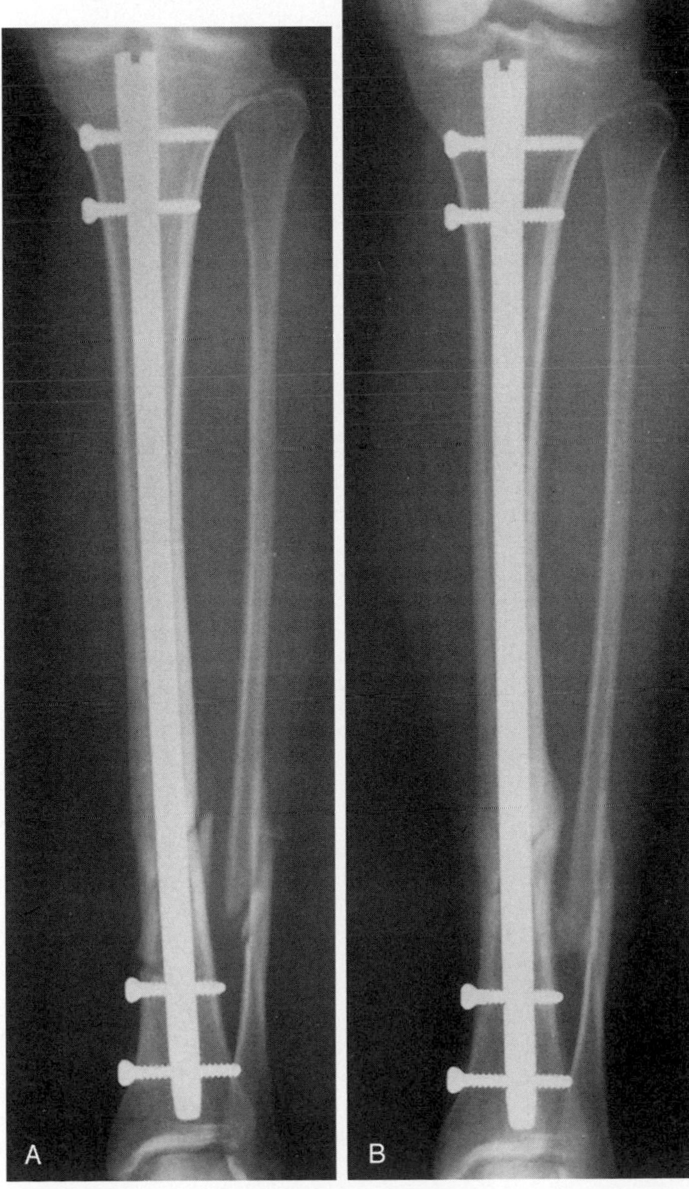

Figure 7–15. Interlocking nail fixation of a tibial fracture. *A*, Intramedullary rod with interlocking screws maintains the normal length of the tibia even with a distal comminuted fracture. *B*, The tibia and fibula fractures have healed with normal alignment without any loss of length 13 weeks later.

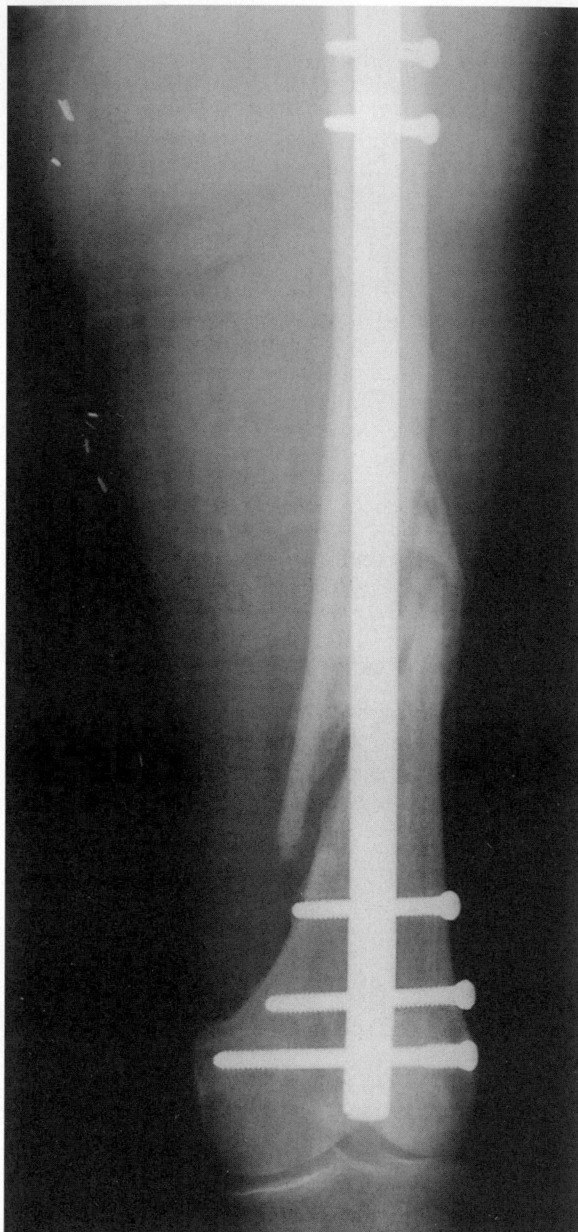

Figure 7–16. Calcified callus bridges the lateral margin of an oblique fracture of the distal femur fixed with an intramedullary rod inserted retrograde through the intercondylar notch. The interlocking screws may be placed more distal with the retrograde rod than with an antegrade rod, allowing fixation of very distal femoral fractures. The rod fits tightly in the medullary canal in the middle third of the femur.

Disadvantages of using interlocking nails include the high cost of tooling up initially to do the procedure. Also, the operative procedure used to insert these rods is demanding and has a significant learning curve.[28, 34] Biplanar (C-arm) fluoroscopic capability is necessary to perform the procedure.

Rods are, in essence, thinner nails. They do not fill the intramedullary cavity. Rush rods (see Fig. 7–8) are round, in cross section measure 2.5 to 6 mm in diameter, and have a hook at one end, and they once (but no longer) were frequently used in the treatment of radius fractures. Ender rods[7, 19] (see Figs. 7–13 and 7–14) are flexible and slightly curved at the ends, and they are used in multiples, usually three or more, to treat fractures of the tibia and femur. The number of rods needed to fill up the medullary cavity of the fractured long bone is used. With the medullary cavity filled with these rods, the fracture cannot displace and therefore is immobilized. The rods are slightly flexible, which allows an amount of motion slight enough to promote a large quantity of callus formation but not sufficient to cause nonunion (see Fig. 7–13).

The devices used for fixation of intertrochanteric fractures are also called nails (Fig. 7–17), consisting of a short rod or nail and a baseplate. The nail is inserted through the greater trochanter toward the femoral head to transfix

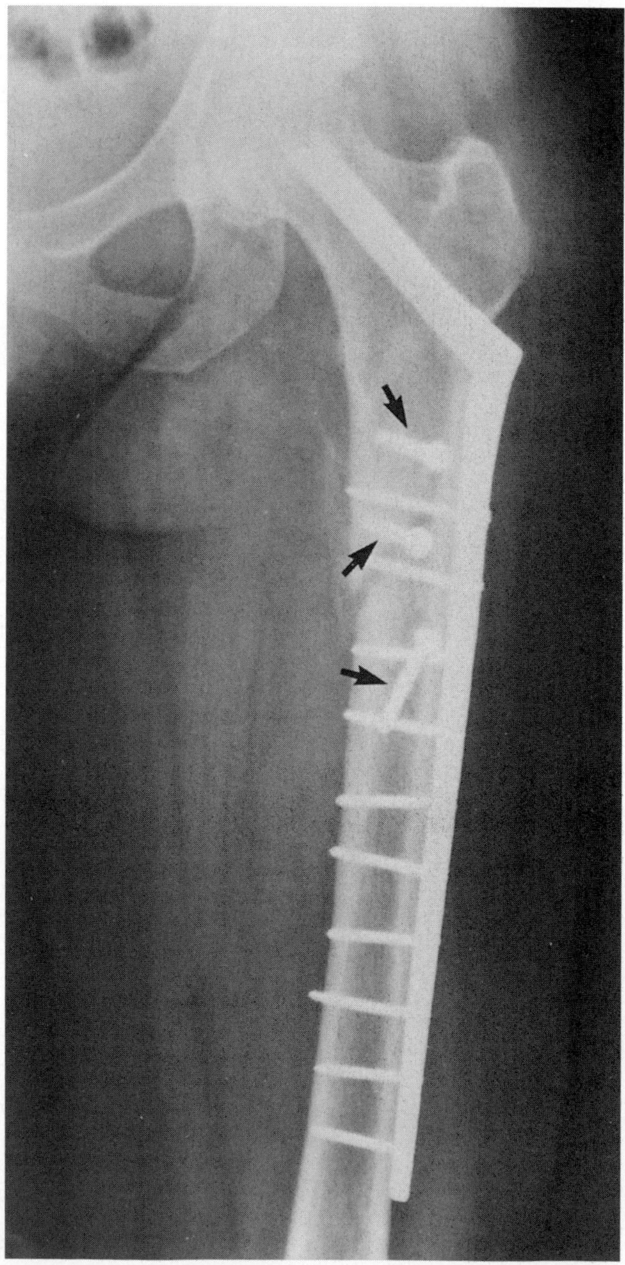

Figure 7–17. A long-bladed Jewett nail used in the treatment of a comminuted subtrochanteric fracture. The screws are machine or cortical screws. In addition to the plate, three cortical screws (*arrows*) were used to transfix comminuted fragments.

the fracture, and the baseplate is fixed to the femoral shaft by screws to hold the nail in place. This type of nail was introduced by Smith-Petersen[65] of Boston in 1931. The nail and plate of the original device were separate; the nail was threaded on one end and fixed to the plate by a nut. The device was later constructed of a single piece.

The *Richard compression screw* and *plate* (Fig. 7–18) have replaced nail and plate fixation of intertrochanteric fractures. Unlike the hip nails, the large thread of the screw rarely cuts through the bone of the femoral head. The shank of the screw slides through the cylinder extension of the proximal end of the plate, which allows the fracture fragments to impact as the screw slides backward through the cylinder. The impaction is controlled and only allowed along the axis of the cylinder. A notch running the full length of the interior of the cylinder fits into a square-bottomed channel in the screw shank and prevents the screw from turning; it only can slide. The impaction of the fracture fragments usually is only slight but leads to rapid fracture healing.

Kirschner introduced the use of thin, 1 to 1.5 mm diameter, stiff wires (Fig. 7–19) to transfix smaller fragments of bone, such as a separated medial epicondyle of the humerus to the humeral shaft, or for intramedullary fixation of small bones such as the phalanges. These wires are commonly referred to as *K wires*.

The use of internal fixation devices is not without complication. Obviously there is the possibility of osteomyelitis. Meticulous sterile technique is mandatory as these devices are being applied or inserted. Excessive stress may lead to bending or fracture of the appliance. Metal fatigue may also lead to fracture of a plate (see Fig. 7–22) or nail. Overly vigorous insertion of an intramedullary nail or appliance may fracture the bone (Fig. 7–20). An attempt to insert too large a nail may result in its becoming jammed in the medullary cavity.

Most appliances must eventually be removed. The screw holes are areas of relative weakness and tend to serve as foci for stress. Fractures may then occur through them. It is necessary to protect the limb following removal of the screws to allow the holes to heal and thereby prevent such fractures.

External Fixation

External fixation relies on pins of 4, 5, or 6 mm in diameter that are inserted through both cortices of the

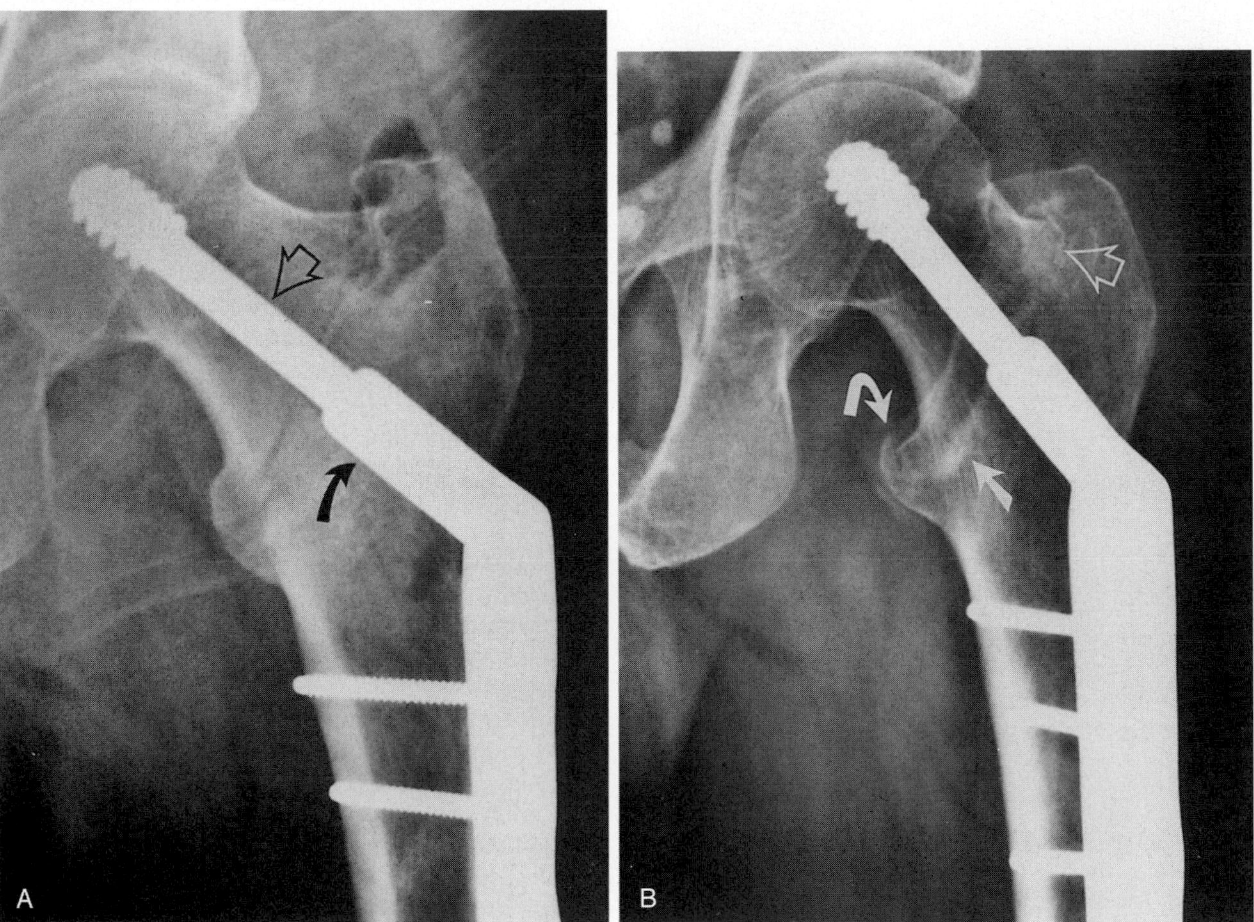

Figure 7–18. Richard screw and plate fixation of an intertrochanteric fracture. *A,* Intertrochanteric fracture without displacement after internal fixation using a Richard screw and plate. The screw shank (*open arrow*) of the appliance slides within the cylinder extension (*black arrow*) of the side plate. *B,* The sliding screw allows impaction of the fracture fragments (*arrows*), which has occurred in the 17 days since the radiograph in *A* was taken. Impacted fractures heal quickly, which is one of the advantages of this appliance.

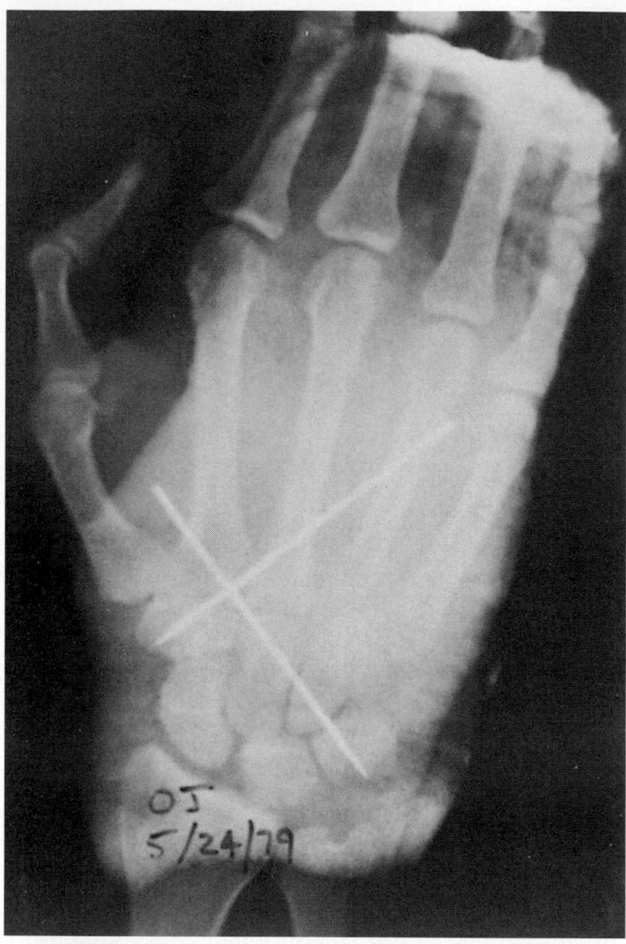

Figure 7–19. Kirschner wires (K wires) used in reduction of a second and third metacarpal-carpal fracture-dislocation. The wires are thin, nonthreaded, and pointed on one end. The hand is in a molded palmar plaster splint.

fractured bone proximal and distal to the fracture site. They may be unilateral, extending through a single skin surface with attachment to a rigid metal rod outside the patient, or they may be bilateral, extending through the skin on both sides of the limb, where they attach to medial and lateral external rods (Fig. 7–21) for stability.[55] The pins are attached to the external rods by special clamps that can be attached to exert either distraction or compression.[4] A hinge is present in some devices to allow correction of fracture angulation.

External fixation is used for static immobilization of a fracture, for compression of a distracted fracture, and for distraction during limb lengthening. It is often used to stabilize open fractures (especially type III), in cases of infected nonunions, when vascular damage is present that needs repair, and when severe soft tissue injury (e.g., a burn) is present superficial to a fracture site.[4] The primary complication has been infection introduction via the pin tracts.[4, 7]

The most recent addition to the external fixation armamentarium has been the introduction of the Ilizarov apparatus from Russia.[34, 35] It consists of multiple rigid metal circular or semicircular rings to which are attached to 1.5- or 1.8-mm diameter Kirschner wires (see Fig. 7–21). The Kirschner wires optimally pass through the bone at approximately 90 degrees to one another, or a third wire may be necessary. They are attached to the metal rings under considerable tension by a special tensioning device. This process converts them into relatively stiff pins. The rings are connected together by threaded rods. Multiple hinges, spacers, posts, support plates, and translation assemblies are also part of the available hardware system.[36] Most of the Kirschner wires are smooth, but some have a welded knob that looks like an olive on a skewer, hence the name *olive wire* (see Fig. 7–21*C*). Olive wires are used when extensive translation of bone is desired. They can be pulled from one end without pulling the wire through the bone (see Fig. 7–21*C–E*).

Ilizarov has greatly expanded the role of external fixation.[35, 36] His apparatus is probably not superior to all other external fixators, but his ideas of what can be done with the apparatus are. His idea that bone can be readily reshaped goes far beyond fracture treatment. His ideas are probably the most important new ideas with current usefulness to the orthopedist dealing with fractures and bone healing in the past two decades. The Ilizarov external fixator is most frequently used for treatment of severely comminuted fractures, nonunion, malunion, replacing segmental defects of fractures, and lengthening of congenitally short limbs.[72] Vigorous physical therapy and use of the limb while the external fixator is in place is advocated irrespective of the reason for its employment. The technique used is as follows for bone lengthening[34–36]:

1. The cortex is cut with a subperiosteal osteotome, taking great care not to damage the blood supply of the periosteum or medullary cavity.
2. At least one but usually two rings of the external fixator are attached both above and below the corticotomy site to eliminate micromotion, except in the axis of the bone.
3. A 3- to 7-day delay is made after surgery before initiating distraction to allow local neovascularization.
4. A distraction rate of 1.0 mm per day is applied contingent on the appearance of bone forming in the distraction gap.
5. Distraction is applied in frequent small increments four or more times per day.
6. After distraction has corrected the abnormality, neutral fixation is used for a time lasting at least as long as the time for limb lengthening or defect correction to permit adequate ossification.
7. Use of the limb and physical therapy are used throughout the time the fixator is in place.

This technique allows a surgeon to create the equivalent of a growth plate anywhere in a long or flat bone.[36] The most important aspects of this procedure are maintenance of rigid fixation and an undisturbed blood supply.[34–36]

Ilizarov's idea that bone is a relatively plastic tissue has allowed him to stretch and reshape it to correct a host of orthopedic problems.[34–36] Prior to Ilizarov's work, fracture healing was thought to occur only in terms of compression loading.[53] The idea of bone formation under tension stress began for Ilizarov in 1956 when he observed bone formation within the distraction site during the course of treat-

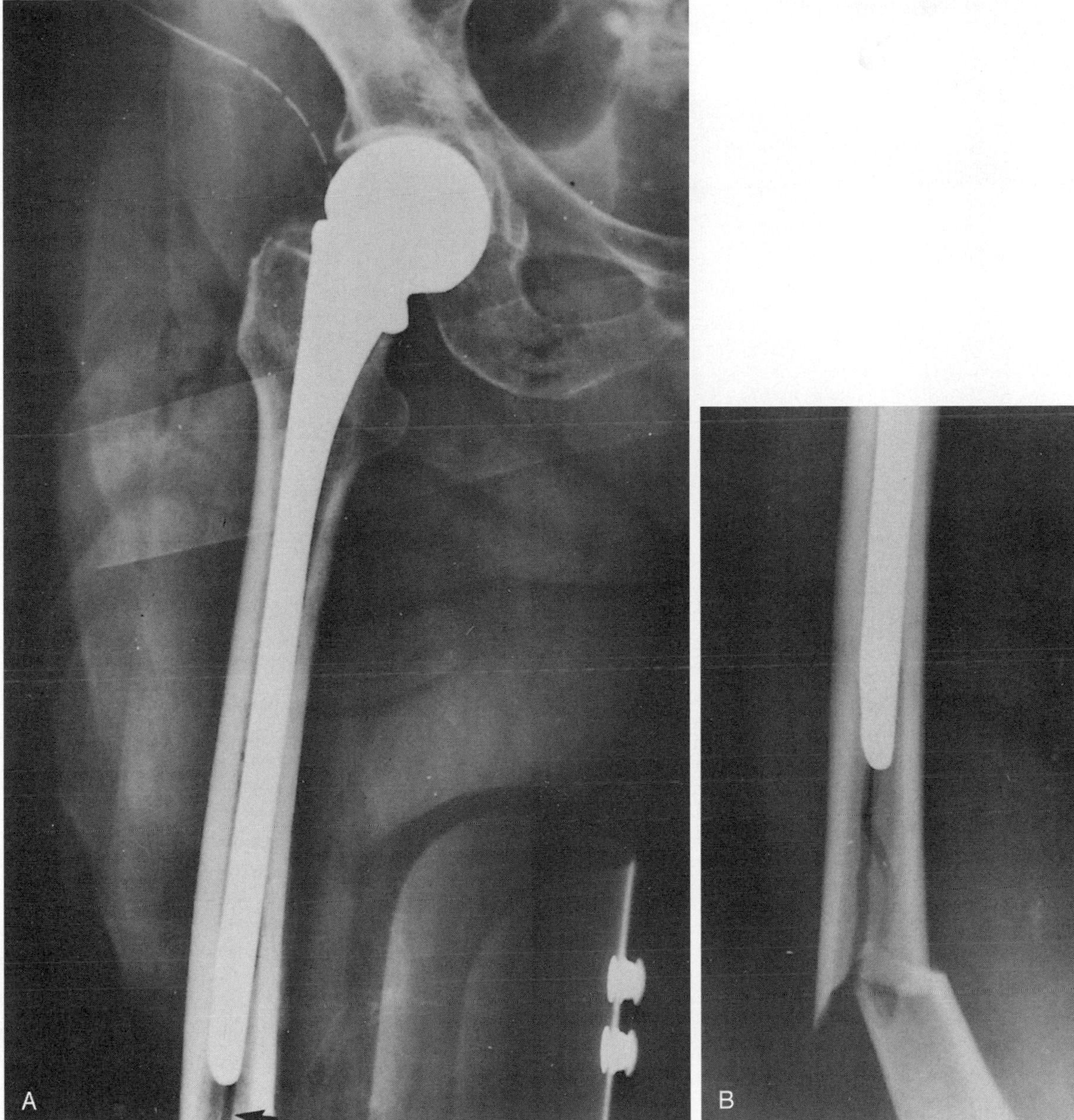

Figure 7–20. Fracture of the distal femoral shaft occurring during insertion of a long-stemmed Thompson femoral head prosthesis for treatment of a displaced fracture of the femoral neck. *A,* At the distal tip of the stem is an abnormal vertical lucent area (*arrow*). *Dashed lines* at the lateral margin of the prosthetic head represent a drain in the surgical wound. This film was obtained at the completion of the operative procedure. *B,* A repeat examination that includes more of the distal femoral shaft reveals that the vertical lucent area seen in *A* is actually the vertical component of a fracture of the femoral shaft that occurred during insertion of the prosthesis. It is important to radiograph and observe the entire length of the prosthetic device immediately after insertion to identify such complications.

ing an ankylosed knee by traditional osteotomy, distraction with external fixation, and bone grafting.[37] Subsequent experiments on canine tibias led to formulation of what he calls the Principle or Law of Tension-Stress. It states that living tissue with normal blood supply under slow, steady traction becomes metabolically activated to stimulate both proliferative and biosynthetic cellular functions.[34–36]

In 1954, Ilizarov was first able to heal pseudarthroses and nonunion fractures by alternating local compression and distraction with his external fixator to convert the interface into new bone,[33] called transformational osteogenesis.[5] A fibrous nonunion is initially treated with distraction to induce osteogenesis. As soon as new bone is seen radiographically, the tension is changed to compression to hasten mineralization and solid fusion.[33] Ilizarov also has successfully treated mobile pseudarthroses by compression of 1 mm per day for 10 to 15 days. This technique is thought to cause local necrosis and stimulate neovascularization. Once local bone resorption is seen radiographically, the compression is changed to distraction to initiate osteogenesis. When new bone formation is seen radiographically in the pseudarthrosis site, compression replaces the distraction to achieve fusion.[37]

Either distraction or compression can be applied with the external fixator, and both have been used by Ilizarov

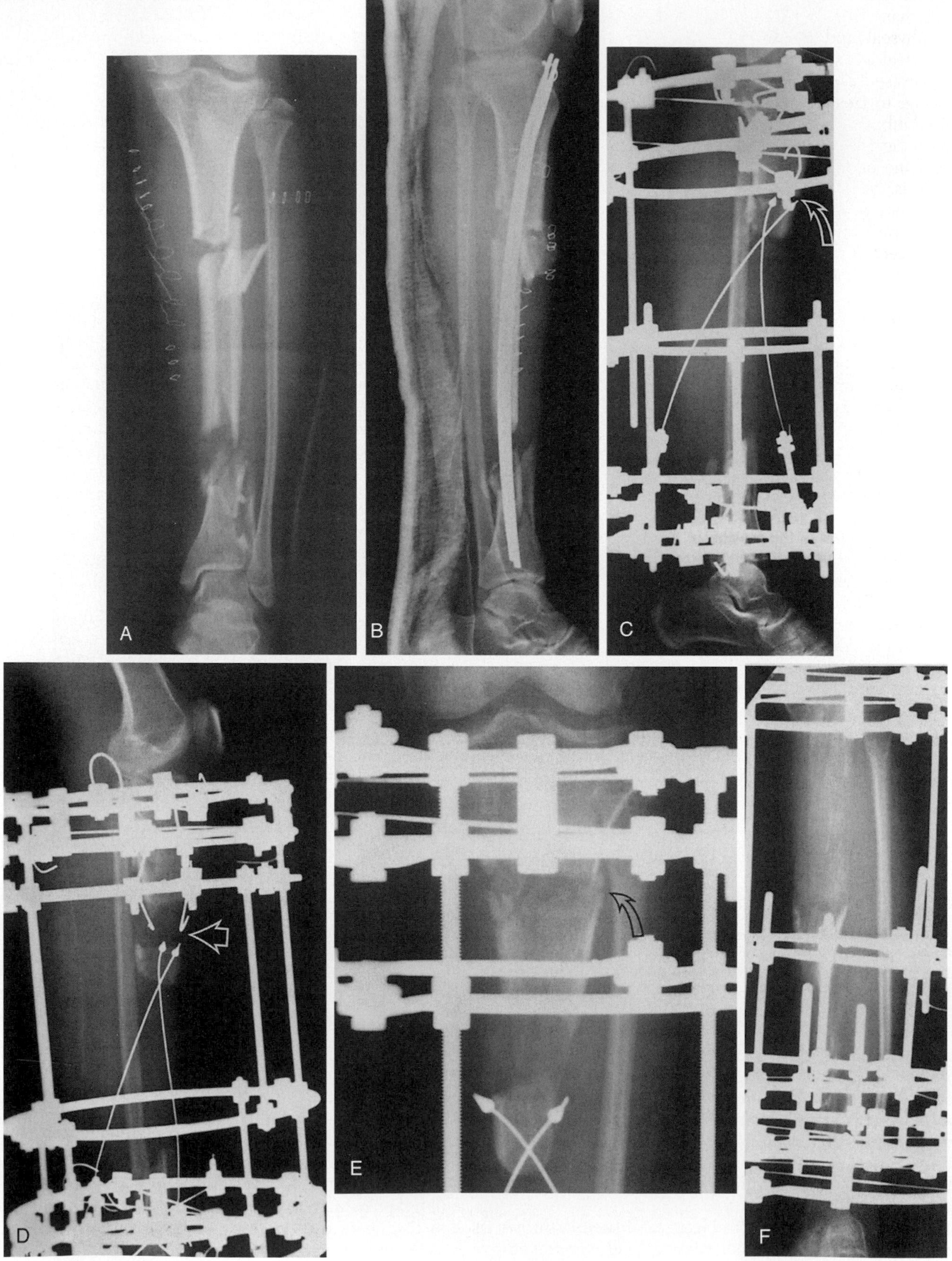

Figure 7–21. *See legend on opposite page.*

in more than 15,000 patients and by others worldwide in more than 300,000 patients[5] to treat all types of closed metaphyseal and diaphyseal (see Fig. 7–7) and many epiphyseal fractures; to repair extensive segmental defects of bone (see Fig. 7–21) and soft tissues without need for grafting; to treat nonunions and pseudarthroses; to perform limb or amputation stump lengthening and bone thickening for cosmetic or functional reasons; to correct long bone or joint deformities; and to perform joint arthrodesis.[34–36] A fibula can be split longitudinally and distracted laterally to increase its diameter to provide it with enough bulk to replace the tibial shaft if the latter has been resected as treatment for infection or trauma.[36]

Using the canine tibia as his experimental model, Ilizarov demonstrated that the most stable configuration of the fixator led to direct osteogenesis without intervening cartilage formation, which resembles intramembranous bone formation. However, the parallel columns of bone that form across the distraction zone are similar to the zone of primary osteoid in a child's physis. Inadequate fixator stability reduces new bone formation, promotes cartilage formation, causes pain, and increases the possibility of wire sepsis.[36]

In the dog tibia experiments, the greater the preservation of bone marrow and periosteum vasculature, the better the quality of new bone formation that occurred in the distraction gap. The rate of distraction that produced the optimal new bone formation was 1 mm per day. Premature osseous fusion occurred at 0.5 mm per day distraction rates, and damage to periosseous soft tissue and poor-quality bone formation occurred with distraction of 2 mm per day. The very best bone formation occurred when the 1 mm of distraction occurred in 60 steps per day using a motorized distractor. Not only does bone respond to the distraction, but the soft tissues also grow. In the area of the limb under distraction, periosteum, nerves, fascia, blood vessels, muscle, and skin were seen with light and electron microscopy to assume characteristic features of cellular growth that are otherwise only seen during embryonic, fetal, and neonatal life.[36]

The results reported by Ilizarov were achieved with the patients under constant hospital supervision throughout their treatment. A vigorous daily physical therapy program was pursued even though it was not always comfortable for the patient. Compliance by outpatients cannot be expected to be of the same quality as Ilizarov's supervised hospital patients. The healing process takes longer when the amount of physical activity is diminished.

Bone Grafting

Bone grafting is the transplantation of bone from one site to another. Although it is infrequently performed in the primary treatment of fractures, bone grafting is often required in the treatment of delayed union or nonunion. This was first successfully accomplished by Macewen,[22, 61] who in 1878 reconstructed the humeral shaft of a youngster using bone removed from six other patients.

Bone grafting is used as part of fracture treatment to enhance osteogenesis and to fill in bone defects.[21] It is used in conjunction with internal fixation of complex fractures, for treatment of nonunions, and to fill in bone defects caused by trauma or débrided infected fractures. Both bone and some bone graft substitutes are used for grafting.[64, 66] Bone stock for grafting can come from the same individual (autograft), from another individual such as a cadaver (allograft or homograft), or from another species (heterograft or xenograft). The bone graft substitutes are produced from coral from a reef using a method that exchanges hydroxyapatite for the calcium carbonate within a piece of coral without altering its structure. The coral has an architecture similar to cancellous bone that can serve as a framework for human osteogenesis.[64] It is mechanically weak and has been used in strips as onlay graft in conjunction with internal fixation of comminuted diaphyseal fractures or as subchondral filler of osseous defects following elevation of depressed articular fragments, such as with tibial plateau fractures.[32] The corallin hydroxyapatite is not as strong as trabecular bone because it lacks a collagen matrix, but it becomes stronger than native bone graft material but less stiff with bone ingrowth into it.[60]

Bone graft material consists of either cortical bone, usually from the tibia, or cancellous bone from the iliac crest. Conventional bone graft material is avascular, but it must eventually establish a vascular supply for incorporation into existing bone to occur. Fresh graft initially becomes surrounded by a hematoma. Cells within an autograft die with the exception of a few on the surface, which remain viable by diffusion of nutrients. The dead bone incites an inflammatory response, and within a few days new vessels invade the periphery of the graft.[21] This invasion is much easier and more complete with cancellous than with cortical graft material. The graft material provides a scaffold for deposition of new bone, and it is thought to release proteins that stimulate bone formation as well. Invasion of cortical bone by vessels occurs through haversian and Volkmann canals, which are enlarged by accompanying osteoclastic activity. Bone resorption occurs in cortical graft with the invasion of vessels and may last for months, causing an osteoporotic radiographic appearance. With cancellous graft, bone is first deposited on the trabeculae and replaced along with the dead trabeculae later.

Allograft material from cadavers typically is treated by deep-freezing the bone to −20°C or −70°C to decrease

Figure 7–21. *A,* Comminuted fracture of the tibia with a large intersegmental fragment was one of multiple fractures sustained in a motor vehicle accident by this 42-year-old woman. *B,* Ender rods were used initially to stabilize the fracture. The fracture site became infected and began to drain. *C,* The infected intersegmental fracture fragment was dead at surgery and was resected as seen here. An Ilizarov external fixator was applied with a corticotomy (*arrow*), performed proximal to the fracture defect. Olive wires, so called because of a knob at their proximal end that prevents their pulling through the bone, allowed traction to be applied to the bone fragment distal to the corticotomy site, and bone transport was begun. *D,* Two months after *C,* the corticotomy site (*arrow*) was distracted almost 30 mm. *E,* Four months after *D,* a second corticotomy (*arrow*) proximal to the first is seen, with the first site showing slightly increased density from early mineralizing bone. *F,* Five months after *E* and 11 months since the first corticotomy was performed, linear spicules of mineralized bone were visible in both corticotomy sites. The entire diaphyseal defect was replaced by transported bone.

its immunogenicity. The lower temperature (−70°C) seems to decrease immunogenicity the most. There has been no reported demonstrable change in the mechanical characteristics of the graft material as a result of freezing, and it becomes incorporated into host bone in the same manner as fresh autografts.[21] Irradiation, autoclaving, and freeze-drying have also been used to reduce immunogenicity of allograft bone, but they also change the mechanical properties of the bone. This is important if the graft must bear a load. Allografts have the advantage of availability in large quantities without morbidity of a patient donor site. Bone banks have been established to preserve allograft bone for grafting.

There has been some interest in using revascularized autografts in special circumstances, as with massive bone loss in a long bone or when the local soft tissues have been compromised and a bone graft is necessary.[56] The bone graft does not become necrotic if its blood supply is reanastomosed immediately. It repairs at each end like a healing fracture rather than like avascular bone of a conventional graft. Use of a vascularized autograft is predicated on adequate vascularity of the donor and recipient sites. It is used to fill a defect 6 cm or longer or to treat a nonunion refractory to conventional bone grafting.[56] The fibula is the most used donor bone, with a maximal straight cortical length of 26 cm available. Although a posterior rib or the iliac crest can also be used, they are restricted by their curved shape and limited strength and length compared with the fibula. One surgical team to obtain the graft and a second to prepare the recipient site are necessary to perform the operation. The bone graft blood supply is reanastomosed outside the area of trauma and is held in place with rigid fixation, with avascular cancellous bone graft added at the graft-bone interface.[56]

Cortical grafts (Fig. 7–22) are not used as often as they once were.[1, 71] The cortical bone is usually obtained from the tibial shaft and then placed and fixed within or upon the bone to be treated. When placed within, it is known as an inlay graft; when placed upon, it is known as an onlay graft. Frequently the graft is transfixed by screws. When originally conceived, prior to the development of acceptable metallic fixation devices, the cortical graft was used to stabilize and fix the fracture as well as serve as a source of new bone. Fixation devices have now largely replaced the need for cortical bone grafting for the purpose of stabilizing fractures.

Cancellous bone grafts,[31, 52, 70, 71] (or, more accurately, corticocancellous bone grafts; Fig. 7–23) are usually obtained by chipping bone or cutting it with a rongeur from

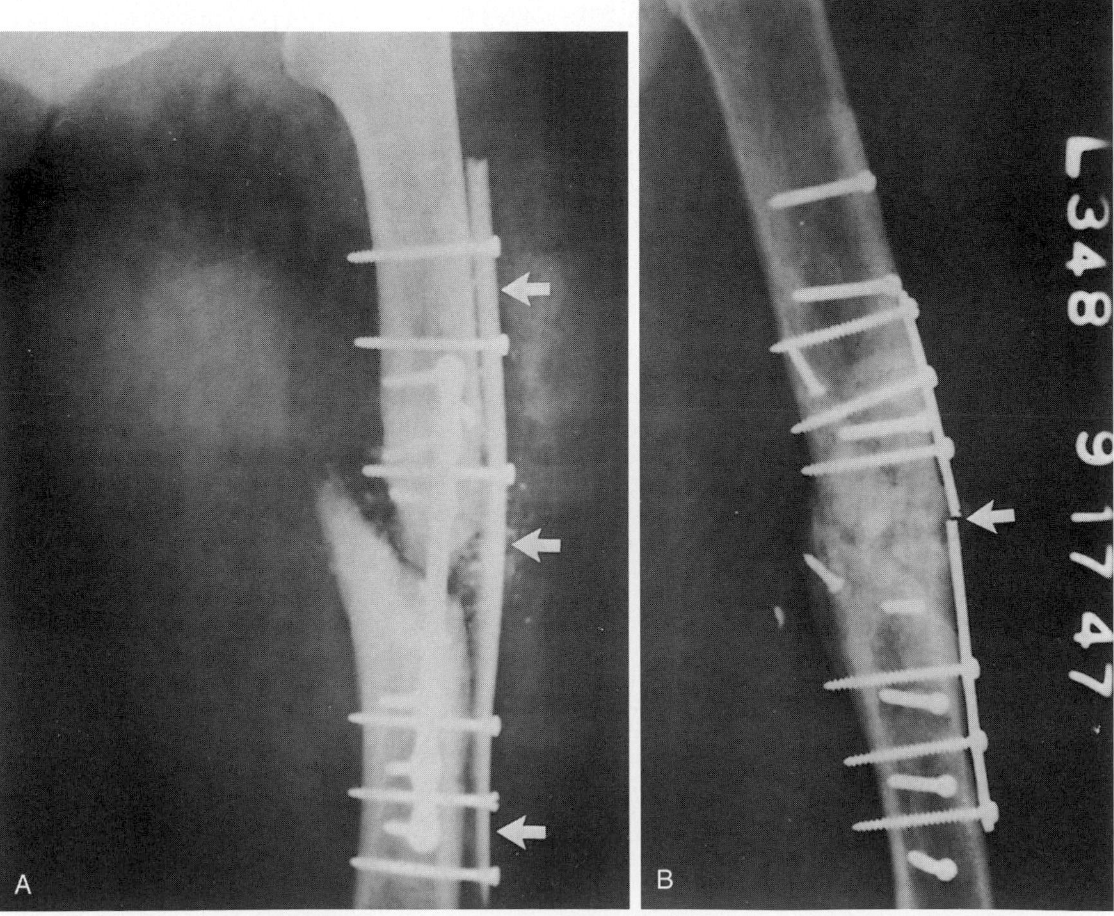

Figure 7–22. Cortical bone graft and plate used in treatment of nonunion of the midshaft of the femur. *A,* A very long tibial cortical graft (*arrows*) was transfixed to the lateral border of the femur by several cortical screws. *B,* Lateral projection obtained 7 months later demonstrates a fracture of the metallic plate (*arrow*). The cortical graft is not well visualized in this projection, but it also has broken. The fracture has not as yet united.

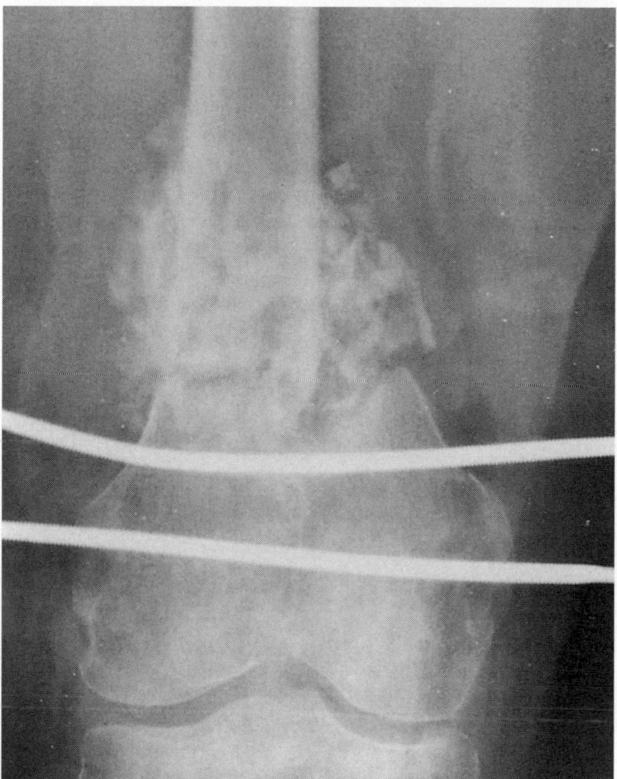

Figure 7–23. Corticocancellous bone graft from the ilium used in the treatment of nonunion of a supracondylar fracture of the femur. Note the multiple irregular fragments of bone about the fracture site. There are two finely threaded pins in the condylar portion of the femur. The patient was placed in an external fixator.

the medullary cavity and posterior cortical surface of the ilium. The bone thus obtained is packed into and about the site to be repaired. Deficits of bone may be filled in this manner. Cancellous bone grafts have been found to have an advantage in the promotion of osteogenesis. More osteogenic cells survive because the grafting material is readily revascularized, thus bone is more promptly laid down than with a cortical graft. This procedure has been in use since it was first reported by Matti[50] in 1931, and its advantages were generally recognized by the mid-1940s.[1] A modification of this technique uses strips of cancellous bone obtained from the iliac crest as an onlay graft.

Electrical Stimulation of Osteogenesis

Use of electrical stimulation has become a popular adjunct in the treatment of fracture-delayed unions and nonunions, osteotomies, and congenital pseudarthroses.[48] How and why electrical currents induce osteogenesis is not known, but nonunions that have not healed with other modes of treatment have healed in more than 70% of patients when electrical stimulation was used.[12, 17, 48] It is known that oxygen is consumed by the cathode to produce hydroxyl radicals according to the equation $2H_2O + O_2 + 4e^- = 4OH^-$. Local tissue oxygen tension is lowered and local tissue pH is elevated by the electrical current.[12] Low tissue oxygen tension and local alkalinity are both favorable to calcification and bone formation. Three to six months of electrical stimulation is used, typically with the extremity immobilized in a non–weight bearing cast for the duration of treatment. Patient cooperation is essential for electrical stimulation to succeed. Special care of percutaneous electrodes is necessary to prevent infection introduction along the wire tract, electrode breakage, or electrode dislodgment.

Three types of electrical stimulation have been used: percutaneous direct current (noninvasive), implanted direct current (invasive), and time-varying magnetic fields (noninvasive).[63] The percutaneous direct current stimulation is provided by an electrode, the cathode, implanted directly into the fracture site. It is attached to a power pack that is external to the patient, and an anode is attached to the skin.[12] Constant currents of 20 μA are typically used.[12, 48] With the implanted direct current, the totally invasive method requiring an operative procedure, the entire battery pack and electrodes are implanted into the treatment area (Fig. 7–24). Less care and patient cooperation are needed with this type of treatment, but infection is a more likely complication than with the other techniques.[48] Time-varying magnetic fields are produced by external coils or capacitor plates embedded in a cast overlying the treatment site.[6, 48] They induce electrical currents in the region of the fracture. These currents are not well understood, and it has not been possible to compute the nature of the locally delivered current. Nevertheless, the healing rate of nonunion fractures treated this way has been similar to that reported with direct current techniques.[6, 17, 48]

Contraindications for electrical stimulation include the presence of a synovial fluid–filled cavity between the fracture fragments as detected by a nuclide bone scan,[17] a bone gap at the nonunion site longer than half the bone diameter at that level, and reactivation of osteomyelitis that was quiescent prior to treatment.[12, 17, 48] The presence of metallic fixation devices at the nonunion site does not compromise the use of electrical stimulation.[12, 17] Connolly[17] believes that inadequate fixation of the nonunion is the most important cause of healing failure after electrical stimulation therapy.

The healing of nonunited fractures achieved with direct current stimulation by multiple investigators[12, 17, 48] does not statistically differ from other reports of nonunion treatment with bone grafting.[39] The lower morbidity and mortality rate with electrical stimulation is a certain advantage. A minor operation or no operative procedure at all is also attractive to patients.

Ultrasound Stimulation of Osteogenesis

Low-intensity pulsed ultrasound (30 mW/cm^2) is capable of accelerating healing of fresh fractures and appears to be useful in treating delayed union and nonunion fractures both in animal and clinical studies.[27] Typically, ultrasound treatment is percutaneous and lasts for 20 minutes per day. It has been shown to influence gene expression, blood flow, tissue remodeling, and activity

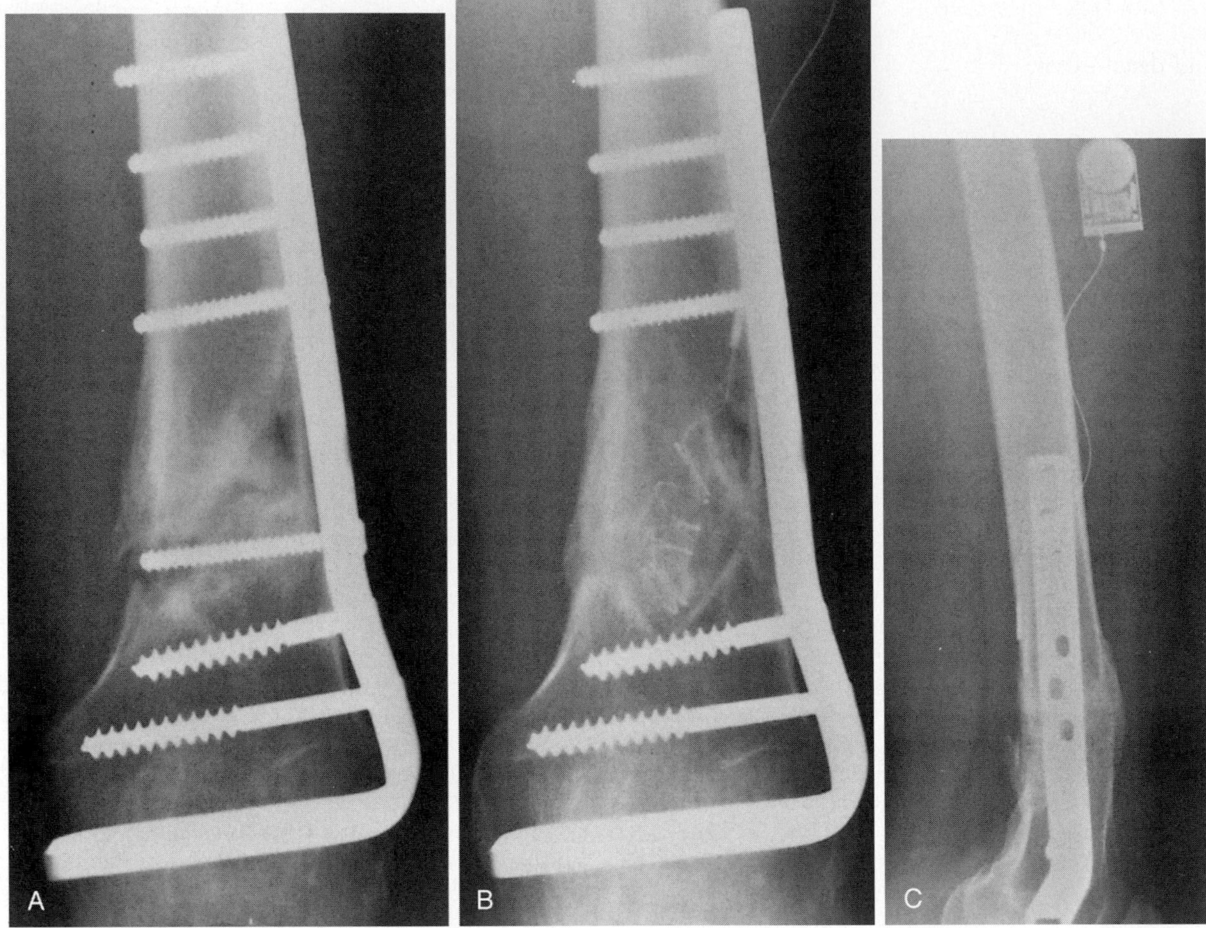

Figure 7–24. *A,* Nonunion of a femoral fracture 10 months after open reduction and internal fixation. *B,* Union of the fracture 6 months later following surgical insertion of an electrical stimulator. The blade plate and screws were left in place during the electrical stimulation. *C,* Lateral view shows the solid bone union and the battery pack in the soft tissues.

of osteoblasts and chondroblasts.[27] Statistically significant reduction of healing time for tibial and distal radius fractures was observed in smokers (by 41% to 51%) and nonsmokers (by 26% to 34%) treated with low-intensity ultrasound as compared with a control placebo device.[18] The mechanism by which ultrasound stimulates fracture healing is unknown, but its energy is absorbed in the soft tissues. Some of the energy is converted into heat, which may affect some enzymatic processes.

Postreduction Radiographs

Postreduction radiographs must be obtained in a minimum of two planes, the anteroposterior and lateral projections, to adequately evaluate reduction of the fracture. Plaster is more radiopaque when wet than when dry; therefore, an additional 8 to 16 kV is required to obtain a satisfactory image. Postreduction radiographs are reported by describing the fracture in a manner similar to the description in the initial examination. The presence of a cast is, of course, recorded, and any modifications, such as a split, bivalve, wedge, or window, are described. These cuts are readily recognized by their characteristic radiolucent course in the plaster. The alignment and degree of apposition of the fracture fragments are described, and any angulation or offset of the fractures is recorded. It is essential that the postreduction radiographs be compared with the prior radiographs so that the changes and corrections brought about by the reduction can be recognized and fully described.[57] Qualitative statements such as "good position and alignment" should be avoided unless the fracture fragments are almost perfectly aligned, with complete apposition and without angulation.

It is particularly important that any separation between fragments be recognized and described. A persistent soft tissue gap between major fragments at the fracture site following attempted reduction suggests either that there is interposition of soft tissue or that a fragment remains impaled in a surrounding muscle. If continuous traction is being used, such a gap indicates or suggests that the traction is excessive and should be reduced.

The report of radiographs obtained following open reduction and fixation should include a full description of the location and type of appliances, wires, and screws. The exact name of the appliance should be used whenever possible (e.g., Jewett nail, Rush rod, Richard's compression plate and screw); otherwise, a general description of the type of appliance is acceptable (e.g., intramedullary nail, blade plate, cortical screw). The proximal and distal extent of nails, rods, and Kirschner wires and location of pins should be noted.[8, 69] It is important that at least the entire length of all appliances, if not the entire length of the bone, be included on the radiograph. Fractures resulting from insertion of intramedullary nails in the femur are most likely to occur in the distal shaft (see Fig. 7–20) or supracondylar area, and they might be overlooked if the knee is not included on the radiograph. Similarly, nails have been known to subsequently migrate and may protrude through the anterior cortex in patients with severe osteopenia. Thus, all follow-up examinations should include two views at right angles of the entire bone. The number and location of all screws should be recorded in relation to the fracture line or lines and the longitudinal axis of the bone. Plates may be described by their length, the number of screws used to fix them, and their position on the surface of the shaft of the bone (e.g., medial, posterior, or anteromedial surface of the distal shaft). The location and type of bone grafts should be noted. Unless there has been open injury with appreciable loss of bone, grafting is infrequently used in the primary treatment of fractures, but it is commonly employed in the treatment of delayed union or nonunion.

References

1. Abbott, L.C., Schottstaedt, E.R., Saunders, J.B.D.M., & Bost, F.C. (1947). The evaluation of cortical and cancellous bone as grafting material. J. Bone J. Surg. [Am.], *29*:381.
2. Alho, A., Stromsoe, K., & Ekeland, A. (1991). Locked intermedullary nailing of femoral shaft fractures. J. Trauma, *31*:49.
3. Allgower, M., Ehrsam, R., Gang, R. et al. (1969). Clinical experience with a new compression plate "DCP." Acta Orthop. Scand. (Suppl.), *125*:45.
4. Alonso, J., Geissler, W., & Hughes, J.L. (1989). External fixation of femoral fractures: Indications and limitations. Clin. Orthop., *241*:83.
5. Aronson, J., Johnson, E., & Harp, J.H. (1988). Local bone transportation for treatment of intercalary defects by the Ilizarov technique. Clin. Orthop., *243*:71.
6. Bassett, C.A.L., Mitchell, S.N., & Schink, M.M. (1982). Treatment of therapeutically resistant non-unions with bone grafts and pulsing electromagnetic fields. J. Bone Joint Surg. [Am.], *64*:1214.
7. Behrens, F., & Searls, K. (1986). External fixation of the tibia. J. Bone Joint Surg. [Br.], *68*:246.
8. Birzle, H., Bergleiter, R., & Kuner, E.G. (1978). Radiology of Trauma. W.B. Saunders Co., Philadelphia.
9. Bostman, O., Varjonen, L., Vainionpaa, S. et al. (1989). Incidence of local complications after intramedullary nailing and after plate fixation of femoral shaft fractures. J. Trauma, *29*:639.
10. Brettle, J. (1970). A survey of the literature on metallic surgical implants. Injury, *2*:26.
11. Brettle, J., Hughes, A.N., & Jordan, B.A. (1971). Metallurgical aspects of surgical implant materials. Injury, *2*:225.
12. Brighton, C.T., Black, J., Friedenberg, Z.B. et al. (1981). A multicenter study of the treatment of non-union with constant direct current. J. Bone Joint Surg. [Am.], *63*:2.
13. Cater, W.H., & Hicks, J.H. (1956). The recent history of corrosion in metal used for internal fixation. Lancet, *2*:871.
14. Chapman, M.W. (1986). The role of intramedullary fixation in open fractures. Clin. Orthop., *212*:26.
15. Chapman, M.W. (1998). The effect of reamed and nonreamed intramedullary nailing on fracture healing. Clin. Orthop. *355S*:230.
16. Collinge, C.A., Sanders, R.W. (2000). Percutaneous plating in the lower extremity. J. Am. Acad. Orthop. Surg., *8*:211.
17. Connolly, J.F. (1984). Electrical treatment of nonunions: Its use and abuse in 100 consecutive fractures. Orthop. Clin. North Am., *15*:89
18. Cook, S.D., Ryaby, J.P., McCabe, J. et al. (1997). Acceleration of tibial and distal radius fracture healing in patients who smoke. Clin. Orthop., *337*:198.
19. Corzatt, R.D., & Basch, A.V. (1978). Internal fixation by the Ender method. J.A.M.A., *240*:1366.
20. Desai, A., Alvai, A., Dalinka, M. et al. (1980). Role of bone scintigraphy in the evaluation and treatment of nonunited fracture: Concise communication. J. Nucl. Med., *21*:931.
21. Friedlaender, G.E. (1987). Current concepts review bone grafts. J. Bone Joint Surg. [Am.], *69*:786.
22. Groves, E.W.H. (1918). Methods and results of transplantation of bone in the repair of defects caused by injury or disease. Br. J. Surg., *5*:185.
23. Gustilo, R.B., & Anderson, J.T. (1976). Prevention of infection in the treatment of one thousand and twenty-five open fractures of long bones: Retrospective and prospective analyses. J. Bone Joint Surg. [Am.], *58*:453.
24. Gustilo, R.B., Gruninger, R.P., & Davis, T. (1987). Classification of type III (severe) open fractures relative to treatment and results. Orthopedics, *10*:1781.
25. Gustilo, R.B., Mendoza, R.M., & Williams, D.N. (1984). Problems in the management of type III (severe) open fractures: A new classification of type III open fractures. J. Trauma, *24*:742.
26. Gustilo, R.B., Merkow, R.L., & Templeman, D. (1990). The management of open fractures. J. Bone Joint Surg [Am.] 72:299.
27. Hadjiargyrou, M., McLeod, K., Ryaby, H.P., & Rubin, C. (1998). Enhancement of fracture healing by low intensity ultrasound. Clin. Orthop., *355S*:216.
28. Henley, M.B. (1989). Intramedullary devices for tibial fracture stabilization. Clin. Orthop., *240*:87.
29. Henry, S.L. (2000). Supracondylar femur fractures treated percutaneously. Clin. Orthop., *375*:52.
30. Hicks, J.H. (1970). The influence of Arbuthnot Lane on fracture treatment. Injury, *2*:314.
31. Higgs, S.L. (1945). The use of cancellous chips in bone-graft surgery. J. Bone Joint Surg. [Am.], *27*:729.
32. Holmes, R.E. (1979). Bone regeneration within a coralline hydroxyapatite implant. Plast. Reconstr. Surg., *63*:626.
33. Ilizarov, G.A. (1975). Basic principles of transosseous compression and distraction osteosynthesis [translated from Russian]. Ortop. Travmatol. Protez., *10*:7.
34. Ilizarov, G.A. (1989). The tension-stress effect on the genesis and growth of tissues: The influence of stability of fixation and soft-tissue preservation. Clin. Orthop., *238*:249
35. Ilizarov, G.A. (1989). The tension-stress effect on the genesis and growth of tissues: the influence of the rate and frequency of distraction. Clin. Orthop., *239*:263
36. Ilizarov, G.A. (1990). Clinical application of the tension-stress effect for limb lengthening. Clin. Orthop., *250*:8.
37. Ilizarov, G.A., Ledyaev, B.I., & Shitin, V.P. (1969). Experimental studies of bone lengthening. Eksp. Khir. Anesteziol., *14*:3.
38. Kempf, I., Grosse, A., & Beck, G. (1985). Closed locked intramedullary nailing: Its application to comminuted fracture of the femur. J. Bone Joint Surg. [Am.], *67*:709.
39. Kirk, N.T. (1924). End results of one hundred fifty-eight consecutive autogenous bone grafts for non-union in long bones (A) in simple fractures: (B) in atrophic bone following war wounds and chronic suppurative osteitis (osteomyelitis). J. Bone Joint Surg., *6*:760
40. Klemm, K.W., & Borner, M. (1986). Interlocking nailing of complex fractures of the femur and tibia. Clin. Orthop., *212*:89.
41. Küntscher, G. (1940). Die Marnagelung Von Knochenbruchen Tierexperimenteller Teil. Klin. Wochenschr., *19*:6.
42. Küntscher, G.B.G. (1958). The Küntscher method of intramedullary fixation. J. Bone Joint Surg. [Am.], *40*:17.
43. Küntscher, G. (1967). Indications for intramedullary nailing of fractures. p. 53. In Practice of Intramedullary Nailing. Charles C Thomas, Springfield, Ill.
44. Küntscher, G. (1967). Principles of bone surgery: Influence of operative procedures on fracture healing. p. 23. In Practice of Intramedullary Nailing. Charles C Thomas, Springfield, Ill.
45. Küntscher, G. (1968). The intramedullary nailing of fractures. Clin. Orthop., *60*:5.
46. Lane, W.A. (1909). The operative treatment of simple fractures. Surg. Gynecol. Obstet., *8*:344.
47. Lange, R.H., Bach, A.W., Hansen, S.T., & Johansen, K.H. (1985). Open tibial fractures with associated vascular injuries: Prognosis for limb salvage. J. Trauma, *25*:203.
48. Lavine, L.S., & Grodzinsky, A.J. (1987). Electrical stimulation of repair of bone. J. Bone Joint Surg. [Am.], *69*:626.
49. Leunig, M., Hertel, R., Siebenrock, K.A. et al. (2000). The evolution of indirect reduction techniques for the treatment of fractures. Clin. Orthop., *375*:7.
50. Matti, H. (1931). Uber Freie Transplantation von Knochenspongiosa. Archiv Klin. Chir., *168*:236.
51. Monro, J.K. (1935). The history of plaster-of-paris in the treatment of fractures. Br. J. Surg., *23*:257.
52. Mowlem, A.R. (1945). Cancellous chip grafts for the restoration of bone defects. Proc. R. Soc. Med., *38*:171.
53. Müller, M.E. (1965). Treatment of nonunions by compression. Clin. Orthop., *43*:83.
54. Müller, M.E., Allgower, M., & Willenegger, H. (1965). Technique of Internal Fixation of Fractures. Springer-Verlag, New York.
55. Murphy, C.P., D'Ambrosia, R.D., Dabezies, D.J. et al. (1988). Complex femur fractures: Treatment with Wagner external fixation device of the Grosse-Kempf interlocking nail. J. Trauma, *28*:1553.

56. Nusbickel, F.R., Dell, P.C., McAndrew, M.P., & Moore, M.M. (1989). Vascularized autografts for reconstruction of skeletal defects following lower extremity trauma. Clin. Orthop., *243*:65.
57. Ogden, J.A., & Southwick, W.O. (1973). Adequate reduction of fractures and dislocations. Radiol. Clin. North Am., *11*:667.
58. Peltier, L.F. (1968). A brief history of traction. J. Bone Joint Surg. [Am.], *50*:1603.
59. Perren, S.M., Russenberger, M., Steinemann, S. et al. (1969). A dynamic compression plate. Acta Orthop. Scand. (Suppl.)., *125*:31.
60. Piecueh, J.F., & Topazian, R.G. (1982). Results of experimental ridge augmentation with porous hydroxyapatite implants: A preliminary report. Acta Stomatol. Int., *3*:67.
61. Rang, M. (1966). Anthology of Orthopaedics. Churchill Livingstone, Edinburgh.
62. Rockwood, C.A., & Green, D.P. (1975). Fractures. Vol. 2. J.B. Lippincott Co., Philadelphia.
63. Ryaby, H.P. (1998). Clinical effects of electromagnetic and electric fields on fracture healing. Clin. Orthop., *355S*:205.
64. Sartoris, D.J., Kusnick, C., & Resnick, D. (1987). New concepts in bone grafting. Orthop. Rev., *16*:53.
65. Smith-Petersen, M.N., Cave, E.F., & Vangorder, G.W. (1931). Intracapsular fractures of the neck of the femur-treatment by internal fixation. Arch. Surg., *23*:715.
66. Stevenson, S. (1998). Enhancement of fracture healing with autogenous and allogeneic bone grafts. Clin. Orthop., *355S*:239.
67. Svenningsen, S., Nesse, O., Finsen, V. et al. (1986). Intramedullary nailing versus AO-plate fixation in femoral shaft fractures. Acta Orthop. Scand., *57*:609.
68. Venable, C.S., & Stuck, W.G. (1948). Results of recent studies and experiments concerning metals used in the internal fixation of fractures. J. Bone Joint Surg. [Am.], *30*:247.
69. Volz, R.G., & Martin, M.D. (1977). Illusory biplane radiographic images. Radiology, *122*:695.
70. Wilson, J.N. (1957). Cancellous strip bone grafting. J. Bone J. Surg. [Br.], *39*:585.
71. Wilson, J.N. (1976). Watson-Jones Fractures and Joint Injuries. 5th Ed. Churchill Livingstone, Edinburgh.
72. Young, J.W.R., Kovelman, H., Resnik, C.S., & Paley, D. (1990). Radiologic assessment of bones after Ilizarov procedures. Radiology, *177*:89.

Chapter 8

FRACTURE HEALING

with Ronald W. Hendrix, MD

It is somewhat surprising to realize that, although fractures are the most common abnormality of bone, the healing process is only partially understood from the standpoint of cellular and biochemical behavior and control. Information available from reports in the past two decades indicates that bone healing is much more complicated than had previously been suspected.[19] Bone is the only tissue in the body that regenerates completely after injury instead of healing with scar.[36, 70] Characteristically, there is a smooth transition from fracture to healing, provided that there is adequate immobilization and vascular supply. A description of this process may be made from any of several vantage points: clinical, radiographic, histologic, or biochemical. Radiographic imaging of the anatomic site aids in the clinical evaluation of healing, especially when the fracture is immobilized in a cast. The bone bridge that must form between the fracture fragments for solid healing to occur is the end result of a cascade of multiple biochemical steps and pathways that stimulate primitive marrow cells to differentiate into all of the necessary cell types to bring about healing and, finally, to turn off the whole process when it is complete.[19] These biochemical reactions control and modulate the generation of cells that form the calcified callus, endosteal ossification, periosteal ossification, and remodeling of the fracture site. The end result of these biochemical reactions can be seen either microscopically as multiple histologic steps or macroscopically as the radiographic progression of the regenerative process ending in the formation of a solid bridge of bone across the osseous defect due to the fracture. The value of histologic knowledge of fracture healing is that it provides a more detailed explanation of what is visible grossly on the radiograph.

Elucidation of the actual biochemical pathways that account for the histologic changes is intriguing in that once the mechanisms are known, it may be possible to manipulate them. For example, it might be possible to restart healing in a nonunion with local injection of a biochemical cocktail, without surgery and bone grafting, or without crushing the site to cause microfractures with an external fixator, as must be done at present.[37, 38] In patients lacking sufficient native bone following multiple joint replacements, osteomyelitis, or traumatic bone loss, perhaps a major part of a given bone or the entire bone with its cartilage could be regenerated de novo, superseding the metal and plastic implants in current use.

The healing process is an evolutionary one that may be separated only arbitrarily into phases for the purposes of study and understanding. It must be recognized that such separation is an abstraction. There is considerable overlap in the sequence of events; many proceed simultaneously.

A discussion of fracture healing needs to include the mechanism of healing insofar as it is understood, because a breakdown in this healing sequence may lead to incomplete, abnormal, or lack of healing. A more complete understanding of fracture healing can be expected to have predictive value in the management of these injuries. If deviation from normal healing can be recognized earlier in the clinical course, appropriate measures can be taken to counteract the abnormality. Thus, such information has pragmatic value if it can lead to earlier determination of when intervention by the physician is needed, and to a more clear-cut determination of when a fracture has healed enough so that the affected body part can be safely used. Unfortunately, our ability to achieve such practical ends is currently far from realized. Nevertheless, the evidence available to date has proved useful in clinical decision-making, as discussed later on.

Some authors[15, 16] have divided fracture healing into three stages (Fig. 8–1), but division into more detailed stages is more useful. Five histologic stages of bone healing were reported by Auxhasen[6] as early as 1907 and have been discussed by other authors since.[2, 30, 31, 67] These

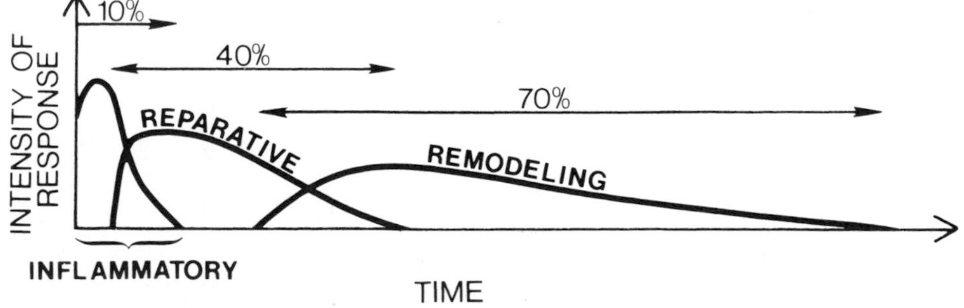

Figure 8–1. Relative intensity of response and duration of the three phases of fracture healing. (Adapted from Cruess, R. L., & Dumont, J. (1975). Current concepts, fracture healing. Can. J. Surg., *18*:403, with permission.)

stages are (1) the occurrence of the fracture, (2) the formation of granulation tissue around the fracture ends, (3) replacement of the granulation tissue by callus, (4) replacement of callus by lamellar bone, and (5) reshaping the bone to normal or near-normal contour.[26] Contemporary reports have appeared elucidating some of the regulatory mechanisms that drive these five histologic stages of healing.[36, 64, 70, 74]

Using recombinant DNA techniques, Wang and coworkers have cloned and sequenced the genes for human bone morphogenetic protein.[74] The bone morphogenetic protein synthesized by these genes was implanted into rats. Cartilage formation followed by bone formation was induced by the protein. Bone formation occurred earlier with larger doses and was seen as early as 5 days. The existence of a class of small proteins that regulate cell proliferation, differentiation, and matrix synthesis during fracture healing was suspected for some time but has only recently been confirmed.[64] Transforming growth factor-β, one of these proteins, was shown to regulate cell proliferation and initiate chondrogenesis and osteogenesis in rat femurs. It appears that transforming growth factor-β is released by platelets into the fracture hematoma, and that chondrocytes and osteoblasts then synthesize it throughout the healing process.[64]

Evidently, a given growth factor is not limited to a single physiologic activity; rather, its action depends on the presence of other molecules and on the stage of differentiation of a target cell. Transforming growth factor-β stimulates growth of fibroblasts in the presence of platelet-derived growth factor but inhibits their growth if epidermal growth factor is present.[64] It is thought that the peptide regulatory molecules are part of a cellular language or alphabet, with different codes spelled out by different combinations. Also, the code is assumed to be contextual (i.e., dependent on what receptors are being acted upon). This specificity accounts for differences in effects with the same peptide in different circumstances.[64]

The significance of these findings is that we are beginning to understand the molecular basis of fracture healing. Once that information is known, we may be able to intelligently set about treating fractures that fail to heal. Injection of a growth factor extract into a nonunited fracture site may be able to induce union. Further investigation of how bone healing is regulated at the molecular level is in order.

The Healing Process

The Fracture

The immediate local effect of injury (Fig. 8–2*A*) caused by the fracture is disruption of a variable amount of surrounding soft tissue, including muscles, tendons, ligaments, and the blood vessels within and about all of these tissues, including those within the bone. Thus, a hematoma is created, and a clot forms[1, 15, 16, 30, 31, 61] as hemostasis is achieved at the fracture site. Tissue destruction is both a direct and an indirect effect of the injury. Tissue may be destroyed directly by the force of the injury and indirectly by devascularization due to the disruption of blood supply.

The fracture damages the mineralized bone, periosteum, bone marrow, and adjacent soft tissue. Some cells from the damaged tissue die, but others are sensitized by local molecules released from the injured cells. This sensitization allows them to respond to local and systemic healing stimuli. In the absence of such sensitization, the response to both local and systemic stimuli would be limited, and healing would proceed very slowly.

In addition, local biochemical messengers are released, some of which cause cells to rapidly proliferate and others which regulate cellular differentiation.[36, 42, 53, 64, 70] Such molecular control or regulation of cell proliferation and differentiation has been partially elucidated for blood cells[60] and is presumed to be similar in bone, although

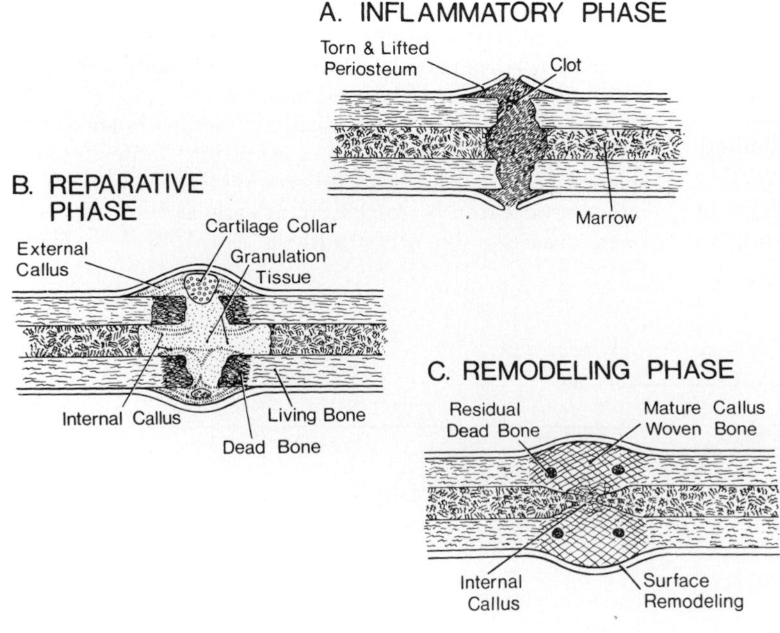

Figure 8–2. Phases of healing. *A*, Inflammatory phase. As the bone is broken the periosteum is torn, and a clot is formed in the line of fracture. *B*, Reparative phase. Granulation tissue is formed within the clot. The periosteum and endosteum form immature callus. Bone deprived of its vascular supply at the margins of the fracture line is devitalized. A ring of cartilage forms at the peripheral margin of the fracture. *C*, During remodeling, the woven bone within the callus is replaced by compact bone in the cortex and cancellous bone within the medullary cavity. The remaining islands of dead bone are resorbed. (Adapted from Ham, A.W., & Harris, W.R. (1971). Repair and transplantation of bone. p. 338. In Boume, G.H. Ed.: The Biochemistry and Physiology of Bone. 2nd Ed. Vol. 3. Academic Press, New York, with permission.)

only some of the regulatory proteins have been isolated and characterized for bone.[42, 64] This first stage of tissue response lasts approximately 7 days.

The extent of damage resulting from the vascular disruption in bone is variable. The periosteal tissue and marrow[57, 58, 69] have a greater blood supply with more collateral channels and therefore are not as severely affected as is the cortical bone. The torn vessels are sealed by the hemostatic mechanisms along their length back to positions of branching and anastomosis. In cortical bone, anastomosis in the haversian systems is relatively infrequent; therefore, the intravascular clotting extends for a greater distance from the fracture line in cortical bone than in other tissues. Thus, a zone of devitalized bone of variable width is created, and this tissue must be resorbed before healing can be completed.

Granulation Tissue Formation

Some of the sensitized local cells rapidly duplicate and differentiate into fibroblasts, new vessels, and other supporting cells. This granulation tissue invades any hematoma that has formed between the fracture fragments (see Fig. 8–2*B*). Macrophages and giant cells from the granulation tissue remove the hematoma. Osteoclasts also appear during this time and resorb dead bone from the opposing fracture surfaces. This stage lasts about 2 weeks.

Callus Formation

Chondroblasts and osteoblasts next begin to appear in large numbers as the organization and differentiation process progresses. They arise from local cells that have the potential to respond to remote mediators and to the various local molecular mediators released by cells damaged by the fracture and from the resulting hematoma.[26, 47] These cells differentiate into all of the many cell types necessary to achieve fracture union.[36, 70] Cartilage and osteoid matrices are produced by some of these cells and begin to mineralize after approximately 1 week. This process of mineralization lasts for several weeks, but early on it can be detected radiographically—faintly at first but with ever-increasing density on serial studies. By the time calcified callus bridges a fracture site, limited use of the affected body part is usually possible. Calcified callus needs to be denser and more completely formed to allow use of weight-bearing bones. Mineralized callus takes approximately 4 to more than 16 weeks to form. It forms more rapidly in spongy bone than in compact bone and more slowly with increasing age.[26] The mineralized bone matrix seen at this time is composed of woven bone. Its trabeculae appear haphazard on microscopic section, as compared with those in compact lamellar bone. Unlike trabeculae of lamellar bone, which are oriented along lines of stress, the trabeculae of woven bone are laid down beside the new capillaries that earlier invaded the area and nourish the trabeculae. Whether cartilage matrix or bone matrix is laid down within and surrounding the fracture site depends on the local availability of oxygen to the cells and the amount of motion at the fracture site. A good oxygen supply favors the formation of bone matrix, and a poor oxygen supply favors cartilage formation.[45] Motion also favors cartilage formation.[36]

Remodeling

The regulatory mechanism for the remodeling stage is not known, but a process is initiated within callus to replace it with discrete cylinders or packets of new bone[26] (see Fig. 8–2*C*). The cellular tissue responsible for the new bone formation and replacement of calcified callus has been termed the basic multicellular unit (BMU) by Frost.[26] This tissue is composed of many cells and of many different cell types. The BMU initially produces osteoclasts, which resorb a cylinder or packet-sized space of callus that is always the same size. This is followed by osteoblast production, which fills the packet-sized space with new bone. What this new bone is like depends on the tissue it replaces. Calcified cartilage is replaced with woven bone, and woven bone or lamellar bone is always replaced with lamellar bone. Thus, calcified cartilage is replaced first by woven bone and at a later time by lamellar bone. The entire process of resorption and replacement effected by a BMU requires 3 or 4 months per BMU.[26] Complete replacement of callus by many BMUs working at a fracture site takes 1 to 4 years. This replacement is rapid for the first third of the process and slows progressively during the last two thirds.[26]

The remodeling process also replaces callus or cartilage between the fractured margins of the compact bone of the cortex with new lamellar bone, which aligns parallel to the stress lines of the bone caused by usage. It also restores the marrow cavity by removing the callus plug.

Modeling

The reshaping of the endosteal and periosteal cortical surfaces of the bone at the fracture site to prefracture shape has been called *modeling* by Frost.[25, 26] His definitions of modeling and remodeling are in current use among bone researchers. Modeling differs from remodeling in that the latter is a process of erosion and replacement of microscopic cavities of bone. Modeling typically causes bone resorption from one cortex of a bone and bone formation in the opposite cortex of the same bone. The modeling process takes place continuously for long periods of time and leads to macro-level changes of bone configuration, such as correction of a fracture deformity; it changes the shape of a bone.[53] Modeling begins about the time at which callus formation ceases (1 to 4 months) and continues for 1 or more years.[26] Bone modeling becomes less effective after skeletal maturation, whereas bone remodeling continues throughout life.[27] The return of a bone to prefracture shape occurs in children and to some degree in young adolescents but not in adults. Modeling is thought to occur in response to local mechanical stress and strain from resumed activity after the callus has matured. It should be noted that callus and young bone are both somewhat plastic and flexible, which may stimulate modeling.

Factors Influencing the Rate of Repair

Not all fractures heal at the same rate. Many factors are at play in determining the time required for healing[34, 75] (Table 8–1). Chief among them are the character of local trauma,[29] general health status of the patient, vascularity of the fracture fragments,[10] pharmacologic effects, and method of treatment.[32] Healing is retarded because of poor vascularity in severely comminuted fractures, in those with extensive associated soft tissue injury, and in fractures distal to the entry point of a nutrient vessel.[10, 29]

Patient physical status includes age, nutritional state,[20] presence of illness (e.g., diabetes, tumor, anemia, chronic disease), deficiency state (hormonal or mineral), and preexisting damage to adjacent soft tissues. A long bone fracture can increase metabolism up to 25%. Lack of adequate calcium and phosphorus slows callus formation, and protein deficiency leads to decreased callus strength. Anemia may cause defective bone healing secondary to a decrease in oxygen tension.[59] Diabetes causes changes in vascularity and in serum glucose levels, and also neuropathy, which adversely affect healing. Previous radiation therapy or soft tissue injury will reduce available blood supply. One or a combination of these factors may be associated with delayed fracture healing. Deficiency of estrogen or growth hormone[49] may also delay healing. The capacity for healing decreases with age. A fracture of the shaft of the femur unites in an infant in 1 month, in an adolescent in 2 months, and in a 50-year-old man in 3 to 4 months.[75]

Table 8–1. Factors Delaying the Rate of Fracture Repair

1. General health status of the patient
   a. Age
   b. Nutritional state
   c. Presence of illness (e.g., diabetes, tumor, anemia, chronic disease)
   d. Deficiency state (hormonal or mineral)
   e. Preexisting soft tissue damage in fracture area
2. Character of the local trauma
   a. Extensive soft tissue injury
   b. Infection
   c. Nerve disruption
3. Vascularity of fracture fragments
   a. Healing is delayed directly with the severity of vascular impairment
   b. Compartment syndrome
   c. Bones with limited blood supply or collateral circulation
4. Pharmacologic factors
   a. Nicotine from smoking
   b. Nonsteroidal anti-inflammatory agents
   c. Corticosteroids
   d. Antibiotics
   e. Anticoagulants
   f. Cytotoxic chemotherapeutic agents
   g. Hormonal influences
5. Type of fracture therapy
   a. Too much motion allowed
   b. Extensive periosteal stripping during open reduction
   c. Delayed manipulation of the fracture site
   d. Cement in the fracture site

Adapted from Gustilo, R.B., Mendoza, R.M., & Williams, D.N. (1984). Problems in the management of type III (severe) open fractures: A new classification of type III open fractures J. Trauma, *24*:742, with permission.

Healing varies directly with the degree of vascularity of the fracture fragments. If both fragments are well supplied, healing is maximized (Fig. 8–3); if one is limited, healing is slowed; if both are limited, healing is impaired; if one fragment is devoid of supply, then healing is greatly impaired. As a generality, there is a greater blood supply in the metaphysis than in the diaphysis; therefore, healing is usually faster at the end of the bone than in the shaft. The distal third of the tibia, ulna, and humerus is limited in collateral circulation.[75] Fractures in the distal third of these bones impairs the distal blood supply because the nutrient artery arises proximally. Therefore, these fractures heal at a slower pace. With segmental fractures a significant disruption in blood supply is more likely, and healing is likely to be impaired. If a segmental fracture occurs in the presence of an already tenuous or limited blood supply, such as the distal tibia, healing is considerably slowed. Fractures resulting in complete obliteration of blood supply to one fragment heal very slowly indeed. Poor healing is frequent in fractures of the carpal scaphoid, wherein the proximal pole is deprived of its blood supply, and all regeneration must arise from the distal fragment. Similarly, displaced fractures of the femoral neck deprive the femoral head of its blood supply. Open fractures with vascular injury have a poor prognosis and heal slowly if at all.[18, 29] A compartment syndrome may also decrease blood flow to a fracture, causing delayed healing.[13]

The loss of bone or separation of fragments (Fig. 8–4), creating a gap at the fracture site, results in significant slowing of healing, because the gap must be filled in with bone. Continued excessive traction also creates gaps, resulting in retardation of healing. An important exception to the traction effect occurs with bone lengthening via a corticotomy and distraction using the technique described by Ilizarov,[37, 38] which is discussed with fracture treatment in Chapter 7.

Delayed healing may also be associated with fracture therapy. A delay of healing may be due to débridement with bone loss, inadequate immobilization, delayed manipulation, use of methylmethacrylate within a fracture site,[21] or overzealous irrigation of the fracture site with leaching out of some of the active biochemical stimulating compounds.[32] Inadequate immobilization allows motion, which produces tissue injury, especially to new vasculature involved in the reparative process, and prolongs the time required for union. The cause may be inadequate external immobilization, such as use of a cast that is too short or too loose; inadequate internal immobilization due to use of a plate of improper length or too-narrow an intramedullary nail; or premature initiation of ambulation or use of the extremity before sufficient healing has taken place. The type of cellular healing seen at the fracture site depends on the type of motion that is permitted by the fixation system.[11] Rigid internal fixation modifies the cellular response to a fracture and to some extent changes the method of fracture healing.[4, 11, 23, 52] With this type of fixation, production of external callus is minimal or does not occur. Most healing is confined to the area between the ends of the fracture. Fracture healing following inter-

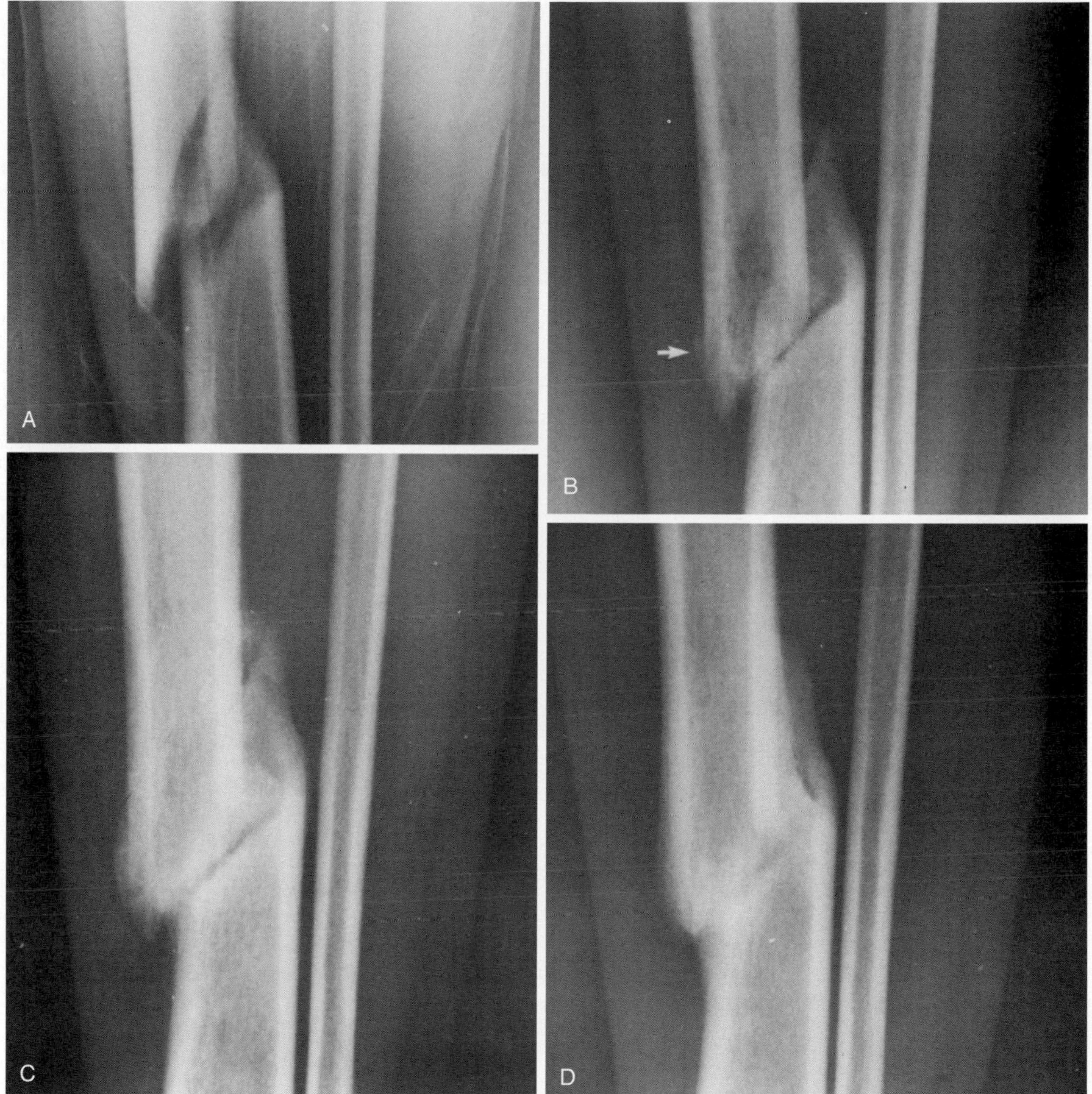

Figure 8–3. Normal healing of fracture of the distal tibia in a 32-year-old woman. *A*, Acute oblique fracture of the distal third of the tibia. The thin radiopaque vertical lines superimposed upon the bones are due to the splint. *B*, Two months after fracture, osteoporosis is manifested by cortical tunneling within both distal and proximal fragments. Bone has been resorbed at the margins of the fracture. Early fluffy callus is evident at the margins of the fracture *(arrow)*. *C*, Four months after fracture, compact callus is evident. The fracture line remains apparent. There is no definite bridging of the fracture line by callus at this time. Disuse osteoporosis, manifested principally by cortical tunneling, is evident in both fragments. *D*, Eight months after fracture, bridging callus is evident. A faint remnant of the fracture line is still evident. Union had been judged to be clinically adequate and the patient had been ambulating for 1 month without a cast at the time this radiograph was obtained.

nal fixation is considered by some authorities to be analogous with the primary healing of soft tissue wounds occurring after approximation of the tissue planes by suture, so-called primary healing.[52] Similarly, treatment by closed techniques has been considered analogous with the secondary healing of a soft tissue wound whose edges have not been approximated, in which the wound is first filled with granulation tissue. The exactness of the analogy is open to question, but internal fixation significantly modifies the manner of healing and in some circumstances shortens the time required for union. The precise reasons for this modification are unknown, although the lack of motion at the fracture site is the one most frequently proposed.[52]

Another major factor affecting the healing rate of fractures is the presence of infection. The humoral and cellular healing mechanisms are diverted from repair of the fracture to the containment and elimination of the infective process. Healing is markedly prolonged but eventually occurs in most cases.

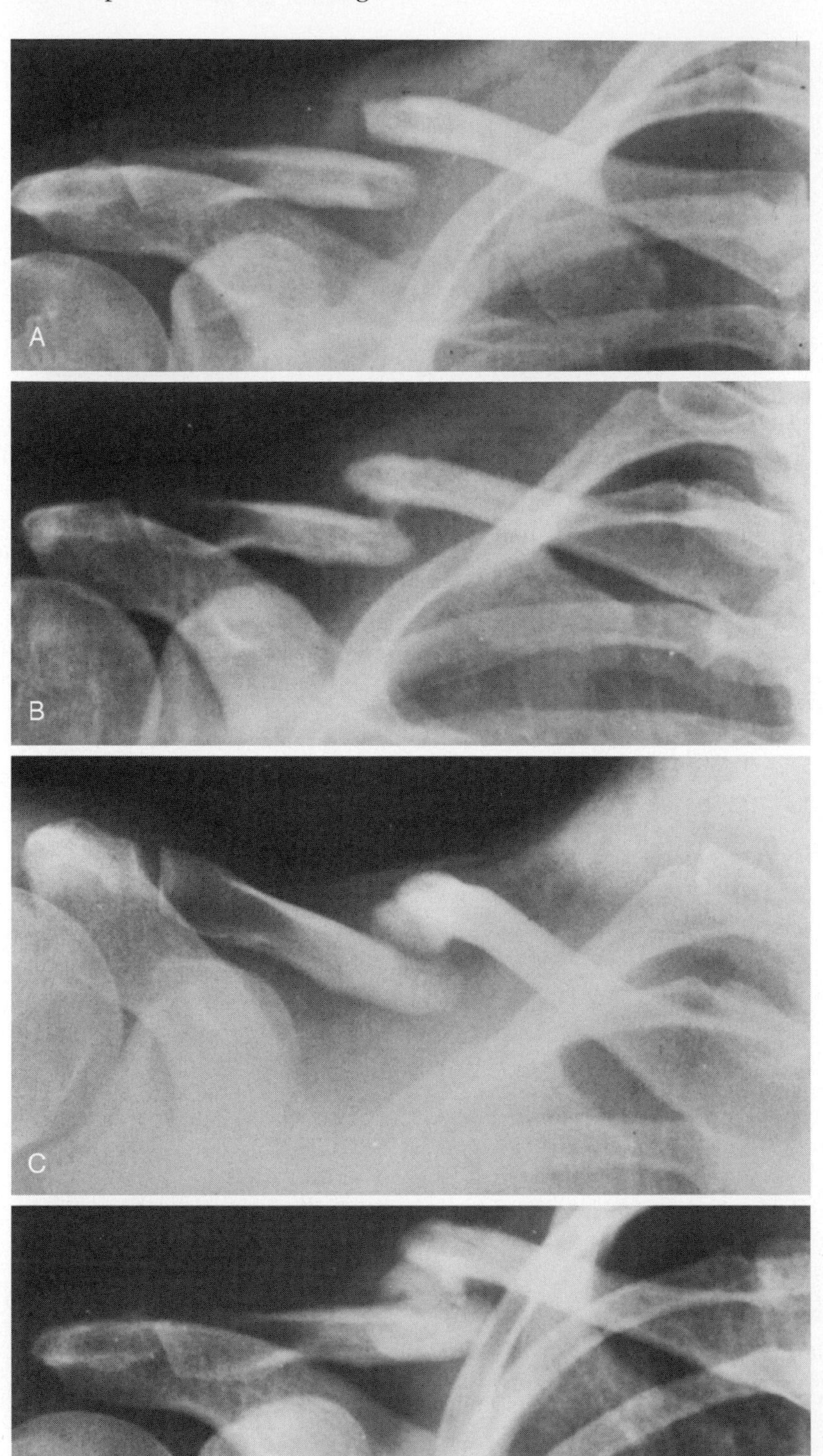

Figure 8–4. Delayed union of a midclavicular fracture in a 28-year-old woman. *A*, The initial radiograph demonstrates a fracture of the midclavicle without apposition of the fracture fragments. The proximal fragment lies 5 mm above the distal fragment. *B*, At 3 months after injury, there is minimal, immature callus lying between the fracture fragments. The margins of the fracture have become rounded. *C*, At 8 months after injury, there has been an increase in callus formation, but as yet no callus bridges the fracture. There was tenderness to palpation and some motion at the fracture site. *D*, At 16 months after injury, mature callus bridges the fracture site. Normally a fracture of the clavicle in an adult would be expected to heal within 3 to 6 months. In this case the union required more than a year.

Healing is also prolonged in the presence of other focal pathologic conditions of bone such as benign and malignant tumors, Paget's disease, fibrous dysplasia, and radiation necrosis. Innervation loss within the fracture site appears to hinder healing as well.[35]

The healing of intra-articular fractures[8] may be affected by the presence of fibrinolysins in the joint fluid, which prohibit clot formation and interfere with the initial stages of callus formation. Furthermore, in intra-articular fractures (i.e., femoral neck, radial head, humeral head, and patella), as compared with fractures of the shaft, the periosteum does not have the same capacity for repair. Healing depends entirely on medullary callus, which arises from pluripotential cells within the marrow-supporting structures. No temporary cartilaginous callus is formed. If a fracture fragment is viable (i.e., has an intact blood supply), the repair response occurs even if the fragment is separated from major fragments. If devitalized and dissociated from a viable contact, the fracture fragment has no potential for repair. The importance of accurate apposition and immobilization is obvious.

Pharmacologic agents such as corticosteroids, anticoagulants, nicotine from smoking, antibiotics, cytotoxic chemotherapeutic agents, and nonsteroidal anti-inflammatory drugs delay fracture healing by various mechanisms. Corticosteroids inhibit differentiation of osteoblasts from mesenchymal cells.[14] Heparin and warfarin sodium (Coumadin) delay healing either by inhibiting clot formation or by diminishing the number of cells at the fracture site.[66] Nicotine is a powerful vasoconstrictor, decreasing oxygen delivery, and also inhibits cell proliferation.[43, 62] Ciprofloxacin has a toxic effect on callus, causing matrix degeneration and decreased cellularity. Methotrexate delays cartilage matrix production to slow healing.[32] The nonsteroidal anti-inflammatory drugs indomethacin and aspirin may delay ossification by diminishing local blood flow or by hindering primitive osteoblasts.[3]

Hormonal influences affecting the healing rate are less well identified.[75] It has been demonstrated experimentally that corticosteroids interfere with healing,[14] and growth hormone promotes healing. Other hormones have lesser effects, but are rarely, if ever, operative to any significant degree in the clinical setting.

Radiographic Manifestations of Fracture Healing

The earliest radiographic manifestation of repair[71, 75] is widening of the fracture line with blurring of the apposing margins of the fragments as a result of resorption of dead bone in the inflammatory (initial) phase of healing. This feature is usually seen within 10 to 14 days of the time of fracture. The second manifestation is the appearance of calcified callus about the fracture site (Fig. 8–5*B*; see also Fig. 8–3*B*). It is fluffy and rather amorphous in outline and is first encountered on the periphery of the bone in the ensheathing callus at a variable distance from the fracture line. Endosteal or intramedullary callus is difficult to identify radiographically.

In time the callus fills in, increasing in density and quantity, and proceeds toward the margins of the fracture (see Figs. 8–3*C* and *D* and 8–5*C* and *D*), the rate of progress depending upon the several factors noted previously. Callus develops the characteristic texture of bone and is then termed mature callus. Bridging of a fracture line by calcified callus is analogous to the insertion of the keystone within an arch. This bridging process cannot be accomplished until an arc of callus is first formed about the fragments on both sides of the fracture. When this is done, bridging of callus occurs between the fragments across the fracture line until the fracture line is closed or filled completely by woven bone. It is common for healing to proceed at an unequal rate about the circumference of the bone (see Fig. 8–8). For example, the extent of periosteal stripping is typically greater on the concave side of the bone when the fracture results from an angulating force. In this case, the subsequent calcified callus is seen first and becomes more extensive on the concave side of the fracture. The periosteum at the apex of the initial angulation is torn without stripping, with subsequent ensheathing callus formation less extensive on that side.

The amount of callus anticipated with normal healing varies from bone to bone and with the position of the fracture within the bone. Long bones develop considerably more peripheral callus than that seen with short bones. The degree of peripheral callus formation is determined in part by the thickness of the cortex at the site of fracture. Diaphyseal fractures have greater callus formation than that noted for metaphyseal fractures. Small irregular bones characteristically heal primarily internally with little, if any, peripheral callus formation. The peripheral callus developed about fractures of bony prominences (i.e., the malleolus) is characteristically minimal. With fractures of the short or irregular bones, such as the scaphoid (Fig. 8–6) or calcaneus, minimal visible external callus develops. These bones have relatively thin cortices and rely chiefly on endosteal callus formation for healing. This process is manifested by gradual obliteration of the fracture line initially by woven bone between the intramedullary portion of the fragments. Callus development is more extensive about comminuted fractures than about simple fractures. The extent of callus is roughly proportional to the amount of separation or gap between the fragments; the greater the gap, the more exuberant the eventual callus. With impacted fractures, peripheral callus formation is minimal. Callus formation is increased by instability or continued motion and by infection at the fracture site. Therefore, greater than normally anticipated amounts of callus should suggest the possibility of these complications.

As compared with closed methods, open reduction with rigid fixation modifies the predicted pattern of healing. Peripheral callus formation is minimal, often practically nonexistent, when open compression plating (Fig. 8–7) or intramedullary rodding with interlocking nailing is utilized. Healing is manifested only by gradual obliteration of the fracture line and the appearance of slight sclerosis at the fracture site. Indeed, if callus formation of any significant degree is demonstrated in fractures managed with these techniques, the possibility of either motion of the fracture site (Fig. 8–8; see also Fig. 8–16*A*) or underlying osteomyelitis must be considered. These two complications are also evidenced by the presence of fine radiolucencies, due to bone resorption, about the screws and other appliances utilized in the fixation. Therefore, in the follow-up examination of fractures treated with open reduction and fixation, it is important to consider the amount of callus formation and to specifically look for fine radiolucencies in the analysis of fracture healing and exclusion of complications.

A precise open reduction may occasionally eliminate any radiographic evidence of a fracture line (see Fig. 7–9). This radiographic appearance may be noted intraoperatively after an exact reduction of the fragments is obtained and maintained by rigid fixation. Absence of a fracture line could easily be misconstrued as evidence of healing, which it obviously is not. It is important to know the circumstances under which the examination was ob-

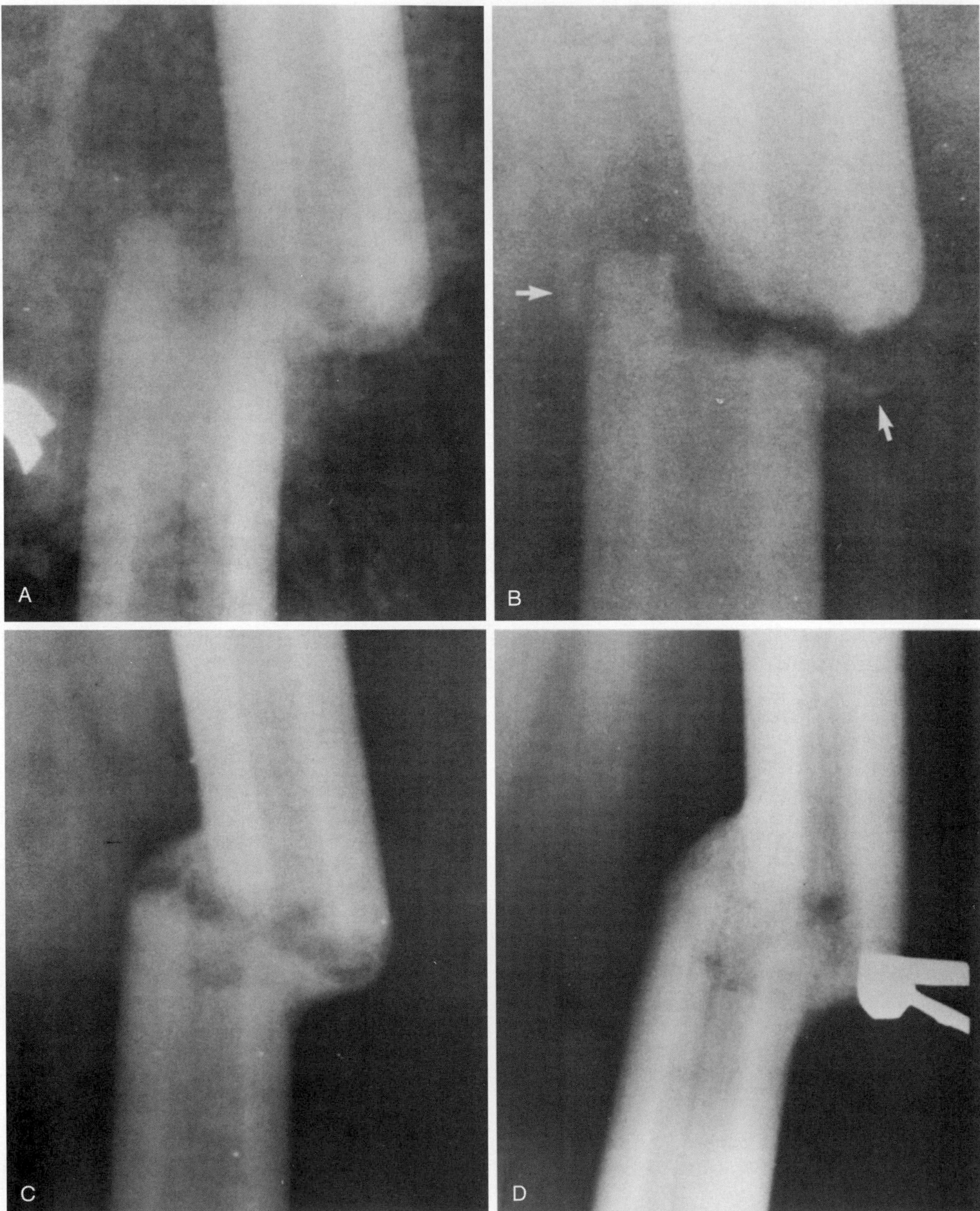

Figure 8–5. Healing of transverse fractures of the midshaft of the femur in a 29-year-old pregnant woman. *A*, Examination through the plaster cast at 7 weeks after injury reveals no definite evidence of callus formation. Early immature callus is easily obscured when viewed through a cast. *B*, The cast was removed and another radiograph was obtained. Fluffy immature callus is now identifiable at the margins of the fracture *(arrows)*. *C*, At 3½ months after injury, the callus is more compact, but the bridging callus between the fracture fragments is incomplete; the fracture line is readily apparent. *D*, At 6½ months after injury, mature callus is present, and the fracture is well healed.

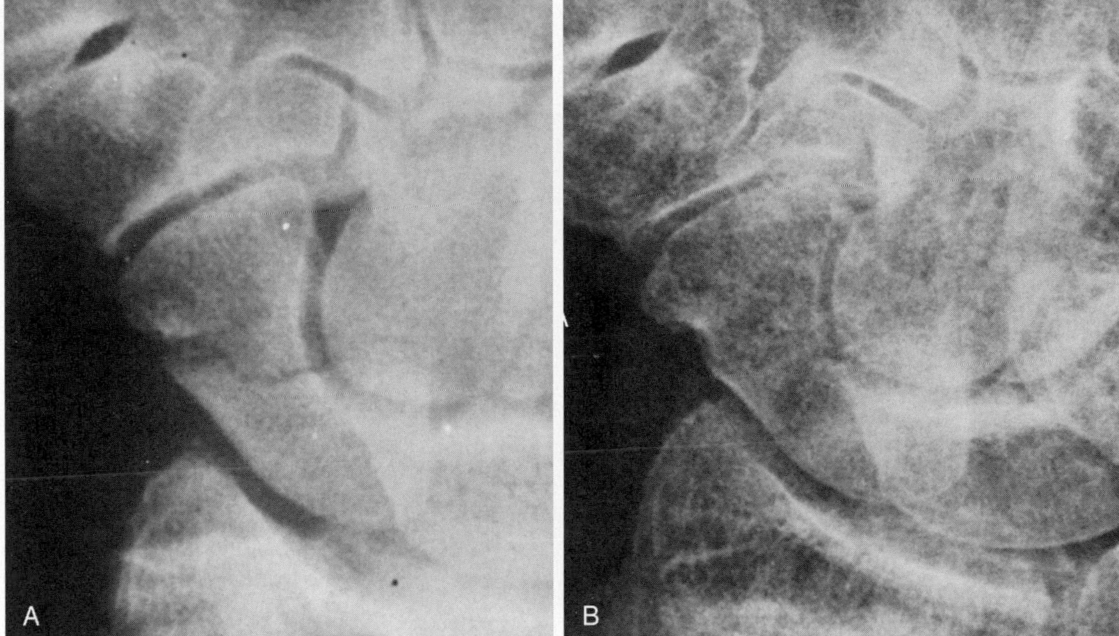

Figure 8–6. Healing of a scaphoid fracture in a 55-year-old man. *A*, There is an undisplaced linear fracture through the waist of the scaphoid, associated with a comminuted fracture of the distal radius. *B*, At 5 months after injury, the scaphoid fracture has healed, without visible external callus. The distal radial fracture has also healed, without visible external callus.

tained and to be aware of this possibility to avoid such an embarrassing error of interpretation.

Disuse Atrophy

Disuse atrophy is an acute form of osteopenia occurring in an extremity because of a lack of use.[28, 33, 41, 65] This condition may result from immobilization following a fracture and occasionally other causes of forced inactivity. The pathologic changes consist of resorption of trabecular and cortical bone in the affected extremity. The pathologic process begins rather abruptly at or immediately proximal to the fracture site and extends to involve all of the bones distal to the fracture (Fig. 8–9). For example, in a fracture of the distal tibia and fibula (Fig. 8–10*B*), the process may involve the entire foot as well as the distal tibia and fibula. The process is reversed, and bone is restored, with resumption of activity after removal of the cast. The resorptive process may be partially prevented by utilizing the extremity while the cast remains in place (i.e., by early ambulation in a walking cast). This acute form of osteopenia can be differentiated from the common chronic form seen in senile osteoporosis.[41, 65] Disuse atrophy is a focal rather than a generalized finding. There are two distinct radiographic features peculiar to disuse atrophy.[41] The first is pronounced resorption on the endosteal surface of the cortical margin of the joints, resulting in a characteristic thin radiolucent line beneath the articular cortex (Figs. 8–11 and 8–12; see also Figs. 8–9 and 8–10). The second is the frequent presence of accentuated resorption across a broader transverse band in the metaphysis extending to the epiphyseal scar in adults (see Figs. 8–9*A* and 8–12*C*). This feature may be seen even in persons older than 40 years of age.

Jones[41] has categorized the radiographic findings in disuse osteoporosis into four patterns: (1) generalized or diffuse osteoporosis, (2) speckled or spotty osteoporosis, (3) linear translucent bands, and (4) cortical changes. There is considerable overlap. The patterns commonly occur in combination (see Figs. 8–9*B* and 8–10*B*). It is important to appreciate the similarities between the findings in this process and those associated with reflex sympathic dystrophy. Full appreciation and understanding of these features allow accurate assessment of the process and avoid the potential for misinterpretations. Radiographic evidence of disuse atrophy is usually present in all patients following 7 to 8 weeks of immobilization. In those under 20 years of age it frequently appears after as little as 4 to 5 weeks.

Generalized osteoporosis is characterized by a loss of finer trabeculae, resulting in a coarsened and blurred radiographic appearance of intramedullary bone (see Figs. 8–9*A*, 8–10*A*, and 8–11). According to Jones,[41] it is the predominant pattern in over half of all patients (52%), particularly in those younger than 20 and older than 50 years of age. Jones states that this is not associated with any perceptible change in cortical thickness.

Speckled or spotty osteoporosis (see Figs. 8–9*B* and 8–10*B*) is found in slightly less than half of all patients[41] (46%) but never in those younger than 15 years of age. Small oval or rounded translucencies first appear in the carpal and tarsal bones and in the bases of the metacarpals and metatarsals; they eventually extend to involve the shafts of long bones but not to the same degree as in the smaller bones. In Jones'[41] series this pattern dominated in 30 patients, none of whom had any clinical evidence of reflex sympathetic dystrophy, the diagnosis of which is based upon the presence of pain, swelling, and dystrophic changes in the skin, not upon the radiographic

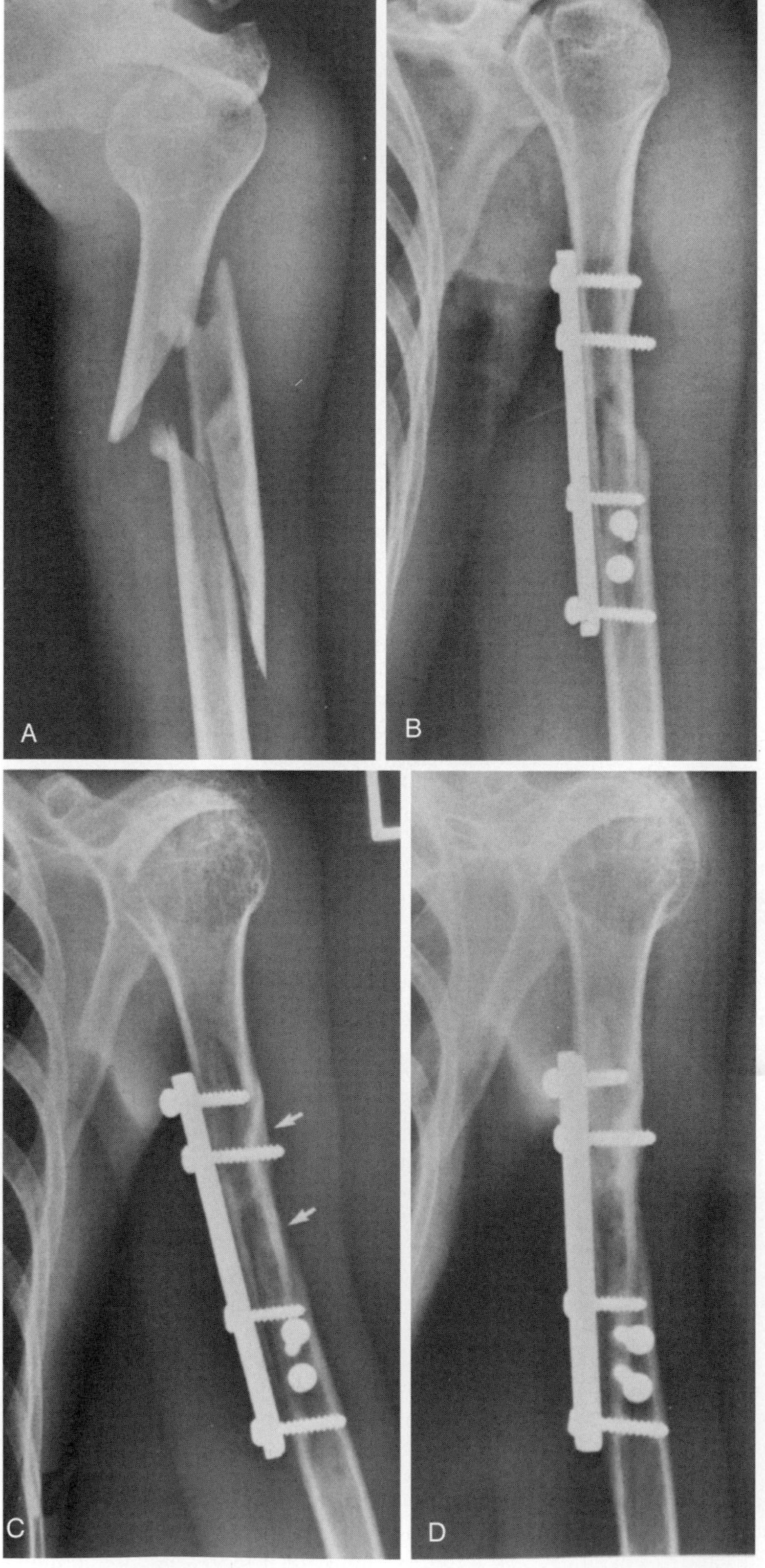

Figure 8–7. Comminuted fracture of the proximal humerus treated by compression plate fixation. *A*, The initial film demonstrates a comminuted fracture with a large butterfly fragment. *B*, A compression plate has been applied with four screws, two proximal and two distal to the principal line of fracture. In addition, two cortical screws were placed within the large butterfly fragment. The apposition of several of the fracture fragments gives the false impression that healing has occurred. This examination was performed at the time of the open reduction and fixation procedure. *C*, At 4 months after injury, there is minimal external callus visible on the lateral margins of the fracture *(arrows)*. The callus bridges the fracture fragments, and clinical union has occurred. *D*, Examination at 7 months demonstrates maturing of the callus. Rigid fixation significantly reduces the extent of external callus formation.

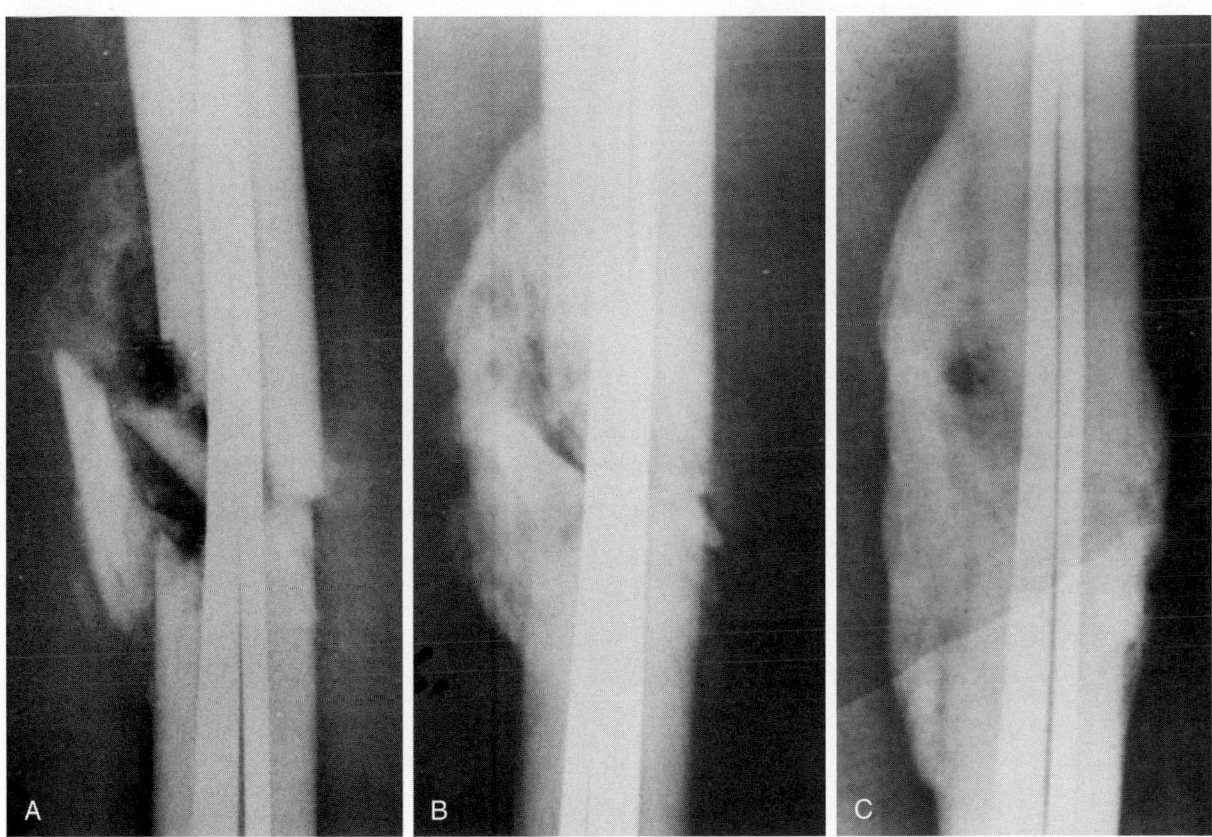

Figure 8–8. Healing femur fracture treated by internal fixation with Ender rods. The patient was a 25-year-old man who sustained bilateral fractures of the femur and fracture of the pelvis in a motorcycle accident. *A*, At 1 month after fracture, the comminuted fracture of the midshaft is evident, with fluffy callus formation at the margins of the fracture. Ender rods are in place. *B*, At 6 weeks, the callus has increased considerably and bridges the fracture line medially but is incomplete laterally. Note the tunneling within the cortex of the distal fragment, indicative of disuse atrophy. Ender rods are slightly flexible allowing some motion at the fracture line, accounting for the exuberant callus formation. *C*, At 5 months after injury, the callus is mature and compact and has bridged and eliminated the line of fracture, except for one circular area of lucency. This area represents the residuum of a large gap created in the fracture line by the comminution of the fracture fragments.

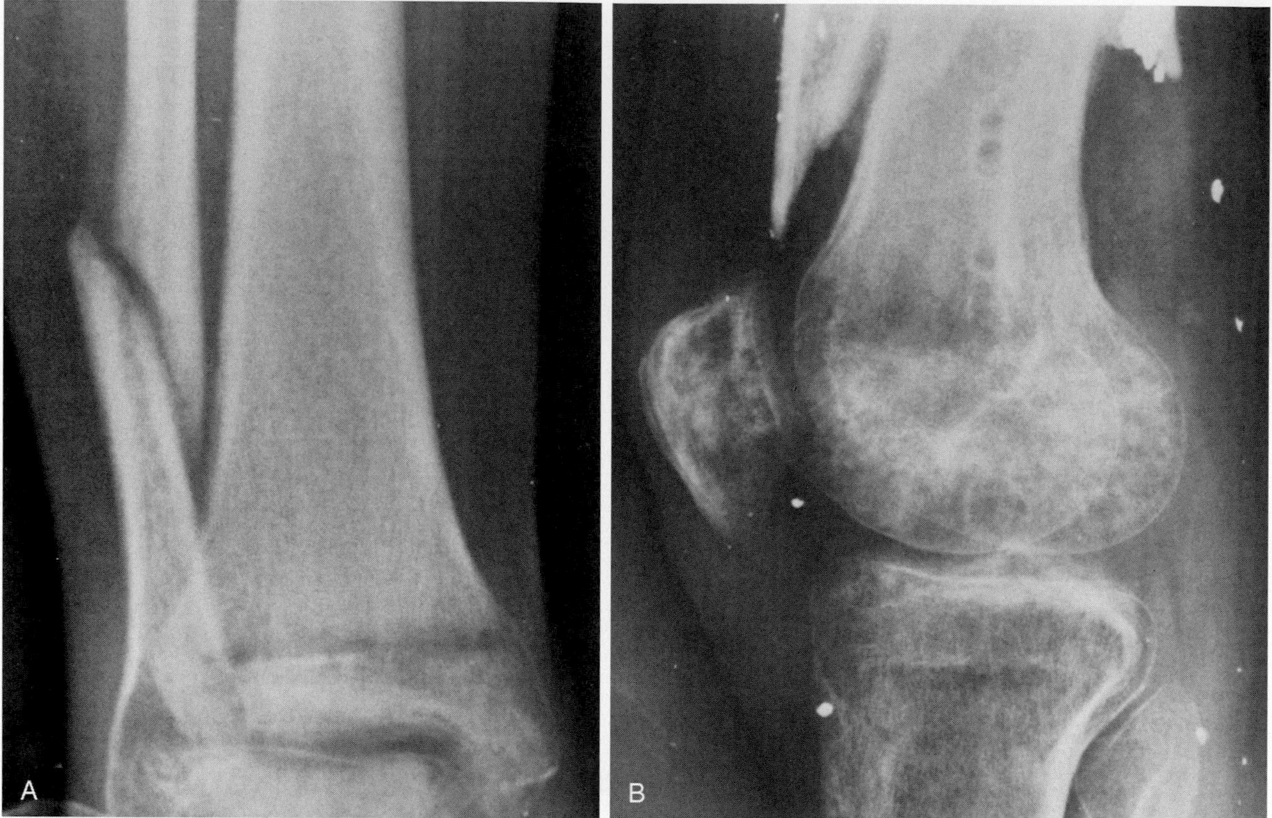

Figure 8–9. Disuse osteoporosis, *A*, In a 25-year-old with a pronation–external rotation fracture of the ankle 7 weeks after injury, there is minimal callus formation at the distal fibular fracture. This examination was performed immediately before open reduction and internal fixation. The disuse atrophy is manifested by coarsening of the trabecular pattern, tunneling within the cortex of the distal tibia, and the presence of linear subcortical lucencies paralleling the joint surface as well as a prominent band-like radiolucency in the metaphysis along the line of the epiphyseal scar. *B*, In this lateral view of the knee of a 24-year-old man, obtained 8½ months after a gunshot wound resulted in a comminuted fracture of the distal femur, spotty or blotchy osteoporosis is present within the patella and femoral condyles. The porosis is accentuated beneath the articular cortex, resulting in a finely etched appearance. Note the faint, rather broad bands of radiolucency in the metaphyseal area of both the distal femur and the proximal tibia.

findings of spotty osteoporosis (see discussion of reflex dystrophy syndromes in Chapter 9). Clinical forms of reflex dystrophy (Sudeck's atrophy) may occur even in the absence of osteoporosis. However, the diagnosis of reflex sympathic dystrophy is suggested by worsening or eventual failure of resolution of spotty osteoporosis following removal of the cast.

Linear translucent bands appear in two forms.[41, 65] The thin, subcortical radiolucent band measuring 1 to 2 mm in width is the earliest and practically a universal radiographic finding in disuse atrophy (see Figs. 8–9 through 8–12). It is frequently the only manifestation of this process. It is often clearly evident through an overlying plaster cast (see Fig. 8–12*B*). The broader translucent bands appear in the metaphysis in the region of the growth plate, in some cases evidenced by the presence of the residual epiphyseal scar. This band extends across the breadth of the shaft. The width of the band varies with the size of the bone involved ranging from roughly 3 to 5 mm in a metacarpal to 10 to 15 mm in the distal tibia. In Jones'[41] series, linear translucent bands were seen in 24%, occurring in patients older than 15 years of age only after epiphyseal fusion.

Cortical changes consist of tunneling (see Figs. 8–3*C* and 8–9*A*), the linear, thin, longitudinal cortical radiolucencies due to enlargement of haversian canals, and scalloping of the outer margin of the cortex. These changes are seen in half of the patients. In older patients the tunneling is particularly evident in the outer third of the cortex and appears to spare the inner two thirds. In Jones' series there was no evidence of decrease in cortical thickness.[41] Evidently, however, thinning of the cortex may occur after prolonged immobilization, and some degree of measurable cortical thinning may persist after complete healing of fractures of major long bones in older persons.

Timing of the reversal of the osteoporotic process and resolution of radiographic changes (see Fig. 8–12) is dependent upon the age of the patient and duration of immobilization. In children, after 5 to 7 weeks in plaster, reversal is noted in approximately 4 weeks and resolution is seen in an additional 6 to 8 weeks. In older persons, longer intervals are required. As has been stated, persistence or worsening of spotty osteoporosis following removal of a cast is suggestive of and consistent with the diagnosis of reflex sympathetic dystrophy.

Not all of the patient's complaints referable to the area of a healing fracture are related directly to the fracture itself. In the elderly, the superimposition of disuse upon preexisting senile osteoporosis may weaken the bone to

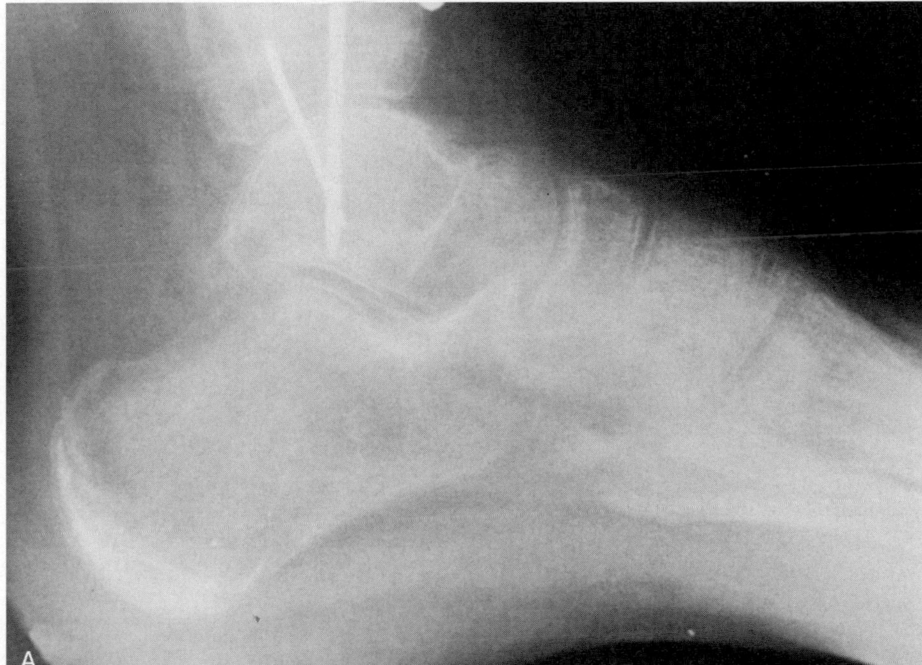

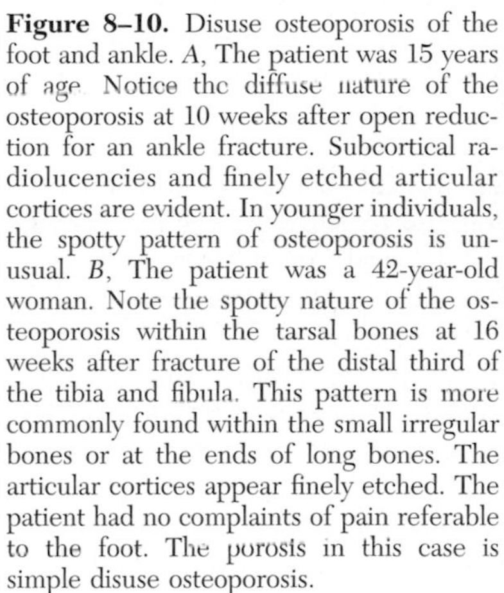

Figure 8–10. Disuse osteoporosis of the foot and ankle. *A*, The patient was 15 years of age. Notice the diffuse nature of the osteoporosis at 10 weeks after open reduction for an ankle fracture. Subcortical radiolucencies and finely etched articular cortices are evident. In younger individuals, the spotty pattern of osteoporosis is unusual. *B*, The patient was a 42-year-old woman. Note the spotty nature of the osteoporosis within the tarsal bones at 16 weeks after fracture of the distal third of the tibia and fibula. This pattern is more commonly found within the small irregular bones or at the ends of long bones. The articular cortices appear finely etched. The patient had no complaints of pain referable to the foot. The porosis in this case is simple disuse osteoporosis.

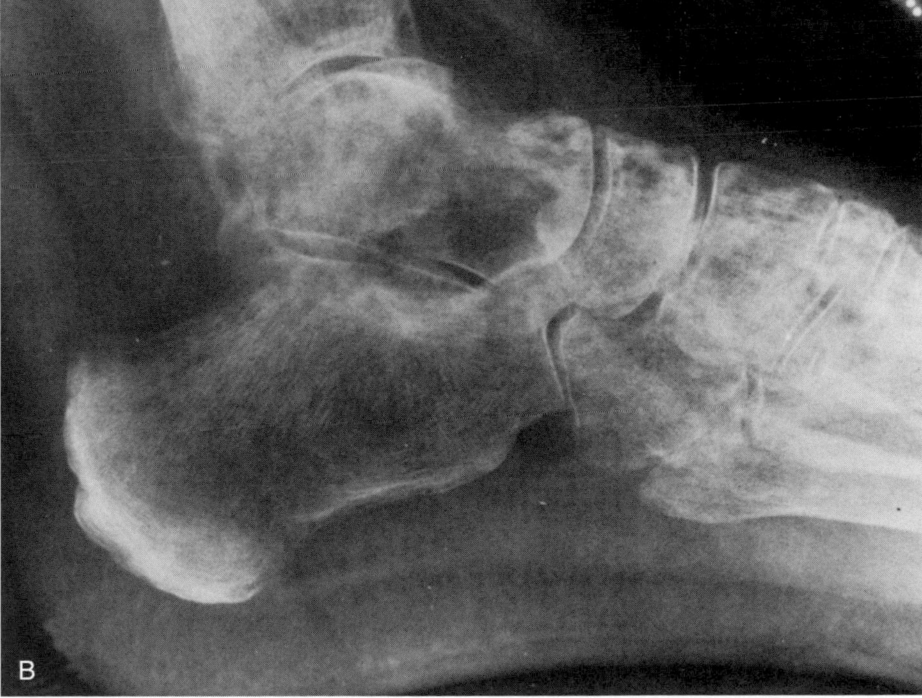

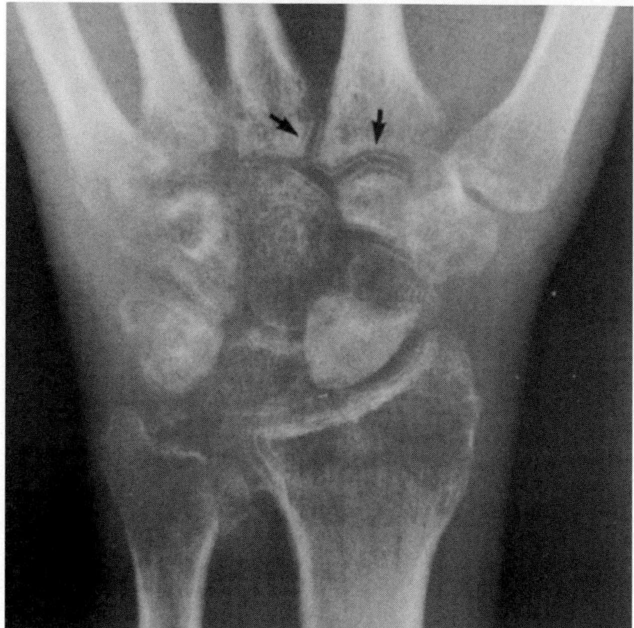

Figure 8–11. Disuse osteoporosis in a 29-year-old man with aseptic necrosis of the proximal pole of the scaphoid. The porosis is present throughout all of the carpal bones and at the base of the metacarpals. There is subarticular resorption with fine radiolucency, particularly at the base of the second and third metacarpals *(arrows)*, an associated fracture of the distal ulna, and calcification within the triangular cartilage. The increased density in the proximal pole of the scaphoid indicates that it is deprived of its blood supply, and therefore no bone has been resorbed. The density of the proximal pole is that of normal bone, whereas the surrounding bone has been resorbed and is radiographically lucent.

such an extent that insufficiency or stress fractures may occur (Fig. 8–13). It is important, under these circumstances, to inspect the entire radiograph and not remain focused on the fracture line to avoid missing additional findings that account for the patient's complaints.

Presumably, the distribution of the vascular supply of bone has some role in the location of the radiographic changes. Hyperemia[28] in the bone in association with osteoporosis has been demonstrated following immobilization.[33, 57, 58, 61] The broad band translucencies in the metaphysis may be evidence of continued hypervascularity in this region. The outer third of the cortex is supplied by periosteal vessels, whereas the inner two thirds is supplied by endosteal branches of the nutrient arteries.[69] This difference in blood supply may account in some way for the difference in the localization of tunneling. Spotty osteoporosis and the thin, subcortical lucencies are less easily explained; the exact explanation remains unknown.[28]

Union

Clinical union of fracture fragments occurs, by the sufficient growth of bone across the fracture line, before radiographic evidence of the fracture line is obliterated (see Fig. 8–3*D*). Union is therefore best determined by clinical means.[34, 75] The clinical indications of fracture healing are stability, as determined by physical examination; lack of pain at the fracture site; and the ability to use the part without external support (e.g., in a fracture of the lower extremity, the ability to walk without cast, crutch, or cane).

The radiographic evidence of union[9, 75] consists of a continuous external bridge of callus across the line of fracture uniting the fracture fragments (see Figs. 8–3*D* and 8–5*D*); the callus is uniformly ossified and approaches the density of normal bone. It is mandatory that these findings be present in at least two views exposed at 90 degrees to one another, commonly an anteroposterior and a lateral projection. Oblique or special views (see Fig. 8–21) may be necessary in some cases for verification or clarification. It is also mandatory that the radiographs be properly exposed. Underexposure is particularly problematic in that the resultant underpenetration may create the illusion of obliteration of the fracture line by bony trabeculae, whereas a properly exposed radiograph will demonstrate the continued presence of the fracture line and the lack of healing. Overlapping of fragments may also give the illusion of union (Fig. 8–14*A*), but this possibility should rarely pose a problem when the examination includes at least two projections. Here again, additional oblique views may be helpful. If the question still persists the use of computed tomography (CT) with multiplanar reconstructed images (Fig. 8–15) may be necessary for clarification.

The time required for clinical union[34, 75] of an uncomplicated fracture varies chiefly with the age of the patient and the bone involved. In an adult, union of a fracture of the clavicle may require 3 to 4 weeks; of the humeral shaft, 6 to 8 weeks; of the tibial shaft, 10 to 12 weeks; and of the femoral shaft, 12 to 14 weeks. However, in a young child, a femoral shaft fracture may be expected to heal within a month, and fractures at other sites in correspondingly shorter times. If there is a question about the solidity of the union, so-called stress films are helpful. Stress films are a series of radiographs obtained with the affected body part in the neutral position and during the application of stress on the distal fragment or part in the plane of suspected motion (Fig. 8–16). Change in the alignment of the fragments before and during the application of stress indicates lack of union. Care must be taken to assure that the proximal fragment is positioned similarly on both the neutral and stress views and that the entire length of the bone is included on the radiograph. These precautions make the determination much easier and more precise.

Viewing the fracture under stress with fluoroscopy has been advocated by Connolly[12] as a quick means of evaluating a fracture for motion. If the amount of motion is small, it may be difficult to interpret radiographs to definitively decide whether a fracture moves with stress. The difficulty arises because the comparative films are taken a few seconds apart, and typically the stress is relaxed between the two radiographs and the patient may be in a slightly different position for the second view. This difference may be enough to make it impossible to decide whether motion is present. The disadvantage of fluoroscopic evaluation is that if the fluoroscopic unit can take spot films, they include only a portion and not the full length of the long bone being evaluated.

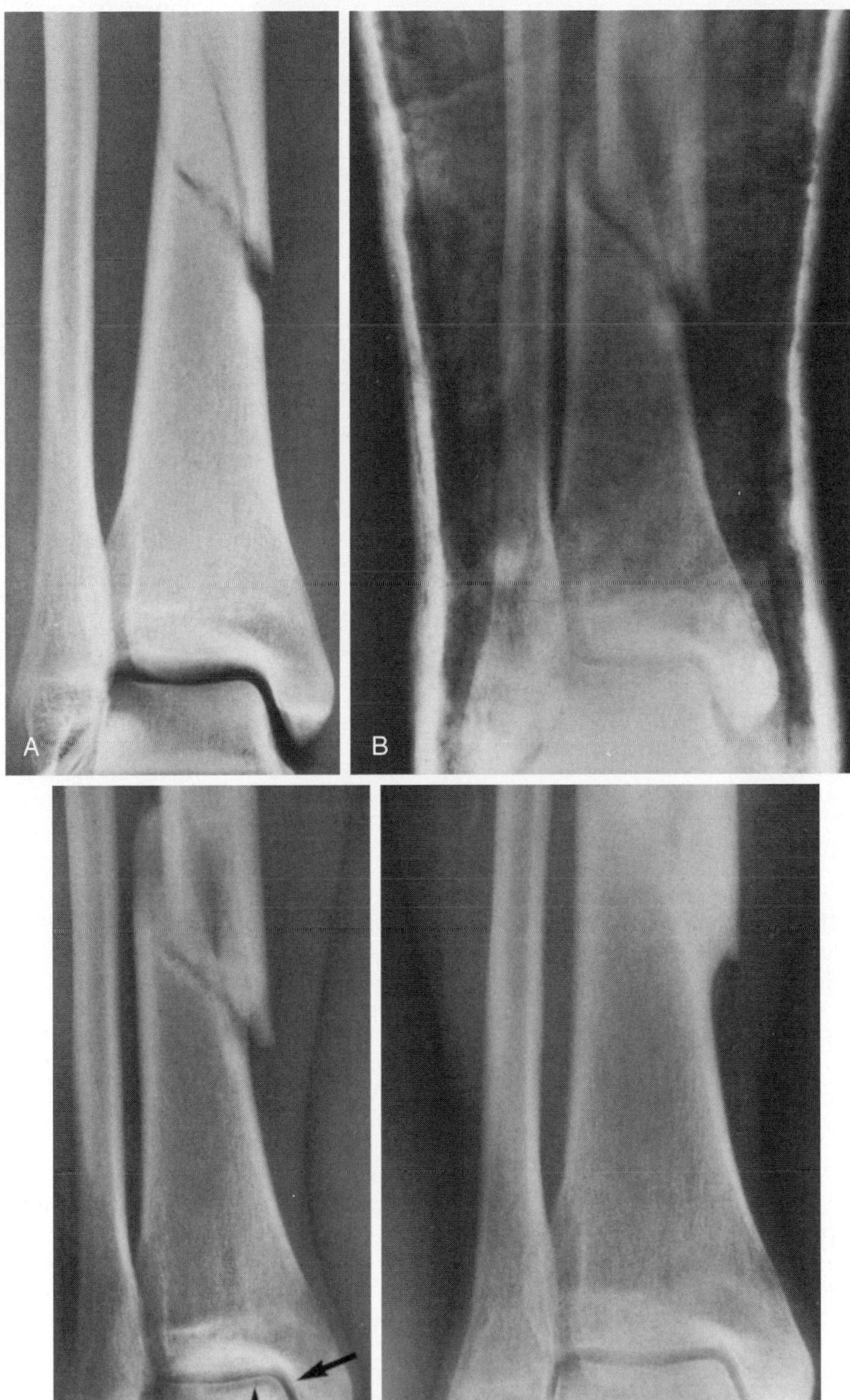

Figure 8–12. Disuse osteoporosis in a 37-year-old woman with fracture of the distal third of the tibia and the proximal third of the fibula. *A*, The initial postreduction radiograph demonstrates an oblique fracture of the distal third of the tibia. *B*, At 2 months after injury, the initial manifestations of disuse osteoporosis are identified through the plaster cast. Note the fine line of subarticular radiolucency of the talus and tibia. *C*, At 10 months after fracture, the subarticular lucencies are clearly evident *(arrows)*, and there is a faint band of radiolucency within the distal tibial metaphysis. *D*, At 2 years after injury, the fracture has healed. There was delayed union. The architecture of the bone has been restored, and the evidence of disuse osteoporosis eliminated.

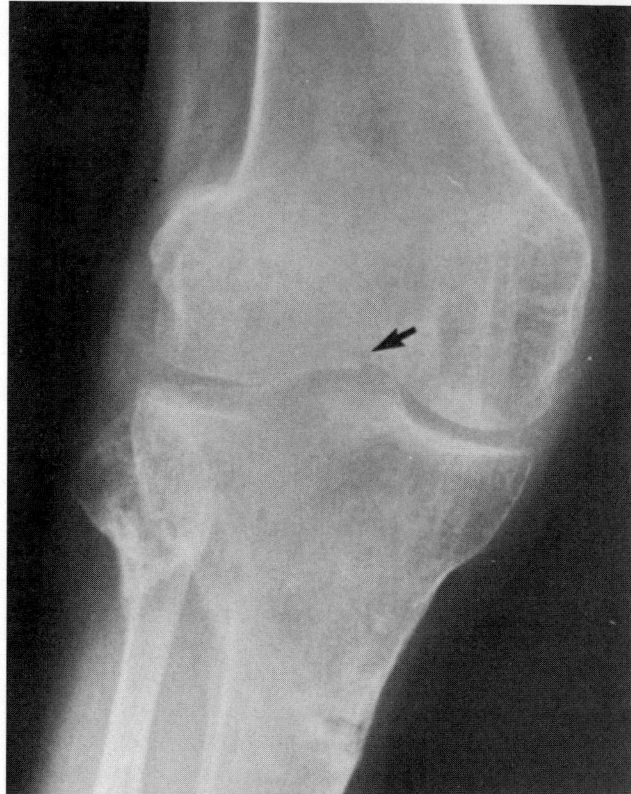

Figure 8–13. Insufficiency fracture of the lateral femoral condyle in an elderly woman with a healing fracture of the proximal tibia and fibula, which she had sustained 7 months previously. Note the marked osteoporosis. She recently began ambulating and complained of pain in the knee. Note the healing fracture of the tibia and fibula and the acute fracture of the lateral femoral condyle. The articular cortex of the lateral condyle and intercondylar notch are disrupted *(arrow)*.

The woven bone of the callus is eventually replaced by haversian bone oriented along lines of stress. Distinct cortical bone and medullary cancellous bone develop at the site of fracture and gradually remodel to form an outline similar to that of the bone before the fracture. In time, the bone may remodel to such a degree that there is no evidence of the previous fracture (Fig. 8–17). Such remodeling occurs frequently in children and adolescents but less commonly in adults.

Malunion

Malunion[34, 75] is the healing of fragments of a fracture in a faulty position (Fig. 8–18). Usually malunion is associated with an excessive rotatory or angular deformity. In a very young child, considerable potential exists for correction of angular deformities with future growth (see Fig. 8–17); therefore, the term may not be appropriate in this age group. No such potential exists in the older child, adolescent, or adult, and surgical correction of significant residual deformity or malunion is required. Angular malunions are usually quite apparent both clinically and radiographically, but rotational deformities are difficult to identify, verify, or exclude on the basis of their radiographic appearance. It is difficult to include a sufficient length of the limb containing an adequate number of identifiable landmarks in the sagittal or coronal plane to conclusively demonstrate the presence of a rotational deformity on a radiograph. These deformities are much more obvious and easier to establish by visual inspection of the limb.

Healing Problems

Failure of bone healing has been divided into three categories: technical failures, biologic failures, and a combination of technical and biologic failures.[27] With technical failures, the biologic healing processes function satisfactorily, but something interferes with them. The interference could be from excessive motion of the fracture site, distraction, poor reduction, loss of local blood supply, or infection. Frost[27] estimated that 70% to 80% of cases of delayed union and nonunion are caused or contributed to by one or a combination of these technical factors. In these cases, radiographs demonstrate adequate callus at the ends of the opposing bone fragments but no callus bridging the fracture line. Nonunion resulting from technical failures has been called hypertrophic nonunion because of adequate or even excessive callus production. Treatment by improving the reduction or fixation and eradicating any infection characteristically leads to successful union of the fracture. In some cases, however, a synovial cavity may form between the fracture ends, or soft tissue may be interposed between the fracture ends.[17] The synovial cavity or soft tissue must be surgically resected to allow bone healing.[12, 17] Radionuclide bone scanning demonstrates a linear or curvilinear area of decreased activity at the fracture site, surrounded on all sides by high-level activity in the opposing fracture fragments.[17]

Biologic failure of the healing process accounts for approximately 20% of cases of nonunion and contributes to another 20%.[27] In most of the cases, cortical bone is involved, and nonunion occurs in spite of proper treatment. Failure to make callus accounts for more than three fourths of these cases of nonunion. Radiation therapy, regional denervation, some cytotoxic agents used for tumor treatment, and some nonsteroidal anti-inflammatory agents, such as indomethacin, can cause failure of callus formation.[27, 36] The failure of callus may be caused by either a local abnormality or a systemic metabolic condition that prevents bone or cartilage matrices from forming. Radiographs of such fractures of a long bone demonstrate a sparse amount of callus or even no callus at 2 months or more after fracture.

Other rare, biologic causes of nonunion and delayed union include abnormalities in remodeling and tissue differentiation.[27] If remodeling breaks down, callus is not replaced in a timely fashion. Callus is not mechanically durable and will become pliable, and deformity will soon develop after weight-bearing begins. Another cause of nonunion is a breakdown in the differentiation of local precursor cells, causing formation of fibroblasts and lipoblasts instead of chondroblasts and osteoblasts. These cells fill the fracture site with scar tissue and fat rather than callus. This abnormality is seen sometimes with fracture distraction, with some metastatic tumors,[5, 39] or

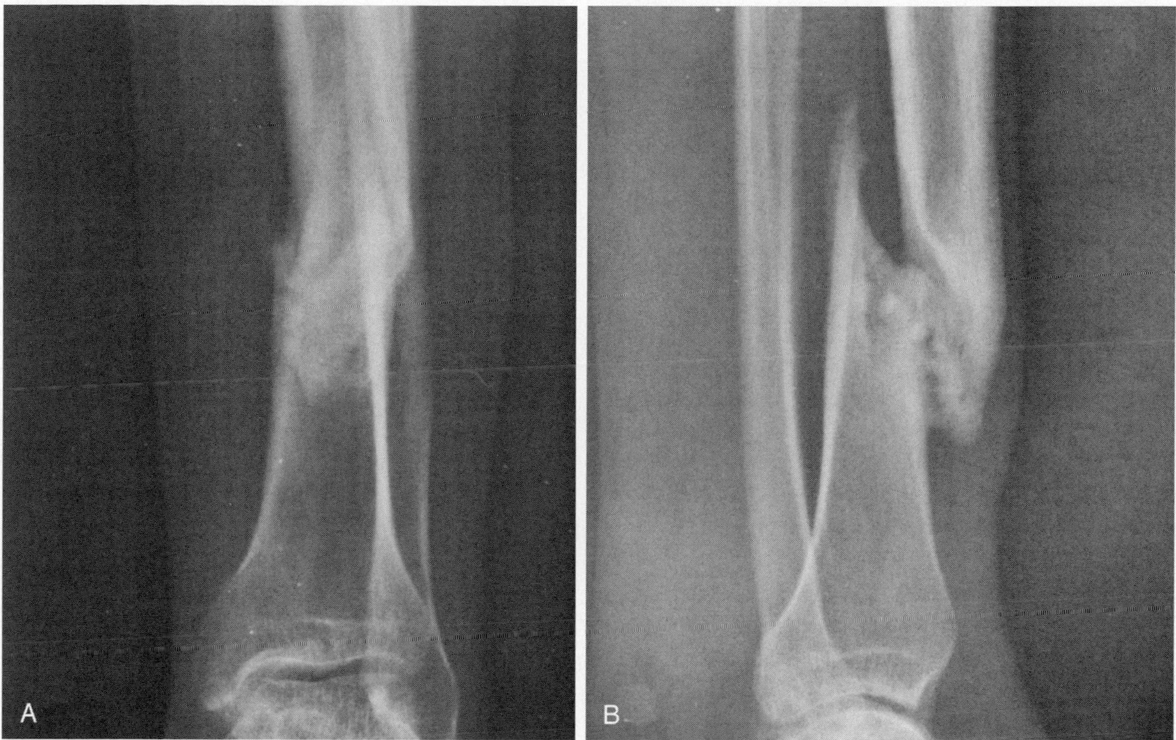

Figure 8–14. Nonunion of fracture of the distal third of the tibia 12 months after injury in a 35-year-old man. The fracture was associated with a fracture of the proximal tibia, which healed. *A*, Anteroposterior projection gives no indication of nonunion. The fracture line is not apparent. *B*, Lateral projection clearly demonstrates a wide separation at the line of fracture. The apposing fracture margins are rounded and smooth, with some sclerosis. Minimal callus is present. The appearance is characteristic of nonunion.

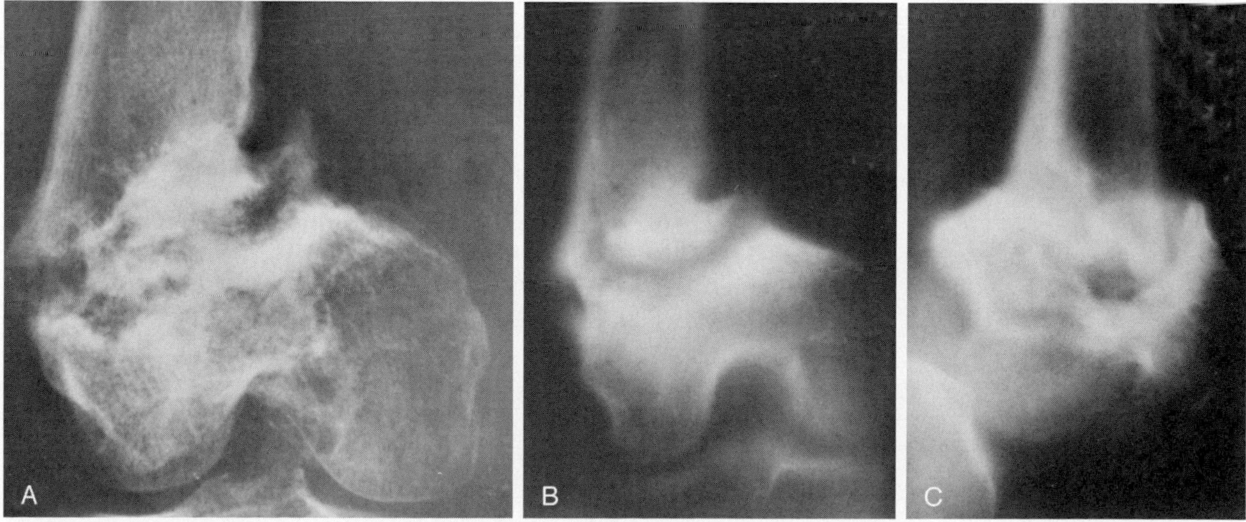

Figure 8–15. Nonunion with pseudarthrosis of a supracondylar fracture of the femur, 17 months after injury. *A*, Anteroposterior projection demonstrates considerable density within the area of the fracture. The peripheral margins of the fracture line are evident. The question of union is not resolved. *B*, Anteroposterior conventional tomogram clearly demonstrates lack of union through the fracture. The apposing margins of the fracture are sclerotic. *C*, Lateral conventional tomogram also demonstrates the lack of union. The fracture line is widened, and the apposing margins of the fracture are sclerotic. The distal margin of the proximal fragment is convex and the apposing margin of the distal fragment concave, findings consistent with pseudarthrosis.

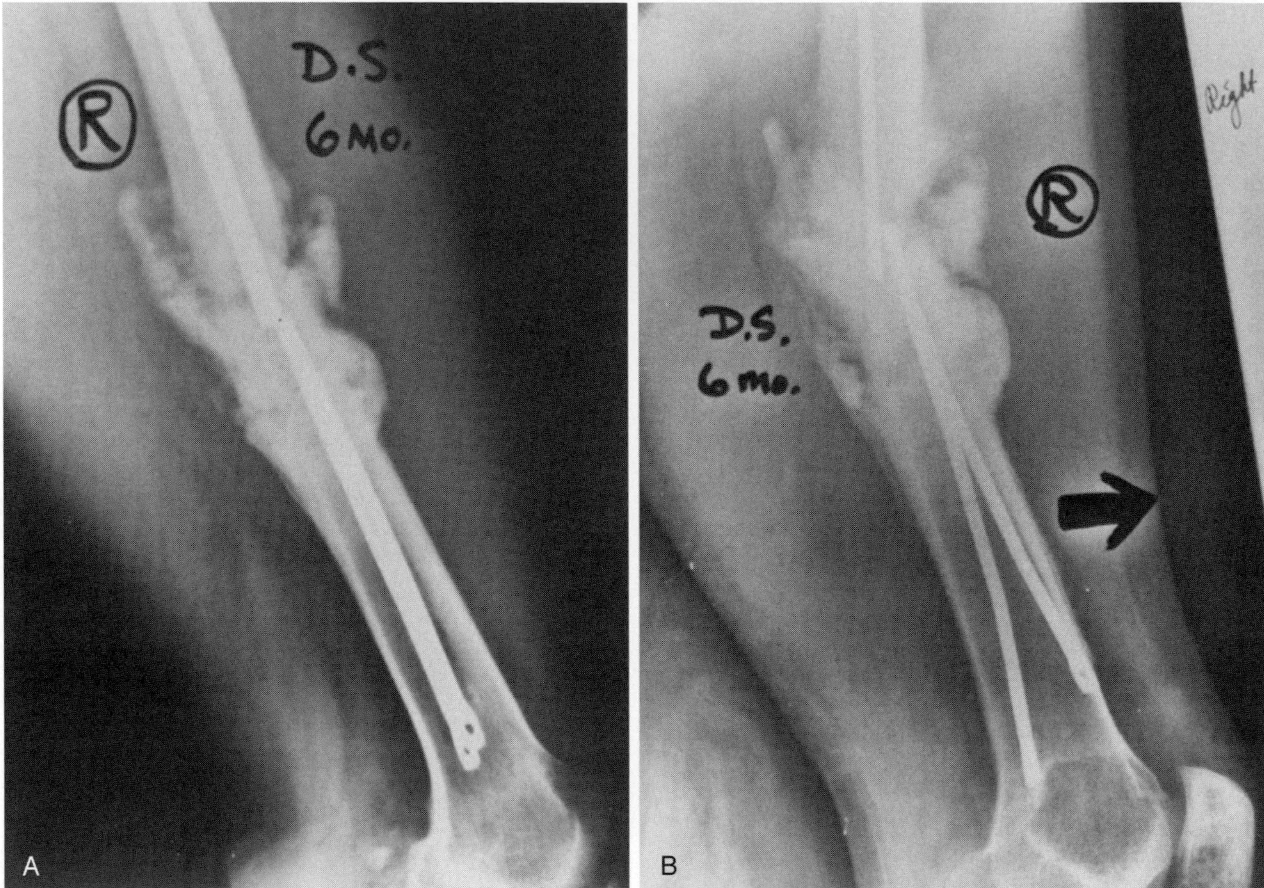

Figure 8–16. Use of stress film. The patient was a 25-year-old man who originally sustained a comminuted fracture of the midshaft of the femur in a motorcycle accident. He was treated primarily with Ender rods. At 4 months he was in another accident that refractured the femur and broke the Ender rods. He was then treated for an additional 3 months. *A*, A lateral view of the femur demonstrates the fractured Ender rods and exuberant callus formation at the fracture site. *B*, Another lateral view obtained while the knee was extended demonstrates motion at the fracture line and lack of union. The patient was subsequently treated with a compression plate.

from no known cause. It also may be seen rarely in the presence of local denervation, chronic primary hyperparathyroidism, congenital pseudarthrosis of the tibia, neurofibromatosis,[68] and diabetic neuropathy.

Delayed Union

Fractures at given anatomic locations are known to heal within a certain average period the duration of which varies chiefly with the severity of the injury and the age of the patient. Failure to heal in a timely manner constitutes delayed union[34, 75] (Fig. 8–19; see also Fig. 8–4). The rate of repair is slower than normal for whatever reason—limited blood supply at the fracture site, inadequate mobilization, loss of bone, presence of infection, or individual idiosyncrasy. The anticipated time for healing is established by experience and clinical judgment. The diagnosis of delayed union is made on the basis of the clinical findings (manipulation produces motion at the fracture

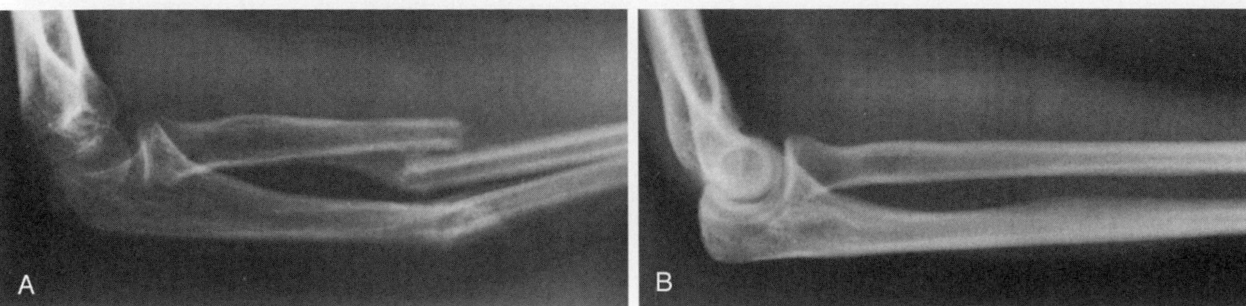

Figure 8–17. Remodeling of both bones fractured in the forearm of an 11-year-old. *A*, The transverse fracture of both bones of the forearm had united at 9 months after injury with considerable overriding of the fracture fragments. *B*, Subsequent examination at age 18 years fails to demonstrate any evidence of abnormality. The bones have completely remodeled.

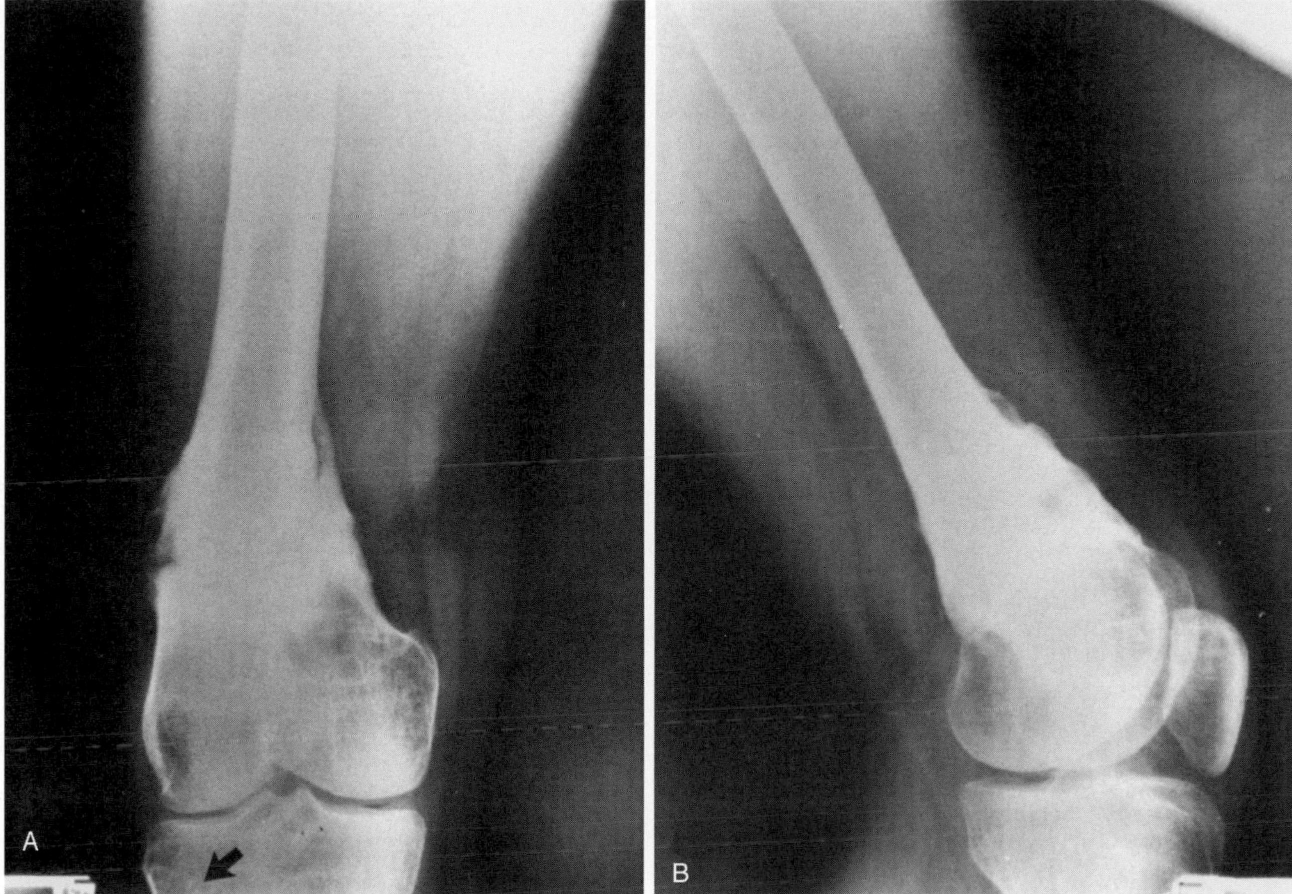

Figure 8–18. Malunion of a supracondylar fracture of the femur in a 21-year-old man. The distorted alignment creates stress within the knee joint that is manifested by the linear lucent crescent of gas within the medial compartment of the joint. *A*, Anteroposterior projection of the right femur. Note the position of the head of the fibula *(arrow)*. The normal medial inclination of the femoral shaft is approximately 10 degrees. In this case, the inclination is actually reversed, with a lateral angulation of the shaft of approximately 5 degrees. *B*, On the lateral projection the distal fragment is healed in flexion, which causes hyperextension of the knee.

line, indicating the lack of union), and the radiographic appearance (persistence of the fracture line and a scarcity or absence of callus formation are demonstrated) substantiates the clinical impression. Union is likely to occur under these circumstances if adequate immobilization is either continued (see Figs. 8–4 and 8–19) or initiated if lacking. A delay of weeks or even months does not mean that union will eventually fail to occur. Healing continues, but at a slower-than-normal pace.

Nonunion

Nonunion[34, 75] exists when the fracture healing process ceases completely, and the fragments remain un-united (Figs. 8–20 through 8–22; see also Fig. 8–14). This problem occurs chiefly in adults; it is uncommon in children. The diagnosis is established by demonstrating continued motion at the fracture site on manipulation and characteristic radiographic findings. There are two types of nonunion: hypertrophic and atrophic. In hypertrophic nonunion, the margins of the fracture become well-defined, smooth, and sclerotic (see Figs. 8–14*B*, 8–20, and 8–21). The medullary canal is occluded by eburnated bone. No callus crosses the fracture line. A false joint or pseudarthrosis[1, 9, 75] may form at the fracture site (Fig. 8–23; see also Fig. 8–22), with one fragment presenting a convex surface that fits into the concave surface of the apposing fragment. In the much less common atrophic type of nonunion, there is a limited amount of sclerosis at the fracture margins—usually a fine line of sclerosis across the medullary canal of the apposing fragments. The gap between the fragments is filled by fibrous tissue attached to the ends of the fragments, oriented in the longitudinal plane of the fracture line. Often a small fluid-filled slit or sac is seen between these two planes of fibrous tissue. The pathologic findings thus mimic a joint: the plug of bone filling the medullary canal serves as articular bone, the fibrous tissue serves as joint cartilage, and the fluid-filled slit mimics the joint space. Radionuclide bone scanning can identify the fluid-filled sac that forms between the bone ends in a nonunion.[17]

With an established nonunion, operative intervention is required to reinitiate the healing process. Some combination of internal fixation, bone grafting, and resection of the fracture line, including the pseudarthrosis, is performed.

A frequent complication of nonunion is the associated failure of an orthopedic appliance used for internal fixation of the fracture (Fig. 8–24). The purpose of the

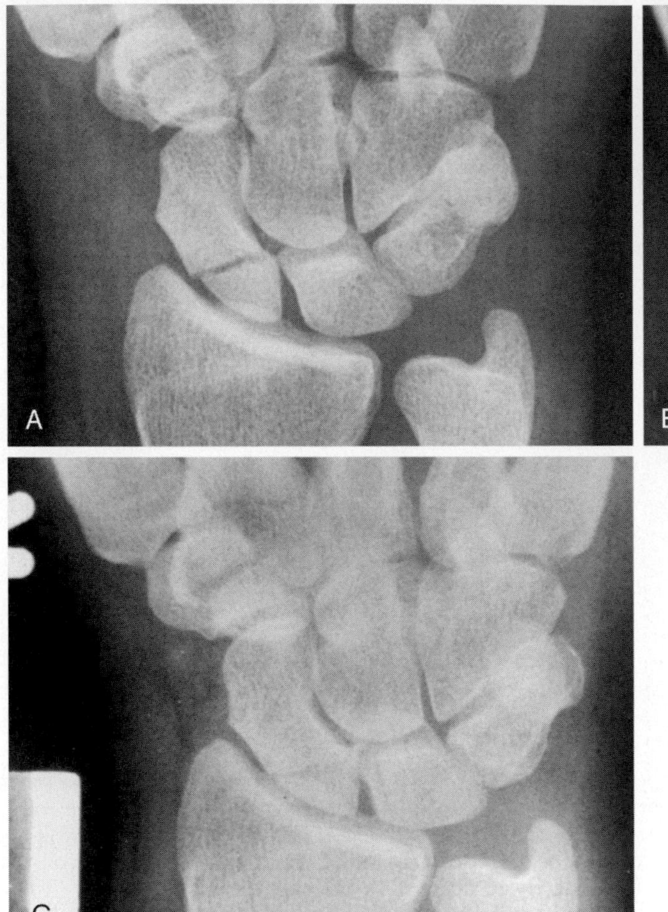

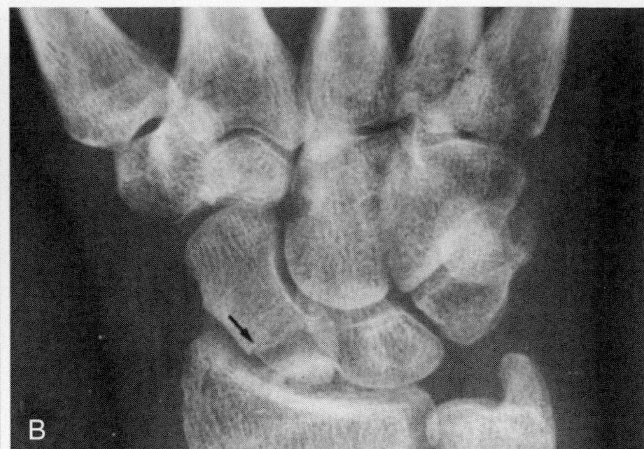

Figure 8–19. Delayed union of a fracture of the proximal pole of the scaphoid in a young man. *A*, The radiograph of the initial injury clearly demonstrates a linear, slightly displaced fracture of the proximal pole of the scaphoid. *B*, At 4 months after fracture, the fracture line is visible *(arrow)*, and the patient experiences pain on motion of the wrist. *C*, At 1 year after fracture, healing has occurred. The fracture line is obliterated. Delayed union and aseptic necrosis, frequent complications of fractures of the proximal pole of the scaphoid, are absent in this patient.

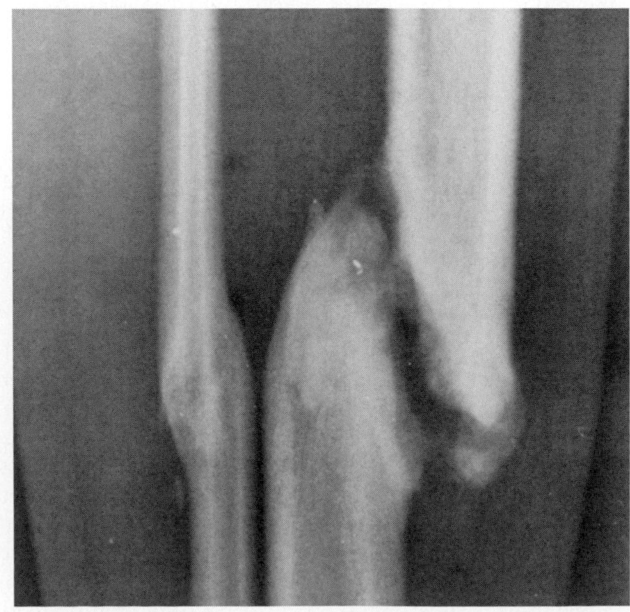

Figure 8–20. Nonunion of a midshaft fracture of the middle third of the tibia 12 months after injury in an 18-year-old girl. Note that the fracture of the fibula has healed. The line of fracture is clearly separated, with rounding and sclerosis of the apposing margins of the fracture. A plug of osseous callus fills the medullary canal of the distal fragment. The radiographic findings are characteristic of nonunion.

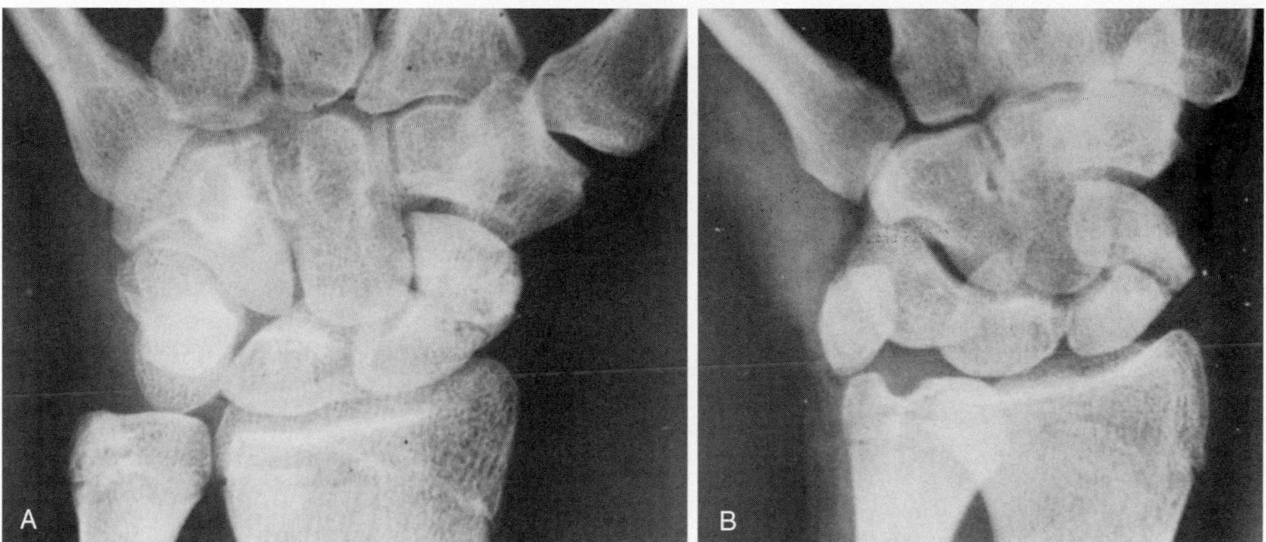

Figure 8–21. Nonunion of a scaphoid fracture in a 20-year-old man. *A*, The standard posteroanterior view of the wrist demonstrates some irregularity in the waist of the scaphoid 14 months after injury. The fracture line is not clearly visualized, and it cannot be determined whether or not union has occurred. *B*, Examination with ulnar deviation clearly demonstrates the line of fracture; the slightly sclerotic, smooth apposing margins are indicative of nonunion.

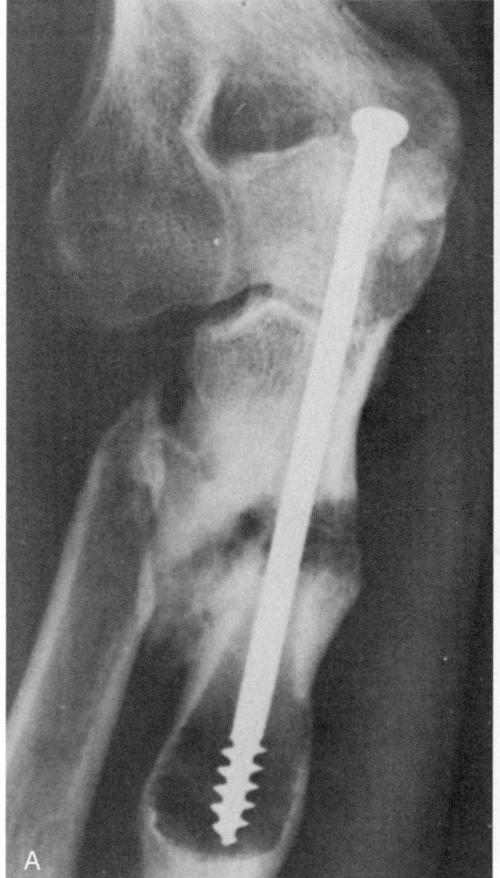

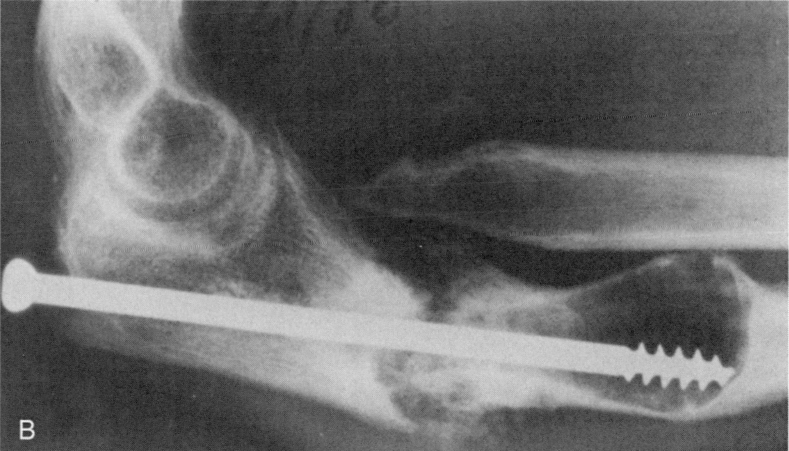

Figure 8–22. Nonunion and pseudarthrosis of a fracture of the proximal end of the ulna. A comminuted fracture of the radial head and neck was originally associated with the ulnar fracture. The radial fracture fragments were excised, and the ulnar fracture was reduced with a long lag screw. *A*, Anteroposterior projection demonstrates a wide band of lucency between the proximal and distal ulnar fragments. A lag screw bridges the fracture site and ends in an expanded area of lucency within the distal fragment. *B*, Lateral view again demonstrates the line of lucency at the fracture site and the presence of the lag screw. The proximal fragment is concave and the distal fragment convex at the fracture line, indicating the presence of a pseudarthrosis. Note the expanded lucency within the distal fragment: Motion at the fracture site has allowed the lag screw to act as a rongeur, hollowing out the shaft of the ulna distally, which accounts for the bulbous lucency. The absence of lucency paralleling the neck of the screw indicates that there is no motion of the screw within the proximal fragment. The distal fragment has rotated about the screw with movement at the pseudarthrosis.

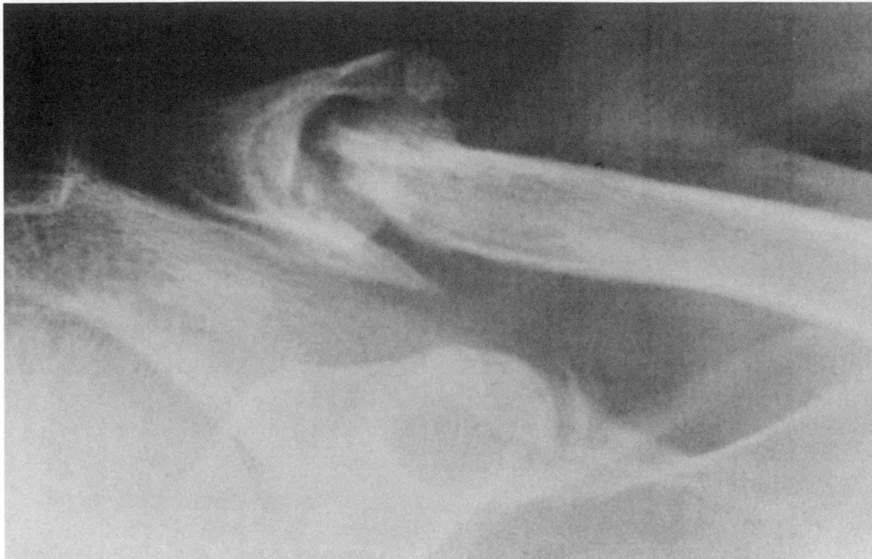

Figure 8–23. Pseudarthrosis of fracture of the distal area of the clavicle in a 43-year-old man. The distal fragment is concave and the proximal fragment convex, and a broad curvilinear band of radiolucency between the two clearly indicates the presence of a pseudarthrosis.

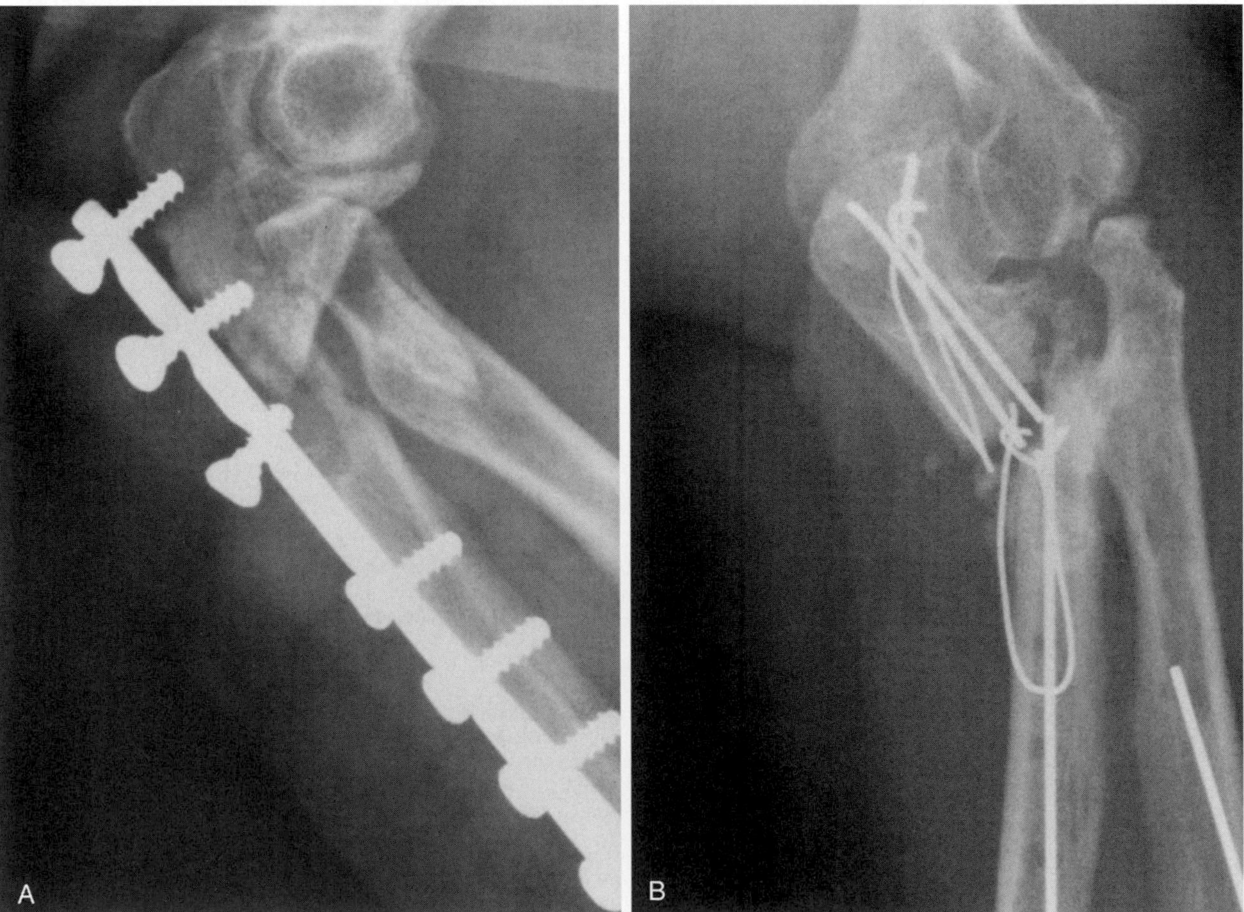

Figure 8–24. Nonunion of fracture of the proximal ulna. Resorption of bone surrounding the proximal three screws has allowed them to back out. There is also a radial head fracture and posterior radial head dislocation. *B*, At 13 months after the compression plate and screws were removed, Kirschner wires and a figure-of-eight wire suture were used for internal fixation of the ulnar fracture, but with similar failure. Note the progressive destruction of the capitellum and radial head.

appliance is to hold the bone fragments in place long enough for fracture healing to occur, but not for an indefinite time. With stress over a long-enough time span, the appliance itself eventually may fracture, or bone may be resorbed around it until it loosens (see Fig. 8–24) and no longer stabilizes the fracture.

Imaging Studies in the Evaluation of Fracture Healing

Plain Radiography

Determination of healing or union of a fracture is principally a clinical decision aided by the radiographic findings. Clinical union may occur while the fracture line is still radiographically apparent. It is usually present before there is radiographic consolidation, with solid ensheathing bony callus and complete obliteration of the fracture line by bony trabeculae. Therefore, the diagnosis of union or absence of union often cannot be made on the basis of radiographic appearance alone. In view of this consideration, and the potential liability surrounding much of the practice of trauma surgery, it is best to avoid use of the designations “union,” “nonunion,” and “delayed union” unless the findings on the radiograph are absolutely characteristic (i.e., an obvious pseudarthrosis), or unless the practitioner making the report is familiar with the clinical findings. Rather, the callus should be completely described with regard to its presence or absence, its nature (i.e., fluffy or mature), its position (i.e., unilateral or encircling), and whether or not it completely bridges the fracture line. When the state of healing is in question, it may be necessary to remove the cast or splint in order to visualize early callus formation, which may appear faint. The appearance of the fracture line should be stated in qualitative terms: readily apparent, partially obliterated, barely perceptible, and the like. It should be remembered that a fracture line may be partially or completely obliterated by precise reduction or by overlap of adjacent fragments. In neither case should this appearance be misconstrued as evidence of healing. The alignment of the principal fragments should be fully described by a method similar to that used with the original fracture. Terms such as “malalignment” and “satisfactory alignment” should be avoided. Angulation is easily determined on a radiograph, but rotation of fragments about the long axis of a bone is at best difficult and often impossible to determine.

To accurately evaluate the progress of healing, comparison with previous radiographs is essential. To make a judgment regarding healing or to render a report without the benefit of previous examinations compromises the value of the examination for both physician and patient.

Computed Tomography

Plain radiographic studies are adequate for determining fracture healing in most situations. However, some fractures are comminuted or spiral, are in planes not easily evaluated with standard radiography, or are in bones with peculiar shapes or axes. With these fractures, the appearance on plain radiographs may be inconclusive than can healing until a large quantity of callus bridges the fracture site. Computed tomography (CT) can detect smaller bone bridges in these instances at an earlier time than can plain radiography. Helical CT scanning is useful in this setting with images obtained in the axial plane and then reconstructed in the coronal and sagittal planes. (Good-quality images are obtained using a pitch of 1.0 or less, as small a field of view as practicable, and image overlap of 50% in the axial plane.)

CT helps the clinician determine at an earlier time

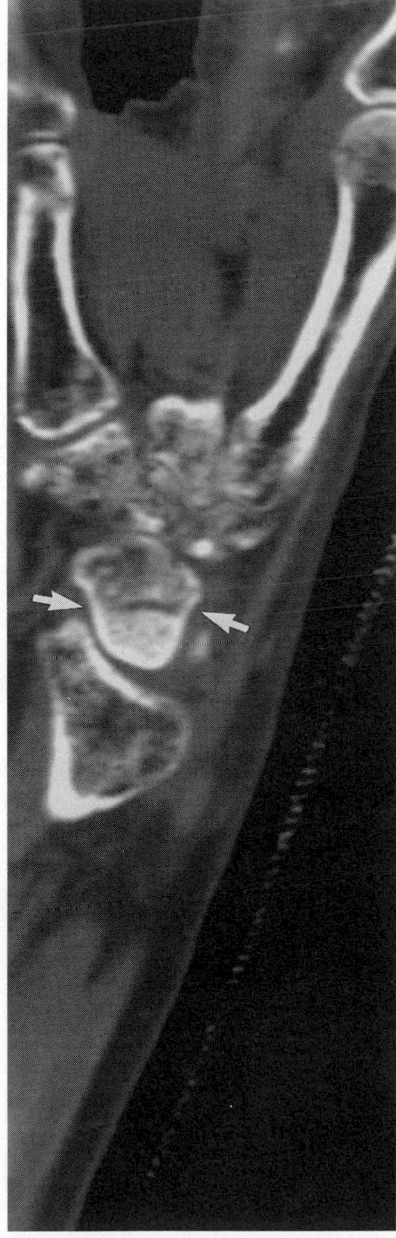

Figure 8–25. Sagittal reconstructed image from a spiral computed tomographic examination of a scaphoid fracture done to evaluate for bone bridging. The fiberglass cast artifact prevented adequate evaluation with plain radiographs. Bone bridging of the scaphoid waist fracture at its cortical margins *(arrows)* is seen, but increased density of the proximal pole indicates that osteonecrosis is also present.

whether additional surgery and bone grafting will be needed or if the fracture will heal on its own if it is left undisturbed. Areas where it may be most useful include the carpal bones (the scaphoid in particular) (Fig. 8–25), tarsal bones (calcaneus most frequently), metacarpal and metatarsal bases, surgical bony fusions especially between carpal or tarsal bones, fractures involving joint articular surfaces (e.g., tibial plateau, ankle pilon, calcaneal fractures) (Fig. 8–26), some elbow fractures, and many comminuted fractures. CT is also used to evaluate healing of complicated fractures of long bones (Fig. 8–27), fractures in the spine, and fractures in the pelvis. An early decision to bone graft has been shown to be important in scaphoid nonunion treatment and possibly carries over to other bones. The success rate in treating scaphoid nonunions was reported to decrease as the duration of nonunion before treatment increased.[63] Early identification of nonunion with CT in other bones hopefully will diminish the overall union time and increase the success rate by initiating earlier bone grafting of those fractures.

Magnetic Resonance Imaging

At present, magnetic resonance imaging (MRI) plays a minimal role in evaluating fracture healing. Bone bruises, bone contusion, occult fractures, and early stress fractures may be detected with MRI or radionuclide bone scintigraphy but not with plain radiography.[22, 48] Usually, stress fractures eventually demonstrate sclerotic healing changes on plain radiographs. It appears that there is a continuum of traumatic injury to bone, the least severe lesion being a bone bruise, or contusion (interchangeable terms), and a displaced, comminuted fracture at the severe end of the spectrum. Occult fractures and impaction fractures are somewhere between the two extremes of the continuum. Bone bruise or contusion and occult fracture cannot be used interchangeably to describe bone marrow edema seen after trauma. A bone bruise is defined by MRI as a geographic, nonlinear area of signal loss in the subcortical bone on T_1-weighted images and increased signal on T_2-weighted images.[48] The overlying cartilage is intact. Occult fractures demonstrate single or multiple linear areas of decreased signal intensity on both T_1-weighted and T_2-weighted images, with a surrounding zone of hemorrhage and edema.[22, 48] Healing of bone bruises and occult fractures must be imaged with MRI or radionuclide bone scintigraphy to evaluate their healing progress when that is desired. An occult fracture presumably reflects a more severe traumatic insult to the bone with fracture of more bone trabeculae than those involved in a bone bruise.[56] Rangger and associates[56] performed biopsies of bone bruises, finding microfractures of cancellous bone, cartilage fragments, and edema and bleeding into the fatty marrow between intact lamellar bone trabeculae on histologic sections. Arthroscopy of the adjacent joint demonstrated no abnormalities of the articular cartilage overlying the bruise, even though some of the deeper cartilage layers were seen to be fragmented on the histologic sections. A typical knee bone bruise meeting the foregoing criteria has been reported to variously heal, with normal bone marrow replacing it, on MRI studies within 2 to 4 months[47] in one study and in 6 to 12 months in another.[73] Bone bruises have been reported to heal without sequelae,[47, 73] but occult fractures may heal with residual cartilage and bone abnormalities.[40] There has been a paucity of reports on follow-up MRI studies of these lesions.[40, 47, 73]

Pre–bone grafting MRI studies were able to predict how scaphoid nonunion fractures would fare following bone grafting.[51] Scaphoid fractures with normal marrow on MRI healed in half the time needed for fractures with abnormal marrow. Scaphoid nonunion fractures with abnormal bone marrow appearance on MR images and cystic changes and trabecular bone loss on plain radiographs did not heal after bone grafting.

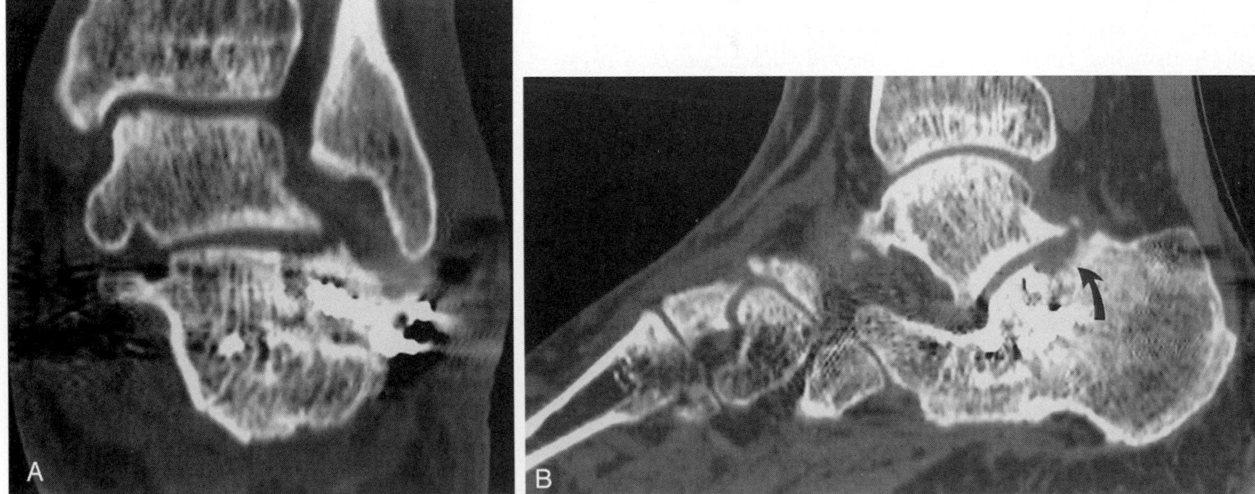

Figure 8–26. Coronal *(A)* and sagittal *(B)* reconstructed images from a spiral computed tomographic study in a patient with a healed comminuted calcaneal fracture and persistent hindfoot pain. There is lack of normal congruity of the articular surfaces of the posterior facet of the subtalar joint *(A)*, as well as a large defect *(B)* in its articular surface *(arrow)*. This feature could not be appreciated with a plain radiographic study. In spite of the presence of metal fixation screws, the bones and articular surfaces can be evaluated with computed tomography.

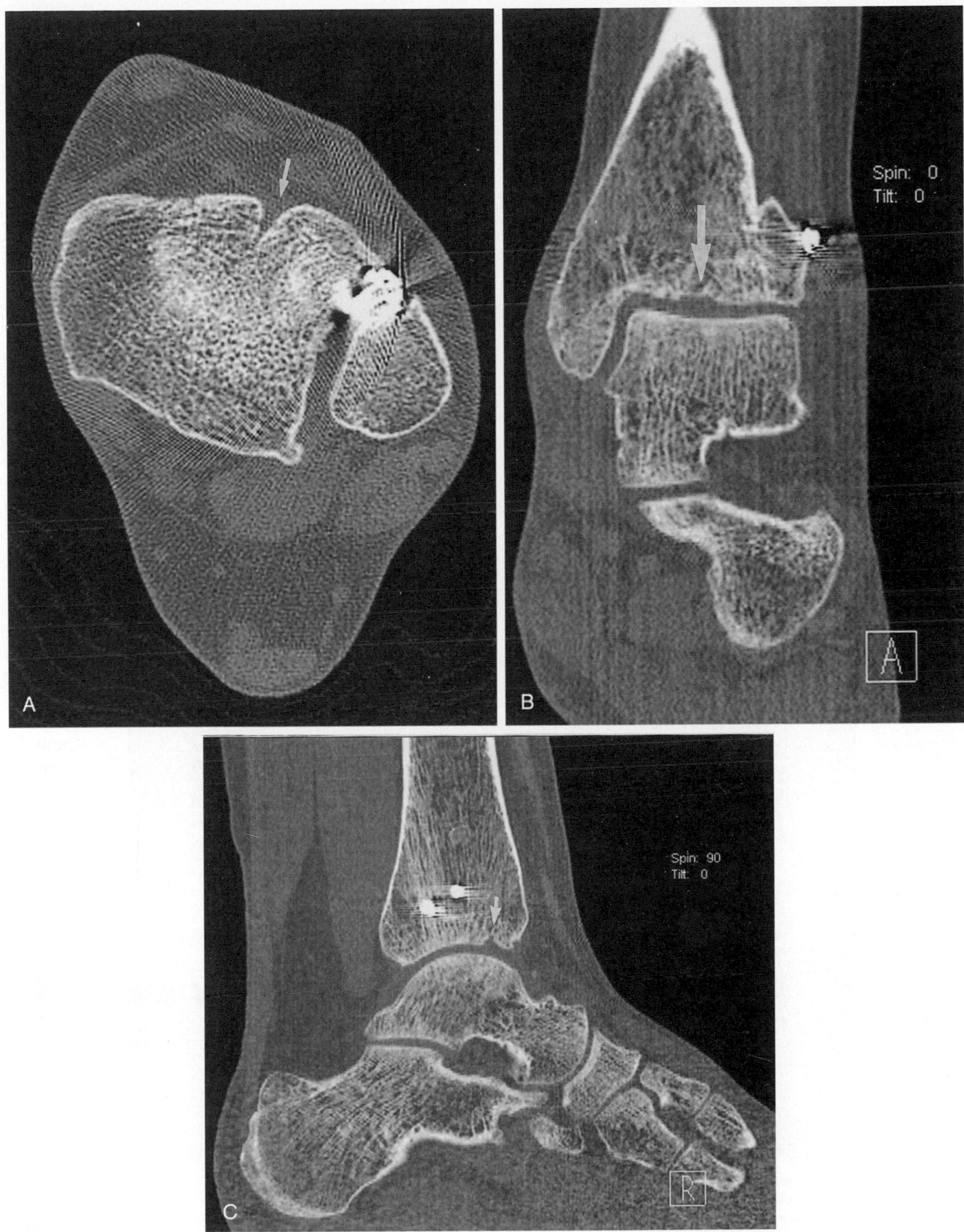

Figure 8–27. Healed pilon fracture evaluated with spiral computed tomography. Axial *(A)*, coronal *(B)*, and sagittal *(C)* images demonstrate a small amount of persistent irregularity of the articular surface of the tibia *(arrows)* and early ankle joint space narrowing *(B)*, accounting for the patient's pain.

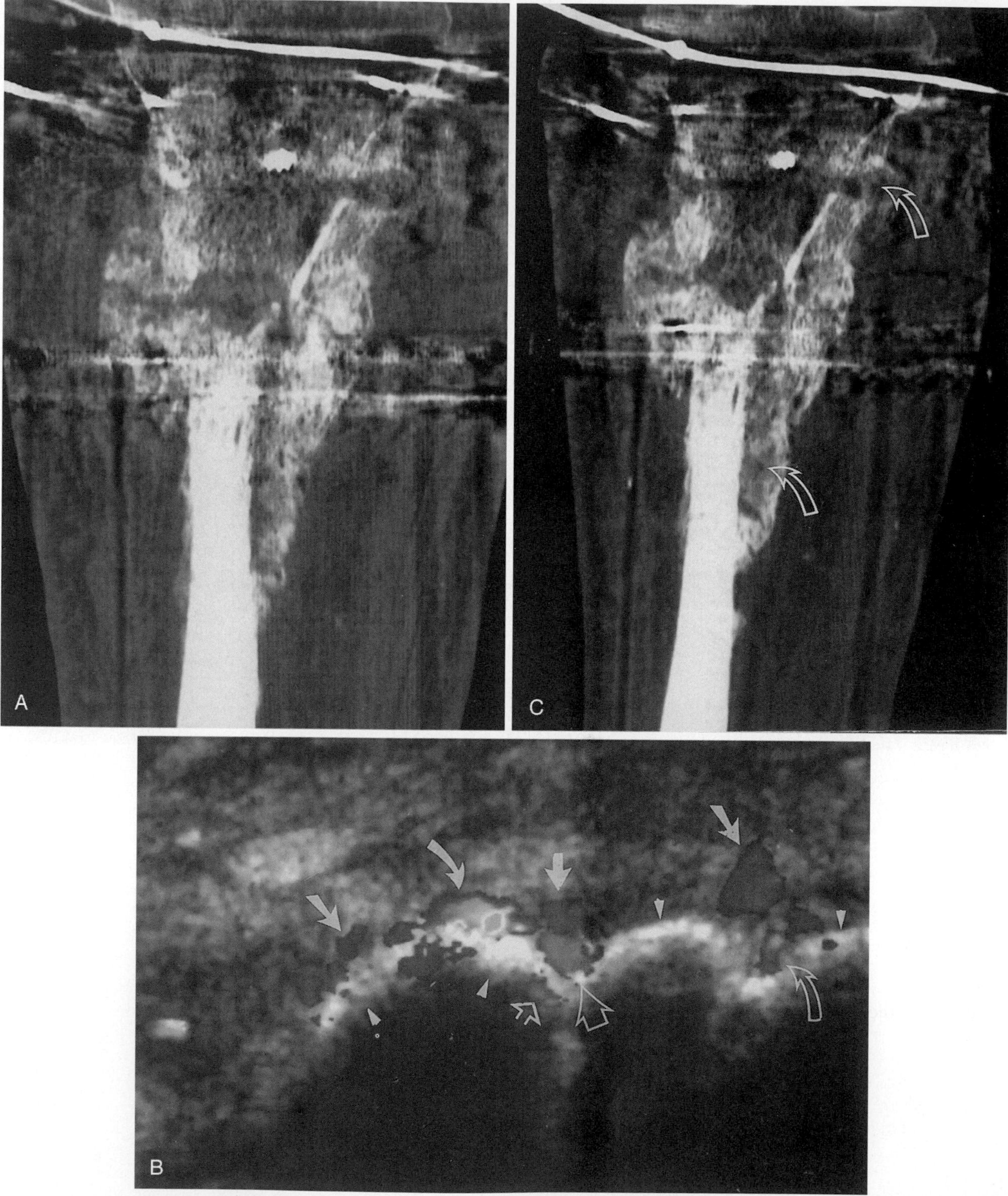

Figure 8–28. *A*, Coronal reconstruction image from a spiral computed tomographic examination done to evaluate a diabetic patient for tibial nonunion. A large amount of calcified callus is present, but unequivocal evidence of bone bridging is lacking. *B*, A color Doppler ultrasound study of the same fracture site in the proximal tibia was done at the same time. The two dimpled areas represent the fracture site. Extensive vascularity *(arrows)* is present at the fracture site, indicating that the fracture will heal. The *solid arrows* indicate blood flow toward and *open arrows* blood flow away from the fracture site, which are represented by different colors in the original images. The Ilizarov external fixator seen in *A* allows access for this ultrasound examination. The *arrowheads* indicate the cortical margin of the tibia. *C*, At 5 weeks later, bone bridging as predicted by the ultrasound study is now beginning to be visible on this computed tomographic image *(arrows)*.

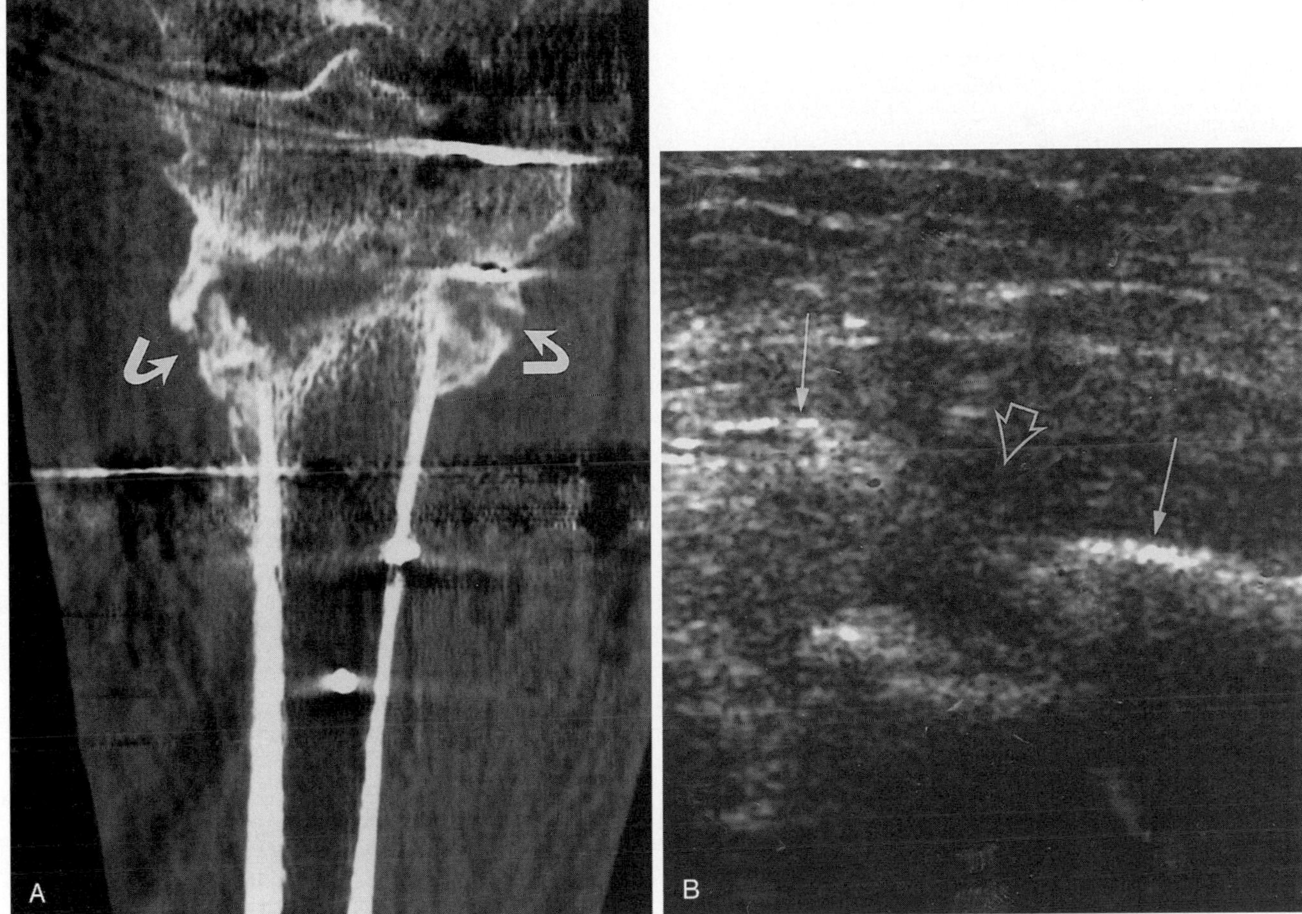

Figure 8–29. *A*, Coronal reconstructed image from a spiral CT study of the tibia done to assess fracture healing in a heavy smoker. The metal wires are from an Ilizarov fixator. Bone bridging was suggested on a plain radiographic examination. A large amount of calcified callus is present, but none bridges the proximal tibial fracture site *(arrows)*. *B*, A color Doppler ultrasound examination done at the same time demonstrates no increase of blood flow, as would be expected in the area of a healing fracture (see Fig. 8–4*A*). The lack of increased vascularity predicts that the fracture will not heal without further intervention, as was borne out by subsequent events. The tibial cortex *(closed arrows)* is interrupted by the fracture defect *(open arrow)*.

Ultrasonography

Ultrasonography currently has no defined role for evaluating fracture healing in the United States. This imaging modality was shown in a small number of patients to be accurate in predicting union or nonunion on the basis of the vascularity present at the fracture site.[50] Color or power Doppler can be superimposed on a gray-scale ultrasound image to demonstrate the vascularity of a fracture site. Color Doppler studies allow differentiation of vessels containing inflowing from outflowing blood from one another. In a normal healing fracture, blood flow to and from the fracture site is increased (Fig. 8–28), whereas blood flow to a nonunion is dramatically diminished (Fig. 8–29), with blood flow similar to that in a section of normal unfractured cortical bone. A serious hindrance to the use of ultrasound studies is that this modality is both operator dependent and labor intensive. At present, most radiology departments have insufficient expertise and personnel to perform these studies routinely.

References

1. Aegerter, E., & Kirkpatrick, J.A. Jr. (1968). Orthopedic Diseases. 3rd Ed. W.B. Saunders Co., Philadelphia.
2. Albright, J.A., & Brand, R.A. Eds. (1987). The Scientific Basis of Orthopaedics. 2nd Ed. Appleton & Lange, Norwalk, Conn.
3. Allen, H.L., Wase, A., & Bear, W.T. (1980). Indomethacin and aspirin: Effect of nonsteroidal anti-inflammatory agents on the rate of fracture repair in the rat. Acta Orthop. Scand, *51*:595.
4. Anderson, L.D. (1965). Compression plate fixation and the effect of different types of internal fixation on fracture healing. J. Bone Joint Surg. [Am.], *47*:191.
5. Anderson, W.A.D., & Kissane, J.M. (1977). Pathology. 7th Ed. C.V. Mosby Co., St. Louis.
6. Auxhasen, G. (1907). Histologische Untershuchunger uber knochen Transplantation am Menschen. Dtsch. Z. Chir., *91*:388.
7. Baltaxe, H.A., Shaw, D.D., & Connolly, J.F. (1980). Assessment of healing of long-bone fractures by intraosseous venography. Radiology, *137*:53.
8. Banks, H.N. (1965). The healing of intra-articular fractures. Clin. Orthop., *40*:17.
9. Birzle, H., Bergleiter, R., & Kuner, E.H. (1978). Radiology of Trauma. W.B. Saunders Co., Philadelphia.
10. Brinker, M.R., & Bailey, D.E. Jr. (1997). Fracture healing in tibial fractures with an associated vascular injury. J. Trauma, *42*:11.
11. Carter, D.R., Beaupre, G.S., Giori, N.J., & Helms, J.A. (1998). Mechanobiology of skeletal regeneration. Clin. Orthop., *355*(Suppl.):41.
12. Connolly, J.F. (1981). Selection, evaluation and indications for electrical stimulation of ununited fractures. Clin. Orthop., *161*:39.
13. Court-Brown, C., & McQueen, M. (1987). Compartment syndrome delays tibial union. Acta Orthop. Scand., *58*:249.

14. Cruess, R.L., & Sakai, T. (1972). The effect of cortisone upon synthesis rates of some components of rat bone matrix. Clin. Orthop., *86*:253.
15. Cruess, R.L., & Dumont, J. (1975). Current concepts, fracture healing. Can. J. Surg., *18*:403.
16. Cruess, R.L., & Dumont, J. (1975). Healing of bone, tendon and ligament, p. 97. In Rockwood, C.A. Jr. & Green, D.P. Eds.: Fractures. Vol. 1. J.B. Lippincott Co., Philadelphia.
17. Desai, A., Alavi, A., Dalinka, M. et al. (1980). Role of bone scintigraphy in the evaluation and treatment of nonunited fractures: Concise communication. J. Nucl. Med., *21*:931.
18. Dickson, K., Katzman, S., Delgado, E., & Contreras, D. (1994). Delayed unions and nonunions of open tibial fractures. Clin. Orthop., *302*:189.
19. Einhorn, T.A. (1998). The cell and molecular biology of fracture healing. Clin. Orthop., *355*(Suppl.):7.
20. Einhorn, T.A., Bonnarens, F., & Burstein, A.H. (1996). The contributions of dietary protein and mineral to the healing of experimental fractures. J. Bone Joint Surg. [Am.], *68*:1389.
21. Enis, J.E., McCollough, N.C. III, Cooper, J.S. (1974). Effects of methylmethacrylate in osteosynthesis. Clin. Orthop., *105*:283.
22. Feldman, F., Staron, R., Zwass, A. et al. (1994). MR imaging: Its role in detecting occult fractures. Skeletal Radiol., *23*:439.
23. Friedenberg, Z.B., & French, G. (1952). The effects of known compression forces on fracture healing. Surg. Gynecol. Obstet., *94*:743.
24. Frost, H.M. (1969). Tetracycline-based histological analysis of bone remodeling. Calcif. Tissue Res., *3*:211.
25. Frost, H.M. (1982). Mechanical determinants of bone modeling. Metab. Bone Dis. Rel. Res., *4*:217.
26. Frost, H.M. (1989). Biology of fracture healing: An overview for clinicians. Part I. Clin. Orthop., *248*:283.
27. Frost, H.M. (1989). Biology of fracture healing: An overview for clinicians. Part II. Clin. Orthop., *248*:294.
28. Geiser, M. (1958). Muscle action, bone rarefaction and bone formation. J. Bone Joint Surg. [Br.], *40*:282.
29. Gustilo, R.B., Mendoza, R.M., & Williams, D.N. (1984). Problems in the management of type III (severe) open fractures: A new classification of type III open fractures. J. Trauma, *24*:742.
30. Ham, A.W. (1974). Histology. 7th Ed. J.B. Lippincott Co., Philadelphia.
31. Ham, A.W., & Harris, W.R. (1971). Repair and transplantation of bone. p. 338. In Bourne, G.H. Ed.: The Biochemistry and Physiology of Bone. 2nd Ed. Vol. 3. Academic Press, New York.
32. Hayda, R.A., Brighton, C.T., & Esterhai, J.L. Jr. (1998). Pathophysiology of delayed healing. Clin. Orthop., *355*(Suppl.):31.
33. Heaney, R.P. (1964). Disuse osteoporosis. In Pearson, O.H., & Joplin, G.F. Eds.: Dynamic Studies of Metabolic Bone Disease. F.A. Davis Co., Philadelphia.
34. Heppenstall, R.B. (1980). Fracture Treatment and Healing. W.B. Saunders Co., Philadelphia.
35. Hukkanen, M., Konttinen, Y.T., Santavirta, S. et al. (1993). Rapid proliferation of calcitonin gene–related peptide–immunoreactive nerves during healing of rat tibial fracture suggests neural involvement in bone growth and remodelling. Neuroscience, *54*:969.
36. Hulth, A. (1989). Current concepts of fracture healing. Clin. Orthop., *249*:265.
37. Ilizarov, G.A. (1989). The tension-stress effect on the genesis and growth of tissues. Part 1. The influence of stability of fixation and soft-tissue preservation. Clin. Orthop., *238*:249.
38. Ilizarov, G.A. (1989). The tension-stress effect on the genesis and growth of tissues. Part 2. The influence of the rate and frequency of distraction. Clin. Orthop., *239*:263.
39. Jaffe, H. (1972). Metabolic, Degenerative and Inflammatory Diseases of Bones and Joints. Lea & Febiger, Philadelphia.
40. Johnson, D.L., Urban, W.P., Caborn, D.N.M. et al. (1998). Articular cartilage changes seen with magnetic resonance imaging-detected bone bruises associated with acute anterior cruciate ligament rupture. Am. J. Sports Med., *26*:409.
41. Jones, G. (1969). Radiological appearance of disuse osteoporosis. Clin. Radiol., *20*:345.
42. Joyce, M.E., Terek, R.M., Jingushi, S., & Bolander, M.E. (1990). Role of transforming growth factor-beta in fracture repair. Ann. N. Y. Acad. Sci., *593*:107.
43. Kwiatkowski, T.C., Hanley, E.N. Jr., Ramp, W.K. (1996). Cigarette smoking and its orthopedic consequences. Am. J. Orthop., *25*:590.
44. Lewis, J.L. (1975). A dynamic model of healing fractured long bone. J. Biomech., *8*:17.
45. McKibbin, B. (1978). The biology of fracture healing in long bones. J. Bone Joint Surg. [Br.], *60*:150.
46. Milch, R.A., Ball, D.P., & Tobie, J.E. (1957). Bone localization of the tetracyclines. J. Natl. Cancer Inst., *19*:87.
47. Miller, M.D., Osborne, J.R., Gordon, W.T. et al. (1998). The natural history of bone bruises. Am. J. Sports Med., *26*:15.
48. Mink, J.H., & Deutsch, A.L. (1991). Occult cartilage and bone injuries of the knee: Detection, classification, and assessment with MR imaging. Radiology, *170*:823.
49. Misol, S., Samaan, N., Ponseti, I.V. (1971). Growth hormone in delayed fracture union. Clin. Orthop., *74*:206.
50. Moed, B.R., Watson, J.T., Goldschmidt, P., & van Holsbeeck, M. (1995). Ultrasound for the early diagnosis of fracture healing after interlocking nailing of the tibia without reaming. Clin. Orthop., *310*:137.
51. Morgan, W.J., Breen, T.F., Courmas, J.M. et al. (1997) Role of magnetic resonance imaging in assessing factors affecting healing in scaphoid nonunions. Clin. Orthop., *336*:240.
52. Muller, M.E., Allgower, M., & Willenegger, H. (1965). Technique of Internal Fixation of Fractures. Springer-Verlag, New York.
53. Parfitt, A.M. (1984). The cellular basis of bone remodeling: The quantum concept reexamined in light of recent advances in the cell biology of bone. Calcif. Tissue Int., *36*(Suppl.):37.
54. Pritchard, J.J. (1946). Repair of fractures of the parietal bone in rats. J. Anat., *80*:55.
55. Pritchard, J.J., & Ruzicka, A.J. (1950). Comparison of fracture repair in the frog, lizard and rat. J Anat., *84*:236.
56. Rangger, C., Kathrein, A., Freund, A. et al. (1998). Bone bruise of the knee. Acta Orthop. Scand., *69*:291.
57. Rhinelander, F.W., & Baragry, R.A. (1962). Microangiography in bone healing. I. Undisplaced closed fractures. J. Bone Joint Surg. [Am.], *44*:1273.
58. Rhinelander, F.W., Phillips, R.S., Steel, W.M., & Beer, J.C. (1968). Microangiography in bone healing. II. Displaced closed fractures. J. Bone Joint Surg. [Am.], *50*:643.
59. Rothman, R.H., Klemek, J.S., & Toton, J.J. (1971). The effect of iron deficiency anemia on fracture healing. Clin. Orthop., *77*:276.
60. Sachs, L. (1987). The molecular control of blood cell development. Science, *238*:1374.
61. Schenk, R., & Willenegger, H. (1967). On the morphological findings in primary fracture healing. Symp. Biol. Hung., *7*:75.
62. Schmitz, M.A., Finnegan, M., Natarajan, R., & Champine, J. (1999). Effect of smoking on tibial shaft fracture healing. Clin. Orthop., *365*:184.
63. Shah, J., & Jones, W.A. (1998). Factors affecting the outcome in 50 cases of scaphoid nonunion treated with Herbert screw fixation. J. Hand Surg. [Br.], *23*:680.
64. Sporn, M.B., & Roberts, A.B. (1988). Peptide growth factors are multifunctional. Nature, *332*:217.
65. Steinbach, H.L. (1964). The roentgen appearance of osteoporosis. Radiol. Clin. North Am., *2*:191.
66. Stinchfield, F.E., Sankaran, B., & Samilson, R. (1956). The effect of anticoagulant therapy on bone repair. J. Bone Joint Surg. [Am.], *38*:270.
67. Sumner-Smith, G. Ed. (1982). Bone in Clinical Orthopaedics. W.B. Saunders Co., Philadelphia.
68. Tachdjian, M.O. (1972). Pediatric Orthopaedics. W.B. Saunders Co., Philadelphia.
69. Trueta, J. (1963). The role of the vessels in osteogenesis. J. Bone Joint Surg. [Br.], *45*:402.
70. Urist, M.R., DeLange, R.J., & Finerman, G.A.M. (1983). Bone cell differentiation and growth factors. Science, *220*:680.
71. Urist, M.R., & Johnson, W. Jr. (1943). Calcification and ossification. IV. The healing of fractures in man under clinical conditions. J. Bone Joint Surg., *25*:375.
72. Urist, M.R., & McLean, F.C. (1941). Calcification and ossification. I. Calcification in the callus in healing fractures in normal rats. J. Bone Joint Surg., *23*:1.
73. Vallet, A.D., Marks, P.H., Fowler, P.J., & Munro, T.G. (1991). Occult posttraumatic osteochondral lesions of the knee: Prevalence, classification, and short-term sequelae evaluated with MR imaging. Radiology, *178*:271.
74. Wang, W.A., Rosen, V., D'Alessandro, J.S. et al. (1990). Recombinant human bone morphogenetic protein induces bone formation. Proc. Natl. Acad. Sci. U. S. A., *87*:2220.
75. Wilson, J.N. Ed. (1976). Watson-Jones Fractures and Joint Injuries. 5th Ed. Churchill Livingstone, Edinburgh.

Chapter 9

COMPLICATIONS OF FRACTURE

with Carol A. Boles, MD, and Ronald W. Hendrix, MD

The complications of fracture are defined here as those abnormalities occurring in association with or as a direct result of a fracture. Abnormalities of healing—delayed union, nonunion, and malunion are considered elsewhere in this book and therefore are not included in the following discussion. Only those complications resulting in abnormal radiographic findings are presented. Complications may be conveniently divided into immediate, intermediate, and delayed complications according to the time of their appearance in relation to the initial injury.

Immediate Complications

Arterial Injury

The association of major vascular injury with fractures is fortunately infrequent in the nonmilitary setting. Less than 0.5%[7, 18] of all fractures resulting from blunt trauma are associated with significant vascular injury. Penetrating injuries account for most civilian arterial injuries. These injuries are chiefly the result of stabbings or gunshot wounds and, to a lesser extent, lacerations by foreign bodies, such as glass. Blunt trauma in association with fractures accounts for only 10% of vascular injuries. Penetrating injuries from gunshot, shrapnel, or other missiles account for the majority of arterial injuries in the military.[21, 22] Approximately 30%[22] of these injuries are associated with fractures.

Certain anatomic sites are more susceptible than others to arterial injury, for either of two reasons.[10, 13, 20, 27] (1) either the artery lies very close to bone, as does the superficial femoral artery to the midshaft of the femur, or (2) the artery is tethered to a point both proximal and distal as it crosses close to a joint, as are the popliteal artery at the knee, the brachial artery at the elbow, and, to a lesser extent, the brachial artery at the shoulder. Because of the proximity of the artery and bone at these locations, the artery may be injured directly by impingement of fracture fragments or indirectly by stretching and kinking of the artery as the fracture or dislocation is created. Arterial injury may also occur as a complication of manipulation or open reduction.[18, 23]

The popliteal is the most commonly injured artery[7, 9, 10, 14, 19] (see Figs. 9–1 and 9–2). Injury occurs in association with fracture of the proximal tibial shaft,[8] dislocation of the knee, and supracondylar fracture of the femur. The incidence of arterial injury is sufficiently high in all of these figures that this possibility should be a primary consideration during initial evaluation and treatment. Next in frequency are fractures of the distal shaft of the femur associated with injury of the superficial femoral (Fig. 9–3) or popliteal (see Fig. 9–2) artery in the region of the adductor canal. Arterial injury may also be iatrogenically induced during reduction and fixation of femoral shaft fractures. Supracondylar fracture of the humerus[13, 26, 30] in children may result in injury to the brachial artery and subsequent ischemia of the forearm, the much-feared Volkmann's contracture. Similar injuries of the brachial artery may occasionally occur in adults from supracondylar fracture or elbow dislocation.[14] Occasionally the brachial artery is injured by an acute anterior dislocation or during reduction of an old anterior dislocation of the shoulder.[14] This type of injury is particularly likely in the elderly. Multiple branches of the iliac arteries and veins are frequently injured in association with fracture of the pelvis, and significant hemorrhage may result.[14]

Mechanism of Injury

Direct impingement by fracture fragments can result in complete transection or laceration of the artery or in creation of a hematoma in the arterial wall, depending on the sharpness of the fracture fragment, force of displacement, and proximity of the artery.[7, 19] Lacerations of an adjacent artery and vein may result in an arteriovenous fistula.[3] An encapsulated hematoma about an arterial laceration may form a false aneurysm.[16]

Partial (see Fig. 9–1) or complete (see Figs. 9–2 and 9–3) occlusions are usually the result of indirect forces applied as the artery is stretched during displacement of the associated fracture or dislocation. It has been shown that stretching of an artery leads initially to tearing of the intima[4, 14] and then subsequently to the media if the force is sufficient. Additional force is required to disrupt the adventitia and completely transect the artery. Usually, only the intima is torn and becomes partially dissected from the arterial wall. A thrombus forms on the surface of the injured intima, and the lumen thus becomes partially (see Fig. 9–1) or completely occluded.

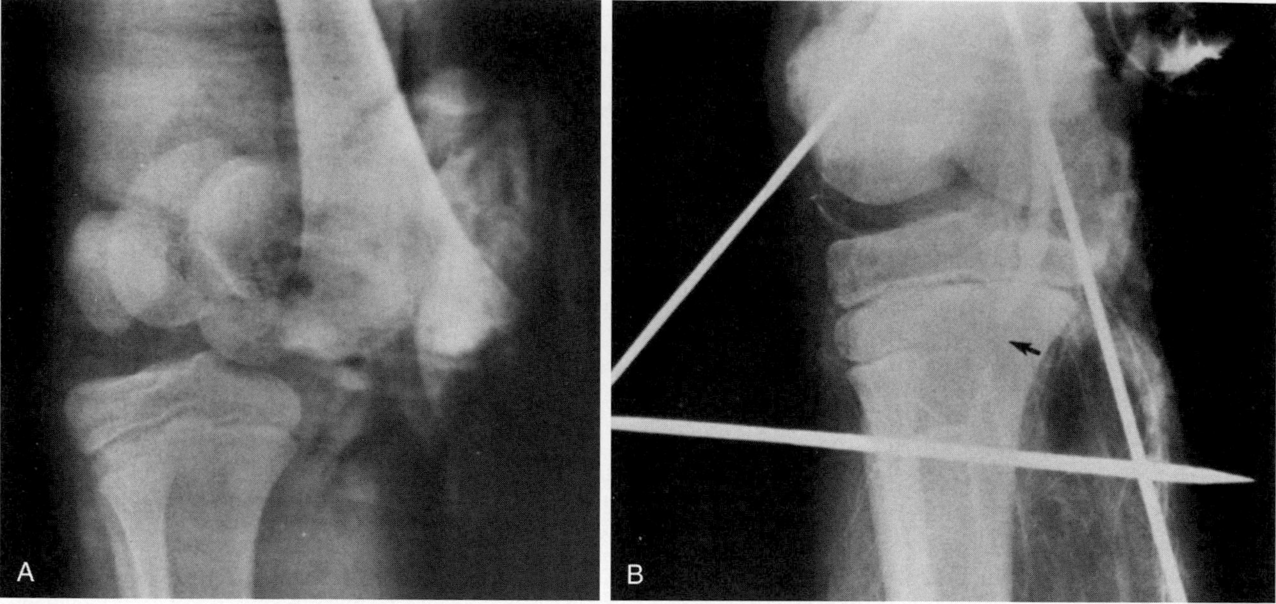

Figure 9–1. Partial occlusion of popliteal artery associated with an open Salter-Harris type I separation of the distal femoral epiphysis. *A*, The metaphysis is widely separated from the femoral condyles, which are rotated at 90 degrees. Note the air within the soft tissues about the femur, indicating the presence of an open wound. *B*, After open reduction and fixation with three threaded pins, an arteriogram was obtained. Note the partial occlusion *(arrow)* of the popliteal artery, which proved to be from a thrombus associated with a tear of the intima.

Arterial spasm is an infrequent cause of partial or complete occlusion.[10] Formerly it was frequently cited to explain arterial insufficiency associated with trauma; however, surgical experience has proved that arterial spasm per se is quite rare. Arteriotomies performed on narrowed or contracted vessels without visible signs of external injury in the presence of arterial insufficiency have usually demonstrated intimal tears, intimal dissections, and associated thrombus formation. Arterial spasm is therefore a diagnosis of exclusion to be invoked only after all other causes have been searched for and ruled out.

Signs and Symptoms

Signs and symptoms of arterial injury depend on the severity of the injury.[9, 10, 14] Complete transection or thrombosis of an artery is manifested by absence of peripheral pulses and coldness of the extremity. Decreased pulses and variable coolness of the distal extremity are manifestations of partial occlusion. In closed injuries there may be considerable swelling, with a warm, tense soft tissue mass, and in open injuries arterial bleeding may be visualized within the wound. Bleeding from a partial laceration is often intermittent, which may lead to dangerous delays in initiation of treatment. The intermittent nature of the bleeding could also account in part for the occasional failure to visualize the site of laceration by angiography. In the presence of a pseudoaneurysm, the distal pulses are intact. A pulsatile mass with a bruit and thrill is present at the site of injury. The pulses are also intact distal to an arteriovenous fistula, and a bruit and thrill can be detected. Venous distention may be present in the distal extremity, depending upon the magnitude of the shunt and adequacy of the valves within the vein.

On occasion, the peripheral pulses may be absent at the time of the initial evaluation but return upon reduction of the fracture or dislocation.[10] If they do return they will do so shortly. Failure of the pulses to return to normal within a short time should be considered evidence of arterial injury and an indication for the institution of appropriate treatment.

Arteriographic Diagnosis

In most clinical situations the presence and probable location of an arterial injury are obvious from the physical examination and location of the fracture.[5, 15, 16, 25] The indications for immediate surgery are equally obvious. There is really no necessity to delay so that formal arteriography[9] can be performed in the radiology department. Arteriographic examination typically requires at least an hour in most hospitals, even in those institutions that have busy trauma and arteriographic services, and considerably longer in other institutions in which personnel are less attuned to and experienced in the management of such patients. In suspected arterial injury, time is of the essence, and obtaining serial films with exquisite detail is a frivolous luxury and potentially dangerous because of the time involved. A single film obtained at surgery after proximal injection of 20 to 40 ml of contrast medium (diatrizoate meglumine and diatrizoate sodium [Renografin-60]) via direct needle puncture of the femoral or brachial artery suffices for the demonstration of most arterial injuries. If long cassettes (14 × 36 in.) and serial film changes are available in surgery, so much the better, but they are not required. Transfer of the patient to a facility that has such equipment and vascular surgical specialists involves a calculated risk because of loss of valuable time.

A complete block to the flow of contrast medium (see Figs. 9–2 and 9–3) indicates the presence of complete

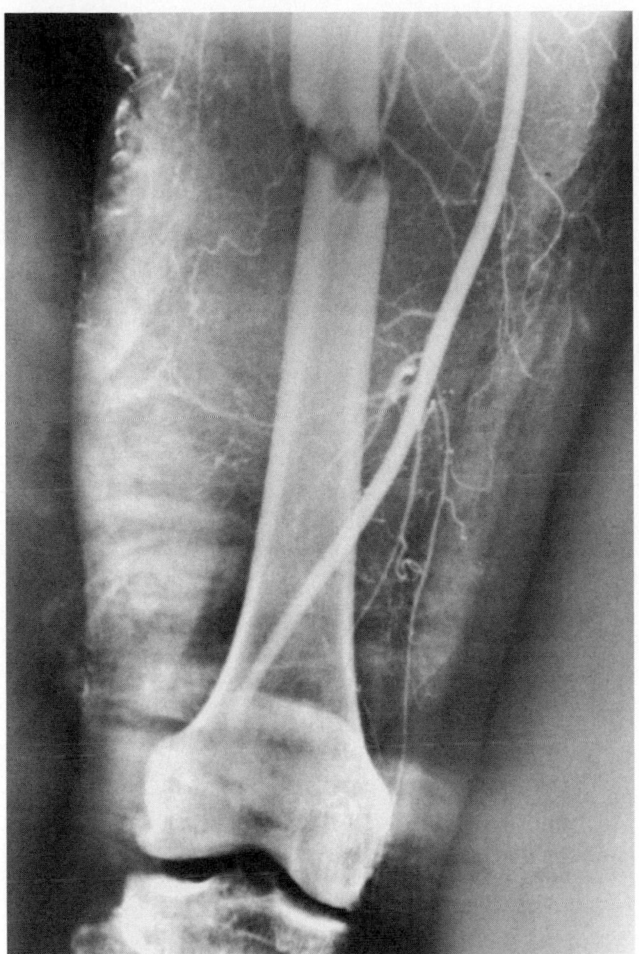

Figure 9–2. Complete occlusion of the popliteal artery in a 64-year-old man who had sustained a fracture of the midshaft of the femur. After injection of 40 ml of contrast material into the femoral artery, it can be seen that the flow is obstructed in the popliteal artery. At surgery, two intimal tears within the popliteal artery were found. The lumen was occluded by a thrombus. The patient had previously undergone fasciotomies in the lower leg for treatment of a compartment syndrome.

transection or thrombosis. The proximal end of the thrombus may be identified as a convex filling defect at the point of occlusion. Collateral branches may be demonstrated immediately after injury[16] in some cases (see Fig. 9–3). Partial transection is manifested by extravasation of contrast medium from the site of injury into the surrounding tissue (Fig. 9–4). If this space is reasonably well defined by clot, it may give the appearance of an aneurysm arising from the side of the vessel. This is termed a false or pseudoaneurysm. In the presence of a traumatic arteriovenous fistula, contrast medium is shunted immediately into an adjoining vein.[3] On occasion the site of laceration is not identified by angiography; rarely, even complete transection may not be visualized. In such situations the column of contrast agent passes through clots in the area of laceration or transection into the distal lumen without demonstrating irregularity or change in caliber of the column. Such false-negative findings are rare, and an anecdotal experience should not be allowed to detract from the general overall accuracy and value of the examination.

Small irregularities in the column of contrast medium with an associated contour defect, which is fixed to the wall of the artery at some point, indicate intimal tears and associated thrombus (see Fig. 9–1). There is probably some element of intimal dissection in all such cases. Small irregularities and complete occlusion are the most common findings. A partial filling defect may also be created by an intramural hematoma, but this is less common.

Most abnormalities are found at the level of the associated fracture, as would be anticipated. In the presence of a partial injury the distal arterial tree should be visualized to exclude the presence of remote thrombi (see Fig. 9–2) or additional arterial injury.

The treatment of arterial injury[10, 22] is resection and end-to-end anastomosis when practical. When this is not possible, repair with an autogenous saphenous vein graft is preferred. Intimal dissections may be resected or occasionally reattached by suturing. A Fogarty balloon cathe-

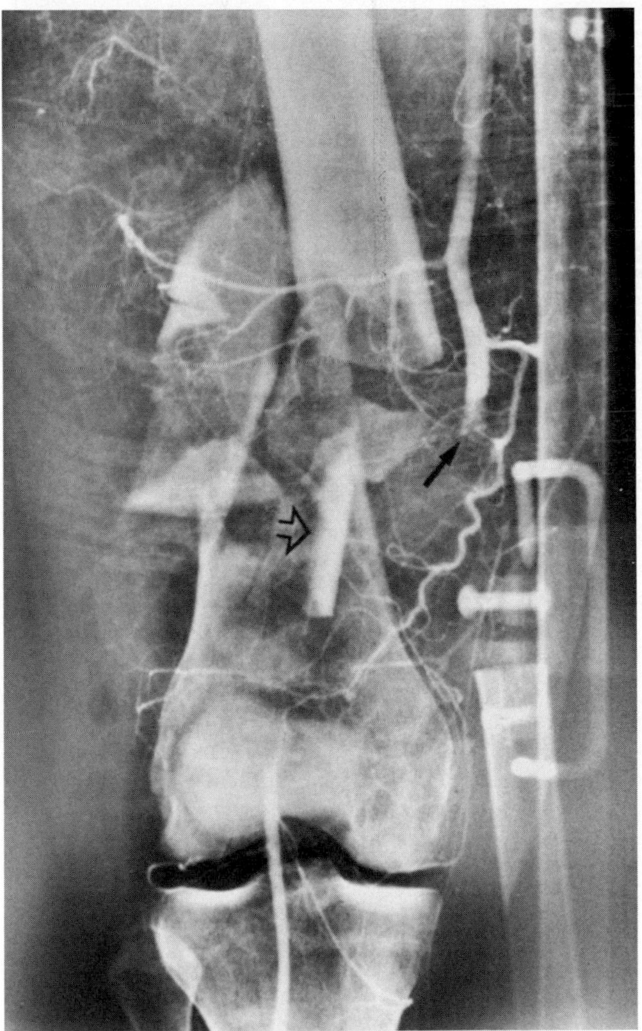

Figure 9–3. Complete obstruction of superficial femoral artery associated with comminuted fracture of the distal shaft of the femur. After injection of 40 ml of contrast medium via catheter into the common iliac artery, complete occlusion of the superficial femoral artery is evident at the level of the adductor canal *(black arrow)*. Note the presence of collateral circulation, which fills the popliteal artery. A bone fragment is seen on end *(open arrow)*.

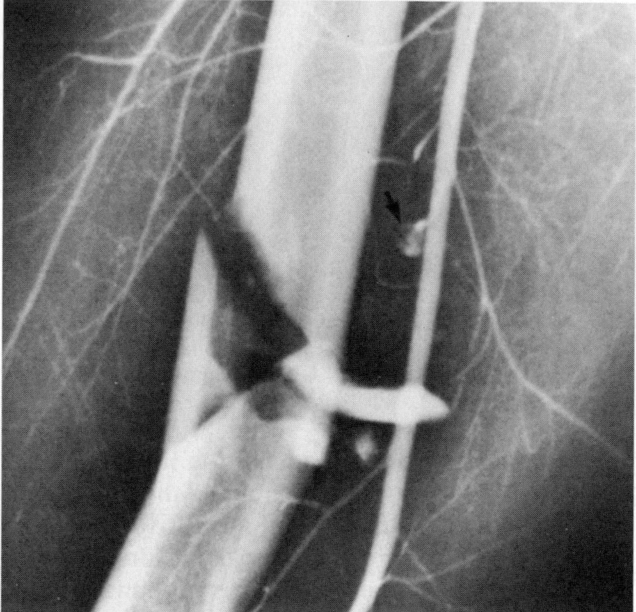

Figure 9–4. Intact superficial femoral artery in a 29-year-old man who had sustained a comminuted fracture of the midshaft of the femur. A large hematoma was present about the fracture site, and the distal pulses were diminished, raising the question of arterial injury. The superficial femoral artery is intact. Bleeding arises from branches of the deep femoral artery. A small pseudoaneurysm *(arrow)* is formed at the site of bleeding from the more inferior of the two small branches.

ter is passed to remove any thrombi that may have formed distal to the site of injury. Prophylactic fasciotomies are performed in the distal compartments to prevent the development of muscle ischemia and necrosis (see "Volkmann's Ischemia and Contracture: Compartment Syndromes"). Arteriospasm is an infrequent cause of arterial insufficiency, and vital time is wasted in waiting for such presumed spasm to clear. The conservative and correct approach is surgical exploration.

Pseudoaneurysm

Pseudoaneurysm presents as apulsatile mass, which results from persistent leakage of blood into the soft tissues from an injured vessel. The vessel wall does not heal, with subsequent fibrous encapsulation of the hematoma. There is a persistent communication with the vessel with blood flow into and out of the space during the cardiac cycle.[31] Pseudoaneurysms may be the result of fracture[32–35] or blunt or penetrating trauma,[36, 37] or may occur after fracture fixation.[38, 39]

Ultrasound Diagnosis

Ultrasound evaluation allows for the accurate diagnosis of a pseudoaneurysm. Duplex Doppler examination reveals a characteristic to-and-fro wave form.[40] Color Doppler imaging demonstrates intra-aneurysmal flow within the pseudoaneurysm that is both toward and away from the transducer, giving a characteristic appearance of alternating color bands or swirls that change during the cardiac cycle (Fig. 9–5). The connection to the artery can also potentially be found, with flow from the vessel to the pulsatile mass.[41]

Volkmann's Ischemia and Contracture: Compartment Syndromes

Volkmann's ischemic contracture is fortunately a rare complication of fracture.[1, 11, 14, 17, 28] It is caused by ischemia of muscle, which results in necrosis and subsequent fibrosis and contracture. Originally it was thought that such contractures were due to associated nerve injury and paralysis. In the 1870s and 1880s, Volkmann recognized and described the underlying vascular nature of the lesion, which therefore became known as Volkmann's contracture.[11]

It is now recognized that processes similar to the muscle contracture of the forearm that follows supracondylar fractures in children[13, 30] can occur elsewhere, particularly in the leg distal to the knee. The anatomic prerequisite is that the muscles be contained in a closed or confined compartment, and the physiologic prerequisite is a sustained increase in tissue pressure. The anterior tibial compartment exemplifies a closed space.[6, 14] It is formed by rigid osseous and fascial boundaries. The tibiofibular interosseus membrane lies posteriorly, the fibula laterally, and the tibia medially, and the deep fascia encloses the space anteriorly. The tibiofibular diarthrosis is superior, and the extensor retinaculum is inferior. These structures are sufficiently rigid that they cannot accommodate any appreciable increase in the size of the structures contained within their boundaries. This compartment contains the anterior tibial, extensor hallucis longus, and extensor digitorum muscles and also the peroneal nerve and the anterior tibial artery. There are similar, though not as sharply defined compartments laterally and posteriorly in the leg and in the forearm.

The increased tissue pressure within the space develops secondary to edema or hemorrhage within the compartment.[12, 17] Tissue edema may be the result of ischemia due to disruption of the proximal arterial supply, such as the popliteal artery in the leg or the brachial artery in the forearm. Alternatively, hemorrhage into the compartment from a bone forming one of its boundaries may account for the increased tissue pressure. It was originally thought that tight bandages, dressings, splints, or casts were the cause of the ischemia. Although constriction from these sources will compound the problem, it is usually of secondary importance to the underlying abnormality. Several nontraumatic causes of the anterior tibial compartment syndrome have been recognized,[12] including arterial embolism, arterial bypass, and even exercise alone.

As the tissue pressure within a compartment increases, the vascular perfusion by the microcirculation is decreased,[10, 17] thereby increasing tissue anoxia and worsening tissue edema. Additional tissue edema further elevates the tissue pressure and further compromises the circulation within the compartment. Thus a vicious circle is established that can be broken only by surgical intervention (i.e., fasciotomy) to afford release of the elevated tissue pressure.

Muscle tissue can tolerate only 4 to 12 hours of ische-

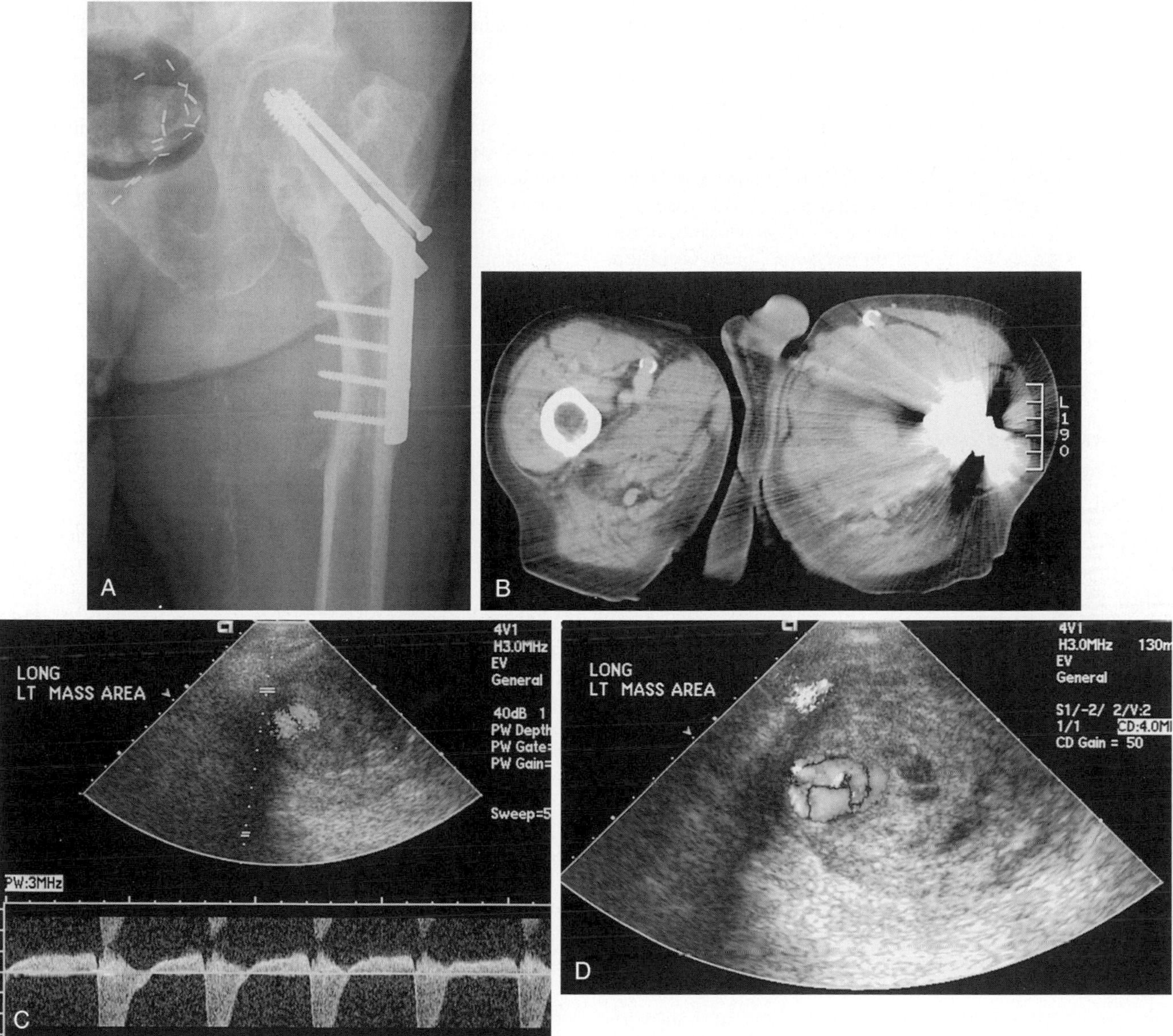

Figure 9–5. Pseudoaneurysm arising from the superficial femoral artery. The patient was an 81-year-old man who presented with a 2-year history of a left thigh mass after proximal femoral fracture treated by fixation. *A*, Anteroposterior view of the hip reveals remodeling of the medial femur and displacement of the calcified superficial femoral artery. *B*, Post-contrast image from a computed tomography study demonstrated the large fluid-density mass with enhanced center. *C* and *D*, Ultrasound examination demonstrates the characteristic to-and-fro flow and swirled color pattern in the pseudoaneurysm.

mia[17] before irreversible necrosis ensues. The nerves are more tolerant, but in this case the ultimate extent of functional recovery is based on the degree of muscle viability. Children seem to have a greater ability to recover function after this type of injury than that noted for adults.[24]

A useful mnemonic,[11, 14, 28] PPPPP (pulselessness, pain, pallor, paralysis, and paresthesia), incorporates all of the signs and symptoms of the various compartment syndromes. Not all need be present, however, to suggest the diagnosis. Any one or any combination of these findings is consistent with the diagnosis and should alert the physician to the potential existence of this complication. The dominant symptom is pain: deep, unremitting pain, poorly localized in the region of the affected compartment, and of a severity out of proportion to that anticipated after the reduction and immobilization of a fracture. The overlying skin is pale, blotchy, or cyanotic. There is often partial paralysis of the affected muscles and a sensory nerve deficit. The distal peripheral pulses are not necessarily absent or even diminished; this point is very important to recognize. The pressure within the compartment needs to be raised only above that required for tissue perfusion to result in tissue necrosis. This threshold is well below arterial pressure; therefore, the pulse may not be affected—that is, may be neither diminished nor absent—in the compartment syndromes and Volkmann's ischemia.

Even though the diagnosis is suspected, no confirmatory test is available other than a direct measure of tissue pressure.[17] This determination is performed by means of a direct needle puncture through the skin and attachment of a manometric system. The critical pressure is approximately 30 to 40 mm Hg.

Treatment of the compartment syndromes[6, 11] consists of a single fasciotomy or multiple ones in the affected compartment or compartments and repair of any associated arterial injury. It is crucial that surgical release be performed as soon as possible after the diagnosis is suspected. The difficulty is that compartment syndromes do not become evident until after the initial reduction and immobilization, when things do not seem quite as urgent and procrastination is easier. The clinician must be aware of the fractures and other injuries with which these syndromes may be associated. Vigilance will avert tragedy.

Gas Gangrene and Anaerobic Soft Tissue Infections: Soft Tissue Emphysema

There are numerous causes of soft tissue emphysema other than gas gangrene.[42, 48, 49] The identification of gas within soft tissues does not automatically indicate the presence of gas gangrene or even infection. The term "*gas gangrene*" should be reserved for invasive anaerobic infections of muscle characterized clinically by profound toxemia, extensive edema, massive tissue necrosis, and gas production within the soft tissue. The differential diagnosis is based more on the character of the associated signs, symptoms, and physical findings and, to a lesser extent, on the clinical history than on the radiographic appearance or presence of gas. The diagnosis of gas gangrene is so crucial that it must be considered one of exclusion; that is, gas gangrene must be considered to be present until proven otherwise. Similarly, in the presence of clinical signs and symptoms pointing to the diagnosis of gas gangrene, the diagnosis should not be ruled out because of the lack of characteristic radiographic findings. The radiographic findings are only ancillary and supportive; they are not specific. Rarely, serious clostridial infections may occur without gas production, or with only minimal gas production.

Gas gangrene is a bacterial infection caused by several species of *Clostridium*, chief among them *C. perfringens*[43] (*C. welchii*). The organisms are ubiquitous in the soil and on clothing and can commonly be found as saprophytes in the gastrointestinal tract or on the skin. Clostridial infection is associated primarily with open, grossly contaminated wounds with concomitant vascular compromise, especially battlefield injuries, but postoperative infections[45–47] have been reported, particularly in immunosuppressed persons. Clostridia are obligate anaerobes, unable to survive in healthy tissues with an adequate oxygen supply. These organisms are virulent only when placed in the proper environment for their growth, that is, in the presence of devascularized necrotic tissue. They produce several forms of toxin that are responsible for the severity of the tissue necrosis and clinical findings. The organisms are introduced into the wound at the time of injury and thrive only if allowed to remain either because of neglect, as in battlefield casualties, in which conditions make it impossible to initiate immediate care, or because of inadequate débridement at the time of treatment.

Classic gas gangrene practically always appears in less than 3 days and usually within 12 to 48 hours after injury.[43] In the military, the site of injury is most commonly the buttock or thigh, less commonly the shoulder or lower extremity. In the civilian population,[43, 45] the lower extremity is most commonly and the forearm less frequently involved. The progress of the disease is characteristically rapid.[43, 44] The patient notes severe pain, and a thin, dark, watery, foul-smelling discharge appears from the wound. The patient then experiences a change in sensorium, is in an extremely toxic state, and subsequently loses consciousness and lapses into coma. On physical examination the skin is noted to be tense and white. Crepitus is present about the wound, and a serous, hemorrhagic exudate and gas bubble up through the wound on deep palpation. Tachycardia is out of proportion to the initial fever. A Gram stain of the exudate reveals gram-positive rods. Surgical exploration is necessary to determine the full extent of muscle invasion and necrosis. The extent of muscle necrosis is greater than indicated by the skin changes.

Radiographs demonstrate the presence of gas bubbles and pockets in the initial wound.[43, 49, 50] The pathologic changes in classic gangrene consist of myonecrosis. Characteristic thin, linear, parallel streaks of gas are seen within the muscle planes (Fig. 9–6), extending out from the initial wound.[43, 48] These streaks measure 1 to 2 mm in width and 1 to 3 cm or more in length.

Another form of clostridial infection is anaerobic cellulitis.[43] This pathologic process appears more than 3 days after injury, the condition of the patient is less toxic, the muscle is not involved, and the gas is confined to the subcutaneous tissues and fascial planes outside of muscle. Admittedly there is some overlap between the cellulitic and myonecrotic forms of clostridial infection.

Clostridial abscesses may form and remain localized to the wound proper, involving no normal surrounding tissues. Other forms of anaerobic infection may occur within the wound and produce gas.[43, 50] Pathogens in these infections include the coliform bacteria, anaerobic streptococci, anaerobic *Bacteroides*, and *Aerobacter aerogenes*. The clinical signs and symptoms are much less severe than those associated with clostridial infections. In such focal infections gas is usually not found in muscle or subcutaneous tissue remote from the initial injury (Fig. 9–7). The gas is characteristically confined to the immediate area of the wound in the form of small bubbles and pockets.[49, 50] Individual bubbles of gas from infection are frequently 2 to 5 or 6 mm in diameter and smooth in outline.

The radiographic identification of gas within a wound does not automatically indicate the presence of an infection.[44, 48, 49] A noninfectious cause is particularly likely for gas identified on the initial radiograph of an open wound (Figs. 9–8 and 9–9) or immediately following operation. Gas may be introduced and trapped within the wound at the time of injury or operation (Fig. 9–10) or may be drawn in with subsequent motion and manipulation. The gas is usually confined to a single pocket, or at most three or four irregular pockets, but the amount may be

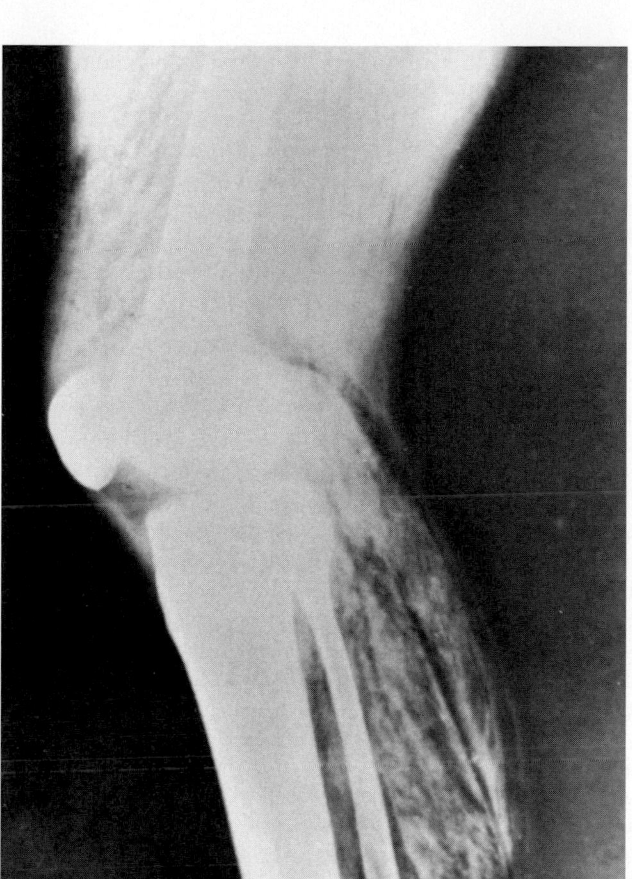

Figure 9–6. Gas gangrene of the lower extremity resulting from a soft tissue wound of the foot. Note the characteristic linear streaks throughout the tissues of the leg. The gas dissects within muscle bundles and in the subcutaneous tissue. The patient was in an extremely toxic state and died.

considerable if the wound is massive. These pockets are larger and more irregular than those associated with infection. Gas trapped within a wound should dissipate over a few days of observation and certainly should not increase in amount unless the wound is manipulated in some way. In the absence of clinical signs and symptoms of infection, serial radiographs are helpful in determining the source of such gas. Air is often seen in the chest wall in association with rib fractures or in the base of the neck following tracheostomy. Air may also be injected into the soft tissues in a wound inflicted by use of compressed-air apparatus.[49] Small bubbles of gas may be introduced during irrigation of the wound, particularly when hydrogen peroxide is utilized.

The primary form of treatment for clostridial infections is extensive débridement of the wound and affected muscle. Amputation is often necessary. Clostridia are penicillin-sensitive organisms, but the infections are frequently mixed, and other antibiotics are required. The prognosis has been greatly improved by the use of hyperbaric oxygen chambers.[43, 50] Other forms of infection are treated by débridement of the wound and administration of appropriate antibiotics.

Fat Embolism Syndrome

Although the occurrence of fat emboli following fracture was first recognized (after a thoracoabdominal crush injury) by Zenker in 1861, the pathophysiology of fat embolism syndrome (FES) remained controversial until relatively recently.[54] Clinically, the syndrome combines the acute respiratory distress syndrome with an associated coagulopathy following a long bone fracture or multiple fractures. Subclinical fat embolization occurs after almost all lower extremity and pelvic fractures.[56] The degree of embolization is the important factor, however, and in only 3% or less[52] of patients who sustain fractures of major bones is the embolization of sufficient magnitude to result

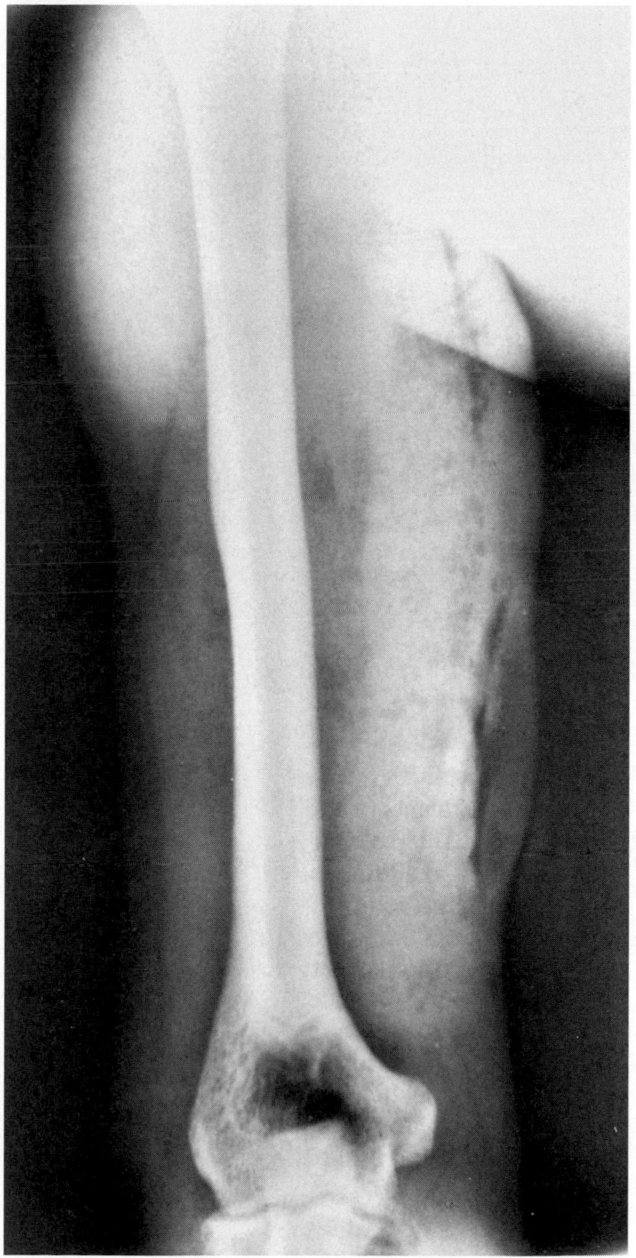

Figure 9–7. Gas in soft tissue from an anaerobic streptococcal infection in a 28-year-old heroin addict. The gas dissects and then bubbles and streaks up the medial aspect of the arm. The cellulitis evident here initiated at the site of previous injections.

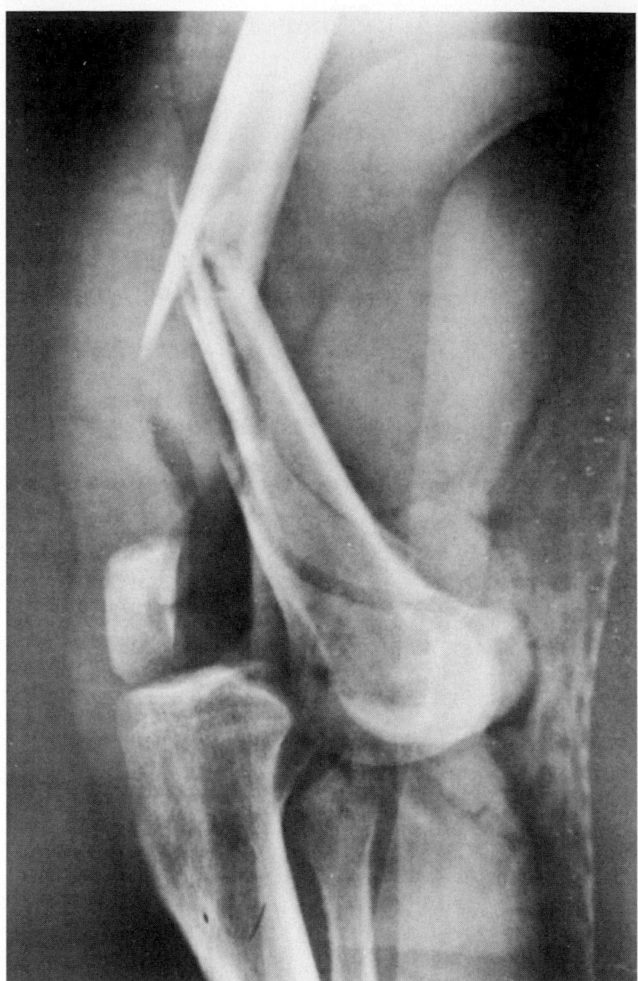

Figure 9–8. Open fracture-dislocation of the knee with air in the joint. Note the large collection of air within the joint, indicating the presence of an open injury. The femur is displaced posteriorly, and the popliteal artery was found to be transected. A severely comminuted open fracture of the distal tibia was also present. An above-the-knee amputation was ultimately performed.

in clinical and radiographic manifestations of FES. The syndrome is more likely to occur with certain fractures. A study of otherwise healthy skiers who sustained isolated fractures of the tibia or femur demonstrated a 23% occurrence of FES.[61] The syndrome is created by the embolization of fat particles initially to the lungs and subsequently throughout the body within a few days after fracture of a major long bone or the pelvis.

The average time to onset of symptoms[52, 55] is approximately 48 hours after the injury, and the usual range is between 1 and 5 days; onset is less common earlier than 24 hours or more than 7 days after the injury. The delay in onset of symptoms is thought to reflect the cumulative effects of vasoactive substances released and the time necessary to hydrolyze neutral fats to toxic free fatty acids.[54] Approximately half of the patients have sustained fractures of multiple bones, including the femur; 30%, fracture of the femur alone; 10%, fracture of the tibia; 5%, pelvic fracture; and the remainder, fracture of smaller bones or soft tissue injury alone without fracture.[55] Thus, the syndrome rarely occurs in the absence of fracture.

The early clinical findings of hypoxia, fever, and tachycardia herald the onset of the syndrome.[54] They are followed by a petechial rash, hemoptysis, and mental status changes ranging from restlessness or lethargy to disorientation, stupor, and coma.[54, 55, 60] Approximately half of the patients will have a petechial rash, most commonly at the base of the neck, upper chest, shoulders, or axillae, but the rash may be generalized on occasion. Hemorrhages may be seen in the conjunctiva and in the retina on funduscopic examination.

There is as yet no specific laboratory test to establish or confirm the diagnosis of FES; rather, the diagnosis is based on the appearance of typical symptoms and signs in association with specific laboratory values and characteristic findings on the chest radiograph. The most characteristic laboratory finding is arterial oxygen desaturation or arterial hypoxemia.[52, 55, 60] Normal values for the partial pressure of oxygen (Po_2) are typically less than 60 mm Hg. Thrombocytopenia and anemia are frequent. Serum lipase activity is increased only after the syndrome is well established. Fat in the urine (lipuria) in the form of triglycerides is noted in half of the patients, and fat may also be found in clotted blood and in specially filtered venous blood. These laboratory findings are nonspecific in the absence of clinical findings, however; identification of such fat is indicative only of the presence of fat emboli and does not necessarily indicate the presence of FES.[51, 55]

The radiographic findings are likewise nonspecific[51–53] (Fig. 9–11). Initially the chest radiograph is normal, and the appearance of pathologic changes generally lags 12 to 24 hours behind the onset of clinical symptoms. A diffuse, combined interstitial and alveolar pattern then appears, accentuated in the perihilar and basilar portions of the lung. This pattern may progress to become quite dense. The apices of the lung are generally spared. Pleural effusions are usually absent but, if present, are and remain minimal. Cardiac size and pulmonary vascularity remain normal. The abnormalities clear in the otherwise uncomplicated case in approximately 7 to 10 days.

The pathophysiology of FES has been disputed in the past but is less so now.[54] Two basic theories have been proposed[51, 52, 55]: one more or less mechanical and the other metabolic. In the mechanical theory the fat emboli are thought to arise from the neutral fats in the injured adipose tissue of the marrow in the region of the fracture. The fat enters the venous system directly through severed veins and capillaries and possibly through the lymphatic system and is transported to the lungs, where most of it forms microemboli in the pulmonary arterioles and capillaries. Some emboli pass through the pulmonary vascular bed to lodge in the brain, skin, and kidneys. Arterial and venous blood samples from patients with isolated femoral fractures have localized the origin of fat macroglobules to the injured extremity.[57] The fatty acids found in the lung most closely resemble those of marrow fat rather than circulating free fatty acids, circulating lipoproteins, or adipose tissue stores.[54] Animal studies using carbon 14–labeled fatty acids fed to the animals or injected into the marrow cavity before fracture also support a bone marrow origin of embolic fat.[54] The metabolic theory holds that the site of injury is not the sole source of emboli. Free fatty acids are mobilized and released into

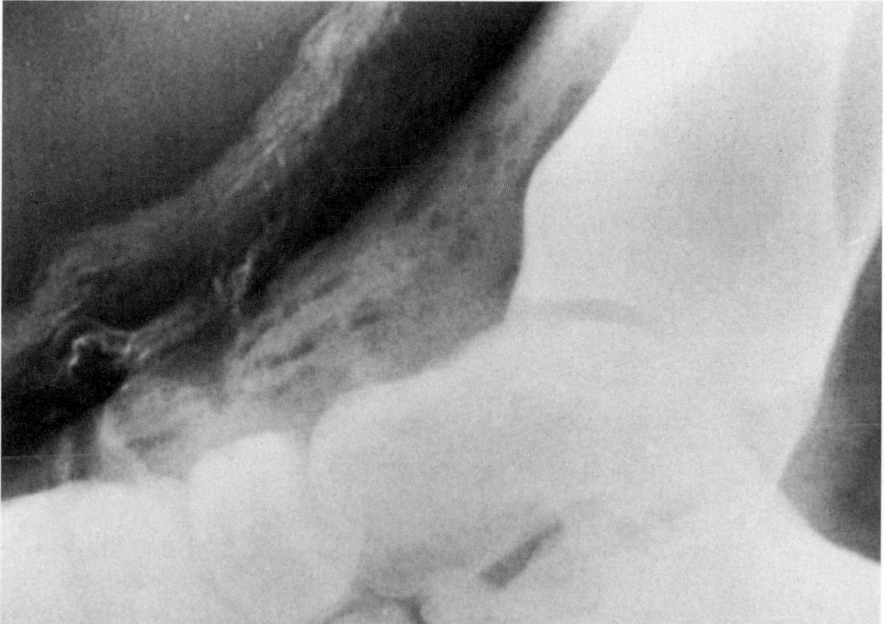

Figure 9–9. Air can be seen trapped in soft tissue over the dorsum of the foot, following a laceration injury.

the blood in response to stress. These fatty acids are esterified or aggregated, or both, into fat globules of sufficient size to embolize in both the pulmonary and the systemic circulations. At present the mechanical theory appears to be correct; however, the metabolic theory may account for the rare case of fat embolism that occurs in the absence of trauma.

Fat emboli cause injury by three principal means[52, 55]: mechanical occlusion of small vessels, aggregation of platelets and stimulation of intravascular coagulation, and chemical injury to vascular walls. Hydrolysis of fat by lipase produces fatty acids that are toxic and capable of causing vascular damage. Lung lipase is activated by fat embolism, and the resultant fatty acids cause local edema, hemorrhage, and loss of surfactant, leading to microatelectasis. A similar chemical process and vascular damage occur at systemic sites of fat embolism. A rise in serum levels of free fatty acids and triglycerides is seen after trauma in humans.[54] The free fatty acids are detergents and are directly toxic to lung parenchyma cells and capillary endothelium and surfactant.[59] They destroy the alveolocapillary membrane, causing interstitial hemorrhage and edema. The loss of surfactant also immediately changes lung compliance. Peltier[59] believes that pneumatocytes produce an increased amount of lipase in response to the embolic fat, with liberation of free fatty acids that are directly toxic to the lung. However, the breakdown of embolic fat to free fatty acids in the lung may not even be necessary to account for the pathologic changes. In addition to fat, other debris lodges in the lung, such as fibrin, platelets, and leukocytes, which can release vasoactive substances as well. Serotonin released by platelets causes vasoconstriction, which leads to vascular congestion. Lysosomal enzymes released from granulocytes destroy lung parenchyma. The complement system activation by intravascular fat results in increased capillary permeability. Histamine release from mast cells causes airway constriction and increases inflammatory response.[54]

Treatment is primarily directed toward correction of the hypoxemia. Oxygen is administered, and other forms of pulmonary support are given as required. High-dose steroid administration is frequently utilized as an anti-inflammation measure and has shown the most promising results to date.[54] Some clinicians advocate the use of heparin; others suggest infusion of dextran of low molecular weight or intravenous administration of alcohol. Heparin not only has not been shown to be useful but may even be harmful, causing bleeding in recently traumatized patients. As yet there is no drug that is specifically effective against or that retards the formation of fat emboli.

The prognosis is directly related to the severity of the pulmonary abnormality. The cerebral symptoms are thought to be related more to the degree of hypoxemia than to the extent of fat embolization within the brain. Death is due to respiratory failure following the development of shock lung[58] or adult respiratory distress syndrome. Approximately 10% to 15%[55] of the patients who develop FES succumb to the disease.

Thromboembolism

Thromboembolic disease is quite common in persons who have sustained fractures of the pelvis and lower extremity, particularly of the hip and femoral shaft. It is well recognized that pulmonary thromboembolism is one of the most underdiagnosed[65] but, at the same time, one of the most prevalent diseases in the hospital population. This limitation in the diagnosis is a testament to the absence or obscure nature of the clinical signs and symptoms and radiologic findings in the disorder. Various studies have demonstrated the incidence of venous thrombosis[1] among patients who have sustained fractures of the hip, pelvis, and lower extremity to be between 15% and 48%, with a mean of 30%. Therefore, it is essential that this possibility be kept in mind in the treatment of these particular patients.

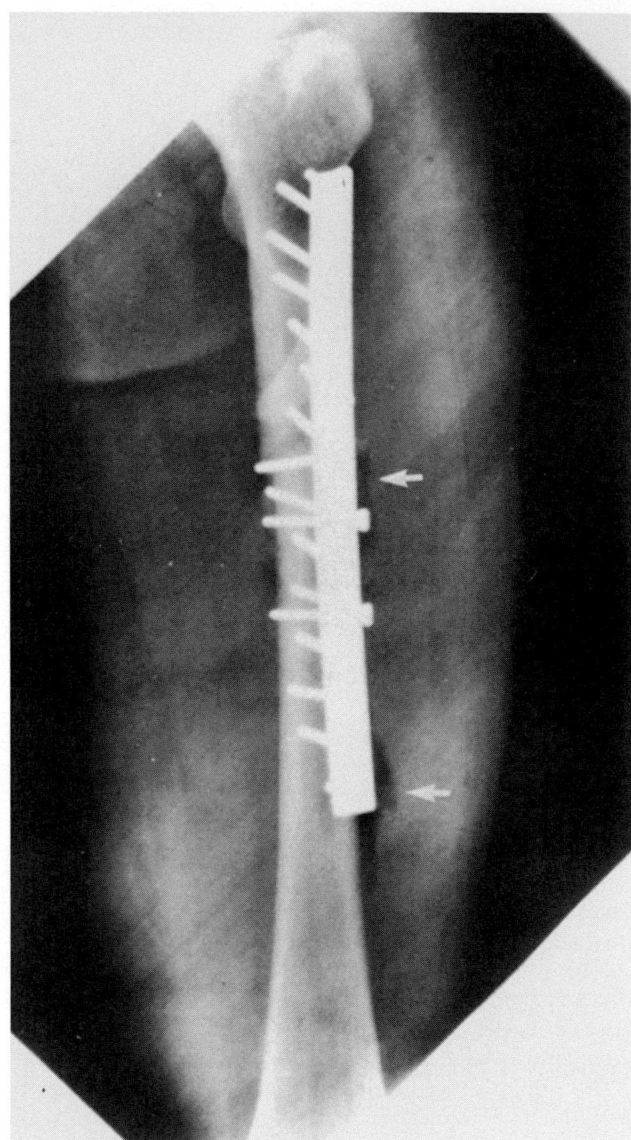

Figure 9–10. Air trapped in a surgical wound. This radiograph was obtained immediately following open reduction and fixation of a comminuted femoral shaft fracture with a compression plate and screws. Note the pockets of gas entrapped within the wound *(arrows)* overlying the compression plate.

The thrombi form in the deep veins of the calf, thigh, and pelvis.[69] They may cause difficulty in two ways. The thrombus may obstruct the venous return in the lower extremity, resulting in edema. However, there are usually sufficient collateral venous channels, so that obstruction is infrequently a significant problem. More important, thrombi may break free and be transported to the lung. Pulmonary embolism is one of the most common causes of death in patients being treated for serious injuries. Autopsy of 161 patients who died after hip fracture showed that 38% died from pulmonary embolism.[1]

The clinical signs and symptoms of deep vein thrombosis—pain, swelling, and tenderness to palpation—are most apparent in the calf, but the diagnosis is frequently difficult to establish. Lower extremity venography may be utilized to confirm the presence of thrombi. This study is performed by injection or infusion of a water-soluble contrast agent into a vein in the foot, while the leg is in the dependent position and after a tourniquet is applied or the lower part of the leg is wrapped in an elastic bandage to assure filling of the deep venous system. The proximal femoral and iliac veins, which cannot be accurately assessed with the use of smaller amounts of contrast material (e.g., 50 ml), are better visualized using greater amounts of contrast (i.e., up to 150 ml).

Real-time duplex ultrasonography and impedance plethysmography have greater than 90% sensitivity in detection of thrombi above the calf, similar to that of venography.[74, 75] These techniques are less accurate in assessing the circulation in the smaller distal veins of the calf but have become the primary methods of evaluation of lower extremity thrombus.

Nuclear medicine evaluation of venous thrombosis has also been utilized. Traditionally use of iodine 125-labeled or technetium 99m (^{99m}Tc)-labeled fibrinogen or albumin microspheres, which adhere to venous thrombi, has provided noniodinated contrast imaging.[68, 69] These methods are almost as accurate as contrast venography in the demonstration of thrombi in the deep veins of the calf but are less accurate in the thigh and pelvis. Furthermore, the isotopes pool in major wounds, so that the technique is inaccurate in assessment of the thrombi in the adjacent venous circulation. For example, presence of a hip fracture precludes evaluation of the status of the adjacent femoral and iliac veins. This technique, however, has largely been supplanted by a new small-peptide radiopharmaceutical, technetium 99m Tc-apcitide, which allows scintigraphic visualization of acute thrombi.[76] Acute clot is characterized by the presence of activated platelets, which have a unique glycoprotein receptor, the GPIIb/IIIA receptor. This receptor binds fibrinogen and also the technetium 99m Tc-apcitide. Imaging is performed at 10, 60, and 120 minutes after injection and is not affected by use of anticoagulants. The sensitivity and specificity are both over 85%.[77] This technique is particularly useful in the evaluation of recurrent thrombosis, when the utility of ultrasonography may be limited.

Computed tomography (CT) and magnetic resonance venography are newer techniques that show promise in evaluation of the presence and extent of deep vein thrombosis. Further study is needed, however.[78]

The real importance of venous thrombi lies in their potential for pulmonary embolization. The formation of venous thrombi with subsequent pulmonary embolization is more likely in elderly, obese persons with preexisting cardiac or pulmonary disease. Standard measures to prevent thrombus formation include the use of elastic stockings and elevating and maintaining mobility of the lower limbs, as possible. Warfarin sodium (Coumadin), an anticoagulant, and low-molecular-weight dextran, an antiplatelet agent, may also be given. Unfortunately, these preventive measures are not or cannot always be taken, and even despite them, pulmonary emboli occur.

The most common signs and symptoms of pulmonary thromboembolism are dyspnea, cough, and chest pain of sudden onset, one or more of these findings are noted in greater than 70% of the patients. Hemoptysis occurs in only 25%. The pain may be either substernal or lateralized in location and is often pleuritic in nature. The most

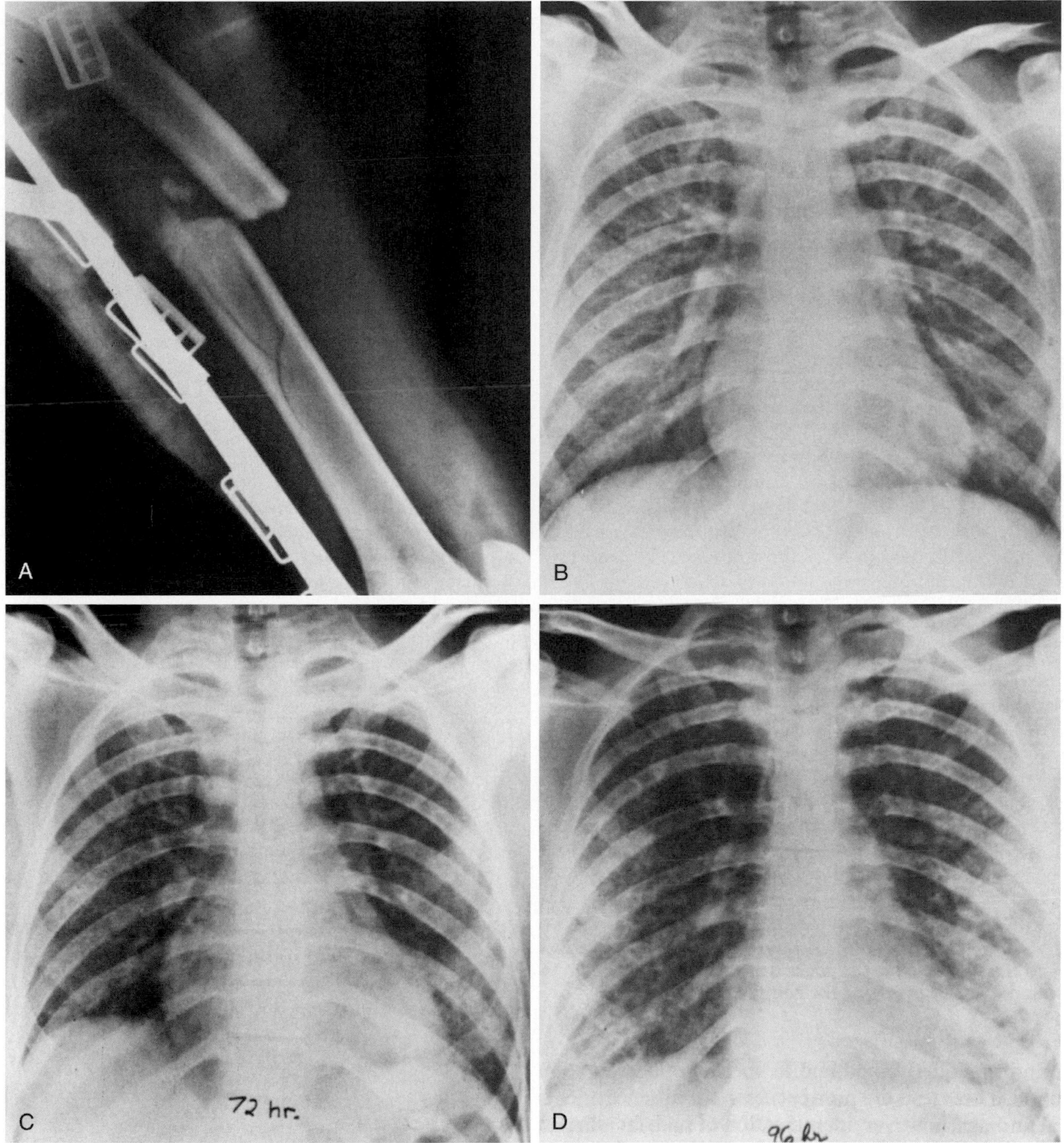

Figure 9–11. Fat embolism syndrome in a 19-year-old with a femoral fracture. *A*, Lateral view demonstrates a transverse, slightly comminuted fracture of the midshaft of the femur, with vertical extensions of the fracture line into the distal fragment. *B*, A chest radiograph at the time of admission is normal. *C*, A chest radiograph at 72 hours after injury shows patchy infiltrates present diffusely throughout both lungs but particularly accentuated in the bases. At this time the patient was dyspneic and delirious. *D*, By 96 hours after injury, the infiltrates have increased but remain more extensive at the base. The infiltrates gradually cleared over the next 6 days. The patient survived.

common physical findings are tachypnea, tachycardia, rales, and fever. Only 50% of patients have identifiable evidence of venous thrombosis in the lower extremity. In many patients the signs, symptoms, and physical findings are not characteristic. To make the diagnosis of a pulmonary thomboembolism, the astute physician must (1) consider the possibility; (2) maintain vigilance in the appropriate clinical setting (for example, with patients who have sustained fractures of the pelvis and lower extremity); and (3) perform the appropriate diagnostic evaluation to substantiate the diagnosis so that treatment may be initiated.

Pathogenesis

The overwhelming majority of pulmonary emboli[69] arise from venous thrombi in the iliac or femoral vein, not those in the deep veins of the calf. Venous thrombi in the deep veins of the pelvis and thigh are difficult[68] to detect on physical examination. The major cause of thrombus formation is thought to be slowing of the venous circulation and sludging of blood within the veins, secondary to immobilization of the trunk and extremity. This reduction in venous circulation is aggravated by obesity, chronic obstructive pulmonary disease, and congestive heart failure, and patients with these disorders have an appreciably higher incidence of both thrombus formation and subsequent pulmonary embolization.

After a thrombus is formed, all or some portion of it may break loose into one or more fragments, which then pass through the systemic circulation and right side of the heart to become lodged in the pulmonary arterial tree. Location of an embolus is directly related to its size: the larger the embolus, the more proximal its location in the pulmonary arterial tree. The obstruction of the artery may be partial or complete and, depending upon the degree of obstruction and the extent of the collateral circulation to the involved segment of lung, may or may not result in an infarction. The degree of obstruction and extent of collateral circulation will determine the reaction of the lung to the presence of the thrombus. If obstruction is only partial and adequate collaterals are present, the lung response is minimal and insufficient to produce radiographic changes. If obstruction is complete or nearly so, edema and hemorrhage may occur, which subsequently clear within a week to 10 days. If complete obstruction occurs in the absence of collaterals, the lung is infarcted and severe tissue necrosis takes place. Edema and hemorrhage persist for up to 3 weeks before clearing. Such infarction occurs in only 10% to 15% of all cases of pulmonary embolization. After the thrombus becomes lodged, it gradually breaks up over a period of a few days and embolizes more distally into the peripheral circulation.[64] As the thrombi pass peripherally, they become more difficult to detect. Therefore, it is important to perform tests early to establish the diagnosis. Delays may result in inconclusive results, and the patient's outcome may be jeopardized.

Radiographic Diagnosis

The chest radiograph is not a reliable indicator of pulmonary embolism; the radiographic appearance is normal in as many as 50% of cases,[53, 67] and when changes are present they are usually nonspecific. The most common findings are diaphragmatic elevation and associated parenchymal consolidation (Fig. 9–12). Often the density is pleural based, and usually the air bronchogram sign is absent.[62] The density may be triangular, with its apex pointing toward the hilus, or the medial margin pointing toward the hilus is rounded—the so-called Hampton's hump. Linear densities of platelike atelectasis are frequent. Identifiable areas of oligemia (Westermark sign) are rare and difficult to visualize. In some cases an enlargement of a pulmonary artery may be demonstrated. Small pleural effusions are frequent.[62]

The most reliable radiographic evidence of pulmonary embolism is provided by a pulmonary arteriogram.[63, 66, 67, 72] This study is performed after placement of a catheter directly into the main pulmonary artery for injection of the contrast material. Selective examination of unilateral, lobar, or segmental pulmonary arteries may be performed if necessary. The thrombi are visualized as filling defects within the column of contrast material.[73] Other signs such as abrupt occlusion of an artery and other forms of perfusion defects are secondary and less reliable. Pulmonary angiography is performed[66, 67, 72] when the combination of findings from the lung scan and chest radiograph is equivocal or in the presence of congestive heart failure, chronic obstructive lung disease, or asthma when the findings from the lung scan may be limited. CT pulmonary angiography has been proved accurate, particularly in the central pulmonary arteries.[79]

Lung Scanning

Radioisotope scanning techniques for identification of pulmonary thrombi were first devised in 1964 and are now accepted procedures for establishment of the diagnosis.[66, 67, 71, 72] Macroaggregates of albumin labeled with various isotopes, most commonly ^{99m}Tc, are injected into a peripheral vein. Ultimately the aggregates become trapped in and temporarily occlude a small fraction of the arteriocapillary pulmonary bed. The scan is best obtained with a gamma camera or scintillation scanner. Views are obtained in multiple projections.

A perfusion defect may involve an entire lobe or be manifested as a wedge-shaped area deficient of radioactivity with its base at the lung periphery or along a lung fissure corresponding to a segment or subsegment of the lung. To be diagnostic, such defects are multiple (see Fig. 9–12*B*). Lobar deficiencies are more reliable[66, 72] than segmental or subsegmental defects (80% versus 30%). Similar defects may be seen in congestive heart failure, asthma, or chronic obstructive pulmonary disease; therefore, the value of this test is limited in the presence of these conditions. The combination of perfusion with ventilation scanning may improve the accuracy.[71, 72] The most common agent, a radioactive inert gas, xenon 133, is inspired, and the distribution of the gas is recorded by a scintillation camera. This technique requires a closed system to prevent the diffusion of radioactive gas into the atmosphere.

Characteristically an area of pulmonary embolism (see Fig. 9–12*B* and *C*) is ventilated normally but not perfused; therefore, defects are demonstrated on the perfusion scan but not on the ventilation scan. This result is termed *ventilation-perfusion mismatch*. Performing a combined ventilation-perfusion examination may not be possible in a severely ill or injured person. The patient must be transported to the laboratory because of the requirements of the ventilation system and should be capable of holding his or her breath for 15 to 20 seconds. The perfusion imaging study can be performed at the bedside if a portable gamma camera is available in the hospital. However, particularly with extensive lung disease, pulmonary angiography may be required to establish the diagnosis of pulmonary thromboembolism in these patients.

Helical CT Pulmonary Angiography

More recently, CT pulmonary angiography has gained acceptance for the initial diagnosis of pulmonary throm-

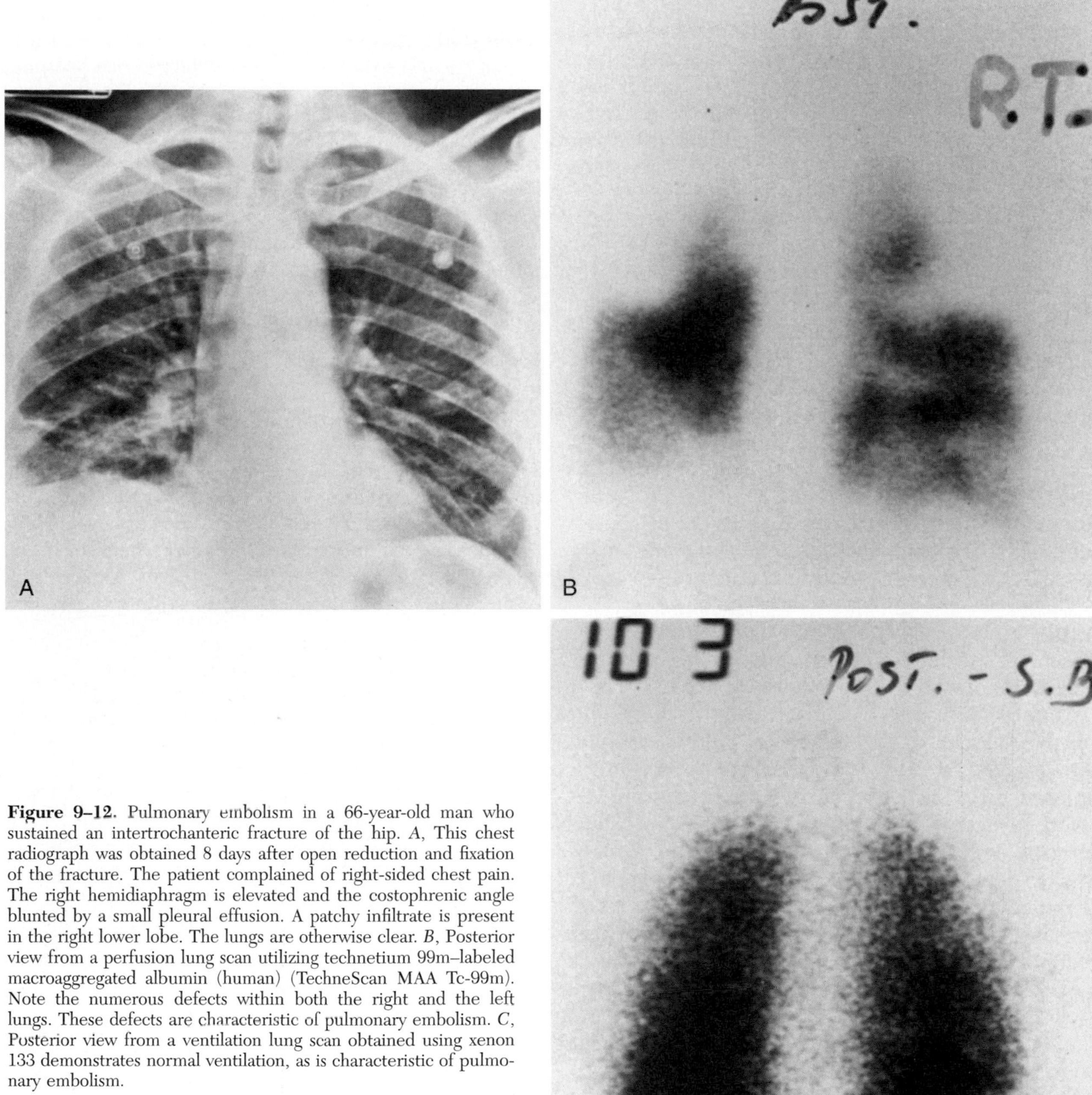

Figure 9–12. Pulmonary embolism in a 66-year-old man who sustained an intertrochanteric fracture of the hip. *A*, This chest radiograph was obtained 8 days after open reduction and fixation of the fracture. The patient complained of right-sided chest pain. The right hemidiaphragm is elevated and the costophrenic angle blunted by a small pleural effusion. A patchy infiltrate is present in the right lower lobe. The lungs are otherwise clear. *B*, Posterior view from a perfusion lung scan utilizing technetium 99m–labeled macroaggregated albumin (human) (TechneScan MAA Tc-99m). Note the numerous defects within both the right and the left lungs. These defects are characteristic of pulmonary embolism. *C*, Posterior view from a ventilation lung scan obtained using xenon 133 demonstrates normal ventilation, as is characteristic of pulmonary embolism.

boembolism.[79] The procedure is performed using a bolus injection of contrast intravenously with spiral acquisition of CT dataset. An embolus is seen as a filling defect in the contrast-filled pulmonary arteries. Sensitivity and specificity are approximately 90% in the central pulmonary vessels. Thin-collimation (2-mm) helical CT improves demonstration of segmental and subsegmental emboli.[80]

In the diagnosis of pulmonary embolism, it is essential to realize that the accuracy of lung scanning and pulmonary angiography—the only real means of establishing the diagnosis—is time dependent. The reliability of these procedures diminishes rapidly as perfusion improves after the embolic event, finally returning to normal or demonstrating a pattern of diagnostic uncertainty.[71] Thus, procrastination in the decision to obtain a scan or an arteriogram increases the likelihood of missing the diagnosis. Demonstration of peripheral thrombus is not necessary to establish the diagnosis of pulmonary thromboembolism. Peripheral venograms are often reserved for patients for whom some form of vena caval interruption is being considered because of repeated episodes of embolism.

Intermediate Complications

Osteomyelitis

The term *osteomyelitis* is a combination of the Greek words *osteo* (bone) and *myelo* (marrow) plus the termination *-itis* (inflammation). Infection is one of the most feared complications of fracture, at the least resulting in additional morbidity and delayed healing and at the worst necessitating amputation or resulting in death. Waldvogel and associates[101] have conveniently divided infections of bone into three categories reflecting the source or pathogenesis of the infection: hematogenous osteomyelitis, osteomyelitis secondary to a contiguous focus of infection,[87, 96] and osteomyelitis associated with peripheral vascular disease. The concern here is with the second category, osteomyelitis secondary to a contiguous focus of infection, including infection introduced at the time of an open fracture, or of soft tissue injury alone or during open reduction and fixation of a closed fracture. In the series of Waldvogel and associates,[101] comprising 247 patients, hematogenous osteomyelitis accounted for 19% of cases; secondary osteomyelitis, 47%; and osteomyelitis secondary to vascular insufficiency, 34%. These figures conclusively demonstrate the importance and frequency of secondary infections.

The incidence of osteomyelitis in open fractures is 12%[100] to 16%,[86] and a similar incidence has been reported in open reduction with plate fixation[84] (Figs. 9–13 and 9–14). The incidence with open reduction utilizing an intramedullary nail with reaming in (Gustilo) 140 type 1 open tibial and femoral fractures (Fig. 9–15) was 7% in the largest reported series.[94] The destruction of medullary blood vessels by an intramedullary rod, especially if ream-

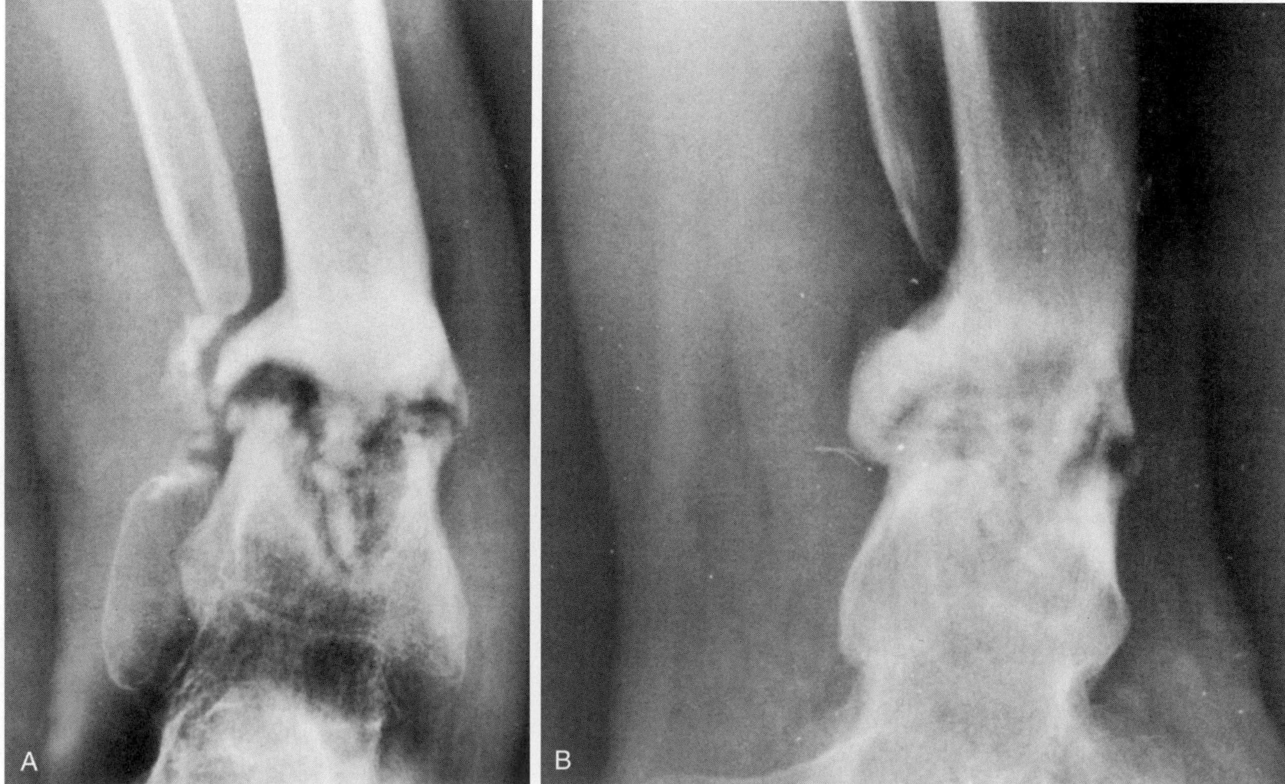

Figure 9–13. Chronic osteomyelitis in nonunion of a fracture of the distal third of the tibia and the fibula. The fracture had been sustained 5 years previously and was treated by open reduction with plate fixation. Osteomyelitis was first noted 4 1/2 months after injury. *A*, Anteroposterior view of the ankle demonstrates obvious nonunion, with a wide line of separation between the proximal and distal fragments. The margin of the proximal fragment is quite sclerotic. Nodules of dense bone (sequestra) are present within the central portion of the fracture line, extending into the excavation within the distal fragment. Fibulectomy had been performed previously. *B*, The line of separation between the fragments is not as obvious on this lateral view. There is partial fusion of the ankle joint. *Pseudomonas* and *Staphylococcus* were cultured from the wound.

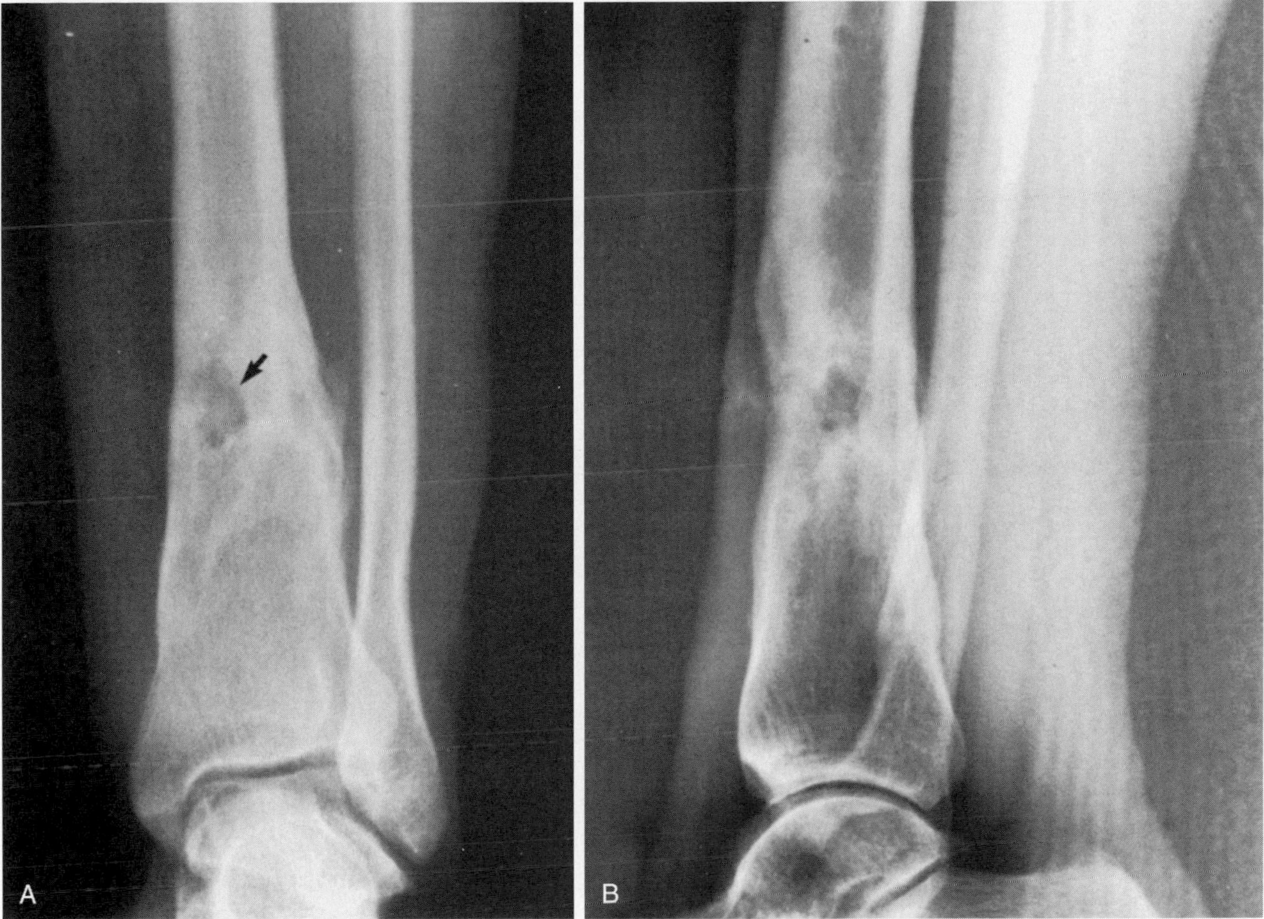

Figure 9–14. Chronic osteomyelitis in an old healed tibial fracture in a 29-year-old woman. The tibial fracture had been sustained 10 years before this examination and was treated by open reduction with plate fixation. There was no prior history of infection. The patient had recently been jogging up to 5 miles a day. Three days before admission, she noted swelling, tenderness, and redness over the old fracture site. *Proteus mirabilis* was cultured after incision and drainage. *A*, A healed fracture of the distal third of the tibia is identified, with distortion of the outlines of the tibia. A 1.5-cm lucency is demonstrated within the fracture line *(arrow)*. *B*, Lateral radiograph demonstrates similar findings, with a central lucency that appears to extend anteriorly to involve the cortex. An uncomplicated healed fracture is unlikely to leave these areas of lucency within the fracture line after such a long time.

ing of the canal is done, is thought to predispose to this high incidence of infection.[97] Other types of management of these type 1 fractures have been reported with an incidence of infection of less than 1%,[90] clearly indicating that intramedullary nailing with reaming should be regarded as a controversial treatment for this grade of fracture. The incidence of fracture infections is greatest in the leg and increases in all open fractures with increasing fracture grade. The fracture grade in turn reflects the severity of associated soft tissue injury.[86]

The femoral shaft, intertrochanteric region (see Fig. 9–18), and femoral neck and tibia (see Figs. 9–13, 9–14, and 9–19) are the most common sites of secondary osteomyelitis,[81, 102] reflecting the occurrence of open fracture or the frequent necessity of open reduction for fractures at these sites, or both. The overall due operating time has been found to be important: the more prolonged the surgical procedure, the more likely the development of osteomyelitis.[100] Although this high risk is in part a reflection of the severity of the injury and the difficulty in achieving adequate reduction, it also underscores the importance of maintaining proper facilities and trained personnel, including radiographic equipment and technicians, so as not to unnecessarily prolong the operative procedure.

Osteomyelitis is a rare complication of closed fracture.[83] All reported cases have occurred in children, were associated with bacterial infections at other sites (pharynx, tonsils, or urinary tract), and were considered to represent a form of hematogenous osteomyelitis.

Pathogenesis

The pathogenesis of secondary infection of bone is easily understood. The simultaneous presence of pathogenic bacteria, vascular stasis, and a favorable tissue environment encourages the establishment of infection.[73] The blood clot and necrotic marrow, muscle, and fat associated with a fracture provide an excellent culture medium for localization and colonization by pathogenic bacteria introduced from the outside by either open fracture or open reduction. Vascular injury and occlusion serve to partially isolate the area from the body defense mechanisms and circulating antibiotics. Any surgical procedure, no matter

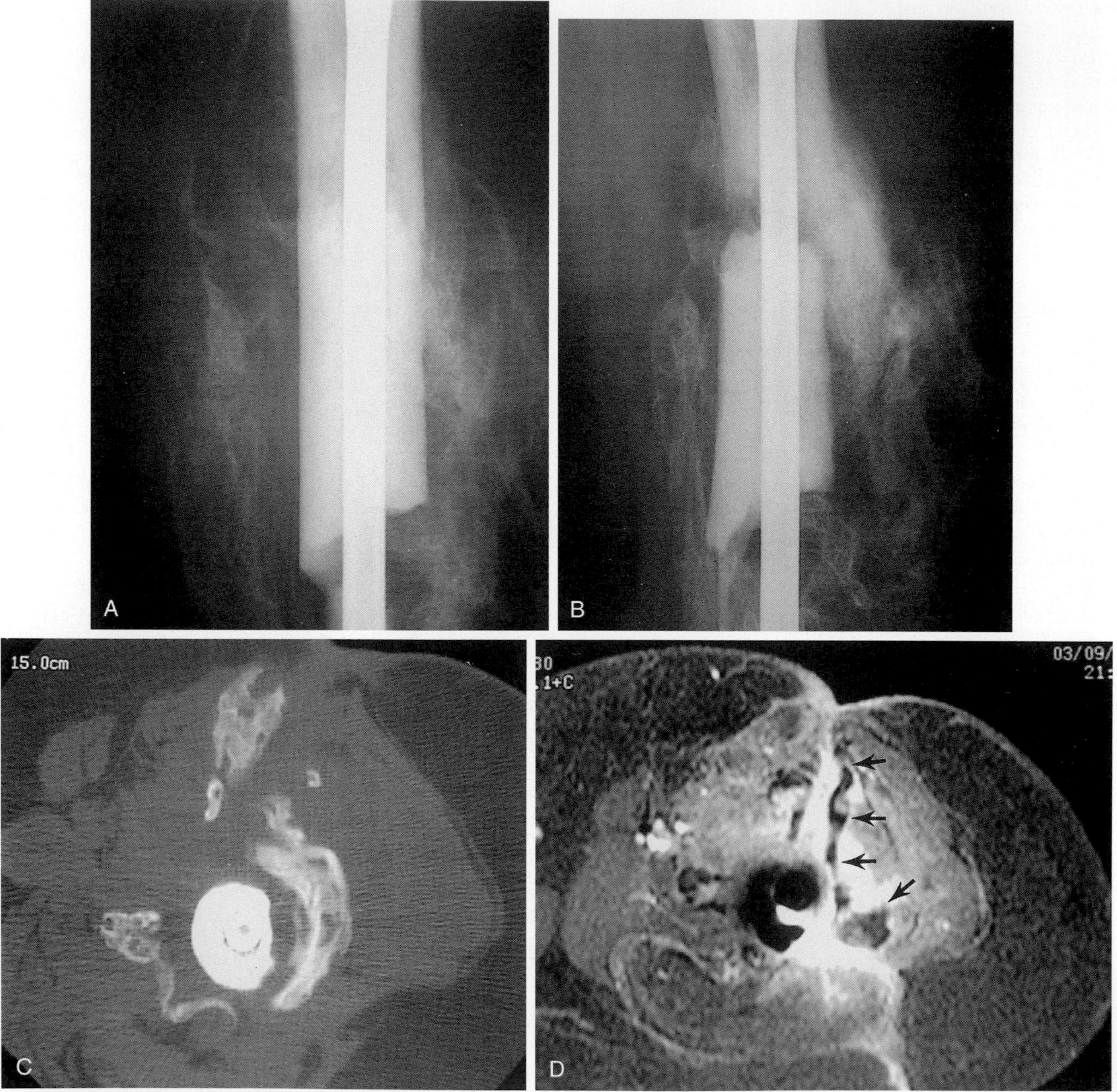

Figure 9–15. Chronic osteomyelitis with sequestrum in the femur of a 15-year-old girl following an all-terrain-vehicle accident. She presented 5 months after the injury with a persistent draining wound despite repeated débridement and irrigation *A*, Anteroposterior view of the femur reveals a densely sclerotic end of the proximal fragment. *B*, One month later, callus has increased, but the sclerotic region of the sequestrum has detached. *C*, Computed tomography study with widened bone windows reveals the dense sclerosis and surrounding new bone. *D*, Post-contrast image from fat-suppressed magnetic resonance study reveals the sinus tract and collection of pus *(arrows)* extending to the intramedullary nail and the sequestrum. Cultures grew enterococci. The intramedullary nail was in place when the patient presented for treatment of the draining wound.

how meticulously performed, results in some degree of ischemia at the operative site.

The infection, once established, provokes a suppurative inflammation, the severity dependent upon the virulence of the organism and the suppressive effects of administered antibiotics. The bacterial enzymes, pH changes, local edema, pus, and resultant increase in local pressure all contribute to the necrosis of tissue and breakdown of bone. The infection extends through the marrow and haversian system of cortical bone, increasing the area of vascular stasis and compromise already existing in the presence of the fracture. Local septic thrombophlebitis of the diaphyseal vessels occurs, obstructing venous return and further increasing local tissue pressure. The pus extends through segments of cortical bone, elevating the periosteum and causing a reaction in the form of periosteal new bone formation. Segments of bone devoid of blood supply remain as sequestra.

Healing of a fracture is delayed but does not necessarily cease in the presence of infection. Healing and union may occur but will take considerably more time than usual. Healing occurs in the presence of metal fixation devices,[95, 105] so they do not necessarily need to be removed. In fact, they aid materially in the healing process as long as they continue to provide stabilization at the fracture site.

The dominant organism is *Staphylococcus aureus*, present in approximately 60% to 70%[100, 101] of cases. Although this organism frequently occurs alone, it is often combined with other organisms. Mixed infections occur in approximately 25% of infections with *S. aureus*, and in most of those of non-staphylococcal etiology.[101] This emphasizes the importance of wound culture. In the more indolent infections, bone biopsy cultures may be necessary. Other organisms include different forms of *Staphylococcus, Streptococcus*, and various gram-negative bacteria including *Pseudomonas, Escherichia coli, Klebsiella*, and *Aerobacter*. Mycobacterial and fungal infections are quite rare.[84, 101] In general the incidence of infection of staphylococcal etiology has been decreasing and that of infection with gram-negative organisms has been increasing.[87]

Most infections are manifest within a month[102] of the occurrence of the open fracture or open reduction and fixation, although a few infections may not appear for several months (Fig. 9–16). The dominant symptom of osteomyelitis is pain. The severity of the pain and the degree of associated fever are usually directly proportional to the virulence of the offending organism. The pain of infection appears after the initial pain of the fracture has subsided and persists despite immobilization. Erythema, swelling, and tenderness at the site vary with the virulence of the organism. Initially it may be difficult to differentiate the findings from those associated with a hematoma. Drainage may not occur from the wound, its ultimate appearance varying with the virulence of the infection. Laboratory findings such as the erythrocyte sedimentation rate and white blood cell count may be

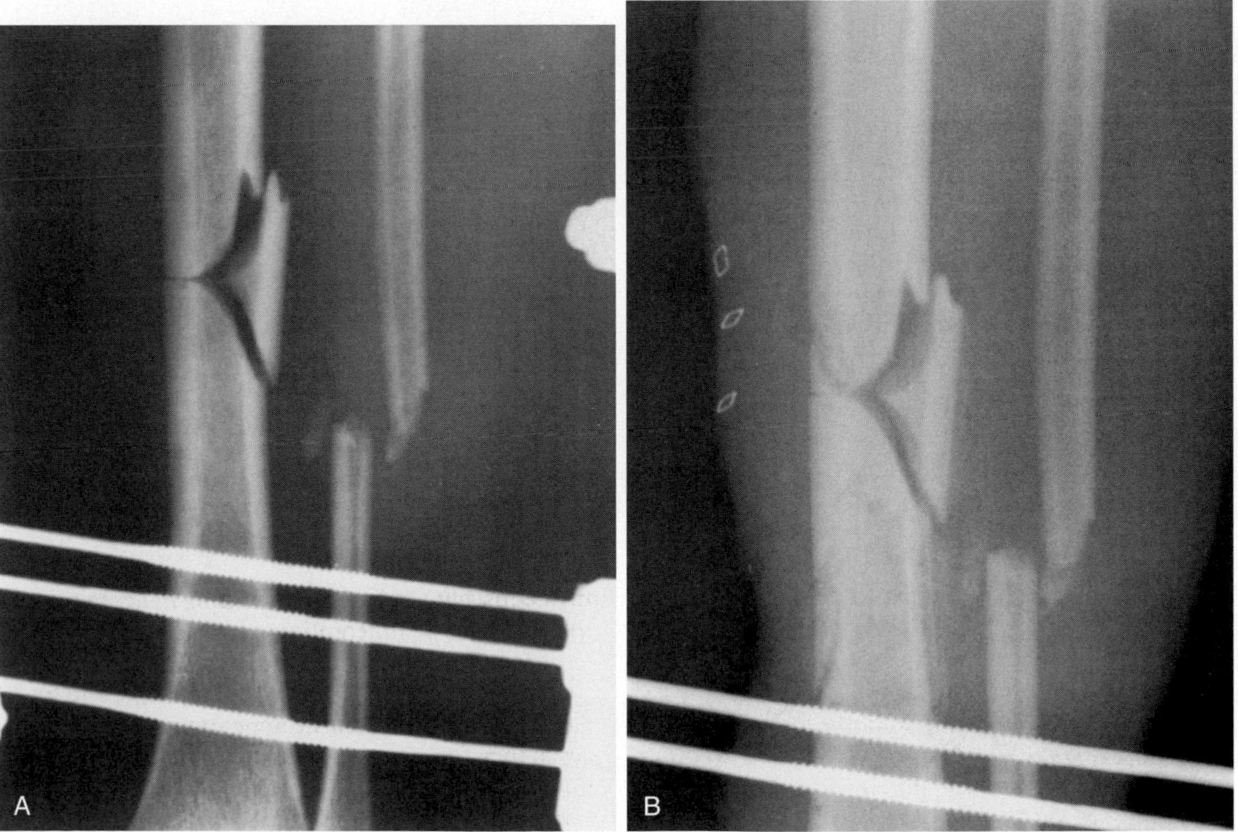

Figure 9–16. *A*, Comminuted fracture of the tibia with a butterfly fragment immobilized by an external fixator. *B*, Four weeks later, bone destruction and periosteal new bone are seen, resulting from acute osteomyelitis originating from a pin tract infection. (From Hendrix, R.W. [1986]. Radiology of bone and joints. In Sider, L. Ed.: Introduction to Diagnostic Imaging. Churchill Livingstone, New York, with permission.)

variable, and values are not always elevated. The ease of diagnosis is therefore dependent upon the virulence of the organism and the degree of the masking effect from administered antibiotics.

If not eliminated by the initial treatment, the infective process may lapse into chronicity with or without more acute intermittent flare-ups. The chronicity varies with the organism or organisms, their response to and the appropriateness of the administered antibiotics, the rigidity of the immobilization, and the presence or absence of sequestra and other foreign bodies within the wound.

Diagnosis

Multiple modalities can be used to evaluate for possible osteomyelitis.[86] Changes of osteomyelitis are seen early with radionuclide bone scanning, although there can be difficulty distinguishing cellulitis from osteomyelitis. The triple-phase technetium bone scan was designed to differentiate between these entities.[89] This study consists of obtaining angiographic images during radiopharmaceutical injection, blood pool images while the agent is being cleared from the circulating blood pool, and delayed images at 2 to 5 hours after injection. Osteomyelitis causes increasing bone uptake of the radiopharmaceutical throughout the study, whereas cellulitis causes initially high soft tissue radionuclide activity that progressively diminishes in later phases of the study compared with normal bone radionuclide activity.[88, 89] In spite of the early detection capability of scintigraphy, conventional radiography is usually the first imaging modality used to evaluate for osteomyelitis.

From the time the infective process begins, 10 to 14 days must pass before the radiographic changes of osteomyelitis become apparent.[85, 102] This period may be prolonged if appropriate antibiotics are administered; in fact, in some patients who receive early treatment with appropriate antibiotics, the radiographic features of infection may never appear. It is therefore imperative that the diagnosis be established on the basis of clinical and laboratory evidence and that treatment be initiated without waiting for radiographic confirmation. Adherence to this approach is essential for all types of osteomyelitis—hematogenous, secondary, or that associated with vascular insufficiency. The problem of radiographic diagnosis is compounded by the presence of a fracture. The principal radiographic features of osteomyelitis[82, 85] are soft tissue changes, periosteal new bone formation, and bone destruction (Fig. 9–17). Of these, only bone destruction is indicative of infection in the presence of a fracture, because such destruction does not result from fracture alone. Soft tissue swelling and the obliteration of fascial planes are normally expected as a result of fracture, and their presence does not allow for distinction between fracture alone and fracture with infection. Periosteal new bone formation mimics the expected callus about a fracture; therefore, its presence cannot always be used as evidence of infection. However, the presence of periosteal new bone formation in a fracture treated by metallic internal fixation with either a plate or nail suggests superimposed osteomyelitis (Fig. 9–18).

It should be remembered that as many as 60% of fractures treated by rigid internal fixation heal without external or peripheral callus formation. When peripheral callus formation does occur, it is usually minimal and is never multilayered. Multilayered periosteal reaction, in the presence of rigid internal fixation devices, must be considered evidence of secondary osteomyelitis until proven otherwise. Callus formation also occurs if there is motion at the fracture site—that is, if the fixation is not rigid—but the periosteal new bone or callus is rarely if ever layered under these circumstances. Under these circumstances, evidence of bone destruction (Fig. 9–19) or rarefaction is probably the most consistent radiographic finding in acute osteomyelitis. This finding can be differentiated from disuse osteoporosis by the localization of the radiographic changes to a limited area adjacent to the fracture site. Initially the radiolucencies are multiple and linear or patchy and moth-eaten in appearance, but as they coalesce they form larger, poorly defined areas of destruction.

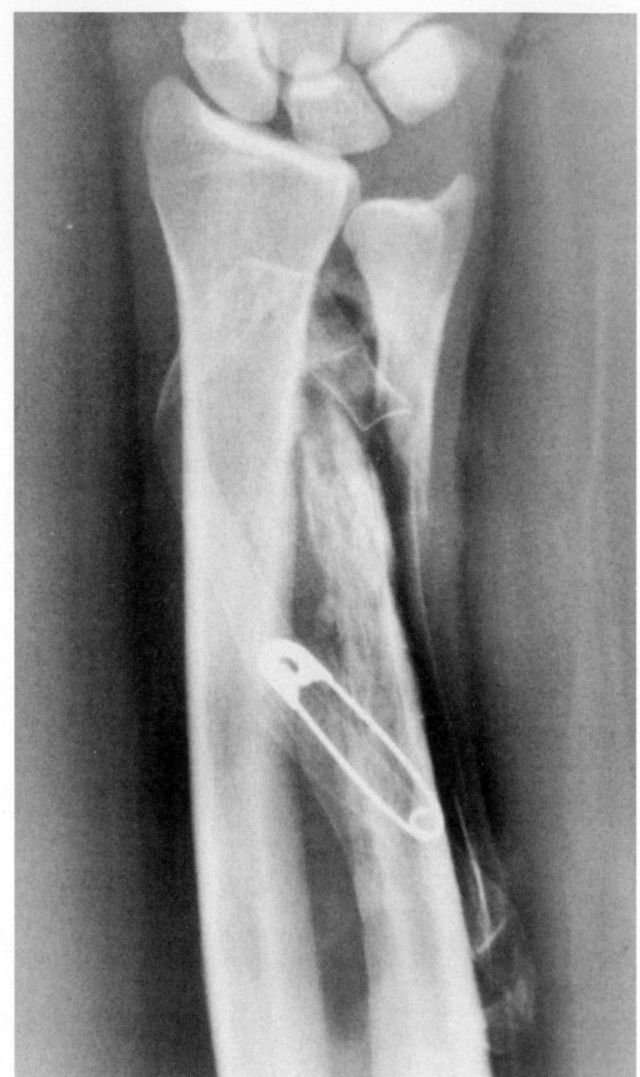

Figure 9–17. Acute osteomyelitis following open fracture of the distal ulna in a 35-year-old man. This radiograph, obtained 6 weeks after injury, demonstrates the lack of healing with irregular lytic destruction of the proximal fragment. Air is present within the wound at the fracture site. A wound culture grew predominantly *Staphylococcus*.

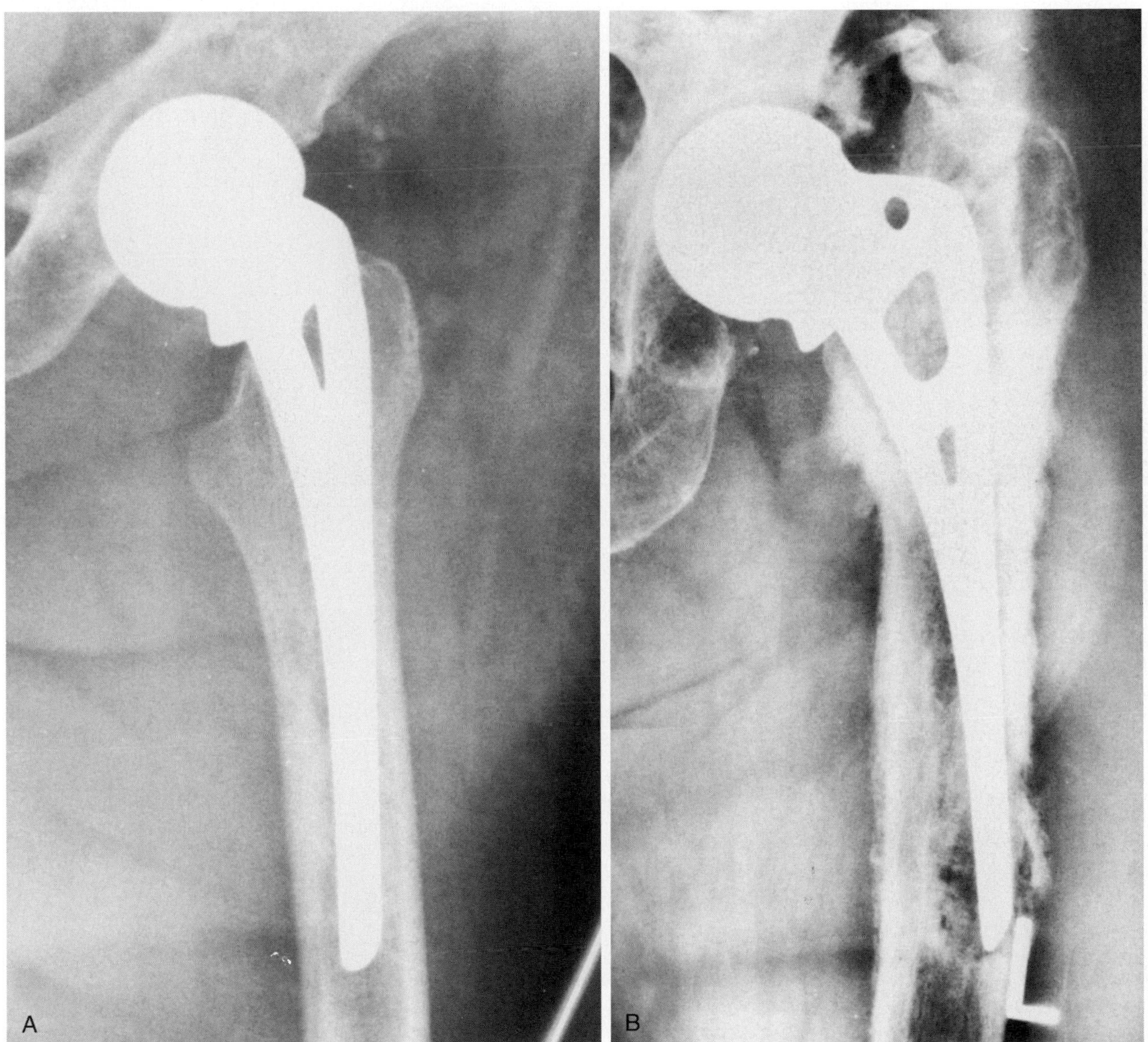

Figure 9–18. Acute osteomyelitis following insertion of an Austin-Moore prosthesis for femoral neck fracture in an 82-year-old woman. *A*, Radiographic examination was performed 5 weeks after insertion of the prosthesis. There is no obvious abnormality. *B*, At 11 weeks, there is extensive bony destruction about the stem of the prosthesis and considerable periosteal new bone formation along the intertrochanteric region and proximal shaft of the femur, findings indicative of acute osteomyelitis. Periarticular ossification is also evident on the superior aspect of the hip joint.

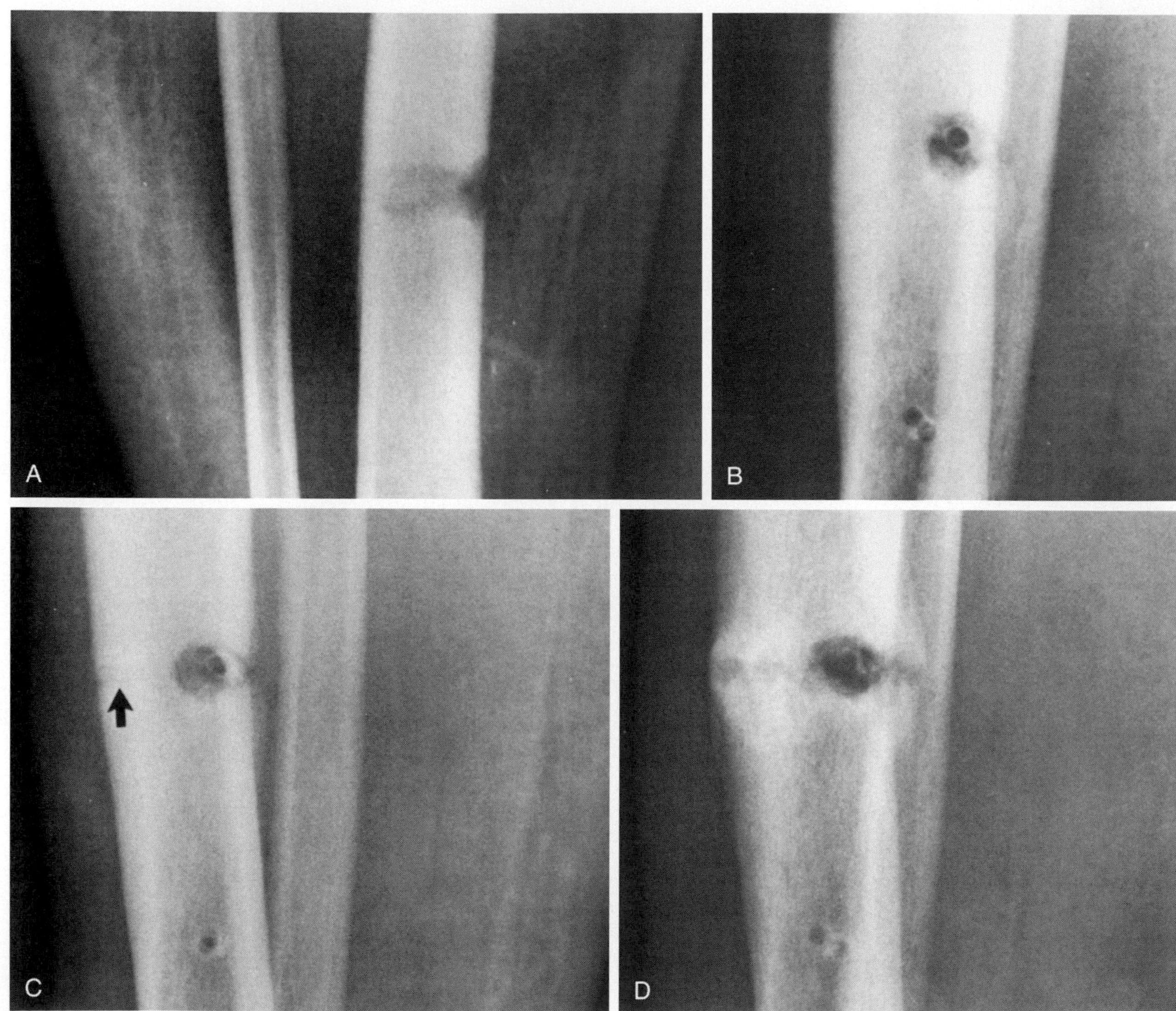

Figure 9–19. Osteomyelitis of the pin tract complicated by subsequent fracture in a 55-year-old man. Steinmann pins had been placed initially as part of the pins-and-plaster technique to treat a comminuted fracture of the distal tibia that extended into the ankle joint. *A*, Anteroposterior radiograph demonstrates a transverse lucency across the tibial shaft. There is soft tissue swelling with obliteration of the surrounding fascial planes. *B*, A lucent area of destruction surrounds the proximal pin tract. The distal pin tract is normal. *C*, Radiographic examination was performed 3 days after *B* was obtained. The patient had felt a "snap" while walking. Note the linear fracture line *(arrow)* extending from the pin tract infection site through the anterior cortex of the tibia. *D*, Lateral view obtained 2 months after *C* was obtained demonstrates that the infection had extended along the fracture line. Callus formation is present both anteriorly and posteriorly. The infection subsequently cleared, and the fracture healed.

Sclerosis (Fig. 9–20; see also Fig. 9–13) and sequestra (see Figs. 9–13*A* and 9–15) are indicative of chronicity. Excessive callus is present. It is often difficult to determine radiologically the state of activity in chronic osteomyelitis (see Fig. 9–14) in the absence of sequestra. The residual deformity of previous disease may be mimicked by chronic infection.

Conventional tomography and sinography[84] may be helpful. Tomography (Fig. 9–21) permits better definition of bone abnormalities than is provided by radiographs. The detail is improved by the removal of plaster splints and casts. The presence of metal reduces the accuracy of the examination by obscuring the visualization of overlying or underlying bone and soft tissue. This problem may be partially compensated for by obtaining radiographic views in two or more projections—at a minimum, an anteroposterior and a lateral projection. CT (see Fig. 9–15*C*) yields similar results.

Sinograms (see Fig. 9–20) are best obtained under fluoroscopic control to determine the most revealing and informative projection of the abnormality and also to better determine the amount of contrast material necessary to fully visualize the entire sinus tract. If the amount of contrast agent to be injected is standardized and only standard projections are obtained, without fluoroscopic monitoring, the entire sinus may not be demonstrated. It is best to utilize a small soft rubber catheter, passing it as far into the wound as it will easily progress before injecting water-soluble contrast material; 30 ml of contrast medium available is usually more than adequate. Methylglucamine salts are better tolerated than sodium salts. Each ostium of each sinus should be identified by taping a metallic marker to the skin.

Contrast material should be injected while the ostium is compressed to prevent backflow, and the injection should be continued as long as additional areas or tracts are visualized. The catheter can then be withdrawn to the ostium, and a small additional amount of contrast injected to fill the entire sinus tract. If multiple sinus tracts are present, each should be filled in turn. The contrast material will usually surround sequestra. Although spot films may be obtained during the filling, it is important to

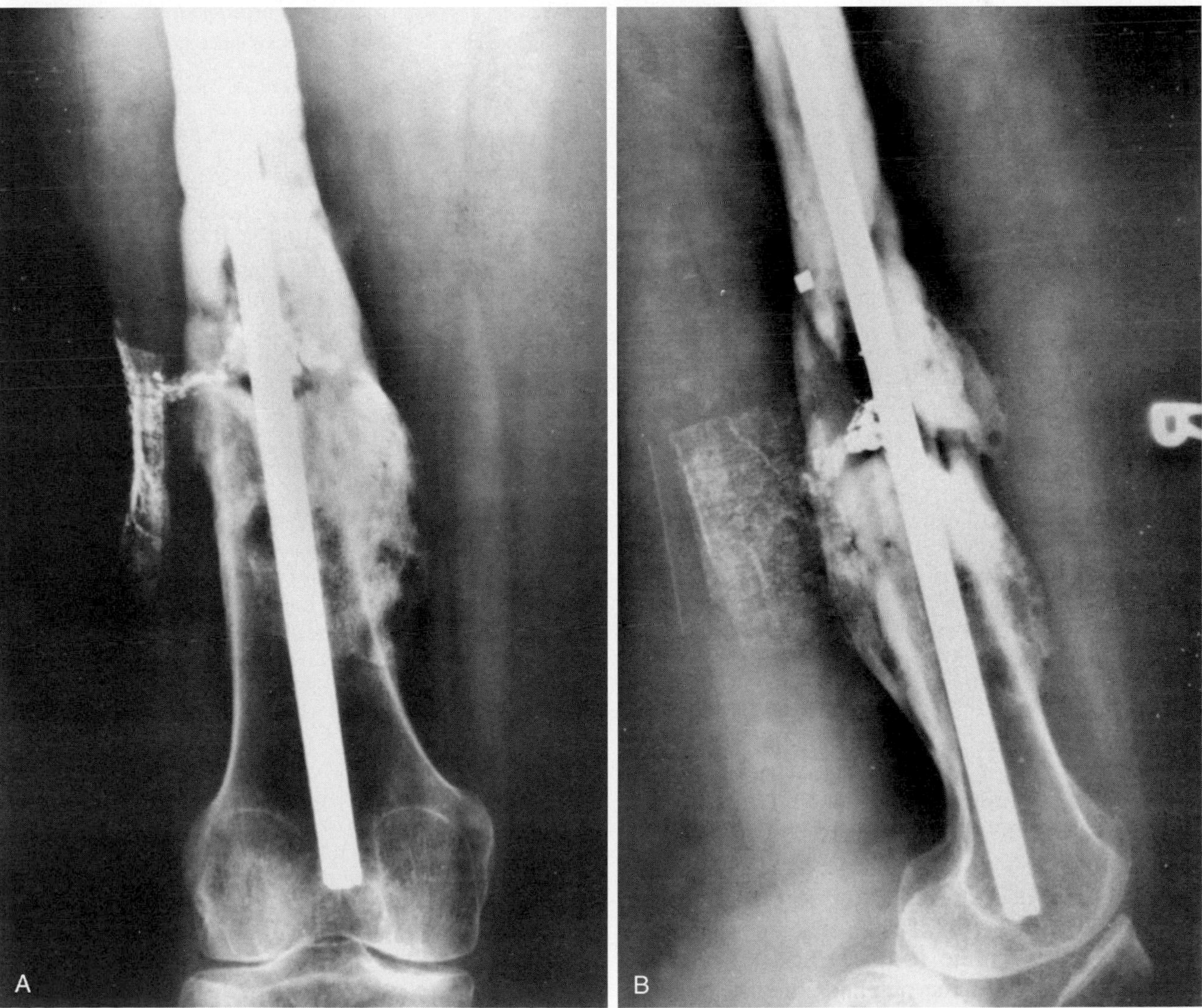

Figure 9–20. Chronic osteomyelitis Kuntscher nail insertion. *A*, Frontal view from a sinogram was obtained after injection of contrast material from the sinus opening situated laterally. The contrast material tracks to and surrounds the nail at the fracture site. *B*, Lateral radiograph demonstrates contrast material within the central lucency surrounding the nail.

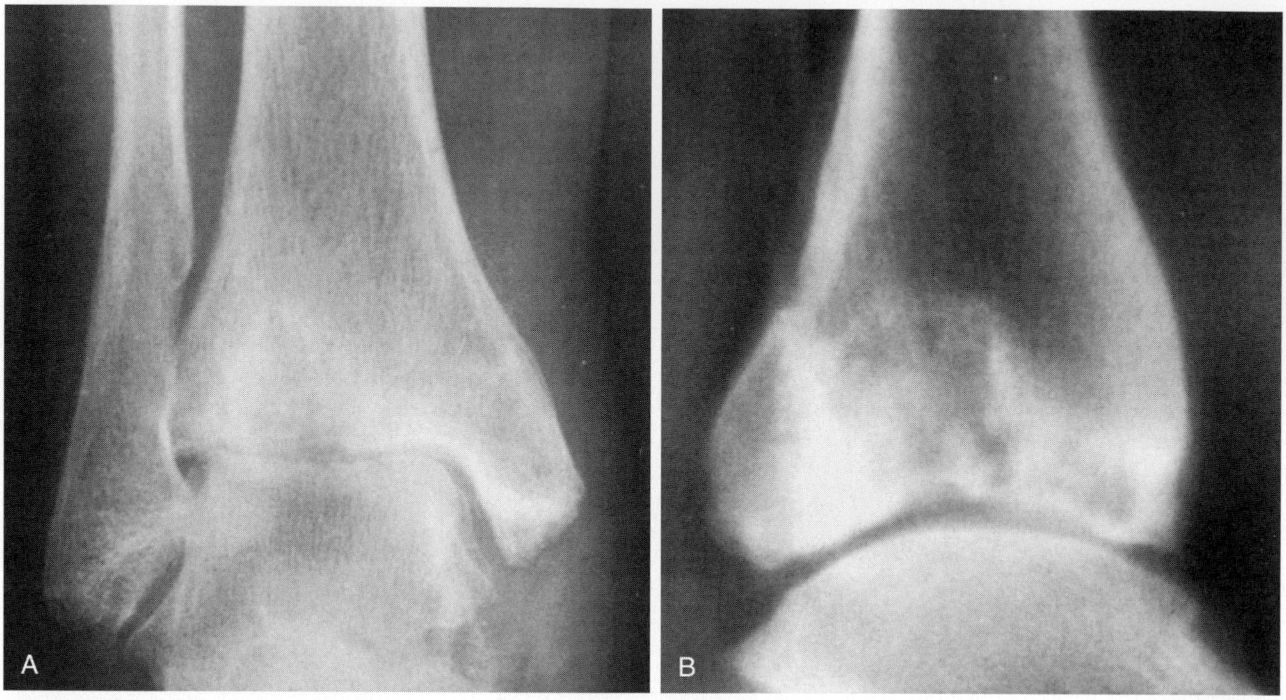

Figure 9–21. Osteomyelitis and septic arthritis 4 years following open reduction and internal fixation of fracture-dislocation of the ankle in a 36-year-old woman. The patient had a 2-year history of pain, swelling, and tenderness. Over the past 6 weeks she had noted an elevated temperature and was treated with antibiotics. *A*, Anteroposterior radiograph of the right ankle demonstrates narrowing of the ankle mortise and an irregular lucency extending into the tibia through the plafond. *B*, Lateral tomogram clearly defines the degree of destruction in the distal tibia. The ankle joint is narrowed. The cultures were sterile at the time of surgery. The patient was treated with suction irrigation and has done well.

obtain at least two large radiographs using projections at 90 degrees to each other, an anteroposterior and lateral, to fully define the sinus tract, its course within the infective process, and its relationship to the surrounding normal anatomy. Small films are confusing, and use of small amounts of contrast material may give misleading results. The sinogram can also be performed in the CT suite, and CT images obtained. This technique requires dilution of the contrast to diminish the occurrence of streak artifacts. It eliminates some of the projectional limitations of fluoroscopy alone.

A diagnostic difficulty can arise when osteomyelitis is suspected at a nonunited fracture site but conventional radiographs do not demonstrate features of osteomyelitis.[98, 99] Seabold and coworkers[99] reported a high specificity and sensitivity for detecting low-grade osteomyelitis at such sites using combined technetium Tc 99m methylene diphosphonate bone scintigraphy and indium 111–labeled leukocyte (^{111}In-WBC) scintigraphy. Compared with ^{111}In-WBC scintigraphy alone, combined scanning significantly improved differentiation of infection in adjacent soft tissues from osteomyelitis at the fracture site.

Treatment

Early in the course of osteomyelitis, the lesion is accessible to antibiotics within the bloodstream, and these agents may completely eradicate the infection. However, as the process becomes chronic, the chance that antibiotics alone will effect a cure decreases, and surgical intervention is required; 15% to 30%[93, 103] of cases of acute osteomyelitis progress to the chronic form. Débridement decompresses the forming abscess and evacuates the pus and infected tissue, including sequestra, and greatly improves the likelihood of cure with prolonged administration of antibiotics.[91, 92, 104] Intra-articular fixation devices such as a femoral head prosthesis should be removed. However, intramedullary devices and plates are left in place until the fracture is healed.[95, 104] It appears that the fixation they provide improves the likelihood of fracture healing. If no metallic fixation devices have been utilized, sequestra are not removed until the fracture fragments are united by involucrum and callus. Removal of the sequestrum prematurely under these circumstances may result in nonunion or in significant shortening of the bone, or both. Closed irrigation with antibiotic-detergent mixtures and administration of hyperbaric oxygen are additional methods of treatment that may be of some value in the treatment of chronic infections. The cornerstone of treatment, however, remains administration of appropriate antibiotics and surgical débridement.[97] Amputation is rarely required.

Chronic osteomyelitis occurs as a complication of fracture and, in turn, rarely can be complicated by squamous cell carcinoma.[155] The tumor arises in the draining sinus tract of long-standing, neglected cases. Aggressive surgical treatment and radiation therapy are necessary to eradicate the tumor, but a one-third mortality rate has been reported in spite of treatment.[156]

Migrating Orthopedic Appliances

Fixation by means of pins and wires is one of the most effective and frequently used methods of managing fractures and dislocations.[2] They are used frequently in the hip, facial bones, proximal humerus, shoulder joint, acromioclavicular joint, clavicle, and sternoclavicular joint, where there have been numerous isolated reports of migrating pins, sometimes causing spectacular complications. Lyons and Rockwood reviewed the orthopedic literature and found 37 reports of 49 cases of complications from the migration of pins from the shoulder and clavicular area.[2] Although pins can migrate from other areas, they rarely have been reported to cause significant complications. A smooth Kirschner wire with an unbent end was the most common offender (see Fig. 15–32), but bent wires and threaded pins were also seen to migrate and cause complications. In Lyons and Rockwood's review,[2] a total of 17 pins migrated to various cardiovascular locations: the heart (4), subclavian artery (2), ascending aorta (6), and pulmonary artery (5). Eight pins migrated to the lung and 10 to the lung and mediastinum. Five pins migrated to the spine, where their tips entered the intervertebral foramen. Two pins traveled through the thorax into the abdomen. One Steinmann pin migrated to the trachea and was coughed up by the patient. Another pin in the clavicle traveled to the contralateral orbit, causing a painful exophthalmos. Two pins migrated to the base of the neck, two to the breast, and one to the proximal arm.

A total of eight deaths were reported. Six of the patients died suddenly of pericardial tamponade, and two died of ventricular fibrillation and acute circulatory collapse shortly after surgical pin removal. All eight of these patients had pin migration from fixation of the sternoclavicular joint within the preceding 3 months. Nonfatal complications included pericardial tamponade, arrhythmia, pericarditis, pneumothorax, hemoptysis, paraplegia, transient hemiplegia, hemianopia, radicular pain, laceration of the subclavian artery, subclavian steal syndrome, splenic hematoma, false aneurysm, aortoinnominate and aortopulmonary fistulas, and dysphagia. Pin migration occurred within 8 months of operation in three fourths of the patients, but the time at which migration was noted ranged from 5 days to 21 years following pin placement. In nine patients, the pin was not removed after migration was recognized, and six of these patients died.

The recommendation of these investigators is that radiographs be obtained intraoperatively to document the placement of the pins. Follow-up radiographs should be obtained every 4 weeks until pin removal, and immediate removal is indicated if any migration is detected on the radiographs[2] (see Fig. 15–32). These authors also think that pin fixation of the sternoclavicular joint is contraindicated because of the gravity of possible complications.

Post-traumatic Reflex Dystrophy Syndrome—Sudeck's Atrophy

Numerous designations[107, 111, 114, 116] exist for post-traumatic reflex dystrophy syndrome. This poorly understood but fortunately infrequent syndrome consists chiefly of pain and tenderness in an extremity associated with hyperesthesia, soft tissue swelling, dystrophic changes of the skin, vasomotor instability, stiffness of joints, and patchy osteoporosis in the affected part. The syndrome was first described by Weir Mitchell and his associates in 1864.[116] They noted the syndrome, which they termed "causalgia," in patients who had sustained injuries of peripheral nerves. In 1902, Sudeck[115] described the clinical and radiographic features of a post-traumatic reflex atrophy of bone that subsequently became known as Sudeck's atrophy. Although the principal interest here is in those syndromes of post-traumatic etiology, it must be recognized that only half or less of dystrophy syndromes are actually due to trauma. The traumatic injury may be soft tissue injury alone (Fig. 9–22), with or without nerve involvement, as well as fracture. Fracture was a component of injury in less than half of those syndromes associated with trauma.[107, 111, 114] Other reported underlying disorders include infection, peripheral neuropathy (Fig. 9–23), thrombophlebitis, myocardial infarction, cervical osteoarthritis, and tendinitis.

The pathogenesis of the syndrome remains theoretical and conjectural.[107, 108, 116] It is generally considered to be due to combinations of reflex arcs initiated by unknown stimuli and transmitted through somatic sensory and possibly efferent sympathetic fibers to the internuncial pool of the spinal cord, resulting in increased sympathetic and parasympathetic activity.

The reflex dystrophy syndromes (also known as complex regional pain syndromes) are divided into several different forms, depending chiefly on their clinical characteristics.[106, 111] Causalgia is characterized by the severe, intractable, excruciating nature of the pain. It usually occurs following injury to a major nerve, as first described by Mitchell and associates.[116] Minor causalgia is pain of lesser severity, which commonly occurs after an injection, thrombophlebitis, or trauma without nerve injury. The shoulder-hand syndrome involves the named joints, sparing the elbow for some reason, and most commonly occurs after myocardial infarction, tendinitis of the shoulder, or minor trauma. On occasion the shoulder-hand syndrome[114] is encountered after a fracture. Reflex sympathetic dystrophy and Sudeck's atrophy are similar in character. The syndrome is often designated "Sudeck's atrophy"[112] when it follows a fracture and "reflex sympathetic dystrophy" when it follows other disorders.

The onset is within 1 week to several months of the inciting event. The clinical course in the reflex dystrophy syndromes is frequently divided into three stages.[107, 111, 114] In the first stage, localized persistent pain, aggravated by movement and other stimuli, is present. The skin is hyperesthetic, and the affected area of limb is tender and swollen. Periarticular swelling and pain lead to limitation of motion. In the second stage, the pain and edema progress proximally. Atrophic changes appear in the skin. Joint stiffness increases, and muscle atrophy is evident. In the third stage, there is definite atrophy of the skin, muscle, and bone.

The radiologic hallmark[108–110] of these syndromes is osteoporosis (see Figs. 9–22*B* and *D* and 9–23), which is likely to be present in all cases associated with fracture. Osteoporosis may be absent in as many as a third of cases of nontraumatic etiology, particularly during the early course or first stage of the disease process. The radiographic appearance of the osteoporosis has been charac-

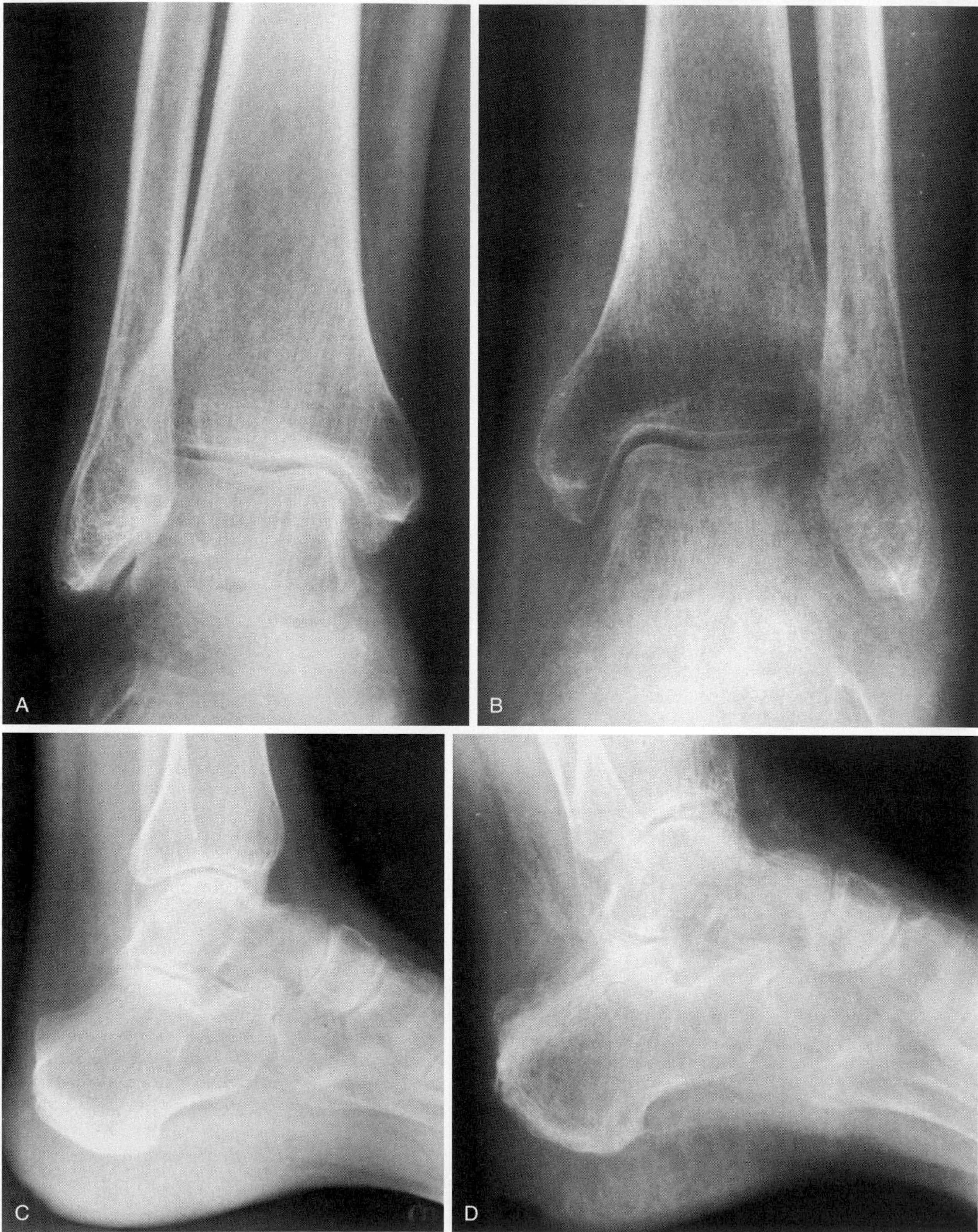

Figure 9–22. Reflex dystrophy syndrome in a 59-year-old woman who twisted her ankle 4 months before this radiographic examination. Beginning 5 days after injury the foot became swollen and tender. The skin is now smooth and atrophic. There was no fracture or dislocation. *A*, Anteroposterior view of the normal right ankle was obtained for comparison. *B*, Anteroposterior view of the left ankle demonstrates soft tissue swelling and blotchy osteoporosis. The subchondral bone within the ankle mortise is sharply defined. *C*, Lateral view of the normal right ankle was obtained for comparison. *D*, Lateral view of the left ankle demonstrates soft tissue swelling and marked diffuse osteoporosis.

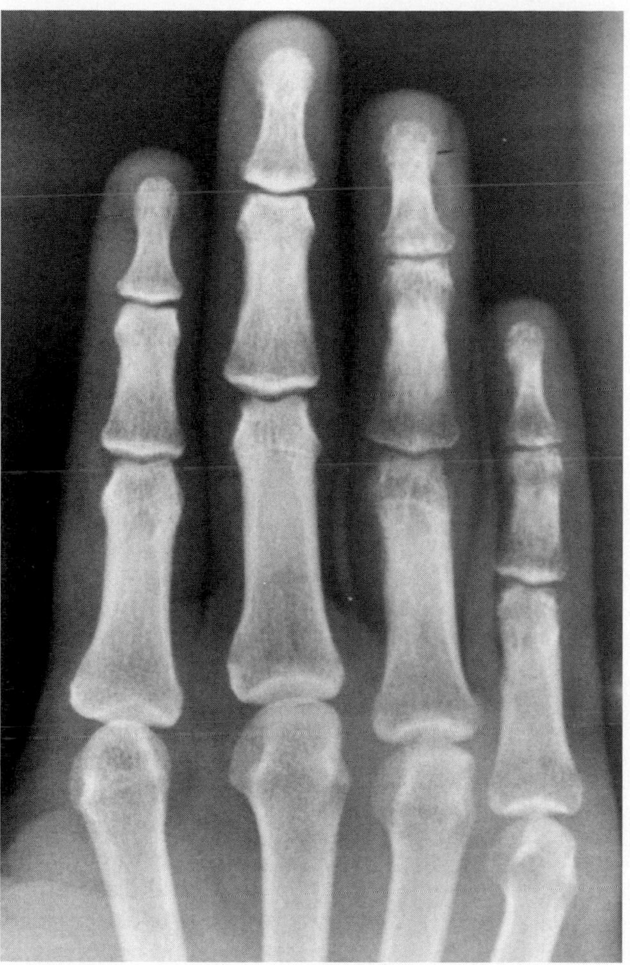

Figure 9–23. Reflex dystrophy syndrome in a 23-year-old man who jammed his ring finger playing basketball approximately 6 weeks prior to this radiograph. One month after injury, pain and swelling in the fourth and fifth digits were noted. The skin is now atrophic. The diagnosis is ulnar neuropathy associated with a reflex dystrophy syndrome. This posteroanterior radiograph demonstrates marked osteoporosis of the phalanges of the fourth and fifth digits with subchondral erosions at the margins of the joints. Cortical tunneling is evident in the proximal phalanges of the affected digits.

terized[108, 110] as spotty or patchy, but in reality it is little different from that of severe disuse osteoporosis. In reflex dystrophy, the osteoporosis is generally more rapidly progressive, however. Periarticular swelling and juxta-articular and subchondral erosions[108] (see Fig. 9–23) are often present in the reflex dystrophies. These features are best demonstrated by fine-detail radiography.[108] The osteoporosis is manifested as thinning of the cortices, loss of finer trabeculae, and tunneling of the cortex due to widening of intracortical haversian canals.

Although reflex dystrophy syndrome may exist in the absence of osteoporosis, the diagnosis of reflex dystrophy or Sudeck's atrophy cannot be made on the basis of the radiographic appearance of the osteoporosis alone, because patchy osteoporosis is seen with disuse alone (see Figs. 8–9*B* and 8–10*B*). The diagnosis requires that the osteoporosis be associated with pain or trophic changes or both.

The course of the disease may be prolonged, or the condition may remit at any stage in the process, although the longer the process continues, the less likely is a subsequent remission. There is no specific treatment. Most therapeutic efforts are directed against the sympathetic nervous system with early integration of physical therapy; spinal cord stimulation, placement of an epidural catheter with continuous analgesia, pharmacologic therapy with agents such as steroids and antidepressants, and surgical sympathectomy all have been utilized.[117–120]

Post-Traumatic Osteolysis

Cases of resorption or osteolysis[122–125] of bone have been reported after either a fracture or single or repeated episodes of minor trauma. The pathologic process begins within 2 months after the traumatic event, is self-limited, and is not associated with any identifiable or apparent metabolic or infectious cause. Pain is mild to absent. The outer end of the clavicle[123–125] appears to be the usual site of this process (Fig. 9–24), although involvement of the distal ulna following fracture of the distal radius has been reported.[122] It can be distinguished from Gorham's disease (massive osteolysis) by its self-limiting nature and the absence of angiomatosis. The largest number of patients (46) with this type of osteolysis has been reported by Cahill[121]; the study population consisted of male athletes, who were found to have osteolytic changes in the distal end of the clavicle. All but one of the patients had a history of an ongoing weight-training program with emphasis on strengthening the upper extremities. Rest or cessation of the weight-training program provided relief for most patients. Nineteen patients chose surgical resection of the distal clavicle; of these, 13 were subsequently able to continue sports activities sports activities with no pain, 4 noted mild discomfort, and 2 experienced moderate pain but not enough to discontinue the sport. In another study, findings on magnetic resonance imaging (MRI) examination consisted primarily of an edema pattern within the distal end of the clavicle (Fig. 9–25).[126] The etiology of post-traumatic osteolysis is unknown.

Refracture

Refracture refers to the occurrence of a second fracture in a previously fractured bone during the healing process (Fig. 9–26); By definition, the second fracture should occur in the original fracture line. Alternatively, a bone may fracture at a different site because of the weakening effects of the original injury, through bone weakened by disuse osteoporosis (see Fig. 8–13), or through a screw hole or pin tract after placement of such appliances for treatment of the original injury. The holes and tracts significantly weaken the bone, and the bone must be protected from excessive stresses until these defects heal. Refractures occur as a result of a second episode of trauma, but because healing is incomplete the force required to create the second fracture is not as great as that for the original injury. Many refractures occur because of inadequate immobilization, allowing the patient to subject the bone to excessive stresses before

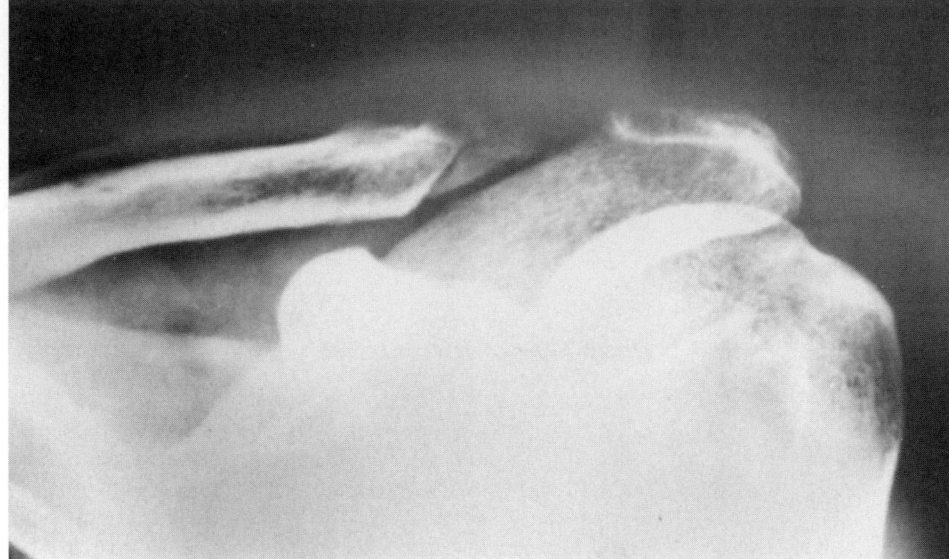

Figure 9–24. Osteolysis of the distal end of the clavicle in a professional hockey player who has sustained numerous injuries to the left shoulder and acromioclavicular joint. Note the resorption of the distal end of the clavicle. The patient was asymptomatic when this radiograph was obtained. (Case courtesy of Joseph Norfray, M.D., Chicago, Ill.)

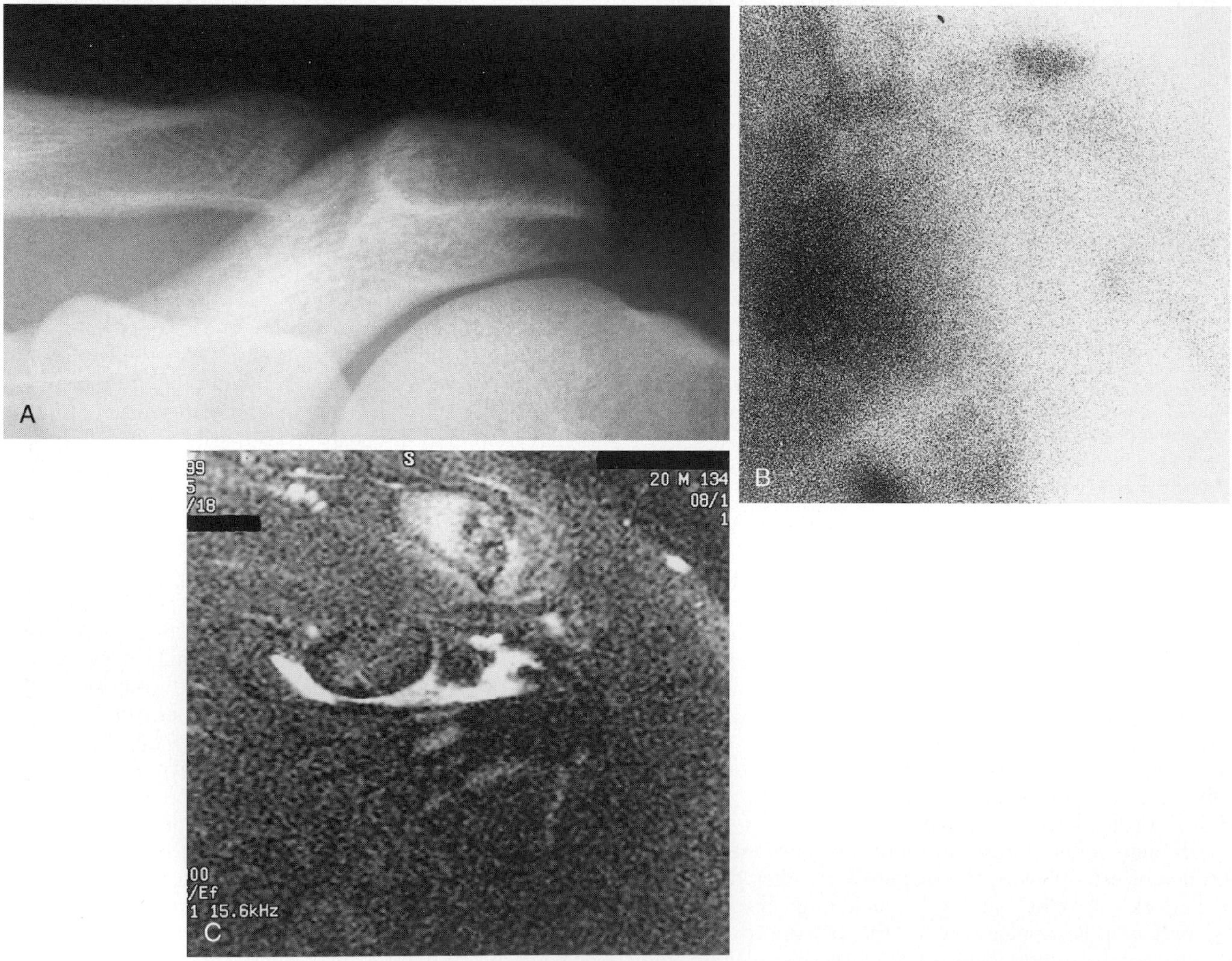

Figure 9–25. Osteolysis of the distal clavicle in a 20-year-old college football player. *A*, Anteroposterior view of the left acromioclavicular joint reveals lucency at the end of the clavicle, with loss of its cortical margin. *B*, Blood pool anterior image from a bone scan reveals focal activity in the distal clavicle. It became more intense on delayed images. *C*, Oblique coronal image from a fat-suppressed T_2-weighted magnetic resonance study demonstrates increased signal of the distal clavicle and the acromioclavicular joint, with sparing of the acromion. The patient reported marked reduction in pain after resection of the distal clavicle.

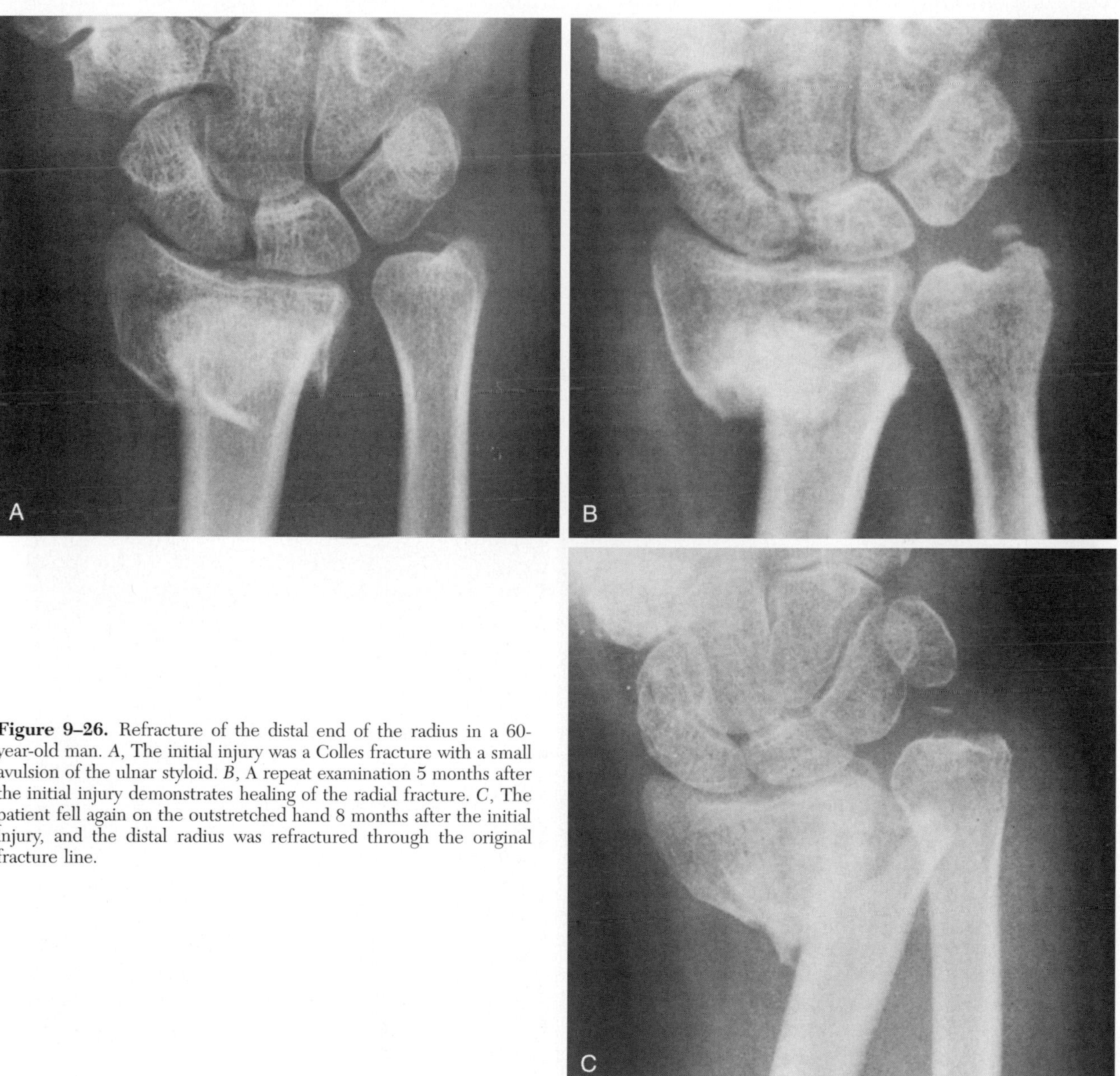

Figure 9–26. Refracture of the distal end of the radius in a 60-year-old man. *A*, The initial injury was a Colles fracture with a small avulsion of the ulnar styloid. *B*, A repeat examination 5 months after the initial injury demonstrates healing of the radial fracture. *C*, The patient fell again on the outstretched hand 8 months after the initial injury, and the distal radius was refractured through the original fracture line.

the healing process is completed. As might be anticipated, refractures occur more commonly in the weight-bearing bones of the lower extremities. Bostman[127] reported refracture in 6 of 62 patients with healed fractures in the distal third of the femur, which had been treated by internal fixation with a blade plate. Removal of the blade plate was done when the fracture was judged to be healed by the surgeon, at a mean time of 28 months after fracture. The average interval between removal of the hardware and refracture was 38 (range 12 to 93) days. In five of six patients, the refracture occurred through a screw hole without preceding trauma, and in one patient, a jump of 50 cm off a stepladder caused the refracture. None of these refractures coincided with the original fracture line. A high percentage (26%) of refractures following plate removal has also been reported with forearm fractures[128] (Fig. 9–27).

A related problem occurs when an orthopedic appliance used for internal fixation of a fracture fatigues and then fractures (Fig. 9–28). Appliance failure is usually seen in the presence of a fracture nonunion. The metallic appliances have a finite life span and, unlike bone, are unable to respond to stress with internal remodeling and repair. They eventually fatigue and fracture after being flexed a certain number of times. Fortunately, under normal circumstances the fracture heals long before the appliance is stressed enough for this complication to occur.

Myositis Ossificans

Myositis ossificans, or heterotopic bone formation, usually occurs as the result of a soft tissue injury without associated fracture of the underlying bone. It is particularly likely to occur in the thigh. A similar process may occur about a joint in association with a dislocation or fracture-dislocation. The most common site is the elbow (Fig. 9–29), less commonly, the hip (Fig. 9–30) and, rarely, other sites are involved. The incidence of myositis ossificans involving the elbow is approximately five times greater following a dislocation than following a fracture without dislocation.[130] The bone formation is increased with delay in treatment and excessive manipulation in the performance of the initial reduction. Generally, calcification appears initially within 4 weeks of the injury, and the bone matures and is partially resorbed over several months. In a small percentage of cases, resorption may be complete. Compared with those of normal adult compact bone, the crystals of heterotopic bone are small, which reflects their substandard crystalline structure and decreases their stability.[129] The small crystals produce a

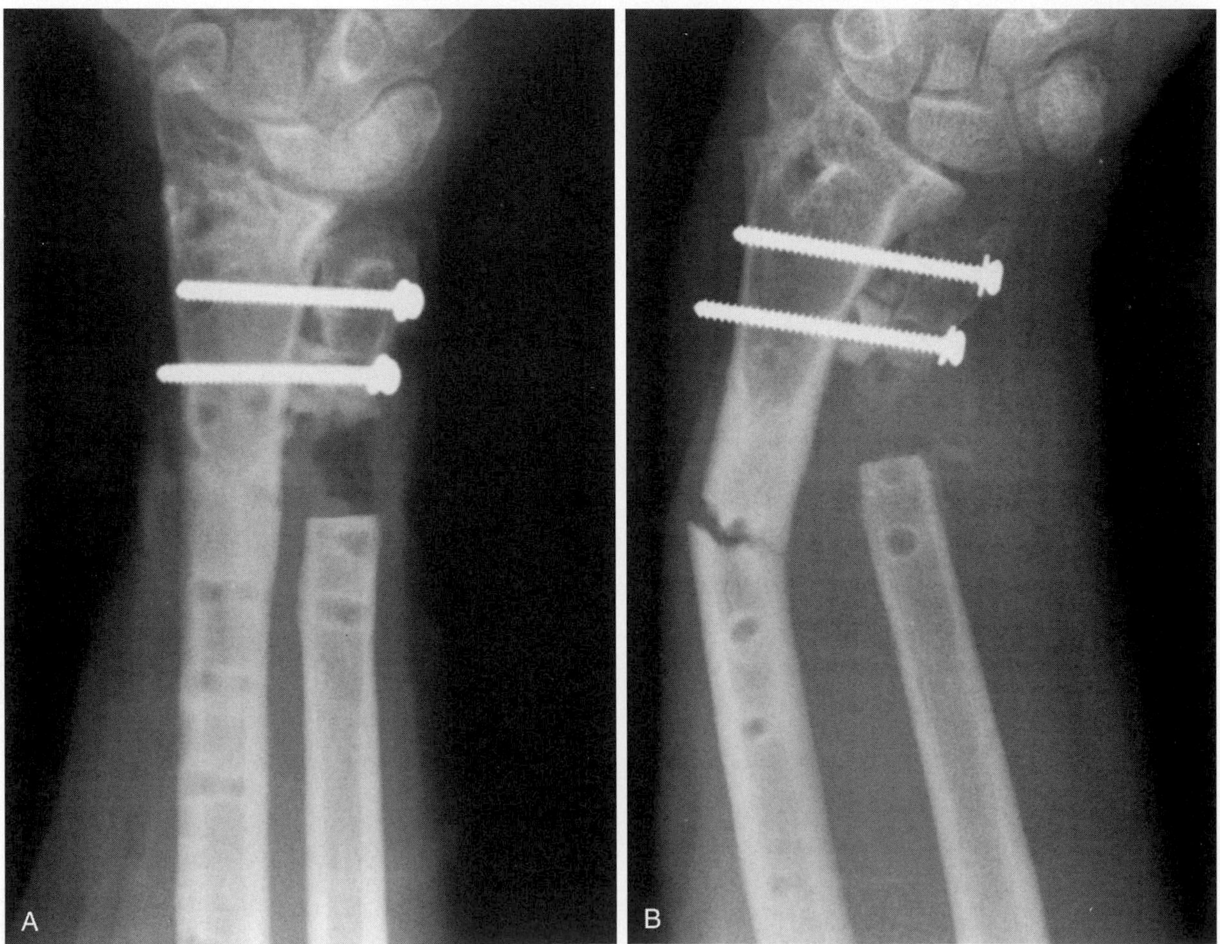

Figure 9–27. *A*, Healed fracture of the radius immediately following removal of the compression plate. *B*, Fracture of the radius through a compression plate screw hole 100 days later.

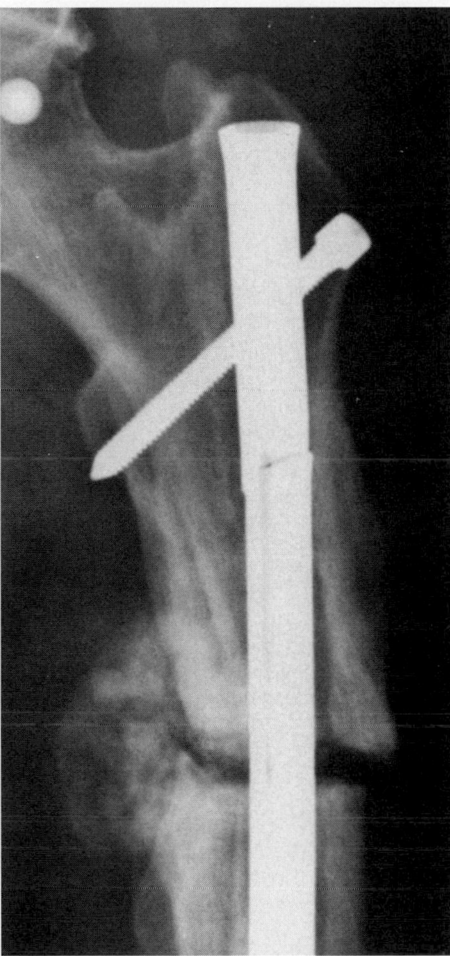

Figure 9–28. Fatigue fracture of an intramedullary rod due to continued stress on the rod when the femoral fracture failed to unite.

large surface area for resorption. Both of these factors contribute to the ease with which the heterotropic bone can be resorbed. The ultimate degree of restriction of joint motion is dependent upon the extent of the residual ossification.

Synostosis

Synostosis refers to the bony fusion between two adjacent bones occurring as a result of an injury to one or both. This complication is most commonly encountered in association with fractures of the proximal third of both bones of the forearm (Fig. 9–31) and may lead to significant limitation of motion. Less commonly, it occurs between the metatarsals or metacarpals but is usually of little functional significance at these sites. Exuberant callus formation may give the false appearance of a synostosis between two adjacent bones. Multiple views may be required to definitively determine the presence of a synostosis. In the forearm the fusion can be identified only with certainty in the anteroposterior and oblique projections. CT can be used to determine the presence of a synostosis if there is any uncertainty about the findings on conventional radiographs. This study is usually most valuable in the proximal forearm.

Delayed Complications

Osteonecrosis

When a portion of the skeleton is deprived of its arterial blood supply, sterile necrosis of bone may result. This process is termed osteonecrosis, avascular necrosis, ischemic necrosis, or aseptic necrosis. Many causes in addition to trauma, including steroid administration, pancreatitis, collagen disease, sickle cell anemia, and Gaucher's disease, can either intrinsically or extrinsically lead to vascular occlusion and subsequent death of bone. The causes that are of concern here are those seen after a fracture, or dislocation or fracture-dislocation.

The most common site of occurrence of avascular necrosis as a result of fracture or dislocation is in the femoral head.[131, 133, 139] It may follow fracture of the femoral neck (Fig. 9–32), dislocation of the femoral head, or, much less commonly, separation of the proximal femoral epiphysis. Structures affected next in frequency are the humeral head (Fig. 9–33), usually following comminuted fractures; or the carpal scaphoid, following fractures of the wrist or proximal pole; and the talus,[141] as a result of fractures of the neck or dislocation or both. Avascular necrosis is less common in the head of the second or third metatarsal (Freiberg's infraction); in the patella, following transverse fracture; and in the head of the second metacarpal, following dislocation of the metacarpophalangeal joint.[137] The specific anatomic relationships that lead to avascular necrosis in each of these injuries are discussed in the chapter devoted to that portion of the anatomy. Here discussion is limited to general principles and findings common to all types of avascular necrosis.

Osteonecrosis involves the end of a bone. At the time of fracture the arteries traversing the region of the line of fracture are torn. In a dislocation the vessels supplying the end of a bone may be torn as the joint is disrupted. Obviously it would be of value to determine the viability of a bone fragment at the time of initial treatment. Many methods have been proposed, but the results are inconsistent and therefore of little clinical use.[144–147]

The subsequent course of events is determined by the degree of vascular disruption and the availability of collateral circulation. In those sites prone to develop avascular necrosis, collateral circulation is limited and the likelihood of avascular necrosis great. The remaining vessels may be sufficient to sustain the viability of only a portion of the fracture fragment, and the remainder must undergo necrosis. Any healing that occurs must come from the apposing viable fragment by bridging the fracture line and subsequently revascularizing adjacent portions of the necrotic fragment.[131] Healing by bridging and revascularization can occur but is usually insufficient to replace the entire volume of bone required, except when the volume is relatively small, as in the proximal pole of the carpal scaphoid, as opposed to the large volume of the femoral head. In some cases, no revascularization occurs, and the entire fragment becomes necrotic.

Immobilization is required to prevent disturbance of the healing process. Similarly, weight-bearing can hinder the revascularization and replacement of bone. Neither immobilization nor refraining from weight-bearing as-

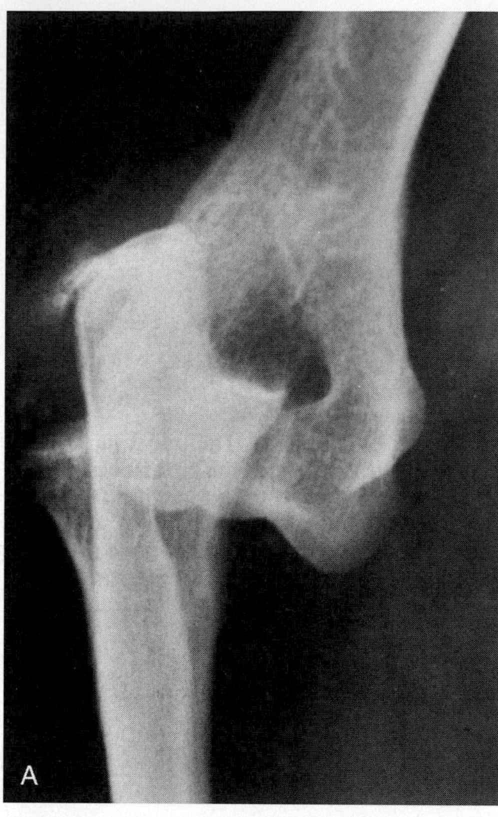

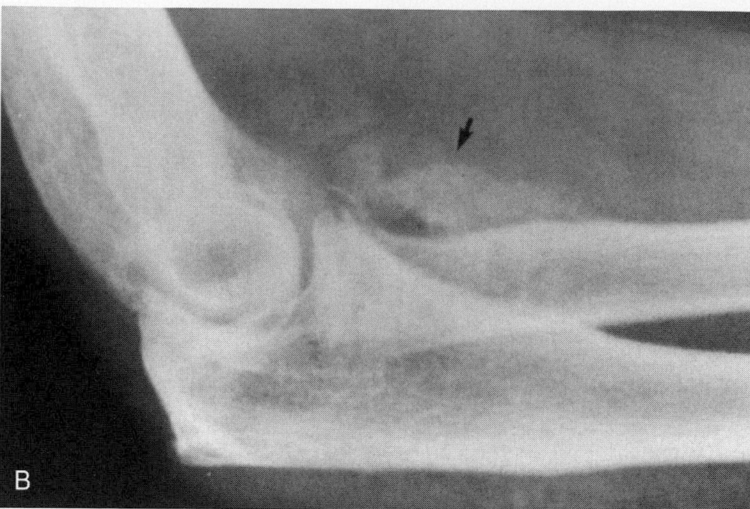

Figure 9–29. Myositis ossificans, or periarticular heterotopic bone formation, following a fracture-dislocation of the elbow. *A*, A posterolateral fracture-dislocation of the elbow is evident. There is a fracture of the radial head. *B*, A lateral radiograph 4 weeks after the injury demonstrates heterotopic bone formation anterior to the elbow joint *(arrow)*. This appearance and location are typical of this process in the elbow.

sures revascularization, however. Usually, the regenerative process in osteonecrosis, particularly in weight-bearing bones, is only partially successful, and finally the variable portion of remaining necrotic bone at the joint margin collapses.

The involved portion of the bone may then present five distinct zones on pathologic examination presupposing partial revascularization[151]: (1) a superficial area of detached articular cartilage and subarticular trabeculae separated by a variable distance from the remainder of the bone; (2) a zone of necrotic bone ranging in extent from a thin band of trabeculae to a sizable segment of the bone; (3) an area of vascular granulation tissue; (4) a zone of repair with new bone formation; and (5) a zone of normal cancellous bone.

The major clinical manifestations of avascular necrosis are pain and limitation of motion. Nonunion or delayed union may well exist, but at times the fracture has united. However, the process still occurs because of insufficient revascularization at the end of the fracture fragment remote from the fracture line. The diagnosis is usually established within 1 year of injury in the smaller bones, but the condition may not become apparent for 3 years or more in the femoral head.

The initial radiographic manifestations[132, 140] of avascular necrosis are sclerotic changes in bone and preservation of the adjacent joint space. As the process continues (see Figs. 9–32*B* and 9–33), irregular radiolucencies appear beneath the joint margin[140] interspersed with other areas of increased density; the bone collapses and the joint surface becomes irregular. The lucencies represent necrotic bone. The characteristic subchondral radiolucency found in the femoral head—the crescent sign—represents a fracture through necrotic bone in this area.

Three different mechanisms have been proposed in the etiology of the sclerosis of bone.[132] First, an absolute increase in the amount of bone substance has been proposed. In the revascularized portion of bone, new trabeculae are laid down directly on old dead trabeculae, thus increasing the density of the involved bone. Second, the increase is conjectured to be, in part, only relative, because the surrounding bone becomes osteoporotic through disuse. The involved bone cannot become osteoporotic because it has been deprived of its blood supply. Third, the increase has been suggested to be caused by impaction of trabecular bone occasioned by the collapse of necrotic bone. There is little or no pathologic evidence to support this last possibility. Therefore, the principal pathogenic mechanism is the absolute increase in bone[132] and, to some extent, osteoporosis of surrounding bone.

Once collapse has occurred, treatment is resection of the involved segment of bone. A prosthesis is used to replace the femoral head. Ankle fusion is required when the talus is removed. The wrist is partially fused when the proximal pole of the scaphoid has collapsed. Core decompression and vascularized bone grafts are generally used before the collapse to promote bone healing.

MRI is the most sensitive imaging modality for detecting changes of ischemic necrosis in bone[96, 138] (Fig. 9–34). This modality is more sensitive in detecting early than in detecting late stages of the disease.[139] In spite of this capability for early detection, avascular necrosis can be demonstrated histologically before it can be detected with any imaging modality.[136] Several patterns of abnormal

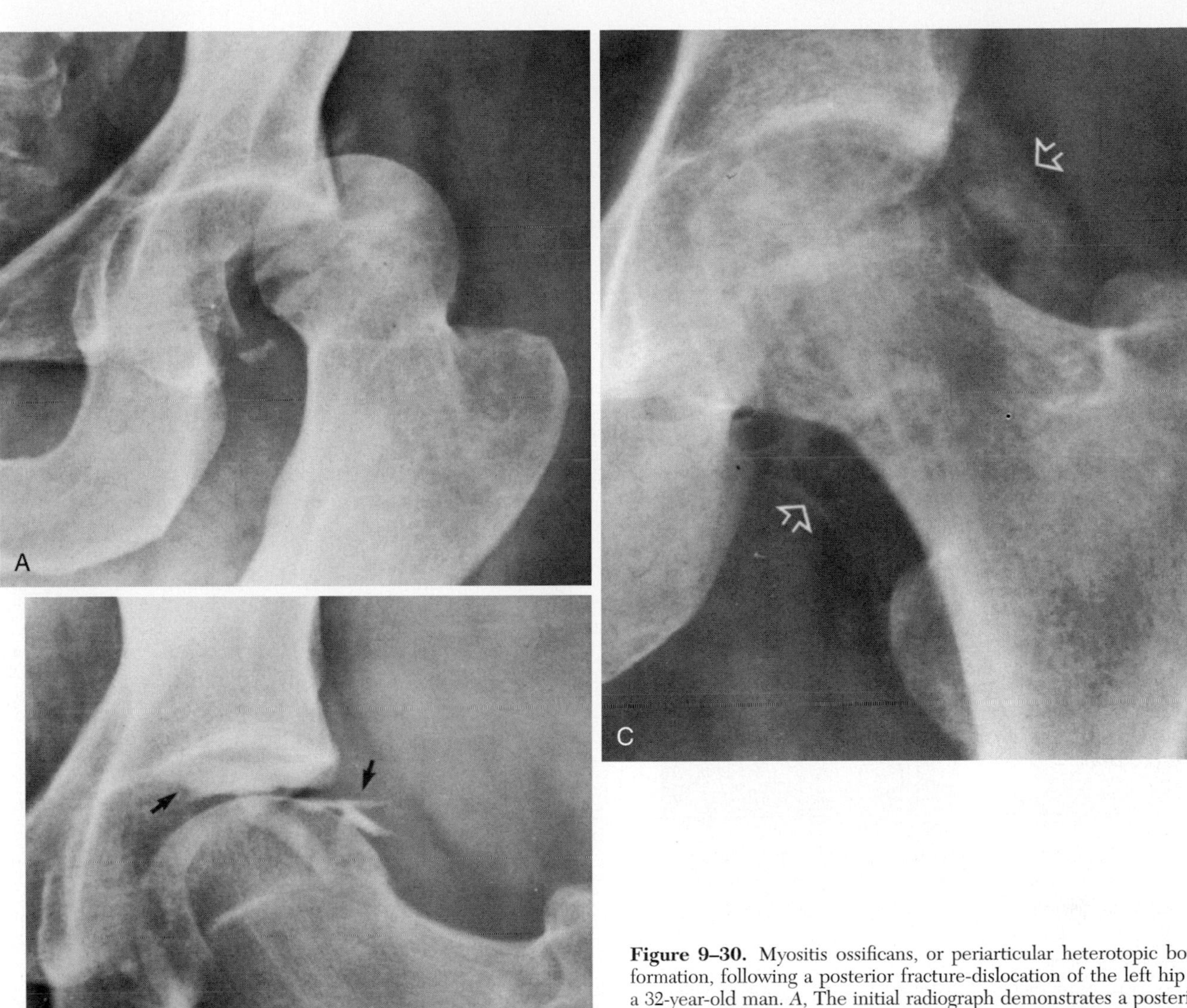

Figure 9–30. Myositis ossificans, or periarticular heterotopic bone formation, following a posterior fracture-dislocation of the left hip in a 32-year-old man. *A*, The initial radiograph demonstrates a posterior dislocation of the hip associated with comminution of the posterior rim of the acetabulum. *B*, Postreduction radiograph demonstrates widening of the joint caused by entrapment of several fragments of bone *(arrows)*. The fragments were removed at surgery. *C*, Examination of the hip 7 weeks after the initial injury demonstrates heterotopic bone formation about the hip *(arrows)*.

signal in hips with avascular necrosis have been reported.[143] MR images reflect changes within the bone marrow. Once the femoral head or part of it loses its blood supply, the marrow cells die. With death of the marrow fat cells the signal decreases in the affected area. Invasion of the area by granulation tissue to replace the dead fat and marrow decreases the MR signal even more.

Avascular necrosis of the femoral head has been classified according to MRI findings into four classes, A through D.[138] At present this classification is most useful for descriptive purposes, and correspondence between its stages and the histologic state of the femoral head still needs some elucidation. The stages of this classification and the one based on conventional radiography outlined in the next paragraph do not correspond stage for stage. The MRI classification is based on the appearance of the central region of signal within the lesion in the femoral head.[138] The central region is surrounded by a peripheral rim of low signal intensity on short and long relaxation time–echo time (TR/TE) sequences. Class A findings in the femoral head are analogous to those for fat, with high signal intensity seen in images with a short TR–short TE interval and intermediate signal intensity in images with a long TR–long TE interval. Class B findings are analogous to blood in the femoral head, with high signal intensity in images with a short TR–short TE interval or with

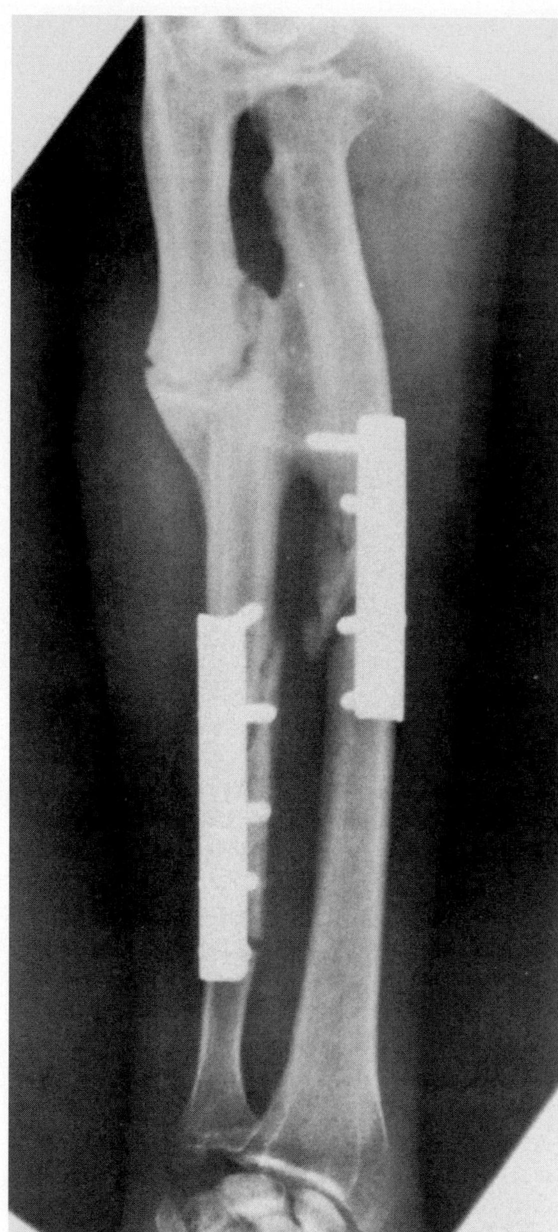

Figure 9–31. Synostosis between the proximal radius and ulna associated with nonunion and pseudarthrosis of the proximal ulna. A broad plate of bone fuses the proximal radius with the ulna distal to the pseudarthrosis. These injuries resulted from the original injury. The patient was subsequently in a fight and sustained oblique fractures of the midshaft of both bones of the forearm distal to the original injury. These fractures were treated with compression plates.

a long TR–long TE interval. Class C findings are analogous to fluid in the femoral head, with low signal intensity in images with a short TR interval–short TE interval and high signal intensity in images with a long TR interval–long TE interval. Class D findings are analogous to fibrous tissue in the femoral head, with low signal intensity in images with short TR–short TE or long TR–long TE intervals.[135, 138]

Avascular necrosis also has been classified into five groups using conventional radiography.[142] In stage 0, both radiographic and radionuclide bone scan findings are normal. In stage I, radiographic findings are normal but abnormal radionuclide bone scan findings are abnormal. In stage II, cystic or sclerotic changes without a crescent sign are seen. In stage III, a crescent sign without flattening of the femoral head is seen in addition to the findings of stage II. In stage IV, findings include subchondral collapse with flattening of the femoral head but without acetabular abnormalities or joint space narrowing. In stage V, all of the foregoing features plus narrowing of the joint are present.

Correlation between the MR and radiographic images

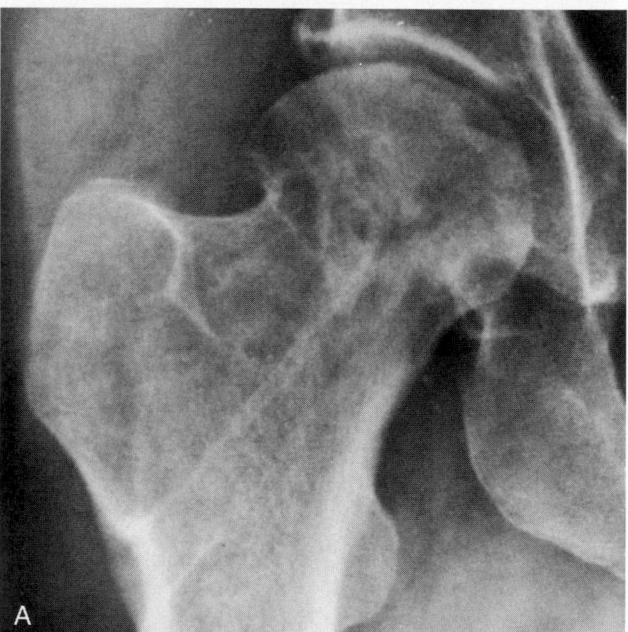

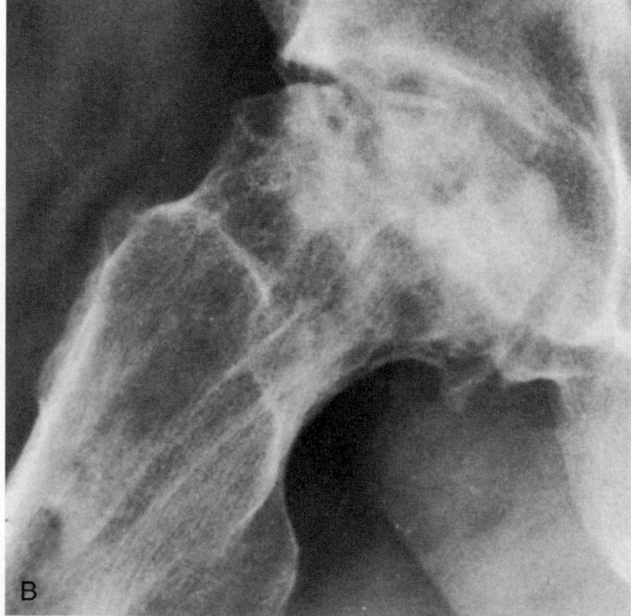

Figure 9–32. Osteonecrosis of the femoral head following a subcapital fracture of the femoral neck. *A*, This radiograph was obtained 4 years after the original injury. The track of the nail utilized in the original treatment is evident as the fine line of bony sclerosis within the intertrochanteric region. *B*, This radiograph, obtained 4 years after the injury, clearly demonstrates the changes of avascular necrosis, manifested as flattening of the head with irregular areas of sclerosis and lucency.

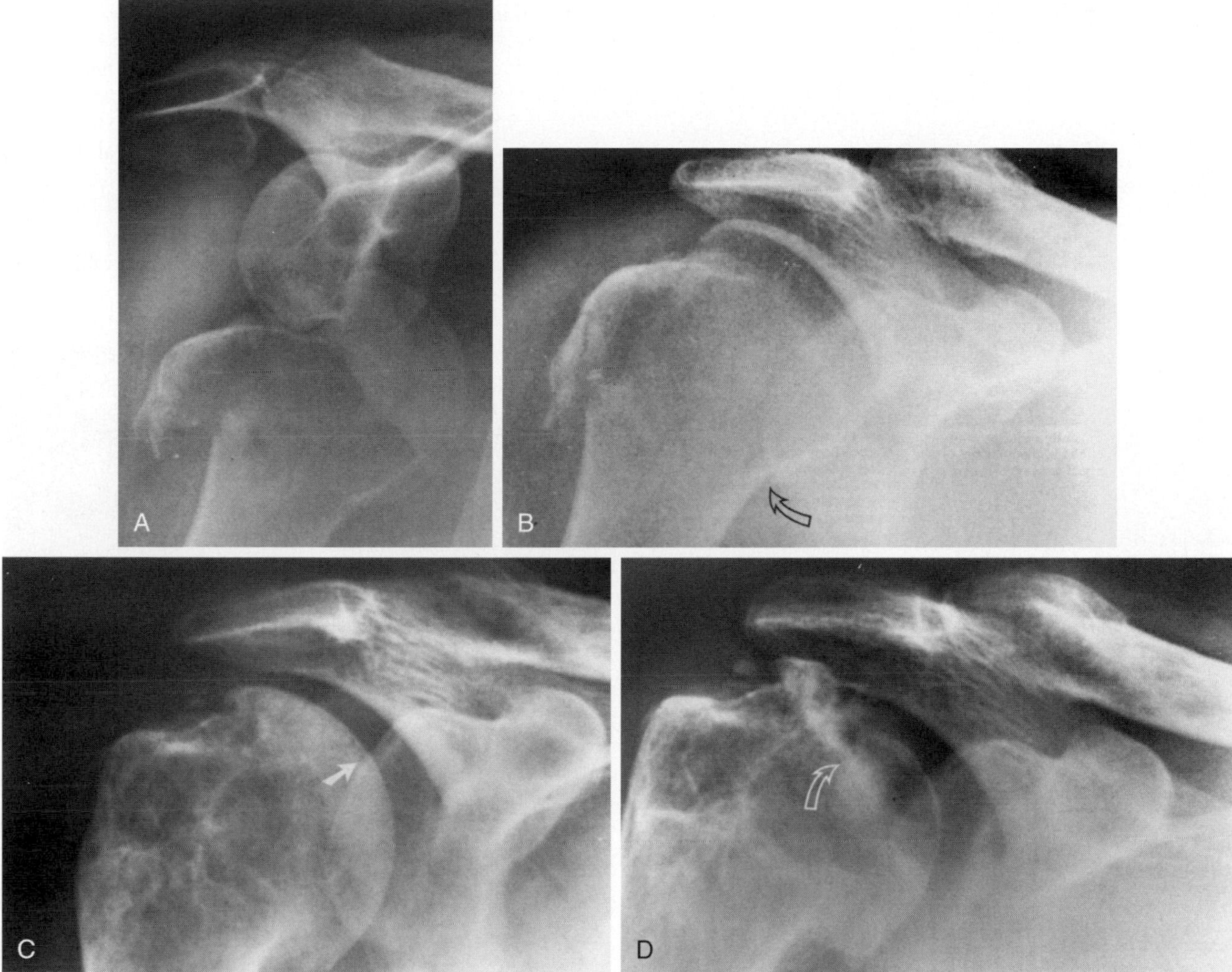

Figure 9–33. *A*, Anterior dislocation of the humeral head with fracture of the greater tuberosity. *B*, Immediately after reduction, the fracture is also seen to include the humeral neck *(arrow)*. *C*, Six months later, the humeral neck fracture has healed, with an intact articular surface. A small focal subarticular lucency *(arrow)* is the first evidence of osteonecrosis. *D*, At 26 months after injury, changes of osteonecrosis are now radiographically obvious but lag far behind the interruption of the blood supply that occurred at the time of fracture. The dense sclerotic line present medially in the humeral head is from collapse of the articular surface.

of avascular necrosis is not exact.[138] Joint space narrowing was frequently seen with MRI but not confirmed with radiographic studies.[138] Better correlation between the two modalities was seen for femoral head flattening. Typical subchondral femoral head fractures in avascular necrosis cases are much more easily seen on radiographs or CT scans than on MR images.[135, 138]

Degenerative Arthritis (Osteoarthritis)

Osteoarthritis is a disorder of diarthrodial joints resulting from changes within the joint cartilage secondary to abnormal mechanical conditions within the joint.[149, 150] There are two forms of this disorder, primary and secondary. The pathologic features of the two are similar; the causes and distribution of involvement differ, however. Primary osteoarthritis is generalized arthritis of unknown etiology involving principally the distal interphalangeal joints of the fingers, the first carpometacarpal joints, the hips, and the knees. Secondary osteoarthritis is focal arthritis resulting from an irregularity in the joint surface or change in the contour of the joint (Fig. 9–35). The joint abnormalities may be brought about by trauma, infection, aseptic necrosis, or other forms of arthritis. The initiating traumatic event may be a fracture extending into the joint, a dislocation, a diastasis, an osteochondral fracture of the joint surface, or a change in the alignment of the joint surfaces due to an angular or rotational deformity of a healed fracture in an adjacent bone.

Joint cartilage is relatively acellular and exists without a direct vascular supply. It is maintained by the nutrients within the synovial fluid. The fluid is absorbed and diffuses throughout the entire joint cartilage, aided by the mechanical pumping action produced by motion of the joint. Cartilage is composed of a ground substance (chondroitin sulfate) containing elastic collagen fibrils. Destruction of these fibrils reduces the elasticity of the joint cartilage. Because of the relative lack of cartilage cells, the potential for repair once an injury has been sustained ranges from very limited to nonexistent.

The principal pathologic features are fibrillation and

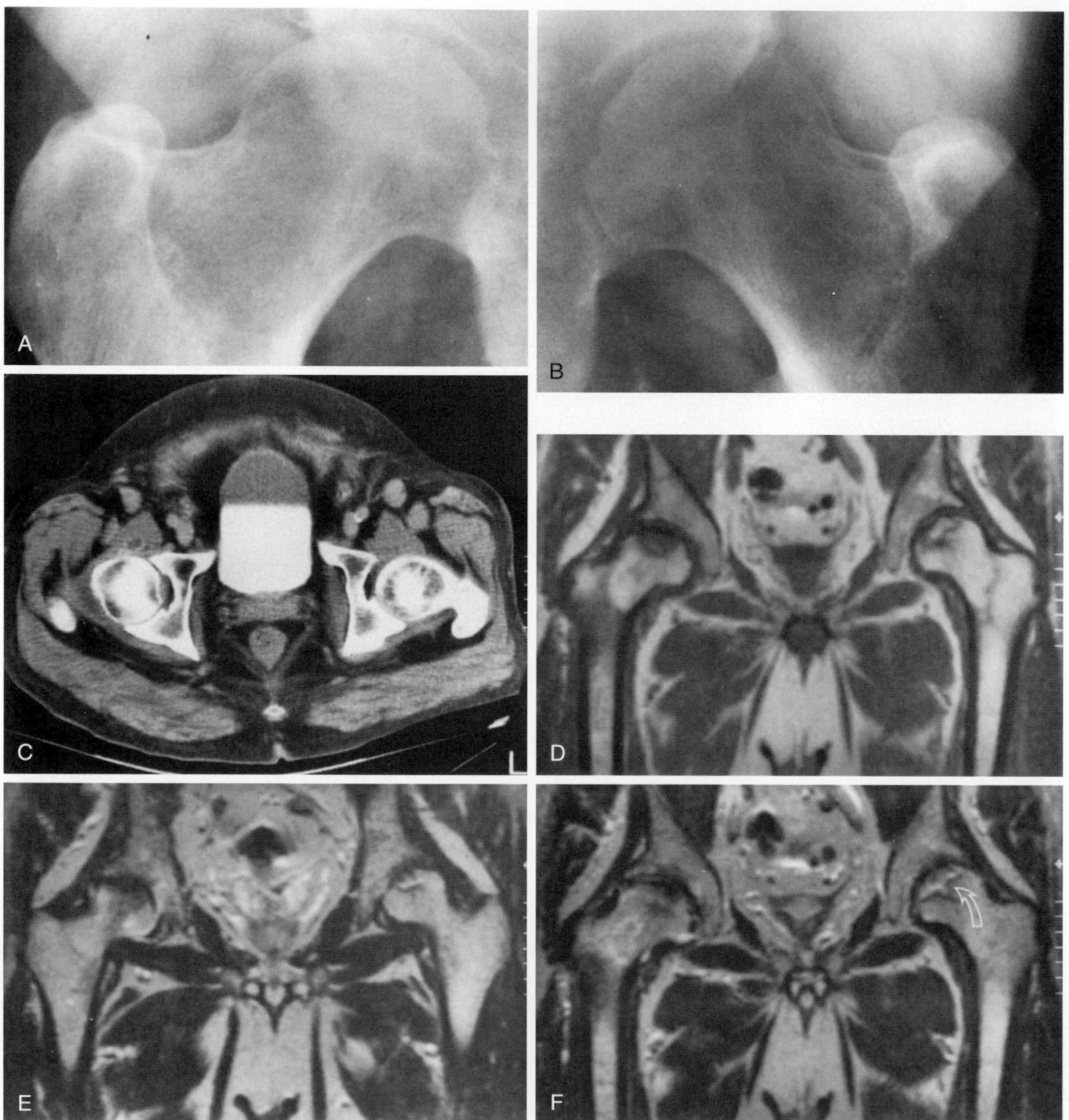

Figure 9–34. *A* and *B*, Anteroposterior views of the right and left hips show vague sclerosis in the superior third of the femoral heads. *C*, This image from a computed tomography scan of both hips demonstrates sclerosis in the superior portion of both femoral heads. *D*, Magnetic resonance image from a spin echo T_1-weighted (TR 416, TE 15) sequence obtained at 1.5 tesla. There is decreased signal intensity in the entire superior third of the right femoral head and fat-intensity signal in the center of the low-signal-intensity band in the left femoral head. *E*, Magnetic resonance image from a T_2-weighted sequence (2216/80) shows a low-signal-intensity band across the femoral head with low signal intensity within the band in the right femoral head and normal signal intensity within the low-signal-intensity band in the left femoral head. This corresponds to a type A osteonecrosis stage on the left and a type D stage on the right. *F*, Double-line sign *(arrow)* in the left femoral head in a different image from the same set of sequences as in *E*.

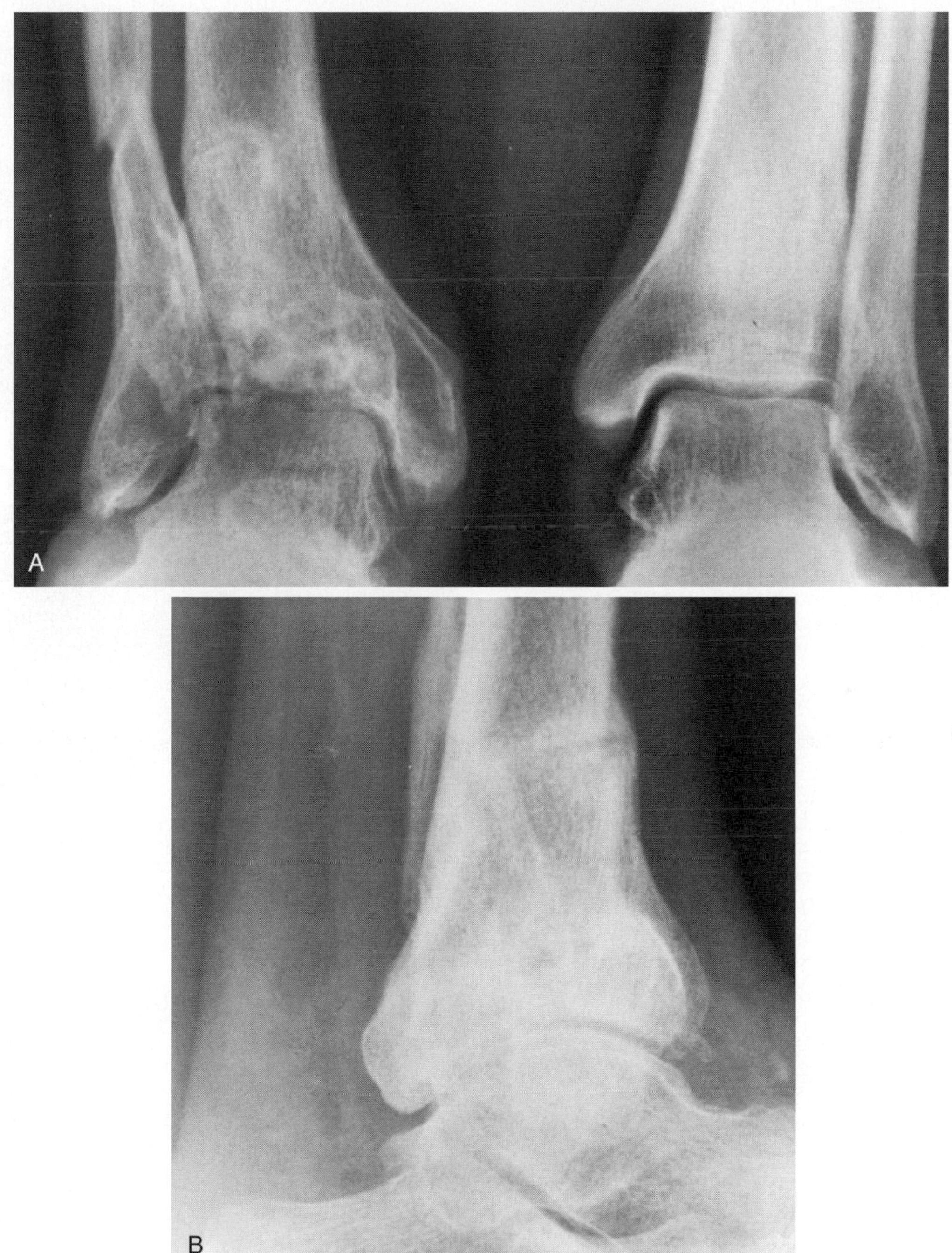

Figure 9–35. Degenerative arthritis 2 years after a comminuted fracture of the distal fibula and tibia that extended into the ankle joint. The patient was 54 years of age. *A*, Anteroposterior radiograph of both ankles clearly demonstrates a narrowing of the right ankle mortise and irregularity of the tibial plafond secondary to the previous fracture. *B*, Lateral view demonstrates irregularity of the tibial joint surface and narrowing of the joint. The findings are indicative of early degenerative arthritis. An ankle fusion was required.

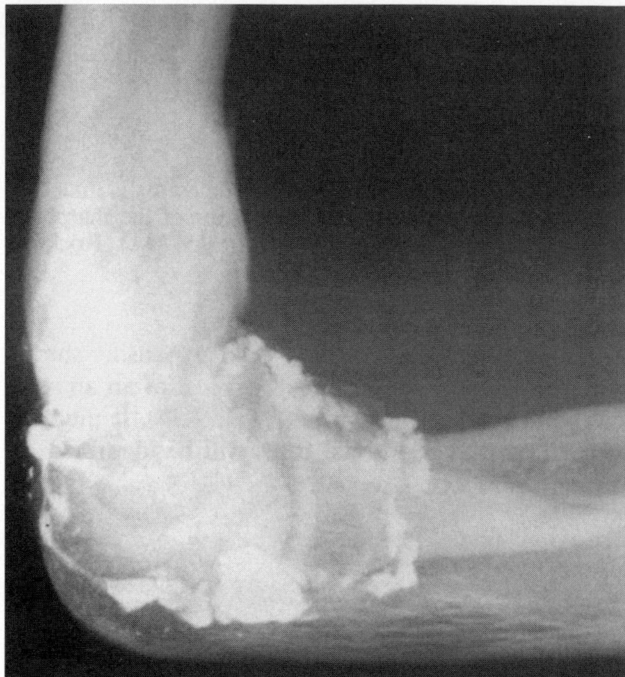

Figure 9–36. Lead arthropathy secondary to a gunshot wound to the elbow sustained several years earlier. Pulverized lead particles line the synovial surface of the joint, greatly increasing the surface from which lead can be dissolved and resorbed. (From Rogers, L.F. [1987]. Metabolic, endocrine, and related bone diseases. In Juhl, J.H., & Krummy, A.B. Eds.: Paul and Juhl Essentials of Radiologic Imaging. 5th Ed. J.B. Lippincott Co., Philadelphia, with permission.)

shredding of the joint surface, leading to fragmentation and, ultimately, denuding of the subchondral bone. The subchondral bone is thickened by appositional growth of new bone. Exposed bone is eburnated. Subchondral cystic areas devoid of trabeculae and marginated by sclerotic bone are seen.[148, 151] These cystic areas may or may not communicate with the joint surface. The cysts are unlined and contain fragments of joint cartilage within synovial fluid or are filled by myxoid and adipose tissue. Bone spurs are present at the margins of the joint. The cortical and medullary bone of these spurs is contiguous with that of the bone from which they arise. The surface of the spur is covered by an extension of cartilage from the joint surface.

The clinical manifestations of osteoarthritis are joint pain, swelling, and limitation of motion. Characteristically, the pain is worse on arising in the morning and gradually subsides to some extent with activity. Weight-bearing intensifies the osteoarthritic process; therefore, involvement of a joint in the lower extremity is associated with greater distress and limitations.

The radiographic features[149–151] are asymmetrical narrowing of the joint space, subchondral sclerosis of bone, subchondral cyst formation, and spur formation at the joint margins. These changes appear in the absence of periarticular osteoporosis. The earliest finding is asymmetrical narrowing of the joint. Narrowing characteristically occurs on the weight-bearing margin of joints in the lower extremity. Fragments of the joint cartilage may form free joint bodies, which become radiographically apparent following degenerative calcification within the cartilage and later appositional bone growth about the cartilaginous nidus.

The medical treatment is symptomatic and nonspecific. Surgical reconstruction, fusion, or joint replacement is often required. Efforts are well spent in averting or preventing subsequent osteoarthritis to the extent possible by prompt recognition of injury, accurate reduction, and sufficient immobilization of fractures, dislocations, diastases, and ligamentous injuries. Because of the serious and complex nature of the disruption of the joint surface in many injuries, it is impossible to prevent subsequent osteoarthritis in all cases. However, in less complex injuries, prompt diagnosis and correct treatment will make a difference.

Lead Arthropathy

A characteristic arthropathy occurs in joints with retained lead fragments. Lead particles become imbedded in the synovium, producing a synovitis that in turn leads

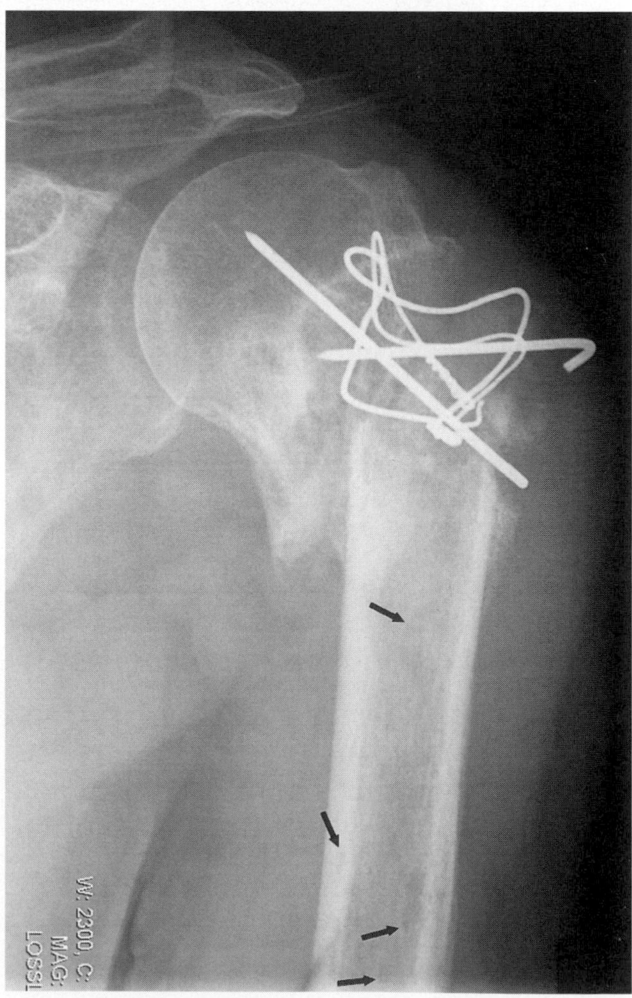

Figure 9–37. Post-traumatic osteoporosis in a 72-year-old man following a left humerus fracture. This anteroposterior view of the left shoulder reveals subtle, predominantly cortical, patchy lucencies *(arrows)* in the humerus 10 months after fracture and 2 months after fixation for nonunion.

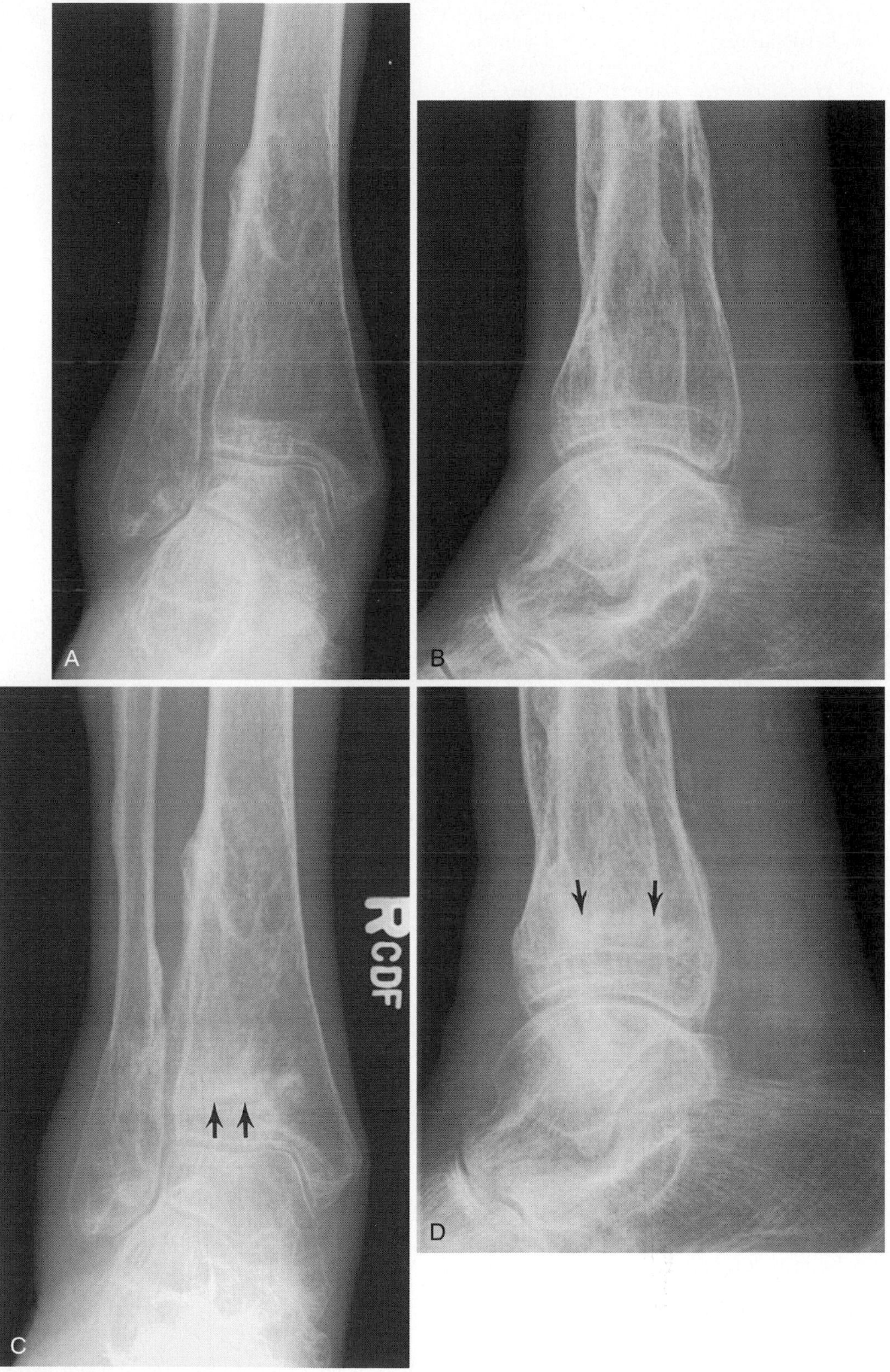

Figure 9–38. Insufficiency fracture in a 67-year-old woman. She had sustained a right ankle fracture 18 years earlier and a right femoral supracondylar fracture 6 months before this radiographic examination. Anterior *(A)* and lateral *(B)* views of the right ankle demonstrate deformity from previous distal tibia and fibula fractures and generalized osteopenia that is more about the ankle. Three months later, the patient presented with pain of 3 weeks' duration, and the radiographic examination was repeated. Anterior *(D)* and lateral *(C)* views reveal the linear sclerosis *(arrows)* typical of the relatively uncommon insufficiency fracture in this location.

to degenerative arthritis (Fig. 9–36). Lead intoxication secondary to retained lead bullet fragments has usually been reported with fragments within or near a joint or with many fragments present (e.g., shotgun pellets) in the soft tissues.[153, 154] The acidity of synovial fluid and the mechanical motion of a joint have been implicated in the resorption of lead and systemic toxicity.[153] In addition, motion fragments the lead, yielding a larger surface area for resorption.

An unusual complication of a fracture nonunion following a 22-caliber gunshot wound to the first metacarpal bone 10 years earlier has been reported.[152] The patient's hand was radiographed because of swelling over the area due to recent trauma. A pseudarthrosis present at the fracture site was demonstrated to contain a 3-mm round lead fragment that moved with positional change of the hand. The patient's serum lead level was twice the upper limit of normal. The pseudarthrosis in this case contained synovial fluid, the same as in a joint, causing dissolution of lead fragments. The possibility of these complications, although rare, arises with fractures caused by gunshot wounds, especially near joints.

Post-traumatic Osteoporosis

A severe form of osteoporosis with a radiographic appearance mimicking that of a malignant neoplasm, myeloma, or metastasis has been reported after a fracture, especially in the humerus. Radiographically, a moth-eaten or permeative destructive process is seen, along with diffuse bone demineralization. Endosteal scalloping and cortical tunneling are features, but no soft tissue mass, periosteal new bone, periosteal scalloping, or expansion of the bone is seen (Fig. 9–37). The onset is typically 7 months to 2 years following trauma. Associated findings in a group of 11 reported patients included metallic internal fixation in 7, ipsilateral cervical root or brachial plexus injury in 6, and predisposition to osteopenia from ethanol abuse, diabetes mellitus, or prednisone use in 7.[157] The history of significant trauma to the area and local neurologic injury help differentiate this process from a malignancy. The cause is unknown.

Post-traumatic osteoporosis may also predispose the patient to the development of insufficiency fractures (Fig. 9–38). A study in rats[158] demonstrated that bones ipsilateral to the side of trauma had a significant reduction in mechanical strength and joint mobility compared with the contralateral side. Blood flow was increased and the amount of bone decreased. The authors could not determine the role that disuse played in this phenomenon. However, a study by Karlsson and colleagues[159] evaluated patients 27 to 43 years following a traumatic fracture of the tibial shaft or ankle. They determined that there was an increased incidence of insufficiency fractures in patients with previous nonosteoporotic fractures early in life.

Post-traumatic Aneurysmal Bone Cysts

It is now recognized that aneurysmal bone cysts are often encountered in association with a variety of benign and malignant lesions of bone.[160] Trauma has been implicated as a cause in the past. Kushner and associates[161] reported a well-documented case of post-traumatic aneurysmal bone cysts localized to the third and fourth ribs. They suggested that after trauma, with or without a fracture, a subperiosteal hematoma is the most likely initiating event. An eccentric, lytic, expansile, sharply demarcated, thin-shelled lesion, typical of an aneurysmal bone cyst, is then formed (Fig. 9–39).

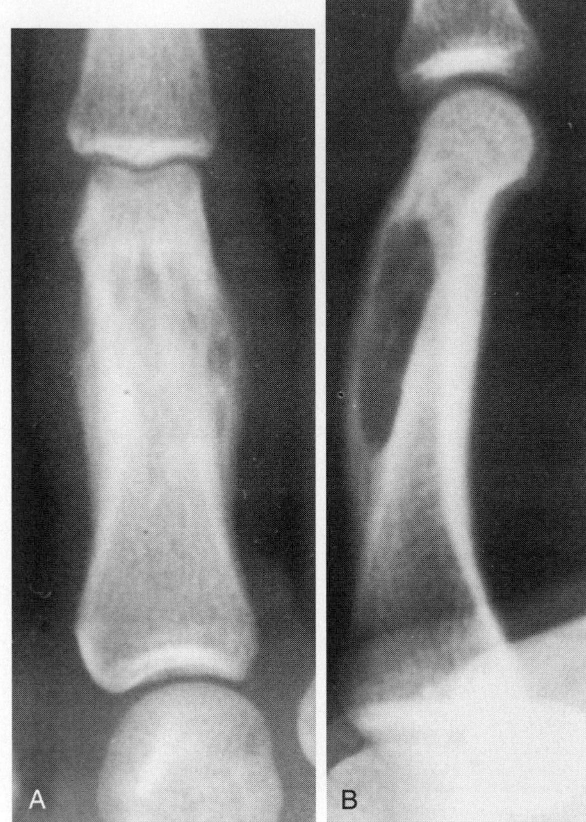

Figure 9–39. Post-traumatic aneurysmal bone cyst of the proximal phalanx of the ring finger 3 months following a crush injury of the hand in a 21-year-old man. Radiographic appearance at the time of injury was normal, without evidence of fracture or other abnormality. *A*, Posteroanterior view demonstrates a lucent expansile lesion involving the distal shaft. The cortex is intact. *B*, Lateral view reveals the eccentric location of the sharply defined lesion. (Case courtesy of Ervin Hrasky, M.D., Rockford, Ill.)

References

General

1. Evarts, C.M. (1975). Complications. p. 156. In Rockwood, C.A., & Green, D.P. Eds.: Fractures. Vol 1. J.B. Lippincott Co., Philadelphia.
2. Lyons, F.A., & Rockwood, C.A. (1990). Migration of pins used in operations on the shoulder. J. Bone Joint Surg. [Am.], 72:1262.

Arterial Injury and Compartment Syndromes

3. Bell, D., & Cockshott, W.P. (1965). Angiography of traumatic arterio-venous fistulae. Clin. Radiol., *16*:241.
4. Bergan, F. (1963). Traumatic intimal rupture of the popliteal artery with acute ischemia of the limb in cases with supracondylar fractures of the femur. J. Cardiovasc. Surg., *4*:300.
5. Berk, M.E. (1963). Arteriography in peripheral trauma. Clin. Radiol., *14*:235.
6. Bradley, E.L. III. (1973). The anterior tibial compartment syndrome. Surg. Gynecol. Obstet., *136*:289.

7. Connolly, J.F., Whittaker, D., & Williams, E. (1971). Femoral and tibial fractures combined with injuries to the femoral or popliteal artery. J. Bone Joint Surg. [Am.], *53*:56.
8. Ellis, H. (1958). Disabilities after tibial shaft fractures. J. Bone Joint Surg. [Br.], *40*:190.
9. Haas, L.M., & Staple, T.W. (1969). Arterial injuries associated with fractures of the proximal tibia following blunt trauma. South. Med. J., *62*:1439.
10. Hoover, N.W. (1961). Injuries of the popliteal artery associated with fractures and dislocations. Surg. Clin. North Am., *41*:1099.
11. Jones, D.A. (1970). Volkmann's ischemia. Surg. Clin. North Am., *50*:329.
12. Leach, R.W., Hammond, G., & Stryker, W.S. (1967). Anterior tibial compartment syndrome. J. Bone Joint Surg. [Am.], *49*:451.
13. Lipscomb, P.R., & Burleson, R.J. (1955). Vascular and neural complications in supracondylar fractures of the humerus in children. J. Bone Joint Surg. [Am.], *37*:487.
14. Lord, R.S.A., & Irani, C.N. (1974). Assessment of arterial injury in limb trauma. J. Trauma, *14*:1042.
15. Love, L. (1970). Arterial trauma. Semin. Roentgenol., *5*:267.
16. Love, L., & Braun, T. (1968). Arteriography of peripheral vascular trauma. A.J.R. Am. J. Roentgenol., *102*:431.
17. Matsen, F.A. (1975). Compartmental syndrome. Clin. Orthop., *113*:8.
18. Porter, M.F. (1968). Delayed arterial occlusion in limb injuries. Report of three cases. J. Bone Joint Surg. [Br.], *50*:138.
19. Pradhan, D.J., Juanteguy, J.M., Wilder, R.J., & Michelson, E. (1972). Arterial injuries of the extremities associated with fractures. Arch. Surg., *105*:582.
20. Rang, M. (1974). Children's Fractures. J.B. Lippincott Co., Philadelphia.
21. Rich, N.M., Baugh, J.H., & Hughes, C.W. (1969). Popliteal artery injuries in Vietnam. Am. J. Surg., *118*:531.
22. Rich, N.M., & Spencer, F.C. (1978). Vascular Trauma. W.B. Saunders Co., Philadelphia.
23. Roper, B.A., & Provan, J.L. (1965). Late thrombosis of the femoral artery complicating fracture of the femur. J. Bone Joint Surg. [Br.], *47*:510.
24. Royle, S.G. (1990). Compartment syndrome following forearm fracture in children. Injury, *21*:73.
25. Saletta, J.D., & Freeark, R.J. (1968). The partially severed artery. Arch. Surg., *97*:198.
26. Staples, O.S. (1965). Dislocation of the brachial artery. J. Bone Joint Surg. [Am.], *47*:1525.
27. Watson-Jones, R. (1976). Vascular injuries, p. 190. In Wilson, J.N. Ed.: Watson-Jones Fractures and Joint Injuries. 5th Ed. Churchill Livingstone, Edinburgh.
28. Whitesides, T.E. (1977). Compartment syndrome. Instr. Course Lect., *26*:179.
29. Willhoite, D.R., & Moll, J.H. (1970). Early recognition and treatment of impending Volkmann's ischemia in the lower extremity. Arch. Surg., *100*:11.
30. Wray, J.B. (1965). Management of supracondylar fracture. Arch. Surg., *90*:279.
31. Kreipke, D.L., Holden, R.W., & Wass, J.L. (1982). Two angiographic signs of pseudoaneurysm: Systolic jet and diastolic washout. Radiology, *144*:79.
32. Ahlgren, S.A., & Eklof, B. (1981). Femur fracture and false aneurysm. Acta Chir. Scand. *147*:377.
33. Shah, A, & Ellis, R.D. (1993). False aneurysm complicating closed femoral fracture in a child. Orthop. Rev., *22*:1265.
34. Cordover, A.M., Israelite, C.L., & Berman, A.T. (1997). Pseudoaneurysm following femoral fracture. Orthopedics, *20*:1086.
35. Dresner, S.M., Banerjee, B., Owen, R., & Lees, T.A. (1999). A popliteal false aneurysm caused by avulsion fracture of the femur; a case presenting with deep venous thrombosis. Eur. J. Vasc. Endovasc. Surg., *17*:180.
36. Crawford, D.L., Yuschak, J.V., & McMombs, P.R. (1997). Pseudoaneurysm of the brachial artery from blunt trauma. J. Trauma, *42*:327.
37. Bapuraj, J.R., Thingnam, S., & Rajak, C.L. (1999). Popliteal artery pseudoaneurysm following penetrating trauma. Australas. Radiol., *43*:116.
38. Braito, W., Montanari, C., Caracciolo, F. et al. (1992). False aneurysm of the anterior tibial artery in lower left leg fracture treated with the Ilizarov external fixator. Case report. Ital. J. Orthop. Traumatol., *18*:135.
39. Vancabeke, M., Heiderich, B., Bellens, B., & Putz, P. (1999). Pseudoaneurysm of the ulnar artery following use of an external fixator—a case report. Acta Orthop. Scand., *70*:522.
40. Abu-Yousef, M.M., Wiese, J.A., & Shamma, A.R. (1988). The "to-and-fro" sign: Duplex Doppler evidence of femoral artery pseudoaneurysm. A.J.R. Am. J. Roentgenol, *150*:632.
41. Mitchell, D.G., Needleman, L., Bezzi, M. et al. (1987). Femoral artery pseudoaneurysm: Diagnosis with conventional duplex and color Doppler US. Radiology, *165*:687.

Gangrene

42. Altemeier, W.A., & Culbertson, W.R. (1948). Acute non-clostridial crepitant cellulitis. Surg. Gynecol. Obstet., *87*:206.
43. Altemeier, W.A., & Fullen, W.D. (1971). Prevention and treatment of gas gangrene. J.A.M.A., *217*:806.
44. Aufranc, O.E., Jones, W.N., & Bierbaum, B.E. (1969). Gas gangrene complicating fracture of the tibia. J.A.M.A., *209*:2045.
45. Colwill, M.R., & Maudsley, R.H. (1968). The management of gas gangrene with hyperbaric oxygen therapy. J. Bone Joint Surg. [Br.], *50*:732.
46. Dehaven, K.E., & Evarts, C.M. (1971). The continuing problem of gas gangrene: A review and report of illustrative cases. J. Trauma, *11*:983.
47. Doty, D.B., Treiman, R.I., Rothschild, P.D., & Gaspar, M.R. (1967). Prevention of gangrene due to fractures. Surg. Gynecol. Obstet., *125*:284.
48. Filler, R.M., Griscom, N.T., & Pappas, A. (1968). Post-traumatic crepitation falsely suggesting gas gangrene. N. Engl. J. Med., *278*:758.
49. Kemp, F.H. (1945). X-rays in diagnosis and localisation of gas-gangrene. Lancet, *1*:332.
50. Pappas, A.M., Filler, R.M., Eraklis, A.J., & Bernhard, W.F. (1971). Clostridial infections (gas gangrene). Clin. Orthop., *76*:177.

Fat Embolism

51. Crawford, W.O. Jr. (1973). Pulmonary injury in thoracic and non-thoracic trauma. Radiol. Clin. North Am., *11*:527.
52. Feldman, F., Ellis, K., & Green, W.M. (1975). The fat embolism syndrome. Radiology, *114*:535.
53. Fraser, R.G., & Pare, J.A.P. (1978). Diagnosis of Diseases of the Chest. 2nd Ed. W.B. Saunders Co., Philadelphia.
54. Gossling, H.R., & Pellegrini, V.D. (1982). Fat embolism syndrome: A review of the pathophysiology and physiological basis of treatment. Clin. Orthop., *165*:68.
55. Gurd, A.R., & Wilson, R.I. (1974). The fat embolism syndrome. J. Bone Joint Surg. [Br.], *56*:408.
56. McCarthy, B., Mammen, E., LeBlanc, L.P., & Wilson, R.F. (1973). Subclinical fat embolism: A prospective study of 50 patients with extremity fractures. J. Trauma, *13*:9.
57. Meek, R.N., Woodruff, M.B., & Allardyce, D.B. (1972). Source of fat macroglobules in fractures of the lower extremity J. Trauma, *12*:432.
58. Ostendorf, P., Birzle, H., Vogel, W., & Mittermayer, C. (1975). Pulmonary radiographic abnormalities in shock. Radiology, *115*:257.
59. Peltier, L.F. (1969). Fat embolism: A current concept. Clin. Orthop., *66*:241.
60. Prys-Roberts, C. (1974). Fat embolism and post-traumatic hypoxaemia. J. Bone Joint Surg. [Br.], *56*:405.
61. Ganong, R.B. (1993). Fat emboli syndrome in isolated fractures of the tibia and femur. Clin. Orthop., *291*:208.

Thromboembolism

62. Bachynski, J.E. (1971). Absence of the air bronchogram sign. Radiology, *100*:547.
63. Chait, A., Summers, D., Krassnow, N., & Wechsler, B.M. (1967). Observations on the fate of large pulmonary emboli. A.J.R. Am. J. Roentgenol., *100*:364.
64. Fred, H.L., Axelrad, M.A., Lewis, J.M., & Alexander, J.K. (1966). Rapid resolution of pulmonary thromboemboli in man. J.A.M.A., *196*:1137.
65. Freiman, D.G., Suyemoto, J., & Wessler, S. (1965). Frequency of pulmonary thromboembolism in man. N. Engl. J. Med., *272*:1278.
66. Gilday, D.L., Poulose, K.P., & DeLand, F.G. (1972). Accuracy of detection of pulmonary embolism by lung scanning correlated with pulmonary angiography. A.J.R. Am. J. Roentgenol., *115*:732.
67. Jackson, D.C., Tyson, J.W., Johnsrude, I.S., & Wilkinson, R.H. Jr. (1975). Pulmonary embolic disease: The roles of angiography and lung scanning in diagnosis. J. Can. Assoc. Radiol., *26*:139.
68. Kakkar, V. (1972). The diagnosis of deep vein thrombosis using the ^{125}I fibrinogen test. Arch. Surg., *104*:152.
69. LeQuesne, L.P. (1974). Relation between deep vein thrombosis and pulmonary embolism in surgical patients (current concepts). N. Engl. J. Med., *291*:1292.
70. Mavor, G.E., & Galloway, J.M.D. (1967). The iliofemoral venous segment as a source of pulmonary emboli. Lancet, *1*:871.
71. MacNeil, B., Holman, B.L., & Adelstein, J. (1974). The scintigraphic definition of pulmonary embolism. J.A.M.A., *227*:753.
72. Moses, D.C., Silver, T.M., & Bookstein, J.J. (1974). The complementary roles of chest radiography, lung scanning, and selective pulmonary angiography in the diagnosis of pulmonary embolism. Circulation, *49*:179.
73. Sagel, S.S., & Greenspan, R.H. (1971). Nonuniform pulmonary arterial perfusion. Radiology, *99*:541.
74. White R.H., McGahan, J.P., Daschbach, M.M., & Hartling, R.P. (1989). Diagnosis of deep-vein thrombosis using duplex ultrasound. Ann. Intern. Med. *88*;382.
75. Montefusco–von Kleist, C.M., Bakal, C., Sprayregen S. et al. (1993). Comparison of duplex ultrasonography and ascending contrast venography in the diagnosis of venous thrombosis. Angiology, *44*:169.
76. Blum, J.E., & Handmaker H. (2000). Role of small-peptide radiopharmaceuticals in the evaluation of deep venous thrombosis. Radiographics, *20*:1187.
77. Taillefer, R., Therasse, E., Turpin, S. et al. (1999). Comparison of early and delayed scintigraphy with ^{99m}Tc-apcitide and correlation with contrast-enhanced venography in detection of acute deep venous thrombosis. J. Nucl. Med., *40*:2029.
78. Laissy, J.P., Cinqualbre, A., Loshkajian, A. et al. (1996). Assessment of deep venous thrombosis in the lower limbs and pelvis: MR venography versus duplex Doppler sonography. A.J.R. Am. J. Roentgenol, *167*;971.
79. van Rossum, A.B., Pattynama, P.M., Ton, E.R. et al. (1996). Pulmonary embolism: Validation of spiral CT angiography in 149 patients. Radiology, *201*:467.

80. Remy-Jardin, M., Remy, J., Baghaie, F. et al. (2000). Clinical value of thin collimation in the diagnostic workup of pulmonary embolism. A.J.R. Am. J. Roentgenol., *175*:407.

Osteomyelitis

81. Altto, A., Koskinen, V.S., & Malmberg, H. (1972). Osteomyelitis in nonoperative and postoperative fracture treatment. Clin. Orthop., *82*:123.
82. Butt, W.P. (1973). The radiology of infection. Clin. Orthop., *96*:20.
83. Canale, S.T., Puhl, J., Watson, F.M., & Gillespie, R. (1975). Acute osteomyelitis following closed fractures. J. Bone Joint Surg. [Am.], *57*:415.
84. Clawson, D.K., & Dunn, A.W. (1967). Management of common bacterial infections of bones and joints. J. Bone Joint Surg. [Am.], *49*:164.
85. Dalinka, M.A., Lally, J.A., Koniver, G., & Coren, G.S. (1975). The radiology of osseous and articular infection. C.R.C. Crit. Rev. Clin. Radiol. Nucl. Med., *7*:1.
86. Dellinger, E.P., Miller, S.D., Wertz, M.J. et al. (1988). Risk of infection after open fracture of the arm or leg. Arch. Surg., *123*:1320.
87. Fitzgerald, R.H., Landells, D.G., & Cowan, J.D.E. (1975). Osteomyelitis in children: Comparison of hematogenous and secondary osteomyelitis. Can. Med. Assoc. J., *112*:116.
88. Gold, R.H., Hawkins, R.A., & Katz, R.D. (1991). Bacterial osteomyelitis: Findings on plain radiography, CT, MR, and scintigraphy. A.J.R. Am. J. Roentgenol., *157*:365.
89. Gupta, N.C., & Prezio, J.A. (1988). Radionuclide imaging in osteomyelitis. Semin. Nucl. Med., *18*:287.
90. Gustilo, R.B., & Anderson, J.T. (1976). Prevention of infection in the treatment of one thousand and twenty-five open fractures of long bones. Retrospective and prospective analyses. J. Bone Joint Surg. [Am.], *58*:453.
91. Horwitz, T. (1973). Surgical treatment of chronic osteomyelitis complicating fractures. Clin. Orthop., *96*:118.
92. Horwitz, T. (1976). Surgical treatment of chronic osteomyelitis complicating fractures (6 year interim follow-up). Clin. Orthop., *114*:207.
93. Kahn, D.S., & Pritzker, P.H. (1973). The pathophysiology of bone infection. Clin. Orthop., *96*:12.
94. Klemm, K.W., & Borner, M. (1986). Interlocking nailing of complex fractures of the femur and tibia. Clin. Orthop., *212*:89.
95. MacAusland, W.R. (1968). Treatment of sepsis after intramedullary nailing of fractures of femur. Clin. Orthop., *60*:87.
96. Resnick, D. (1976). Osteomyelitis and septic arthritis complicating hand injuries and infections: Pathogenesis of roentgenographic abnormalities. J. Can. Assoc. Radiol., *27*:21.
97. Roesgen, M., Hierholzer, G., & Hax, P.M. (1989). Post-traumatic osteomyelitis. Arch. Orthop. Trauma Surg., *108*:1.
98. Schauwecker, D.S. (1989). Osteomyelitis: Diagnosis with ^{111}In-labeled leukocytes. Radiology, *171*:141.
99. Seabold, J.E., Nepola, J.V., Conrad, G.R. et al. (1989). Detection of osteomyelitis at fracture nonunion sites: Comparison of two scintigraphic methods. A.J.R. Am. J. Roentgenol., *152*:1021.
100. Stevens, D.B. (1964). Postoperative orthopaedic infections. J. Bone Joint Surg. [Am.], *46*:96.
101. Waldvogel, F.A., Medoff, G., & Swartz, M.N. (1970). Osteomyelitis: A review of clinical features, therapeutic considerations and unusual aspects (first of three parts). N. Engl. J. Med., *282*:198.
102. Waldvogel, F.A., Medoff, G., & Swartz, M.N. (1970). Osteomyelitis: A review of clinical features, therapeutic considerations and unusual aspects (second of three parts). N. Engl. J. Med., *282*:260.
103. Waldvogel, F.A., Medoff, G., & Swartz, M.N. (1970). Osteomyelitis: A review of clinical features, therapeutic considerations and unusual aspects (third of three parts). N. Engl. J. Med., *282*:316.
104. Watson-Jones, R. (1976). Open and infected injuries of bones and joints. p. 391. In Wilson, J.N. Ed.: Watson-Jones Fractures and Joint Injuries. 5th Ed. Churchill Livingstone, Edinburgh.
105. Wilson, J.N. (1966). The management of infection after Kuntscher nailing of the femur. J. Bone Joint Surg. [Br.], 48:112.

Reflex Dystrophy Syndrome—Sudeck's Atrophy

106. Coller, F.A., Campbell, K.N., Berry, R.E.L. et al. (1947). Tetra-ethyl-ammonium as an adjunct in the treatment of peripheral vascular disease and other painful states. Ann. Surg., *125*:729.
107. Drucker, W.R., Hubay, C.A., Holden, W.D., & Bukovnic, J.A. (1959). Pathogenesis of post-traumatic sympathetic dystrophy. Am. J. Surg., *97*:454.
108. Genant, H.K., Kozin, F., Bekerman, C. et al. (1975). The reflex sympathetic dystrophy syndrome. A comprehensive analysis using fine-detail radiography, photon absorptiometry, and bone and joint scintigraphy. Radiology, *117*:21.
109. Helms, C.A., OBrien, E.T., & Katzberg, R.W. (1980). Segmental reflex sympathetic dystrophy syndrome. Radiology, *135*:67.
110. Herrmann, L.G., Reineke, H.G., & Caldwell, J.A. (1942). Post-traumatic painful osteoporosis. A.J.R. Am. J. Roentgenol., *47*:353.
111. Pak, T.J., Martin, G.M., Magness, J.L., & Kavanaugh, G.J. (1970). Reflex sympathetic dystrophy. Minn. Med., *53*:507.
112. Plewes, L.W. (1956). Sudeck's atrophy in the hand. J. Bone Joint Surg. [Br.], *38*:195.
113. Seale, K. (1989). Reflex sympathetic dystrophy of the lower extremity. Clin. Orthop., *243*:80.
114. Steinbrocker, O., & Argyros, T.G. (1958). The shoulder-hand syndrome: Present status as a diagnostic and therapeutic entity. Med. Clin. North Am., *42*:1533.
115. Sudeck, P. (1902). Ueber die akute (trophoneurotische) Knochenatrophie nach Entzundungen und Traumen der Extremitaten. Dtsch. Med. Wochenschr., *28*:336.
116. Takats, G. de. (1965). Sympathetic reflex dystrophy. Med. Clin. North Am., *49*:117.
117. Kemler, M.A., Barendse G.A., van Kleef, M. et al. (2000). Spinal cord stimulation in patients with chronic reflex sympathetic dystrophy. N. Engl. J. Med., *343*:618.
118. Buchheit, T., & Crews, J.C. (2000). Lateral cervical epidural catheter placement for continuous unilateral upper extremity analgesia and sympathetic block. Reg. Anesth. Pain Med., *25*:313.
119. Vecht, C.J. (2000). [Treatment of posttraumatic dystrophy]. Ned. Tijdschr. Geneeskd., *144*:1620.
120. Gellman, H. (2000). Reflex sympathetic dystrophy: Alternative modalities for pain management. Inst. Course Lect., *49*:549.

Post-Traumatic Osteolysis

121. Cahill, B.R. (1982). Osteolysis of the distal part of the clavicle in male athletes. J. Bone Joint Surg. [Am.], *64*:1053.
122. Halaby, M.F., & DiSalvo, E.I. (1965). Osteolysis: A complication of trauma. A.J.R. Am. J. Roentgenol., *94*:591.
123. Levine, A.H., Pais, M.J., & Schwartz, E.E. (1976). Posttraumatic osteolysis of the distal clavicle with emphasis on early radiologic changes. A.J.R. Am. J. Roentgenol., *127*:781.
124. Madsen, B. (1963). Osteolysis of the acromial end of the clavicle following trauma. Br. J. Radiol., *36*:822.
125. Seymour, E.Q. (1977). Osteolysis of the clavicular tip associated with repeated minor trauma to the shoulder. Radiology, *123*:56.
126. de la Puente, R., Boutin, R.D., Theodorou, D.J. et al. (1999). Post-traumatic and stress-induced osteolysis of the distal clavicle: MR imaging findings in 17 patients. Skeletal Radiol. *28*:202.

Refracture

127. Bostman, O.M. (1990). Refracture after removal of a condylar plate from the distal third of the femur. J. Bone Joint Surg. [Am.], *72*:1013.
128. Hidaka, S., & Gustilo, R.B. (1984). Refracture of bones of the forearm after plate removal. J. Bone Joint Surg. [Am.], *66*:1241.

Ectopic Ossification

129. Chantraine, A., Very, J.M., & Baud, C.A. (1990). A biophysical study of posttraumatic ectopic ossification. Clin. Orthop., *255*:289.
130. Thompson, H.C., & Garcia, A. (1967). Myositis ossificans: Aftermath of elbow injuries. Clin. Orthop., *50*:129.

Osteonecrosis

131. Banks, H.H. (1965). A study of healing and non-union in femoral-neck fractures. J. Bone Joint Surg. [Am.], *47*:1675.
132. Bobechko, W.P., & Harris, W.R. (1960). The radiographic density of vascular bone. J. Bone Joint Surg. [Br.], *42*:626.
133. Catto, M. (1965). A histological study of avascular necrosis of the femoral head after transcervical fracture. J. Bone Joint Surg. [Br.], *47*:749.
134. Catto, M. (1965). The histological appearance of late segmental collapse of the femoral head after transcervical fracture. J. Bone Joint Surg. [Br.], *47*:777.
135. Coleman, B.C., Kressel, H.V., Dalinka, M.K. et al. (1988). Radiographically negative avascular necrosis: Detection with MR imaging. Radiology, *168*:525.
136. Genez, B.M., Wilson, M.R., Houk, R.W. et al. (1988). Early osteonecrosis of the femoral head: Detection in high-risk patients with MR imaging. Radiology, *168*:521.
137. Gilsanz, V., Cleveland, R.H. & Wilkinson, R.H. (1977). Aseptic necrosis: A complication of dislocation of the metacarpophalangeal joint. A.J.R. Am. J. Roentgenol., *129*:737.
138. Mitchell, D.G., Rao, V.J., Dalinka, M.K. et al. (1987). Femoral head avascular necrosis: Correlation of MR imaging, radiographic staging, radionuclide imaging, and clinical findings. Radiology, *162*:709.
139. Mitchell, M.D., Kundel, H.L., Steinberg, M.E. et al. (1986). Avascular necrosis of the hip: Comparison of MR, CT, and scintigraphy. A.J.R. Am. J. Roentgenol., *147*:67.
140. Norman, A., & Bullough, P. (1963). The radiolucent crescent sign—an early diagnostic sign of avascular necrosis of the femoral head. Bull. Hosp. Jt. Dis., *24*:99.
141. Palmia, C., & Volterrani, F. (1971). The radiologic picture of post-traumatic necrosis of the astragalus. Radiol. Med., *57*:177.
142. Steinberg, M.E., Brighton, C.T., Hayken, G.D. et al. (1984). Early results in the treatment of avascular necrosis of the femoral head with electrical stimulation. Orthop. Clin. North Am., *15*:163.
143. Totty, W.G., Murphy, W.A., Ganz, W.I. et al. (1984). Magnetic resonance

imaging of the normal and ischemic femoral head. A.J.R. Am. J. Roentgenol., *143*:1273.

144. Lucie, R.S., Fuller, S., Burdick, D.C., & Johnston, R.M. (1981). Early prediction of avascular necrosis of the femoral head following femoral neck fractures. Clin. Orthop., *161*:207.
145. Brunner, S., Christiansen, J., & Kristensen, J.K. (1967). Arteriographic prediction of femoral head viability in medial femoral neck fractures. Acta Chir. Scand., *133*:449.
146. Gill, T.J., Sledge, J.B., Ekkernkamp, A., & Ganz, R. (1998). Intraoperative assessment of femoral head vascularity after femoral neck fracture. J. Orthop. Trauma, *12*:474.
147. Ruland, L.J. III, Wang, G.J., Teates C.D. et al. (1992). A comparison of magnetic resonance imaging to bone scintigraphy in early traumatic ischemia of the femoral head. Clin. Orthop., *285*:30.

Osteoarthritis

148. Collins, D.H. (1953). Osteoarthritis. J. Bone Joint Surg. [Br.], *35*:518.
149. Edeiken, J., & Hodes, P.J. (1973). Roentgen Diagnosis of Diseases of Bone. Vol. 2. p. 804. Williams & Wilkins Co., Baltimore.
150. Murray, R.O., & Jacobson, H.G. (1977). Fundamentals of skeletal radiology. p. 318. In Murray, R.O. Ed. The Radiology of Skeletal Disorders. Vol. 1. Churchill Livingstone, Edinburgh.
151. Resnick, D., Niwayama, G., & Coutts, R.D. (1977). Subchondral cysts (geodes) in arthritic disorders: Pathologic and radiographic appearance of the hip joint. A.J.R. Am. J. Roentgenol., *128*:799.

Lead Arthropathy

152. Jensen, S.P., Richardson, M.L., Conrad, E.J., & Lazerte, G.D. (1990). Case report 608. Skeletal Radiol., *19*:233.
153. Dillman, P.O., Crumb, C.K., & Lidsky, M.J. (1979). Lead poisoning from a gunshot wound: Report of a case and review of the literature. Am. J. Med., *66*:509.
154. Linden, M.A., Manton, W.I., Stewart, R.M. et al. (1982). Lead poisoning from retained bullets: Pathogenesis, diagnosis, and management. Ann. Surg., *195*:305.

Post-Traumatic Tumor or Tumorlike Lesion

155. Fitzgerald, R.H., Brewer, N.S., & Dahlin, D.C. (1976). Squamous-cell carcinoma complicating chronic osteomyelitis. J. Bone Joint Surg. [Am.], *58*:1146.
156. Lifeso, R.M., Rooney, R.J., & El-Shaker, M. (1990). Post-traumatic squamous-cell carcinoma. J. Bone Joint Surg. [Am.], *72*:12.
157. Kattapuram, S.V., Khurana, J.S., Ehara, S., & Ragozzino, M. (1988). Aggressive posttraumatic osteoporosis of the humerus simulating a malignant neoplasm. Cancer, *62*:2525.
158. Kirkeby, O.J., Larsen, T.B., Nordsletten, L. et al. (1993). Fracture weakens ipsilateral long bones: Mechanical and metabolic changes after femoral or tibial injury in rats. J. Orthop. Trauma, *7*:343.
159. Karlsson, M.K., Hasserius, R., & Obrant, K.J. (1993). Individuals who sustain nonosteoporotic fractures continue to also sustain fragility fractures. Calcif. Tissue Int., *53*:229.

Post-Traumatic Aneurysmal Bone Cyst

160. Bonakdarpour, A., Levy, W.M., & Aegerter, E. (1978). Primary and secondary aneurysmal bone cyst: A radiological study of 75 cases. Radiology, *126*:75.
161. Kushner, D.C., Vance, Z., & Kirkpatrick, J.A. Jr. (1979). Post-traumatic aneurysmal bone cyst affecting third and fourth ribs. Skeletal Radiol., *4*:240.

Chapter 10

THE SKULL

with Curtis A. Given II, MD, and Daniel W. Williams III, MD

Contemplation of the possibility of a skull fracture conjures up considerable anxiety in the mind of the layperson, the conviction being that a skull fracture is attendant with dire consequences. This common misconception permeates even the minds of health care professionals. It is a misconception born of the belief that a skull fracture is invariably associated with significant intracranial injury (and, conversely, that the absence of a fracture excludes such injury). Such an association does not exist.

There is a low incidence of fracture on skull radiographs obtained for trauma,[8–10, 12, 50, 69, 83] with an overall incidence of less than 10%.[47, 83] Many skull radiographs may be obtained for medicolegal purposes[15, 19] or at the demand of the patient or family members.

Skull radiography established itself in the evaluation of trauma patients on the basis of the false assumption that significant intracranial injury would be reflected by the presence or absence of injury to the cranial vault.[14, 57, 59, 82] This is clearly not the case. Only 15% of patients with subdural hematomas have an associated calvarial fracture.[23] More important, intracerebral hematoma or contusion can occur without a skull fracture.[23] Around 90%[73, 98, 179] of epidural hematomas are associated with fractures, which are often depressed. When severe intracranial injury is present, there is a 65% to 80% chance of skull fracture, in which case the fracture is generally depressed.[13, 23, 47] The side of the fracture is not necessarily related to the side of the hematoma. Fractures that cross the dural sinus are at times associated with venous thrombosis.

In actual practice, skull radiographs significantly affect patient management only if a depressed skull fracture, foreign body, pneumocephalus, or mass effect is demonstrated. It is infrequent that detection of a linear skull fracture per se significantly changes or affects the treatment of the patient. More important, it should be emphasized that skull radiography is no substitute for a good history and physical examination in the evaluation of patients with a head injury.

There is a significant correlation between certain clinical factors and the presence of a fracture.[6, 7, 15, 16, 26, 50] These factors include abnormal neurologic findings (i.e., loss of consciousness, abnormal reflexes, and focal sensory or motor abnormalities); abnormal physical findings (i.e., palpable defect, discharge from the ear, and eardrum discoloration); and abnormal historical findings (i.e., loss of consciousness, retrograde amnesia, and vomiting). With these findings either alone or in combination, the incidence of fracture is between 15% and 45%. When the examining physician believes that a fracture is unlikely, the incidence of fracture approaches 1%[47]; thus, from an economic and medical viewpoint, skull radiography seems unjustified.[3, 8, 27, 28]

Criteria for Skull Radiographic and Computed Tomographic Examinations after Head Trauma

Since the publication of the landmark paper by Bell and Loop[50] in 1971, considerable effort has been expended on determining the efficacy of skull radiography after head trauma.[3, 6, 10, 11, 20, 25–27, 29] Initially, studies were directed toward disclosure of skull fractures alone, but more recent studies have focused on intracranial abnormalities as well.

These studies culminated in the publication of recommendations by a multidisciplinary skull x-ray referral criteria panel[16] supported by the Center for Devices and Radiologic Health of the Food and Drug Administration (Table 10–1), which divided patients into three risk groups: low, moderate, and high. In the low-risk group, it is recommended that the patient simply be observed; no skull radiograph is required. In the moderate-risk group, computed tomography (CT) examination and skull radiographic series may be considered under some circumstances, and in the high-risk group, CT examination is recommended.

The skull x-ray referral criteria study comprised 7035 patients. Skull radiographs were obtained in 53% of the low-risk patients, 70% of the moderate-risk patients, and 84% of the high-risk patients. Among these patients, 21.5% of the high-risk, 4.2% of the moderate-risk, and only 0.4% of the low-risk patients had fractures. None of the low-risk patients had an intracranial injury, whereas 4% of the moderate-risk and 24% of the high-risk patients had an intracranial injury. More than half of the 7035 patients with head injuries underwent skull radiography, and of these 1.7% of adults and 4.25% of children up to the age of 10 were found to have skull fractures. As a part of the same study a large series of over 22,000 patients was reviewed. In this series, 91% of the patients with skull fractures did not have an associated intracranial injury, and 51% of the patients with an intracranial injury did not have a skull fracture. These findings validate the

Table 10–1. Management Strategy for Radiographic Imaging in Patients with Head Trauma*

Low-Risk Group	Moderate-Risk Group	High-Risk Group
Possible findings		
Asymptomatic Headache Dizziness Scalp hematoma Scalp laceration Scalp contusion or abrasion Absence of moderate-risk or high-risk criteria	History of change of consciousness at the time of injury or subsequently History of progressive headache Alcohol or drug intoxication Unreliable or inadequate history of injury Age less than 2 yr (unless injury very trivial) Post-traumatic seizure Vomiting Post-traumatic amnesia Multiple trauma Serious facial injury Signs of basilar fracture† Possible skull penetration or depressed fracture‡ Suspected physical child abuse	Depressed level of consciousness not clearly due to alcohol, drugs, or other cause (e.g., metabolic and seizure disorders) Focal neurologic signs Decreasing level of consciousness Penetrating skull injury or palpable depressed fracture
Recommendations		
Observation alone: discharge patients with head-injury information sheet (listing subdural precautions) and a second person to observe them.	Extended close observation (watch for signs characteristic of high-risk group). Consider computed tomography examination and neurosurgical consultation. Skull series may (rarely) be helpful, if positive, but do not exclude intracranial injury if normal.	Patient is a candidate for neurosurgical consultation or emergency computed tomography examination or both.

*Physical assessment of the severity of injury may warrant reassignment to a higher risk group. Any single criterion from a higher risk group warrants assignment of the patient to the highest risk group applicable.

†Signs of basilar fracture include drainage from ear, drainage of cerebrospinal fluid from nose, hematotympanum, Battle's sign, and "raccoon eyes."

‡Factors associated with open and depressed fracture include gunshot, missile, or shrapnel wounds; scalp injury from firm, pointed object (including animal teeth); penetrating injury of eyelid or globe; object stuck in the head; assault (definite or suspected) with any object; leakage of cerebrospinal fluid; and sign of basilar fracture.

From Masters, S. J., McClean, P. M., Arcarese, J. S. et al. (1987). Skull x-ray examination after head trauma. N. Engl. J. Med., *316*:84, with permission.

use of the risk criteria. The use of these criteria would substantially reduce the cost without compromising the care of any head-injured patient. By utilizing clinical criteria, it is possible to reduce the use of skull radiographs by 50% to 65% without missing any significant intracranial injury.

The real conundrum is posed by the use of CT versus skull radiography.[22] The primary concern regarding the presence or absence of intracranial injury so outweighs the presence or absence of skull fracture that it seems reasonable that if any imaging examination is to be performed at all, it should be a CT examination. Indeed, the American College of Radiology[1] endorses CT as the initial imaging examination in the setting of most acute head injuries, followed by magnetic resonance imaging (MRI), and then skull radiography. Although a small number of skull fractures may be missed on axial CT images,[6, 17] this number can be reduced by including digital scout radiographs of the skull in the frontal and lateral projections with each examination. If a CT examination is to be done, skull radiography is superfluous and can be safely omitted or at least delayed pending the results of the CT study.

Pathomechanics of Injury

Appreciation of the physical characteristics of the skull and the cranial contents and awareness of the dynamics of craniocerebral trauma[68, 89] are fundamental to understanding the relationship between clinical factors and the presence of a fracture (Fig. 10–1). The skull is a semielastic ball containing the brain, a gelatinous mass suspended in a thin layer of cerebrospinal fluid. The two main mechanical forces involved in most head injuries are acceleration-deceleration and deformation. At impact, the head moves or is suddenly stopped, the skull is bent, and the shape of the brain is distorted. Just as the skull and brain differ in consistency and shape, each has its own particular inertial properties. When the head is set in motion by a blow, the brain moves independently within the cranium because of these differences in inertia. Because the skull is elastic, it is bent inward at the site of the blow (inbending) and simultaneously bent outward at all points surrounding this site (outbending).[68] A fracture occurs only if the tensile strength of the skull is exceeded. A linear fracture originates in an area of outbending and then may extend toward the point of impact and in the opposite direction. Low-velocity forces of large mass create this type of linear fracture. High-velocity forces of small mass may exceed the tensile strength of the skull at the point of impact and result in a depressed fracture. In general, the higher the velocity and the smaller the mass of the object, the more likely is a depressed fracture.

As the skull is bent inward the brain may be contused. More important, the brain is set in motion by the accelerating forces. Such movement may easily be accomplished without fracturing the skull. The movement of the brain within the cranium may shear the dural veins traversing the subarachnoid space, resulting in a subdural hematoma.[58, 92] The inbending and outbending of the skull may tear the meningeal arteries and veins, creating an epidural hematoma.[85] As the brain slides across the rough surfaces of the floor of the anterior and middle fossae and against

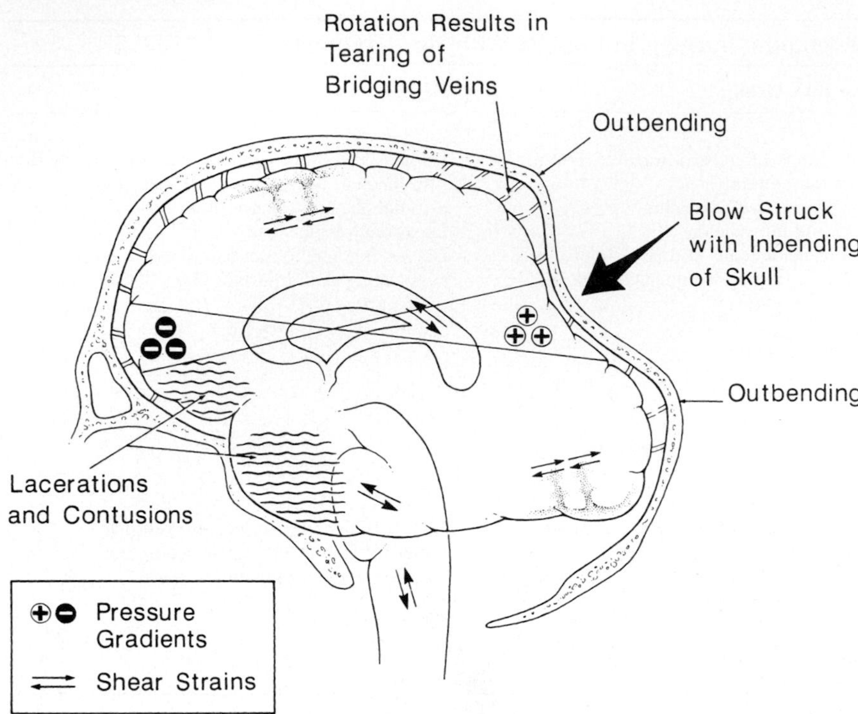

Figure 10–1. Mechanisms of cerebral injury.

the sharp edge of the sphenoid ridge, the frontal and temporal lobes may be contused, or intracerebral hematomas may form.[68, 77, 91] The latter may occur on the side opposite the impact (i.e., contrecoup injury) (see Fig. 10–9). The smooth inner surface of the calvaria prevents intracerebral injury of the parietal lobes and upper surface of the frontal lobe. Thus, intracerebral hematomas are far more frequent in the anterior portion of the temporal lobes and base of the frontal lobes.

As the skull is bent inward, there is elevation of the pressure in the adjacent brain.[65, 67, 68, 89] This increase is accompanied by a decrease in pressure or negative pressure in the brain opposite the point of impact. The negative pressure may exceed the vapor pressure of the brain, causing focal cavitation. This cavitation disrupts both the brain tissue and the capillaries and results in formation of focal edema or hemorrhage. Thus, injury may occur in the brain tissue opposite the point of impact. The skull rebounds at the point of impact, and the pressure in the underlying brain is quickly reduced from positive to negative: then cavitation, focal edema, and hemorrhage may occur beneath the point of impact. The pressure changes are reverberated within the cranial cavity after impact; therefore, it is possible for focal changes to occur at any point within the brain tissue. These pressure changes are frequently focused about the foramen magnum, resulting in edema and focal hemorrhage within the brain stem and medulla.[53] If edema and hemorrhage are of sufficient severity, loss of consciousness may result. Injury may occur either directly, as the result of increased pressure, or indirectly, as the result of a negative pressure with cavitation.

Shear strain deformation is characterized by a change in shape without a change in volume (see Fig. 10–1). It is created by linear and rotational acceleration and deceleration. Rotational forces are particularly devastating because they produce shear strains at the junction or interface of tissues of different rigidity (e.g., gray matter–white matter, dura mater–brain, brain–cerebrospinal fluid), resulting in focal hemorrhages at these locations (see Fig. 10–18).[43, 45, 46, 52, 78, 86, 100] Shear strains may also give rise to focal hemorrhage in the brain stem and the corpus callosum, often in the body and splenium. The superior soft tissue contrast afforded by MRI, particularly within the posterior fossa and brain stem, makes this modality superb for evaluating these shear-type injuries.

It therefore is obvious that considerable anatomic and physiologic abnormalities occur in response to a blow to the head that are not reflected in a radiograph of the skull.

Children differ from adults in the nature of their response to injury.[38, 42] Newborn infants and young children have open sutures and a thin calvaria, resulting in a more flexible skull capable of absorbing a greater impact than is the case with the skull of an adult. Poor myelination contributes to the greater plasticity of the infant's cerebral hemispheres. Calvarial flexibility and cerebral plasticity also permit severe distortion between the skull and dura on the one hand and the cerebral vessels and brain on the other. These distortions produce lesions rarely seen in adults, such as interhemispheric subdural hematomas (see Fig. 10–49) and tentorium–dural sinus tears. The child's brain is subject to a rapid increase in cerebral blood flow, presumably owing to vasodilation, which may result in acute, diffuse cerebral swelling.[38, 42] The incidence of acute interhemispheric subdural hematomas is six times higher in children than in adults and that of depressed fractures is three and one-half times greater in children than adults.[38, 42] Adults have a fourfold greater incidence of acute subdural hematomas, a threefold greater incidence of intracerebral hematomas, and a twofold greater incidence of hemorrhagic contusion. These factors are most important between birth and 2 years of age, the period in which the risk of intracranial damage is the highest. Between the ages of 2 and 6 to 8 years the brain matures rapidly, and by 8 to 10 years the skull and intracranial structures in children respond to trauma as do those of adults.

Imaging Techniques

In the discussion that follows, the question of whether to perform a CT examination versus plain radiography of the skull versus MRI in the setting of head trauma is set aside, and the imaging techniques of the various modalities are reviewed.

Computed Tomography

When CT is readily accessible and there is a possibility of intracranial injury, it is best to proceed directly with a CT examination[1, 54, 72, 80, 84, 96] and to forego the plain film examination of the skull. Adding a digital image of the skull in both the lateral and frontal projections will probably disclose any linear fractures that are inapparent on axial CT images.

Widespread availability and technicologic advances have established CT as the modality of choice in the initial evaluation of patients who have sustained head trauma. Numerous examination protocols have been developed, but the majority incorporate thinner section (5- to 6-mm) axial images through the posterior fossa with thicker (10-mm) slices through the supratentorial region (Fig. 10–2). The orientation of the axial plane can be manipulated to reduce bone artifact within the posterior fossa; this is best achieved choosing an inclination of 5 degrees below the infraorbitomeatal line (Reid baseline).[21] After acquisition of the data, postprocessing should include both standard soft tissue and high-spatial-resolution (e.g., bone) reconstruction algorithms. Simply viewing the calvaria in a bone window display of the standard soft tissue algorithm does not afford the edge detail necessary to evaluate for subtle fractures (Fig. 10–3). Images should be filmed or viewed at a workstation with soft tissue (e.g., window width 100, center 40 Hounsfield units [HU]), subdural (e.g., window width 150, center 50 HU), and bone (e.g., window width 4000, center 750 HU) windows. Subdural window images utilize a slightly wider window than the standard soft tissue settings, allowing visual separation of hemorrhage from the adjacent dense bone and increasing the conspicuity of small extra-axial collections (Fig. 10–4).

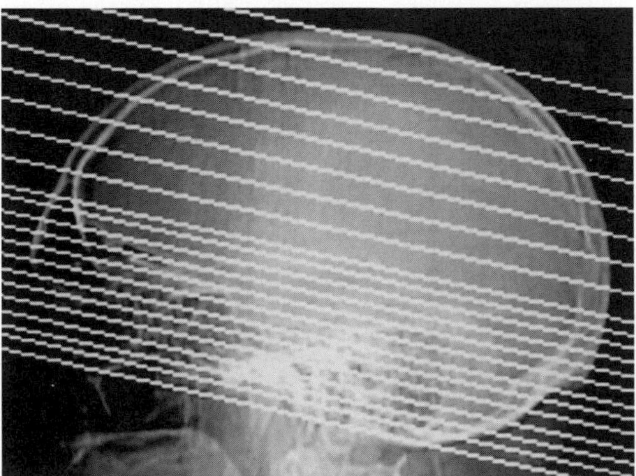

Figure 10–2. Digital radiograph from a CT examination demonstrates alignment of the axial plane at approximately 5 degrees below the infraorbitomeatal line. The slice thickness is 5 mm through the posterior fossa and 10 mm throughout the supratentorial region.

Spiral (helical) technology and multislice scanners have significantly reduced acquisition time and motion artifacts while improving image quality. These advances have had the largest impact in abdominal and vascular imaging. However, the utility of spiral CTs in the evaluation of head trauma remains limited. Spiral applications serve to reduce scan time and motion artifacts but also introduce several new volume-averaging artifacts. The vertex of the skull is particularly susceptible to artifacts that may simulate extra-axial or subarachnoid hemorrhages[2] (Fig. 10–5). Thus, incremental CT protocols remain the current standard, with spiral imaging reserved for only the most noncompliant patient.

The largest impact of spiral technology in the setting of head trauma lies in permitting high-quality multiplanar reconstructions of skull and facial fractures. Utilizing thin-section axial slices through the face and head, reconstructions can be generated in any desired plane. Nearly all protocols employ imaging in the axial plane with 1- to 3-mm thick sections, often with overlapping slices. This approach allows for rapid thin-section acquisitions while minimizing patient motion and respiration artifacts— particularly beneficial in traumatized patients, who often cannot undergo direct coronal imaging at the time of initial evaluation (see Fig. 10–31). Both two-dimensional and three-dimensional (S-D) reconstruction images can aid in the recognition and surgical planning of skull and facial fractures (Fig. 10–6).[24, 76]

CT[57, 74, 97] provides a noninvasive technique to directly demonstrate all forms of intracerebral injury, including subdural (see Fig. 10–4) and epidural hematomas (Figs. 10–7 and 10–8), cerebral contusion (Figs. 10–9 and 10–10), and subarachnoid bleeding. Although the full evaluation of intracranial pathology is beyond the scope of this chapter, a few key points are worth mentioning. In evaluating intracranial injuries, the first observation is for symmetry in size and shape of the ventricular system and the density of the brain. Acute blood generally appears or an area of high absorption density (white) on CT scans at the soft tissue window setting, secondary to formation of blood clot.[87, 98] In rare instances such as in anemic patients (hemoglobin levels of 8 to 10 g/dL) and in disseminated intravascular coagulation, acute hemorrhage may appear hypodense or isodense to adjacent brain parenchyma.[51] In addition, acute extra-axial hematomas may have a mixed density (see Fig. 10–8) secondary to active hemorrhage with areas of unclotted blood, clot retraction with serum extrusion, or cerebrospinal fluid admixture in the clot secondary to a tear of the arachnoid.[64, 87, 98] Extra-axial hematomas are often associated with a considerable midline shift to the contralateral side and distortion of

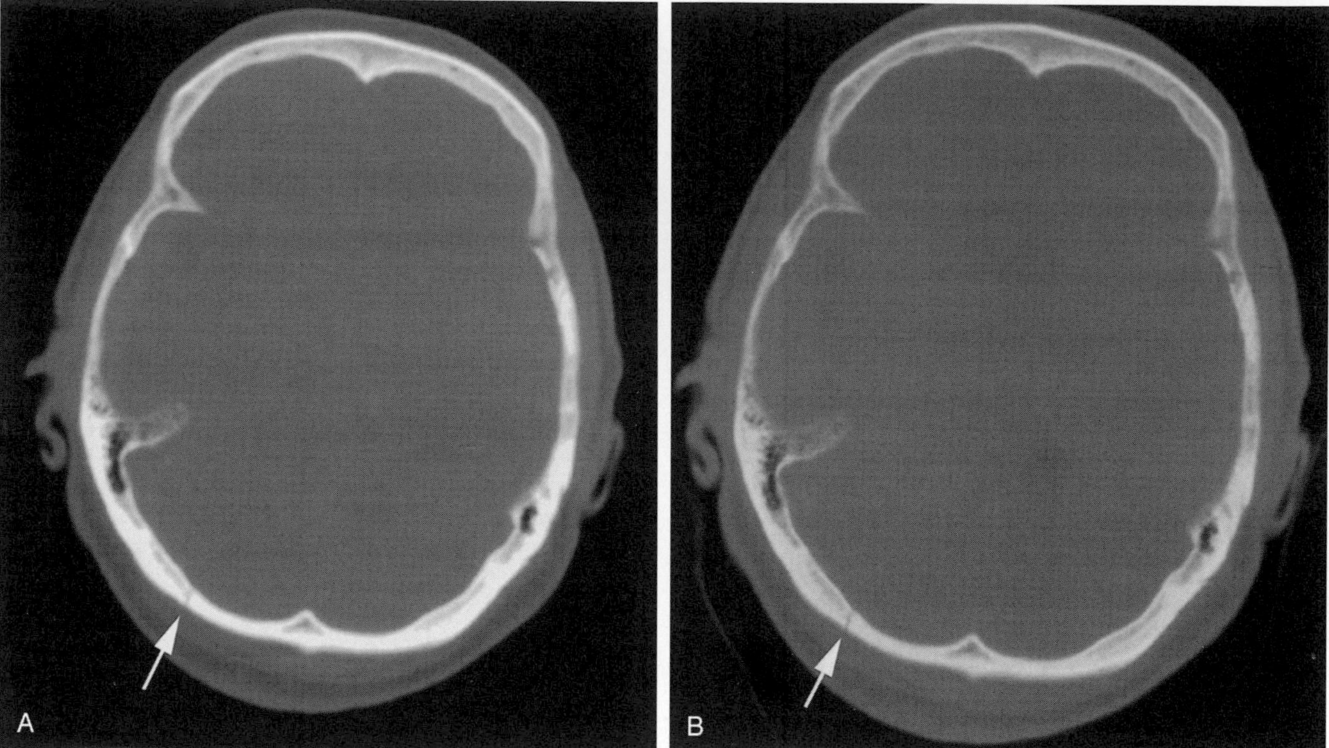

Figure 10–3. Right occipital fracture (*arrow*) displayed on CT obtained with bone window settings using standard soft tissue (*A*) and high-resolution bone (*B*) reconstruction algorithms. The fracture line is better defined on the image reformatted utilizing the bone algorithm.

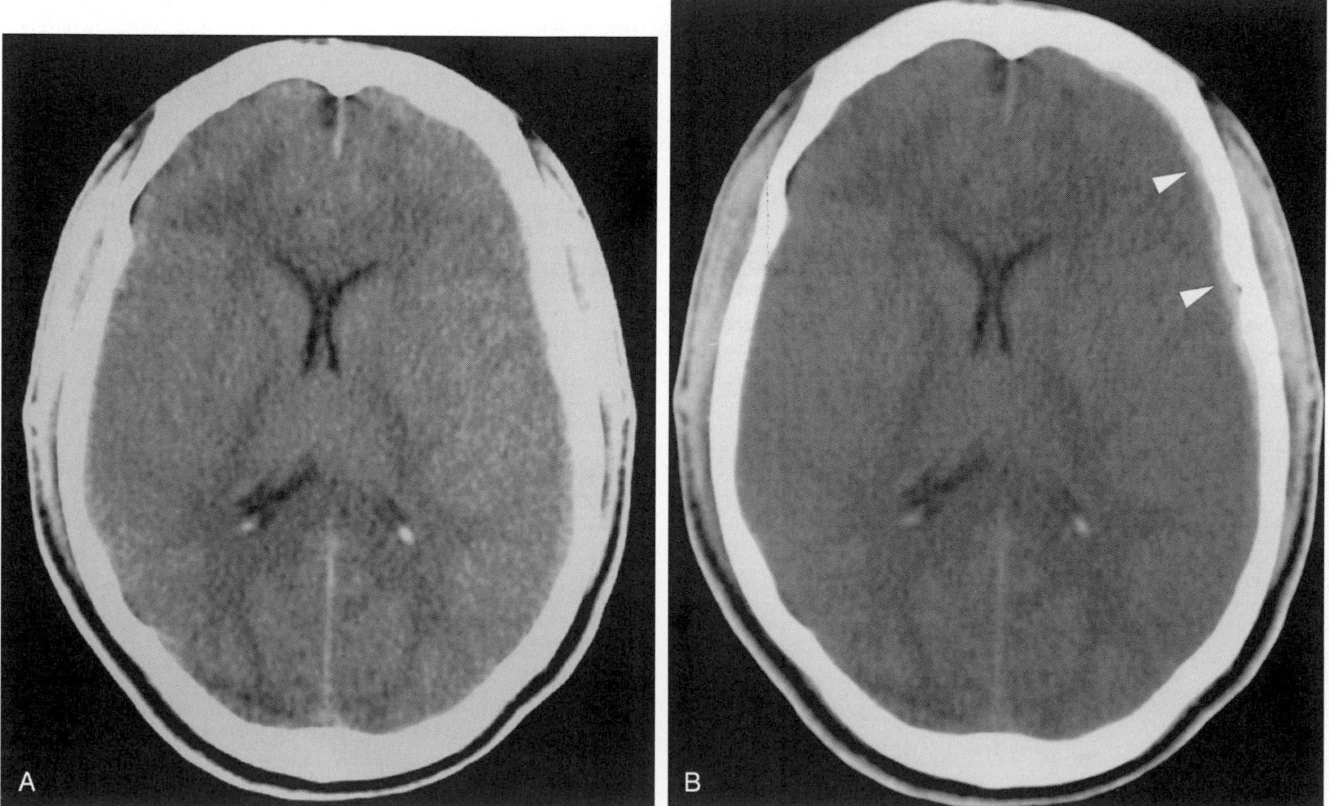

Figure 10–4. Thin left frontal subdural hematoma in *B* displayed on CT with brain (*A*) and subdural (*B*) window settings. The wider window settings of the subdural window increase the conspicuity of the hemorrhage (*arrowheads* in *B*). Although a small amount of midline shift is present, the hemorrhage might have been overlooked if viewed using only brain window settings.

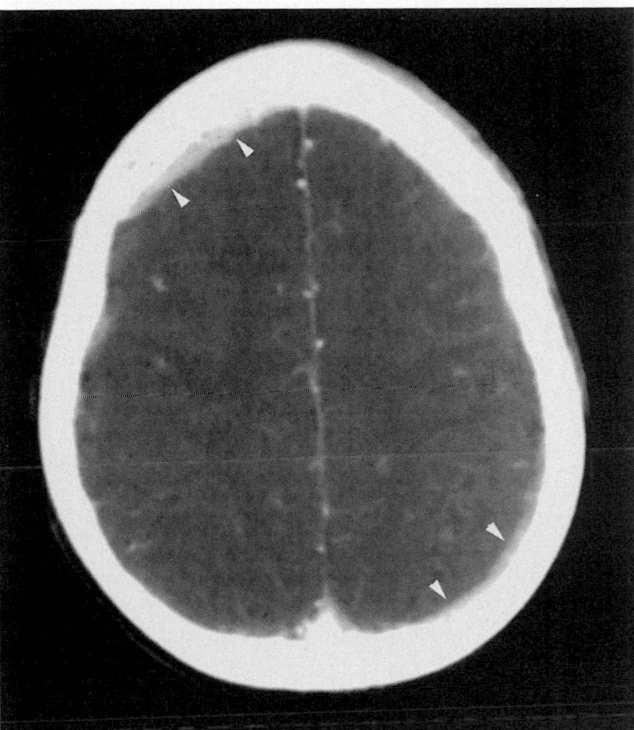

Figure 10–5. Volume-averaging artifacts mimicking a thin subdural hemorrhage (*arrowheads*) on this contrast-enhanced computed tomography image acquired using spiral technique.

the underlying brain (see Figs 10–8 and 10–12). Bilateral subdural hematomas may impose symmetrical pressures on the underlying brain and thus not be associated with significant (if any) shift of the midline structures (Fig. 10–11). Subdural hemorrhages are characteristically convex on their external surfaces and concave on their internal surfaces. The natural evolution of subdural hematomas involves lysis of red blood cells and resorption of clot[73]; as a result, there is a subacute stage (10 days to 3 weeks) during which subdural hemorrhages may be isodense to the adjacent parenchyma (Fig. 10–12). However, signs of mass effect with effacement of the lateral ventricle and inward displacement of gray-white matter junction will remain present and aid in identification of the *isodense subdural hematoma*.

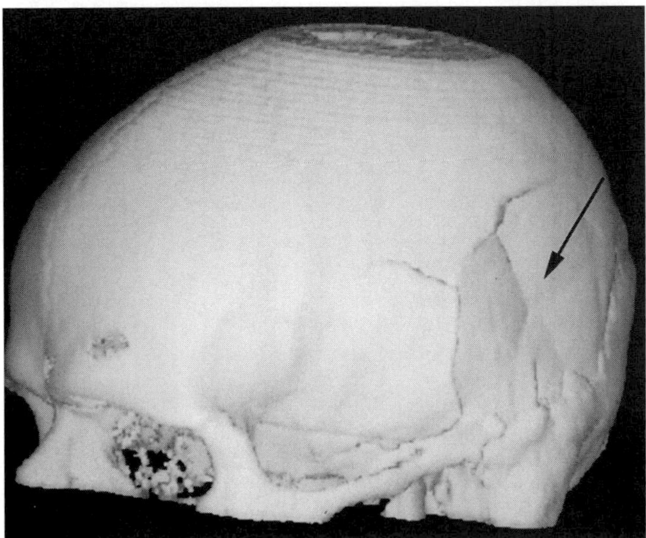

Figure 10–6. Surface-shaded three-dimensional image reconstructed from contiguous 2-mm-thick slices of the skull in a left anterior oblique projection, demonstrates a comminuted, depressed fracture (*arrow*) in the left parietal region.

Epidural hematomas are smaller in volume, biconvex in configuration, and usually accompanied by less shift (see Fig. 10–7). Once identified, epidural hematomas should be scrutinized for the presence of areas of low attenuation within the hematoma (see Fig. 10–8), as this appearance suggests unclotted blotted and active hemorrhage, possibly requiring emergency surgical management.[64, 98]

Cerebral contusions occur more commonly in the base of the frontal lobes and in the temporal poles, manifested by areas of patchy increased absorption and surrounding edema (see Figs. 10–9 and 10–10). Subarachnoid hemorrhage is confined to the surface of the brain and follows the configuration of the sulci and gyri.

In order to demonstrate fractures of the skull, it is mandatory to view images in bone window settings, preferably utilizing a high-resolution ("bone") reconstruction algorithm. Depressed fractures are nicely displayed in the axial plane (Fig. 10–13). The only exception is a depressed fracture at the vertex in or about the sagittal suture, which requires a "hanging head" coronal examination for optimal depiction. The digital scout radiographs accompanying the CT examination will help identify these fractures (Fig. 10–14) and indicate those requiring imaging in the coronal plane. The uncertainty of cervical spinal injury often prohibits direct coronal examination in trauma patients; in these instances, coronal reconstruction images obtained from thin-section (3-mm-thick slices) axial data will usually suffice.

Vertically oriented, linear fractures are readily visualized (see Fig. 10–10), but volume-averaging artifacts may render a significant number of horizontally oriented fractures invisible in the axial plane (Fig. 10–15). Some studies have estimated that only 20% of all skull fractures are visualized with standard axial projections.[52] However, the addition of digital radiographs in both the frontal and lateral projections will allow detection of most if not all linear fractures.[6] It is best to begin the evaluation by looking at the digital radiographs to identify or rule out linear fractures, which may not be evident in the axial projection.

Skull Radiography

The widespread availability of CT and its ability to evaluate for intracranial injury have rendered skull radiography a secondary modality in the evaluation of most acute head trauma. Skull radiographs are often obtained for medicolegal purposes or to reassure anxious patients or family members when a low clinical suspicion for injury exists.[15, 19] When the presence or absence of a subtle linear fracture is of utmost importance, such as in suspected cases of nonaccidental trauma (child abuse), skull radiographs maintain a role in the radiologic evaluation.

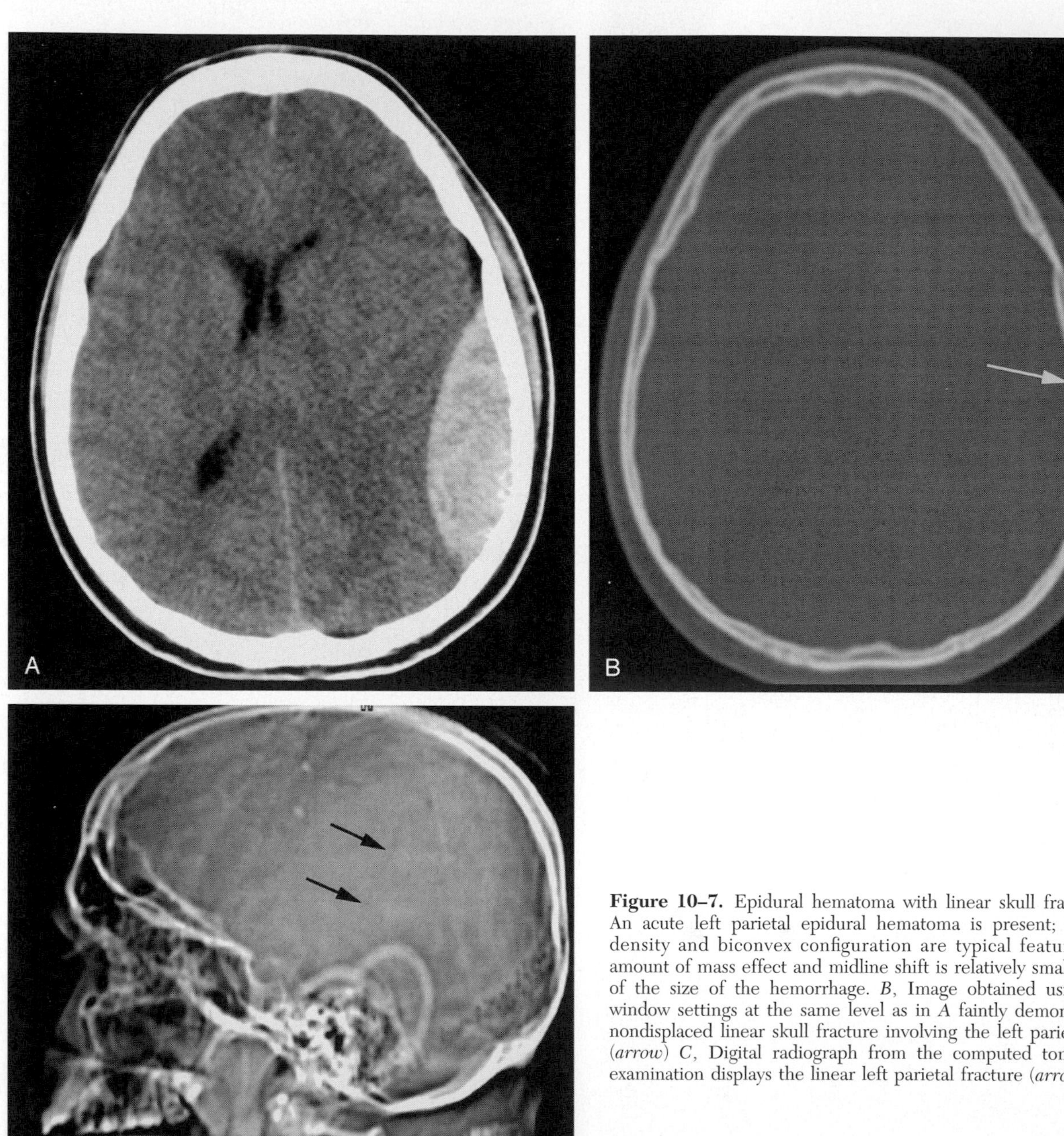

Figure 10–7. Epidural hematoma with linear skull fracture. *A*, An acute left parietal epidural hematoma is present; the high density and biconvex configuration are typical features. The amount of mass effect and midline shift is relatively small in view of the size of the hemorrhage. *B*, Image obtained using bone window settings at the same level as in *A* faintly demonstrates a nondisplaced linear skull fracture involving the left parietal bone (*arrow*) *C*, Digital radiograph from the computed tomography examination displays the linear left parietal fracture (*arrows*).

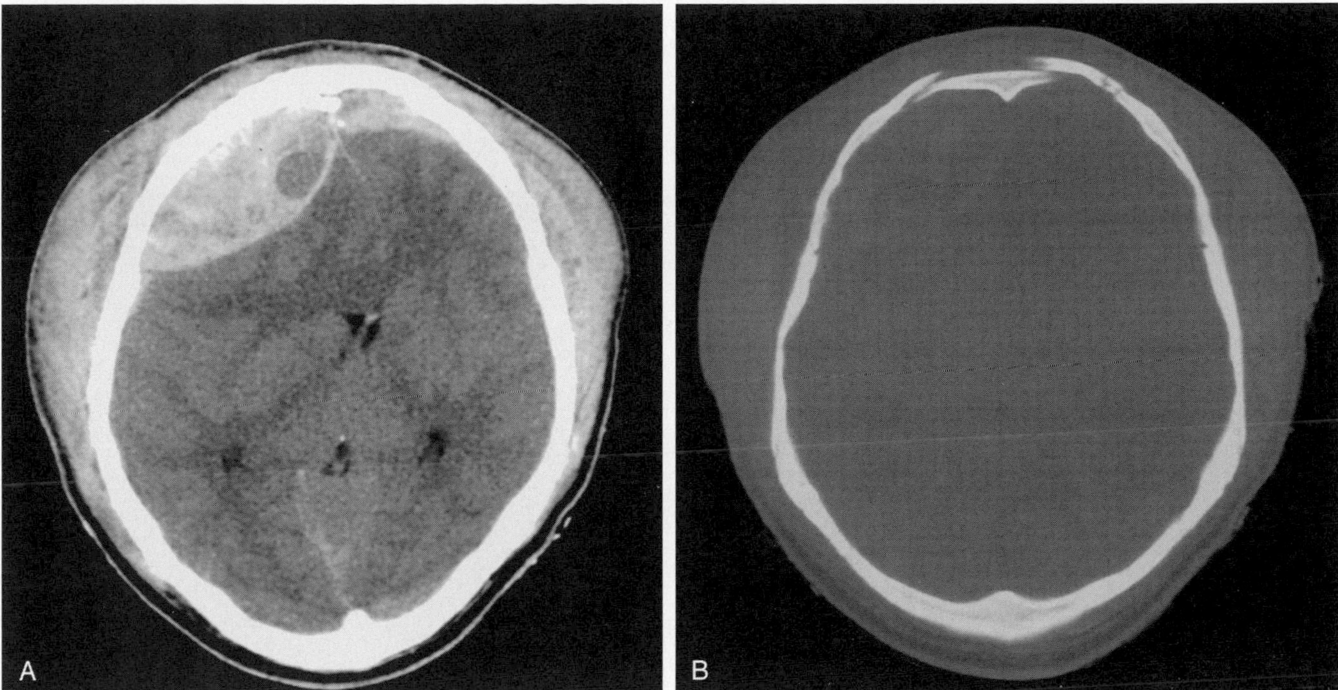

Figure 10–8. Active hemorrhage within an epidural hematoma. *A*, An acute epidural hematoma located predominantly in the right frontal region, with a biconvex configuration and considerable mass effect with subfalcine herniation. The hematoma is markedly larger then it was 2 hours earlier as seen on a previous study. The low-attenuation regions within the hematoma represent areas of unclotted blood (active hemorrhage). *B*, Image obtained using bone window settings at the same level as in *A* demonstrates a comminuted, depressed bifrontal skull fracture.

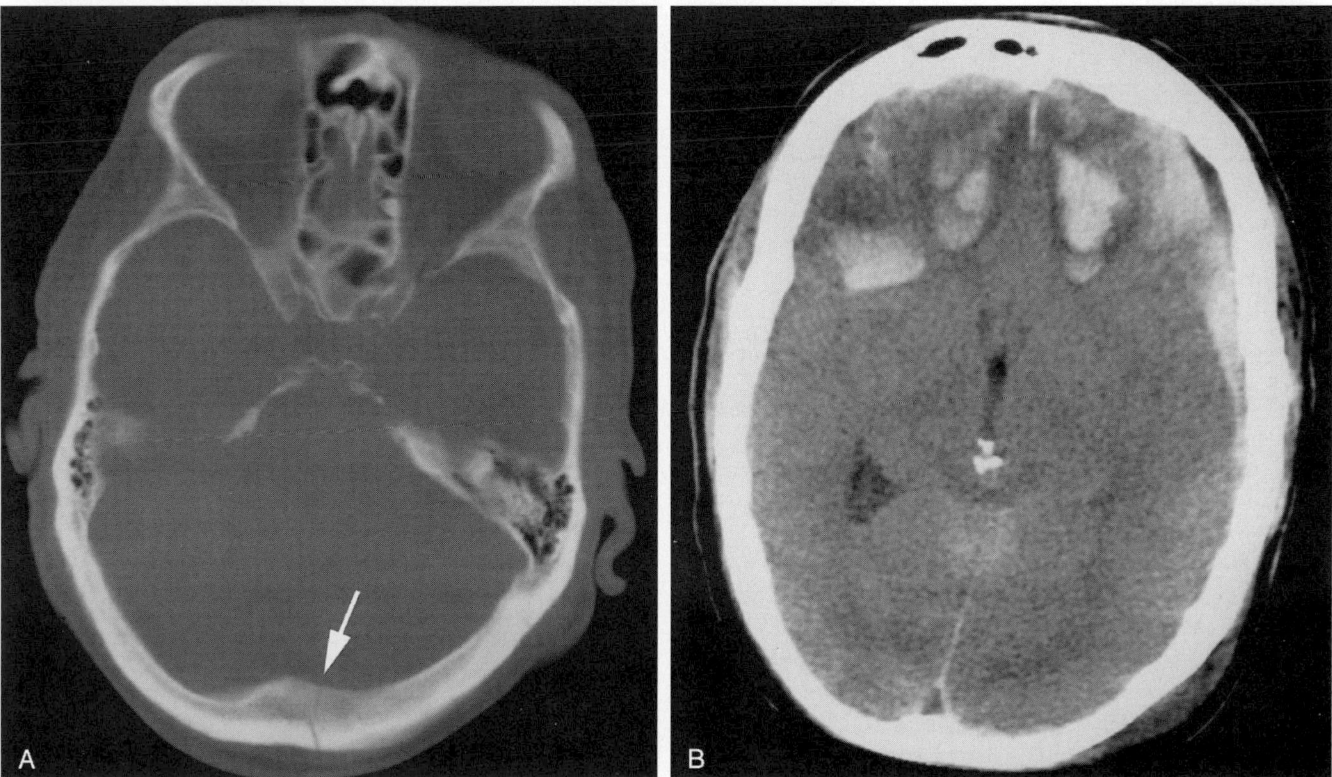

Figure 10–9. Occipital skull fracture with contre coup injury. *A*, CT reveals a nondisplaced occipital fracture (*arrow*). *B*, Image obtained using brain window settings at a slightly higher level than in *A* reveals a contre coup injury with bifrontal parenchymal hematomas and a left frontal subdural hemorrhage.

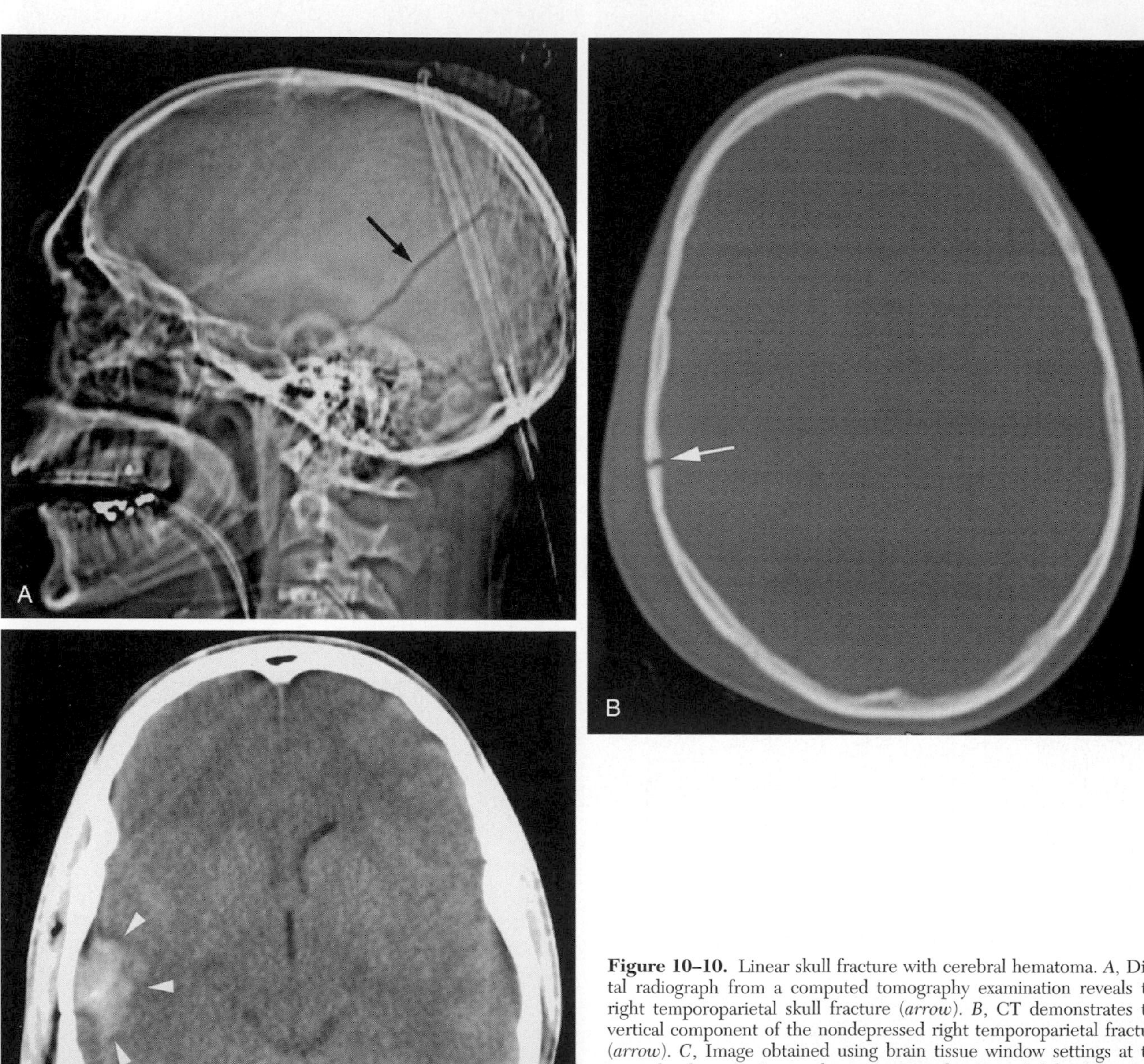

Figure 10–10. Linear skull fracture with cerebral hematoma. *A*, Digital radiograph from a computed tomography examination reveals the right temporoparietal skull fracture (*arrow*). *B*, CT demonstrates the vertical component of the nondepressed right temporoparietal fracture (*arrow*). *C*, Image obtained using brain tissue window settings at the same level as in *B* reveals an associated temporal lobe hematoma (*arrowheads*).

Short of a few such instances, the digital radiographs accompanying CT examinations are usually an acceptable alternative.

The number of radiographic projections obtained in the evaluation will depend upon the condition of the patient. If the patient is ambulatory, it may be possible to perform the radiologic examination with a standard skull radiographic unit in the upright position and with the patient sitting. Under these circumstances, the minimum radiographic projections required include anteroposterior, posteroanterior, both right and left lateral, and Towne's projections of the skull. These views should allow adequate visualization and localization of any fractures (Fig. 10–16). In addition, the pineal gland and choroid plexus calcifications are demonstrated and may serve as evidence of a significant mass lesion when these structures are displaced. However, caution should be exercised in evaluating for intracranial mass effects on skull radiography. A midline position of the pineal gland calcification does not exclude significant intracranial injury or mass effect, as bilateral mass lesions (e.g., subdural hemorrhages) may be present and prevent significant displacement (see Fig. 10–11).

In contradistinction to the ambulatory patient, the unconscious, severely injured patient requires significant modification in the radiographic examination. Initial radiographs should include a cross-table lateral, frontal, and Towne's projections with the patient in a supine position on a stretcher or radiographic table. The patient's head should never be manipulated until injury to the cervical spine and craniocervical junction has been excluded.

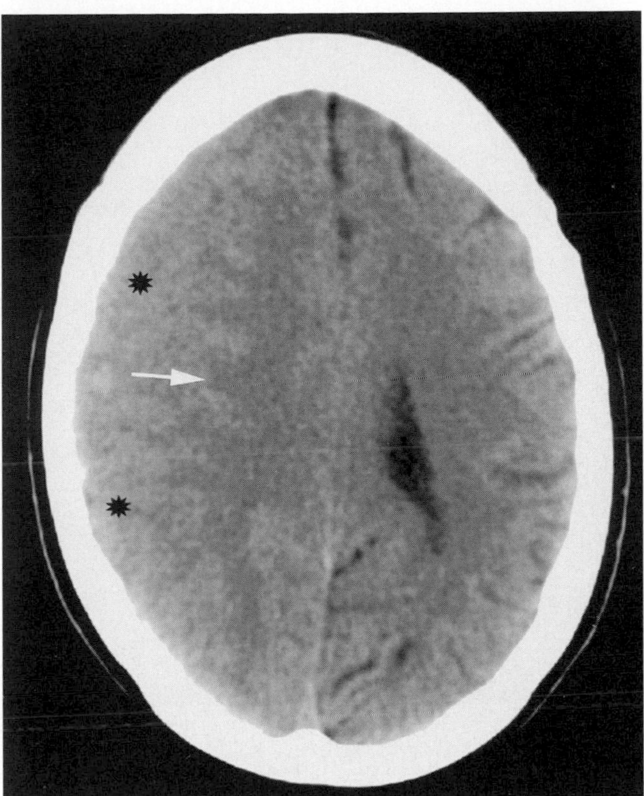

Figure 10–12. CT viewed with brain window settings reveals a right isodense subdural hematoma (*asterisks*). The patient had been involved in a bicycle accident 13 days earlier. There is considerable mass effect, with compression of the ipsilateral lateral ventricle, sulcal effacement, and inward displacement of the gray matter–white matter junction (*arrow*).

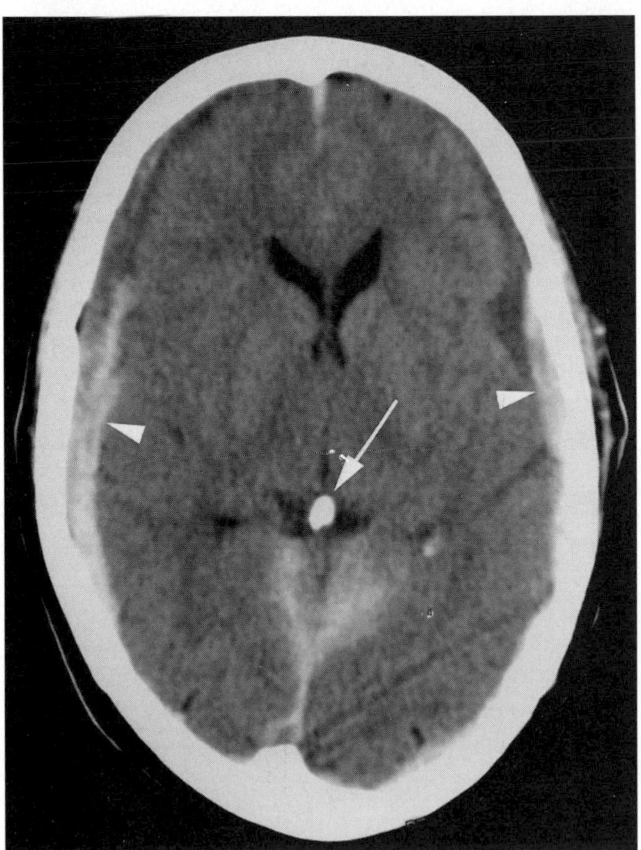

Figure 10–11. CT reveals bilateral subdural hematomas (*arrowheads*). Despite the size of the hemorrhages, their bilateral nature permits only minimal midline shift, with no significant displacement of the calcified pineal gland (*arrow*).

Magnetic Resonance Imaging

MRI provides an exquisitely detailed demonstration of cerebral anatomy and traumatic abnormalities* but poses problems in the initial evaluation of trauma that may preclude examination of the seriously injured or comatose patient.[71] Although a significant number of MRI-compatible life support devices (e.g., ventilation/monitoring systems) have become widely available, such compatibility still remains an issue with several surgical devices that often accompany trauma patients. The majority of MRI scanners are located remotely from the emergency department or intensive care unit; although, "open" bore scanners may become central to the emergency department in the future, increasing the utility of MRI in the setting of acute head injury. Technologic advances with stronger gradients have significantly reduced imaging times, but motion artifact and image quality remain limitations in the traumatized patient. Last, MRI poorly visualizes cortical bone compared with CT, and fractures are notoriously difficult to demonstrate (Fig. 10–17).

Text continued on page 286

*See references 55, 56, 60, 61, 63, 70, 71, 90, 95, 97, 99.

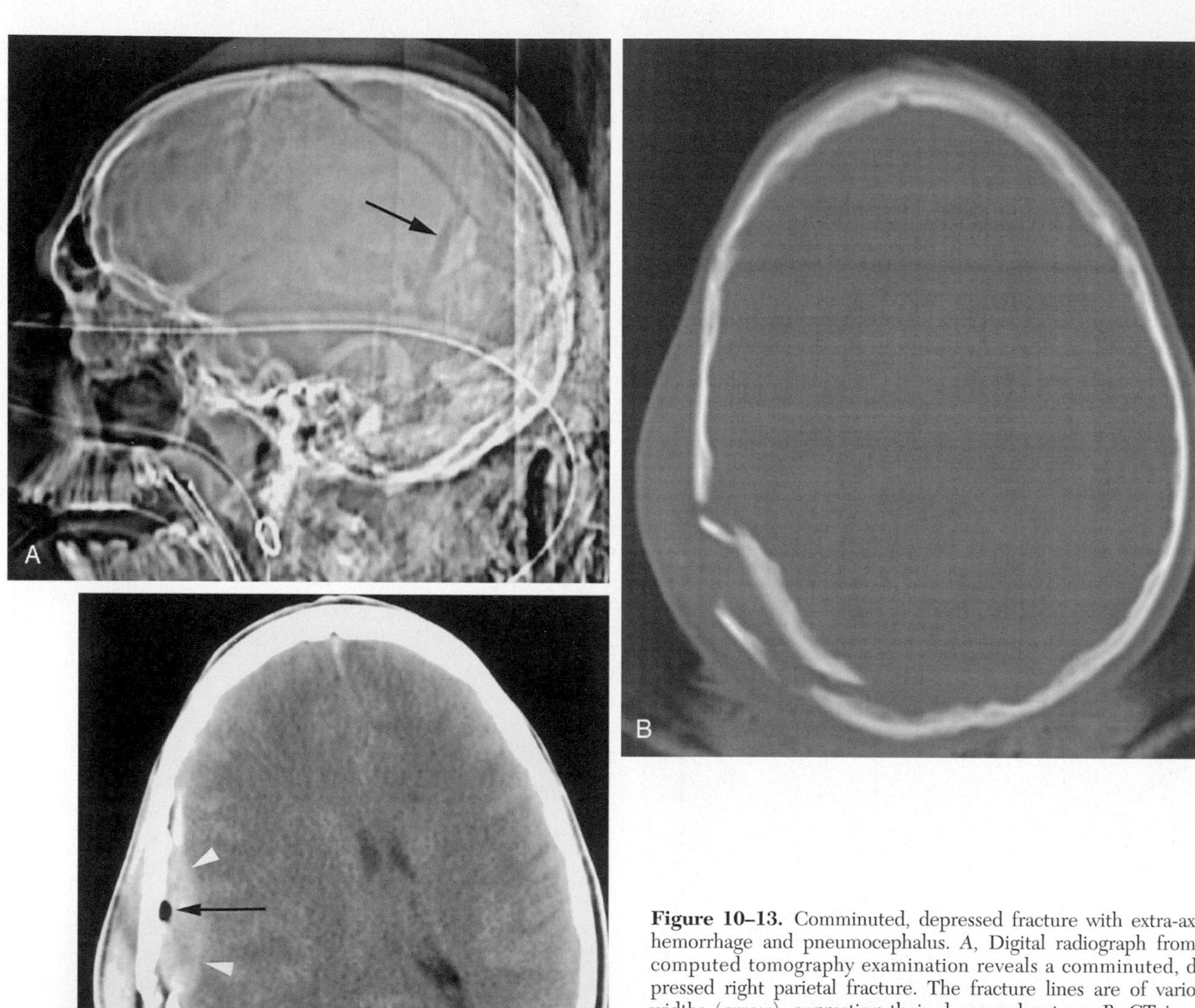

Figure 10–13. Comminuted, depressed fracture with extra-axial hemorrhage and pneumocephalus. *A*, Digital radiograph from a computed tomography examination reveals a comminuted, depressed right parietal fracture. The fracture lines are of various widths (*arrow*), suggesting their depressed nature. *B*, CT image confirms the depressed nauture of the fracture. *C*, Image obtained using brain window settings at the same level as in *B* reveals an associated extra-axial hemorrhage (*arrowheads*) and a small amount of pneumocephalus (*arrow*).

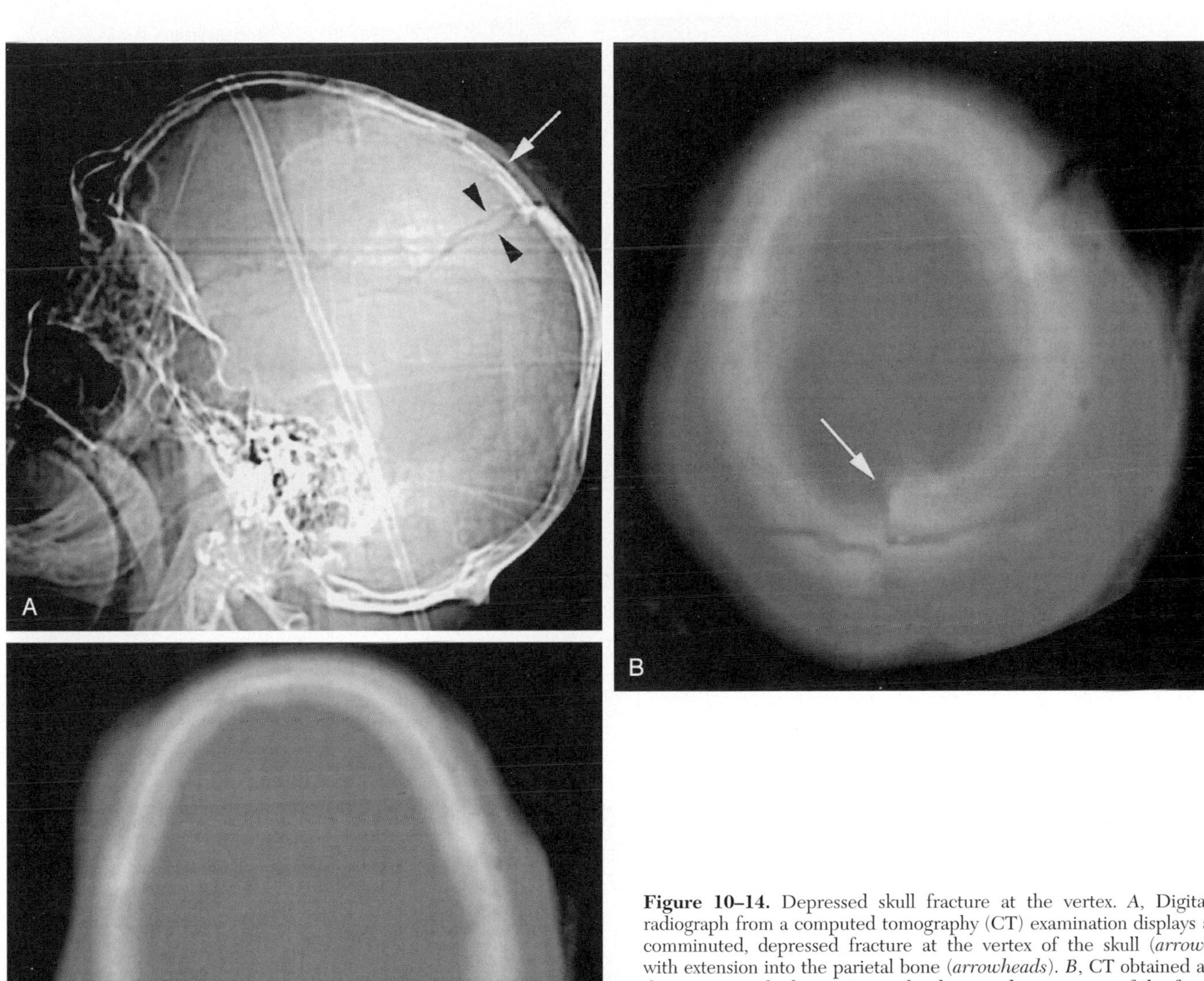

Figure 10–14. Depressed skull fracture at the vertex. *A*, Digital radiograph from a computed tomography (CT) examination displays a comminuted, depressed fracture at the vertex of the skull (*arrow*) with extension into the parietal bone (*arrowheads*). *B*, CT obtained at the vertex poorly demonstrates the depressed component of the fracture (*arrow*) when compared with the digital radiograph. *C*, CT obtained at a slightly lower level than in *B* confirms the bilateral parietal bone fractures (*arrows*).

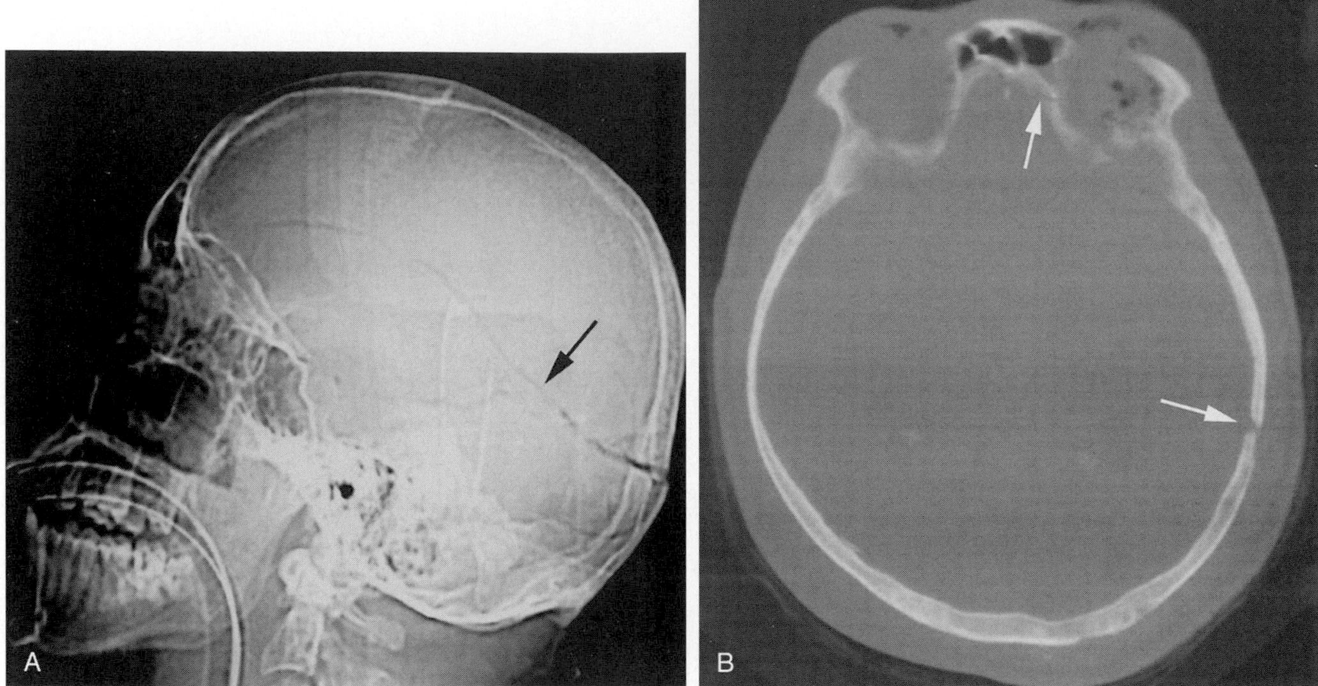

Figure 10–15. Comminuted left skull fracture oriented in the axial plane. *A*, Digital radiograph from a computed tomography examination clearly demonstrates a fracture (*arrow*) extending through the frontal, parietal, and occipital regions. *B*, CT demonstrates only a small component of the fracture (*arrows*), because the majority of the fracture lies within the axial imaging plane.

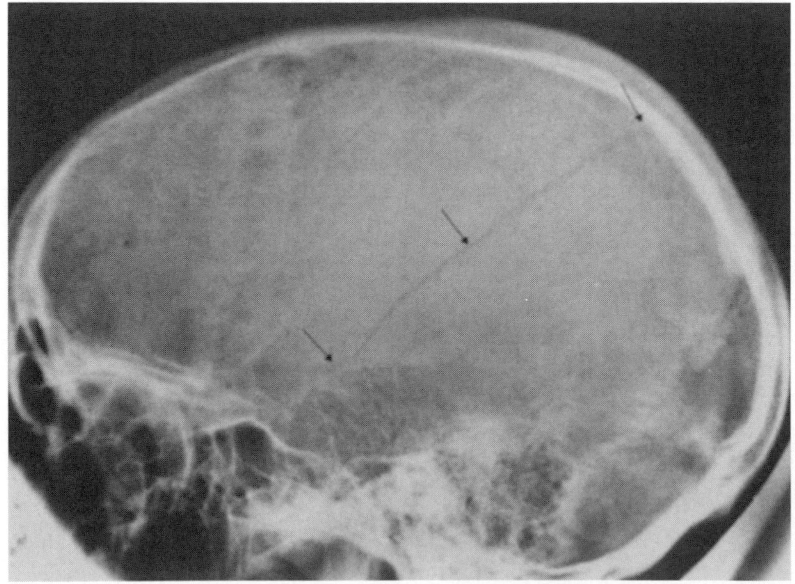

Figure 10–16. Linear fracture (*arrows*) and vascular grooves of the skull. The long linear fracture of the parietal and temporal bones appears as a single lucent line inferiorly, but more superiorly, two roughly parallel lines are visualized because of involvement of the outer and inner tables at slightly separate levels. Note that the fracture line is more lucent than are the vascular markings and cranial sutures.

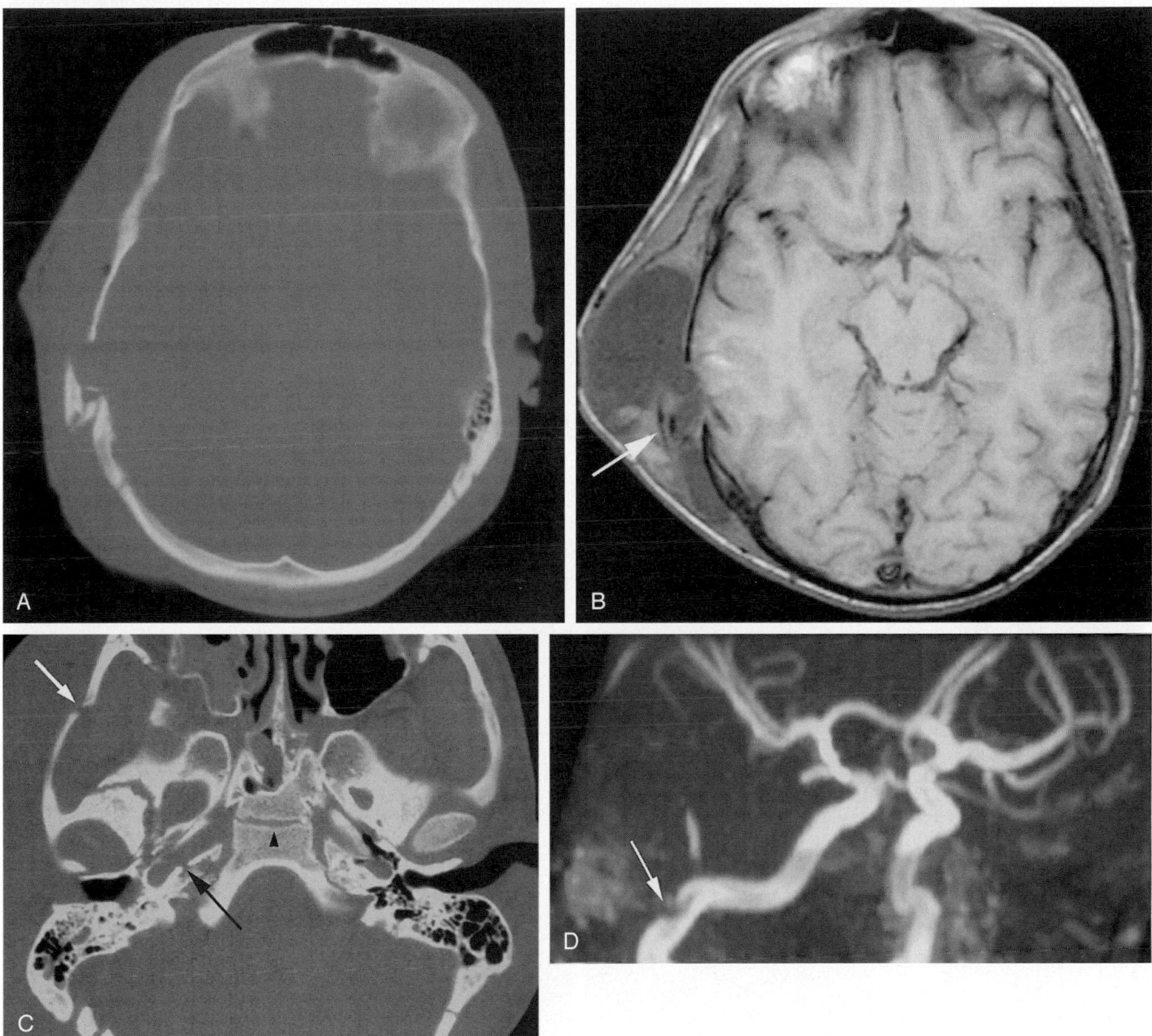

Figure 10–17. Comminuted temporal fracture with skull base extension and vascular injury in a 17-year-old boy involved in a motor vehicle accident. *A*, CT displays a comminuted right temporal bone fracture. *B*, T_1-weighted magnetic-resonance image obtained at a level comparable to that in *A* shows the displaced bone fragment (*arrow*), with soft tissue swelling and a scalp cerebrospinal fluid collection. *C*, CT obtained through the skull base demonstrates a fracture extending through the right zygomatic arch (*white arrow*), skull base, and the carotid canal (*black arrow*). The normal sphenoidal synchondrosis is illustrated (*arrowhead*). *D*, Attenuated flow with a focal dissection (*arrow*) is demonstrated within the petrous right internal carotid artery on this right anterior oblique projection image from a three-dimentional time-of-flight magnetic resonance angiogram.

Although MRI is an excellent means of evaluating the subacute and late effects of intracranial injury, at present its use as an emergency procedure in the evaluation of the acutely injured patient is limited. MRI does demonstrate intra-axial lesions with great clarity. These lesions have been classified as diffuse axonal injury (DAI) at the gray matter at white matter interface, cortical contusions, subcortical gray matter injury, and primary brain stem injury.[60] Of these, DAI is the most common (accounting for 48% of intra-axial lesions), followed closely by cortical contusion (accounting for 44%). Gradient echo imaging is associated with increased susceptibility to calcification and products of hemorrhage, allowing increased conspicuity of DAI lesions secondary to the "blooming" effect of the blood products (Fig. 10–18). Magnetic resonance arteriography and venography are beneficial in evaluating the integrity of and injury to the vasculature in fractures involving the skull base and those crossing cranial sutures (see Fig. 10–17).

Indirect Radiographic and Computed Tomographic Signs of Cranial and Intracranial Injuries

Indirect evidence of cranial injury consists of scalp soft tissue swelling overlying the cranium (Fig. 10–19); opacification or air-fluid levels within the sinuses or mastoid air cells (see Fig. 10–39), suggesting the presence of hemorrhage and implying a fracture in these structures; and pneumocephalus (Fig. 10–20; see also Fig. 10–44), indicating direct communication of the cranial contents with the exterior through a paranasal sinus or mastoid air cell. In some cases, air may be seen to extend directly to the outside through the external auditory canal or through the eustachian tube into the nasopharynx.

When a fracture line is not immediately obvious, attention may be directed to it by the presence of overlying soft tissue swelling or hematoma. This abnormality is usually apparent on the soft tissue window displays of the CT examination but is less obvious on the bone window display or on a skull radiograph. Opacification of the paranasal sinuses is particularly meaningful in the case of fractures involving the ethmoid and sphenoid sinuses.[117, 118] It is unlikely that either the ethmoid or the sphenoid sinuses will be completely opacified just from intranasal hemorrhage associated with a nasal fracture, facial fracture, or contusion. Opacification of these sinuses is more likely to be the result of a fracture involving one or more of the sinus walls. In contradistinction, the maxillary sinuses may fill with fluid simply from rhinorrhea or nasal hemorrhage of any cause (including nasal intubation). Therefore, opacification in the maxillary antrum is not a reliable indication of maxillary fracture.

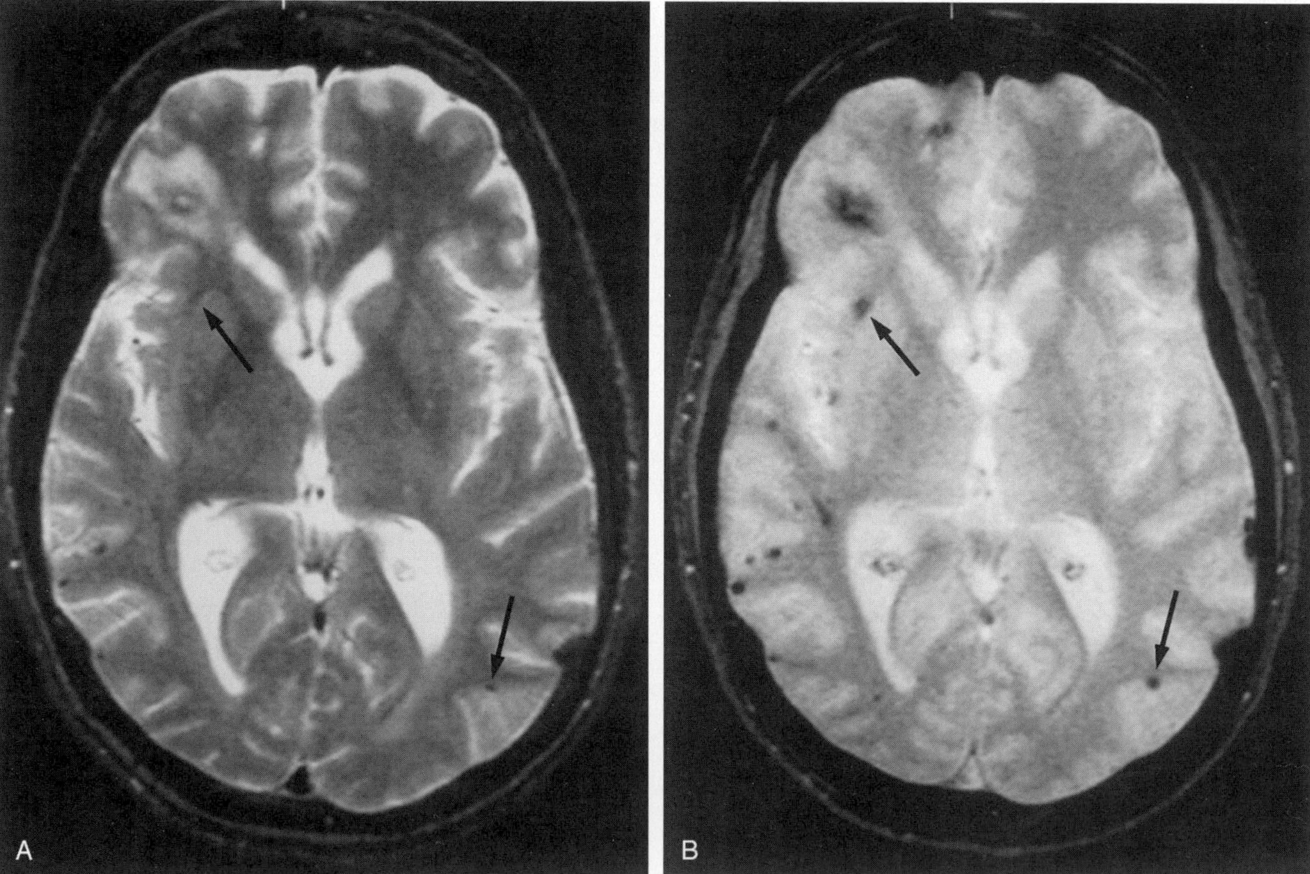

Figure 10–18. Diffuse axonal injury. *A*, Spin-echo T_2-weighted image shows an area of edema and contusion within the right frontal lobe and a few subtle areas of hypointensity at the gray matter–white matter junction (*arrows*), the degree of injury being greater on the right than on the left. *B*, The hypointensities (*arrows*) identified on the spin echo T_2-weighted image are much more obvious on a gradient-echo T_2-weighted image obtained at the same level as in *A*, secondary to the "blooming" effect of blood products.

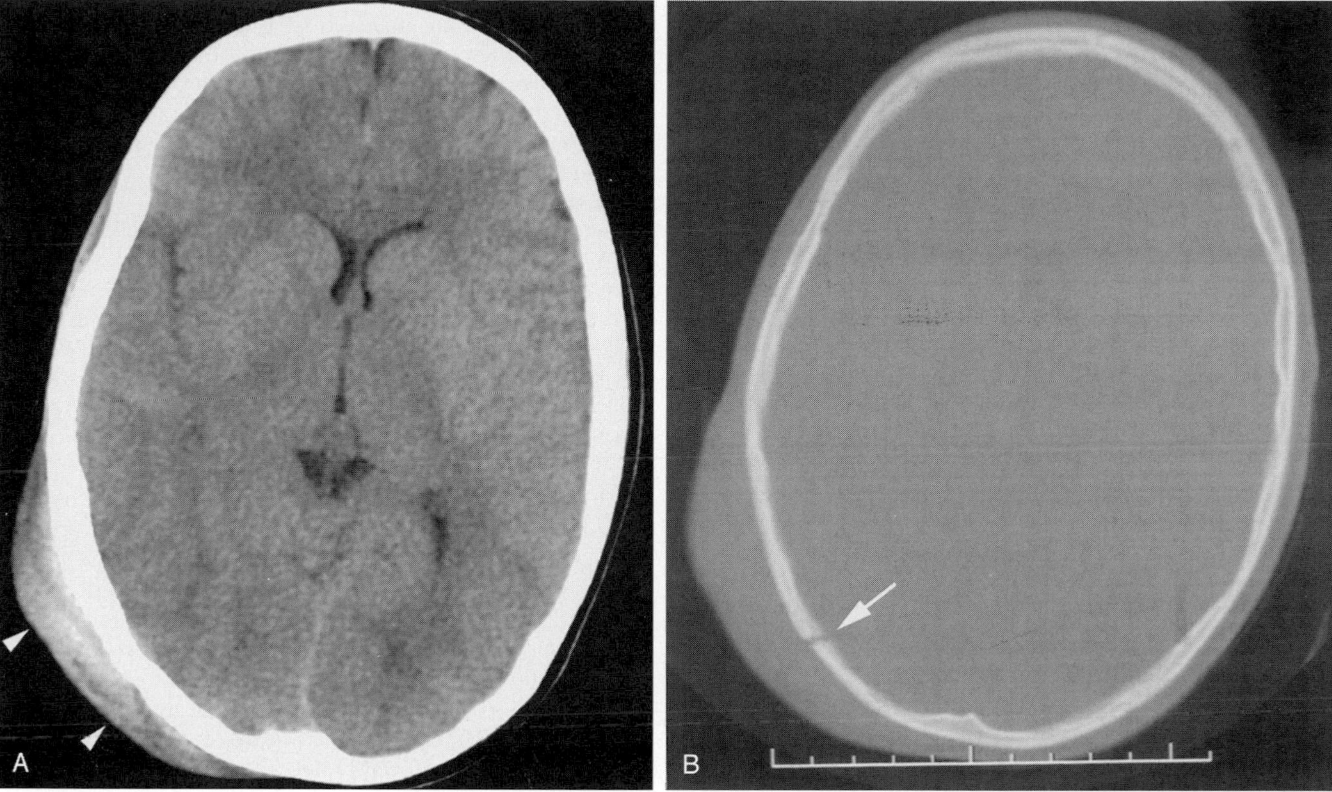

Figure 10–19. Soft tissue swelling and fracture without intracranial injury. *A*, CT reveals soft tissue swelling (*arrowheads*) over the right parietal region but no intracranial injury. *B*, Image obtained using bone window settings at the same level as in *A* reveals a nondisplaced right parietal skull fracture (*arrow*).

Pneumocephalus may be found within the subarachnoid space with air outlining the cerebral sulci (see Fig. 10–20), the ventricular system (see Fig. 10–20), or more frequently the basal cisterns about the sella turcica, and occasionally in extra-axial fluid collections on CT (see Fig. 10–13).[142, 146, 148] The anatomic distribution of the air does not allow a specific designation of its point of origin; it simply indicates that an open injury exists. CT is much more sensitive to the detection of pneumocephalus than is plain radiography, with as little as 0.5 mL of air identifiable on CT images.[158] The air usually congregates adjacent or in close proximity to an underlying fracture.

CT has the distinct advantage of directly demonstrating intracranial injury, whereas there is no direct evidence of intracranial injury on a skull radiograph. Skull radiography is no substitute for CT in the evaluation of intracranial injury, but on occasion, indirect signs of intracranial injury are apparent on skull radiographs. Indirect radiographic evidence of intracranial injury includes shifts in the calcified pineal gland or choroid plexus. However, calcification of the pineal gland and choroid plexus varies with age, and asymmetry of choroid plexus size and location is common. Although CT has relegated skull radiography to a place of merely historical interest in the evaluation of intracranial lesions, pineal calcification shifts of greater than 2 mm are considered significant for the presence of a mass lesion. Unfortunately, the detection of pineal calcification shift is somewhat unreliable owing to head rotation. In addition, a small number of subdural hemorrhages will be bilateral, with balanced mass effect on the cerebral hemispheres negating any midline shift of the pineal gland.

The most important observation, with immediate surgical implications, is the presence of a depressed fracture, because approximately one third of these are associated with dural tears and must be repaired. The importance of identifying a foreign body is obvious. Pneumocephalus signifies the presence of an open injury and is an indication for prophylactic administration of antibiotics but does not imply the necessity for immediate surgery. Fortunately, most of these open injuries heal spontaneously, and surgical treatment is not required.

Fractures of the Calvaria

Linear fractures account for approximately 80% of all skull fractures. Diastatic fractures (i.e., traumatic splitting of the sutures) account for 5% and are usually merely extensions of a linear fracture. The remaining 15% of skull fractures are depressed.

Linear Fractures

Linear fractures present as fine, lucent lines having sharp margins without sclerosis on skull radiographs (see Figs. 10–10 and 10–16). Some fractures are short, as short as even 1 cm; they usually occur in the thin bones, particularly on either side of the squamosal suture, and

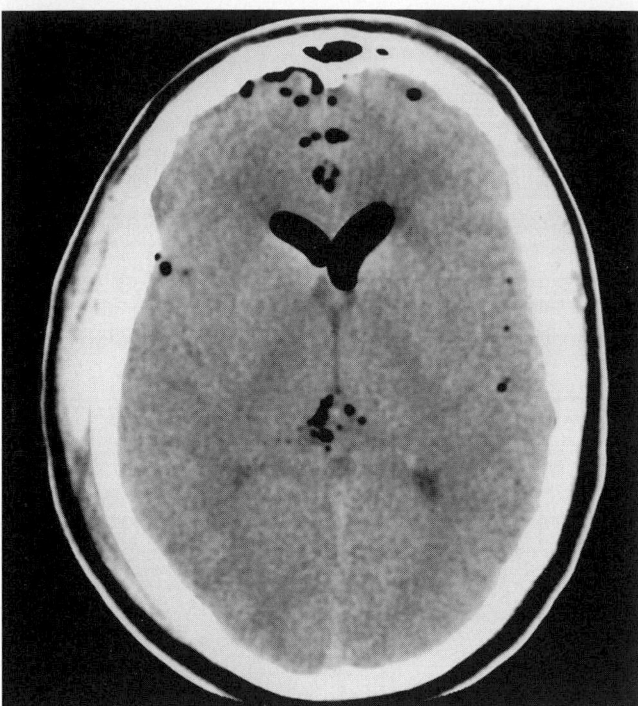

Figure 10–20. Axial computed tomography image viewed with brain window settings demonstrates extensive pneumocephalus, with intraventricular and subarachnoid air. The patient had sustained a skull base fracture (not shown).

are often overlooked. More often, fracture lines are several centimeters in length, and frequently their entire length cannot be determined, particularly in the case of vertically oriented fractures that disappear into the dense structures of the skull base. A linear fracture is somewhat irregular when it changes course significantly. It is more likely to form an angle than a smooth, gentle curve. The fracture line crosses vascular grooves and sutures and does not branch. The lucency is formed by the superimposition of fracture lines involving both the inner and outer tables of the skull.

Linear fractures present on CT images as linear radiolucencies disrupting both the inner and outer tables (see Figs 10–9 and 10–19). Vertically oriented fractures run perpendicular to the plane of the axial section and are readily demonstrated (see Fig. 10–10), whereas the more common horizontally oriented fractures lying within the plane of the axial section may be obscured by volume averaging (see Fig. 10–15). However, most of these fractures will be apparent on digital scout radiographs accompanying the CT examination.

In some cases it is quite difficult to differentiate between a linear fracture and a vascular groove[101–103] on a skull film or digital radiograph obtained at CT examination. The fracture is more lucent than a vascular groove because it involves both the inner and outer tables of the skull, whereas a vascular groove consists of an impression of varying depth on either the inner or the outer table. The distinction is easily made on CT examination when the depth of the groove is sufficient to be visualized, but usually a vascular impression is of insufficient depth to be identified with certainty.

The impressions made by the meningeal arteries on the inner table and those made by the superficial arterial branches on the outer table of the temporal and frontal bones are particularly confusing. In general, these branches have predictable location, are less radiolucent because they involve only a portion of one table, have a fine sclerotic margin, and frequently branch. The grooves created by the diploic veins are usually relatively wide and tortuous, have a distinct sclerotic margin, and taper rather abruptly, so that they are readily differentiated from fractures on plain films. The diploic veins within the parietal bone may be particularly bothersome, with a stellate appearance, but these dilemmas are easily resolved with CT, by which the lucencies are shown to reside within the diploë and the adjacent inner and outer tables of the skull are intact.

Cranial sutures and developmental fissures within the cranial bones may also be mistaken for fractures. A basic understanding of the sutural anatomy is essential before interpretation of radiographs of the skull is undertaken. The problem is particularly evident in young children in whom numerous variations and normal sutures and fissures are encountered within or about the occipital bone. Sutures have a characteristic serpentine appearance with sclerotic edges (Fig. 10–21). Sutures and developmental fissures are almost always bilateral, with the exception of the sagittal and metopic sutures; therefore, comparison with the opposite side is most helpful.

The developmental anatomy of the occiput is rather complex, and during the course of development, numerous fissures and sutures appear.[4] Mendosal sutures are commonly encountered in the neonatal skull. These are oblique sutures extending from within the occipital bone to the lambdoid suture in the region of the asterion, the junction of the squamosal, lambdoidal, and occipitomastoid sutures. The mendosal sutures are frequently bilateral and may persist into adult life. Lateral fissures extending from the posterior margin of the foramen magnum are frequent. Occipital fissures represent another developmental variation presenting as a parasagittal lucency extending from just lateral to the posterior portion of the foramen magnum into the occipital bone. There is often a similar lucency on the contralateral side. Fortunately, most of the developmental structures are paired and can be identified on the contralateral side. The sphenoidal synchondrosis (see Fig. 10–17) extends roughly perpendicular to the clivus and should present no diagnostic problem.

Occasional difficulty is encountered in distinguishing recent from old fractures, similar to the problem in differentiating old fractures from vascular channels on skull radiographs. In children, simple fractures usually heal in time, whereas in adults, they may remain visible for months or even years. As a fracture line heals, it becomes less distinct, and its margin shows a smoothness or rounding that may allow it to be distinguished from a recent fracture. In some cases in adults, because of the lack of healing, it may be impossible to make a radiographic distinction between a recent and an old fracture; the distinction must be based on the physical examination and history. The margins of a craniotomy flap may present

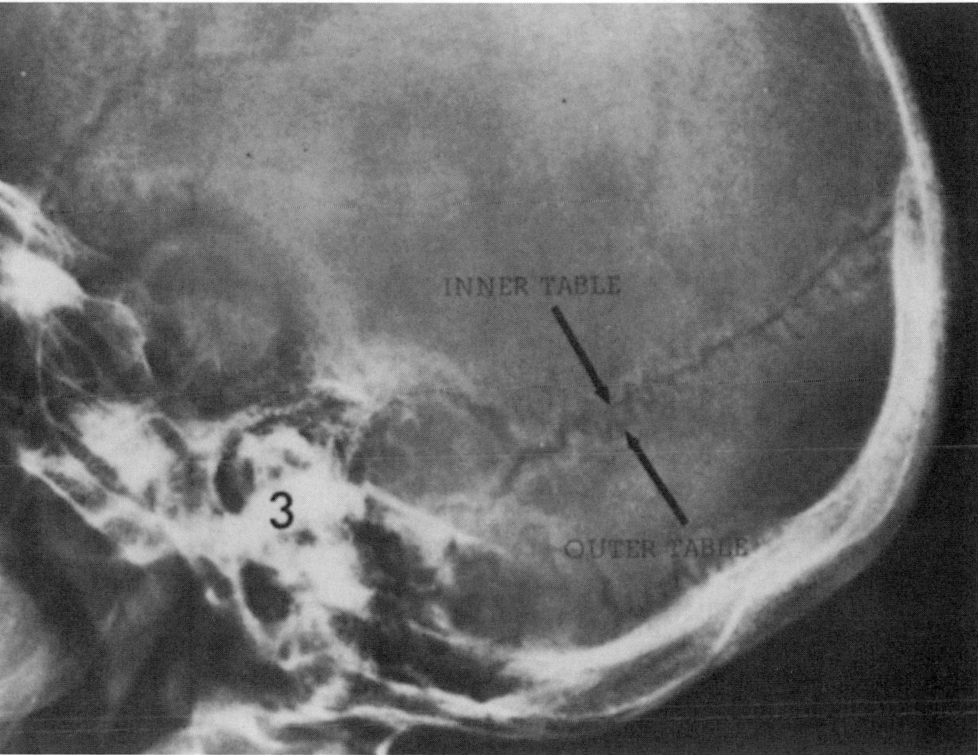

Figure 10–21. Interdigitation of lambdoid suture. Note the wavy contour of the outer margin of the suture and the linear course of the suture on the inner table (*arrows*). The latter could be mistaken for a fracture line. (Case courtesy of J. Powell Williams, MD, Mobile, Ala.)

similar difficulties. These are usually accompanied by burr holes and should present less of a problem.

Various artifactual densities may be confused with fractures on plain radiographs of the skull but pose no problems in CT. Chief among these is air trapped within a scalp laceration. Such lucencies are usually wider than fracture lines. If there is any question of their identity, the examination can be repeated following closure of the laceration, which usually eliminates the lucency. Hair braids, bandages, and straps or bands placed on the head for immobilization at times may result in a lucent appearance, suggesting fracture, or in radiodensity, suggesting the possibility of depressed fragments. These entities are usually identified on only a single view, and if there is any question, the troublesome projection should be repeated.

Diastatic Fractures

Diastatic fractures are the result of traumatic widening of a cranial suture and account for approximately 5% of all cranial fractures.[18, 23, 66, 93] These fractures are usually associated with and represent an extension of a linear fracture of the skull (Fig. 10–22), although they may be seen with elevated intracranial pressures resulting in "splitting" of the sutures.[35] These fractures most frequently involve the lambdoid and less frequently the sagittal sutures (Fig 10–23) and are usually found in younger persons before closure of the intracranial sutures. At times the diagnosis may be difficult, but if the sutures are separated by more than 2 mm and are clearly asymmetrical, the diagnosis is reasonably certain. Depression of the diastatic fracture is uncommon.

Multiple and Comminuted Fractures

Occasionally the skull may sustain multiple linear fractures in various positions, often two linear fractures on opposite sides of the skull. Correct localization of these fractures may be difficult on plain radiographs but poses no difficulty on the CT examination (see Fig. 10–14). Comminuted fractures are usually stellate, or the fracture lines form a mosaic in the involved portion of the skull. They are almost always depressed to some extent as demonstrated on CT images or a skull radiograph obtained tangential to the area in question. In children, multiple and comminuted fractures are more often a result of abuse or nonaccidental trauma.[37, 39]

Depressed Fractures

Depressed fractures are the result of impact by a small mass of high velocity, such as a direct blow with a hammer, and are almost always located within the cranial vault.[18, 23, 67] The depression may involve a single fragment, but usually there are several fragments forming a mosaic that is angulated inward (see Figs. 10–13 and 10–14). On plain films and digital radiographs the fracture lines between the fragments appear as lucencies of varying widths (see Fig. 10–13), usually wider than those associated with a linear fracture because of the displacement. The displacement and angulation of the fragments may result in an increase in bone density, as the fragments are seen obliquely or on end. In the evaluation of head injuries, all areas of increased density projected within the skull on plain or digital radiographs should be suspect, and appropriate views must be obtained to exclude the possibility of a depressed fracture.

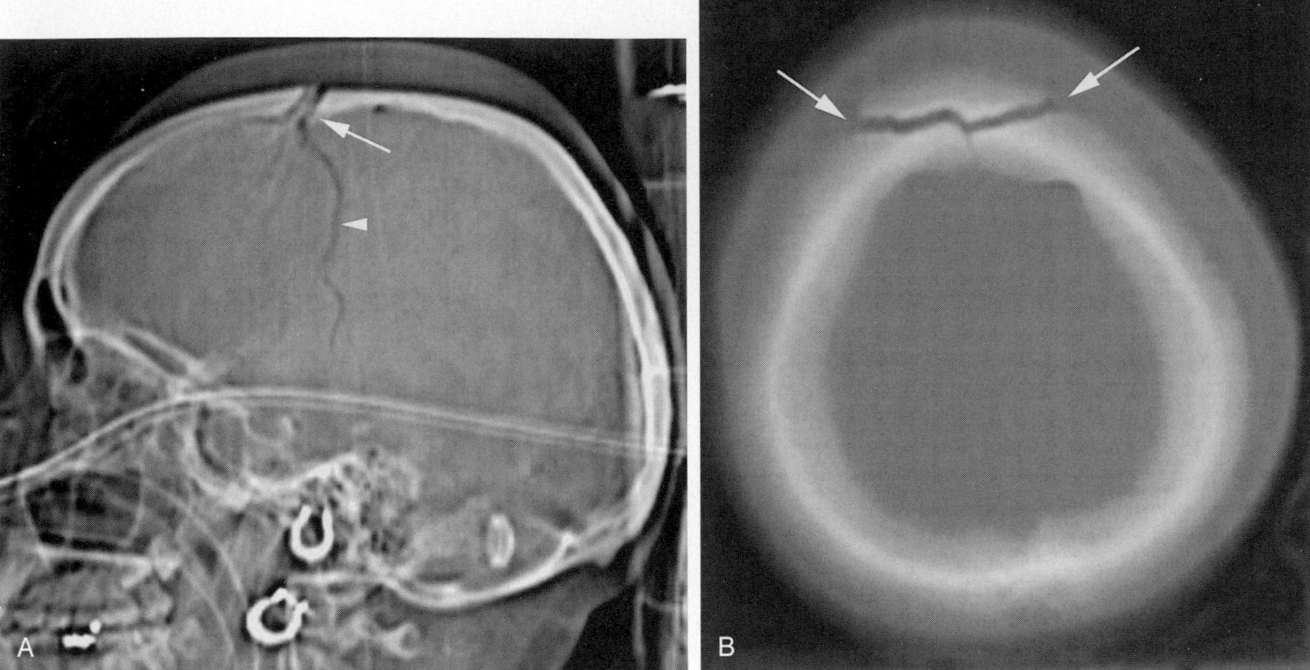

Figure 10–22. Diastasis of the coronal suture in a 36-year-old-woman involved in a motor vehicle accident. *A*, Digital radiograph from a computed tomography examination reveals a linear fracture of the parietal bone (*arrowhead*) with extension into and diastasis of the coronal suture (*arrow*). *B*, Axial image from computed tomography study obtained near the vertex of the skull illustrates the diastatic coronal sutures (*arrows*).

Approximately one third of depressed fragments are associated with dural tears that require surgical repair. The probability of a dural tear is related to the depth of the displacement of the fragments. The usual indication for repair is displacement of 5 mm or more or depression beyond the inner table.[23] CT is the modality of choice for evaluating suspected depressed skull fractures, as it can provide information regarding the depth of fracture displacement and assess for concurrent intracranial abnormalities. Most depressed skull fractures lie laterally in the frontoparietal region or, less commonly, anteriorly about the frontal sinuses. Most are tangential or perpendicular to the plane of an axial CT section and are well demonstrated by this method (see Fig. 10–13). Less commonly, depressed fractures occur at the vertex in and about the sagittal suture, parallel to the axial plane, and are difficult to visualize on CT (see Fig. 10–14). These are better demonstrated on images obtained in the coronal plane with the patient either in the hanging head position or in the supine position with the neck flexed and the CT gantry angulated, or with coronal reconstruction images of the axial data.

A unique variety of depressed skull fracture is the *orbital blow-in fracture* (Fig. 10–24). These fractures result from a sudden, extreme rise in the intracranial pressure associated with a shear strain injury to the temporal region.[49, 88] The rapid rise in intracranial pressure is decompressed through fracture and depression of the orbital roofs into the orbit.[49, 88] Long-term complications of orbital blow-in fractures include herniation of brain tissue into the defect (encephaloceles), pulsatile proptosis,[49] cerebrospinal fluid rhinorrhea, and pneumocephalus.[81] It may be difficult to appreciate this type of fracture on either skull radiographs or CT images acquired in the axial plane; these fractures are best demonstrated with thin-section coronal CT images. Patients involved in trauma are often unable to undergo direct coronal CT imaging, and reconstructed images in the coronal plane will usually be adequate at characterizing these fractures.

There is one exception to the rule that all depressed fractures are comminuted. The skull may sustain a depression without an associated overt fracture; this type of fracture is usually seen in newborns and very young children, in whom the skull is very soft and pliable[4] (Figs. 10–25 and 10–26). This has been termed a "ping-pong fracture" because it mimics the indentation that can be produced by the fingers in a Ping-Pong ball. These fractures are at times difficult to visualize when seen in *en face* projections because of the large area involved and the relatively small degree of associated depression. They may be visualized on CT images or in profile on skull radiographs, and because they usually involve the lateral aspects of the skull, they are usually visualized in the frontal projection.

Depressed fractures are three and one-half times more common in children than in adults.[38, 42] This increased frequency is explained by the relative plasticity of the skull under the age of 10 years. A depressed fracture of the fetal skull in utero has been reported.[30] Spontaneous reduction of closed, depressed skull fractures occasionally occurs in children.[32] Because of the plasticity of the young skull, iatrogenic depressions of the cranial vault also have been described—for instance, from the use of head clamps in immobilizing infants for skull radiography.[40] Localized depressions of the skull have been described in the neonate without associated trauma,[33, 34] presumably

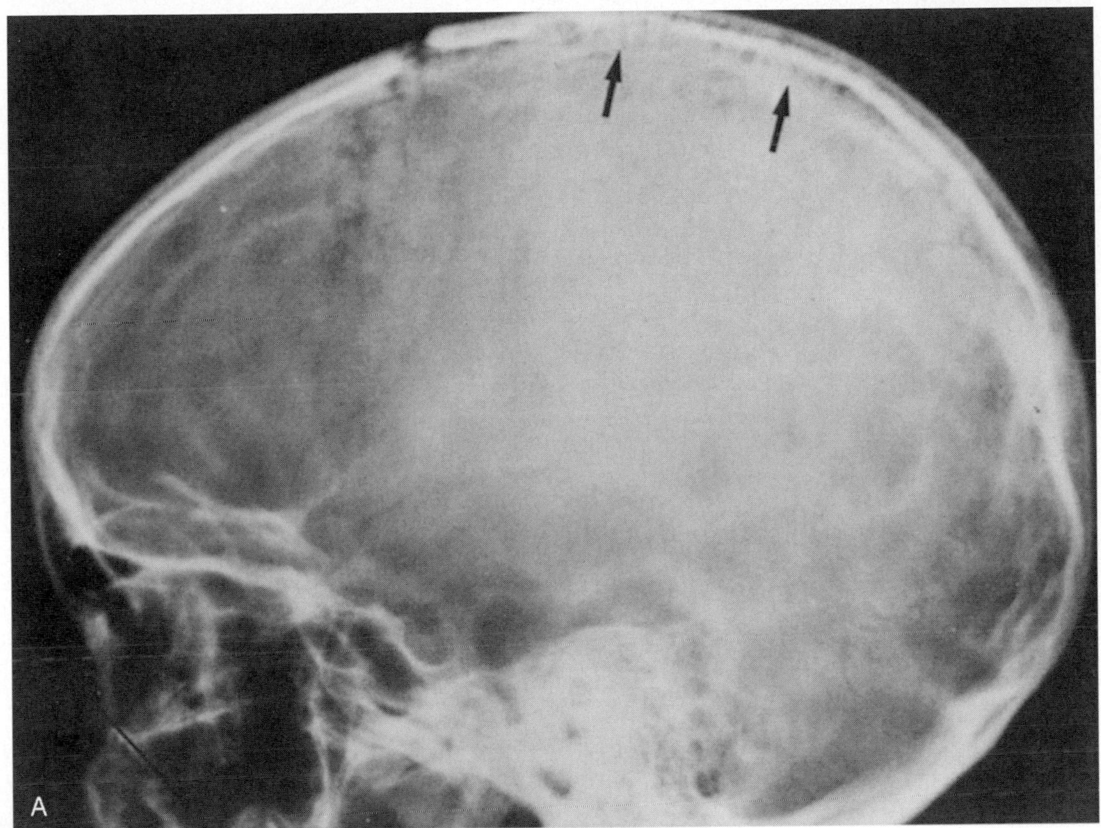

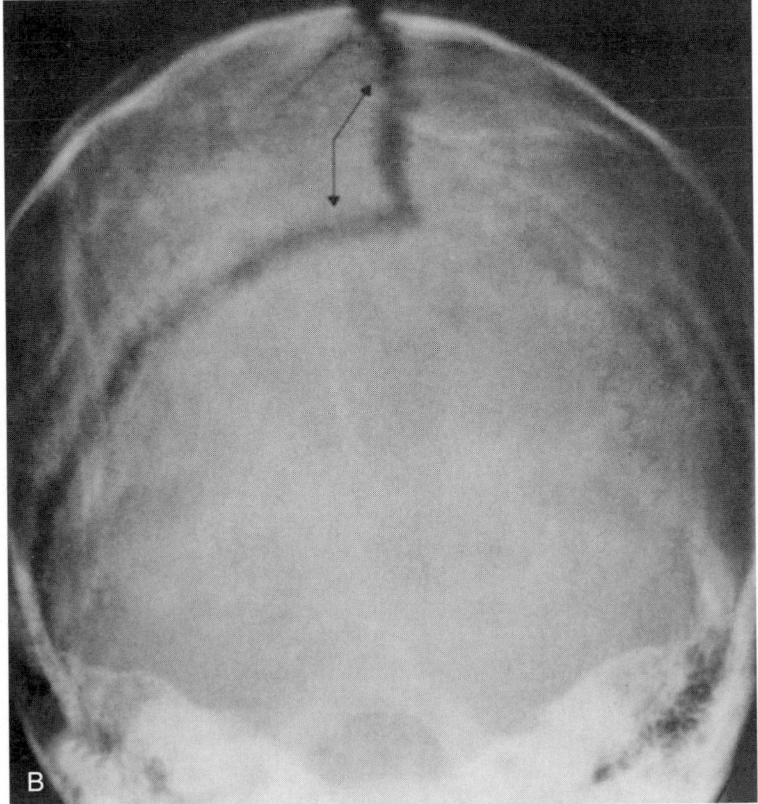

Figure 10–23. Diastasis of the sagittal and coronal sutures in a 9-year-old girl. *A*, Lateral view of the skull demonstrates irregularities at the vertex (*arrows*) and gap at the junction of the coronal and sagittal sutures. There is only a suggestion of widening of the coronal suture. *B*, Towne's view clearly demonstrates widening of the sagittal and right coronal sutures (*arrows*).

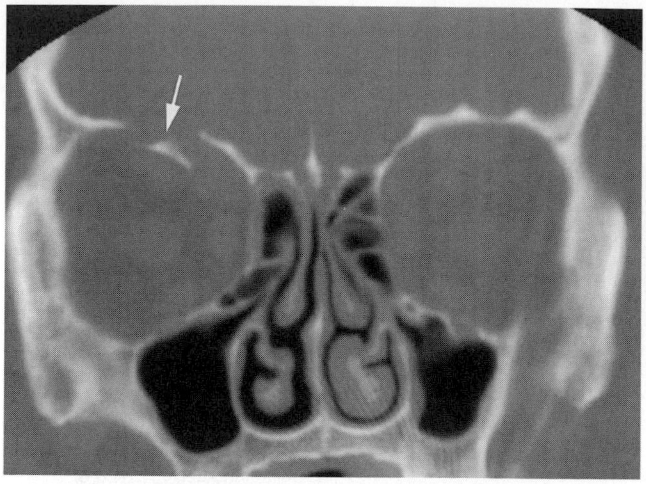

Figure 10–24. Orbital "blow-in" fracture. Coronal computed tomography image reveals a depressed fracture of the anterior cranial fossa floor (*arrow*), with displacement of the fracture fragment into the upper orbit.

caused by pressure of the fetal skull on a bony prominence, such as the sacral promontory, pubic rami, or some form of pelvic deformity, and, less probably by a uterine fibroid or a hand or foot of the fetus. These have been called "congenital intrauterine depressed skull fractures"[24] but are probably better termed *intrauterine moldings* of the skull. They may resolve spontaneously without complication. CT of the head would be helpful to exclude the presence of an underlying hematoma or cortical abnormality, but these problems are unlikely in the absence of trauma.

Foreign Bodies

Most foreign bodies within the cranium are the result of gunshot wounds. The site of entrance, course, and site of exit, if any, of the missile are easily identified by the metallic fragments left along the bullet track (Fig. 10–27). Bone fragments are carried into the wound beneath the site of entrance for various distances along the track and can also be identified (see Fig. 10–27). The entry and exit sites can normally be determined by analyzing the defects within the calvaria. The inner table is beveled at the entry site, whereas the outer table is beveled at the exit site (see Fig. 10–27).[105] The exit site is usually larger and associated with a greater degree of bone destruction.[105] It cannot be presumed that because a bullet fragment is visualized on plain or digital skull radiographs that it necessarily lies within the cranium (Fig. 10–28). On occasion a bullet of very low velocity will only penetrate the skin and pass beneath the scalp or into the subgaleal tissues for a variable distance around the skull. In such a case, although the bullet fragment is identified, there is no associated skull fracture. Rarely, a penetrating object such as a knife blade or possibly a nail may have penetrated the skull and then broken off or removed without leaving any visible external evidence except a soft tissue wound (Fig. 10–29). Records of such oddities are usually found in the files of larger teaching institutions. They are as infrequent as they are amazing.

Wooden foreign bodies pose a particular dilemma in the evaluation of intracranial injury. Plain radiographs of the skull are often normal, and wood has a strikingly low attenuation value on CT when displayed at the standard soft tissue windows and may mimic intracranial air.[104] However, when viewed with bone window settings, these foreign bodies are easily differentiated from intracranial air and possess a characteristic striated appearance (Fig. 10–30).[104] Identification of these and other foreign bodies is vitally important, as a strong association exists with infection and abscess formation.[106]

Fractures of the Frontal, Ethmoid, and Sphenoid Sinuses

Problems in identifying and managing fractures of the frontal, ethmoid, and sphenoid sinuses are inextricably bound up with problems related to basal skull fractures in general, cerebrospinal fluid rhinorrhea, and pneumocephalus. Each of these is discussed in a separate section later in this chapter.

Fractures of the frontal sinus are easily demonstrated on skull radiographs, but direct visualization of sphenoid and ethmoid fractures is exceedingly difficult. The latter are generally easily identified with thin-section (2- to 3-mm-thick slices) CT imaging in the axial projection. Additional information can be obtained with either direct coronal CT imaging or coronal reconstructions of the axial acquisition. As a result, CT has largely replaced skull radiography in the evaluation of suspected sinus fractures. On either plain films or CT scans, the indirect signs of fracture consist of opacification and the presence of air-fluid levels within the sinuses (see Fig. 10–39). At times the fracture line is very thin and nondisplaced and may be overlooked. In such cases, opacification of the sinuses and occasionally pneumocephalus alert the radiologist to the possibility of fractures. Small bubbles of air may also be identified in epidural and subdural hematomas adjacent to fractures of the frontal and ethmoid sinuses.

Fractures involving the sphenoid and ethmoid sinuses are often extensions of linear fractures of the vault. While experimentally creating linear fractures of the cranial vault in the parietal area, Gurdjian and coworkers[67] noted that these fractures were at times associated with separate fractures across the floor of the anterior fossa (Fig. 10–31). The bone that forms the floor of the anterior fossa and the roof of the orbits and surrounds the cribriform plate is quite thin and less able to withstand distortion than are the thicker portions of the skull. On the basis of this experimental evidence, it seems likely, therefore, that fractures involving the ethmoid may be the result of a blow sustained at any position on the vault.

Fractures of the floor of the middle or anterior cranial fossa are often difficult to visualize with conventional radiographic techniques. The variations in bone density, the irregularity of the bone, and the presence of multiple, overlapping anatomic structures make it extremely difficult to identify linear fractures at the base of the skull on plain radiographs. Although there may be difficulty in

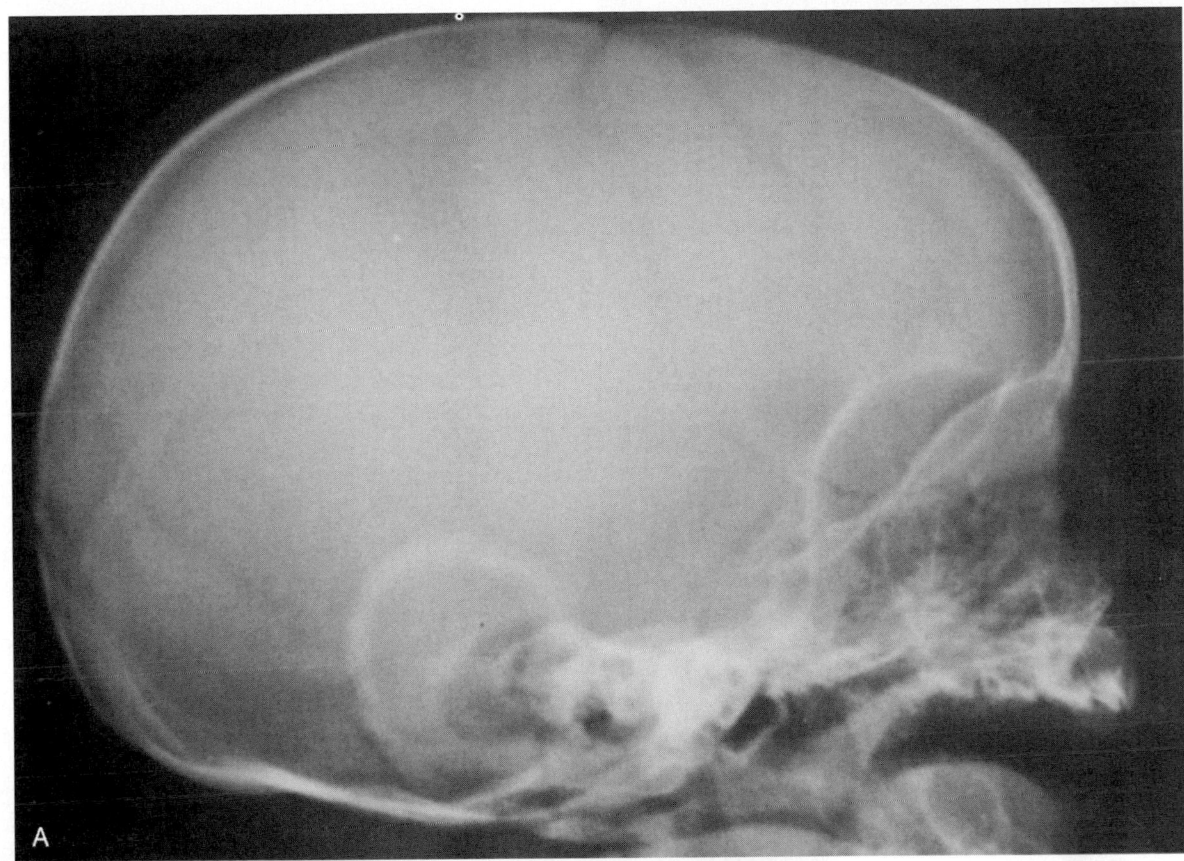

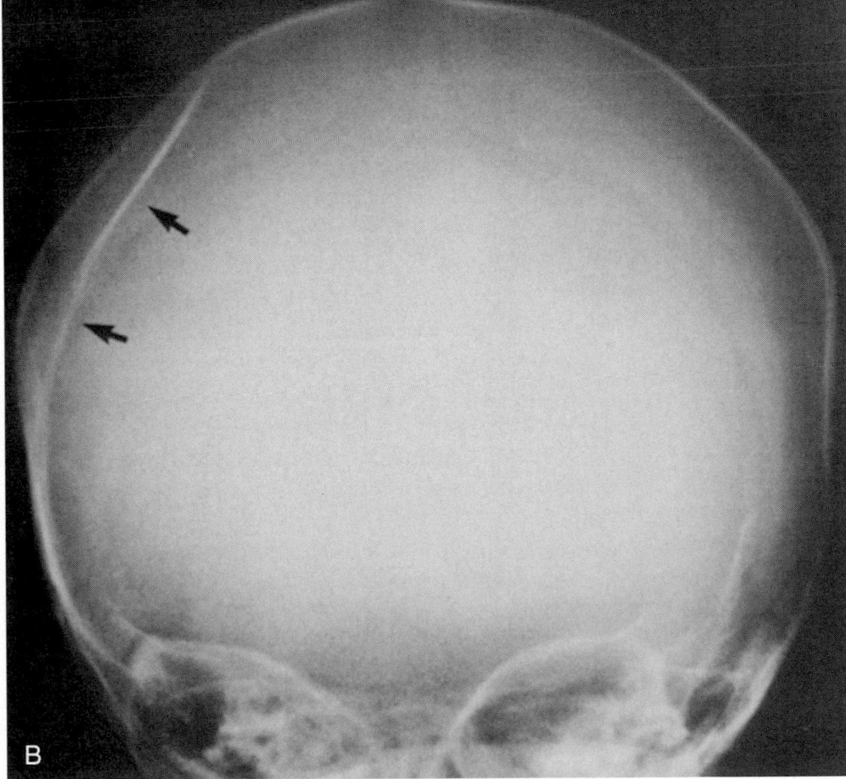

Figure 10–25. "Ping-pong" depressed fracture of the right parietal bone in a 4-month-old girl. *A*, Lateral view fails to demonstrate any evidence of abnormality. The depression in this type of fracture is very broad and therefore poorly defined unless seen tangentially. *B*, Frontal projection demonstrates the depressed fracture (*arrows*). The "ping-pong" type of depression is due to the softness of the infant's skull.

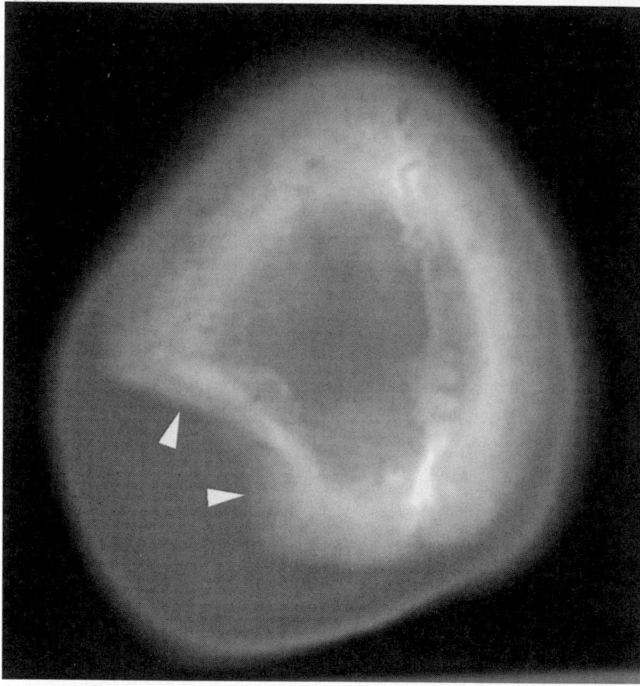

Figure 10–26. Axial computed tomography image obtained at the vertex of the skull demonstrates a "ping-pong" fracture with a focal depression (*arrowheads*) of the right parietal bone in a 26-year-old man who sustained trauma to the skull. This type of fracture is an unusual in the adult population; the overlying soft tissue swelling confirms the acute nature of the injury.

evaluating the anterior fossa because its plane is similar to the axial projection and volume averaging potentially may obscure fractures, there is generally a vertical or transverse component that is easily identified with CT.

In contradistinction to the sphenoid and ethmoid sinuses, fracture lines can readily be visualized in the frontal sinus by either plain radiography or CT (Fig. 10–32). The fracture may involve either the anterior wall or both the anterior and posterior walls of the sinus. Obviously, this distinction is crucial, because fracture of the posterior wall of the sinus is by definition an open injury. Comminuted and depressed fractures of the frontal portion of

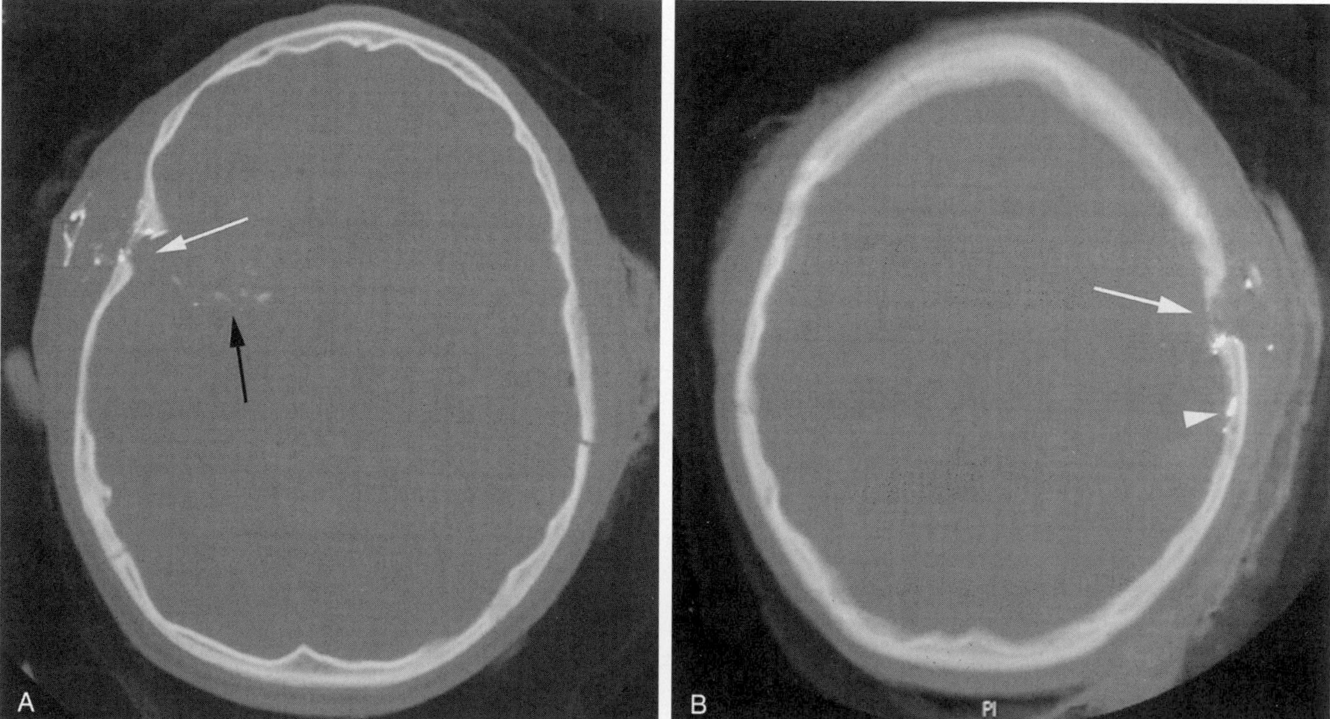

Figure 10–27. Gunshot injury to the skull. *A*, Axial computed tomography image illustrates the typical appearance of the entrance site, with a beveled inner table (*white arrow*). Bullet and bone fragments are carried along the path of the bullet (*black arrow*). *B*, Axial image obtained at a slightly higher level than in *A* displays the typical appearance of the exit site, with a beveled outer table (*arrow*). Small bullet fragments are lodged against the inner margin of the calvaria (*arrowhead*).

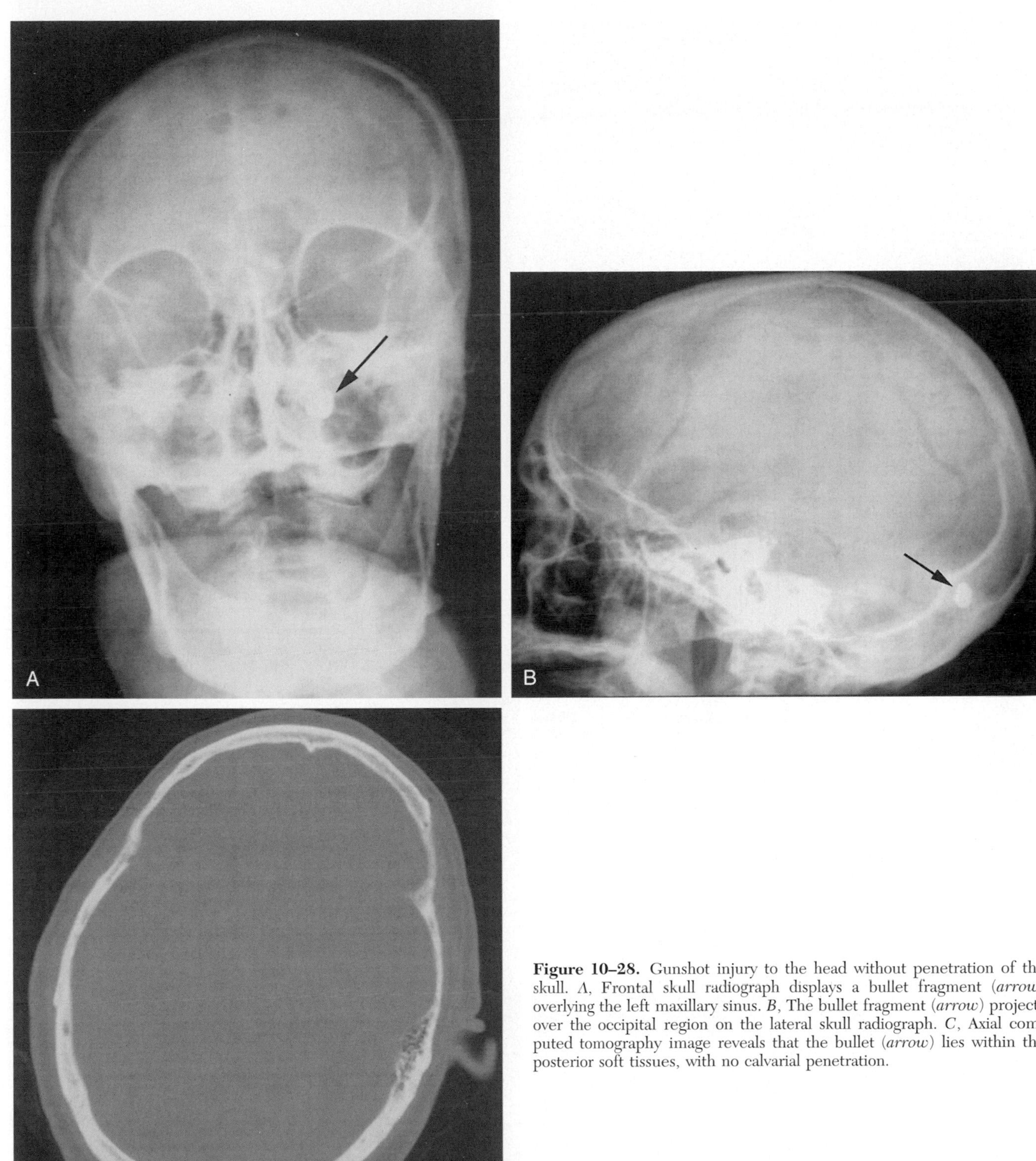

Figure 10–28. Gunshot injury to the head without penetration of the skull. *A*, Frontal skull radiograph displays a bullet fragment (*arrow*) overlying the left maxillary sinus. *B*, The bullet fragment (*arrow*) projects over the occipital region on the lateral skull radiograph. *C*, Axial computed tomography image reveals that the bullet (*arrow*) lies within the posterior soft tissues, with no calvarial penetration.

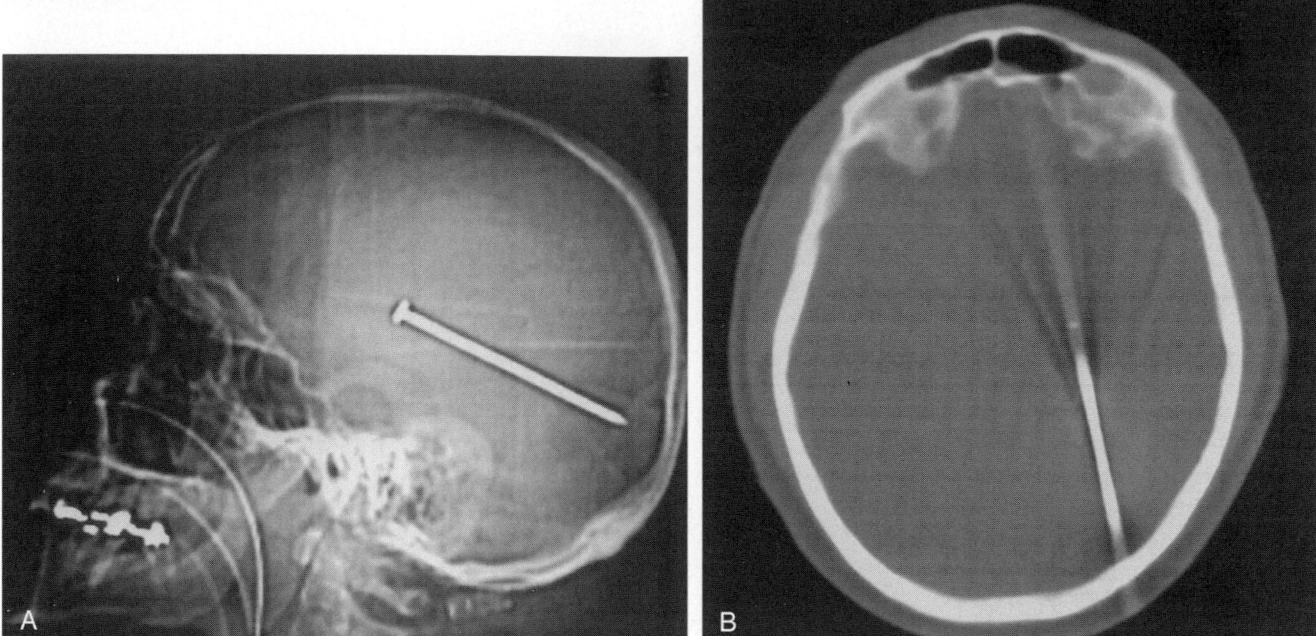

Figure 10–29. Penetrating foreign body (nail) within the calvaria. *A*, Digital radiograph from a computed tomography examination demonstrates a nail projecting over the calvaria. *B*, Axial image from a computed tomography study obtained with bone window settings demonstrates the intracranial location of the foreign body.

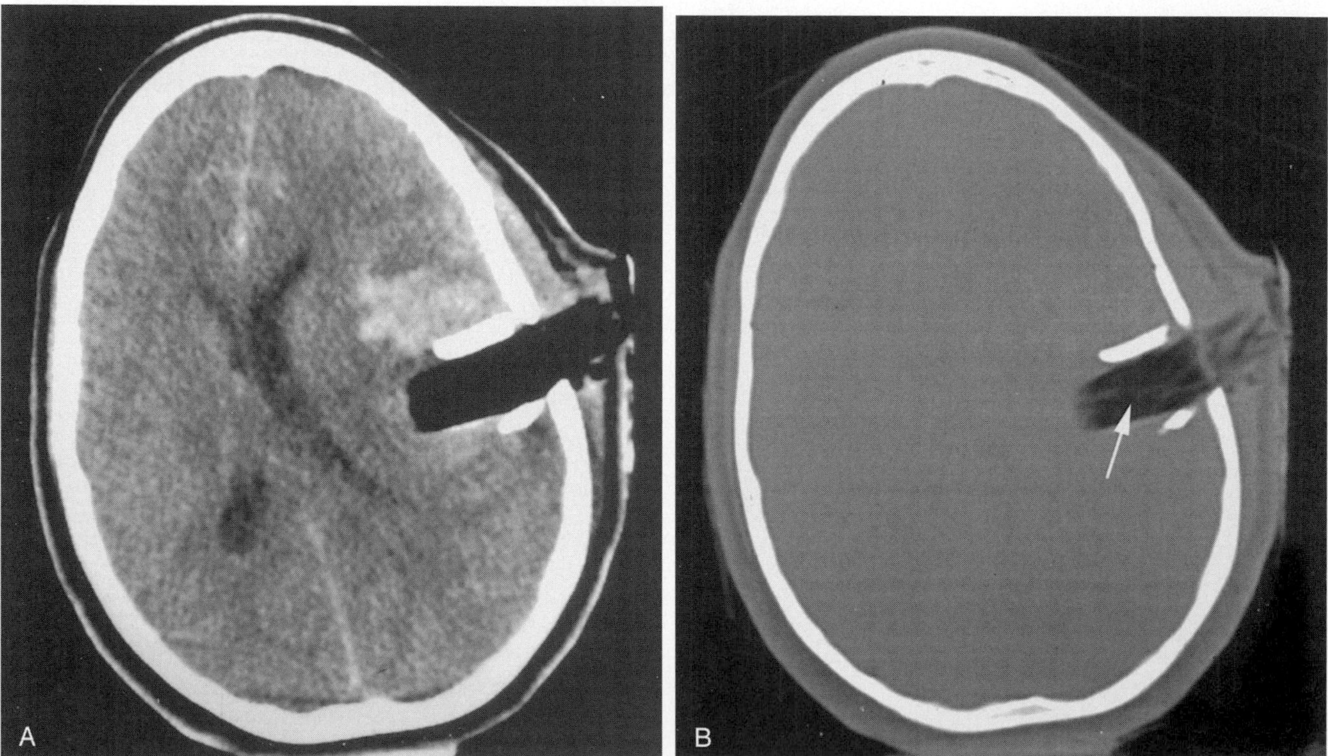

Figure 10–30. Wooden foreign body in the skull of a young man ejected from an automobile and impaled on a picket fence. *A*, Axial computed tomography image viewed with brain window settings shows depressed bone fragments, parenchymal/subarachnoid hemorrhage, and an air density "object" traversing the calvaria. *B*, Image obtained with bone window settings at the same level as in *A* demonstrates that the hypodense area is of a higher density than the surrounding air, with the characteristic striated appearance (*arrow*) of wood. (Case courtesy of Charles Kenney III, MD, Lexington, Ky.)

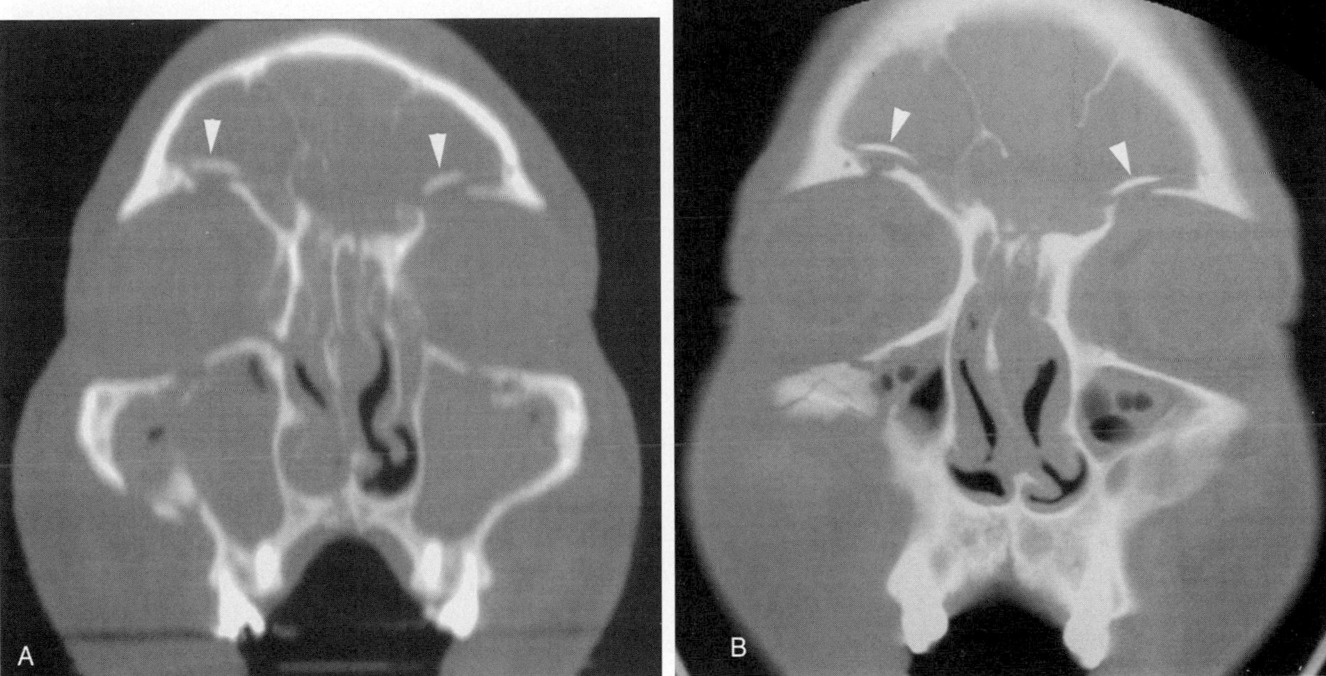

Figure 10–31. Skull and ethmoid sinus fractures with reconstruction images. *A*, Reformatted image reconstructed in the coronal plane from a thin-section axial computed tomography examination reveals multiple facial fractures involving the nasoethmoidal complex, maxillary sinuses, and the floor of the anterior cranial fossa (*arrowheads*). *B*, An image acquired in the coronal plane at a comparable position to that in *A* demonstrates the fractures with better detail but adds no diagnostic information.

the skull frequently extend into the frontal sinuses and usually involve both the anterior and posterior walls; thus, most depressed fractures of the frontal portion of the skull are also open injuries.

Basilar Skull Fractures and Sphenoid Effusion

Usually, basilar skull fractures (Fig. 10–33) are the result of a blow to the front of the skull and are accompanied by signs of soft tissue or other injuries of the fore-

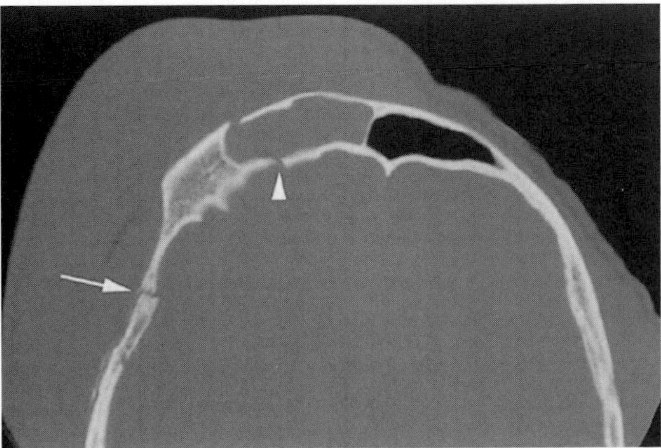

Figure 10–32. Axial thin-section CT image displays a comminuted right frontal skull fracture (*arrow*) with involvement of the anterior and posterior (*arrowhead*) walls of the frontal sinus. Massive soft tissue swelling is noted over the frontal region.

head. Radiologic demonstration of fractures of the base of the skull is notoriously difficult.[18, 23, 108, 117] Thin section, high-resolution CT is much more sensitive to the detection of basilar skull fractures than is plain radiography. The true incidence of basilar skull fractures has never been established, although they have been estimated to occur in approximately 20% of all head injuries.[62] Demonstration of an air-fluid level or opacification of the sphenoid sinus (see Fig. 10–39) has been found to be a reliable indication of such fractures, however.[117, 118] In the presence of sphenoid effusion or air-fluid level, fractures have been demonstrated radiologically in two thirds to three fourths of patients, and additional patients have been noted to have a fracture at operation or on postmortem examination.[118]

CT in the axial projection readily demonstrates air-fluid levels because the patient is examined in the supine, brow-up position. Although the maxillary sinus can fill from adjacent nasofacial hemorrhage, the sphenoid sinus is less capable of doing so because of its small size and the position of its ostium. Although hemorrhage has been shown to accumulate within the sphenoid sinus in patients with epistaxis and nasal packing,[114] demonstration of an air-fluid level or opacification in the sphenoid sinus in the setting of trauma should be regarded as highly suspicious for a basilar skull fracture and an indication for a dedicated CT examination of the skull base.[115]

Fractures of the body of the sphenoid bone (including clivus) are either transverse or longitudinally oriented (see Fig. 10–33). Transverse fractures often extend into the long axis of one or both petrous pyramids.[110] Longitudinal fractures of the sphenoid commonly extend anteriorly to involve the floor of the frontal fossa in or about the

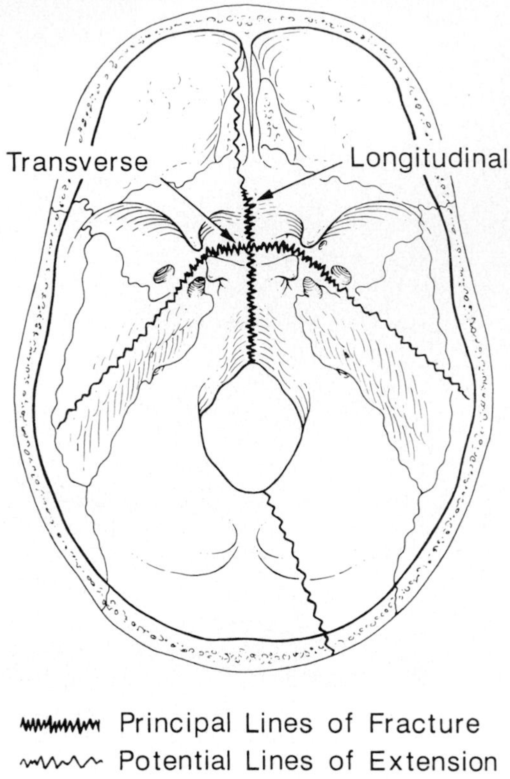

Figure 10–33. Principal direction of fractures involving the base of the skull. Transverse fractures of the sphenoid bone often extend laterally and become longitudinal fractures of the temporal bone. Longitudinal fractures of the sphenoid bone often extend anteriorly to involve the floor of the frontal fossa adjacent to the midline and traverse the foramen magnum posteriorly as sagittal fractures of the occipital bone.

midline and posteriorly through the foramen magnum into the occipital bone (see Fig. 10–33).[110] The fracture may appear to jump the foramen magnum. Fractures of the occiput that extend to the foramen magnum commonly traverse the foramen to continue on the opposite side. Transverse sphenoid fractures are often associated with vascular injuries (Fig. 10–34), most notably injury to the carotid artery in the form of pseudoaneurysm,[116, 119] intimal injury[116, 119] and dissection, or carotid artery–cavernous sinus fistula formation.[107, 110] Sphenoid (and other skull base) fractures are estimated to involve the carotid canal in 24% of cases.[116] With extension of a skull base fracture into the carotid canal, a concomitant injury to the carotid artery is present 18% of the time.[116] Massive epistaxis in the setting of head trauma and sphenoid sinus fracture warrants interrogation of the carotid vasculature for the presence of a traumatic pseudoaneurysm.[120] Longitudinally oriented fractures are often fatal because of associated vertebral-basilar artery occlusion (Fig. 10–35) or occasionally vertebral artery entrapment.[107, 110] Alternatively, these fractures may result in venous sinus thrombosis[112] or cerebrospinal fluid fistulas.[110] Other components of the sphenoid bone may also be fractured, including the clinoids, greater and lesser wings, and margins of the optic canals.[111] Optic canal margin fractures may be associated with blindness. Associated intracerebral and extracerebral hematomas are frequent.[115]

Fractures of the occipital condyles were once thought to be a rare occurrence owing to their strong association with fatal atlanto-occipital dislocations and difficulties in identifying the fractures with skull radiographs and polytomography.[75] These fractures are occasionally identified on "odontoid" views of the cervical spine, but CT affords a greater detection rate of occipital condyle fractures (Fig. 10–36) and is the modality of choice for their evaluation.[75, 79] Coronal and sagittal reformatted images (Fig. 10–37) of the craniocervical junction are particularly useful in detecting and classifying occipital condyle fractures. In one study, occipital condyle fractures were discovered in approximately 4% of patients with substantial head trauma.[79] Various combinations of axial loading, rotational stress, and direct blows to the skull are implicated as mechanisms of injury.[94] Several classification schemes[48, 94] have been proposed, with the most recent based upon the presence or absence of displaced fragments.[94] In addition to the association with atlantooccipital dislocations, displaced fragments from occipital condyle fractures may produce injury to adjacent structures such as the vertebral arteries, medulla oblongata, and the cranial nerves.[75]

Fractures of the skull base are often identifiable on standard head CT examinations, but thin (1 to 3 mm) sections processed using a bone algorithm are often necessary to demonstrate the full extent of the fracture and to identify them with certainty.[110] Opacification of the sphenoid sinus or mastoid air cells and pneumocephalus, particularly in the basilar and perisellar cisterns, serve as clues to an underlying fracture and indicate the necessity for dedicated imaging of the skull base with CT. Pneumorrhachis (air within the spinal canal) visualized on a lateral radiograph of the cervical spine has also been reported in the setting of skull base fracture.[113] Air in the cavernous sinus as a result of sphenoid fracture has been described[146, 109]; the air probably entered through a tear in the adjacent dura. However, caution should be exercised, as air can be visualized within the cavernous sinus from nontraumatic causes such as septic cavernous sinus thrombosis or may be iatrogenically related to intravenous injections.[109] When a longitudinal fracture of the mastoid is identified, the sphenoid bone should be examined closely for evidence of extension of the fracture into the base of the skull (see Fig. 10–39).[110]

Fractures Involving the Mastoid and Petrous Pyramid of the Temporal Bone

Blows to the head may produce fractures of the mastoid or petrous pyramid or result in dislocation of the ossicles.[129, 136] The direction of fracture lines extending through and into the mastoid and petrous portion of the temporal bone is variable, and the fractures are minimally displaced.[127, 136] Classically, the fractures are described[121, 123, 136, 138] (Fig. 10–38) as either longitudinal (Fig. 10–39), along the long axis of the petrous bone as an extension of a fracture in the squamous portion of the temporal or parietal bones, or transverse (Fig. 10–40), across the petrous bone as an extension from a fracture of the occiput. However, thin-section CT has revealed that the majority of fractures are "mixed" and lie within an oblique plane,

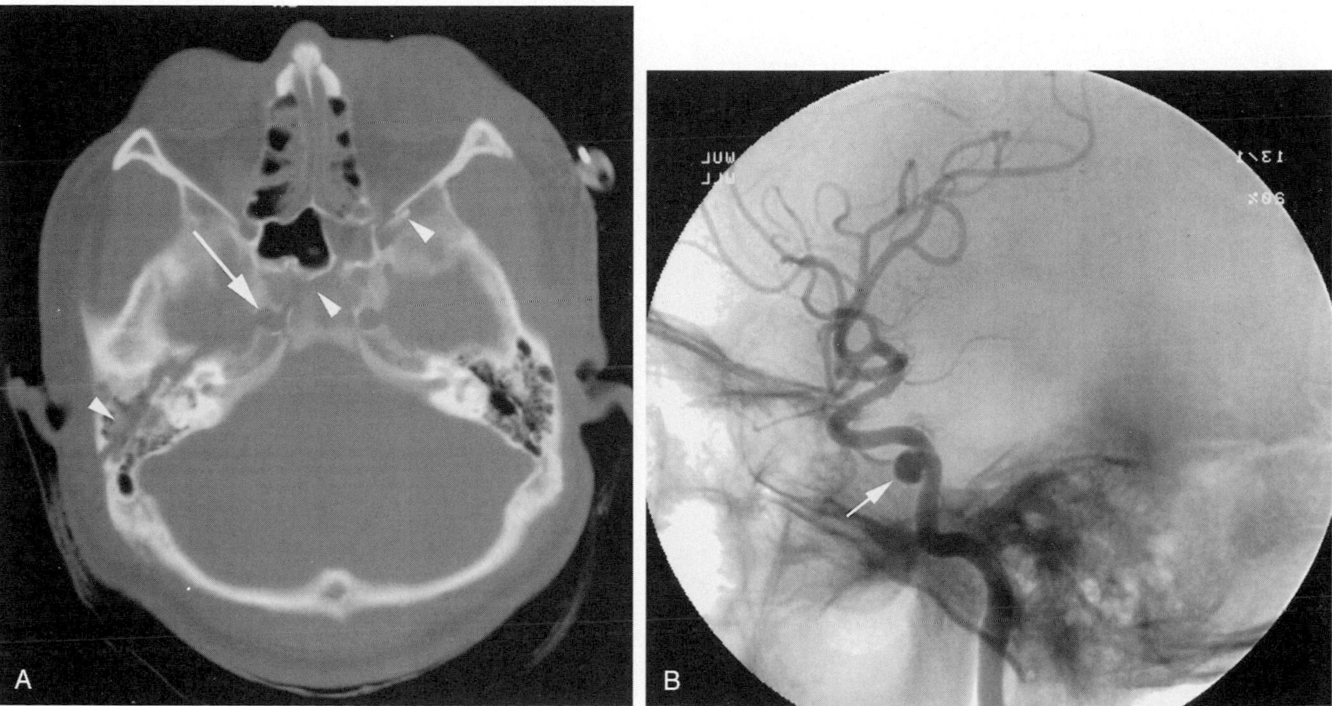

Figure 10–34. Longitudinal temporal bone fracture extending through the skull base with associated vascular injury. *A*, Axial computed tomography image displays a longitudinal fracture of the right temporal bone (*arrowheads*), with extension anteriorly through the sphenoid sinus and on into the left orbital apex. The fracture line crosses through the right carotid canal (*arrow*). *B*, Lateral view from a right internal carotid arteriogram demonstrates a pseudoaneurysm (*arrow*) arising from the pre–cavernous sinus portions of the internal carotid artery as it passes through the skull base.

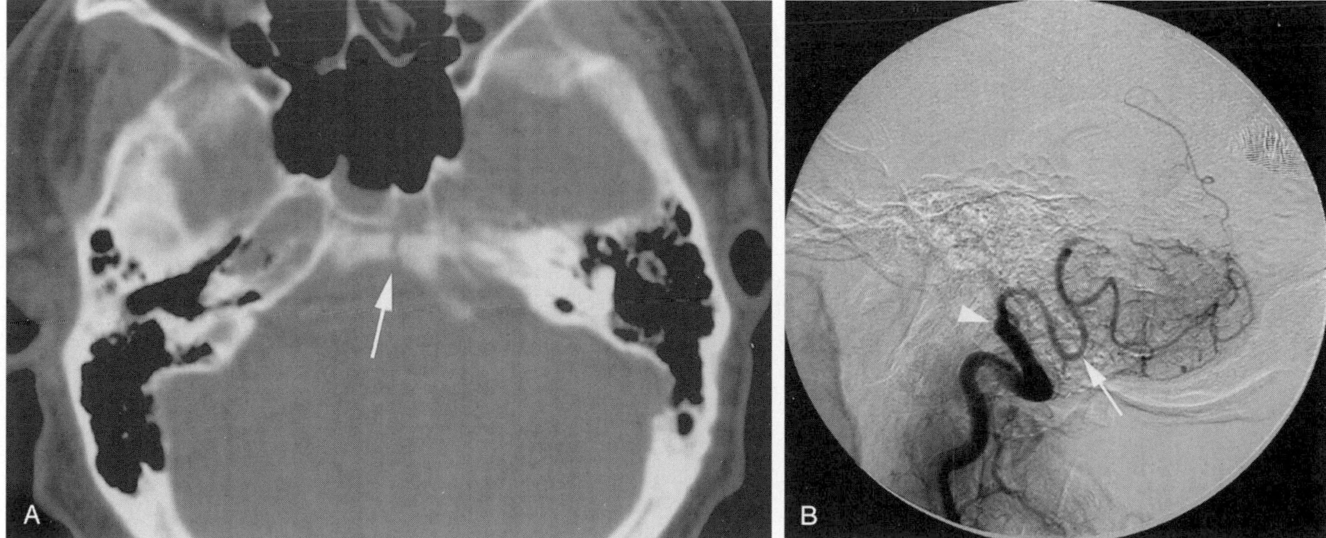

Figure 10–35. Clivus fracture with associated vascular injury. *A* Axial image of the skull base from a routine head computed tomography examination demonstrates a longitudinally oriented fracture of the clivus (arrow). *B*, Lateral view from a digital subtraction left vertebral arteriogram reveals traumatic occlusion of the proximal basilar artery (*arrowhead*); the posterior inferior cerebellar artery (*arrow*) is normal. (Case courtesy of P. Pearse Morris, MD, Winston-Salem, N.C.)

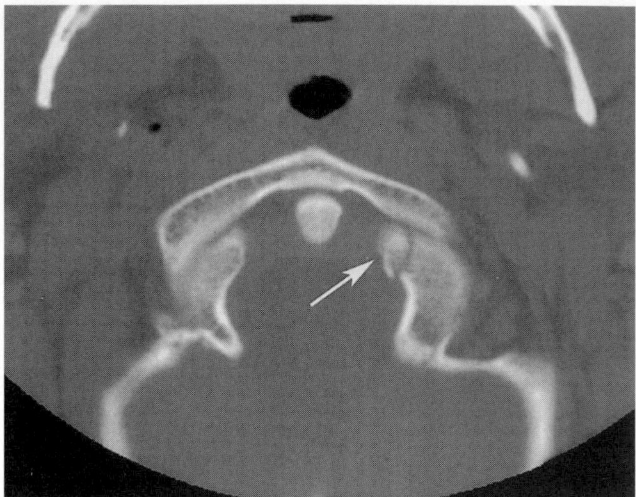

Figure 10–36. Axial CT image through the skull base demonstrates a minimally displaced fracture of the left occipital condyle *(arrow)*.

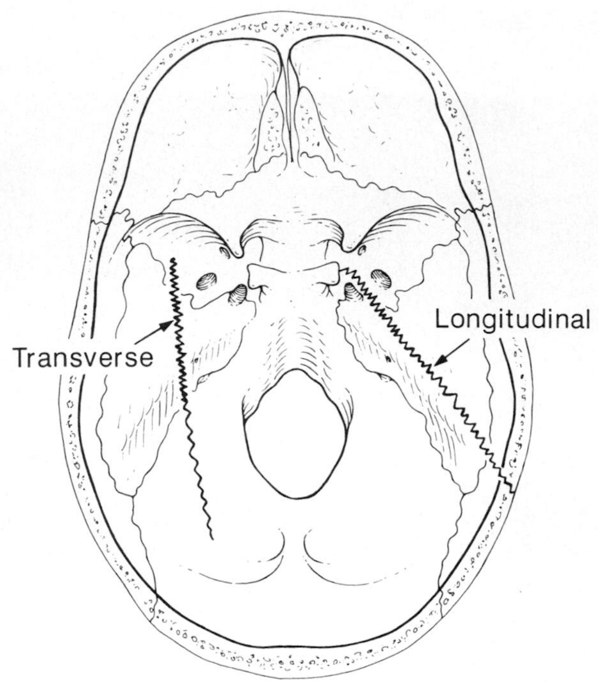

Figure 10–38. Principal direction of fractures of the temporal bone. Longitudinal fractures (*left*) may extend anteriorly to become transverse fractures of the sphenoid bone. Transverse fractures of the temporal bone often extend into the occipital bone.

true longitudinal and transverse fractures being quite rare.[125, 140] Longitudinal and oblique fractures both course parallel to the long axis of the petrous bone, but they are differentiated by their course through the external skull.[125, 140] The oblique fractures traverse the petrotympanic fissure and often extend into the mandibular fossa without involvement of the undersurface of the skull base, whereas true longitudinal fractures course through the petrosphenoid suture to the base of the skull.[125, 140] Thus, oblique fractures are best differentiated from the more rare longitudinal fractures by analyzing their external course on thin-section CT, and 3-D surface-shaded reconstructions may aid in the correct categorization.[125] The optimum surgical approach to temporal bone fractures is dependent upon the correct categorization of the fracture.[125]

Longitudinal and oblique fractures are generally associated with bleeding from the external ear or conductive hearing loss from abnormalities of the middle ear. This conductive hearing loss commonly results from hemorrhage within the middle ear or disruption of the ossicular chain (Fig. 10–41; see also Fig. 10–39), seen in approximately 20% of cases.[128] Injury to the facial nerve (Fig. 10–41) may be seen with longitudinal or oblique fractures but is most commonly associated with transverse fractures of the temporal bone. Transverse fractures may also result

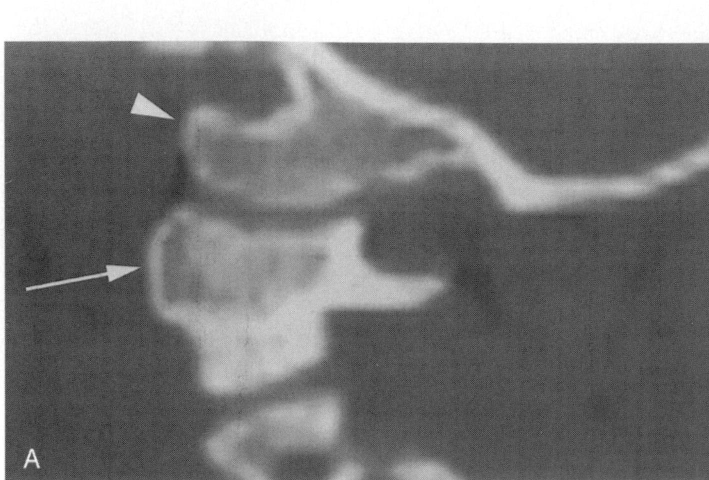

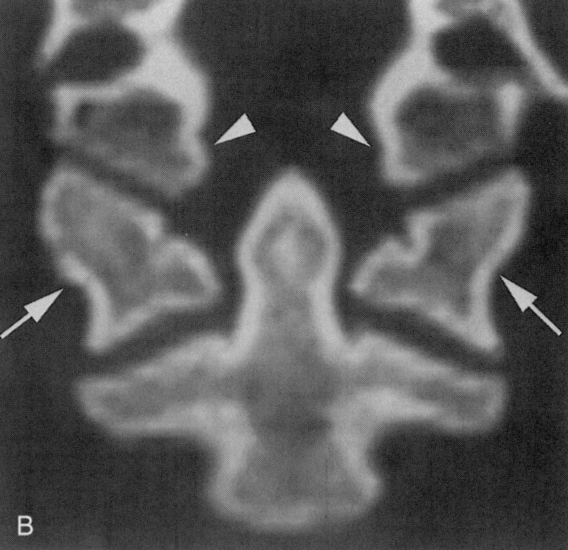

Figure 10–37. Normal occipital condyle on reformatted images. Sagittal (*A*) and coronal (*B*) reconstructed images from a thin-section axial computed tomography examination of the craniocervical junction demonstrate a normal appearance of the occipital condyles (*arrowheads*) and their relationship to the lateral masses of the C1 vertebral body (*arrow*).

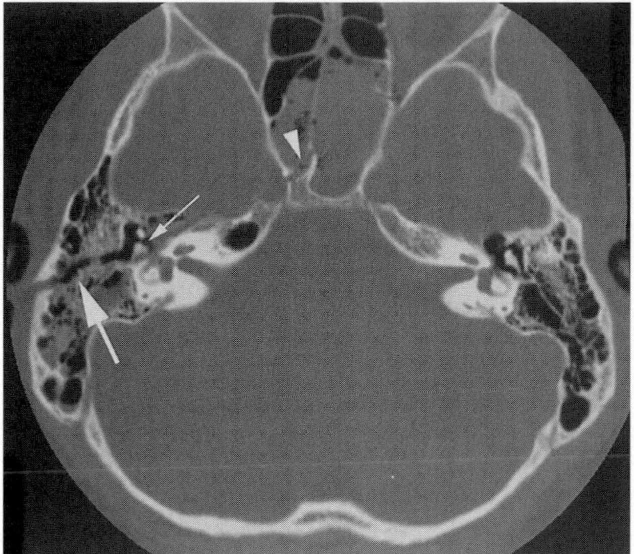

Figure 10–39. Axial image from a high-resolution temporal bone computed tomography examination reveals a longitudinal fracture of the right temporal bone (*large white arrow*), with extension across the sphenoid sinuses (*arrowhead*). There is associated traumatic ossicular disruption (*small white arrow*).

in neurosensory hearing loss secondary to injuries of the eighth nerve, cochlea, vestibule (see Fig. 10–40), or labyrinth.[131]

Because of the lack of displacement and their oblique course, suspected temporal bone fractures are infrequently visualized on standard or specialized radiographic projections. CT images of the head obtained with 1-cm-thick slices fail to demonstrate nearly 60% of temporal bone fractures.[128] Consequently, thin-section (using 1- to 2-mm-thick slices) CT is the modality of choice in identifying and categorizing fractures of the temporal bones[124, 126, 128, 130, 137] and should be performed in all cases in which a fracture of the mastoid or petrous pyramid is suspected. If the patient's condition permits direct coronal imaging, this examination should also be performed; however, coronal imaging may be impossible in the acutely injured patient, and reformatted images from the axial plane may be an acceptable alternative.

Temporal bone fractures are often unsuspected and are identified because of air space opacification or local pneumocephalus[139] on routine thick-section axial CT images of the skull. Air space opacification may involve the external auditory canal, middle ear, or mastoid air cells[128] (see Figs. 10–34 and 10–39). The presence of air within the temporomandibular joint is an additional sign of temporal bone fracture (Fig. 10–42), found in slightly greater than 20% of cases.[122] Two thirds of patients with temporal bone fractures have associated extra-axial hematomas or intracerebral injuries.[123] Such injuries are often on the side opposite the temporal bone fracture and may draw attention away from the temporal bone injury itself.

Pneumolabyrinth (air within the vestibule and cochlea) has been described in association with temporal bone fractures (Fig. 10–43).[132, 133, 135] One fracture was identified at the time of surgery at the footplate of the stapes, and a second involved the ponticulus just posterior to the round window. Pneumolabyrinth may be seen in both transverse and longitudinal fractures.

Small bubbles of air have been identified in acute epidural hematomas associated with contiguous longitudinal fractures of the mastoids, with the air entering through a tear in the adjacent dura. This appears to be a unique association; when air is identified in an epidural hematoma contiguous with the temporal bone, it implies the presence of an underlying fracture.[142]

Pneumocephalus has also been reported as a consequence of barotrauma in a scuba diver. Presumably, pressure within the middle ear leads to disruption of the tegmen tympani, allowing air to escape into the subdural space.[151]

To date, MRI has had limited application in the evaluation of acute temporal bone fractures.[141] However, tech-

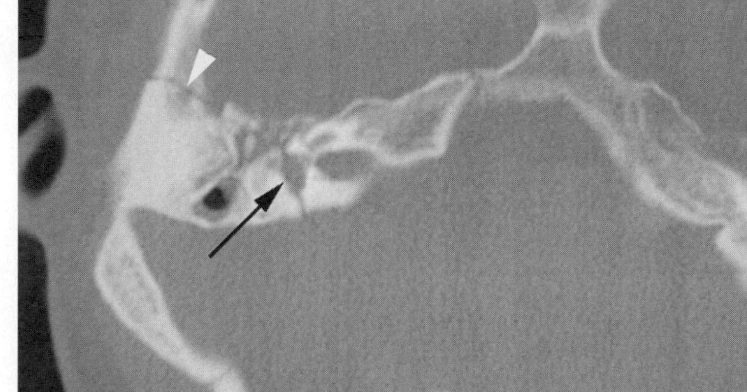

igure 10–40. Axial image from a high-resolution temporal bone computed tomography examination reveals a transverse fracture of the right temporal bone (*arrowhead*), with extension through the vestibule (*arrow*).

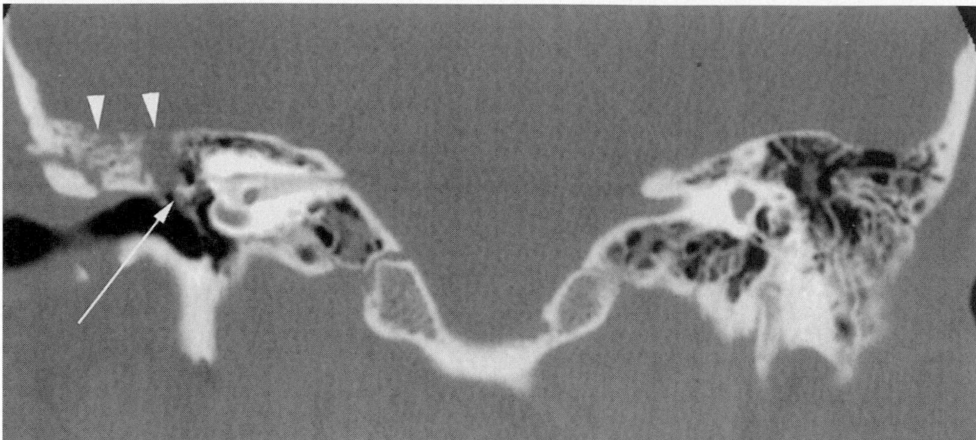

Figure 10–41. Coronal image from a high-resolution temporal bone computed tomography examination displays a complex right temporal bone fracture with disruption of the tegmen tympani (*arrowheads*) and ossicular disruption. The patient had symptoms of a distal facial nerve injury following tumour. The incus is inferiorly displaced (*arrow*) and encroaches on the facial nerve canal.

nologic advances with thinner section images and improved resolution permits direct visualization of the cranial nerves, and as a result, MRI may have a utility in evaluating patients with a neurosensory hearing loss following trauma.

The location of a fracture of the mastoid or petrous pyramid is dependent upon the signs and symptoms resulting from the injury. *Bleeding* from the external ear is frequently associated with a fracture involving the posterior wall of the external auditory canal. The presence of a *conductive hearing loss* is due either to fluid in the middle ear or to dislocation of the ossicles.[123, 134, 136] Ossicular dislocation may occur indirectly as a result of a blow on the head with or without an associated longitudinal fracture of the mastoid (see Fig. 10–39 and 10–41), or more directly by placement of a foreign body such as a hairpin or golf tee into the external auditory canal. Iatrogenic dislocations may occur during attempts to dislodge foreign bodies from the external canal. In 80% of cases the incudostapedial joint is separated, often with marked dislocation of the incus.[136] *Cerebrospinal fluid otorrhea* is due to fracture of the roof of the middle ear or tegmen tympani (see Fig. 10–41).[136] However, caution is advised in searching for fractures of the tegmen tympani, as this structure is often imperceptibly thin and may appear to be fractured when it is intact. On occasion the tegmen may shatter, with herniation of the temporal lobe into the mastoid.[126, 130] This herniation plugs the defect in the roof of the mastoid and prevents otorrhea. *Neurosensory hearing loss* is due to fracture in the inner ear, involving either the internal auditory canal or the labyrinth capsule, including the vestibule, semicircular canals, and cochlea.[123, 134] The localization of a fracture associated with facial nerve paralysis is dependent upon the signs and symptoms of the seventh nerve injury.[136] If taste and lacrimation both are affected, the fracture lies proximal to the geniculate ganglion in either the labyrinth or the internal auditory canal. If taste is affected but lacrimation

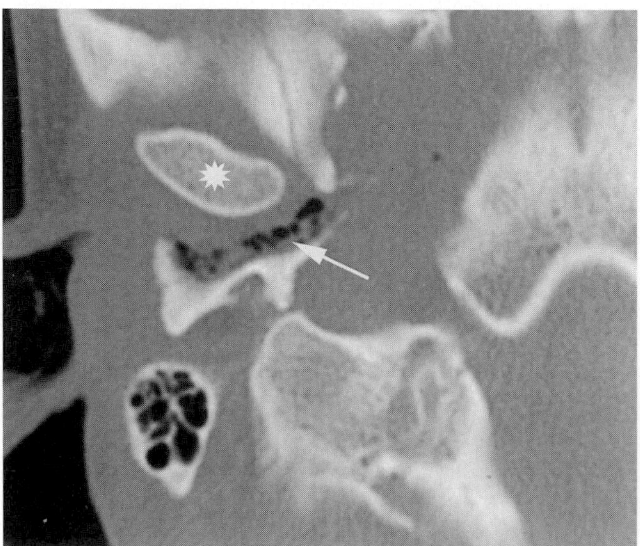

Figure 10–42. Axial image from a high-resolution temporal bone computed tomography examination in a patient with an oblique temporal bone fracture (not shown) reveals air (*arrow*) within the temporomandibular joint. The mandibular condyle (*asterisk*) remains located within the glenoid (mandibular) fossa.

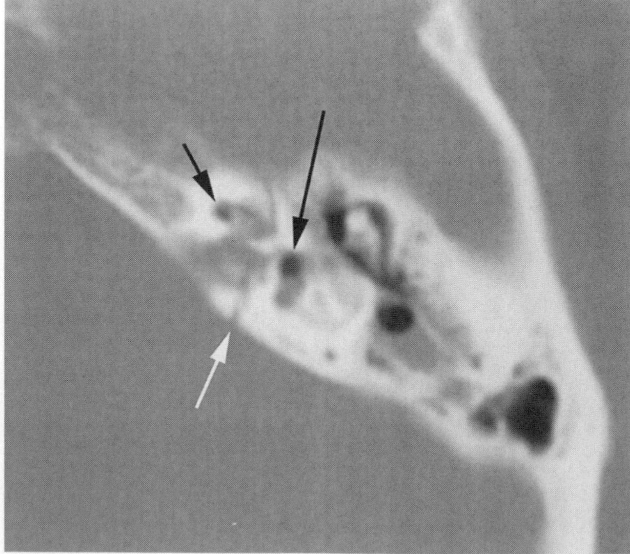

Figure 10–43. Axial image from a high-resolution temporal bone computed tomography examination reveals a transverse temporal bone fracture (*white arrow*) with associated pneumolabyrinth. Air is present within both the cochlea (*shorter black arrow*) and the vestibule (*longer black arrow*).

is not disturbed, then the fracture is distal to the geniculate ganglion either within the horizontal or the vertical portions of the facial canal.

Complications of Skull Fracture

Exclusive of direct injury to the brain, the immediate complications of skull fractures are pneumocephalus, cerebrospinal fluid rhinorrhea, vascular injury, and growing skull fractures.

Pneumocephalus

Pneumocephalus results from disruption of a bony wall of a paranasal sinus or mastoid air cell contiguous with the cranial cavity. There is usually simultaneous disruption of the dura, and air may pass freely from the affected sinus or mastoid into the cranium. Other causes for pneumocephalus include penetrating injury, such as with gunshot wounds, and iatrogenic causes such as after a myelogram.

Chiari first recognized intracranial pneumocephalus in 1884.[154, 157] The second case reported, by Luckett in 1913,[143, 157] was diagnosed on the basis of a radiographic examination. The air may be located in one or more of the intracranial compartments[143, 157]: epidural, subdural (see Fig. 10–13), subarachnoid (see Fig. 10–20), ventricular (see Fig. 10–20), or intracerebral. Subdural and subarachnoid collections are most common. Epidural collections are uncommon.

Trauma is by far the most frequent cause of pneumocephalus, accounting for approximately 74% of cases. It was the chance visualization of intraventricular air on the radiographs of the skull in a person who had sustained skull trauma that suggested to Dandy[149] the possibility of intentionally introducing air in evaluation of the central nervous system. Among other causes of pneumocephalus, neoplasms[142, 145, 159] are responsible for 13% of the cases, infections for 9%, and previous surgery for the remaining 4%.[157] Two cases without any identifiable cause have been reported.[157]

Less than 3% of all skull fractures[157] are associated with pneumocephalus, but approximately 8% of fractures of the paranasal sinuses result in pneumocephalus. Depressed fractures of the frontal sinus are the most common, followed by fractures of the ethmoid and sphenoid sinuses. Fractures of the mastoid are the least frequent. Pneumocephalus secondary to tension pneumothorax associated with a comminuted fracture of the midthoracic spine has been described.[155]

CT is more sensitive than plain radiography in detecting pneumocephalus. As little as 0.5 mL of air can be identified by CT, whereas more than 2 mL of air must be present before it is apparent on a skull radiograph.[158]

Two mechanisms have been suggested to explain the entry of air into the cranial cavity.[154, 157] They are not mutually exclusive, and it is likely that either or both may be operative in any case. The first is a ball-valve mechanism. Air is forced through the dural laceration by coughing, sneezing, or straining. Between such episodes the brain compresses the tear. The second mechanism is based upon a vacuum phenomenon, wherein air is drawn into the cranium by negative intracranial pressures created by loss of cerebrospinal fluid. This machanism is analogous to the filling of a bottle with air as it is emptied of its fluid content. However, cerebrospinal fluid rhinorrhea is apparent in only half of the cases of pneumocephalus.[157] Whether this is a reflection of the mechanism by which the air has entered or of other factors is unknown. In any event, cerebrospinal fluid rhinorrhea is not an invariable accompaniment of pneumocephalus.

It is of interest to note the frequent delay in onset of pneumocephalus[150, 155] (Fig. 10–44). Initial evaluation reveals evidence of intracranial air in only 25% of cases. The pneumocephalus is usually evident within 4 or 5 days, but in one third of cases, delays of up to 6 months and longer have been encountered.

Diagnosis is dependent on recognition and proper interpretation of findings on the radiographic examination[150] of the skull, examination of the head by CT,[158] or both. Air in the subarachnoid space and ventricular system has the same appearance as in pneumoencephalography. The air commonly resides in the perisellar basal cisterns or in the sulci over the convexity of the brain. Air is thought to enter the ventricular system through the foramina of Luschka and Magendie. When it does so, the lateral ventricles are most commonly visualized, the third ventricle less frequently, and the fourth ventricle rarely, if ever. Subdural air is distributed over the hemispheres, commonly along the falx and tentorium. In contradistinction to subdural and subarachnoid air, epidural air is limited in distribution, is usually unilateral, and fails to migrate with changes in the positioning of the skull. Intracerebral air is characteristically manifested by an air-fluid level (an aerocele) in the frontal lobes.[152] These commonly communicate with the lateral ventricles (see Fig. 10–44). For an intracranial aerocele to form, the brain must become adherent to the edges of the dural defect. Because of this adherence, air cannot enter either the subdural or subarachnoid space.

The appearance of intracranial air on CT images is quite characteristic; it has a very low attenuation, and its distribution and outline are dependent upon its location.[158] Epidural air appears as a biconvex air pocket that does not change with position. Small bubbles of air may enter extra-axial hematomas through adjacent fractures of the frontal and ethmoid sinuses or mastoid air cells.[142, 146, 148] Subdural air is usually thin and convex on its outer margin and concave on its inner margin. Subdural air moves freely and characteristically shifts with changing head position. Most CT images are obtained with the patient in the supine, brow-up position; therefore, air is located anteriorly. An air-fluid level is usually identified. If the subdural collection is of sufficient size, it may result in "tension pneumocephalus," with a mass effect (Fig. 10–45). Subarachnoid air is identified as small, nonconfluent bubbles conforming to the sulci and cerebrospinal fluid cisterns. Intracerebral air and intraventricular air are seen as collections of gas within the cerebral substance and ventricle, respectively, often with an air-fluid level.[147, 156]

Air also collects extracranially, although much less fre-

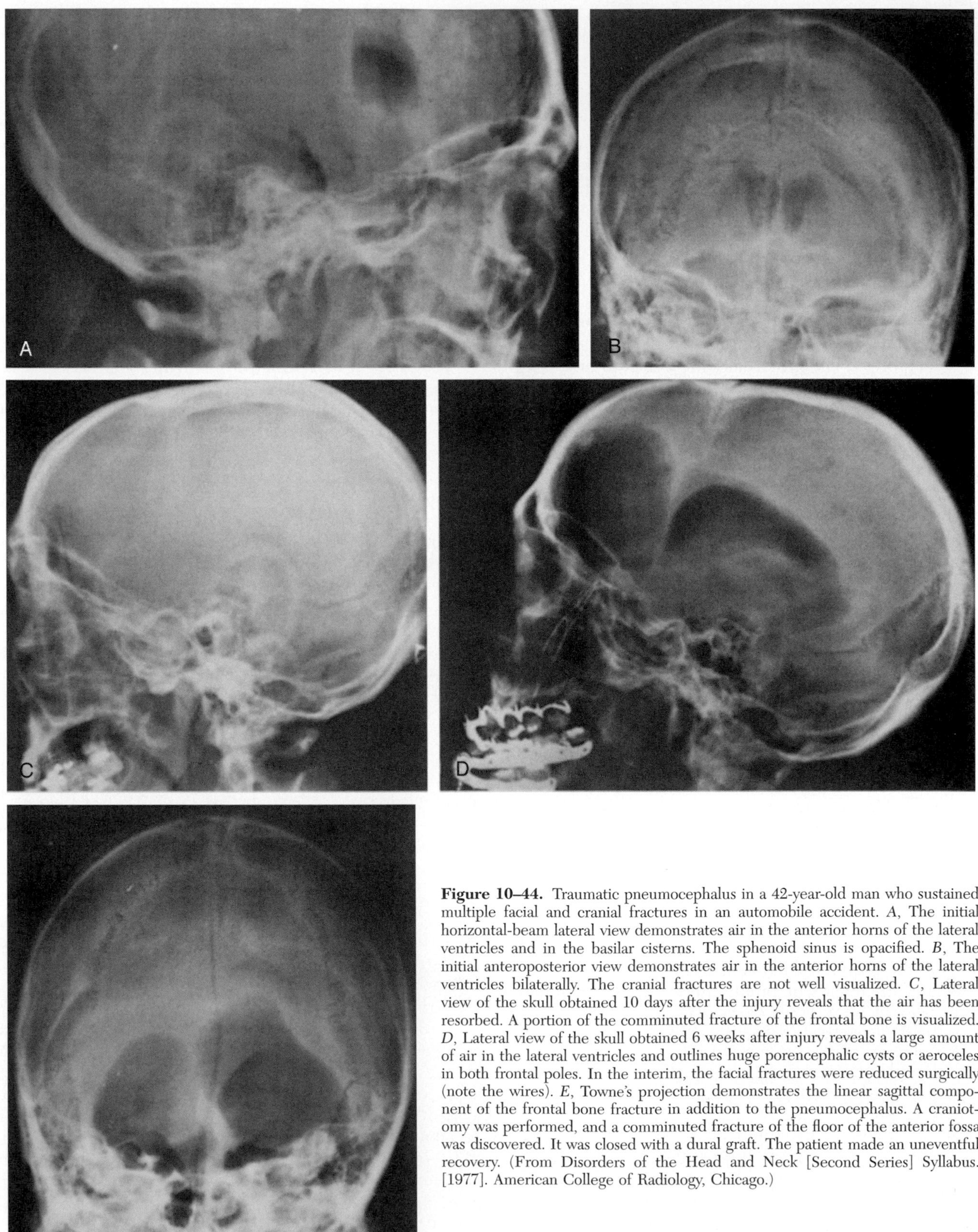

Figure 10–44. Traumatic pneumocephalus in a 42-year-old man who sustained multiple facial and cranial fractures in an automobile accident. *A*, The initial horizontal-beam lateral view demonstrates air in the anterior horns of the lateral ventricles and in the basilar cisterns. The sphenoid sinus is opacified. *B*, The initial anteroposterior view demonstrates air in the anterior horns of the lateral ventricles bilaterally. The cranial fractures are not well visualized. *C*, Lateral view of the skull obtained 10 days after the injury reveals that the air has been resorbed. A portion of the comminuted fracture of the frontal bone is visualized. *D*, Lateral view of the skull obtained 6 weeks after injury reveals a large amount of air in the lateral ventricles and outlines huge porencephalic cysts or aeroceles in both frontal poles. In the interim, the facial fractures were reduced surgically (note the wires). *E*, Towne's projection demonstrates the linear sagittal component of the frontal bone fracture in addition to the pneumocephalus. A craniotomy was performed, and a comminuted fracture of the floor of the anterior fossa was discovered. It was closed with a dural graft. The patient made an uneventful recovery. (From Disorders of the Head and Neck [Second Series] Syllabus. [1977]. American College of Radiology, Chicago.)

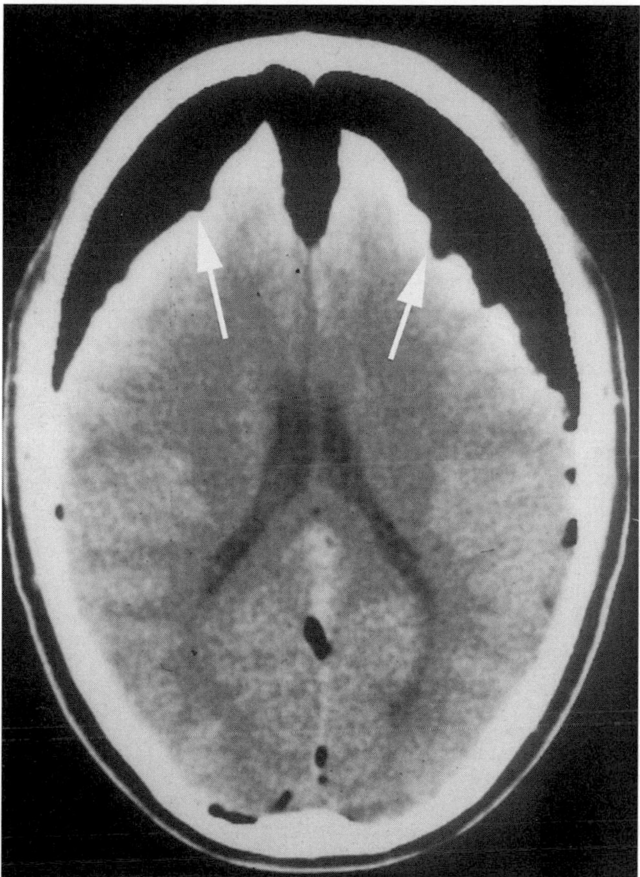

Figure 10–45. Axial computed tomography image demonstrates tension pneumocephalus in a patient who suffered a complication during sinonasal surgery. Note the mass effect, with a pointed configuration (*arrows*) of the frontal lobes.

quently than intracranially. The air collects in the subaponeurotic space of the scalp and has been termed a *subgaleal aerocele*. These lesions usually arise from a defect in the skull over the mastoids[57] but have also occurred over the frontal sinus. They may be secondary to fracture or infection.

Because a fistula exists between the exterior and the brain, the presence of pneumocephalus implies the presence of an open wound. Accordingly, there is considerable potential for bacterial contamination[153, 154, 157] with development of meningitis or brain abscess. These complications occur in up to 25% of cases.[157] Despite antibiotic therapy, the mortality remains appreciable, approximately 15%.[157]

As soon as pneumocephalus is recognized, antibiotic therapy is initiated to prevent meningitis and brain abscess. Should the tear of the meninges fail to heal, as manifested by persistence of the pneumocephalus, surgical treatment is indicated. It consists of repair of the dural tear, utilizing pericranium or fascia lata.

Cerebrospinal Fluid Rhinorrhea and Otorrhea

Leakage of cerebrospinal fluid through either the nose or the ear following trauma can be a vexing problem. Leakage of cerebrospinal fluid has probably been known since antiquity, but Bidloo of Holland first described it in 1700, and its first description in the English literature was in 1826 by Miller.[157, 170] Thompson coined the term *cerebrospinal fluid rhinorrhea* in 1879.[164] Fortunately, most of the associated dural tears heal spontaneously, and the exact identification of the site of injury and surgical repair are not required. When surgical repairs are required because of persistent leakage, it may be very difficult to identify the exact site of injury.[170]

The majority of fractures[170, 172, 174] resulting in cerebrospinal fluid rhinorrhea involve the floor of the anterior cranial fossa in either the frontal or ethmoid sinus. The ethmoid sinuses have the largest share of fractures. The roof of the ethmoid air cells (fovea ethomoidalis) is quite thin on either side of the cribriform plate. The cribriform plate and the crista galli are relatively stronger and tend to remain intact. Fractures involving the ethmoid labyrinth may therefore surround the cribriform plate, leaving it isolated. It is uncommon for fractures to actually traverse the plate. Fractures of the sphenoid sinus (Fig. 10–46) are a much less common cause of cerebrospinal fluid rhinorrhea. On rare occasions a fracture may extend through the temporal bone or mastoid air cells in association with a dural tear, allowing cerebrospinal fluid to enter the middle ear, flow into the eustachian tube, and then exit through the nasal cavity.

Initially, because of bleeding, it may be difficult if not impossible to recognize the presence of cerebrospinal fluid rhinorrhea. Once hemorrhage and bleeding stop, the condition becomes obvious. The sinuses are completely separate on each side, and because of the lack of continuity, the cerebrospinal fluid will exit through only one side

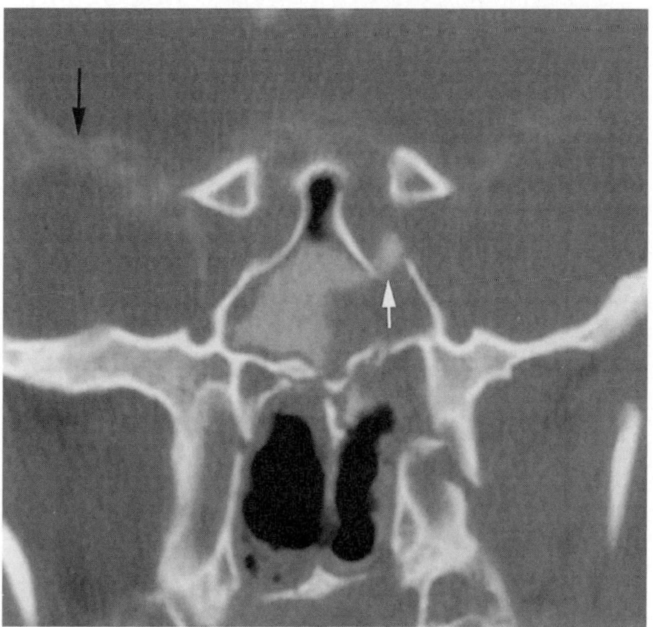

Figure 10–46. Coronal image from a high-resolution computed tomography cisternogram reveals a displaced fracture, with spillage of contrast material (*white arrow*) into the sphenoid sinus. The patient had post-traumatic cerebrospinal fluid rhinorrhea. Note the high-density contrast within the subarachnoid spaces following intrathecal contrast administration (*black arrow*).

of the nose. This accurately identifies the side of the associated fracture.

Demonstration of the actual fracture resulting in the cerebrospinal fluid rhinorrhea may be difficult. Such fractures are rarely demonstrated on routine radiographs. Even CT is unable to demonstrate all of them. The fractures usually involve the posterior walls of the frontal sinuses or the roof of the ethmoid air cells in the region of the cribriform plate. The thinness of the bone in these locations makes the evaluation difficult.

Fortunately, most dural tears heal spontaneously.[171] In 70% to 80% of cases, cerebrospinal fluid rhinorrhea will cease spontaneously within 2 weeks, and in 80% to 95% of cases, cerebrospinal fluid otorrhea will also cease spontaneously. In the remaining small percentage, surgical repair will more than likely be required and is aided materially by precise demonstration of the fistula preoperatively. Such localization is obviously difficult, as suggested by the many methods proposed and utilized for their purposes.[166, 167, 169, 172, 173] These methods include injection of dyes into the cerebrospinal fluid,[172] and the use of contrast myelography,[167, 172] nuclear medicine radioisotopic cisternography,[172] CT cisternography,[160, 162, 165, 168] and MRI cisternography. However, radioisotopic and CT cisternography are methods that have proved to have the most utility in localizing fracture sites.[166] When pneumocephalus is extensive, the site of leakage may be found by simply tracking the course of air through the defect into the sinus.[163] All these methods have met with varying degrees of success, but none is wholly satisfactory.

CT cisternography provides the best definition of the site and extent of dural disruption but is not infallible. The success of CT cisternography is dependent upon the presence of active leakage of cerebrospinal fluid during the examination; it is beneficial to scan the patient in any position that augments the leak, if possible. Typically, approximately 3 to 5 mL of 200 to 300 mmol/L nonionic contrast medium is inserted into the thecal sac via routine lumbar puncture after obtaining a preprocedural thin-section CT image in the coronal (and often axial) plane. The patient is then placed in a head-down position for approximately 1 to 2 minutes to allow the contrast to flow intracranially. High-resolution, thin-section coronal and axial images are obtained with the patient positioned to augment any cerebrospinal fluid leak. Despite meticulous attention to technique, identifying contrast passing through a fistulous defect in the bone (see Fig. 10–46) is an unusual occurrence.[166] In addition, it is rare to document contrast accumulation within a sinus without visualization of a bony defect or at least an air-fluid level on the precontrast portion of the CT examination.[166]

Magnetic resonance cisternography techniques employing a fat-suppressed T_2-weighted image are utilized to visualize the fistulous communication between the sinus and anterior cranial fossa.[166] However, MRI is hampered by relatively poor depiction of the bony abnormalities as compared with CT. Nuclear medicine radioisotope cisternography employing nasal cavity pledgets can often identify the side of cerebrospinal fluid leakage within the nasal cavity but does not depict the exact site of leakage or identify the bony disruption. Despite using a combination of the aforementioned techniques, the exact site of the fistula may not be identified preoperatively in some cases.

The complications of cerebrospinal fluid rhinorrhea and otorrhea are those of an open injury.[171] Meningitis[171] occurs in 25% of cases of cerebrospinal fluid rhinorrhea. A smaller percentage of cases may be complicated by intracerebral abscess. Meningitis is a less common complication of cerebrospinal fluid otorrhea, occurring in 2% to 5%[171] of cases. Once cerebrospinal fluid rhinorrhea or otorrhea is identified, antibiotics are indicated. Other potential complications of cerebrospinal fluid leak include low-pressure headaches and subdural fluid collections from intracranial hypotension.[161] Fortunately, most of the injuries will heal spontaneously[170, 171]; surgical treatment will not be required. When surgery is required, attempts should be made to identify the exact site of the fistula. Such localization may be quite difficult and at times prove impossible.

Growing Skull Fractures

The dura may be torn in association with an otherwise simple linear fracture, uncommonly resulting in a growing skull fracture. The estimated occurrence of such fractures is 0.05% to 0.7%.[178] Other entities associated with growing skull fractures include leptomeningeal cysts, cranial burst fractures,[175] growing cranial fracture,[177] cephalohydrocele,[177] and post-traumatic porencephaly.[175, 177] Growing skull fracture is most common in infants and young children and is usually suspected clinically when a pulsatile bulging mass is observed at the site of a prior skull fracture or surgical defect.[171] The parietal region is most frequently affected.[176, 178] The pathogenesis of this unique complication remains unclear, but several mechanisms for its development have been proposed. The skull and brain are undergoing rapid growth in infants and young children, and MRI reveals an association of cortical brain herniation with the development of the growing skull fracture.[175, 178] Other factors implicated in the development of growing skull fractures include elevated intracranial pressure,[175, 178] leptomeningeal cysts, and cortical injury.[175] Leptomeningeal cysts arise when adhesions of the arachnoid are interposed in the fracture line and develop into incomplete cysts. The cerebrospinal fluid pulsation within the cyst may lead to erosive changes at the fracture site, although recent studies indicate that pulsation of the herniated brain tissue itself is probably the more important contributor to skull fracture growth.[176, 178] In addition, leptomeningeal cysts have been identified in only a minority of growing skull fractures.[176, 178]

Patients may initially be asymptomatic but may have a delayed presentation, with developmental delay, headache, hemiparesis, and seizure.[177, 178] Growing skull fractures are manifested on skull radiographs as progressive erosion of bone and widening of the fracture, usually with diastasis greater than 4 mm.[175, 178] CT not only demonstrates the fracture line but also provides additional information regarding any underlying brain injury (Fig. 10–47). However, CT is less than optimal in identifying the underlying dural tear.[175] MRI has shown great utility in identifying the dural disruption and defining associated

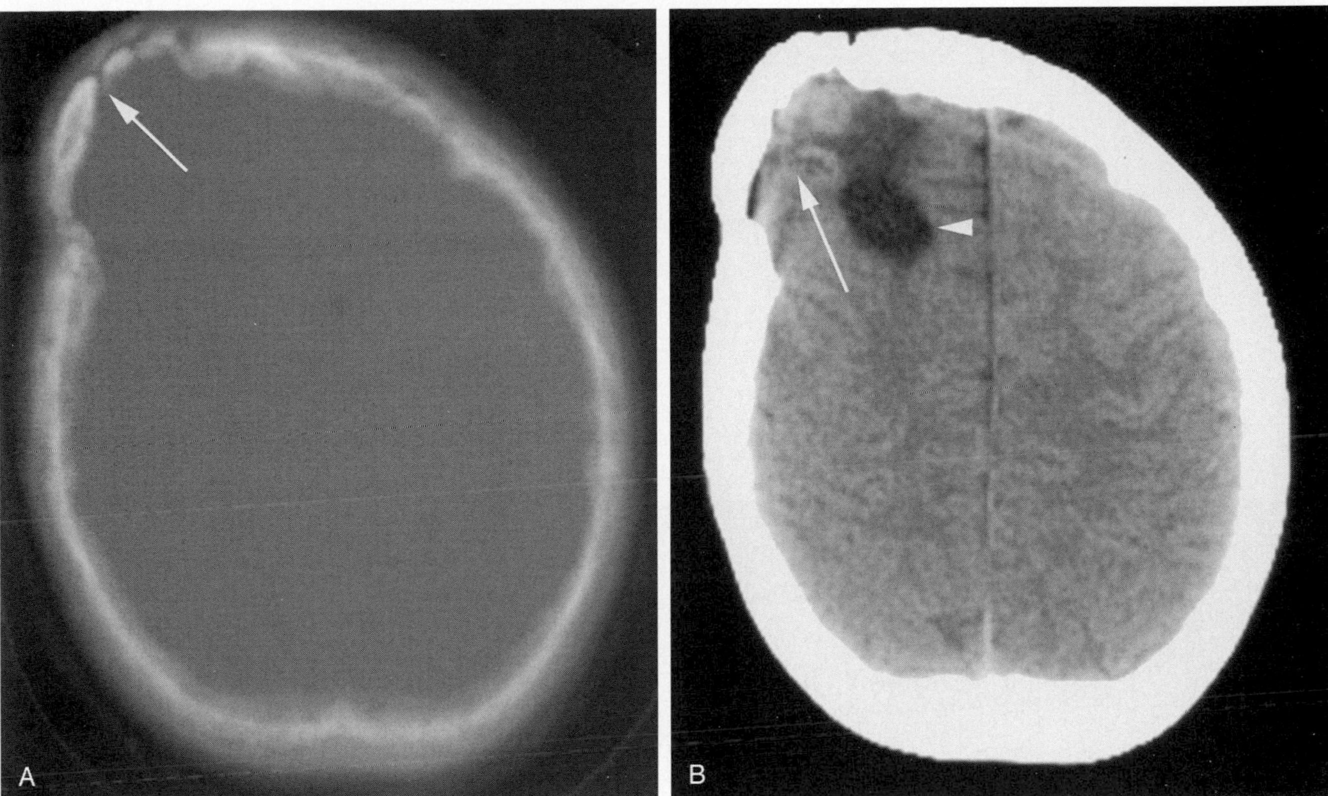

Figure 10–47. Growing skull fracture in a child who had sustained a skull fracture several years earlier. *A*, Axial computed tomography image obtained with bone window settings demonstrates thinning and expansion of the right frontal bone with an area of bony nonunion (*arrow*) at the prior fracture site. *B*, Image obtained with brain window settings at the same level as in *A* reveals herniation of the underlying parenchyma through the calvarial defect (*arrow*), with an underlying area of gliosis (*arrowhead*).

cerebrospinal fluid or brain herniation.[175, 176] A significant number of affected patients will develop delayed neurologic symptoms (e.g., seizure, headache), leading some authorities[175] to advocate early evaluation with MRI to identify those fractures at risk for developing into growing skull fractures. Once those fractures are identified, early surgical repair may be indicated.[175, 177]

Child Abuse

Child abuse, more properly termed *nonaccidental trauma*, accounts for approximately 90% of all life-threatening head injuries in children.[179] It has been estimated that 30%[31] to 45%[179] of cases of nonaccidental trauma will have associated skull fractures, and one half of those with skull fractures will have concomitant intracranial abnormalities.[39] Accidental skull fractures, such as those from falling on a hard surface, are generally simple fractures of the parietal region.[39] Nonaccidental trauma should be suspected when the child has multiple and bilateral fractures, especially if the fracture is complex with a stellate appearance (Fig. 10–48) and involves the occipital region.[39, 179] Although the majority of skull fractures will be demonstrated on the axial CT image or the accompanying digital radiograph, plain skull radiography may also be indicated in cases of suspected abuse to maximize detection of subtle fractures.[31]

Intracranial injuries account for the majority of morbidity and mortality associated with nonaccidental trauma,[36] most commonly in the form of subarachnoid hemorrhages, subdural hemorrhages, parenchymal hematomas and contusions, and diffuse axonal injury.[31] Although not specific for nonaccidental trauma, a posterior interhemispheric subdural hematoma (Fig. 10–49) in a child should be regarded as highly suspicious for abuse.[41] If the head CT is normal but the clinical scenario is strongly suggestive of abuse, MRI is more sensitive for the detection of intracranial pathologic processes and may prove useful in the radiologic evaluation.[179]

Summary

The likelihood of a skull fracture is dependent on the nature and severity of the clinical signs and symptoms of injury. The more severe the injury and prominent the signs, the more likely it is that a fracture will be demonstrated. Clinical criteria can be quite useful in determining the need for a head CT examination or possibly a skull radiograph. From the standpoint of clinical relevance, the possibility of an intracerebral injury far exceeds the presence or absence of a fracture of the calvaria. If intracerebral injury is suspected, it is advantageous to proceed directly with a CT examination and forego plain radiographic evaluation of the skull. MRI is an excellent means of demonstrating and clarifying intracerebral injury in the subacute (Fig. 10–50) and chronic stages. Linear

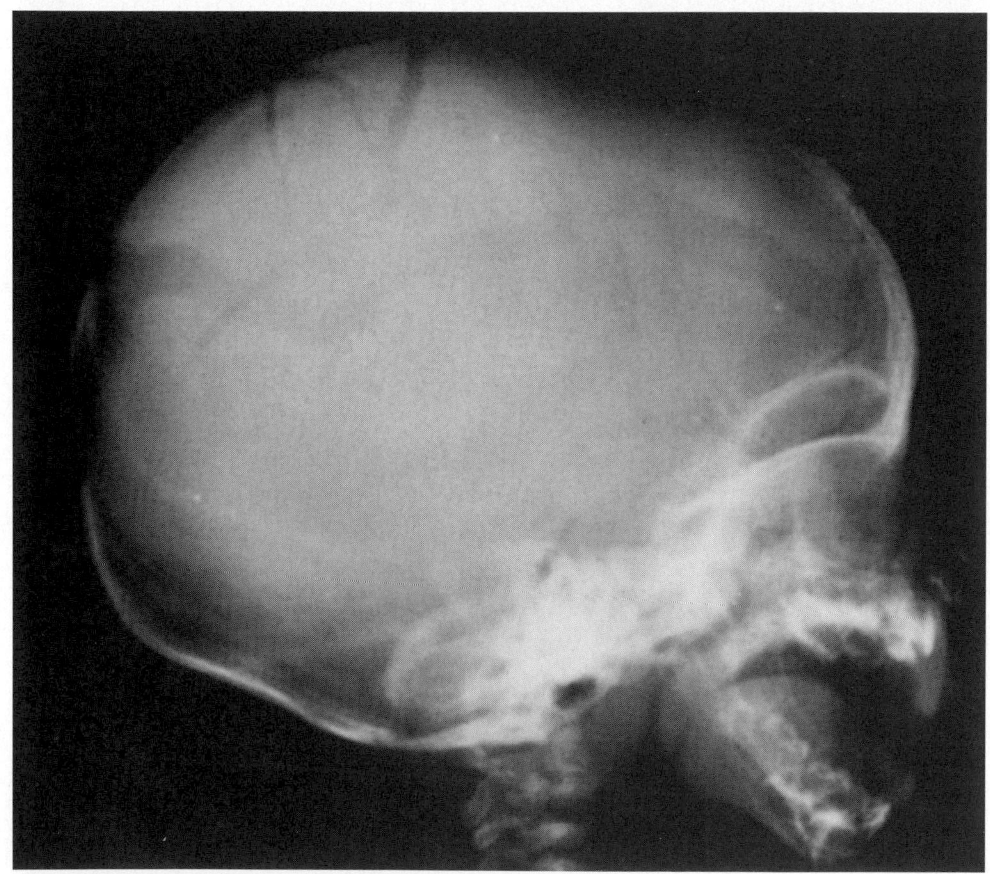

Figure 10–48. Multiple fractures of the skull in a 3-month-old infant subjected to physical abuse. Multiple fractures of the skull in a young infant are characteristic of child abuse. (Case courtesy of Mary Ann Radkowski, MD, Chicago.)

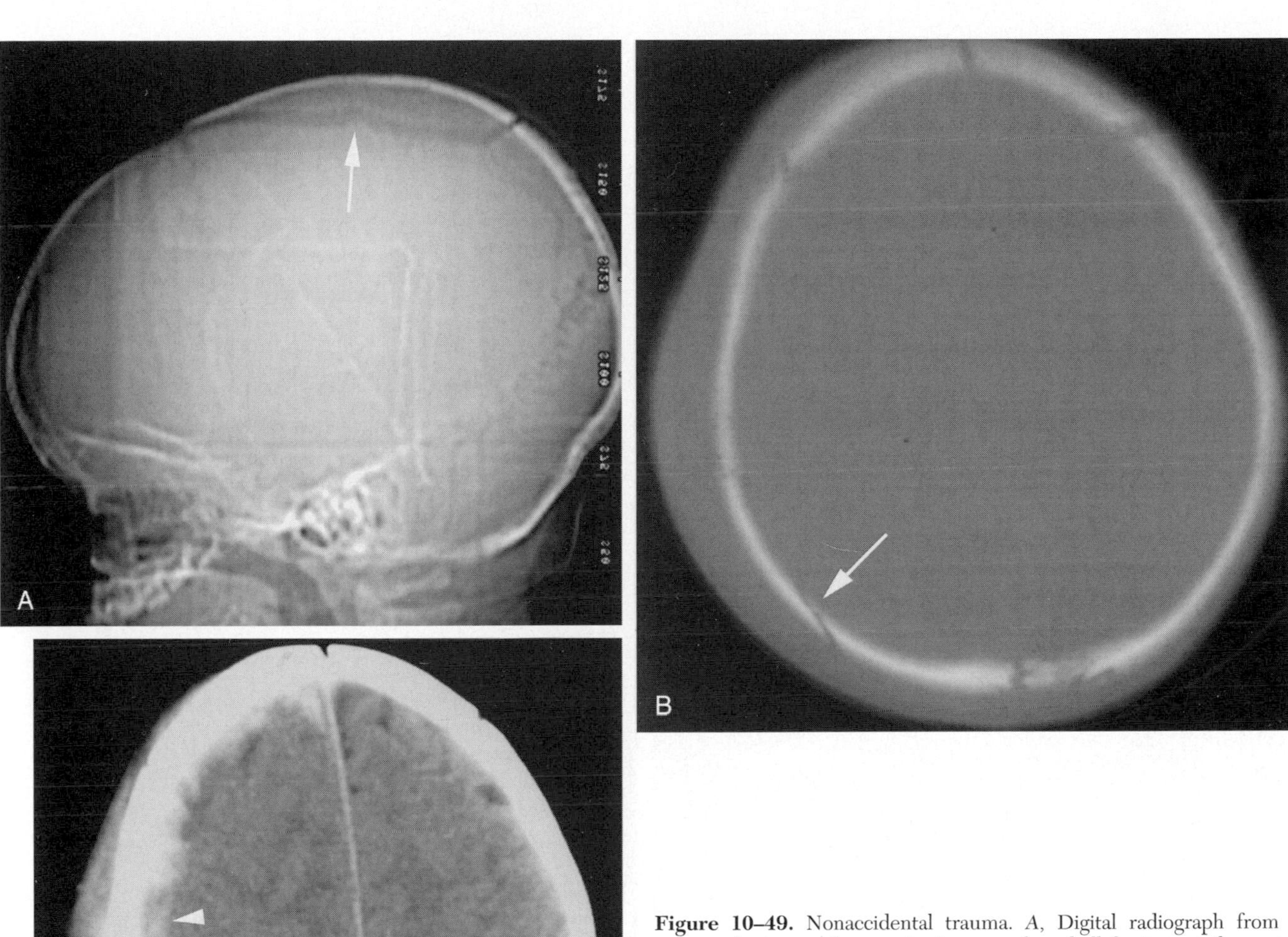

Figure 10–49. Nonaccidental trauma. *A*, Digital radiograph from a computed tomography examination reveals a skull fracture at the vertex (*arrow*). *B*, Axial image from the study demonstrates the right parietal fracture (*arrow*) with overlying soft tissue swelling. *C*, Image obtained with brain window settings at the same level as in *B* displays both convexity (*arrowhead*) and interhemispheric (*arrow*) subdural hemorrhages.

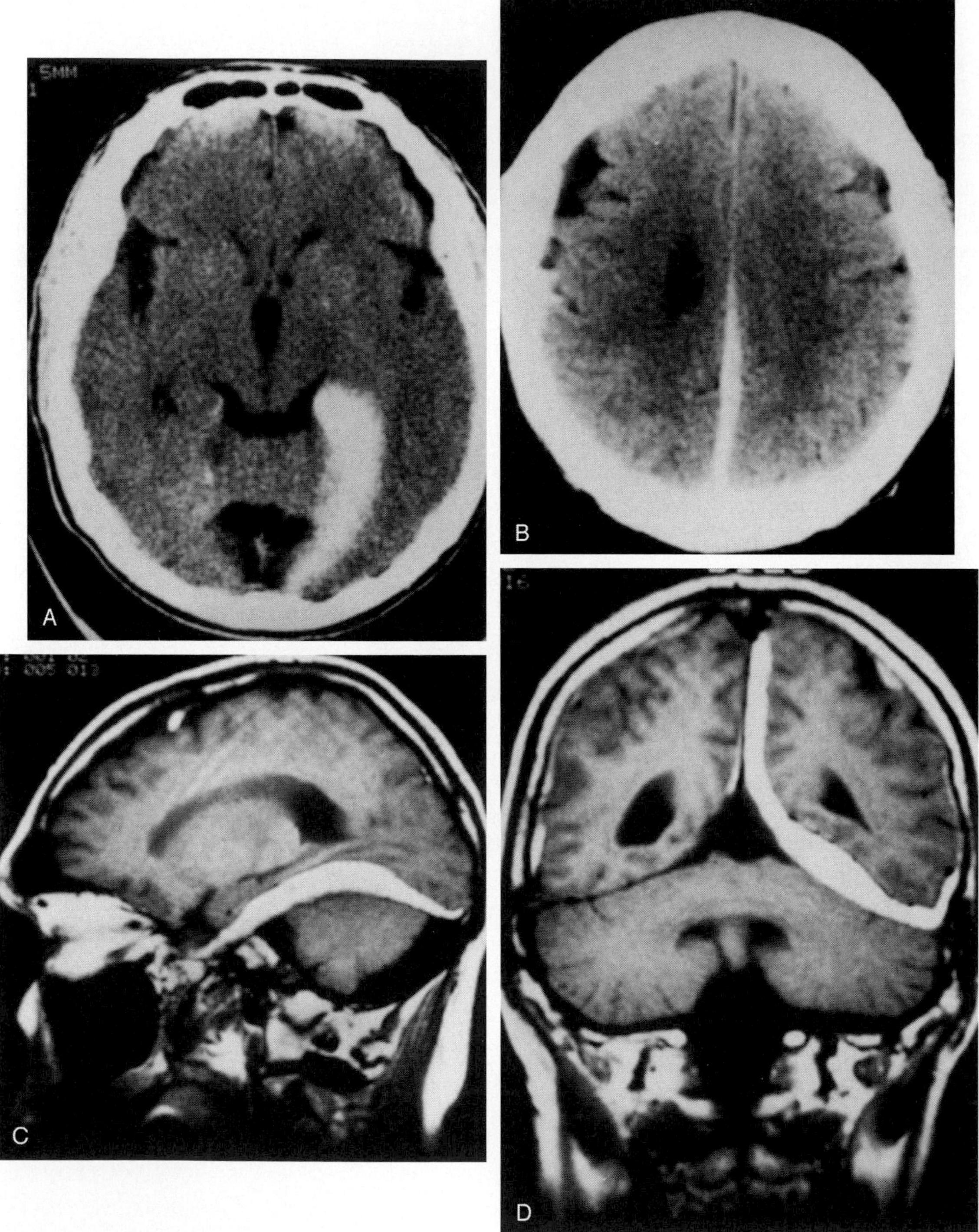

Figure 10–50. Tentorial and interhemispheric subdural hematoma in a 78-year-old man. *A*, This image from a computed tomography examination demonstrates a region of high absorption along the course of the tentorium on the left. Brain atrophy and a large cisterna magna are noted. *B*, Higher cut at the convexity shows similar density in the interhemispheric region posteriorly. *C*, A T_1-weighted sagittal magnetic resonance image demonstrates the tentorial subdural hematoma to excellent advantage. *D*, A coronal T_1-weighted magnetic resonance image shows that the tentorial and interhemispheric subdural hematomas are contiguous.

fractures that cross the meningeal grooves are particularly important because of their association with epidural hemorrhages. Most comminuted fractures are depressed, and the degree of depression correlates with the likelihood of intracranial injury.

Pneumocephalus is indicative of an open injury, usually through the frontal or ethmoid sinuses, and is manifested by air in the ventricles or subarachnoid space. The most frequent location for this air is in the basal cisterns about the sella turcica. Opacification or an air-fluid level within the sphenoid sinuses is an important indicator of basilar skull fracture. The sphenoid sinus and perisellar areas should be scrutinized in every examination of the skull for the evaluation of trauma for the express purpose of identifying these significant findings.

References

General

1. American College of Radiology. (2001). ACR Appropriateness Criteria Head Trauma. Available at http://www.acr.org
2. Bahner, M.L., Reith, W., Zuna, I. et al. (1998). Spiral CT vs. incremental CT: Is spiral CT superior in imaging the brain? Eur. Radiol., *8*:416.
3. Bligh, A.S., Dawson, J.M., Davies, E.R. et al. (1983). A national study by the Royal College of Radiologists. Patient selection for skull radiography in uncomplicated head injury. Lancet, *1*:115.
4. Caffey, J. (1972). Pediatric X-Ray Diagnosis. 6th Ed. Year Book Medical Publishers, Chicago, Ill.
5. Clarke, J.A., & Adams, J.E. (1989). Skull radiographs after head injury. Lancet, *2*:457.
6. Cromwell, L.D., Mack, L.A., & Loop, J.W. (1982). CT scoutview for skull fracture: Substitute for skull films? A.J.N.R. Am. J. Neuroradiol., *3*:421.
7. Cummins, R.O. (1980). Clinician's reasons for overuse of skull radiographs. A.J.N.R. Am. J. Neuroradiol., *1*:339.
8. DeCampo, J., & Petty, P.G. (1980). How useful is the skull x-ray examination in trauma? Med. J. Australia, *2*:553.
9. DeLacey, G., Guilding, A., Wignall, B. et al. (1980). Mild head injuries: A source of excessive radiography? (Analysis of a series and review of the literature.) J. Clin. Radiol., *31*:457.
10. Eyes, B., & Evans, A.F. (1987). Post-traumatic skull radiographs. Time for a reappraisal. Lancet, *2*:85.
11. Fowkes, F.G., Evans, R.C., Williams, L.A. et al. (1984). Implementation of guidelines for the use of skull radiographs in patients with head injuries. Lancet, *2*:795.
12. Jennett, B. (1980). Skull x-rays after recent head injury. Clin. Radiol., *31*:463.
13. Jennett, B., Teasdale, G., & Galbraith, S. (1977). Severe head injuries in three countries. J. Neurol. Neurosurg. Psychiatry, *40*:291.
14. Lehman, L.B. (1988). Skull fractures. Dispelling some misconceptions affecting management. Postgrad. Med., *83*:53.
15. Masters, S.J. (1980). Evaluation of head trauma: Efficacy of skull films. A.J.R. Am. J. Roentgenol., *135*:539.
16. Masters, S.J., McClean, P.M., Arcarese, J.S. et al. (1987). Skull x-ray examination after head trauma. (N. Engl. J. Med., *316*:84.
17. Macpherson, P., & Teasdale, E. (1989). Can computed tomography be relied upon to detect skull fractures? Clin. Radiol., *40*:22.
18. Newton, T.H., & Potts, D.G. (1971). Radiology of the Skull and Brain. The Skull. C.V. Mosby Co., St. Louis, Mo.
19. Phillips, L.A. (1979). Skull radiography and professional liability. West. J. Med., *131*:82.
20. Rathbun, P.E. (1981). Skull radiography after trauma. A.J.R. Am. J. Roentgenol., *136*:632.
21. Rozeik, C., Kotterer, O., Preiss, J. et al. (1991). Cranial CT artifacts and gantry angulation. J. Comput. Assist. Tomogr., *15*:381.
22. Servadei, F., Ciucci, G., Pagano, F. et al. (1988). Skull fractures as a risk factor of intracranial complications in minor head injuries: A prospective CT study in a series of 98 adult patients. J. Neurol. Neurosurg. Psychiatry, *51*:526.
23. Taveras, J.M., & Wood, E.H. (1976). Diagnostic Neuroradiology, 2nd Ed. Williams & Wilkins, Baltimore, Md.
24. Tello, R., Suojanen, J., Costello, P., & McGinnes, A. (1994). Comparison of spiral CT and conventional CT in 3D visualization of facial trauma: Work in progress. Comp. Med. Imaging Graph., *18*:423.
25. Thornbury, J.R., Cambell, J.A., Masters, S.J., & Fryback, D.G. (1984). Skull fracture and the low risk of intracranial sequelae in minor head trauma. A.J.N.R. Am. J. Neuroradiol., *5*:459.
26. Thornbury, J.R., Masters, S.J., & Campbell, J.A. (1987). Imaging recommendations for head trauma: A new comprehensive strategy. A.J.R. Am. J. Roentgenol., *149*:781.
27. Tunturi, T., Neiminen, R., Paetiaelae, H. et al. (1982). Head injuries and skull radiography: Clinical factors predicting a fracture. Injury, *13*:478.
28. Vydareny, K.H., Harle, T.S., & Potchen, E.J. (1983). An algorithmic approach to the roentgenographic evaluation of head trauma: Medical and financial implications. Invest. Radiol., *18*:390.
29. White, J.D. (1987). Skull x-ray examination after head trauma. N. Engl. J. Med., *317*:316.

Skull Fractures in Infants and Children

30. Bowdler, N., Faix, R.G., & Elkins, T. (1987). Fetal skull fracture and brain injury after a maternal automobile accident. A case report. J. Report. Med., *32*:375.
31. Cohen, R.A., Kaufman, R.A., Myers, P.A., & Towbin, R.B. (1986). Cranial computed tomography in the abused child with head injury. A.J.R. Am. J. Roentgenol., *146*:97.
32. Cozzens, J.W., & Eller, T.W. (1987). Spontaneous reduction of a closed depressed skull fracture: A case report. Neurosurgery, *20*:771.
33. Eisenberg, D., Kirchner, S.G., & Perrin, E.C. (1984). Neonatal skull depression associated with birth trauma. A.J.R. Am. J. Roentgenol., *143*:1063.
34. Garza-Mercado, R. (1982). Intrauterine depressed skull fractures of the newborn. Neurosurgery, *10*:694.
35. Holmes, R.D., Kuhns, L.R., & Oliver, W.J. (1977). Widened sutures in childhood meningitis: Unrecognized sign of an acute illness. A.J.R. Am. J. Roentgenol., *128*:977.
36. Kleinman, P.K. (1990). Diagnostic imaging in infant abuse. A.J.R. Am. J. Roentgenol., *155*:703.
37. Meservy, C.J., Towbin, R., McLaurin, R.L. et al. (1987). Radiographic characteristics of skull fractures resulting from child abuse. A.J.N.R. Am. J. Neuroradiol., *8*:455.
38. Mohsenipour, I., Gabl, M., Kostron, H. et al. (1987). Kindliche impressionsfrakturen. Unfallchirurg, *90*:27.
39. Petitti, N., & Williams, D.W., III. (1998). CT and MR imaging in nonaccidental pediatric head trauma. Acad. Radiol., *5*:215.
40. Rosenblum, J., Yousefzadeh, D.K., Ramilo, J.L. (1986). Skull radiography in infants: Potential hazards of the use of head clamps. Radiology, *161*:367.
41. Zimmerman, R.A., Bilaniuk, L.T., Bruce, D. et al. (1978). Interhemispheric acute subdural hematoma: A computed tomographic manifestation of child abuse by shaking. Neuroradiology, *16*:39.
42. Zimmerman, R.A., & Bilaniuk, L.T. (1981). Computed tomography in pediatric head trauma. Neuroradiology, *8*:257.

Skull and Brain Trauma

43. Adams, J.H., Gennarelli, T.A., & Graham, D.I. (1982). Brain damage in nonmissile head injury: Observations in man and subhuman primates. In Smith, W.T., & Cavanah, J.B. Eds.: Recent Advances in Neuropathology. Vol. 2. Churchill Livingstone, Edinburgh.
44. Adams, J.H., Graham, D.L., Murray, L.S., & Scott, G. (1982). Diffuse axonal injury in humans: An analysis of 45 cases. Ann. Neurol., *12*:557.
45. Adams, J.H., Graham, D.I., & Scott, G. (1980). Brain damage in fatal nonmissile head injury. J. Clin. Pathol., *33*:1132.
46. Adams, J.H., Mitchell, D.E., Graham, D.I., & Doyle, D. (1977). Diffuse brain damage of immediate impact type: Its relationship to primary brainstem damage in head injury. Brain, *100*:489.
47. Alker, G.J., Oh, Y.S., Leslie, E.V. et al. (1975). Postmortem radiology of head and neck injuries in fatal traffic accidents. Radiology, *114*:611.
48. Anderson, P.S., & Montesano, X.P. (1988). Morphology and treatment of occipital condylar fractures. Spine, *13*:731.
49. Antworth, M.V., & Beck, R.W. (1989). Traumatic orbital encephalocele. Can. J. Ophthalmol., *24*:129.
50. Bell, R.S., & Loop, J.W. (1971). The utility and futility of radiographic skull examination for trauma. N. Engl. J. Med., *284*:236.
51. Boyko, O.B., Cooper, D.F., & Grossman, C.B. (1991). Contrast-enhanced CT of acute isodense subdural hematoma. A.J.N.R. Am. J. Neuroradiol., *12*:341.
52. Clark, J.M. (1974). Distribution of microglial clusters in the brain after head injury. J. Neurol. Neurosurg. Psychiatry, *37*:463.
53. Cooper, P.R., Maravilla, K., Kirkpatrick, J. et al. (1979). Traumatically induced brainstem hemorrhage and the computerized tomographic scan: Clinical, pathological, and experimental observations. Neurosurgery, *4*:115.
54. Cooper, P.W., & Kassel, E.E. (1983). CT of the cranium in head injury. J. Can. Assoc. Radiol., *34*:167.
55. DeLaPaz, R.L., New, P.F., Buonanno, F.S. et al. (1984). NMR imaging of intracranial hemorrhage. J. Comput. Assist. Tomogr., *8*:599.
56. Dooms, G.C., Uske, A., Brant-Zawadzki, M. et al. (1986). Spin-echo MR imaging of intracranial hemorrhage. Neuroradiology, *28*:132.
57. Dublin, A.B., French, B.N., & Rennick, J.M. (1977). Computed tomography in head trauma. Radiology, *122*:365.
58. Gennarelli, T.A., & Thibault, L.E. (1982). Biomechanics of acute subdural hematoma. J. Trauma, *22*:680.
59. Gentry, L.R., Thompson, B., & Godersky, J.C. (1988). Trauma to the corpus callosum: MR features. A.J.N.R. Am. J. Neuroradiol., *9*:1129.
60. Gentry, L.R., Godersky, J.C., & Thompson, B. (1988). MR imaging of head trauma: Review of the distribution and radiopathologic features of traumatic lesions. A.J.N.R. Am. J. Neuroradiol., *9*:101. A.J.R. Am. J. Roentgenol., *150*:663.
61. Gentry, L.R., Godersky, J.C., Thompson, B., & Dunn, V.D. (1988). Prospective comparative study of intermediate-field MR and CT in the evaluation of closed head trauma. A.J.N.R. Am. J. Neuroradiol., *9*:91. A.J.R. Am. J. Roentgenol., *150*:673.
62. Goh, K.Y., Ahuja, A., Walkden, S.B., & Poon, W.S. (1997). Is routine computed tomographic (CT) scanning necessary in suspected basal skull fractures? Injury, *28*:353.
63. Gomori, J.M., Grossman, R.I., Goldberg, H.I. et al. (1985). Intracranial hematomas: Imaging by high field MR. Radiology, *157*:87.
64. Greenberg, J., Cohen, W.A., & Cooper, P.R. (1985). The "hyperacute" extraaxial intracranial hematoma: Computed tomographic findings and clinical significance. Neurosurgery, *17*:48.
65. Gross, A.G. (1958). A new theory on the dynamics of brain concussion and brain injury. J. Neurosurg., *15*:548.

66. Grossart, K.W., & Samuel, E. (1961). Traumatic diastasis of cranial sutures. Clin. Radiol., *12*:164.
67. Gurdjian, E.S., Lissner, H.R., Hodgson, V.R., & Patrick, L.M. (1974). Mechanism of head injury. Clin. Neurosurg., *12*:112.
68. Gurdjian, E.S., Webster, J.E., & Lissner, H.R. (1955). Observations on the mechanism of brain concussion, contusion, and laceration. Surg. Gynecol. Obstet., *101*:680.
69. Harwood-Nash, D.C., Hendrick, E.B., & Hudson, A.R. (1971). The significance of skull fractures in children. A study of 1,187 patients. Radiology, *101*:151.
70. Jenkins, A., Teasdale, G., Hadley, M.D. et al. (1986). Brain lesions detected by magnetic resonance in mild and severe head injuries. Lancet, *2*:445.
71. Kelly, A.B., Zimmerman, R.D., Snow, R.B. et al. (1988). Head trauma: Comparison of MR and CT—experience in 100 patients. A.J.N.R. Am. J. Neuroradiol., *9*:699.
72. Klein, F.C. (1982). Silent epidemic: Head injuries, often difficult to diagnose, get rising attention. Wall Street Journal, LXIII(30):1.
73. Klufas, R.A., Liangge, H., Patel, M.R., & Schwartz, R.B. (1996). Unusual manifestations of head trauma. A.J.R. Am. J. Roentgenol., *166*:675.
74. Koo, A.H., & LaRoque, R.L. (1977). Evaluation of head trauma by computed tomography. Radiology, *123*:345.
75. Leone, A., Cerase, A., Colosimo, C. et al. (2000). Occipital condylar fractures: A review. Radiology, *216*:635.
76. Levy, R.A., Edwards, W.T., Meye, J.R., & Rosenbaum, A.E. (1992). Facial trauma and 3-D reconstructive imaging: Insufficiencies and correctives. A.J.N.R. Am. J. Neuroradiol., *13*:885.
77. Lindenberg, R. (1966). Significance of the tentorium in head injuries from blunt forces. Clin. Neurosurg., *12*:129.
78. Lindenberg, R., & Freytag, E. (1960). The mechanism of cerebral contusions: A pathologic-anatomic study. Arch. Pathol. Lab. Med., *69*:440.
79. Link, T.M., Schuierer, G., Hufendiek, M.S. et al. (1995). Substantial head trauma: Value of routine CT examination of the cervicocranium. Radiology, *196*:741.
80. Lipper, M.H., Kishore, P.R., Enas, G.G. et al. (1985). Computed tomography in the prediction of outcome in head injury. A.J.N.R. Am. J. Neuroradiol., *6*:7. A.J.R. Am. J. Roentgenol., *144*:483.
81. Manfre, L., Nicoletti, G., Lombardo, M. et al. (1993). Orbital "blow-in" fracture: MRI. Neuroradiology, *35*:612.
82. McRae, D.L. (1966). The role of radiology in the management of the head injured patient. p. 111. In Caveness, W.F., & Walker, A.E. Eds.: Head Injury: Conference Proceedings. J.B. Lippincott Co., Philadelphia.
83. Roberts, F., & Shopner, C.E. (1972). Plain skull roentgenograms in children with head trauma. A.J.R. Am. J. Roentgenol., *114*:230.
84. Peyster, R.G., & Hoover, E.D. (1982). CT in head trauma. J. Trauma, *22*:25.
85. Piepmeier, J.M., & Wagner, F.C. Jr. (1982). Delayed post-traumatic extracerebral hematomas. J. Trauma, *22*:455.
86. Pilz, P. (1983). Axonal injury in head injury. Acta Neurochir. Suppl. (Wien), *32*:119.
87. Reed, D., Robertson, W.D., Graeb, D.A. et al. (1986). Acute subdural hematomas: Atypical CT findings. A.J.N.R. Am. J. Neuroradiol., *7*:417.
88. Sato, O., Kamitani, H., & Kokunai, T. (1978). Blow-in fracture of both orbital roofs caused by shear strain to the skull. Case report. J. Neurosurg., *49*:734.
89. Shigemori, M., Kojyo, N., Yuge, T. et al. (1986). Massive traumatic hematoma of the corpus callosum. Acta Neurochir., *81*:36.
90. Snow, R.B., Zimmerman, R.D., Gandy, S.E., & Deck, M.D. (1986). Comparison of magnetic resonance imaging and computed tomography in the evaluation of head injury. Neurosurgery, *18*:45.
91. Soloniuk, D., Pitts, L.H., Lovely, M., & Bartkowski, H. (1986). Traumatic intracerebral hematomas: Timing of appearance and indications for operative removal. J. Trauma, *26*:787.
92. Stone, J.L., Lowe, R.J., Jonasson, O. et al. (1986). Acute subdural hematoma: Direct admission to a trauma center yields improved results. J. Trauma, *26*:445.
93. Tomsick, T.A., Chambers, A.A., & Lukin, R.R. (1978). Skull fractures. Semin Roentgenol., *8*:27.
94. Tuli, S., Tator, C.H., Fehlings, M.G., & Mackay, M. (1997). Occipital condyle fractures. Neurosurgery, *41*:368.
95. Wilberger, J.E., Deeb, Z., & Rothfus, W. (1987). Magnetic resonance imaging in cases of severe head injury. Neurosurgery, *20*:571.
96. Zimmerman, R.A., Bilaniuk, L.T., Gennarelli, T.G. et al. (1978). Cranial computed tomography in diagnosis and management of acute head trauma. A.J.R. Am. J. Roentgenol., *131*:27.
97. Zimmerman, R.A., Bilaniuk, L.T., & Gennarelli, T.G. (1978). Computed tomography of shearing injuries of the cerebral white matter. Radiology, *127*:393.
98. Zimmerman, R.A., & Bilaniuk, L.T. (1982). Computed tomographic staging of traumatic epidural bleeding. Radiology, *144*:809.
99. Zimmerman, R.A., Bilaniuk, L.T., Hackney, D.B. et al. (1986). Head injury: Early results comparing CT and high-field MR. A.J.N.R. Am. J. Neuroradiol., *7*:757. A.J.R. Am. J. Roentgenol., *147*:1215.
100. Zimmerman, R.A., & Bilaniuk, L.T. (1979). Computed tomography in diffuse traumatic cerebral injury. p 253. In Popp, A.J., Bourke, R.S., Nelson, L.R., & Kimelberg, H.K. Eds.: Neural Trauma. Raven Press, New York.

Cranial Sutures and Vascular Grooves

101. Allen, W.E., Kier, E.L., & Rothman, S.L. (1973). Pitfalls in the evaluation of skull trauma (a review). Radiol. Clin. North Am., *11*:479.
102. Santagati, F. (1939). Anatomia radografica dei solchi e dei canali vascolari del cranio. Radiol. Med., *26*:317.
103. Schunk, H., & Maruyama, Y. (1960). Two vascular grooves of the external table of the skull which simulate fractures. Acta Radiol., *54*:186.

Foreign Bodies

104. Ginsberg, L.E., Williams D.W. III, & Mathews, V.P. (1993). CT in penetrating craniocervical injury by wooden foreign bodies: Reminder of a pitfall. A.J.N.R. Am. J. Neuroradiol., *14*:892.
105. Hollerman, J.J., Fackler, M.L., Coldwell, D.M., & Ben-Menachem, Y. (1990). Gunshot wounds: Parts I and II: Bullets, ballistics, and mechanisms of injury. A.J.R. Am. J. Roentgenol., *155*:685.
106. Miller, C.F., Brodkey, J.S., & Colombi, B.J. (1977). The danger of intracranial wood. Surg. Neurol., *7*:95.

Sphenoid Fractures

107. Archer, C.R., & Sundaram, M. (1976). Uncommon sphenoid fractures and their sequelae. Radiology, *122*:157.
108. Carlson, G.O., Haverling, M., & Molin, C. (1973). Isolated fracture of the base of the skull within the sella region. Acta Radiol., *14*:662.
109. Chen, S.S., Shao, K.N., Chiang, J.H., et al. (2000). Cavernous sinus gas. Zhonghua Yi Xue Za Zhi (Taipei), *63*:586.
110. Joslyn, J.N., Mirvis, S.E., & Markowitz, B. (1988). Complex fractures of the clivus: Diagnosis with CT and clinical outcome in 11 patients. Radiology, *166*:817.
111. Ghobrial, W., Amstrutz, S., & Mathog, R.H. (1986). Fractures of the sphenoid bone. Head Neck Surg., *8*:447.
112. Hasso, A.N., Lasjaunias, P., Thompson, J.R., & Hinshaw, D.B. Jr. (1979). Venous occlusions of the cavernous area—a complication of crushing fractures of the sphenoid bone. Radiology, *132*:375.
113. Newbold, R.G., Wiener, M.D., Vogler, J.B. III, & Martinez, S. (1987). Traumatic pneumorrhachis. A.J.R. Am. J. Roentgenol., *148*:615.
114. Ogawa, T.K., Bergeron, R.T., Whitaker, C.W. et al. (1976). Air-fluid levels in the sphenoid sinus in epistaxis and nasal packing. Radiology, *118*:351.
115. Quinn, S.F., & Smathers, R.L. (1984). The diagnostic significance of posttraumatic sphenoid sinus effusions: Correlation with head computed tomography. CT, *8*:61.
116. Resnick, D.R., Subach, B.R., & Marion, D.W. (1997). The significance of carotid canal involvement in basilar cranial fracture. Neurosurgery, *40*:1177.
117. Reynolds, D.F. (1961). Traumatic effusion of the sphenoid sinus. Clin. Radiol., *12*:171.
118. Robinson, A.E., Meares, B.M., & Goree, J.A. (1967). Traumatic sphenoid sinus effusion: An analysis of 50 cases. A.J.R. Am. J. Roentgenol., *101*:795.
119. Tartara, F., Regolo, P., Servadei, F., et al. (2000). Fatal carotid dissection after blunt head trauma. J. Neurosurg. Sci., *44*:103.
120. Uzan, M., Cantasdemir, M., Seckin, M.S. et al. (1998). Traumatic intracranial carotid tree aneurysms. Neurosurgery, *43*:1314.

Temporal Bone Trauma

121. Aguilar, E.A., III, Yeakley, J.W., Ghorayeb, B.Y. et al. (1987). High resolution CT scan of temporal bone fractures: Association of facial nerve paralysis with temporal bone fractures. Head Neck Surg., *9*:162.
122. Bradford, W.B., & Wiener, M.D. (1991). Air in the temporomandibular joint fossa: CT sign of temporal bone fractures. Radiology, *180*:463.
123. Cannon, C.R., & Jahrsdoerfer, R.A. (1983). Temporal bone fractures. Arch. Otolaryngol., *109*:285.
124. Chakeres, D.W., & Spiegel, P.K. (1983). A systematic technique for comprehensive evaluation of the temporal bone by computed tomography. Radiology, *146*:97.
125. Ghorayeb, B.Y., & Yeakley, J.W. (1992). Temporal bone fractures: Longitudinal or oblique? The case for oblique temporal bone fractures. Laryngoscope, *102*:129.
126. Grobovaschek, M., & Oberascher, G. (1988). Dislocations and fractures of the ossicles—HR-CT of the injured petrous bone. Digit. Bilddiagn., *8*:78.
127. Grove, W.E. (1939). Skull fractures involving the ear. A clinical study of 211 cases. Laryngoscope, *49*:678.
128. Holland, B.A., & Brant-Zawadzki, M. (1984). High-resolution CT of temporal bone trauma. A.J.R. Am. J. Roentgenol., *143*:391.
129. Hough, J.D., & Stuart, W.D. (1968). Middle ear injuries in skull trauma. Laryngoscope, *78*:899.
130. Johnson, D.W., Hasso, A.N., Stewart, C.E. III et al. (1984). Temporal bone trauma: High resolution computed tomographic evaluation. Radiology, *151*:411.
131. Li, S.T., & Baxter, A.B. (2000). Traumatic ossicular disruption. A.J.R. Am. J. Roentgenol., *174*:1296.
132. Lipkin, A.F., Bryan, R.N., & Jenkins, H.A. (1985). Pneumolabyrinth after temporal bone fracture: Documentation by high-resolution CT. A.J.N.R. Am. J. Neuroradiol., *6*:294.
133. Mafee, M.F., Valvassori, G.E., Kumar, A. et al. (1984). Pneumolabyrinth: A new radiologic sign for fracture of the stapes footplate. Am. J. Otol., *5*:374.
134. Momose, K.J., Davis, K.R., & Rhea, J.T. (1983). Hearing loss in skull fractures. A.J.N.R. Am. J. Neuroradiol., *4*:781.

135. Nurre, J.W., Miller, G.W., Ball, J.B. Jr. (1988). Pneumolabyrinth as a late sequela of temporal bone fracture. Am. J. Otol., *9*:489.
136. Potter, G.D. (1969). Trauma to the temporal bone. Semin. Roentgenol., *4*:143.
137. Shaffer, K.A., Haughton, V.M., & Wilson, C.R. (1980). High resolution computed tomography of the temporal bone. Radiology, *134*:404.
138. Wiet, R.J., Valvassori, G.E., Kotsanis, C.A., & Parahy, C. (1985). Temporal bone fractures. State of the art review. Am. J. Otol., *6*:207.
139. Woodrow, P.K. (1981). CT detection of subarachnoid pneumocephalus secondary to mastoid fracture. CT, *5*:199.
140. Yeakley, J.W. (1999). Temporal bone fractures. Curr. Probl. Diagn. Radiol., *28*:65.
141. Zimmerman, R.A., Bilaniuk, L.T., Hackney, D.B. et al. (1987). Magnetic resonance in temporal bone fracture. Neuroradiology, *29*:246.

Pneumocephalus

142. Aoki, N. (1986). Air in acute epidural hematomas. Report of two cases. J. Neurosurg., *65*:555.
143. Azar-Kia, B., Sarwar, M., Batinitzky, S., & Schechter, M.M. (1975). Radiology of intracranial gas. A.J.R. Am. J. Roentgenol., *124*:315.
144. Barth, E.E., & Irwin, G.E. Jr, (1950). Traumatic pneumocephalus. Radiology, *54*:424.
145. Bartlett, J.R. (1971). Intracranial neurological complications of frontal and ethmoidal osteomas. Br. J. Surg., *58*:607.
146. Bartynski, W.S., & Wang, A.M. (1988). Cavernous sinus air in a patient with basilar skull fracture: CT identification. J. Comput. Assist. Tomogr., *12*:141.
147. Bhimani, S., Virapongse, C., Sabshin, J.K. et al. (1985). Intracerebral pneumatocele: CT findings. Radiology, *154*:111.
148. Cervantes, L.A. (1983). Concurrent delayed temporal and posterior fossa epidural hematomas. Case report. J. Neurosurg., *59*:351.
149. Dandy, W.E. (1926). Pneumocephalus (intracranial, pneumatocele or aerocele). Arch. Surg., *12*:949.
150. Eaglesham, D.C. (1945). Radiological aspects of intracranial pneumocephalus. Br. J. Radiol., *18*:335.
151. Goldmann, R.W. (1986). Pneumocephalus as a consequence of barotrauma. J.A.M.A., *255*:315.
152. Jones, H.M. (1970). Cranial pneumatocele. Proc. R. Soc. Med., *63*:257.
153. Kahn, R.J., & Daywitt, A.L. (1963). Traumatic pneumocephalus. A.J.R. Am. J. Roentgenol., *90*:1171.
154. Markham, J.W. (1967). The clinical features of pneumocephalus based upon a survey of 284 cases with report of 11 additional cases. Acta Neurochir, 161.
155. McCall, C.S., Nguyen, T.Q., Vines, F.S., & Brenner, A.M. (1986). Pneumocephalus secondary to tension pneumothorax associated with comminuted fracture of the thoracic spine. Neurosurgery, *19*:120.
156. Mendelsohn, D., & Hertzanu, Y. (1985). Intracerebral pneumatoceles following facial trauma: CT findings. Radiology, *154*:115.
157. North, J.W. (1971). On the importance of intracranial air. Br. J. Surg., *58*:826.
158. Osborn, A.G., Daines, J.H., Wing, S.D., & Anderson, R.E. (1978). Intracranial air on computerized tomography. J. Neurosurg., *48*:355.
159. Sage, M.R., & McAllister, V.L. (1974). Spontaneous intracranial "aerocele" with chromophobe adenoma. Br. J. Radiol., *47*:727.

Cerebrospinal Fluid Rhinorrhea

160. Ahmadi, J., Weiss, M.H., Segall, H.D. et al. (1985). Evaluation of cerebrospinal fluid rhinorrhea by metrizamide computed tomographic cisternography. Neurosurgery, *16*:54.
161. Christoforidis, G.A., Mehta, B.A., Landi, I.L. et al. (1998). Spontaneous intracranial hypotension: Report of four cases and review of the literature. Neuroradiology, *40*:636.
162. Drayer, B.P., Wilkins, R.H., Boehnke, M. et al. (1977). Cerebrospinal fluid rhinorrhea demonstrated by metrizamide CT cisternography. A.J.R. Am. J. Roentgenol., *129*:149.
163. Fox, J.L., & Schiebel, F.G. (1979). Intracranial air bubbles localizing cerebrospinal fluid fistula. J. Comput. Assist. Tomogr., *3*:832.
164. Gissane, W., & Rank, B.K. (1940). Post-traumatic cerebrospinal rhinorrhea with case report. Br. J. Surg., *27*:717.
165. Ghoshhajra, K. (1980). Metrizamide CT cisternography in the diagnosis and localization of cerebrospinal fluid rhinorrhea. J. Comput. Assist. Tomogr., *4*:306.
166. Hudgins, P.A. (1999, May). Evaluation of the patient with a CSF leak. Presented at the American Society of Head and Neck Radiology Symposium: Clinical Problem Focused Imaging in the Head and Neck, San Diego, Calif.
167. Jungmann, A., & Peyser, E. (1963). Roentgen visualization of cerebrospinal fluid fistula with contrast medium. Radiology, *80*:92.
168. Manelfe, C., Cellerier, P., Soble, D. et al. (1982). Cerebrospinal fluid rhinorrhea: Evaluation with metrizamide cisternography. A.J.N.R. Am. J. Neuroradiol., *3*:25.
169. Marc, J.A., & Schechter, M.M. (1973). The significance of fluid gas displacement in the sphenoid sinus in post-traumatic cerebrospinal fluid rhinorrhea. Radiology, *108*:603.
170. Morley, T.P., & Hetherington, R.F. (1957). Traumatic cerebrospinal fluid rhinorrhea and otorrhea, pneumocephalus, and meningitis. Surg. Gynecol. Obstet., *104*:88.
171. Raaf, J. (1967). Post-traumatic cerebrospinal fluid leaks. Arch. Surg., *95*:648.
172. Ray, B.S., & Bergland, R.M. (1969). Cerebrospinal fluid fistula: Clinical aspects, techniques of localization, and methods of closure. J. Neurosurg., *30*:339.
173. Teng, P., & Edalatpour, N. (1963). Cerebrospinal fluid rhinorrhea with demonstration of cranionasal fistula with Pantopaque. Radiology, *81*:802.
174. Ware, M., Swinscow, T.D., & Thwaites, J.G. (1969). CSF rhinorrhoea. Br. J. Radiol., *1*:137.

Growing Skull Fractures

175. Ellis, T.S., Gilbert, L.G., & Donahue D.J. (2000). Acute identification of cranial burst practure: Comparison between CT and MR imaging findings. A.J.N.R. Am. J. Neuroradiol., *21*:795.
176. Husson, B., Pariente, D., Tammam, S., & Zerah, M. (1996). The value of MRI in the early diagnosis of growing skull fracture. Pediatr. Radiol., *26*:744.
177. Kutlay, M., Demircon, N., Niyazi, O., & Basekim, C. (1998). Untreated growing cranial eractures detected in late stage. Neurosurgery, *43*:72.
178. Muhonen, M.G., Piper, J.G., & Menezes, A.H. (1995). Pathogenesis and treatment of growing skull fractures. Surg. Neurol., *43*:67.
179. Murray, J.G., Gean, A.D., & Evans, S.J. (1996). Imaging of Acute Head Injury. Semin. Ultrasound CT MR, *17*:185.

Chapter 11

THE FACE

with James T. Rhea, MD, Mark E. Mullins, MD, and Robert A. Novelline, MD

Facial trauma is a common clinical problem in emergency medicine centers. In the United States, most injuries result from motor vehicle collisions, fights, and assaults. Motor vehicle collisions are the most common cause of serious facial injury.[14] Most of these injuries are limited to the soft tissue, but many include fractures of the facial skeleton. Traffic accidents and blows sustained during assaults together account for 80% of all injuries to the facial skeleton. The ratio[13, 19, 23] of accidents to blows, ranging from 4:1 to 1:4, depends on the series. The remainder of injuries in most series (15% to 20%) are due to falls, sports activities, and, in smaller numbers, industrial accidents and gunshot wounds. Facial fractures occur in about a third of injuries from powered watercraft collisions, a third of injuries from street bicycle accidents, and over half of injuries from mountain bike accidents.[164, 165] About 40% of patients with skiing injuries sustain facial fracture.[166] In the multitrauma patient, facial fracture frequently is not suspected clinically and is initially identified on computed tomography (CT) examination of the patient's head.[167]

The distribution of fractures within the facial skeleton also varies with the mechanism of injury. McCoy and associates[46] reported a series of 855 patients with fractures of the face; 41% had fractures in the middle third of the face, 38% had fractures limited to the mandible, and 22% had fractures limited to the nasal bones. Of those patients who had fractures of the middle third of the face, 12% also had fractures of the mandible, and 8% had nasal fractures. Fractures of the middle third of the face are more likely to occur as the result of automobile accidents, and the ratio of fractures of the middle third of the face to fractures of the mandible is expected to be higher in reported series including a high percentage of auto accidents. Some investigations exclude outpatients, which results in a lower percentage of nasal fractures.

The most common fracture of the midface is the zygomatic complex (ZMC) fracture. ZMC fractures account for approximately 40%[13, 19, 23] of all midfacial fractures. Fractures limited to the zygomatic arch account for an additional 10% of midfacial fractures. Another 5% of midfacial fractures are limited to the alveolar process of the maxilla. The remaining 45% are complex fractures. The LeFort classification is commonly utilized to describe midfacial fractures, but precise definition of these complicated injuries is frequently difficult.[39, 40, 42, 54] As a rough approximation, it can be said that 15% of the complex fractures are basically LeFort I injuries, whereas LeFort II and LeFort III injuries are found in 10%, respectively; the remainder are highly comminuted fractures—so-called smash injuries, defying classification.

Less than 10% of all facial fractures occur in children, and children tend to be less seriously injured than adults.[2] Falls are by far the most common cause of these injuries, followed by traffic collisions, usually involving a bicycle. The middle portion of the face is less prominent in children, and the sinuses are less pneumatized in younger children, resulting in relatively fewer fractures involving this portion of the face than in adults.[177] For example, classic LeFort fractures are not seen. A fracture across the middle of the face may occur, but the fracture plane tends to be oblique when the relative areas of weakness and strength seen in the adult have not yet developed.[195] Bone in children is more elastic, and greenstick-type fractures may be seen, especially in the condylar process of the mandible.[126, 128, 132] Fractures that are more frequent in children than in adults include fractures of the mandibular condyle and the orbital roof.[192]

Most facial fractures represent a shearing off of one portion of the facial skeleton from the remainder. The separated fragment is frequently called the principal fragment. Blows from a small mass moving at a high velocity, such as from a club, bat, or pipe, may result in fractures confined to the site of impact, as with depressed fractures of the skull. These injuries are most likely to occur at the orbital rim, particularly superiorly, in the zygomatic arch, or in the nasofrontal region. Blows from a relatively greater mass with a lesser velocity, as from a fist, have a broader impact. Comminution at the point of impact is less likely than is rotational displacement of a larger bone fragment. This type of injury is exemplified by the ZMC fracture, which is frequently sustained from a blow on the cheek or malar eminence. High-speed forces of broader impact create fractures along the lines of weakness described by LeFort.[43, 55] Initially the force is absorbed at the point of impact, often resulting in comminution, but then it is dispersed along the lines of weakness as a shearing force producing fractures remote from the point of impact.

The possibility of facial injury should be carefully evaluated on the CT study of the head in a multitrauma patient because some injuries may compromise vision if not immediately recognized. If there is evidence of a facial injury in a stable patient, obtaining a facial CT examination takes little additional time when the patient is already in the scanner. If vision is not in jeopardy, surgical repair of facial fractures can safely be deferred until the patient's condition stabilizes, swelling of the face subsides, and other more pressing and serious injuries have been treated.

Injuries of other parts of the body associated with facial fracture are frequent,[13, 19, 23] occurring in one third to one half of patients. Extremity injury accounts for the majority. Skull fractures are reported in 3% to 14%, and cervical spine fractures, in 1% to 4%.[145] In contrast, 20% of patients with cervical spine fractures have facial injuries, just under half of which are facial fractures.[17]

A chest radiograph may show evidence of problems directly related to facial injuries. Fractures involving the alveolar processes of the mandible or maxilla may result in aspiration of teeth, which may be identified initially within the airway or may result in associated atelectasis. Occasionally, pneumomediastinum[53, 56, 82, 140] is seen as a result of facial fractures involving the sinuses. Pneumomediastinum has also been reported after a nasal fracture.[205] Air enters the mediastinum via communication with the retropharyngeal soft tissues. Because pneumomediastinum suggests the possibility of rupture of the bronchus or trachea or of the esophagus, these injuries should be clinically and radiologically excluded before facial fracture is accepted as the cause of mediastinal air.

The diagnosis of facial trauma has been greatly improved by the use of CT. On plain radiography, superimposition of facial structures and the thinness of some of the facial bones often interfere with accurate assessment. With CT, the facial bones and soft tissues are displayed in exquisite detail. To most effectively utilize CT in facial trauma diagnosis, the examiner should be familiar with facial anatomy as well as the types of injuries that can occur.

The purpose of imaging is to identify fractures, fragment displacement and rotation, and any soft tissue injuries. In addition to injury, imaging should also identify the presence of stable bone for use in surgical repair. CT examination in axial and coronal planes is optimal for diagnosis of fractured and stable bone, whereas three-dimensional (3-D) CT is useful in showing rotation and displacement.[21] Three-dimensional CT has proved useful in orbital reconstruction with restoration of orbital volume.[204] Stereoscopic 3-D CT has been described in the evaluation of facial trauma.[216]

Normal Facial Anatomy

The facial bones are irregularly shaped and may contain protrusions or processes that extend toward adjacent bones. A process is named for a bone with which there is a suture. For example, the frontal process of the zygoma joins the frontal bone at the zygomaticofrontal suture. Flat portions of facial bones are often referred to as plates. For example, the orbital plate of the ethmoid (lamina papyracea) forms part of the medial orbital wall. Normal skeletal anatomy of the facial bones is depicted in Figure 11–1, and the anatomy of the eye, in Figure 11–2.

The nasal bones are small and quadrilateral in shape. The left and right nasal bones have a suture between them in the midline and are bound by sutures with the frontal bone and the frontal process of the maxilla. In the midline the nasal bones and the frontal bone articulate with the perpendicular plate of the ethmoid, which with the vomer forms the bony nasal septum.

The orbital rim is composed of relatively thicker bone compared with that of the walls of the orbit. The medial orbital rim is composed largely of the frontal process of the maxilla, with frontal bone contributing superiorly. The superior rim is formed by the frontal bone. The lateral rim is composed of the frontal process of the zygoma and the zygomatic process of the frontal bone. The inferior rim is formed by the zygoma and maxilla.

The orbital space is bound by its medial and lateral walls and the roof and floor. Extending posteriorly from the nasal bone and frontal process of the maxilla are the bones of the medial wall of the orbit: the lacrimal bone and the orbital plate of the ethmoid bone (lamina papyracea). The lacrimal bone contains the lacrimal duct; injury to this structure may result in poor drainage of tears from the orbit. The floor of the orbit is composed largely of the orbital plates of the maxilla and zygoma, with a small contribution posteriorly from the orbital plate of the palatine bone. The floor is bound by the inferior orbital fissure laterally. The inferior orbital groove runs through the floor and contains the infraorbital nerve, which innervates the cheek. The lateral orbital wall is formed by the orbital plate of the zygoma and the greater wing of the sphenoid. The superior orbital fissure separates the greater wing of the sphenoid from the lesser wing of the sphenoid and the orbital plate of the ethmoid medially. The roof of the orbit is formed by the orbital plate of the frontal bone.

The body of the zygoma forms the prominence of the cheek, the malar eminence. The zygoma extends across the lateral wall of the orbit to articulate with the sphenoid bone and across the orbital floor and upper portion of the maxillary sinus to articulate with the maxilla. The zygoma has two processes: the frontal process, which forms the lateral orbital rim, and the temporal process, which forms the anterior portion of the zygomaticotemporal (zygomatic) arch. The posterior portion of the arch is formed by the zygomatic process of the temporal bone. The suture of the zygoma with the temporal bone is located near the middle of the arch. The body of the zygoma is supported by the inferior orbital rim, the lateral orbital rim, and the zygomatic arch.

The maxilla is composed of the hard palate, the alveolar process that supports the maxillary teeth, the inferior portion of the maxillary sinuses, the floor of the orbit medially, and the frontal process. The frontal process of the maxilla articulates with the nasal bone, the frontal bone, and the lacrimal bone. The maxilla forms the medial part of the floor of the orbit and articulates with the ethmoid medially and the zygoma laterally. Posteriorly, the maxilla articulates with the pterygoid processes of the sphenoid and with the palatine bone, which forms the posterior part of the hard palate. In the midline, the maxilla articulates with the vomer, which is the inferior portion of the nasal septum. The anterior nasal spine of the maxilla is at the anterior aspect of the hard palate in the midline.

The mandible has no sutures with other bones. The

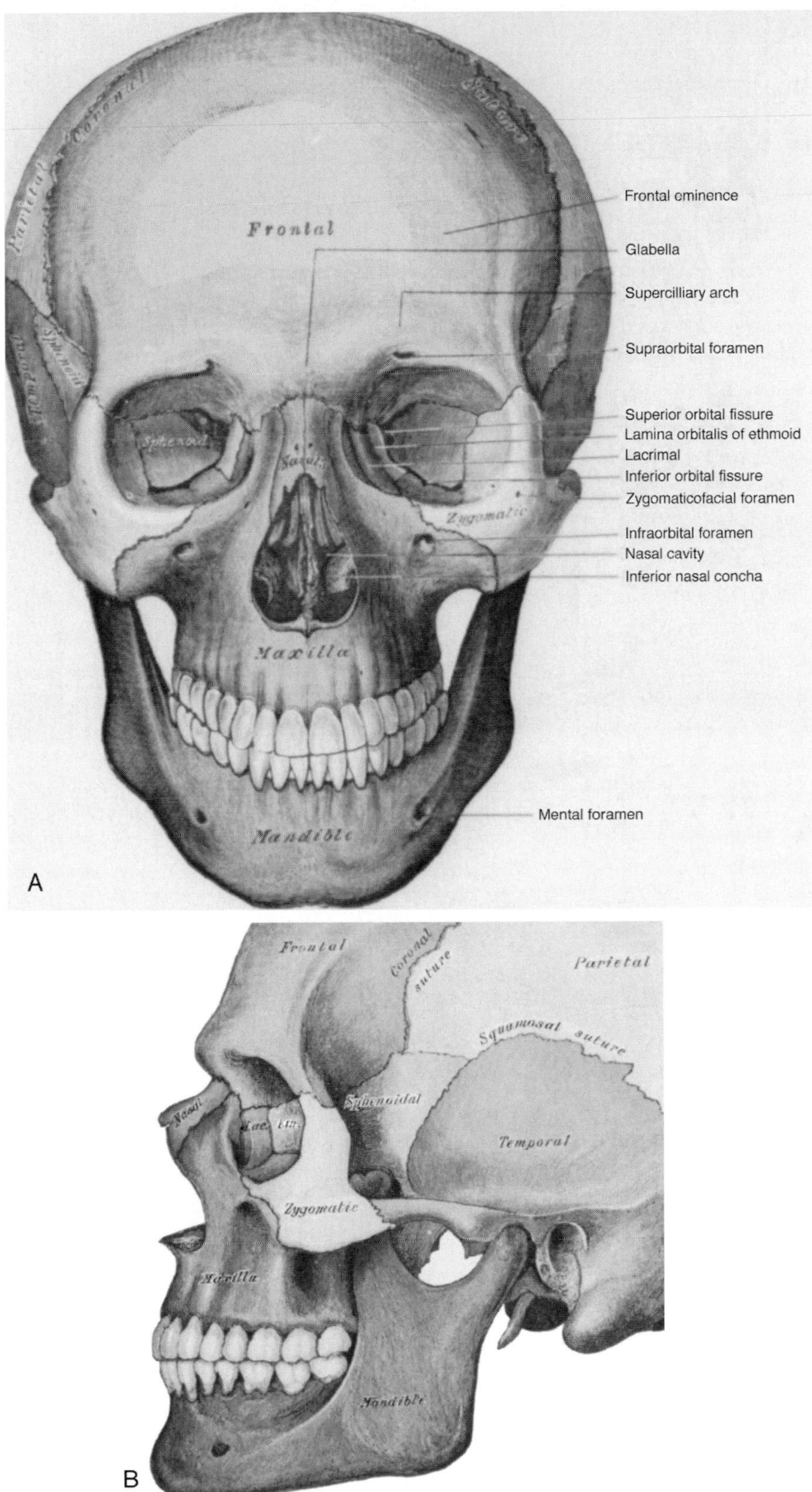

Figure 11–1. The facial skeleton. *A*, Frontal view of the facial skeleton. The bones at the anterior surface of the face—the frontal, nasal, zygomatic, maxillary, and mandibular bones—are nearly always involved in facial fractures, either singly or in combination with other adjacent bones. Exceptions to this rule include some blow-out and blow-in fractures of the orbit. *B*, Lateral view of the facial skeleton. The strongest bony structures of the face are the body of the zygoma, the alveolar process of the maxilla, and the frontal process of the maxilla (see Fig. 11–3). LeFort showed that fractures tend to skirt around these strongest areas. On the lateral view the lacrimal bone (Lac.) and orbital plate of the ethmoid (Eth.) are seen articulating with the maxilla and frontal bones. With the frontal process of the maxilla, the lacrimal bone and orbital plate of ethmoid bone form the medial wall of the orbit. Note the position of the zygomaticotemporal suture: within the middle third of the zygomatic arch, which is formed by the temporal process of the zygoma and the zygomatic process of the temporal bone.

Illustration continued on following page

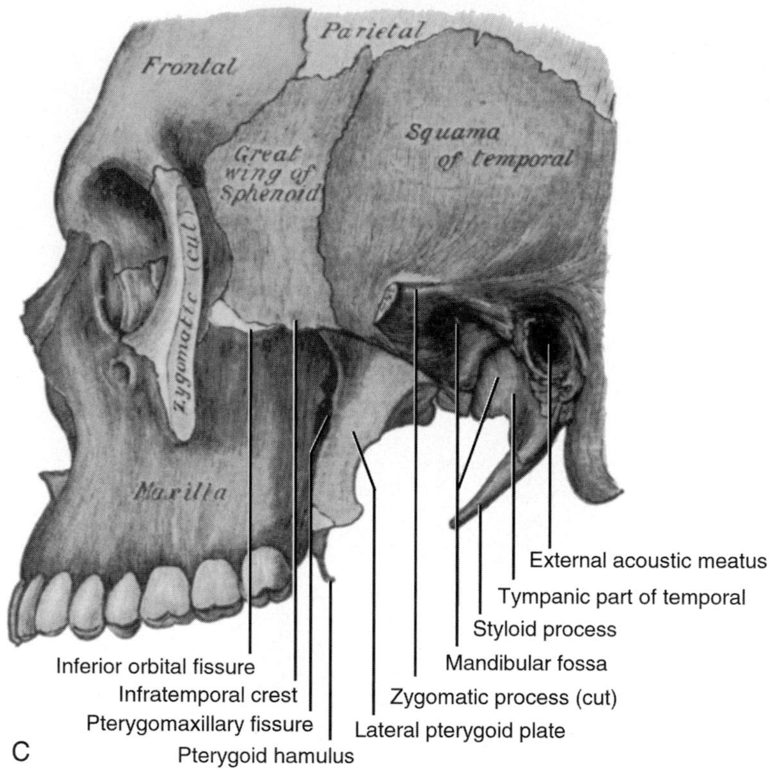

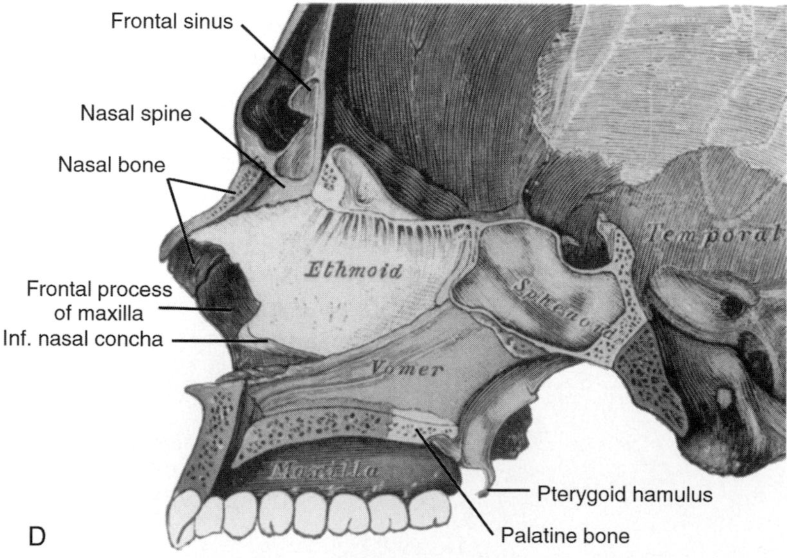

Figure 11–1 *Continued. C,* Lateral view of the facial skeleton with the posterior portion of the zygoma and mandible removed, revealing the position of the pterygoid processes of the sphenoid bone. The pterygoid processes are located posterior to the maxillary sinuses and attach to the base of the skull superiorly. These processes and the posterior portion of the maxilla are fractured in all of the LeFort fractures. There is a space between the pterygoid processes and the maxilla, the pterygomaxillary fissure, which is readily seen on a lateral plain film or axial computed tomographic image. The contribution of the greater wing of the sphenoid to the lateral wall of the orbit is seen in this projection as well as in *A. D,* Sagittal view of the facial skeleton near the midline. The bony nasal septum is composed of the perpendicular plate of the ethmoid superiorly and the vomer inferiorly. The vomer forms a suture with the palatine crest of the hard palate. The hard palate is separated by a sagittal suture into right and left halves, and there is a coronally oriented suture between the maxilla anteriorly and the palatine bone posteriorly. Note the suture between the nasal bone and the frontal process of the maxilla.

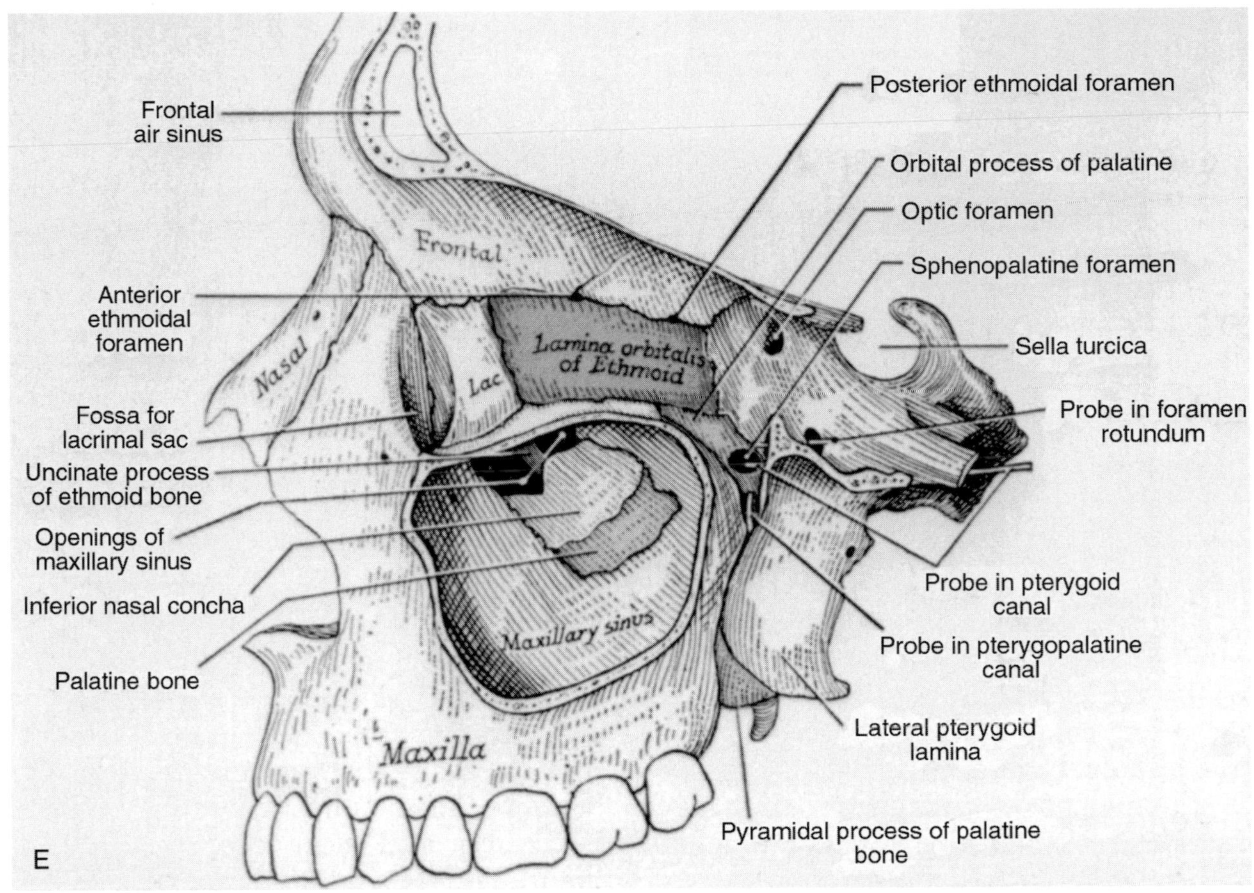

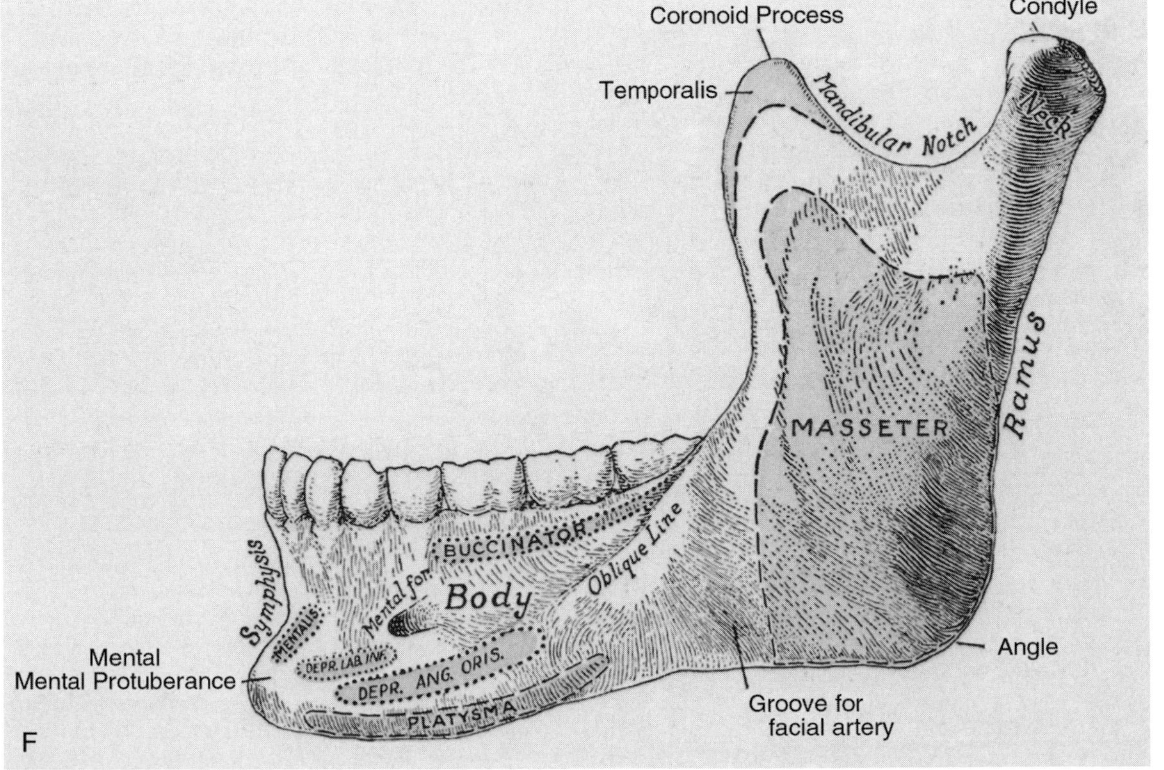

Figure 11–1 *Continued. E,* Medial wall of the orbit and maxillary sinus. Various foramina, the orifice of the maxillary sinus, and the fossa for the lacrimal sac at the cephalic opening of the nasolacrimal duct are shown. These anatomic features may be seen at computed tomographic examination and should not be confused with fracture. The frontal sinus has three surfaces: the anterior and posterior walls and a floor. A break in the posterior wall would communicate with the intracranial space. *F,* Lateral view of the mandible. The mandible articulates with the temporal bone at the condyle. There are no sutures with other bones. The insertions of the muscles of mastication are shown. The major portions of the mandible are the symphysis at the midline, the body between the symphysis and the angle, and the ramus between the angle and the coronoid process and the neck of the condyle.

Illustration continued on following page

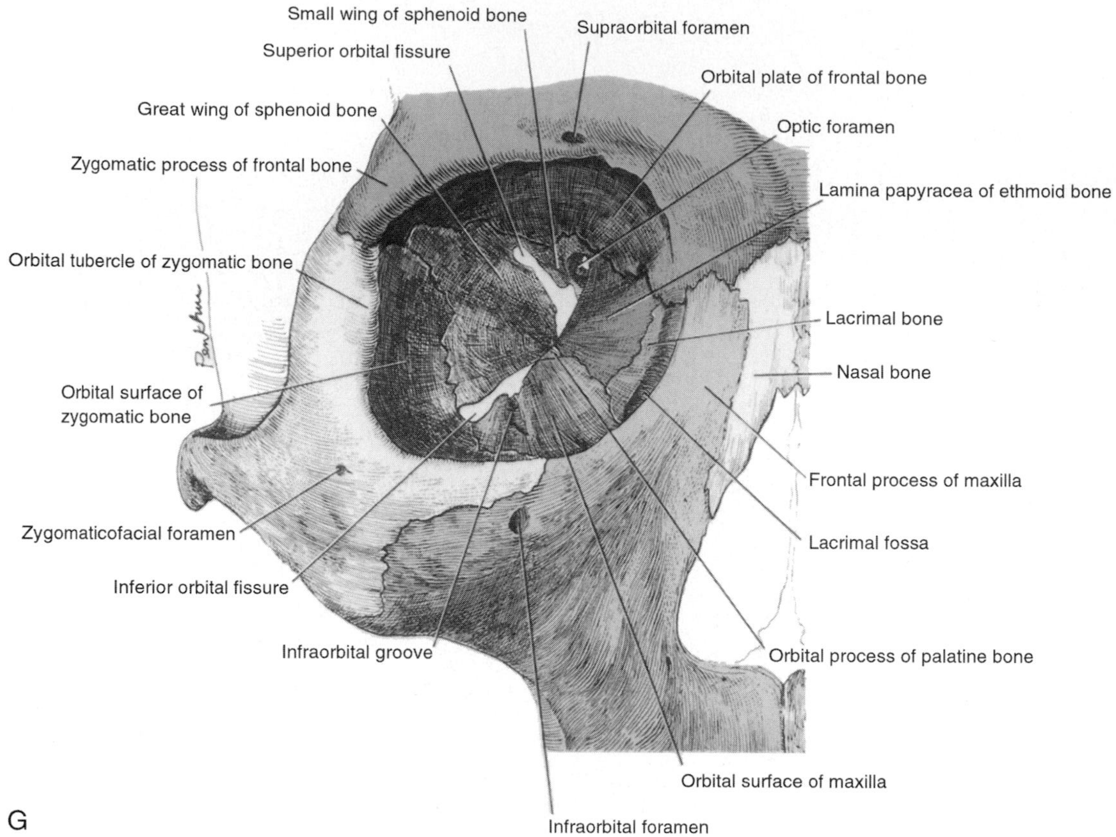

Figure 11–1 *Continued. G,* The bony orbit. The bones of the right orbit are shown. (*A* through *G,* From Gray's Anatomy, 29th American Edition, 1973, by permission of the publisher Churchill Livingstone.)

mandibular condyles articulate with the skull at the temporomandibular joints. It is an arc-shaped bone whose halves join in the midline anteriorly at the symphysis. From the symphysis the body extends posteriorly to the angle of the mandible, where the bone curves cephalad. The portion between the angle and the condyle is called the ramus. The coronoid process extends superiorly and anteriorly from the ramus and serves as a point of attachment for the temporalis muscle and the deep portion of the masseter muscle.

Facial Imaging for Trauma

Specific regions of the face—the nasal, zygomatic, maxillary, orbital, and mandibular regions—may be fractured as separate entities while the remainder of the face remains intact. The frontal sinuses may be fractured as a separate entity as well. Multiple regions may be fractured together in the more complex fractures. The nasal region includes not only the nasal bones but also the frontal processes of the maxillae and the structures immediately posterior to them: the ethmoid air cells, the medial walls of the orbits, and the nasal cavity. The left and right orbital regions are composed of those bones that form the rim and cone-shaped walls of the orbit. The frontal sinus region is composed entirely of the frontal bone. Most facial fractures fall into only a few fracture patterns that involve these regions.[208]

The identification of any facial fracture should prompt a search for the regions involved. For example, a fracture of the zygomatic arch may involve only the zygomatic region or may involve both the zygomatic region and adjacent regions. If the arch fracture is limited to the zygomatic region, there are two possibilities: an isolated arch fracture or a ZMC fracture. Thus, recognition of an arch fracture should prompt a search for the other components of a ZMC fracture such as fractures of the inferior orbital rim and the frontal process of the zygoma. If the arch fracture is a component of fractures that involve regions in addition to the zygoma, one classification to consider is a LeFort III fracture. Identification of an arch fracture, therefore, should also prompt examination of the pterygoid processes, because the pterygoid processes are always fractured in any LeFort fracture. Intact pterygoid processes serve to exclude a LeFort III fracture.

Analysis of the images using the foregoing approach permits determination of whether a region has sustained an isolated injury or whether an injury is a component of a combination of injuries of adjacent regions. The recognition and classification of injury then become simplified based on knowledge of the isolated and combined injuries as described subsequently.

A more detailed conceptualization of facial anatomy may be based on the way the face is suspended from the skull and on the planes of relatively thick bones that act as major areas of support, or buttresses.[158, 190] These buttresses are used in surgical fixation of facial fractures. The facial skeleton[7, 50] is attached to and suspended from

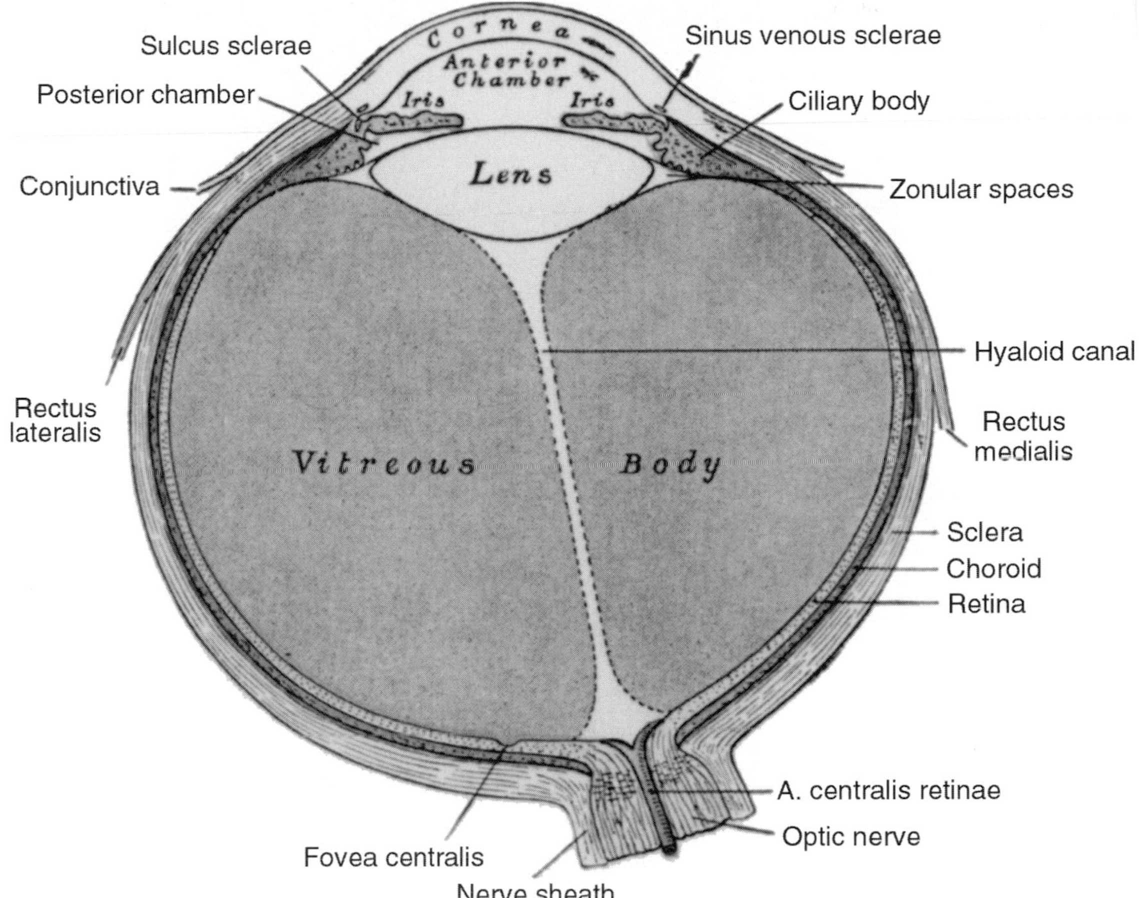

Figure 11–2. The eyeball. Note that both the anterior and posterior chambers are anterior to the lens and are separated by the iris. Behind the lens is the vitreous chamber. The lens is held in place by zonular fibers that are present in the zonular spaces labeled above. The zonular fibers attach the lens to the ciliary body. (From Gray's Anatomy, 29th American Edition, 1973, by permission of the publisher Churchill Livingstone.)

the skull by the medial and lateral walls of the orbit, the zygomatic arch, and the pterygoid processes of the sphenoid bone. The two halves of the face and the two maxillary sinuses are connected by the hard palate inferiorly and separated by the nasal fossa lying between them. The face is supported centrally by the bony nasal septum, consisting of the perpendicular plate of the ethmoid bone and the vomer.

Relative areas of strength within this supporting structure[7, 43, 50, 55] tend to be spared by fractures. LeFort described three such areas of relative strength[34, 43, 55] within the facial skeleton: the alveolar process of the maxilla, the frontal process of the maxilla, and the body of the zygoma or malar eminence (Fig. 11–3). Lines of fracture tend to avoid these areas of strength; most facial fractures run either peripheral to or between these areas. Therefore, the search for fractures should be concentrated at their boundaries—that is, the frontal process of the zygoma, the zygomatic arch, the inferior orbital rim, the lateral wall of the maxillary sinuses, and the medial wall of the orbits in the region of the nasion.

Gentry and associates[11, 12] developed a geometric concept of facial anatomy in which the face is viewed as a series of interconnected osseous struts in the horizontal, sagittal, and coronal planes (Fig. 11–4). An analysis of each strut for fracture and adjacent soft tissue injury facilitates evaluation of facial trauma.

The horizontal plane consists of the superior, middle, and inferior horizontal struts. The superior horizontal strut includes the roofs of the orbits, fovea ethmoidalis, and cribriform plate of the ethmoid bone. The middle horizontal strut is made up of the floor of the orbits and the zygomatic arches. The inferior horizontal strut is the hard palate.

In the sagittal plane there are a midline sagittal, two parasagittal, and two lateral facial struts. The midline strut is the nasal septum formed by the vomer, the perpendicular plate of the ethmoid, and the cartilaginous nasal septum. Each parasagittal strut consists of the medial wall of the orbit and the maxillary sinus. Each lateral facial strut is composed of the lateral part of the maxillary alveolar process and the lateral walls of the maxillary sinus and orbit.

There are two struts in the coronal plane, the anterior and posterior. The anterior coronal strut has many components, including the vertical portion of the frontal bone, zygomaticofrontal buttresses, nasofrontal complex, anterior walls of the maxillary sinuses, and anterior part of the alveolar process. The posterior strut is composed of the posterior walls of the maxillary sinuses and the medial and lateral pterygoid plates.

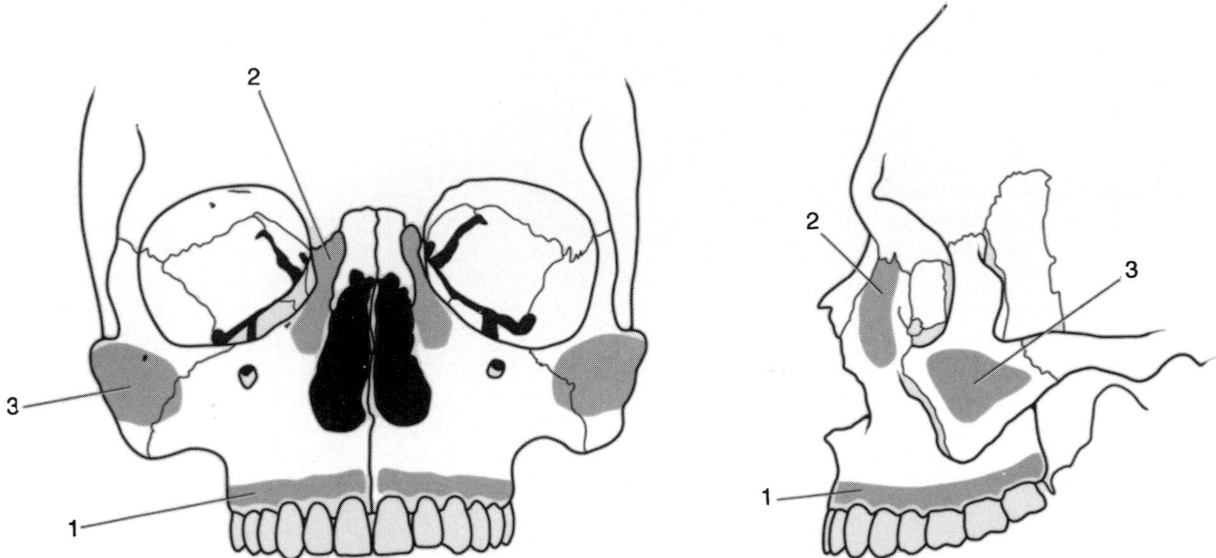

Figure 11–3. Areas of relative strength within the facial skeleton: the alveolar process of the maxilla (1); the frontal process of the maxilla (2); and the body of the zygoma, or malar eminence (3).

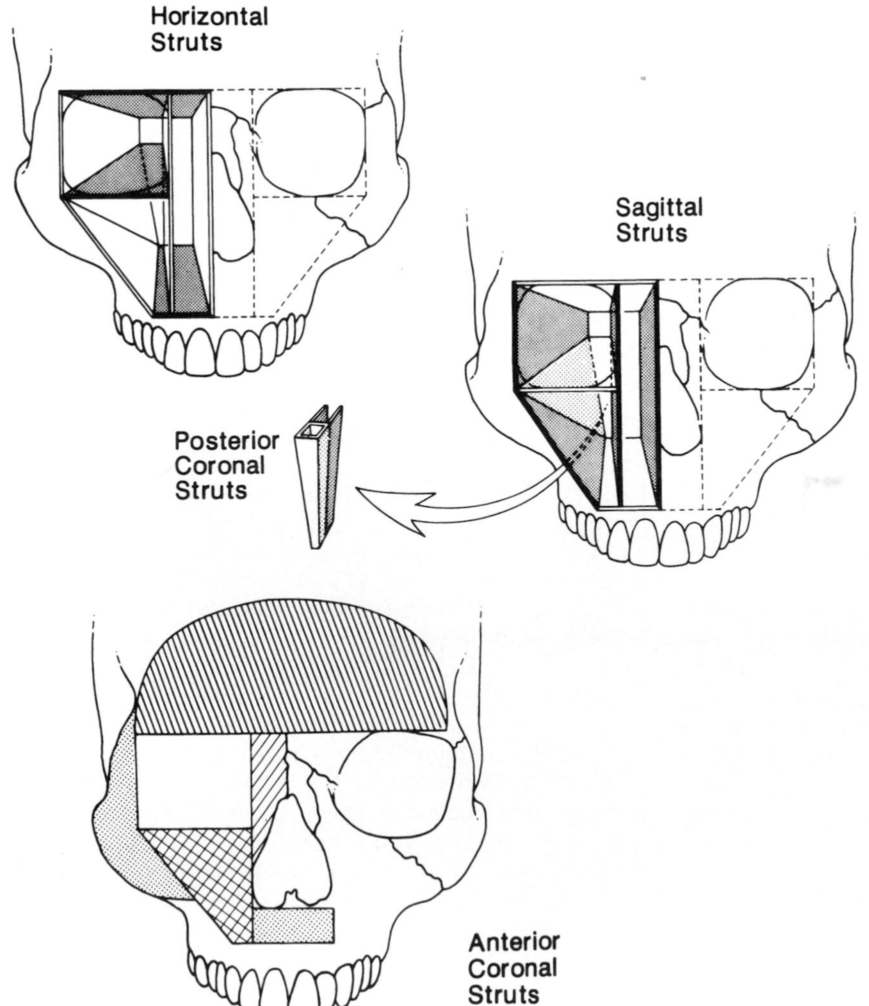

Figure 11–4. Facial struts. The concept of struts in the horizontal, sagittal, and coronal planes was developed to help organize the facial anatomy. These struts support the three-dimensional configuration of the face. The horizontal struts (superior, middle, and inferior) support the face in the anterior-posterior and medial-lateral dimensions. The sagittal struts give support in the anterior-posterior and cranial-caudal dimensions. The coronal struts support the face in the cranial-caudal and medial-lateral dimensions.

Computed Tomography

CT is the preferred modality for imaging the face in patients suspected to have soft tissue or bone injury[154, 186] (Figs. 11–5 through 11–7). CT detects fractures that are not apparent on plain film radiographs and shows significant soft tissue injury such as rupture of the eyeball. Also, CT can be performed more easily and quickly than plain radiography, especially in the multitrauma patient.[198] Three-dimensional CT may be useful in presurgical planning, especially for demonstration of displacement and rotation of fragments and for showing the pattern of complex injuries.[161, 167, 179, 191, 199, 211, 224] Other advantages of CT include visualization of fine detail free of the overlapping structures encountered in plain film radiography, as well as a low radiation dose.[1, 3, 15, 16, 20, 24, 26, 28] An investigation by Storrs and Byrd showed an average dose to the lens of 4.2 rads (range 0.47–6.29 rads) using nonhelical scanning with 5-mm collimation, 120 kilovolts peak (kVp), 140 or 170 milliamperes (mA), and 2-second scan time. For comparison, production of cataracts requires a minimal single dose of 200 rads and a fractionated dose of 550 rads.[221]

Ideally, CT scans in both the axial and the coronal planes are obtained. Direct coronal imaging requires hyperextension of the cervical spine, which may not be possible in some trauma patients. Of those patients with facial fracture, 1% to 4% are found to have cervical spine injury. Optimal coronal and axial images are obtained at 90 degrees and 0 degrees, respectively, to the orbitomeatal line (Reid's baseline)[28] (see Fig. 11–5). Structures that are aligned parallel to the plane of imaging are not well visualized on CT examination. Thus, structures such as the floor of the orbit are not well evaluated on axial images. However, when a structure is perpendicular to the plane of imaging, visualization is optimal. Therefore, the floor of the orbit is best seen on coronally oriented images.

CT scanning in the coronal plane (see Fig. 11–6) accurately detects horizontally directed fractures and corresponds to the traditional way in which facial anatomy has been viewed, so that the nature and extent of the injury can be best appreciated. Coronal images are better for evaluation of the orbital floor, orbital roof, cribriform plate, and pterygoid processes. Axial images are better for evaluation of the nasolacrimal duct, zygomatic arch, and posterior walls of the maxillary and frontal sinuses (see Fig. 11–7). Axial images are useful in judging the degree of posterior displacement in LeFort fractures and ZMC fractures.

If the patient is unable to extend the neck, images in the coronal plane may be obtained by reformatting the axial images. With a helical scanner, coronally reformatted images are obtained by reconstructing the thicker image spacing (e.g., 3 mm) to thin (e.g., 1 mm) image spacing. Thinner spacing allows reformatting in the coronal plane with fewer artifacts than if thicker image spacing is used. With a nonhelical scanner, primary acquisition of thinner images results in better coronal reformatted images. Nonetheless, the resolution of reformatted images is degraded with either axial or helical data acquisition. With a multi-slice scanner, reconstruction in any plane is possible without relative loss of information when thin collimation is used.

Whether provided as hard copy or by a picture archival and communication system (PACS), CT scans should always be viewed in bone and soft tissue window settings for thorough evaluation of both bone and soft tissue structures. In some cases it is useful to view the images using a lung window setting. Use of lung window settings may help to differentiate orbital emphysema from fat, and also some wooden foreign bodies from air.

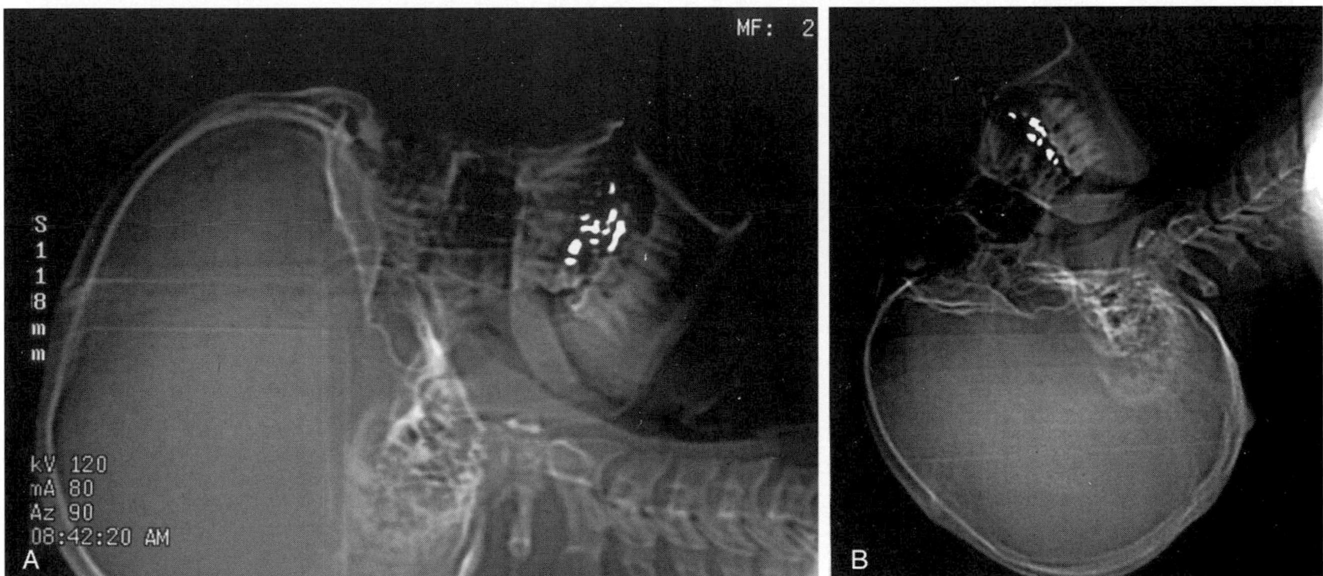

Figure 11–5. Scout images for CT examination. *A,* Axial images are obtained with the patient lying supine with the back of the head on the examination table. The gantry may be tilted so that the central ray is aligned with the orbitomeatal line (Reid's baseline). *B,* Directly obtained coronal images require hyperextension of the neck; therefore, the cervical spine must be "cleared" of injury in the polytrauma patient before these studies are obtained. Extension is accomplished by placing support under the shoulders with the patient lying supine.

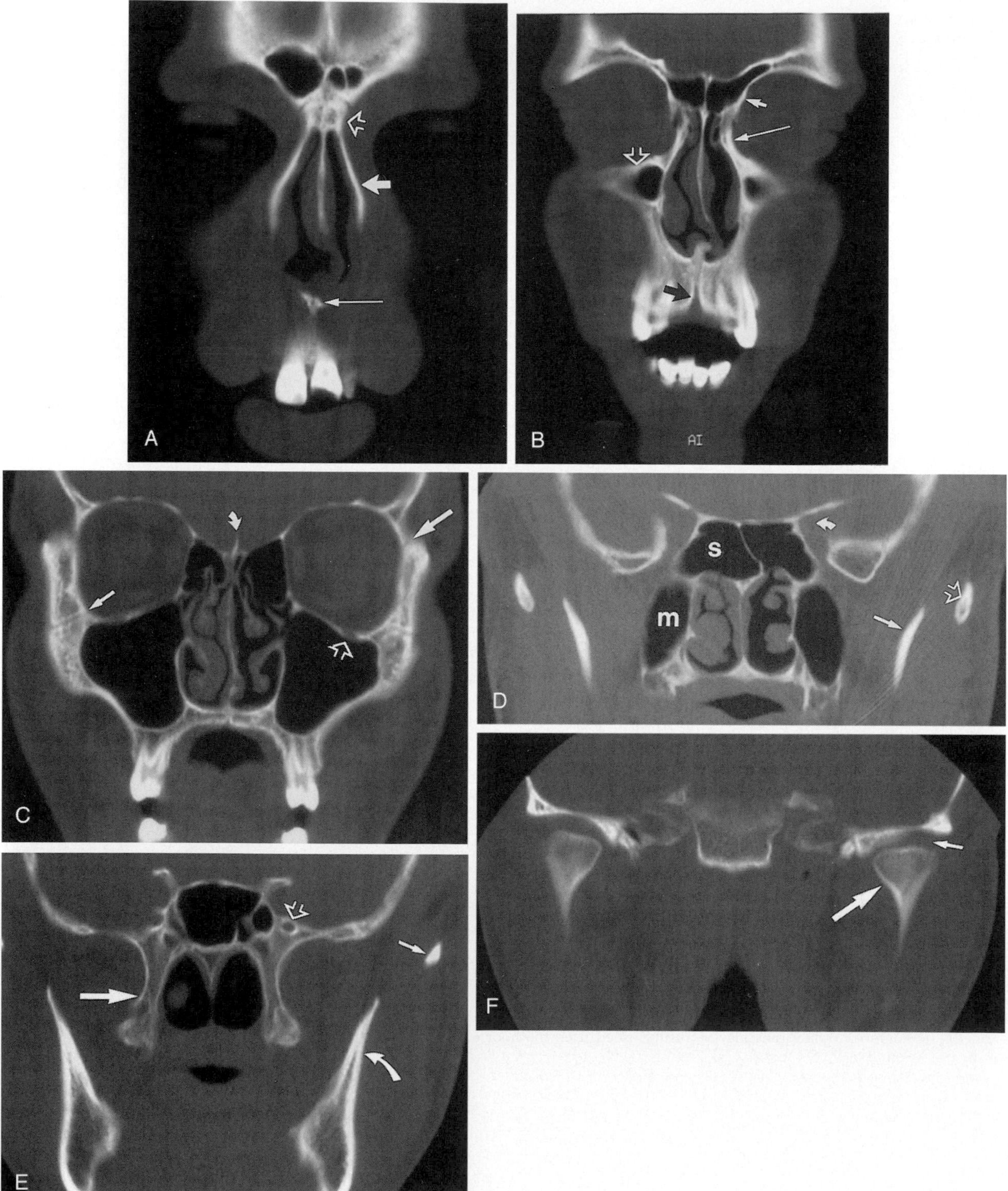

Figure 11–6 *See legend on opposite page*

Table 11–1. Common Soft Tissue Injuries Accompanying Facial Fractures

Intracranial and Frontal Region Injury
Brain contusion, laceration, or hemorrhage
Pneumocephalus
Carotid artery injury
Carotid artery–cavernous sinus fistula
Open frontal sinus fracture
Cerebrospinal fluid leak via cribriform plate

Orbital and Zygomatic Region Injury
Eyeball rupture
Corneal avulsion
Lens subluxation/dislocation
Choroidal hemorrhage
Vitreous hemorrhage
Retinal detachment
Optic nerve injury
Extraocular muscle entrapment
Enophthalmos
Injury to lacrimal structures
Orbital compartment syndrome
Orbital emphysema
Injury to infraorbital nerve
Injury to trochlea, resulting in superior oblique tendon sheath syndrome
Disruption of lateral canthal ligament
Superior orbital fissure syndrome
Disruption of medial canthal ligament, resulting in telecanthus and epiphora
Injury to supraorbital or infraorbital nerve

Nasal Region Injury
Nasal septal hematoma
Interruption of normal maxillary sinus drainage
Injury to the nasofrontal duct

Maxillary Region Injury
Injury to neurovascular structures in pterygomaxillary fissure and pterygopalatine fossa
Compromise of eustachian tube
Hematoma compromising airway

Mandibular Region Injury
Posterior displacement of tongue compromising airway
Displacement of condyle into temporal fossa
Damage to temporomandibular joint cartilage

Although identification of fractures is important, detection of soft tissue injuries may be potentially of greater urgency (Table 11–1). Fractures through the orbital roof may be associated with injury to the dura, frontal lobe, or upper extraocular muscles. Fractures may extend into the optic canal, thus predisposing to injury of the optic nerve. Cerebrospinal fluid rhinorrhea can accompany fractures of the cribriform plate. Hematomas of the frontal lobe and pneumocephalus may also be identified in patients with facial fractures (see Fig. 11–23). Fractures of the orbital floor may be associated with orbital emphysema, entrapment of inferior rectus or oblique muscles, herniation of orbital fat into the maxillary sinus, or injuries to the optic nerve, eyeball, or lens. Fractures of the nasal septum are often associated with hematomas, which may be difficult to identify clinically, especially when situated posteriorly. Resorption of the septum and perforation may occur if the hematoma is not evacuated. Fractures of the medial orbital wall are commonly associated with herniation of orbital fat and may occasionally be the cause of herniation of the medial rectus muscle into the ethmoid sinuses. Fractures of the anterior part of the medial wall may be associated with damage to the nasolacrimal duct. Fractures through the frontal bones may extend into the frontal sinus. It is important to determine whether both the anterior and the posterior walls of the sinus are involved, because fracture of the posterior wall provides communication to the intracranial space. Fractures at the inferior and posterior aspects of the face may extend into the base of the skull, temporal bone, or proximal tips of the petrous bone to involve the eustachian canal. Retropharyngeal hematomas also may occur with posterior fractures.

A thorough familiarity with normal anatomy is essential in evaluation of facial trauma because sutures, foramina, fissures, poorly mineralized bony septa, and partial volume averaging of sloping surfaces all result in discontinuities of bone that may be mistaken for fractures (Table 11–2).

Plain Radiography

If CT is not immediately available, plain films can be obtained to screen for facial injury (Fig. 11–8). If plain films identify a fracture other than a simple nasal bone fracture, further evaluation by CT is indicated.[8] Proper positioning of the patient is essential for adequate evaluation of the facial skeleton. The majority of projections are aligned by reference to an imaginary topographic line drawn from the outer canthus to the external auditory meatus—the canthomeatal line. Proper positioning of the patient's head relative to the cassette and proper alignment of the central x-ray beam in relation to the canthomeatal line ensure a correct projection.

Figure 11–6. Normal CT appearance on coronal images. Coronal images should be obtained from a point anterior to the nasal bones to a point posterior to the mandibular condyles. *A,* Anterior image shows the normal nasofrontal suture, nasal bones (*open arrow*), frontal process of maxilla (*short solid arrow*), bony nasal septum, and anterior maxillary spine (*long solid arrow*). The frontal sinuses contain no air-fluid levels or membrane thickening. *B,* The inferior orbital rims may be distinguished from the floor of the orbit because the rims are seen on the first image posterior to the soft tissues (*open arrow*). The bony nasal septum is curved—a normal finding. The gap between the superior and inferior parts of the septum, which consist of the perpendicular plate of ethmoid and vomer, respectively, is also normal when this area is viewed anteriorly. The area of fusion of the two halves of the hard palate is seen (*black arrow*). The medial orbital rim is formed by the frontal bone superiorly (*short white arrow*) and by the frontal process of the maxilla inferiorly (*long white arrow*). *C,* The walls of the maxillary sinuses and orbits are seen to good advantage on this image just posterior to the eyeball. The canal for the infraorbital nerve is almost always seen (*open arrow*). Fractures of the orbital floor may damage the infraorbital nerve that runs through this canal. The zygomaticofrontal suture is noted on the left in the upper portion of the lateral orbital rim (*large straight arrow*). The thick body of the zygoma is seen, and a canal with cortical margins extends through the zygoma bilaterally (*small straight arrow*). This canal ends laterally in the zygomaticofacial foramen, as seen in Figure 11–1A. In the midline the crista galli (*curved arrow*) is seen just above the cribriform plates. *D,* In this image obtained through the posterior portion of the maxillary sinuses (m) and sphenoid sinuses (s), the lateral wall of the maxillary sinuses can be seen faintly. The posterolateral wall of the maxillary sinus runs oblique to the axial plane and thus is not as well seen as the medial wall, which is perpendicular to the axial plane. The coronoid process of the mandible (*solid arrow*) and the zygomatic arch (*open arrow*) are seen laterally. Just lateral to the sphenoid sinus is the orbital apex (*curved arrow*), just anterior to the optic foramen. *E,* The pterygoid processes including medial and lateral plates (*large straight arrow*) are well seen in the coronal plane. The optic nerve runs just under the anterior clinoid processes. The foramen rotundum (*open arrow*) is well seen on the left. The ramus of the mandible (*curved arrow*) and posterior portion of the zygomatic arch (*small straight arrow*) are seen inferiorly and laterally. *F,* The temporomandibular joints (*small arrow*) are well seen, as is the condyle of the mandible (*large arrow*).

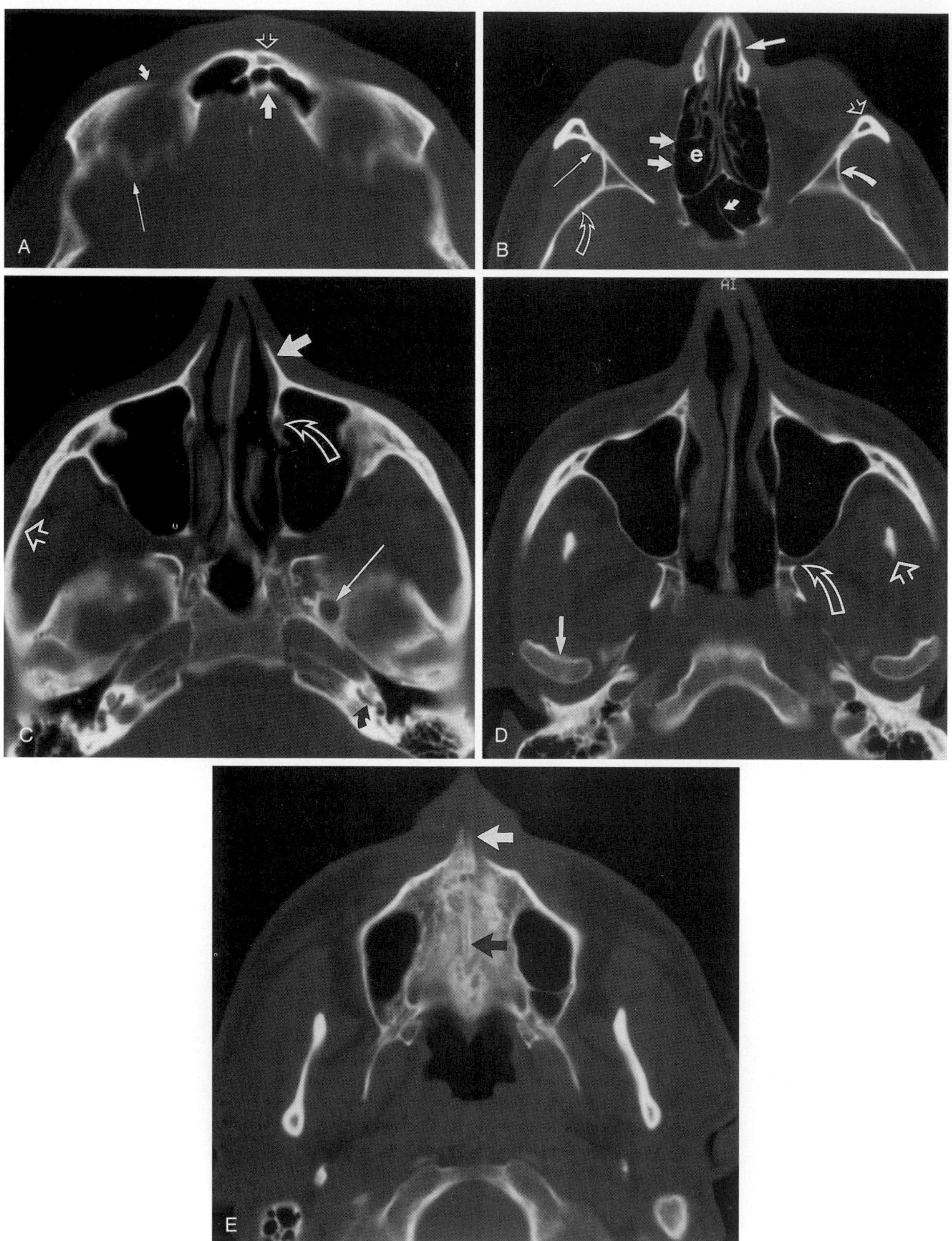

Figure 11–7 *See legend on opposite page*

Table 11–2. Normal Discontinuities of Bone That May Mimic Fracture on Computed Tomography Images

Coronal Plane
Sutures
- Nasofrontal
- Internasal
- Nasomaxillary
- Zygomaticofrontal
- Zygomaticomaxillary

Nasolacrimal duct
Perforation of cribriform plate
Intraorbital canal in orbital floor
Posterior superior alveolar canal in lateral wall of maxillary sinus
Ostia of maxillary sinus
Pterygomaxillary fissure and sphenopalatine foramen

Axial Plane
Sutures
- Nasofrontal
- Nasomaxillary
- Zygomaticofrontal
- Vomer—perpendicular plate of ethmoid in nasal septum

Intraorbital canal in orbital floor
Incisive foramen in hard palate
Greater and lesser palatine foramina of hard palate
Cribriform plate
Incomplete frontal sinus septum

The facial skeletal anatomy is quite complex, even in a dry skull specimen. The complexities are compounded when this anatomy is seen in two dimensions, as in radiographs. The overlapping of many variably shaped structures significantly obscures anatomic detail. The standard views have been selected because they minimize this overlap and allow visualization of certain important individual anatomic features as free of overlying structures as is possible. Despite the fact that the anatomy is complicated, it becomes quite familiar on the standard views. This radiographic familiarity is reduced, and the quality of the interpretation compromised, with improper positioning of the patient.

The overlying soft tissues cast companion shadows, and it is important to be familiar with them. Swelling of the soft tissues directs attention to the possibility of underlying skeletal injury. However, it is possible to confuse some companion shadows for fractures if the examiner is not aware of their appearance.

When the cortical bone is visualized end on, it is seen as a fine line of increased bone density. The radiographic appearance may not correspond precisely to the full width of an anatomic structure; it often represents only that portion of the structure viewed on edge. Some portions of the facial anatomy are normally visualized in this manner. However, in a fracture, fragments of bone may be displaced or rotated so that they are visualized end on[35, 48] and similarly present as fine cortical lines. Abnormal linear radiodensities are particularly common in fractures involving the floor of the orbit. It is necessary to be familiar with the position and appearance of the normal lines in order to recognize those that are abnormal.

As complicated as it is, the bony facial anatomy is fairly symmetrical, allowing comparison of one side with the other. Such comparative examinations must be done routinely. Freimanis[10] pointed out the importance of remembering the elementary fact that on well-positioned frontal views, the two sides of the face are quite symmetrical. Normal radiodensities are frequently bilateral, and abnormal radiodensities are unilateral. Symmetry is usual, and asymmetry is suspect.

Fractures of the facial skeleton are frequently multiple. There is a natural tendency for attention to be drawn to and remain with the obvious. Less obvious but equally or even more important findings may then go unnoticed. It is important to develop a disciplined, routine pattern of search to prevent such oversights. This pattern should be based on easily followed anatomic lines and encompass all of the more frequent sites of injury.

The direct signs of fracture are obviously cortical disruption and displacement of bone fragments. These signs may not be immediately obvious, and attention is directed to them by indirect signs involving the paranasal sinuses or soft tissues.[89, 92] Hemorrhage related to a fracture may manifest as opacification, mucosal thickening, a polypoid mass, or an air-fluid level within a sinus. Fluid in a paranasal sinus is almost always present when the patient has sustained a fracture that involves a sinus wall.[180] Obviously, these findings are not absolute indications of trauma because they also may be due to coincidental inflammatory disease. The sinuses may also appear opaci-

Figure 11–7. Normal anatomy on axial CT images. Axial CT images should be obtained from above the frontal sinuses to a point below the hard palate. If mandible fracture is also a clinical concern, then the scan should be extended inferiorly to include the mandible. *A*, Axial CT images show the anterior (*open arrow*) and posterior (*thick arrow*) walls of the frontal sinuses to better advantage than is possible with coronal images. The superior orbital rim (*curved arrow*) is seen, and the roof of the orbit is just coming into view. Parts of the roof (*long arrow*) are only faintly seen because of volume averaging. *B*, The ethmoid air cells (e) and medial walls of the orbits (*paired arrows*) are well visualized. The septum separating the right and left sphenoid sinuses may normally be curved (*small curved arrow*). The nasomaxillary suture (*large straight arrow*) is seen between the nasal bones and frontal processes of maxillae. Laterally, the frontal process of zygoma forms the lateral orbital rim (*open straight arrow*). The suture in the lateral orbital wall between the zygoma and the greater wing of the sphenoid (*thin straight arrow*) is well shown on the right. Posteriorly, the suture between the greater wing of the sphenoid and the temporal bone is seen (*large curved open arrow*). The cortical surface of the sphenoid bone, which runs from anterior to posterior, is the surface that forms the innominate line seen on plain films (*solid curved arrow*). *C*, Axial imaging plane obtained through the maxillary sinuses shows the zygomatic arches (*open straight arrow*) that run from the temporal bone to the body of the zygoma. This image is inferior to the nasal bones, and the anterior nasal structures are the frontal processes of the maxillae (*short solid arrow*). The nasolacrimal duct (*curved open white arrow*) is seen coursing through the medial wall of the maxillary sinus. Posteriorly, the mastoid air cells, semicircular canals of the inner ear (*curved black arrow*), and foramen ovale (*long solid white arrow*) are seen. *D*, The mandibular condyles (*solid arrow*) are seen in normal position. The coronoid process of the mandible (*open straight arrow*) is medial to the zygomatic arch. The upper portions of the pterygoid processes are separated from the posterior walls of the maxillary sinuses by the pterygopalatine canal (*curved open arrow*). *E*, As an incidental finding, the suture between the two halves of the hard palate has a sclerotic margin (*black arrow*). The anterior spines of the maxillae (*white arrow*) are noted anteriorly.

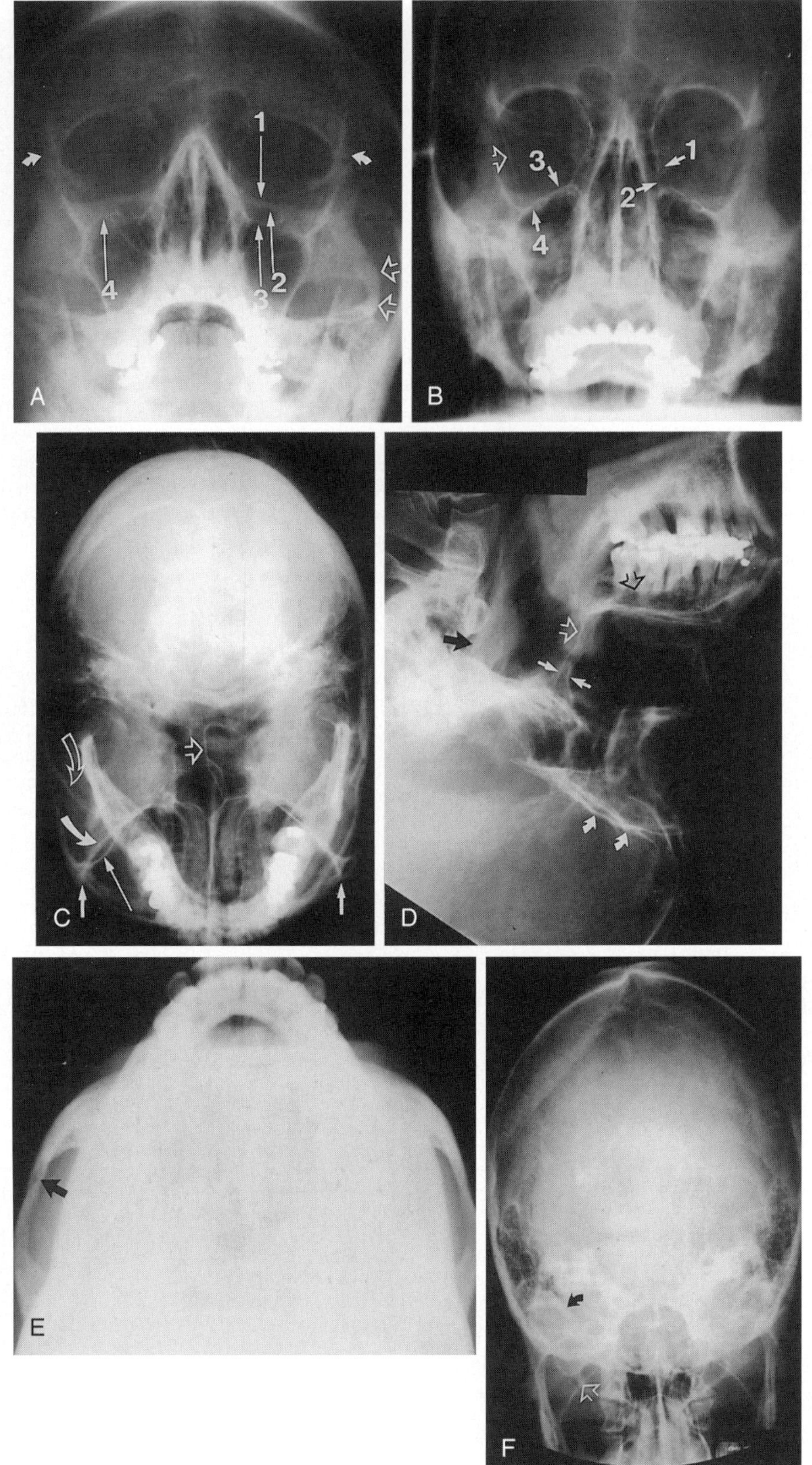

Figure 11–8 *See legend on opposite page*

fied because of overlying soft tissue swelling or underdevelopment. Radiographically apparent soft tissue swelling is seen over the malar eminence and the lip and about the orbit. Hemorrhage associated with midfacial fractures may extend into the retropharyngeal or nasopharyngeal tissues and manifest as soft tissue prominence in these areas on the lateral view.

Orbital emphysema or air within the soft tissues of the face suggests the presence of an open injury of an adjacent sinus (see Figs. 11–15 and 11–16). Lloyd[88] reported a series of 129 patients with orbital emphysema; 40% of cases were associated with a medial orbital wall fracture, 34% with a blow-out fracture of the floor of the orbit, and 5% with a combined fracture involving the maxillary sinus and ethmoid air cells. Eleven percent were associated with zygomatic fractures, and 8% were due to frontal sinus fractures. Significant orbital emphysema may increase intraconal pressure, resulting in transient or permanent loss of vision.[172]

Penetrating wounds from sharp objects[67, 100] may extend through the adjacent sinuses and communicate with the middle or anterior cranial fossa, resulting in pneumocephalus. Radiographic evidence of pneumocephalus[100] is often delayed in appearance; therefore, the air may not be detected on the initial examination. Penetrating injuries through the orbits[67] have also resulted in false aneurysms of the intracranial portions of the carotid artery and its branches.

The standard radiographic evaluation of facial trauma includes five views[8, 22, 25]: the Waters, Caldwell, lateral, base (submentovertex), and Towne views (see Fig. 11–8). All of these views should encompass the entire facial skeleton, including the mandible. If the patient is conscious and ambulatory, use of a standard skull or upright Bucky radiographic unit may be possible so that all views can be obtained with the patient sitting erect. If the patient is unsteady or there is any question about the patient's ability to assume an erect position, the examination should be performed with the patient lying on the radiographic examination table. If there are either extensive injuries of the facial skeleton or significant associated injuries, the entire examination may be performed with the patient in the supine position. A cross-table lateral view of the facial skeleton may be obtained; also, an anteroposterior view of the face may be substituted for the Caldwell view, and an anteroposterior reverse view, for the standard Waters view. Although the face is farther away from the film in an anteroposterior projection, so that the structures are magnified and the sharpness of the detail is reduced, it is still possible to obtain a satisfactory evaluation in this manner. A standard examination with greater detail may be performed at a later time when the patient's condition permits.

The views described in the following discussion are those obtained in the general evaluation of facial trauma. There are numerous projections for evaluation of specific areas. Panoramic views of the mandible and facial structures can be obtained with special radiographic equipment, either the Panorex or the Orthopantograph devices[30, 37, 52] (see Fig. 11–66). Linear or multiplanar tomography can be performed in the anteroposterior projection[15, 16] (see Fig. 11–21).

Waters' View

Waters' view[47] is obtained by aligning the central ray with the junction of the patient's upper lip and nose at an angle of 37 degrees with the canthomeatal line (see Fig. 11–8*A*). This arrangement places the alveolar process of the maxilla just above the petrous portion of the temporal bone so that the entire maxillary sinus is projected clear of the petrous bone. This projection affords an excellent view of the maxilla and maxillary sinus, the zygoma and the zygomatic arches, the rims of the orbits, and the nasal bones.

Figure 11–8. Normal anatomy on plain radiographs. *A,* Waters' view. The alignment of the nasal bones is well seen in the Waters view. The inferior orbital rim (1) projects above the two lines of the floor of the orbit that are seen medially. The upper line is the posterior part of the floor (2). The lower line is the anterior part of the floor (3). A single line from the floor is seen laterally (4). The zygomaticofrontal sutures (*curved arrows*) are symmetrical. The zygomatic arches (*open arrows*) are foreshortened, but a displaced fracture would be well seen. The lateral walls of the maxillary sinuses are seen as a sharp cortical line. *B,* Caldwell's view. The ethmoid air cells are filled with air. The orbital rim is well seen in its entirety except, on occasion, parts of the medial rim, which may not be well shown. Because of the conical shape of the orbit, the posterior part of the medial wall (1) projects lateral to the anterior part of the medial wall (2). Also, the posterior part of the floor (3) projects above the orbital rim and the anterior part of the floor. Laterally, the floor is short and flat and is seen as a single line (4) projected inferior to the orbital rim. The cortical line (*open arrow*) that projects through the lateral aspect of the orbit is caller the innominate line and is formed by the sphenoid bone as noted in Figure 11–7*B*. *C,* Base view. The base view can be obtained only if the patient's neck can be hyperextended. In some patients, the zygomatic arches are well seen lateral to the temporal bone. In other patients, special "jughandle" views, which are taken in the base projection with slight tilts to each side, are necessary to visualize the arch. The arch joins the body of the zygoma anteriorly. The two zygoma bones (*short straight arrows*) should project at a similar point anteriorly. Asymmetry in the position of the bodies of the zygoma bones suggests posterior displacement of one side. The sphenoid sinuses with a septum (*open straight arrow*) between them are seen. Just lateral and anterior to the sphenoid sinus three lines can be seen that superimpose. The sigmoid-shaped line represents the posterolateral wall of the maxillary sinus (*long solid arrow*). The line that is convex posteriorly is the posterolateral wall of the orbit (*solid curved arrow*). The line that is convex anteriorly (*open curved arrow*) is the anterior wall of the middle cranial fossa. These latter two lines are formed by the sphenoid bone and join medially at a point corresponding to the origin of the innominate line. *D,* Lateral view. The two halves of the mandible should superimpose. The condyles and necks (*solid black arrow*) are well seen, and a dislocation of the condyle anteriorly can be noted on this view. The pterygoid processes (*posterior solid white arrow*), pterygomaxillary fissure (*space between solid white arrows*), and posterior walls of the maxillary sinuses (*anterior solid white arrow*) should form smooth intact lines. The inferior portion of the pterygoid processes fuses with the maxillary sinus walls (*open white arrow*). The orbital roofs superimpose with the frontal sinuses and slope posteriorly and inferiorly. Frequently the maxillary tooth roots project through the inferior portion of the maxillary sinuses (*open black arrow*). Using lighter technique (see Fig. 11–41), the nasal bones, the frontal process of the maxilla, and the anterior spine of the maxilla are well seen. *E,* Base view to show the zygomatic arches. With hyperextension of the neck, a light technique shows the zygomatic arches to excellent advantage. On the right, the zygomaticotemporal suture is seen (*arrow*). *F,* Towne's view. The mandibular condyles (*black arrow*) are seen in the mandibular fossa of the temporal bone. Medial displacement of the condyle should not be seen. The posterolateral wall of the maxillary sinus (*white arrow*), which also forms the margin of the inferior orbital fissure, is seen. Using a "bright light," the zygomatic arches may be seen laterally.

Dolan and Jacoby[7] have described three imaginary lines of bone continuity that are very helpful in visualization of bone contours and identification of fractures (Fig. 11–9). The first line begins at the inner surface of the zygomaticofrontal suture and follows the orbital surface of the zygoma, the orbital surface of the maxilla, the frontal process of the maxilla, and the arch produced by the nasal bones and then follows the same course on the opposite orbit. The line has the contour of a "lazy W" or the outlines of half-frame reading glasses. The second line begins at the outer surface of the zygomaticofrontal suture and runs downward along the orbital process of the zygoma and along the upper and outer surfaces of the zygomatic arch and curves medially to the glenoid fossa of the temporomandibular joint on each side. The third line begins at the lateral and inferior margins of the maxilla and extends along the lateral wall of the maxillary sinuses and the inferior surface of the zygomatic arch to the glenoid fossa. Dolan and Jacoby[7] have also noted that the second and third lines together form a figure that resembles the side view of an elephant's head and trunk. Any disruption in the continuity of these lines probably indicates the presence of a fracture, and any difference in contour between the two sides is suggestive of a fracture and warrants closer evaluation.

The rim of the orbit is smaller in circumference than the anterior portion of the orbit immediately behind it. As a consequence of this expansion, the inferior rim of the orbit is projected above the floor of the orbit or roof of the maxillary sinus on the Waters view. The orbital floor is roughly parallel with the orbital rim. The infraorbital foramen is identified just below the midportion of the orbital rim. The palpable lateral and superior lateral margins of the orbit are visualized as sharp, cortical linear densities. The superior medial and medial walls of the orbits are not well visualized. The extent of visualization of the superior orbital rim is dependent on the degree of pneumatization within the frontal sinus. The orbital rim adjacent to the frontal sinus tends to be less sharply defined. Because the orbit is shaped like a pyramid or cone, with its base at the orbital rim, the posterior ethmoid air cells are visualized lateral to the medial portion of the orbital rim.

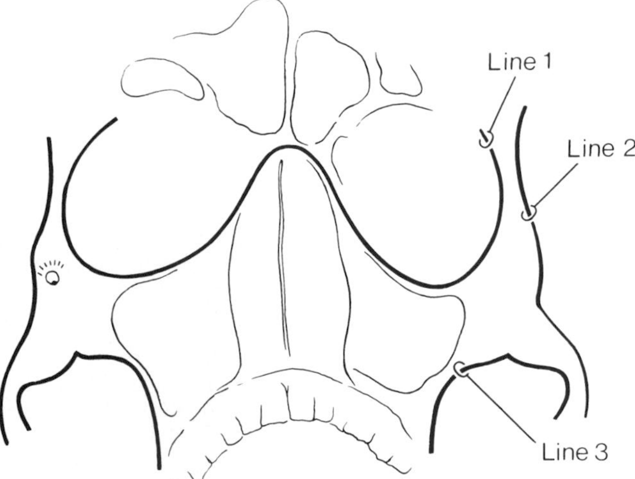

Figure 11–9. Dolan's lines of reference on a Waters view. These lines form a shape like that of an elephant's head and trunk on the Waters view. The head is the body of the zygoma. The trunk is the zygomatic arch. The back is the interior orbital rim, and the lateral orbital rim forms the ear. The front legs are the lateral walls of the maxillary sinus. Almost any fracture of the midface will disrupt one of these lines.

A thin cortical oblique, almost vertical line is noted in the lateral aspect of the orbit, extending from above the superior rim and inferiorly into the maxillary sinuses. It is known as the *lateral oblique line* or *innominate line* of the orbit. A portion of the sphenoid bone creates this line (see Fig. 11–7*B*). In some cases it ends abruptly within the sinuses after curving or hooking medially.

In approximately 15% of persons, a groove[34] containing the posterior superior alveolar nerve and accompanying maxillary artery is identifiable on the lateral wall of the maxillary sinus just above the alveolar process. This groove may be confused with a fracture. However, a fracture will be seen to extend entirely through the lateral maxillary wall, whereas a thin layer of cortical bone is noted beneath the lucency formed by the canal containing this nerve. The lucency of the canal is accentuated by opacification in the sinuses. There is also a groove for the anterior superior alveolar nerve that runs diagonally from the nasal fossa toward the infraorbital foramen but does not extend through the orbital rim, thus distinguishing it from a fracture. It is also more likely to be visualized when the sinus is opacified.

Caldwell's View

The Caldwell view is obtained by passing the central ray through the nasion at an angle of 15 degrees with the canthomeatal line (see Fig. 11–8*B*). This projection affords an excellent view of the entire rim of the orbit, with the superior-medial portion of the rim better seen than on other routine facial projections. On the Caldwell view the palpable margin of the superior orbital rim is seen inferior to the thin cortical density of the roof of the orbit. This appearance is similar to that for the floor of the orbit and the inferior palpable margin, as shown on Waters' view. The bony nasal septum formed by the perpendicular plate of the ethmoid and the vomer is demonstrated. The innominate line is seen in the outer portion of the orbit.

The Caldwell view provides good visualization of the orbital floor if the petrous bones are projected just below the inferior orbital rim. Because the medial part of the floor is sigmoid in shape, two lines from the floor are seen medially. The lower line is the anterior part of the floor; the higher line is the posterior part. Laterally, the floor is comparatively short and straight from just behind the orbital rim to the inferior orbital fissure. Thus, a single line representing the orbital floor is seen laterally.

The ethmoid air cells bounded by fine septations are seen on the Caldwell view with less superimposition of the nose than on the Waters view. The Caldwell view shows the opacification of the ethmoid sinus caused by adjacent fracture and bleeding into the sinus. The septations of the air cells will not be apparent when these structures are adjacent to blood. The best view of the ethmoid air cells is on the posteroanterior view, which may not be routinely obtained as part of a radiographic facial series.

Lateral View

It is important that the patient's head be placed in a true lateral position so that the structures on each side are superimposed. The canthomeatal line is placed parallel to the superior and inferior margins of the cassette, and the central ray passes through the outer canthus at an angle of 90 degrees with the film. Proper exposure of the facial skeleton requires approximately 10 kVp less than that used for the lateral skull film (see Fig. 11–8*C*).

The lateral view[4, 61] visualizes the anterior wall of the frontal sinus, floor of the anterior fossa, lateral rims of the orbit, anterior and posterior walls of the maxilla, hard palate, pterygoid process of the sphenoid bone, sphenoid sinus, mandible, retropharygeal soft tissues, and nasopharynx. To visualize the nasal bones, an additional lateral view using a soft tissue exposure is necessary. Both the anterior nasal spine and the nasal bones are demonstrated with this technique.

The lateral view allows evaluation of posterior displacement of midfacial fractures. It is helpful to use Dolan's lines of reference, which emphasize several important relationships.[7] An anterior vertical line connects the surface of the frontal sinus and the anterior surface of the hard palate and should parallel a posterior vertical line connecting the sphenoidal wing and the posterior edge of the hard palate. A horizontal line extended from the planum sphenoidale should parallel the nasal surface of the hard palate. These four lines approximate a square (Fig. 11–10). This square is disrupted by displacements of the palate and facial structures associated with LeFort injuries. Displacements are also suggested by an abnormal relationship of the central incisors. Normally, of course, the upper central incisors are anterior to the lower central incisors.

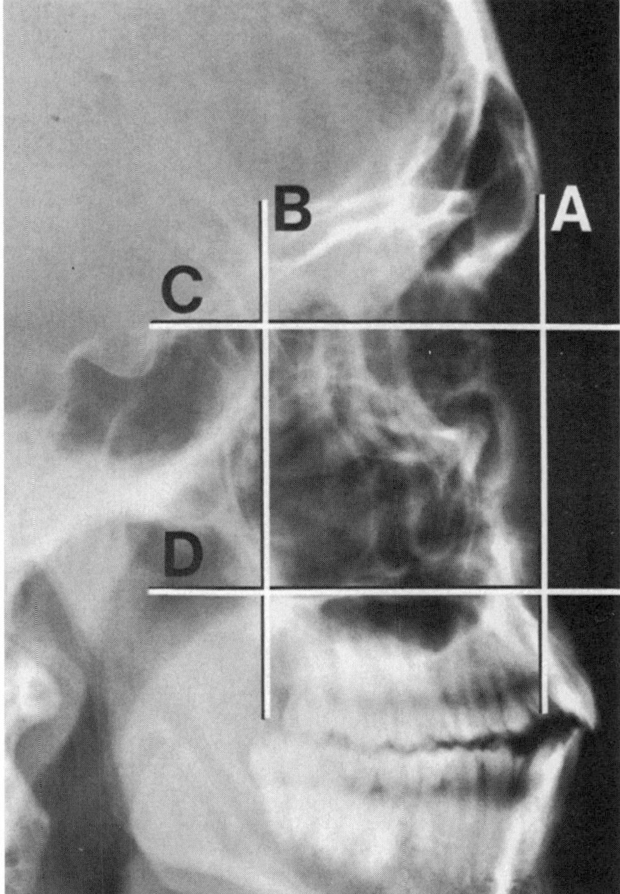

Figure 11–10. Dolan's lines of reference on a lateral view. Lines A and B and lines C and D should be almost parallel. Line A connects the anterior surface of the frontal sinus and the anterior surface of the hard palate. Line B connects the sphenoid wing (anterior wall of temporal fossa) and the posterior edge of the hard palate. Line C extends along the planum sphenoidale. Line D is drawn through the hard palate.

Base View

To obtain a submentovertex or base view of the skull it is necessary to hyperextend the patient's head on the neck. This maneuver should not be done unless injuries of the cervical spine are excluded on the basis of the clinical evaluation or have been excluded radiographically. The head is extended until the orbitomeatal line is parallel to the film cassette. The central ray is placed perpendicular to the canthomeatal line at a point 1 to 2 cm anterior to the external auditory meatus (see Fig. 11–8*D*).

Ideally, the symphysis of the mandible should overlie the frontal sinus on this view, but in practice, extension of the head may be insufficient to accomplish the ideal. This projection affords an excellent view of the anterior and lateral walls of the maxillary sinuses, the lateral walls of the orbits, the sphenoid and ethmoid sinuses, the nasal fossa, the nasopharynx, and the anterior wall of the middle fossa. The zygomatic arches are not well shown because they are overexposed on the routine examination. A soft tissue technique using a lighter exposure is necessary to show them properly (see Fig. 11–8*E*).

Three important cortical lines are shown on the base view. They were named the *triple line shadows* by Dodd and associates.[33] These lines converge at the lateral posterior margin of the nasal fossa at about the level of the posterior border of the bony septum. Whalen and Berne[58] noted that each has a characteristic shape. Two lines extend from this convergence anteriorly and laterally. The straighter of the two represents the posterolateral wall of the orbit, and the sigmoid line represents the posterolateral wall of the maxillary sinus. The semicircular line extending laterally from the convergence represents the sphenoidal surface of the temporal fossa, the anterior border of the middle cranial fossa.

Towne's View

On Towne's view, the projection is oriented so that the facial structures are not superimposed on the calvaria (see Fig. 11–8*F*). The mandibular condyle is normally positioned in the temporomandibular joint. If the condyle is displaced medially, which is frequently the case owing to muscular traction, an abnormal position may be seen.

The posterolateral wall of the maxillary sinus is seen adjacent to the inferior orbital fissure. The opposite side of the fissure is bounded by the sphenoid bone forming the lateral wall of the orbit.

The zygomatic arches are seen obliquely, and a depressed fracture may be apparent. A "bright light" is usually needed to see the arches.

Facial Fractures

Orbital Fractures

The orbit is displayed in exquisite detail by CT. This imaging modality demonstrates orbital wall fractures more accurately than plain film radiography, which is associated with a 7% to 30% false-negative rate.[173] In addition to the axial and coronal planes, the orbit can be displayed in the sagittal plane by using a special oblique sagittal projection.[65, 66] This projection as originally described requires the patient to extend the neck against a special positioning bolster, which may not be possible if the patient is severely injured. The high quality of reformatted images obtained in the sagittal projection using modern scanners renders unnecessary this unusual patient positioning (see Fig. 11–18*C*).

Fractures of the floor and entrapment of the inferior rectus and inferior oblique muscles are best shown in the coronal projection and are difficult to show in the axial plane. The axial image may also show fractures of the medial wall of the orbit, hemorrhage into the underlying ethmoid sinuses, and occasional entrapment of the medial rectus muscle. Fractures involving the nasolacrimal duct are best visualized on the coronal projection but may also be shown in the axial projection. Fractures of the optic canals and intraorbital hematomas are seen in both projections. Injuries of the eyeball,[94] including rare injuries such as avulsion of the optic nerve and extraocular muscles[176] and prolapse of the eyeball into the maxillary sinus[212] or the ethmoid sinus,[194] are well seen in either projection. Traumatic optic neuropathy from hemorrhage or impingement by a fracture fragment is well shown by CT.[226]

With plain film radiography the orbit is visualized best on Caldwell's and Waters' views. On the Waters view, the superior, lateral, and inferior portions of the orbital rim are well shown. The superior and medial orbital rims are best shown on a Caldwell view. The lateral wall of the orbit is best seen on the base view. Portions of the orbital floor are visualized on both Caldwell's and Waters' views and on the lateral view of the face, but standard radiographs do not demonstrate the orbital floor in its entirety.

Two unique types of orbital fractures are (1) *blow-out fractures,* in which bone is displaced away from the orbit, and (2) *blow-in fractures,* in which bone is displaced into the orbit. Fractures of the orbit also may be conveniently divided according to site of involvement: the orbital rim, the orbital floor, the orbital roof, the medial or lateral walls of the orbit, and the orbital apex.

Blow-out Fractures

Blow-out fractures may involve the roof, floor, and medial or lateral walls of the orbit (Figs. 11–11 through

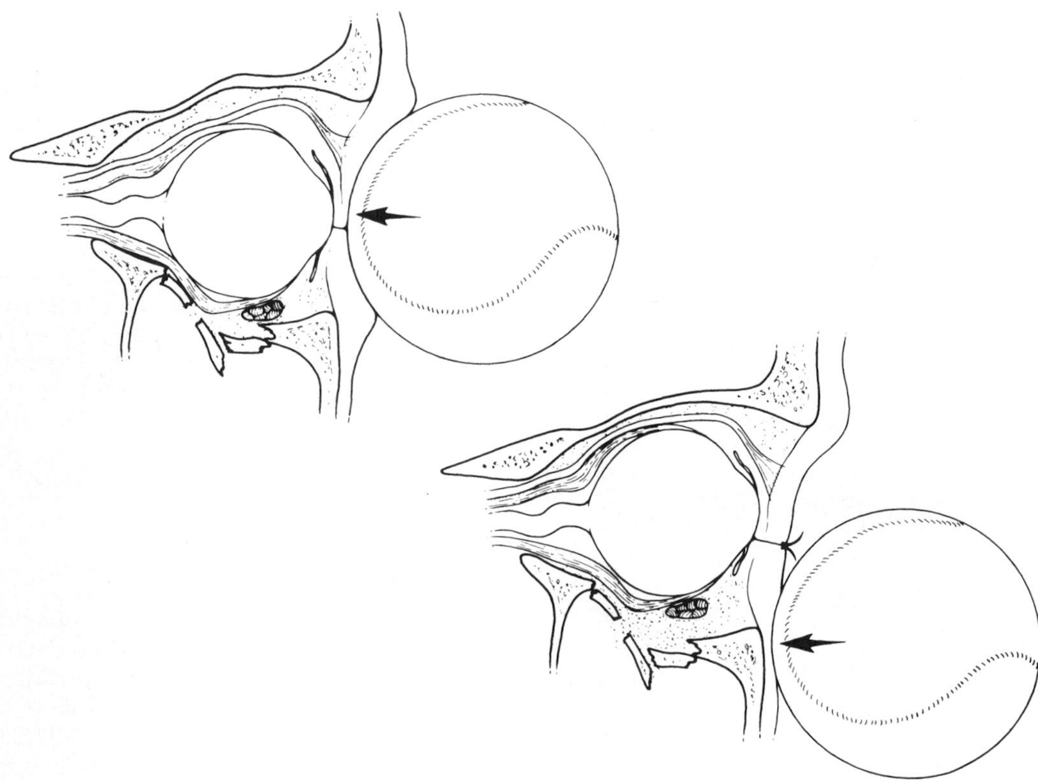

Figure 11–11. Proposed mechanisms of blow-out fracture. *Upper left,* Hydraulic mechanism: An object hits the soft tissues anteriorly, compressing contents of the orbit and resulting in a fracture of the orbital floor. *Lower right,* Buckling mechanism: An object encounters the inferior orbital rim, compressing the orbital floor and leading to a comminuted fracture of the orbital floor. The inferior orbital rim springs back into its normal position, without sustaining a fracture.

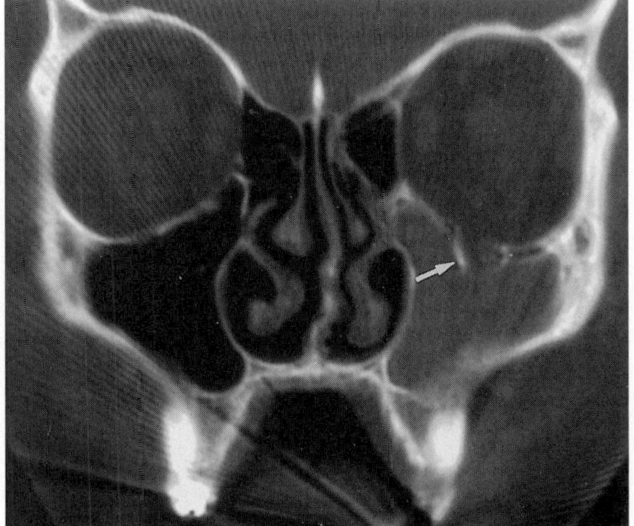

Figure 11–12. Blow-out fracture of the left orbital floor: CT findings. Coronal CT image reveals a small fracture in the middle portion of the left orbital floor. A bone fragment has hinged downward (*arrow*) into the maxillary sinus. Other images reveal that the inferior orbital rim is intact. The left maxillary sinus is filled with blood.

11–18). The orbital rim is intact in a classic blow-out fracture. Blow-out fractures most commonly involve the floor. Medial wall blow-out fracture involving the orbital plate of ethmoid bone may occur as an isolated injury in about 10% of patients with medial wall fracture[73, 74, 88, 89, 93, 97, 198] (see Fig. 11–14). The orbital plate of the ethmoid is extremely thin, and it is reasonable to question why the blow-out mechanism—described in the next paragraph—does not preferentially result in fractures of this area. The exact explanation is unknown, but the combination of blow-out fractures of the orbital floor and of the medial wall involving the orbital plate of the ethmoid is rather frequent[79, 83] (see Fig. 11–16). Dodick and associates[74] reported a series of 15 blow-out fractures, in 8 of which there were concomitant fractures of the orbital plate of the ethmoid of the medial orbital wall. In most series the combination occurs in 20% to 50% of cases.[28] In fact, Smith and Regan[95] noted that such a fracture of the medial wall accompanied orbital floor fracture produced experimentally.

Two mechanisms of injury for blow-out fractures have been proposed: a hydraulic mechanism and a buckling

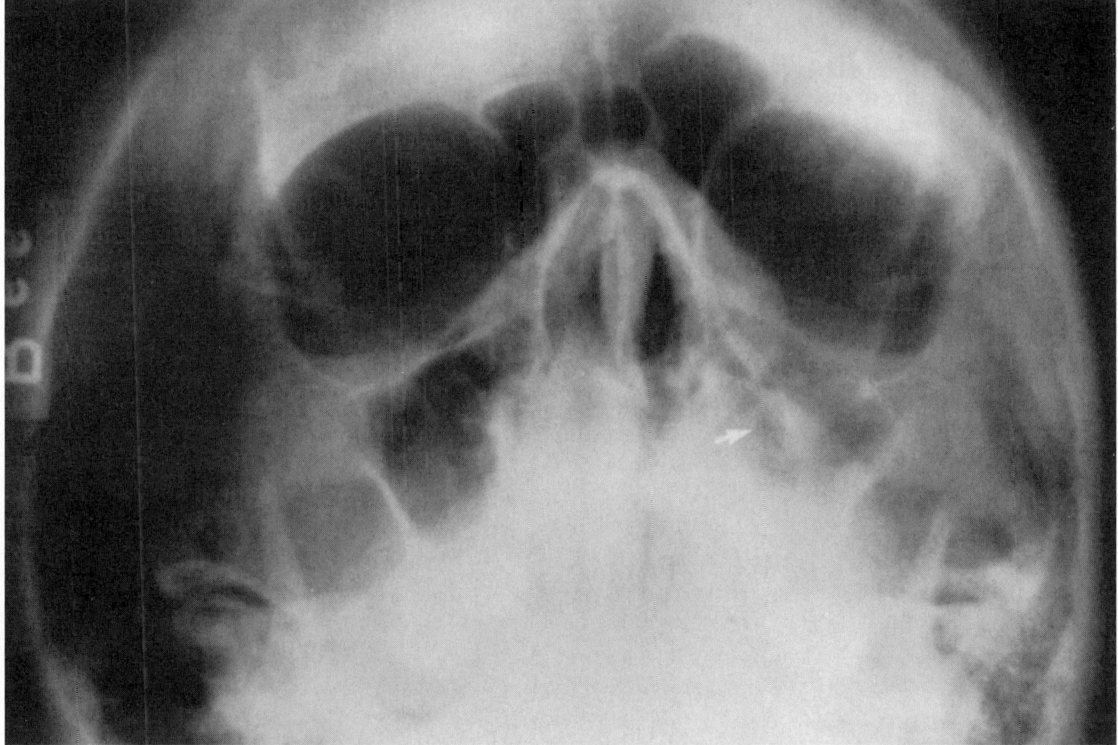

Figure 11–13. Blow-out fracture of the left orbital floor: Waters' view. This view shows opacification of the left maxillary antrum with an apparent bony spicule (*arrow*) in its midportion. There is soft tissue swelling over the left malar eminence and the lateral aspect of the nose. The orbital rim and remainder of the facial skeleton are intact.

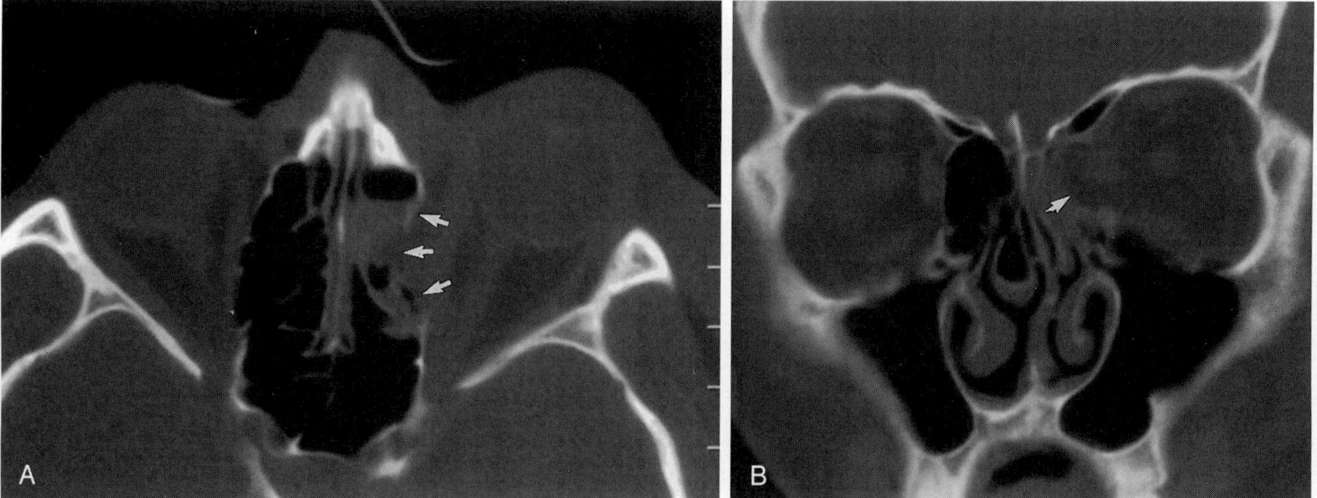

Figure 11–14. Blow-out fracture of the left medial orbital wall: CT findings. *A,* Axial CT image shows a large fracture (*arrows*) of the medial wall. There is blood in the ethmoid air cells adjacent to the fracture. *B,* Coronal CT image shows the defect in the medial wall with herniation of orbital fat (*arrow*) into the ethmoid air cells. The orbital floor is intact.

mechanism[78, 85, 86] (see Fig. 11–11). King and Samuel first described the blow-out fracture in 1944 (as noted by Zizmor and coauthors).[103] Smith and Regan[95] in 1957 showed a mechanism of injury and named the fracture. They experimentally produced injuries in cadavers by placing a hurling ball on the eye and striking the ball with a mallet. Subsequent examination revealed that although the blow created a fracture of the orbital floor, the orbital rim remained intact, and the adjacent intraorbital contents, periorbital fat, and inferior rectus muscle prolapsed through the defect in the floor. These investigators postulated a hydraulic mechanism: The pressure on the eyeball increased the intraorbital pressure, and the orbit then ruptured at its weakest point—that is, in the thin floor. Most blow-out fractures are the result of a blow by a fist, although a blow from any other small object, such as a ball, may result in this injury. An appreciable percentage of blow-out fractures (as many as 30% of cases[87, 91]) are associated with other forms of ocular injury,[72] which tends to support the mechanism of injury proposed by Smith and Regan.

A blow to the inferior orbital rim can displace it inward, leading to fractures of the adjacent thin orbital floor. This finding has led to the proposal of a second theory of the mechanism of injury, the buckling mechanism.[78, 85, 86] The comminuted fragments may be displaced inferiorly into the sinus, as occurs with a classic blow-out fracture. The inferior rim is more resilient and rebounds without sustaining a fracture. Indirect support for this mechanism of fracture has been given by Potter,[92]

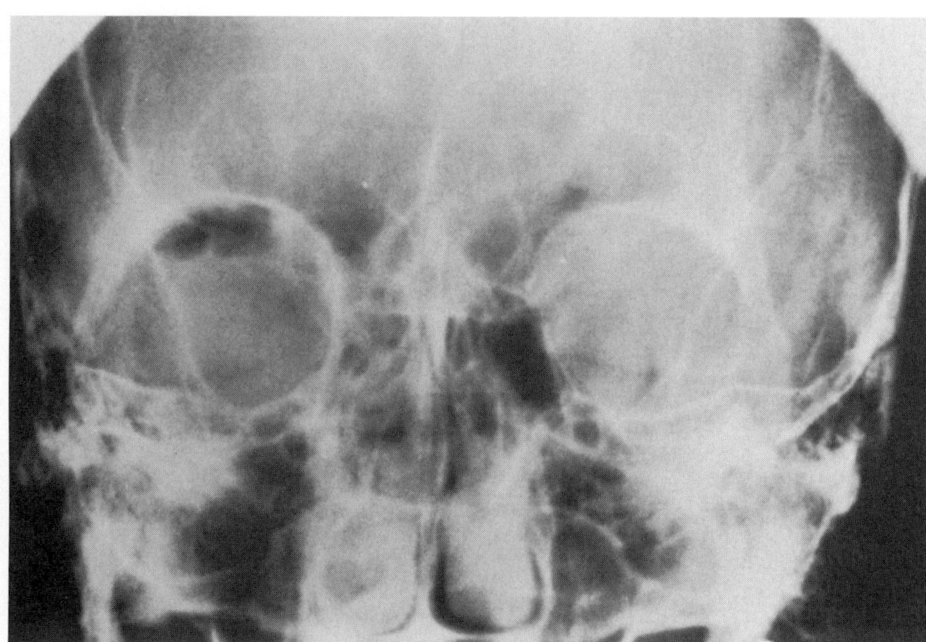

Figure 11–15. Blow-out fracture of the right medial orbital wall: Caldwell's view. This view shows emphysema of the right orbit and opacification of the right ethmoid air cells. The actual bony fracture may not be apparent on plain films. (Case courtesy of Paul E. Ross, MD, Columbia, S.C.)

out fractures of the floor[69, 77, 84, 89, 92, 103] are opacification of the maxillary sinus associated with an inverted dome–like or polypoid mass protruding from the roof of the maxillary sinus and often containing a thin spicule of bone. These features may be accompanied by intraorbital emphysema. The findings are most easily appreciated on a Waters projection. In the classic blow-out fracture the inferior orbital rim is intact. The opacification of the maxillary sinus is due to hemorrhage (see Fig. 11–13). Medial wall blow-out will result in opacification of the ethmoid air cells (see Fig. 11–15). Blow-out fractures may also be shown on magnetic resonance imaging (MRI) scans.[90, 96]

The inverted dome or polypoid mass protruding from the roof of the sinus may represent the herniated orbital contents, periorbital fat, and the inferior rectus muscle. A soft tissue mass in the roof of the maxillary sinus does not always represent herniated periorbital contents[70, 76] associated with a fracture, however. A hematoma[76] may dissect beneath the periosteum or sinus mucosa, either without an associated fracture of the floor or in association with a nondisplaced fracture of the floor, simulating soft tissue herniation. The protrusion may also represent a coincidental polyp or retention cyst in the sinus. On occasion, the mucosal lining of the roof of the sinus may remain intact; in such cases the maxillary sinus is clear except for the soft tissue density protruding from the roof of the sinus.

The thin spicule of bone often seen within the mass is the depressed portion of the orbital floor. The bone spicule may or may not be apparent, depending on the angle of the fragment in relation to the x-ray exposure beam. Unless the fragment is oriented parallel to the beam, it may not be visualized. The depth of the depression of the orbital fragment should not be estimated on the basis of its apparent displacement on a Waters view.[69] With this projection, the floor of the orbit is tilted; therefore, measurement of the distance between the fragment and the inferior orbital rim is misleading. Blow-out fracture of the medial wall may show only bleeding into the ethmoid air cells without visualization of bone fragments on plain radiographs.

Blow-in Fractures

Blow-in fractures occur when bone fragments are displaced into the orbit and intraorbital volume is decreased.[70, 139] A blow-in fracture may involve the medial wall, lateral wall, floor, or roof of the orbit (Figs. 11–19 through 11–21). Dingman and Natvig originally described this entity in 1964 in a patient with such a fracture of the orbital floor.[157] Blow-in fractures are called "pure" if the orbital rim is intact.[139] One mechanism in a pure blow-in fracture is similar to that for the buckling theory suggested for blow-out fractures. Compression of the orbital rim results in slight posterior bending; the rim does not break, but the transmitted force is sufficient to fracture the orbital wall. Another proposed mechanism is trauma resulting in increased pressure in an adjacent sinus sufficient to "blow in" the medial wall, floor, or anterior part of the roof.[139] The fractured bone is displaced toward the eyeball. A fracture with displacement of bone into the orbit, which also involves the orbital rim, has been called an "impure" blow-in fracture. This injury may be the result of a segmental isolated rim fracture. Associated injuries that may involve the rim with a blow-in fracture include naso-orbital-ethmoidal (NOE) fractures, ZMC fractures, frontal bone fractures, and more complex combination injuries.

Clinical findings in blow-in fractures result from decreased orbital volume or direct trauma to the eyeball or optic nerve. Exophthalmos may occur because of the decreased orbital volume.[163] Decrease in visual acuity may occur secondary to eyeball trauma or traumatic optic neuropathy.[220] The loss of visual acuity may be transient or may be permanent, especially if the optic canal is fractured. Blindness has occurred with damage to the optic nerve associated with orbital apex fracture. Ocular mobility limitation may also follow a blow-in fracture. The limitation usually is due to mechanical interference with ocular motion, although injury to the extraocular muscles or superior orbital fissure syndrome with injury to the nerves supplying the extraocular muscles may also be the cause.[150, 231] Rupture of the eyeball due to perforation by a bony fragment has been reported.[182] Orbital compartment syndrome may occur if post-traumatic edema or hemorrhage results in sufficiently increased intraorbital pressure to result in ischemia of the optic nerve. In addition to intraorbital injury, blow-in fractures of the orbital roof are associated with brain injury such as contusions, hemorrhage, and herniation and with delayed meningitis.[189]

Imaging of blow-in fracture is best performed with CT, which can exactly define the site and extent of fractures as well as the position of fracture fragments.[175] If there is orbital roof fracture with herniation of frontal lobe, MRI may be useful because it may be better than CT in distinguishing herniated brain from hematoma.[187] If plain radiography findings suggest a fracture fragment within the orbit, CT should be performed.

Orbital Rim Fractures

A direct blow to the orbital rim by a high-velocity object with a small surface, such as a club or bat, may result in an isolated fracture of the orbital rim (see Fig. 11–34). These fractures are most likely to involve the superior or superior lateral margin of the orbit. Fractures of the superior rim are frequently associated with fractures of the roof of the orbit and may involve the frontal sinus (see Fig. 11–48). Fractures of the inferior rim are usually associated with zygomatic or NOE fractures (Fig. 11–22). Fracture of the lateral rim of the orbit is usually a component of a more significant fracture involving the zygomatic region, either a ZMC fracture (see Fig. 11–36) or a more complex fracture of the LeFort variety.

Fractures of the medial orbital rim are associated with opacification of the underlying ethmoid air cells and may extend through the lacrimal duct, resulting in pathologic tearing or epiphora. They may also be associated with separation of the medial canthal ligament, which results in an unacceptable cosmetic appearance with laxity of the lids and lateral displacement of the medial canthus (pseudohypertelorism). Fractures involving the medial

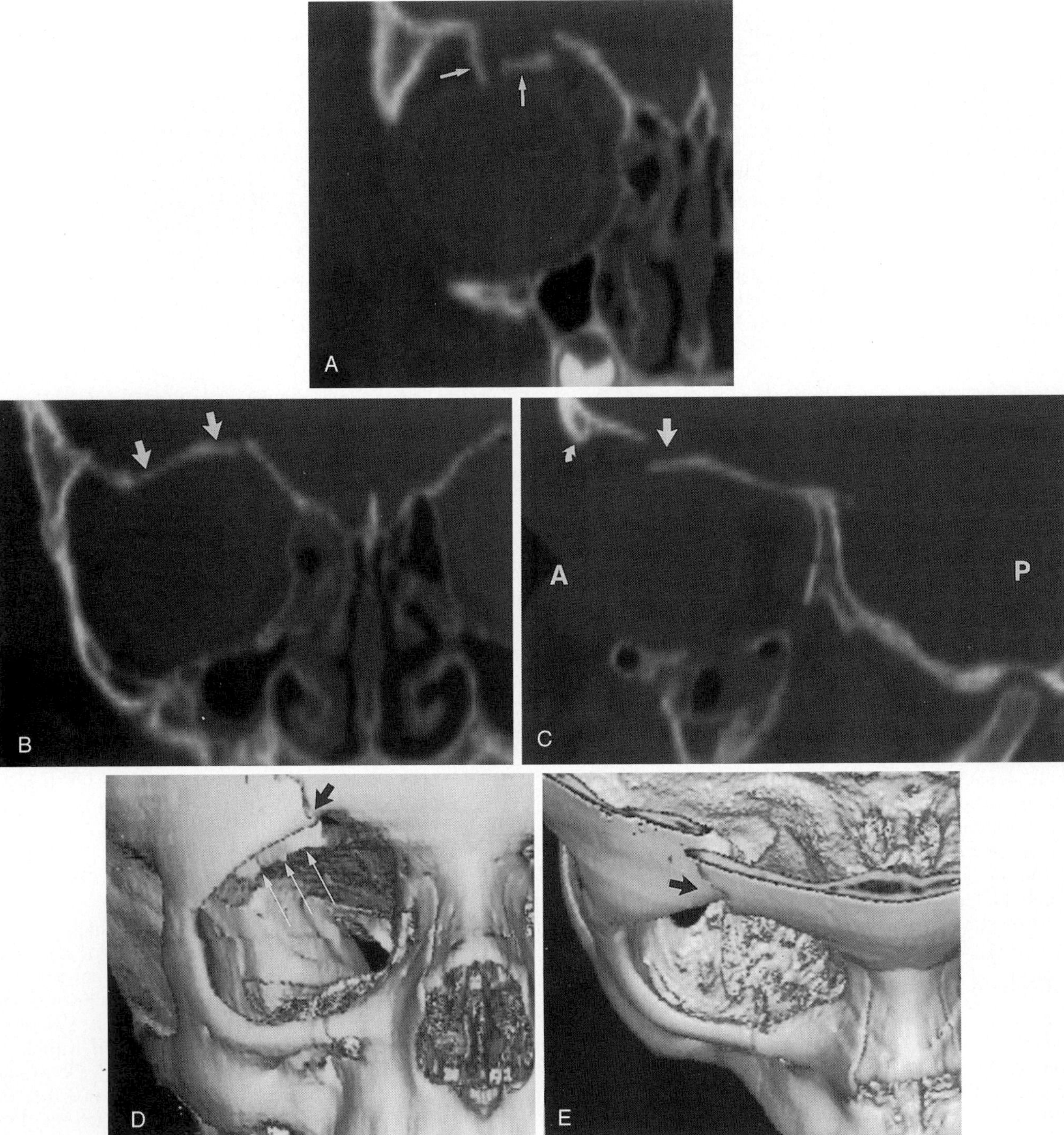

Figure 11–19. Blow-in fracture of the orbital roof. *A,* Coronal CT view just posterior to the superior orbital rim shows fragments from the roof (*arrows*) displaced toward the eyeball. Such a fracture of the roof may be present with an intact superior orbital rim (pure roof blow-in) or may be seen in association with a fracture of the rim (impure blow-in fracture). *B,* Coronal CT view obtained slightly posterior to Figure 11–18*A* indicates that a wider portion of the orbital roof is involved and displaced toward the eye (*arrows*). *C,* On this sagittal reformatted image obtained through the orbit, anterior (A) is to the left and posterior (P) is to the right. The depressed fragment from the roof (*straight arrow*) is seen just posterior to the superior orbital rim (*curved arrow*). *D,* Frontal view with 3-D reformatting shows that the superior orbital rim and frontal bone are fractured (*black arrow*). A fragment from the roof (*white arrows*) can be seen projected just inferior to the rim. *E,* Towne's view with 3-D reformatting shows the posterior displacement of the lateral aspect of the superior orbital rim and frontal bone (*arrow*). These three-dimensional images are superior to the other images in showing the displacement and rotation of the rim and piece of frontal bone.

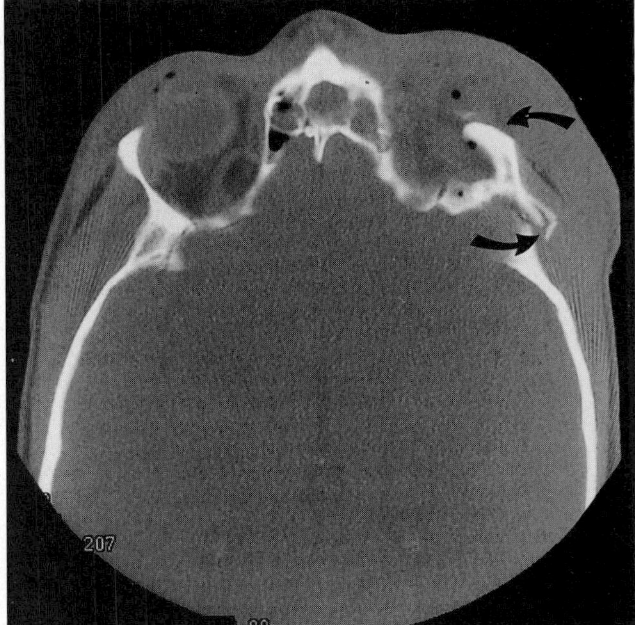

Figure 11–20. Blow-in fracture of the lateral orbital rim and wall. The lateral blow-in fracture is usually associated with fractures of the zygoma. In this case the superior portion of the left frontal process of zygoma and the attached lateral wall have rotated medially (*anterior arrow*). The posterior portion of the fragment has rotated laterally (*posterior arrow*). Such displacement toward the eyeball results in decreased orbital volume.

rim[63] may be components of more complex NOE fractures. Such fractures may be limited to one side but are commonly midline fractures involving the medial rim and wall of both orbits and usually include the bony margins of the nasolacrimal ducts. They are shown by CT examination in both the coronal and axial projections.

Orbital Floor Fractures

The floor is the most common portion of the orbit to sustain a fracture. Orbital floor fractures may be seen as components of the common ZMC fracture (see Fig. 11–36) and LeFort II and LeFort III fractures (see Fig. 11–55), and as isolated entities in orbital blow-out fractures (see Fig. 11–12). Crumley and associates,[70] in reviewing 363 fractures of the orbital floor, found that 46% were associated with ZMC fractures and 35% with complex facial fractures, including the LeFort variety; 8% involved the inferior orbital rim and adjacent floor; and 11% were isolated fractures of the orbital floor of the blow-out variety. As many as 25% to 50% of orbital floor fractures are associated with fractures of the medial wall of the orbit, involving the orbital plate of the ethmoid and extending into the ethmoid air cells[79, 83] (see Fig. 11–16). Such fractures can be visualized in both the coronal and axial projections and are manifested by bone disruption and opacification of the ethmoid air cells. Rarely, there is an associated fracture of the orbital roof.[65, 66]

Fractures of the orbital floor may be linear, comminuted, or segmental. With segmental fractures, bone is likely to be depressed into the maxillary sinus, either partially, in the manner of a hinge or trap door, or completely, as a circumscribed fragment free from attachment to adjacent bone.[147] With comminuted fractures, portions of involved bone may be similarly depressed. The importance of this distinction lies in the possibility of herniation of the intraorbital contents and muscle entrapment in association with depression of orbital floor fragments. This possibility is unlikely with simple linear fractures. The orbital floor component of a ZMC fracture is usually linear. The orbital floor component of complex facial fractures is frequently linear but may be segmental. Blow-out fractures of the orbital floor are usually segmental, with at least partial fragment depression.

The best means of evaluation and confirmation of orbital floor fractures is CT. Because of the oblique horizontal course of the floor of the orbit, this structure is best seen in the coronal projection. The axial projection will delineate associated fractures of the medial wall of the orbit. CT shows to good advantage the position, degree of displacement, and comminution of fracture fragments. CT also can show that the floor of the orbit is intact, thereby excluding injury. Evaluation of a fracture of the floor of the orbit should address the following: (1) the size of the fracture fragments and the degree of their depression, which determines the magnitude of expansion of the orbit; (2) whether the inferior rectus muscle is free or hooked, or entrapped; (3) the presence or absence of other associated fractures, particularly of the medial wall and roof of the orbit; and (4) the presence or absence of injuries of the eyeball and other intraorbital structures.

Surgery is not necessary in every case of fracture of the orbital floor.[68, 150] The principal determinants of the need for surgery are the possibility of subsequent enophthalmos and persistent diplopia. Significantly depressed, large, or comminuted fragments greatly expand the orbit, so that enophthalmos is very likely. In contrast, linear fractures and minimally depressed fractures of the orbital floor with minimal orbital expansion are less likely to result in enophthalmos. CT findings that indicate the need for surgery include involvement of 50% or more of the floor with fracture and combined floor and medial wall fractures with soft tissue herniation.[218]

The course of the inferior rectus muscle should be identified on the coronal image and followed over the length of the fracture. Persistent diplopia is likely if the

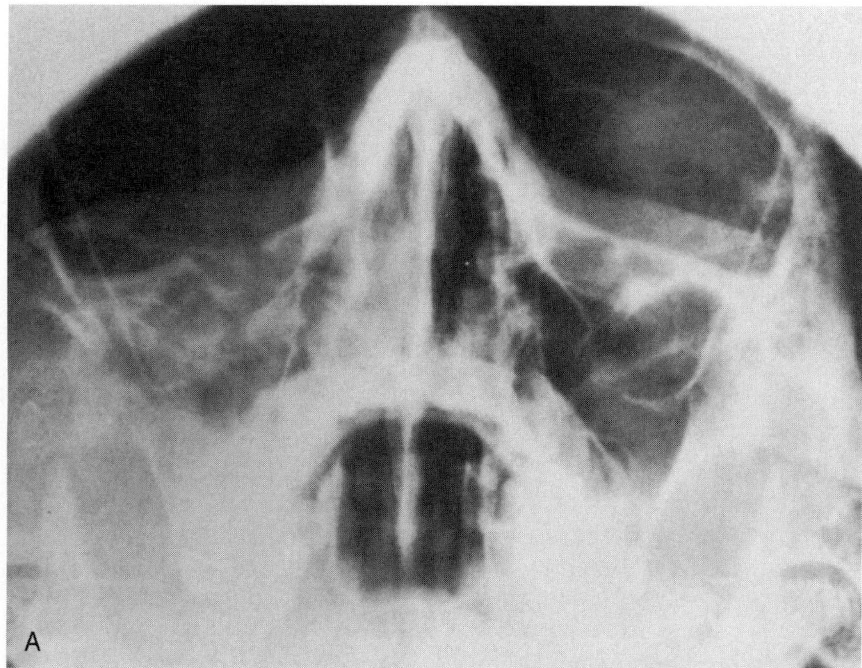

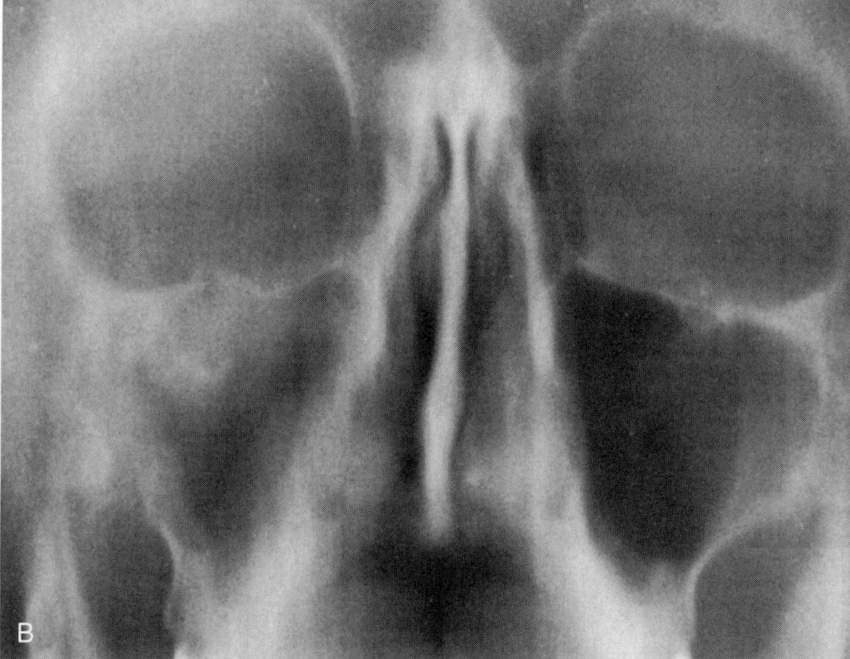

Figure 11–21. Inferior orbital rim fracture: Plain films. *A,* Waters' view shows a fracture of the orbital rim and a soft tissue density in the roof of the maxillary sinus. There is a depressed fragment of the orbital floor within the soft tissue density. Fluid is present at the base of the maxillary sinus. *B,* Conventional linear tomogram obtained in the posteroanterior projection clearly shows the fracture of the orbital floor and depressed fragment within the soft tissue density of the roof of the right maxillary sinus. The term "blow-out fracture" implies that the rim is intact. This fracture should be called a "rim and floor fracture." Orbital rim fractures extend into the adjacent wall with or without displacement.

fracture fragments entrap the inferior rectus muscle (see Fig. 11–18). This problem can be identified in either the coronal or oblique sagittal projection by an acute buckling of the muscle trapped and held between adjacent fracture fragments. In some cases the muscle is herniated between the fragments into the maxillary sinus, so that it is difficult to identify with certainty. If the muscle is not visible in a series of three consecutive thin-section coronal CT images, a safe conclusion is that it is herniated and entrapped.[62] The muscle is said to be hooked when it is only pinched in one portion by the fracture margins. In most cases in which the muscle is hooked, diplopia is only transient and ultimately resolves without surgery.

Medial Wall Fractures

Medial wall fracture occurs as an isolated injury in about 10% of patients in whom the medial wall is fractured. Medial wall fracture also occurs in conjunction with blow-out fracture of the floor in 36% of patients (see Fig. 11–16), with involvement of the zygoma and floor in 28% and with more complex fractures in 26%[198] (see Fig. 11–55). The medial wall is fractured in LeFort II, LeFort III, and NOE fractures.

CT is required to show the site of the fracture. Good visualization is possible in both the coronal and axial projections.[102] In rare cases, the medial rectus muscle becomes hooked (see Fig. 11–18) or entrapped[97, 102]

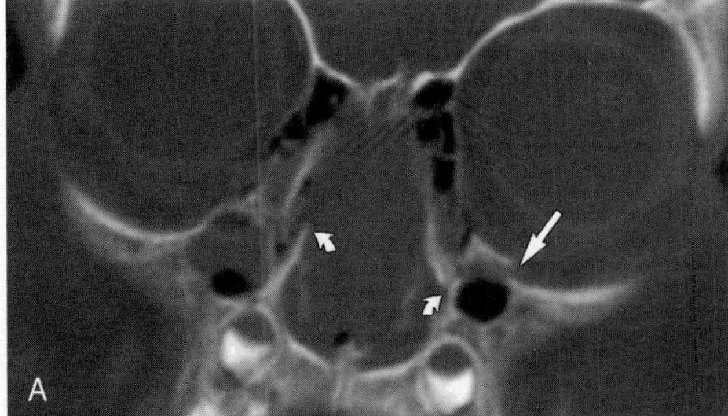

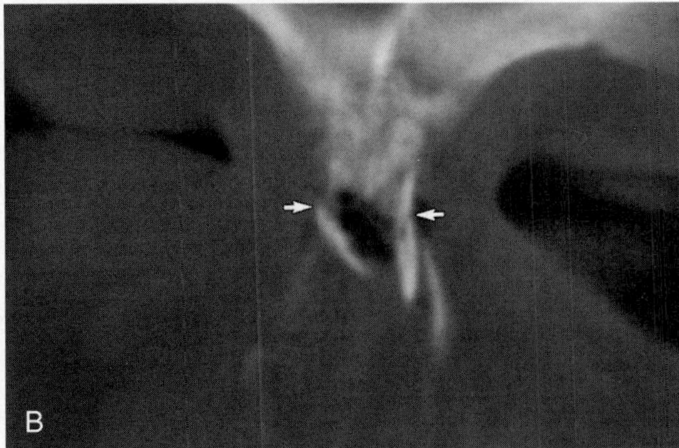

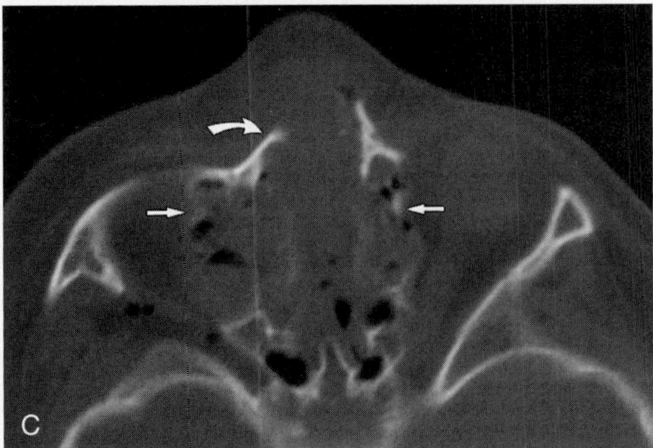

Figure 11–22. Inferior orbital rim fracture: CT findings. *A,* A fracture of the left inferior orbital rim (*straight arrow*) is seen on this coronal CT view and is a component of a more complex naso-orbital-ethmoidal fracture. There are fractures involving the maxilla at the lateral borders of the nasal fossa (*curved arrows*). *B,* Coronal CT view shows that the nasal bones are broken bilaterally (*arrows*). *C,* The frontal process of the maxilla and the lacrimal bone on the right appear to be rotated (*curved arrow*) on this axial CT view, and the medial orbital walls are disrupted bilaterally (*straight arrows*).

within the defect, resulting in limitation of lateral motion of the eye. Entrapment may be suspected on the basis of the CT appearance. Medial wall fractures are manifested radiographically by the presence of orbital emphysema, opacification of the involved ethmoid air cells, or both on a Caldwell view. It is difficult to visualize fractures of the orbital plate of ethmoid bones on the standard projections.

Lateral Wall Fractures

With lateral orbital wall fractures, there may be displacement of fragments either toward or away from the eyeball.[41] Lateral wall fracture is rarely an isolated fracture; rather, it is usually a component of a LeFort III or ZMC fracture (see Fig. 11–36).

A classification has been suggested for lateral wall blow-in fractures by Stanley and colleagues.[220] In type 1, the frontal process of the zygoma is displaced medially and posteriorly to a position between the eyeball and greater wing of the sphenoid. Type 2 involves lateral and posterior displacement of the frontal process of the zygoma with medial displacement of a fragment from the orbital plate of the greater wing of the sphenoid. Type 3 lateral blow-in fracture is characterized by impaction of the entire greater wing of the sphenoid toward the orbital apex and possibly into the middle cranial fossa. In type 4, the greater wing of the sphenoid is displaced across the orbital apex, with possible involvement of the lesser sphenoid wing. Although the intraorbital portion of the optic nerve may be involved with any lateral wall blow-in fracture, the intracanilicular portion of the nerve is more likely to be involved in type 4.

Orbital Roof Fractures

Fractures of the orbital roof occur in 5% to 9% of patients with facial fractures.[163, 189] They are rarely isolated injuries but are commonly associated with fractures of the superior orbital rim, with severely comminuted facial fractures, and occasionally with fractures of the orbital floor (see Figs. 11–19, 11–49, and 11–60). Isolated blow-in fractures of the roof may occur with blunt trauma to the frontal bone.[153, 175] The fracture fragment may "blow in" into the orbit or "blow out" into the anterior cranial fossa.[71, 99] Intracerebral injuries to the bases of the frontal lobes adjacent to the roof may be encountered. In similar fashion, herniation of brain into the orbit may occur and is especially well shown by MRI.[187] Pneumocephalus may occur with orbital roof fractures, and tension pneumocephalus has been reported.[228]

Orbital fractures are best evaluated by CT examination in the coronal or oblique sagittal projections, both of which will also reveal injuries of the adjacent frontal lobe. Three-dimensional CT may be particularly useful in preoperative assessment of bone displacement and in displaying the position and alignment of fracture fragments.[153, 175]

Orbital Apex Fractures

Fractures of the orbital apex usually occur as extensions of fractures of the face, base of the skull, or other orbital fractures, particularly those involving the orbital roof. They are seldom isolated injuries[98] (Figs. 11–23 and 11–24), and they may be associated with traumatic blindness. The optic canal and related fractures are best delineated by CT examination in the axial projection. Fractures traversing the optic canal commonly extend medially and inferiorly into the sphenoid sinus.[81] Fractures of the optic canal may be associated with concomitant injuries of the carotid artery and should suggest the

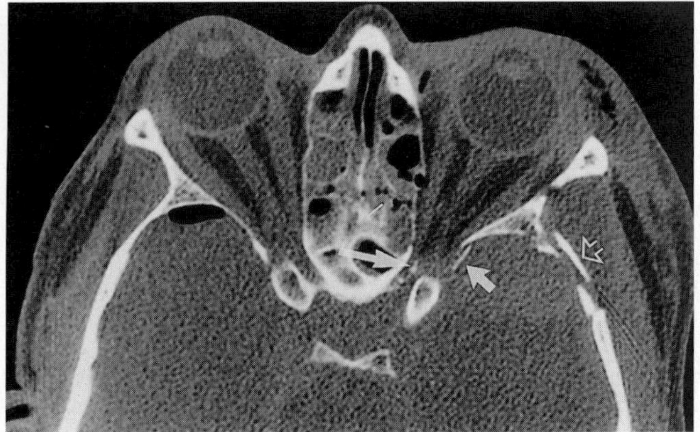

Figure 11–23. Orbital apex fracture: Sphenoid fracture. Axial CT image shows fractures at the apex (*solid small arrow*) of the pyramidally shaped orbit. A fragment of bone lies within the optic canal (*large solid arrow*), adjacent to the optic nerve. Injury to the optic nerve from the orbital apex fracture is a cause of blindness. There is fracture of the greater wing of the sphenoid laterally (*open arrow*). Pneumocephalus is noted on the right. (Reprinted with permission from Rhea, J.T., Rao, P.M., & Novelline, R.N. (1999). Helical CT and three-dimensional CT of facial and orbital injury. Radiol. Clin. North Am., 37:489.)

need for arteriography. Carotid artery–cavernous sinus fistula may also occur with orbital apex fractures.

Soft Tissue Injuries of the Orbit

Soft tissue injuries of the orbit may occur in the presence or absence of orbital fractures. They are best shown by CT, which can diagnose rupture of the eyeball, lens injuries, intraorbital hemorrhage, and intraorbital foreign bodies. The CT appearance may be suggestive of orbital compartment syndrome.

Eyeball Rupture

Rupture of the eyeball may occur without fracture from either perforating or blunt trauma (Figs. 11–25 and 11–26). Perforation may be from a foreign body or a bone fragment in a blow-in fracture.[139, 169] With rupture, there is usually extrusion of the vitreous, because intraocular pressure is normally higher than intraorbital pressure.[219] Extrusion leads to reduction in ocular volume, resulting in two signs of rupture at CT. One sign is flattening of the posterior wall of the eyeball—the "flat tire" sign described by Sevel and associates.[217] Anteriorly, the convexity of the eye surface tends to be maintained if the anterior chamber is intact and if the attachment of the orbital septum remains intact. Posteriorly, the surface of the eye is not tethered, and thus that portion of the eyeball "deflates."

Another sign of rupture is "deepening" of the anterior chamber.[227] The lens moves slightly posteriorly as the normal pressure in the vitreous is decreased. The normal anterior chamber measures 2 to 3.5 mm in depth from the cornea to the lens in the midline. With rupture, this depth increases to about 5 mm.[227]

Lens Injury: Subluxation, Dislocation, and Traumatic Cataract

Zonular fibers hold the lens in place, attaching the lens to the ciliary muscle. These fibers may be partially or completely torn during trauma. A partial tear on one side allows subluxation of the lens, and a complete tear results in dislocation of the lens (Figs. 11–27 and 11–28). The lens is denser than the vitreous and thus will move dependently through the vitreous. With subluxation, the intact zonular fibers hold one side in place, allowing it to swing posteriorly from the unattached side, like a trap door. With dislocation, the lens may sink through the vitreous and come to lie on top of the retina.

With traumatic cataract, the lens becomes acutely edematous.[214] Influx of fluid into the lens lowers its CT density. This change may be detected by comparison with the unaffected eye; the abnormal lens is of a lower density, often by 30 Hounsfield units (HU), than that of the normal lens.[146] Of note, a traumatic cataract may not be apparent clinically.

Orbital Compartment Syndrome

The clinical findings in orbital compartment syndrome are caused by increased intraorbital pressure and include proptosis, blindness, immobile eyeball, and dilated pupil. To ensure full recovery, this condition should be diagnosed and treated within 2 hours.[181, 183] Increased postseptal pressure may compromise vascular supply to the optic nerve or retina, resulting in transient or permanent loss of vision.[182] The increase in pressure, following trauma, may occur because of hemorrhage or postseptal emphysema with a ball-valve mechanism. Blow-in fractures may result in a decrease in orbital volume with a concomitant increase in pressure.[139]

Intraorbital Hemorrhage

Vitreous hemorrhage appears on CT scans as an area of hyperdensity that forms an acute angle if located adjacent to the wall of the eye (Fig. 11–29). Choroidal or subretinal hemorrhage is of approximately the same density as the sclera and may be differentiated from vitreous hemorrhage by its mound shape and the obtuse angle formed between the area of hemorrhage and the vitreous (Fig. 11–30).

Hemorrhage may occur into the sheath of the optic nerve. Ischemic damage to the nerve may result from hemorrhage, as well as from any cause of increased intraorbital pressure. CT may show hemorrhage into the sheath as an asymmetrical bulging contour on comparison with the normal side. Hemorrhage may also occur adjacent to the optic nerve (Fig. 11–31).

Intraorbital Foreign Body

Almost any intraorbital foreign body is detectable by CT (Figs. 11–32 through 11–34). The location of the

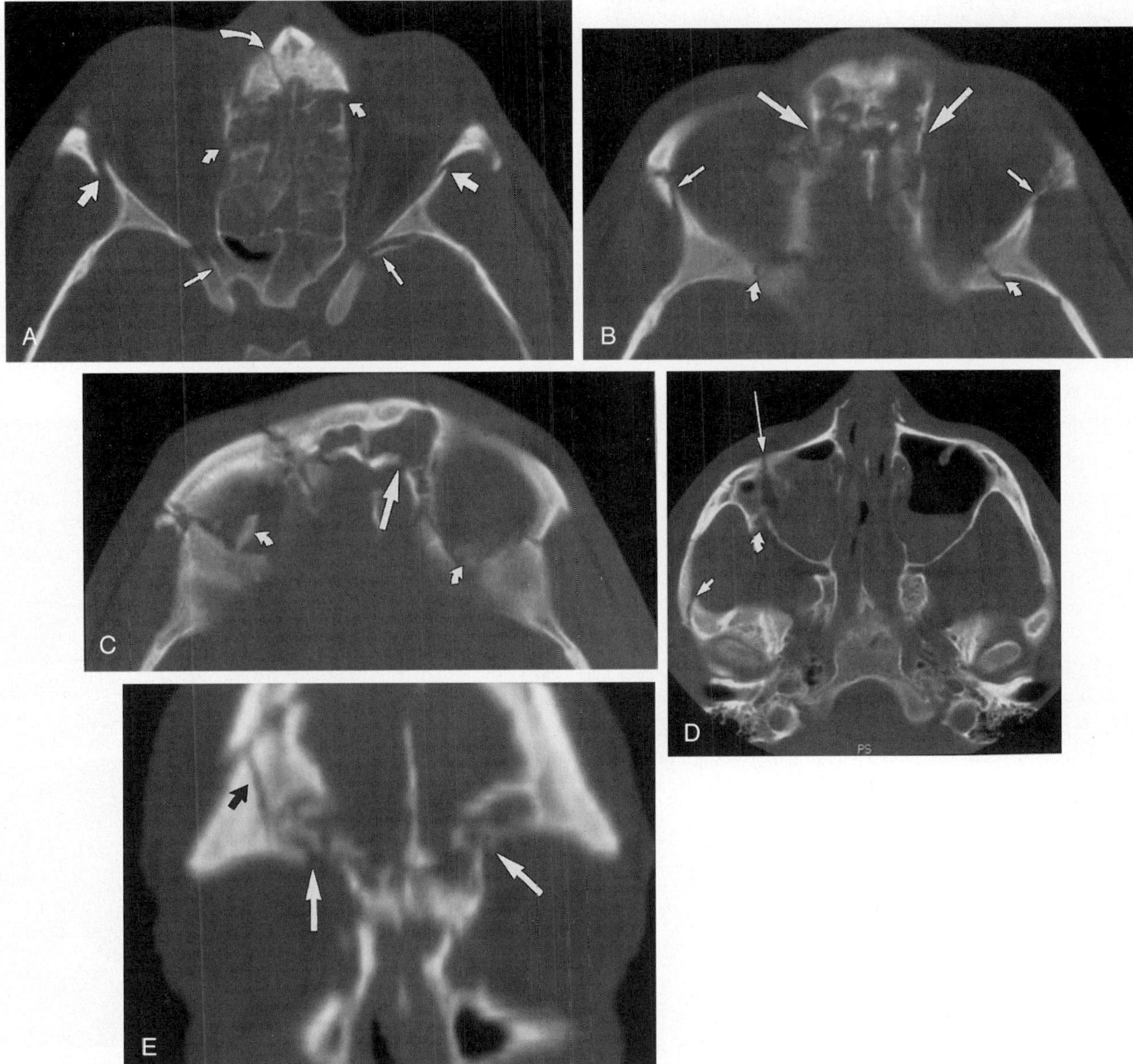

Figure 11–24. Orbital apex fracture: Multiple associated fractures. Complex fractures such as fractures of the frontal sinuses and orbital roofs, naso-orbital-ethmoidal fractures, and zygomatic fractures may extend to the orbital apex. *A,* Bilateral fractures of the greater wing of sphenoid at the orbital apex are seen (*thin straight arrows*). On the right, a fragment of bone impinges on the optic canal. There are also fractures of the nasal bone (*large curved arrow*) and bilateral medial orbital walls (*small curved arrows*) from a naso-orbital-ethmoidal fracture. Also present are bilateral fractures of the lateral orbital walls (*thick straight arrows*). *B,* On an image obtained cephalad to *A,* fractures of the posterior portion of the orbital roofs (*curved arrows*), lateral orbital walls (*small straight arrows*), and medial orbital walls (*large straight arrows*) are present. There is posterior displacement of the anterior nasal structures into the ethmoid air cells. *C,* On an image obtained further cephalad to *B,* there are fractures of both orbital roofs (*curved arrows*) and of the posterior wall of the frontal sinus (*straight arrow*). *D,* Fractures of the zygomatic arch (*short straight arrow*), the posterior wall of the right maxillary sinus (*curved arrow*), and the anterior wall of this sinus (*long straight arrow*) just below the inferior orbital rim are seen. These fractures, in addition to the evidence of displacement of the frontal process of the zygoma in *A,* constitute a zygomatic complex fracture on the right. *E,* Coronal CT images were reformatted. Anteriorly, fractures of the superior orbital rims are noted extending into the frontal sinuses (*white arrows*), and the fracture on the right extends to the frontal bone (*black arrow*). A summary description of these fractures in *A* through *D* would be as follows: "There are bilateral orbital roof fractures extending to the apex of both orbits with impingement of the optic nerve on the right. The posterior wall of the frontal sinus is fractured. There are bilateral naso-orbital-ethmoidal fractures with posterior displacement, and there is a right zygomatic complex fracture without displacement."

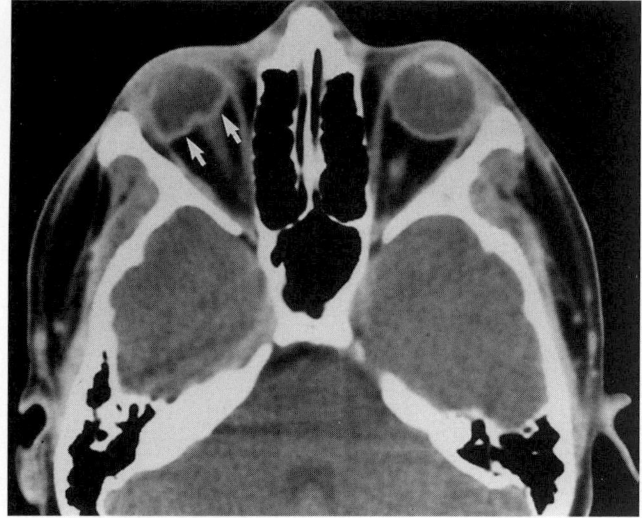

Figure 11–25. Rupture of the eyeball: "Flat tire." A "flat tire" sign is seen on the right after rupture of the eyeball due to scleral laceration and extrusion of vitreous. This sign refers to the flattening of the posterior surface of the eyeball (*arrows*). The anterior margin of the eye maintains its convex shape in many cases of decompression of the eyeball. The optic nerve is slack in the neutral position and does not tether the posterior surface of the eye.

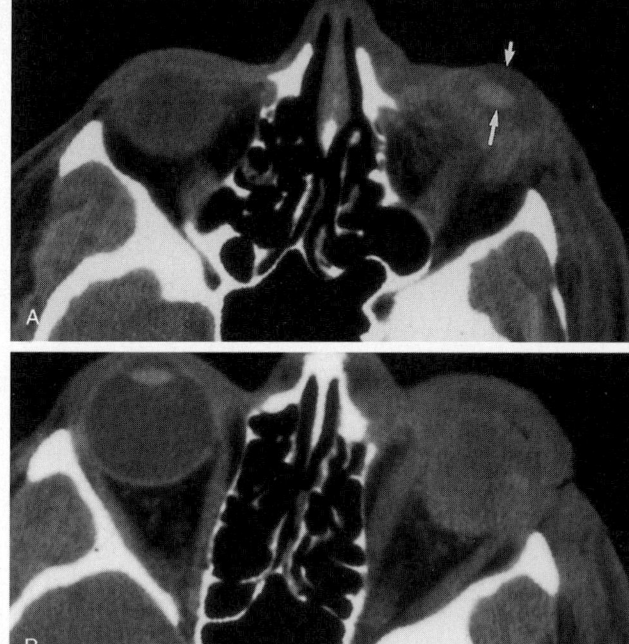

Figure 11–26. Rupture of the eyeball: Deep anterior chamber. The left lens (*long arrow*) appears abnormally posterior to the cornea (*short arrow*) in *A*, compared with the right lens shown in *B*. This finding has been called the "deep anterior chamber sign" and may be the result of posterior sagging of the lens with relaxation of the zonular fibers. The difference in depth of the anterior chamber from eye to eye should be no more than 2 mm.

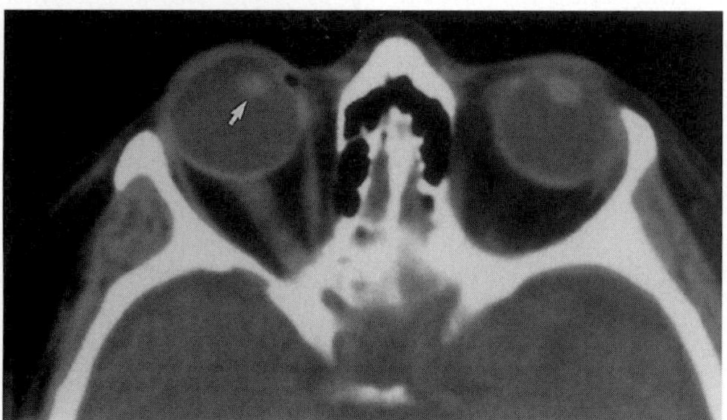

Figure 11–27. Lens subluxation. On the right, the lens (*arrow*) had displaced (subluxated) toward the medial aspect of the eyeball. Subluxation occurs when there is tearing of a portion of the circumferential zonular fibers. A subluxated lens may hinge posteriorly, like a trap door, if enough fibers have been disrupted, or as in this case, the lens may be displaced only medially or laterally.

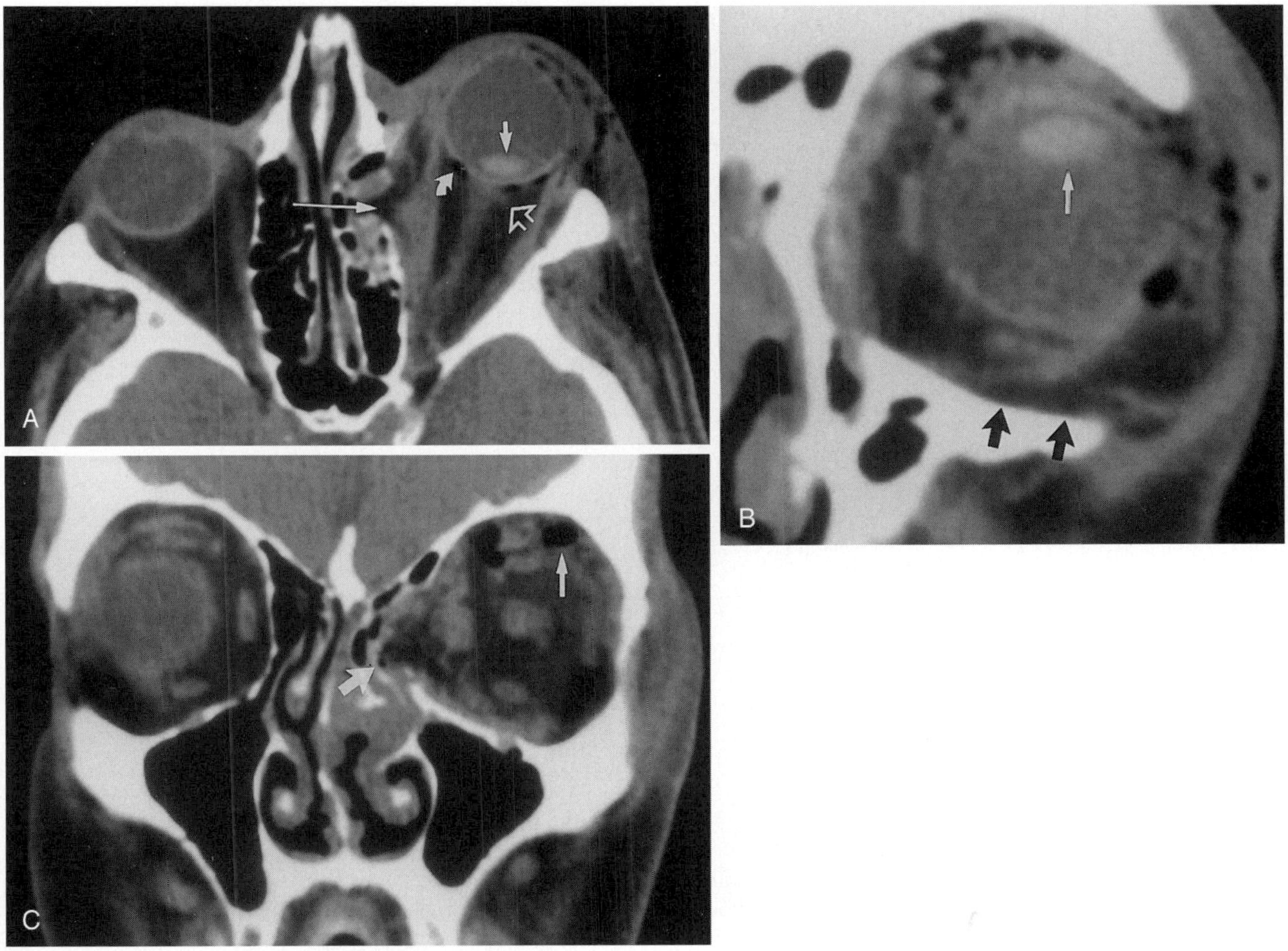

Figure 11–28. Lens dislocation. Lens dislocation occurs when all the supporting zonular fibers are torn, allowing complete displacement of the lens. The patient sustained a medial blow-out fracture of the left eye with a lens dislocation. *A,* Soft tissue window setting shows that the dislocated lens (*short arrow*) has settled in a dependent position in the eye on this supine axial CT image. There is intraconal orbital emphysema (*curved arrow*) signifying a fracture into an adjacent sinus—in this case, of the medial wall into ethmoid air cells (*long arrow*). There is herniation of fat into the fracture with displacement of the medial rectus muscle. A small amount of blood (*open arrow*) is noted around the optic nerve, and the increased width of the optic nerve at its attachment with the eyeball suggests hemorrhage into the optic nerve sheath. *B,* The patient's neck was extended for direct coronal CT images, and the lens (*white arrow*) is seen to move to the dependent superior surface of the eyeball. The inferior orbital rim (*black arrows*) is intact. *C,* Coronal CT image posterior to the eyeball shows the medial blow-out fracture with herniation of fat (*thick arrow*). Orbital emphysema is noted (*thin arrow*).

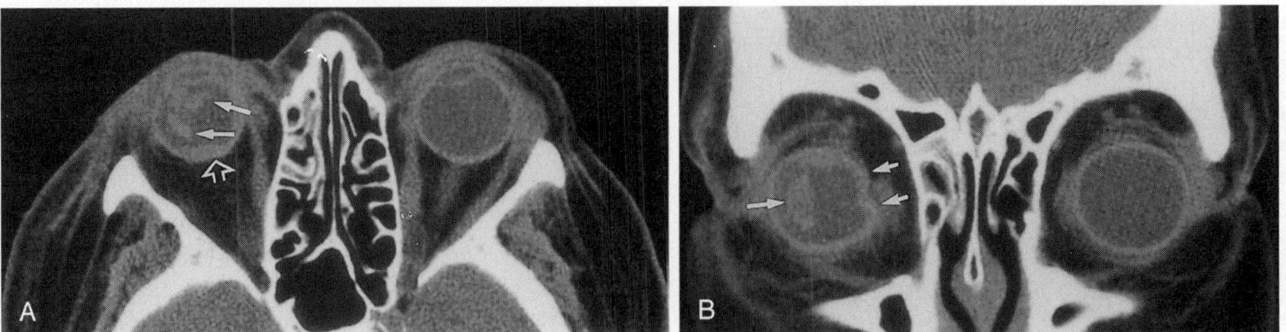

Figure 11–29. Vitreous hemorrhage. *A,* The higher density material in the vitreous (*solid arrows*) represents blood. The patient had a history of cataract surgery. Where the blood is adjacent to the choroid layer, an acute angle may be seen; this finding helps to differentiate this entity from choroidal hemorrhage under the retina. There is slight flattening of the posterior surface of the eye with adjacent subretinal hemorrhage (*open arrow*). *B,* In addition to the vitreous hemorrhage (*long arrow*), there is a scleral laceration with decompression and loss of the outward convexity of the medial surface of the eyeball (*short arrows*), as seen on this coronal image.

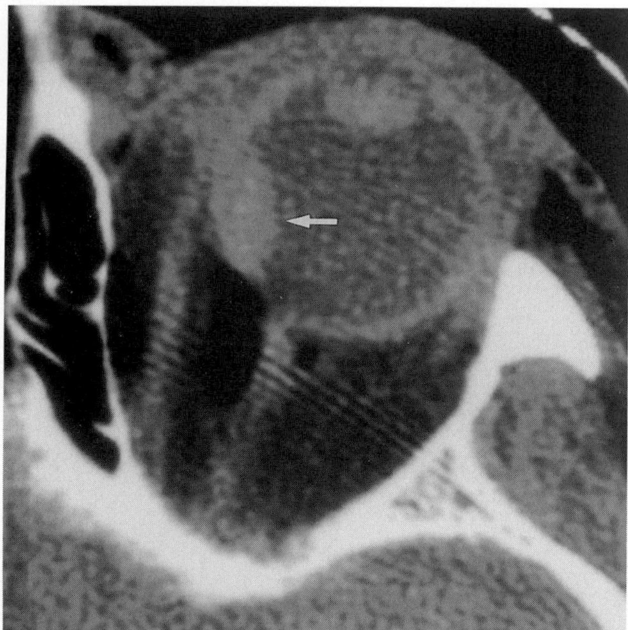

Figure 11–30. Choroidal hemorrhage. The hemorrhage is seen as a mound-shaped density in the wall of the eyeball (*arrow*). The interface of this density with the adjacent wall and the vitreous makes an obtuse angle, suggesting that the hemorrhage is not within the vitreous.

foreign body is important to specify, although it may be difficult to discern whether a foreign body is immediately adjacent to or within the sclera, owing to artifact.[178] Foreign bodies are usually best shown on soft tissue windows at CT, especially those made of metal and glass.[152] A lung window may be required to show a wood or plastic foreign body. The density of wood and plastic is usually 0 HU or less (negative HU value).[197] Not all foreign bodies need to be removed. Small metal, glass, and stone foreign bodies usually are inert, although copper may incite inflammation. Infection is frequent with organic materials.[159]

Zygomatic Fractures

Zygomatic Complex Fracture

The ZMC fracture (Figs. 11–35 through 11–38) is usually the result of a blow over the malar eminence. The principal lines of fracture involve the three distinct components of the zygomatic bone: the orbital process, the zygomatic arch, and the inferior orbital rim. The term *tripod fracture*[40, 51] has been used to refer to ZMC fractures because these three limbs supporting the body of the zygoma are broken. The ZMC fracture is also known as the *trimalar* and *malar eminence fracture*.[36, 38]

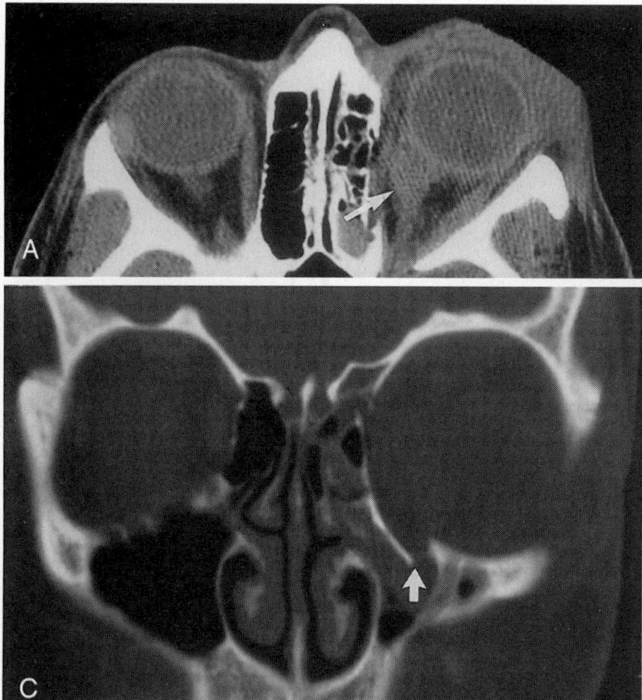

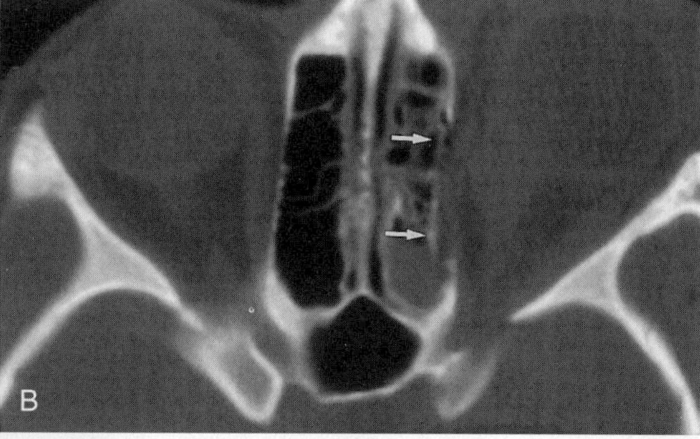

Figure 11–31. Perioptic hematoma. *A*, Multiple axial CT images show blood (*arrow*) adjacent to the optic nerve. The optic nerve is obscured by the hemorrhage. On this image the course of the optic nerve appears medially displaced relative to its expected course. These findings raise the question of optic nerve avulsion, a rare entity. *B*, Better shown on the bone window setting of *A* is a medial blow-out fracture (*arrows*). *C*, Coronal CT image shows an additional blow-out fracture of the orbital floor (*arrow*).

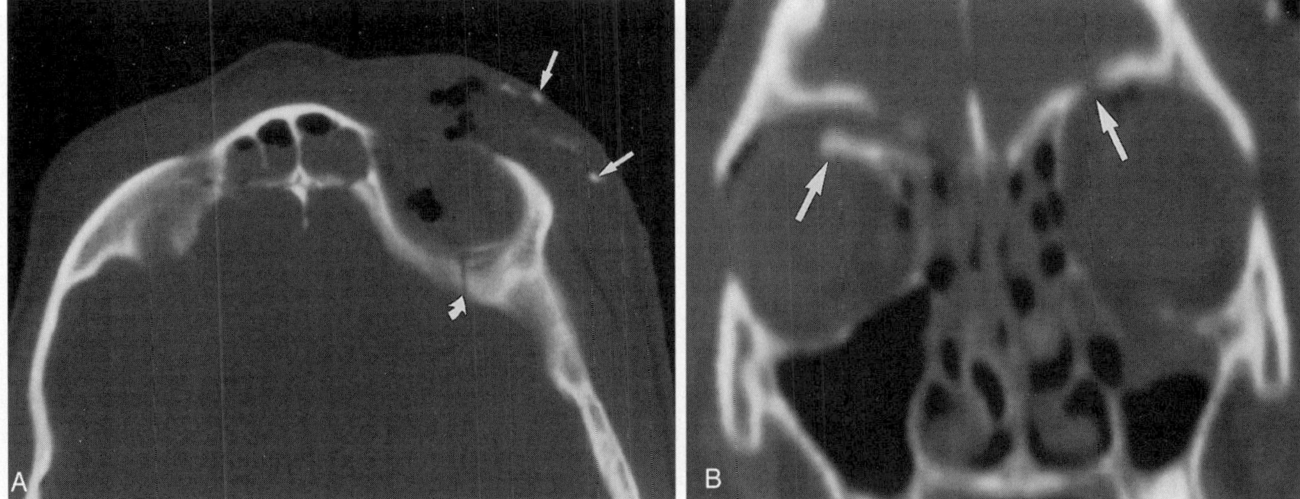

Figure 11–32. Glass foreign bodies. *A,* Glass foreign bodies (*straight arrows*) are seen in the soft tissues anterior to the left eye. Glass is usually well shown by computed tomography. The patient also had bilateral orbital roof fractures; only the left is shown in this image (*curved arrow*). *B,* The coronal reformatted CT image shows a nondisplaced fracture of the left orbital roof and a blow-in fracture of the right orbital roof (*arrows*).

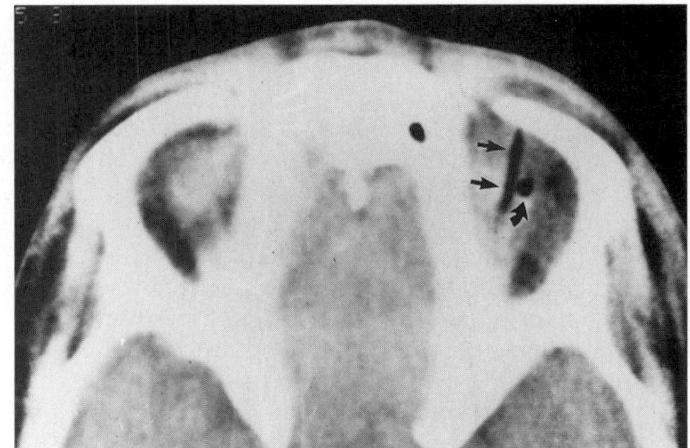

Figure 11–33. Wooden foreign body. There is a wooden splinter in the left orbit (*straight arrows*). The linear configuration of the splinter helps to differentiate it from orbital emphysema, which forms round bubbles, seen as rounded lucent areas (*curved arrow*) in this image. Use of a lung window setting may actually show striations in wood. (Reprinted with permission from Rhea, J.T., Rao, P.M., & Novelline RN. [1999] Helical CT and three-dimensional CT of facial and orbital injury. Radiol. Clin. North Am., *37*:489.)

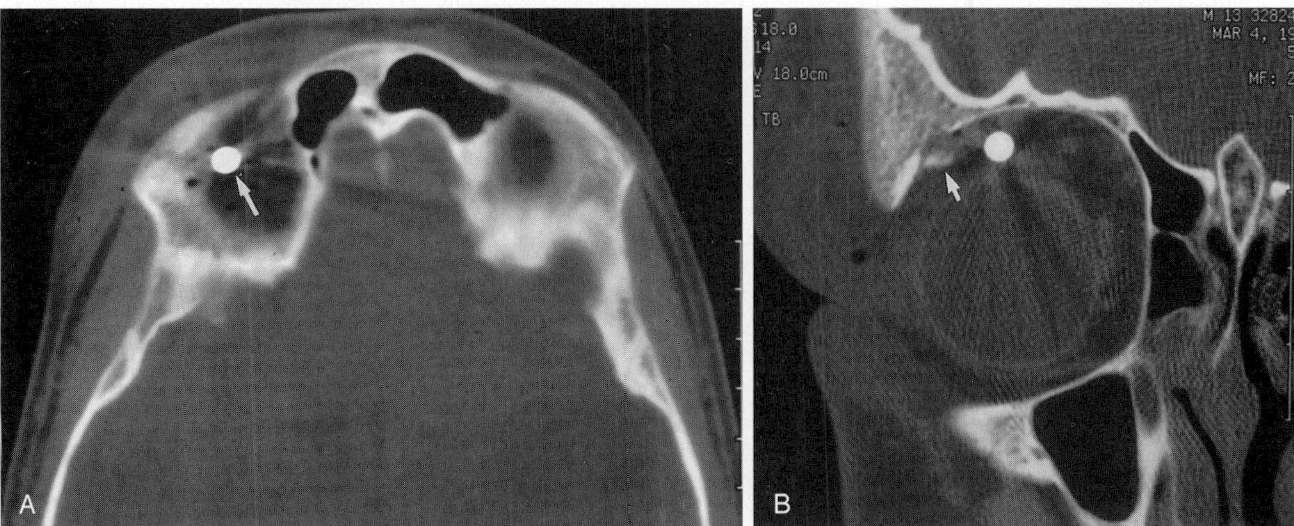

Figure 11–34. Metal foreign body. *A,* Metallic orbital foreign bodies are characteristically dense on computed tomographic images. When such a foreign body (*arrow*) is present, its location should be specified relative to the orbital contents, and the eyeball should be carefully examined for signs of rupture. Both coronal and axial images are necessary for exact localization. *B,* On the coronal CT image there is an isolated fracture of the superior orbital rim (*arrow*) lateral to the foreign body.

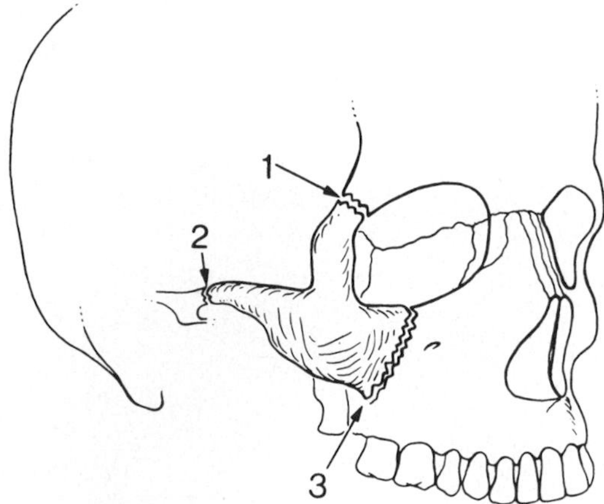

Figure 11–35. Zygomatic complex fracture: Drawing. This fracture usually consists of separation of the zygomaticofrontal suture (1), fracture of the zygomatic arch (2), and fracture of the zygomaticomaxillary suture, which includes a fracture of the inferior orbital rim extending through the anterior and posterolateral walls of the maxillary sinus (3). The location of the actual fracture lines may vary; for example, instead of separation of the zygomaticofrontal suture, there may be fracture of the frontal process of the zygoma. The term "tripod fracture" has been used to describe this fracture because there is disruption of the three major supports of the body of the zygoma: the rim inferiorly, the rim laterally, and the arch.

Components of ZMC fractures include separation of the zygomaticofrontal suture, fracture of the inferior orbital rim medially in the area of the zygomaticomaxillary suture, and a separate fracture of the zygomatic arch posteriorly or in the area of the zygomaticotemporal suture. The orbital portion of the zygoma is frequently separated along its sutures with the sphenoid and maxillary bones. The line of fracture runs inferiorly and laterally across the anterior and lateral walls of the maxillary sinus. Thus, the principal fragment is the zygoma, which has become separated from its three areas of attachment.

Over 75% of ZMC fractures require surgical reduction.[222] Successful treatment may require stabilization of the zygomaticosphenoid fracture line in addition to the frontal process, orbital rim, and zygomatic arch.[148] Zygomatic fractures most often are reduced and fixed in place with miniplates and screws; less frequently, wiring is used.[191, 209] Restoration of function and appearance is more successful if repair is performed within 3 weeks of injury rather than later.[151]

CT well depicts ZMC fractures in the axial plane and constitutes the "gold standard" imaging method for diagnosis and surgical planning[222] (see Figs. 11–36 and 11–38). Posterior displacement and rotation of the body of the zygoma and fractures of the zygomatic arch are readily appreciated. Coronal scans best show associated fractures of the orbital floor. The zygomatic arch component of a ZMC fracture may consist of only a bending of the arch without a distinct break in the cortex and is readily shown by CT. The coronal scan may also show diastasis of the zygomaticofrontal suture.

The position of fractures of the lateral orbit accompanying ZMC fractures may vary. In some cases, the frontal process of the zygoma is involved in association with fractures of the lateral orbital wall instead of a diastasis of the zygomaticofrontal suture. In other cases, fractures of the orbit may extend posteriorly to involve the orbital apex and optic canals. Both the frontal process of the zygoma and the lateral orbital wall may move medially, constituting a blow-in fracture of the orbit.[220, 231]

In depressed zygomatic fractures, bone may impinge on the coronoid process and restrict motion of the mandible. Less commonly, fractures of the base of the zygomatic arch may extend into the temporomandibular joint or be associated with tears of the joint capsule. Even intracranial impaction of the zygoma has been reported.[201]

Plain radiographic signs of this injury include soft tissue swelling over the malar eminence, opacification of the maxillary sinus, widening of the zygomaticofrontal suture, and disruption in the inferior orbital rim, usually in the medial half (see Fig. 11–37). These are best shown on the Waters view.[7, 57, 92] Closer inspection will then reveal the fracture of the thin portion of the lateral sinus wall above the alveolar process and the associated fracture of the zygomatic arch. The fracture of the lateral wall may be manifested only by angular distortion because of overlap of the zygomatic fragment without clear demonstration of a fracture line. With medial or lateral displacement of the frontal process of the zygoma and depression of the lateral margin of the inferior orbital rim, the fragment is usually rotated. The infraorbital foramen may not be visualized on the affected side because of rotational displacement of the zygoma.

The separation of the zygomaticofrontal suture in the lateral rim of the orbit is often best appreciated on the Caldwell view. Also on this projection, the inferior margin of the lateral wall of the maxillary sinus is projected beneath the petrous bone, and in some cases the fracture involving the lateral wall may be best shown in this view.

Posterior displacement[60] is quite common and is best visualized on the base view by comparing the positions of the anterior walls of the maxillary sinuses. This same view shows the fracture within the zygomatic arch. Posterior displacement of fractures of the zygomatic arch is well visualized by CT examination in the axial plane. In rare cases, a clinically obvious ZMC fracture may not be demonstrable on Waters' view, particularly when there is posterior displacement of the zygoma fragments without significant rotation. The fracture will be seen on the base view or on CT scans, however, manifested as the posterior displacement and the obvious asymmetry of the anterior maxillary sinus walls.

Isolated Fracture of the Zygomatic Arch

A direct blow by a small blunt object may result in a fracture limited to the zygomatic arch (Figs. 11–39 and 11–40). This injury commonly consists of three fractures through the arch: one at each extremity and a third fracture in the center with depression of the fracture fragments.

Zygomatic arch fractures are clearly shown by CT examination in the axial plane (see Fig. 11–39). If the displaced arch impinges on the coronoid process of the mandible, this abnormality is readily apparent on both the coronal and axial images. Impingement may result in limitation of mandibular motion. Mandibular motion may also be limited, because the masseter muscle arises from the zygomatic arch.

Text continued on page 353

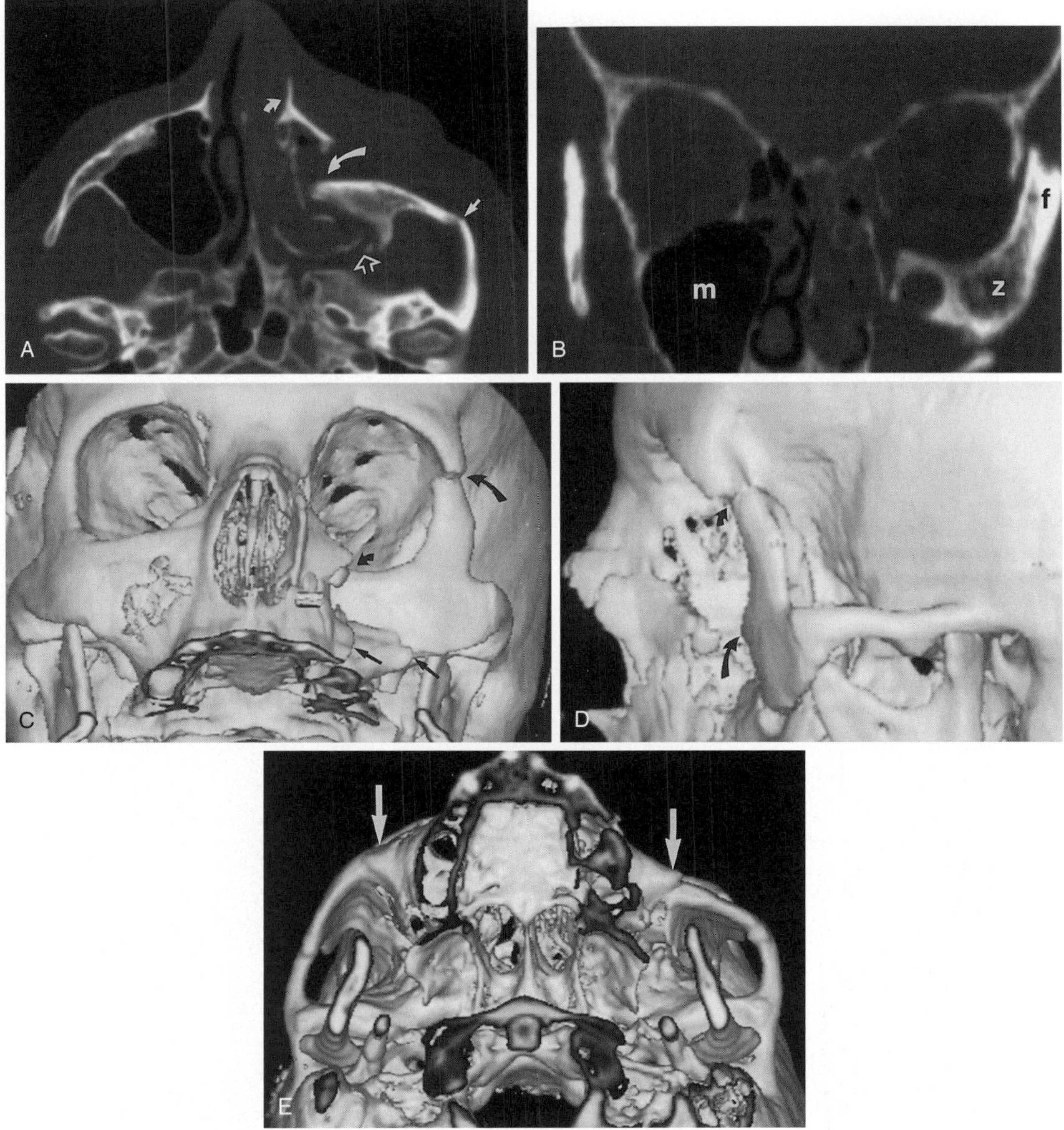

Figure 11–36. Zygomatic complex fracture: CT findings. *A,* Axial CT image obtained at the level of the body of the zygoma shows a fracture of the inferior orbital rim (*large curved arrow*) and zygomatic arch (*straight arrow*) with marked posterior displacement of the body of the zygoma on the left. As would be expected as part of a zygomatic complex fracture, there is fracture of the posterolateral wall of the maxillary sinus (*open arrow*); as an unexpected finding, there is also rotation of the frontal process of the maxilla (*small curved arrow*). *B,* Coronal CT image shows the displaced body (z) and frontal process (f) of the zygoma on the left. The body is displaced into the left maxillary sinus relative to the right (m). *C,* Waters' view from a three-dimensional reformatting shows the separation of the zygomaticofrontal suture (*large curved arrow*). The frontal process of the zygoma is medially displaced; the inferior rim is inferiorly displaced (*small curved arrow*). The displacement is consistent with counterclockwise rotation of the major fragment in the coronal plane. There are fractures of the anterior wall of the maxillary sinus (*straight arrows*). *D,* Left lateral view from a three-dimensional reformatting shows the extent of posterior displacement of the zygomatic body (*large arrow*) and lesser degree of posterior displacement of the frontal process of the zygoma (*small arrow*). *E,* Inferior view from a three-dimensional reformatting shows the extent of posterior displacement of the left body of the zygoma compared with the right (*arrows*). The configuration of the fractured left zygomatic arch is well visualized.

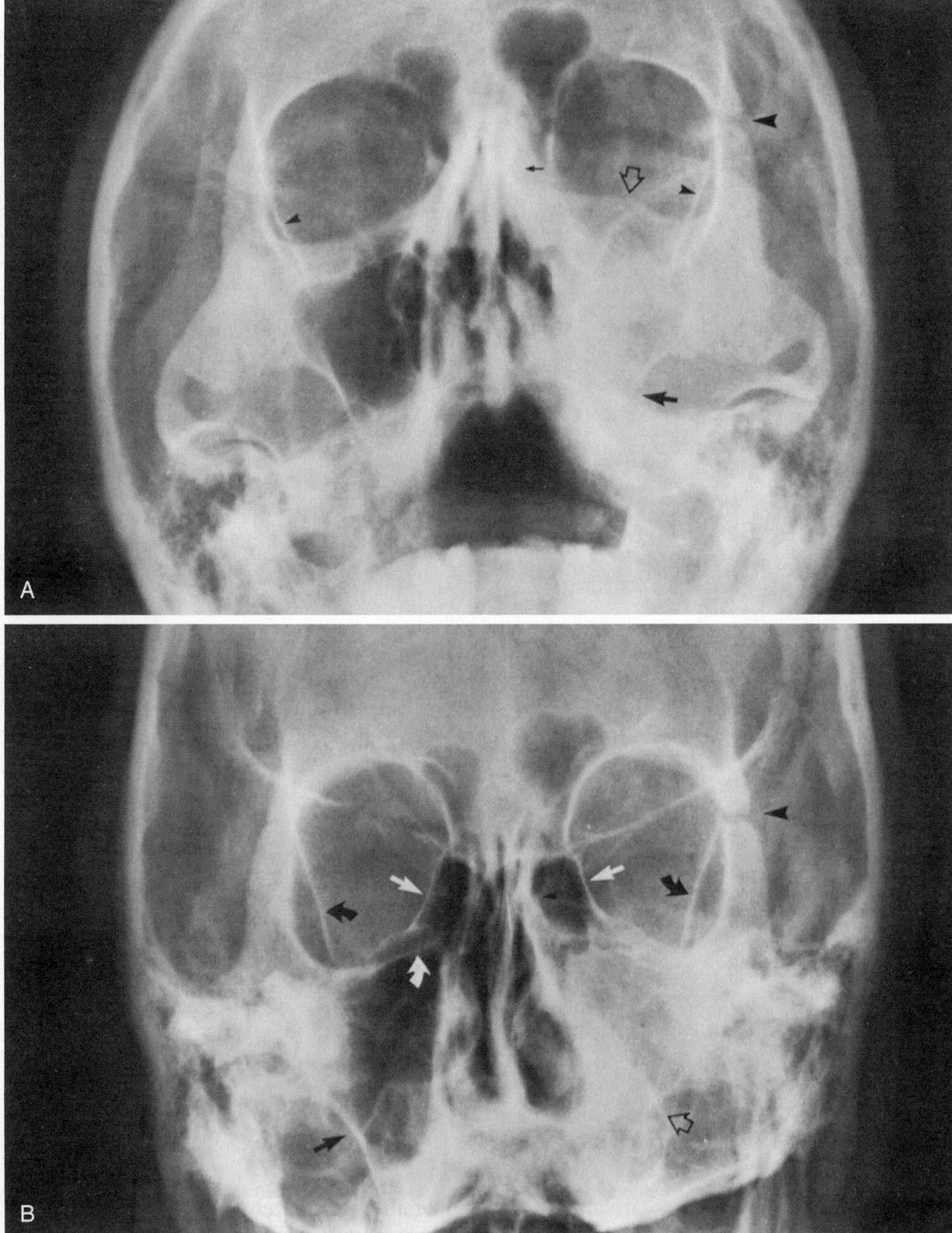

Figure 11–37. Zygomatic complex fracture: Plain films. *A,* Waters' view shows fracture of the lateral wall of the left maxillary sinus (*large arrow*) and the left inferior orbital rim (*open arrow*) and separation of the left zygomaticofrontal suture (*large arrowhead*). There is an associated fracture of the left nasal bone (*small arrow*). The left maxillary sinus is opacified. Note the soft tissue swelling over the left malar eminence. The innominate lines of the orbit are well visualized (*small arrowheads*). *B,* Caldwell's view shows the separation of the left zygomaticofrontal suture to better advantage (*large arrowhead*). The lateral walls of the maxillary sinuses are also visualized. Note the intact sinus on the right (*straight black arrow*) and the fracture of the inferior wall of the maxillary sinus on the left (*open arrow*). The nasal fracture is also shown (*small arrowhead*), as are the innominate lines of the orbit (*curved black arrow*), inferomedial portion of the orbital rim (*curved white arrow*), and lateral margin of the posterior ethmoids (*straight white arrows*).

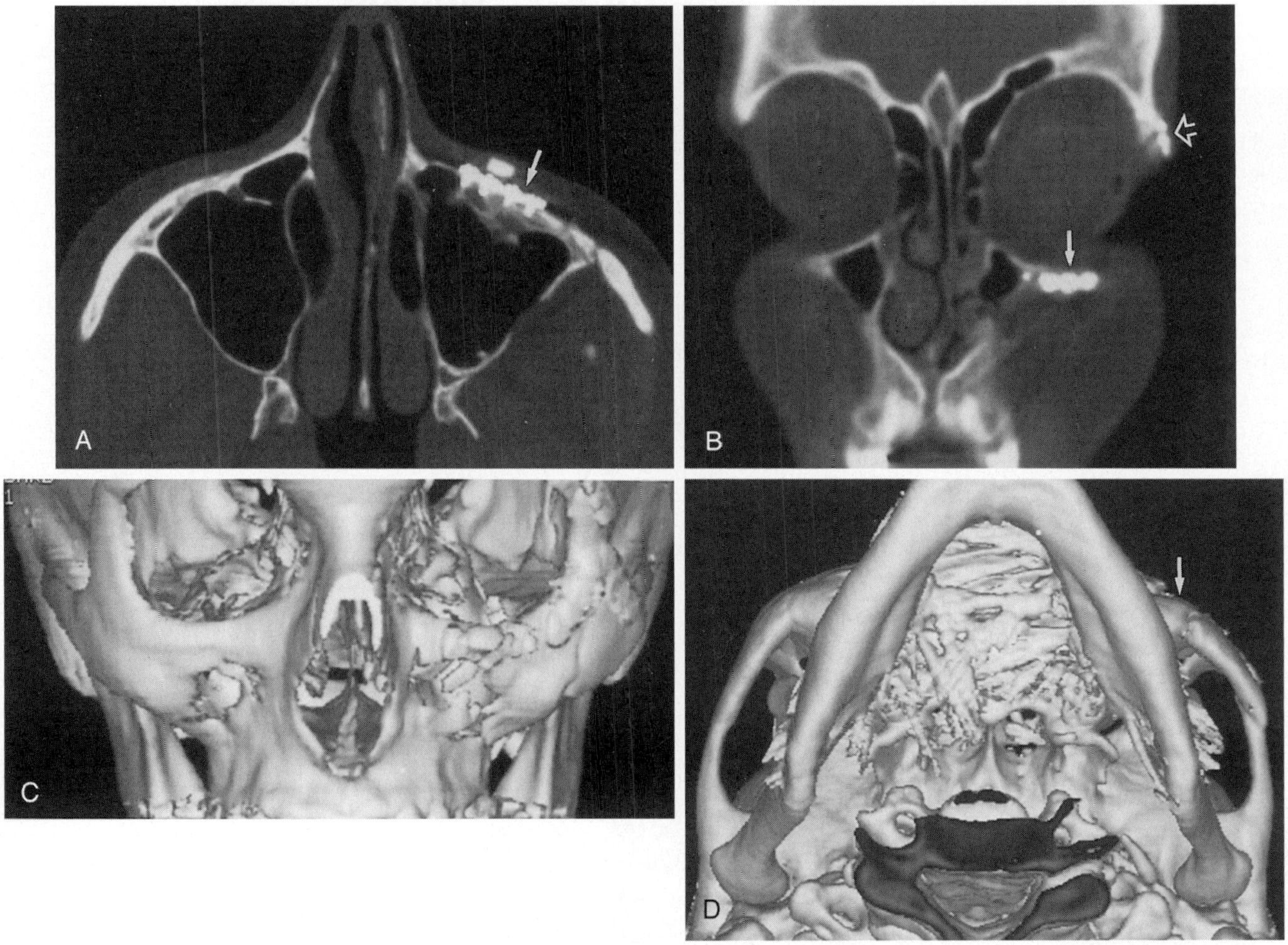

Figure 11–38. Postoperative examination following zygomatic complex repair. *A* and *B*, Axial and coronal CT views show miniplate and screws along the inferior orbital rim (*solid arrows* on *A* and *B*) and zygomaticofrontal suture (*open arrow* on *B*). *C*, Frontal view from a three-dimensional reformatting shows no rotation of the zygoma in the coronal plane. *D*, Inferior view from a three-dimensional reformatting shows minimal residual posterior displacement of the body of the zygoma (*arrow*) compared with the right side.

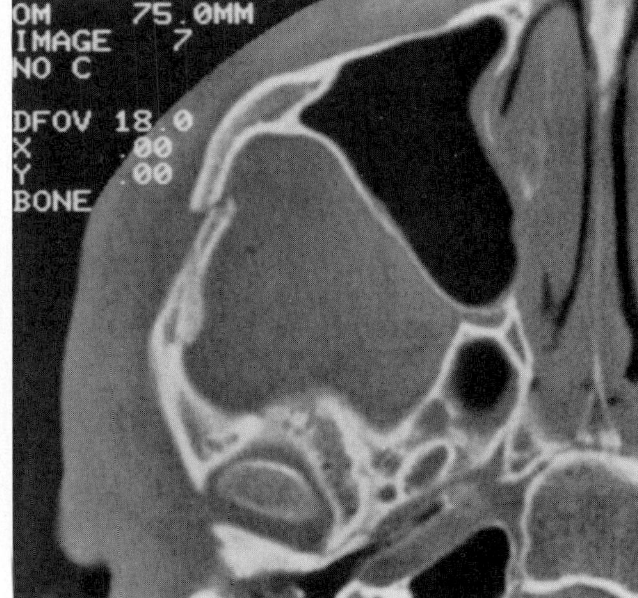

Figure 11–39. Isolated zygomatic arch fracture: CT findings. Axial CT shows comminuted fracture of the arch without other fractures. There is slight medial displacement of the central fragment.

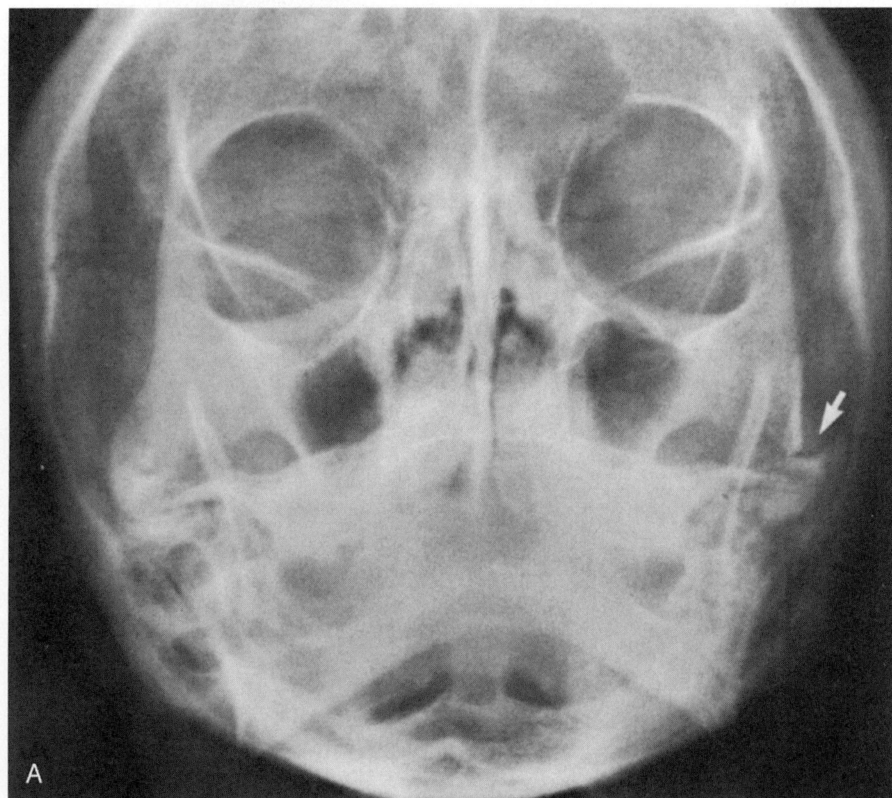

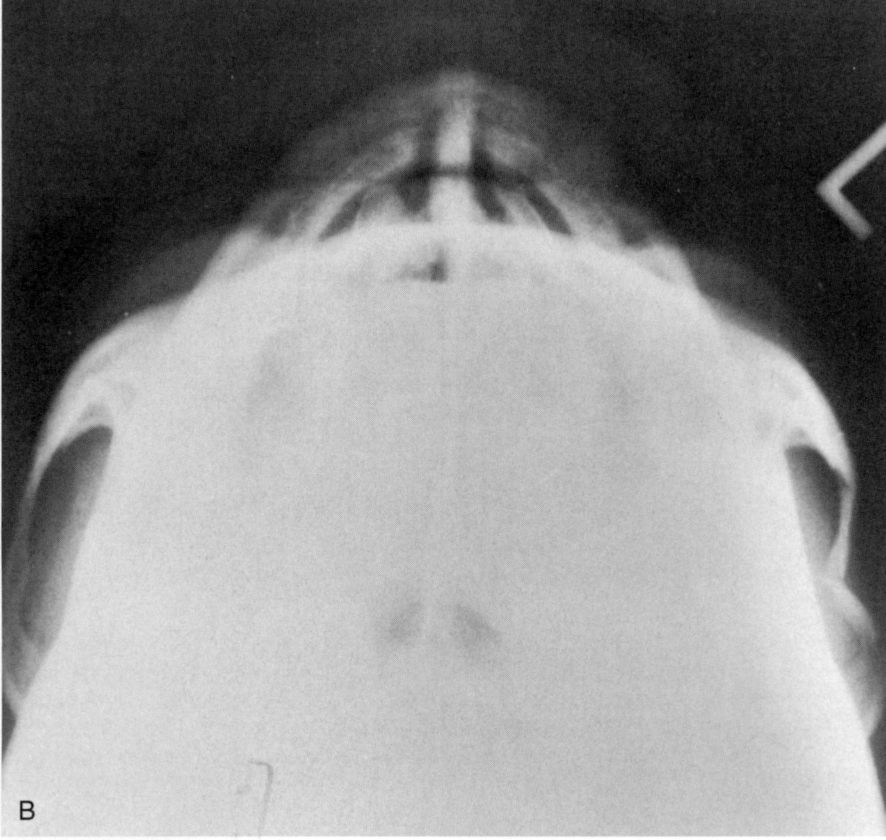

Figure 11–40. Isolated zygomatic arch fracture: Plain films. *A,* Waters' view demonstrates distortion of the "elephant's trunk" (*arrow*). The linear density just medial to the *arrow* is a sign of depression of a portion of the arch, which is viewed end on. *B,* Base view shows three fractures of the arch with depression of the central fracture.

With plain radiographs, the zygomatic arch fractures are best shown on the base view and may be overlooked on the Waters and Caldwell views (see Fig. 11–40). Angular distortion of the elephant's trunk[7] and asymmetry as visualized on Waters' view are clues to the presence of this injury. Yanagisawa and Greenspan[59] described another clue that was identified in 76% of isolated fractures of the zygomatic arch but in only 6% of ZMC fractures. Depression of the anterior fragment creates an oval or rectangular vertical area of increased density in the region of the lateral part of the zygomatic bone, as shown on either a Waters or Caldwell view. This finding is the result of displacement of the fragment, which is visualized end on, leading to an appearance of increased density.

Nasal Fractures

With plain films, the nasal bones are best seen on the lateral view[6, 7, 10] using a soft tissue technique (Figs. 11–41 and 11–42). This view shows both the nasal bones and the anterior nasal spine, an anterior projection of the maxilla at the base of the cartilaginous nasal septum. Most fractures are transverse and tend to depress the distal portion of the nasal bones, but longitudinal fractures do occur. The nasomaxillary suture is normally seen on the lateral view as extending the length of the nasal bone on its lateral border. Frequently seen on lateral plain films are fine, longitudinally oriented grooves within the nasal bone that contain branches of the nasociliary nerves. These grooves should not be mistaken for fractures. Both the sutures and the nasociliary grooves are less lucent than would be expected with a longitudinal fracture. A longitudinal fracture usually results in medial displacement of the nasal bones; this abnormality can be verified on Waters' projection. Fractures of the anterior nasal spine often result in considerable swelling of the upper lip and are associated with disruption of the cartilaginous portion of the anterior nasal septum.

An axial plain radiographic view of the nasal bones may be obtained by placing an occlusal film between the teeth and directing the central x-ray beam vertically across the forehead through the nose onto the occlusal radiograph. This examination is more easily accomplished when the nose is prominent, but even then the view obtained visualizes only the anterior portion of the nasal bones. In smaller noses and in children, it may be impossible to show more than the very anterior tip of the nasal bones by this method.

Although isolated fractures of the nasal bones may be seen on plain films,[31, 32, 44] the frontal process of the maxilla may not be well visualized, and depression of the frontal process can lead to facial deformity. Johnson and associates[174] reported that fracture of the frontal process of the maxilla was missed on plain films in more than 75% of the patients in one small series. All nasal structures are well visualized with CT (Fig. 11–43).

Naso-orbital-ethmoidal Fractures

Nasal fractures may be associated with more complex fractures[44] involving the ethmoid and frontal sinuses. NOE fractures are sustained with direct impact of high-velocity forces on the upper nose, resulting in fractures of the medial orbit, nose, and ethmoid sinuses[18, 75, 110, 112] (Figs. 11–44 through 11–47). These fractures involve the interorbital space, which is limited superiorly by the cribriform plate and roof of the ethmoid sinuses and laterally by the medial orbital walls, inferiorly by the lower border of the ethmoid sinuses, and anteriorly by the nasal bones and frontal process of maxilla. Most bones in this region are thin, have a low tolerance to impact, and are readily fractured and displaced. The medial canthal ligament attaches to the frontal process of the maxilla.[170] Posterior and lateral displacement creates an increased distance

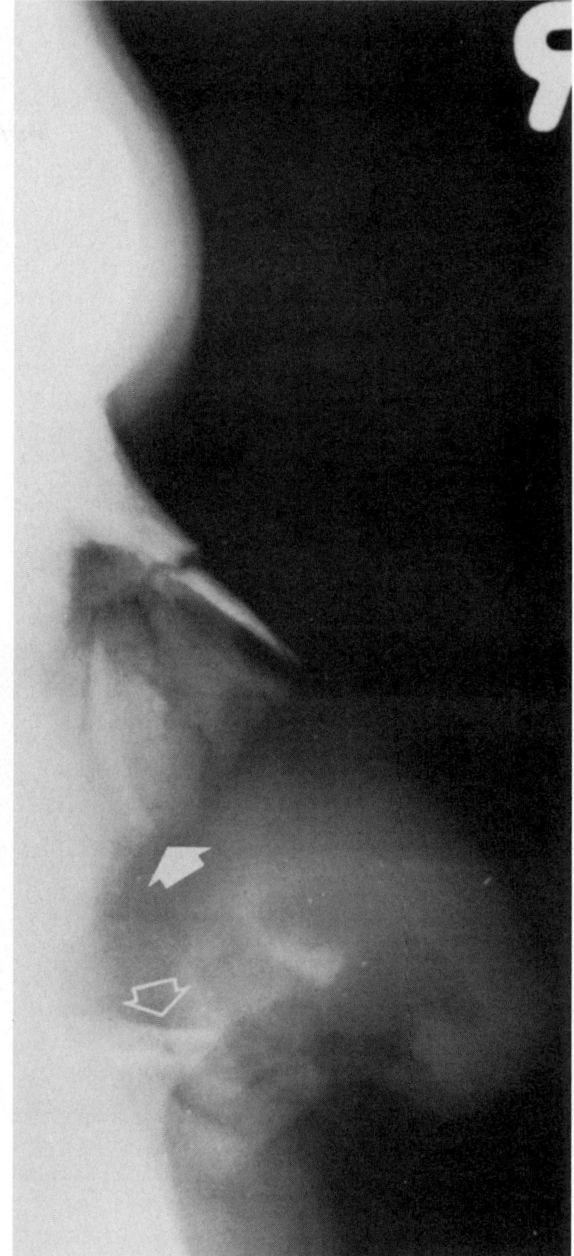

Figure 11–41. Nasal and anterior nasal spine fractures. There is a depressed fracture of the nasal bones anteriorly and a fracture of the frontal process of the maxilla (*solid arrow*) evidenced by a band of increased density representing overlap of the fracture fragments. Note also a fracture of the anterior nasal spine of the maxilla (*open arrow*). (Case courtesy of Michael Siegel, MD, Brooklyn, N.Y.)

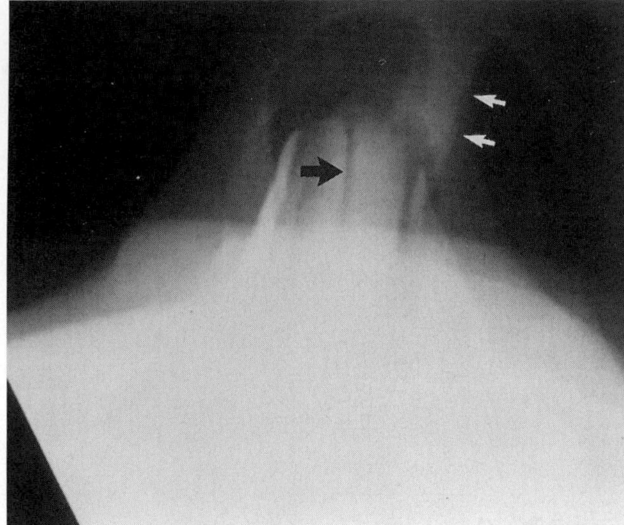

Figure 11–42. Dislocation of the nasal cartilage. This occlusal view was obtained by placing a film between the patient's teeth and directing the central ray in the cephalocaudal direction from above. The displacement of the nasal cartilage (*white arrows*) to the left is evident on comparison with the other midline structures such as the intranasal suture (*black arrow*).

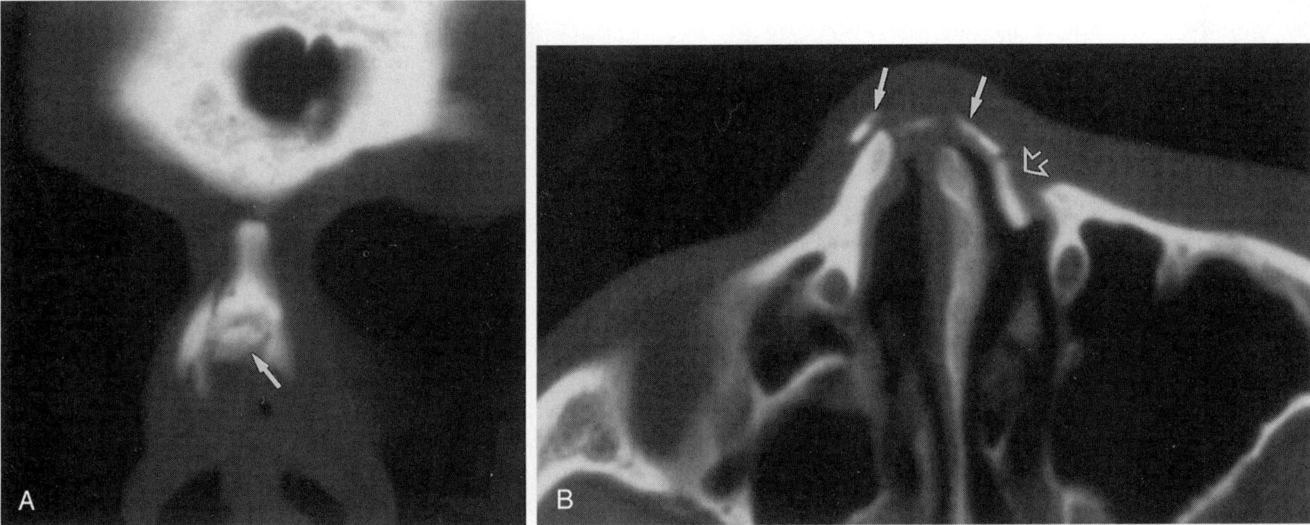

Figure 11–43. Nasal fracture. *A*, Coronal CT image shows a comminuted fracture of the nasal bones with slight displacement to the right (*arrow*). *B*, Axial CT image shows posterior displacement of the nasal bones (*solid arrows*) and fracture with displacement to the right of the left frontal process of the maxilla (*open arrow*).

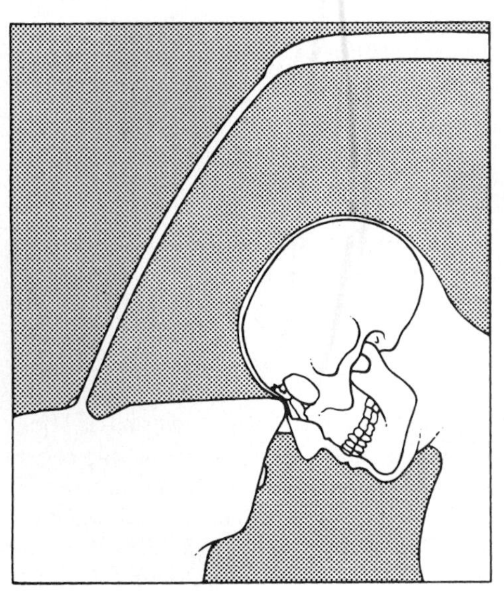

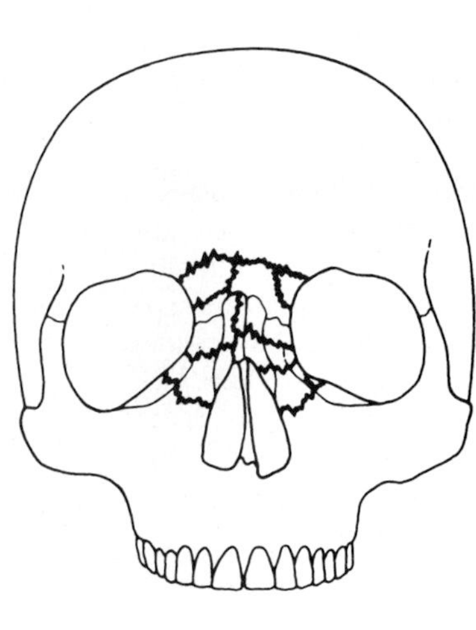

Figure 11–44. Naso-orbital-ethmoidal fractures. A sharp blow to the nasion (*left*) can result in a comminuted fracture involving the medial walls of both orbits, the nasal bones, and the frontal processes of the maxillae (*right*). Naso-orbital-ethmoidal fractures may extend into the floor of the orbit, the inferior orbital rim, the frontal sinuses, and the orbital apex.

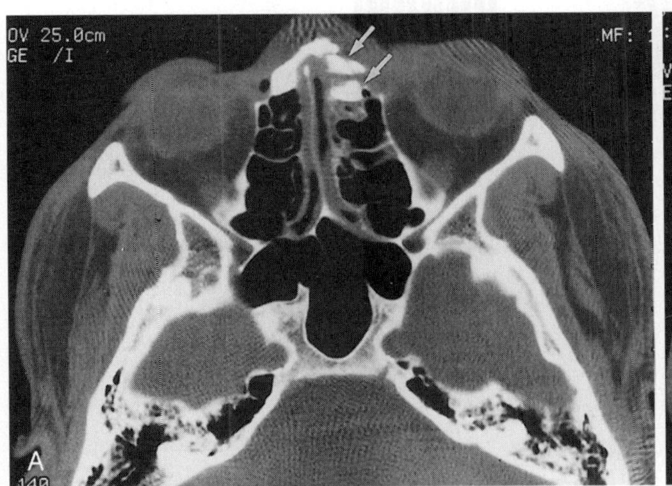

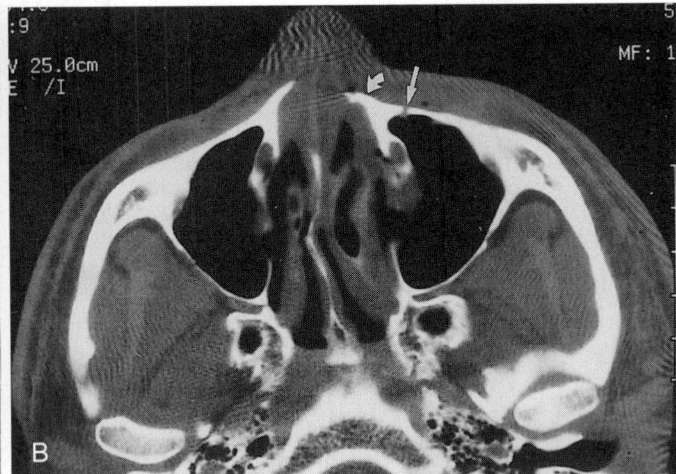

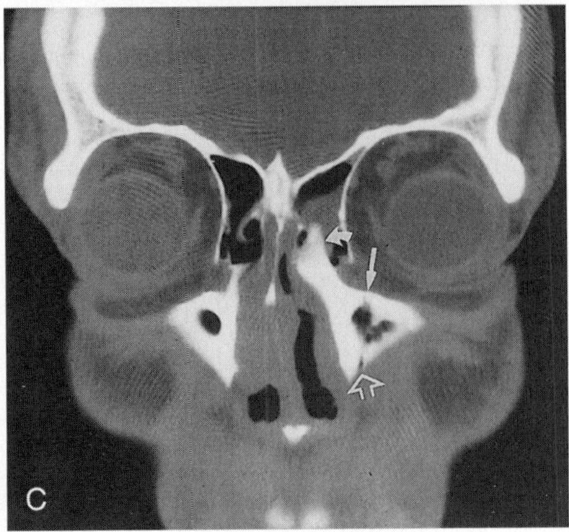

Figure 11–45. Unilateral naso-orbital-ethmoidal fracture: CT findings. *A,* Axial CT image shows fractures of the left nasal bone and the left frontal process of the maxilla, with posterior displacement of fragments into the left ethmoid sinus (*arrows*). *B,* Lower axial CT image reveals medial rotation of the left frontal process of the maxilla (*curved arrow*). There is also a fracture of the anterior wall of the left maxillary sinus (*straight arrow*). *C,* Coronal CT image shows medial rotation of the left frontal process of the maxilla (*curved arrow*), fracture through the left inferior orbital rim (*straight solid arrow*), and fracture of the anterior wall of the left maxillary sinus (*open arrow*).

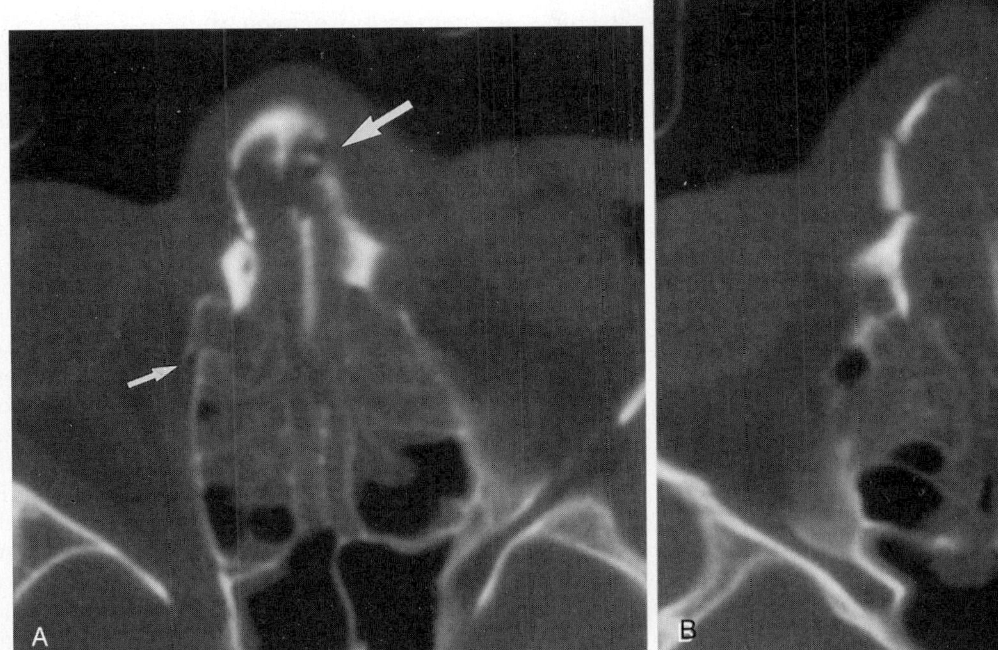

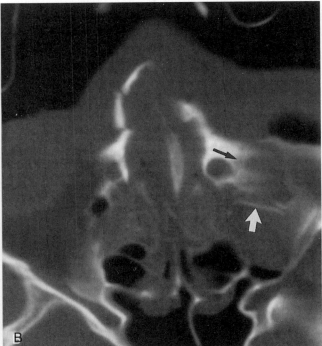

Figure 11–46. Bilateral naso-orbital-ethmoidal fractures: CT findings. *A,* These are fractures of both nasal bones and both frontal processes of maxillae, which are displaced posteriorly and to the right (*large arrow*). These are fractures of both medial orbital walls; the *small arrow* points to the fracture on the right. *B,* Slightly lower image again shows multiple fractures involving the nasal bones, the frontal processes of the maxillae, and the lacrimal bones. *Black arrow* indicates fracture running into the nasolacrimal duct. *White arrow* indicates an additional left orbital floor fracture.

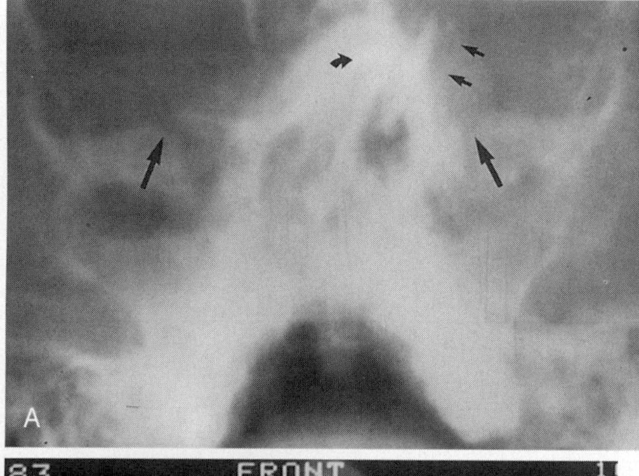

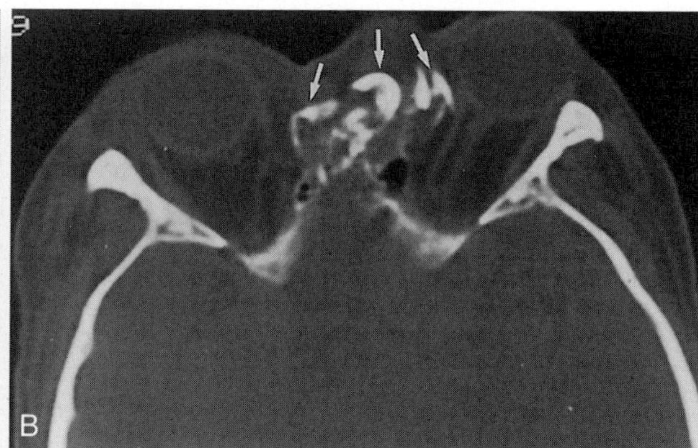

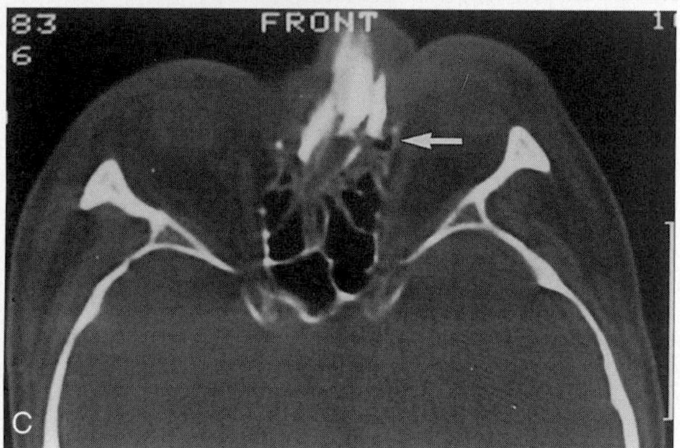

Figure 11–47. Bilateral naso-orbital-ethmoidal fractures: Plain film and CT findings. *A,* Waters' plain film shows deviation of the nasal structures to the left (*curved arrow*). A faint line that may represent the medial wall of the left orbit (*small arrows*) appears somewhat laterally displaced. There are also fractures of both inferior orbital rims (*large arrows*). *B* and *C,* Computed tomographic images. *B,* Axial CT image shows both posterior and leftward displacement of fracture fragments (*arrows*). *C,* Axial CT image shows the lateral displacement of the medial wall of the orbit (*arrow*) on the left.

between the medial canthi, resulting in telecanthus. The medial wall of the orbit is composed anteriorly of the lacrimal bone and posteriorly of the orbital plate of the ethmoid. These structures are extremely thin and fragile, and fractures involving them are invariably comminuted. Fractures of the medial orbital wall may be associated with direct ocular injury. Fractures extending into the cribriform plate may result in cerebrospinal fluid rhinorrhea. When the thin perpendicular plate of the ethmoid, the upper component of the nasal septum, and the ethmoid air cells are involved in NOE fractures, the bone fragments are readily comminuted and displaced posteriorly. The nasolacrimal duct drains the lacrimal sac, located in the lacrimal fossa just posterior to the medial canthal ligament. The duct courses through the lacrimal bone to drain into the nasal fossa beneath the inferior turbinate. The nasolacrimal sac or duct may be injured in NOE fractures and in about 20% of midfacial fractures.[202]

NOE injury is rarely isolated and is typically the result of a high-velocity vehicular collision. One third of patients with NOE fractures have associated injuries of the thorax or abdomen, and 50% have intracranial injuries.[18] Seventy percent of patients with NOE fractures have associated complex maxillary fractures. Fractures of the inferior orbital rim or floor occur in nearly 100%, and 30% have ocular injury, either eyeball perforation or optic nerve injury. Optic nerve injury usually occurs with associated fractures that extend posteriorly.[170] In half of NOE injuries, open fracture is present, and hemorrhagic complications may occur.[9]

The patterns of NOE injuries are often complex, and several classifications have been proposed.[111, 113] Simple classifications divide the fractures into unilateral and bilateral (see Figs. 11–45 and 11–46) and into those isolated to the medial orbital rim or extended to other portions of the orbit and maxilla. Approximately one third of the fractures are unilateral. Common patterns of extension include the frontal bone, supraorbital rim, lower orbit, and zygoma. NOE fractures may occur as a component of LeFort fractures of the midface or complex smash fractures involving the entire facial skeleton. Gruss[111] proposed a classification of five types. In type 1, there is a fracture of the nasal bones, and a portion of the medial orbital wall is telescoped backward into the interorbital space. The bone fragments may be impacted and displaced laterally, resulting in traumatic telecanthus. In type 2, in addition to fractures of the NOE region, there is extensive comminution of the perpendicular plate of the ethmoid and central maxilla, with crushing of the cartilaginous and bony nasal support, resulting in a prolapse of the distal nose—a finding pathognomonic of this type of injury. Injuries may extend laterally to involve one or both maxillae. In type 3, the injuries either extend superiorly to involve the base of the skull or are associated with LeFort II or LeFort III fractures. Type 4 fractures are associated with an inferior displacement of a portion of the orbit. Type 5 fractures are severe injuries with bone destruction and a loss of some portion of bone through skin or mucosal lacerations.

CT is the best method for depicting NOE fractures[155] (see Figs. 11–45 and 11–46). Both axial and coronal images are necessary to fully define the fracture extent. The axial image is particularly valuable in showing the degree of posterior displacement and any associated intraorbital injury. Fractures of the cribriform plate, base of the skull, medial orbital wall, and nasal septum are well visualized in the coronal plane. Three-dimensional CT with reformatting may be of use in surgical planning and to establish a preoperative baseline. If radiographs are obtained, the Waters and Caldwell views show fractures in the NOE region, and posterior displacement may be suggested on lateral or base views of the skull (see Fig. 11–47).

Fractures of the Frontal Sinus

Fracture of the frontal sinus may be linear and nondisplaced or comminuted and depressed[27, 61, 67, 149] (Figs. 11–48 through 11–51). It is necessary to determine whether the posterior wall is involved,[105, 106] because such involvement indicates the presence of an open injury that may result in meningitis, cerebrospinal fluid rhinorrhea, or pneumocephalus. It is vital that open injuries be disclosed. Therefore, when a fracture of the frontal sinuses is encountered, CT should be performed in both the coronal and axial projections to confirm the presence or absence of a fracture of the posterior wall of the sinus[107] (see Figs. 11–48 and 11–49). The posterior wall of the frontal sinus is best evaluated in the axial projection, whereas associated intracranial injury and pneumocephalus are best shown in the coronal projection.

On plain radiographs, frontal fractures are almost always associated with sinus opacification. The opacification may be total, or there may be an air-fluid level or mucosal thickening secondary to hemorrhage within the mucosal lining. Frontal fractures are best visualized on the Caldwell and lateral views. They may be limited to the anterior wall or involve both the anterior and posterior walls simultaneously[104, 108, 109] (see Figs. 11–50 and 11–51).

A blow by a relatively sharp object may result in a comminuted fracture limited to the anterior wall. Extensive comminuted fractures in the NOE region commonly extend into the base of the frontal sinuses and typically involve the nasolacrimal duct. Fractures of the medial and superior aspects of the orbital rim frequently involve

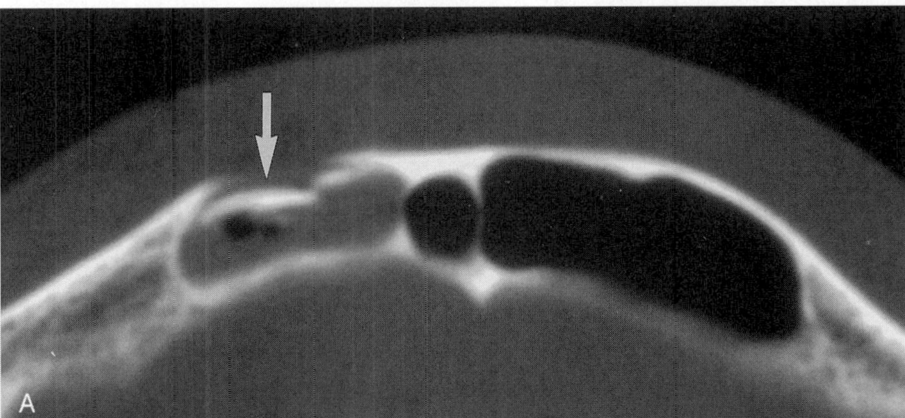

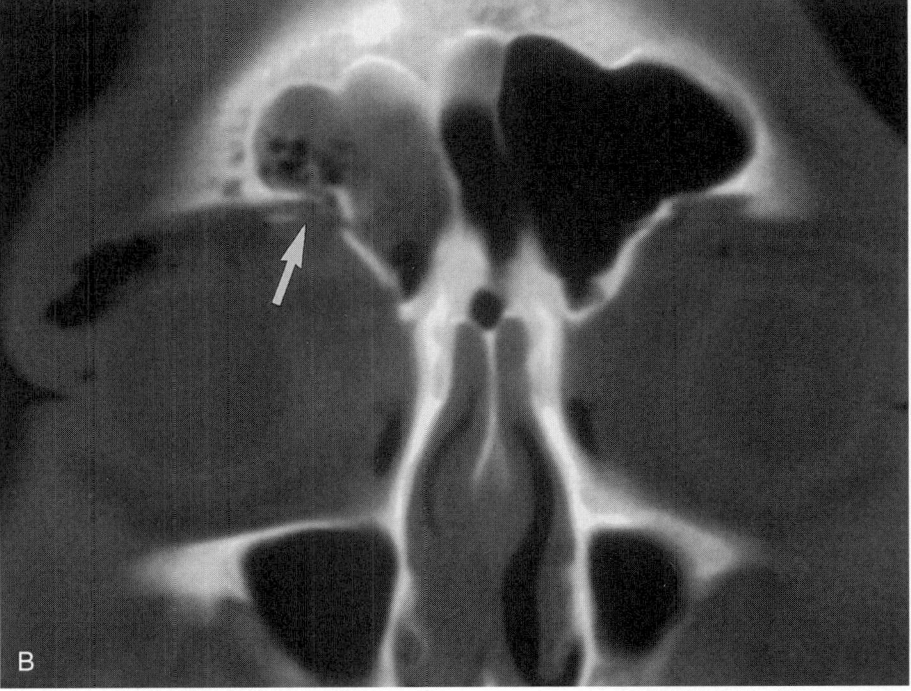

Figure 11–48. Fracture of the anterior wall of frontal sinus: CT findings. *A,* Axial CT image shows fracture of the anterior wall of the right frontal sinus (*arrow*). *B,* Coronal CT image shows that the orbital roof or floor of the frontal sinus is involved (*arrow*).

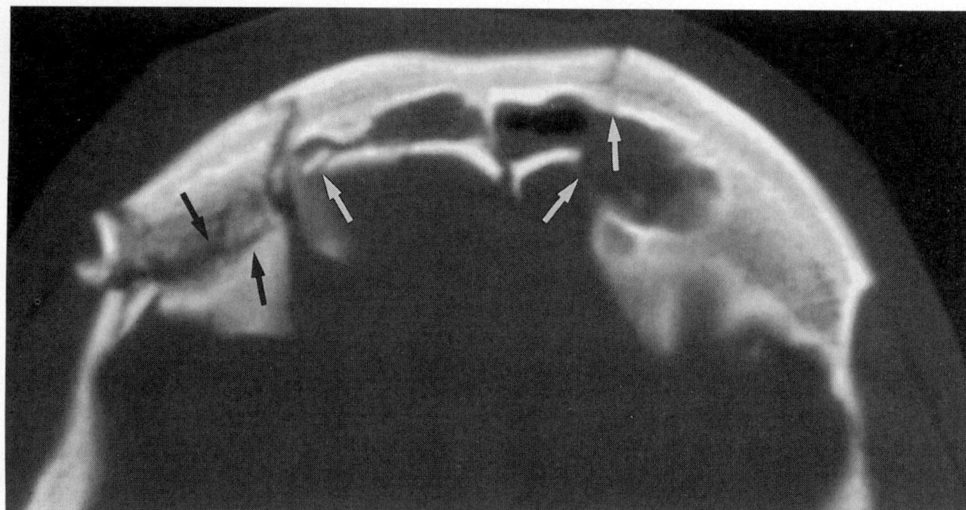

Figure 11–49. Fracture of the anterior and posterior walls of the frontal sinuses: CT findings. Both the anterior and posterior walls of the frontal sinus have been fractured (*white arrows*); therefore, this injury constitutes an open fracture. The fracture extends into the right orbital roof (*black arrows*).

a portion of the frontal sinuses. Such fractures represent another form of open injury, because the intraorbital contents then freely communicate with the exterior through the sinus and nasal cavity.

Maxillary Fractures

Isolated Alveolar Process Fracture

Isolated fracture of the alveolar process[29] is evidenced clinically by malalignment and displacement of the teeth contained within the fractured segment (Fig. 11–52), or teeth may be broken or absent.[184] The fracture may involve any portion of the alveolar process. With these fractures, findings on CT examination may be subtle, and both axial and coronal images should be perused closely so that the fracture is not overlooked.

On Waters' view, the teeth form a smooth arch. Any disruption in this arch or displacement of the teeth is suggestive of a fracture of the alveolar process and warrants further evaluation. There may be associated opacification of the maxillary sinus if the fracture extends into

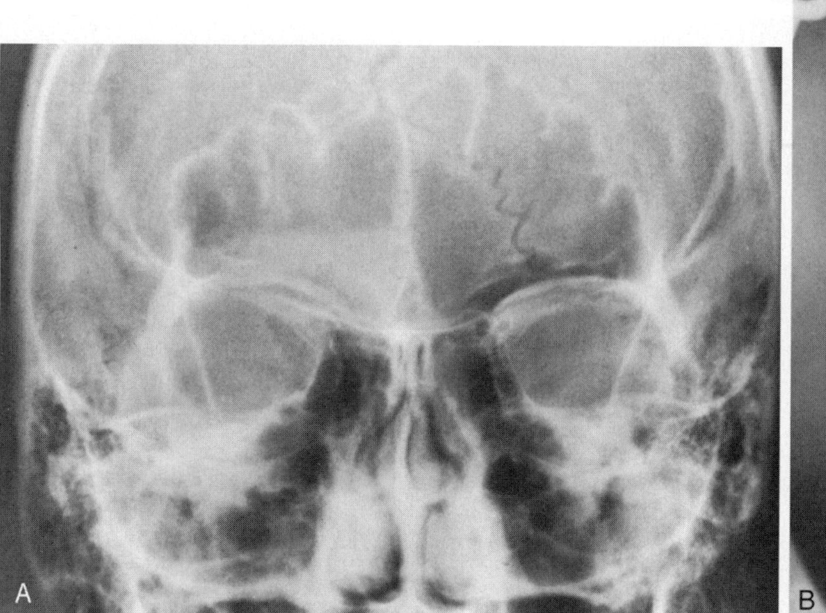

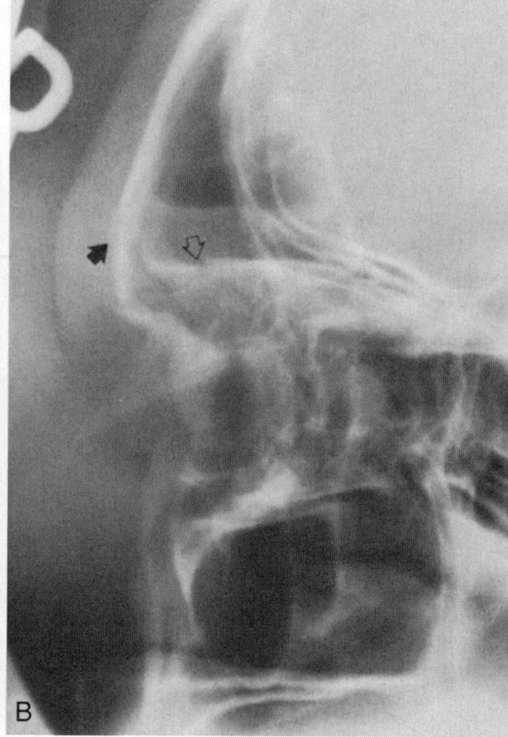

Figure 11–50. Fracture of the anterior wall of the frontal sinus: Plain films. *A,* Upright Caldwell's view shows an air-fluid level within the right frontal sinus. *B,* Upright lateral view shows a fracture of the anterior wall (*black arrow*) and floor (*open arrow*) of the frontal sinus. An air-fluid level is present within the sinus. The posterior wall is intact.

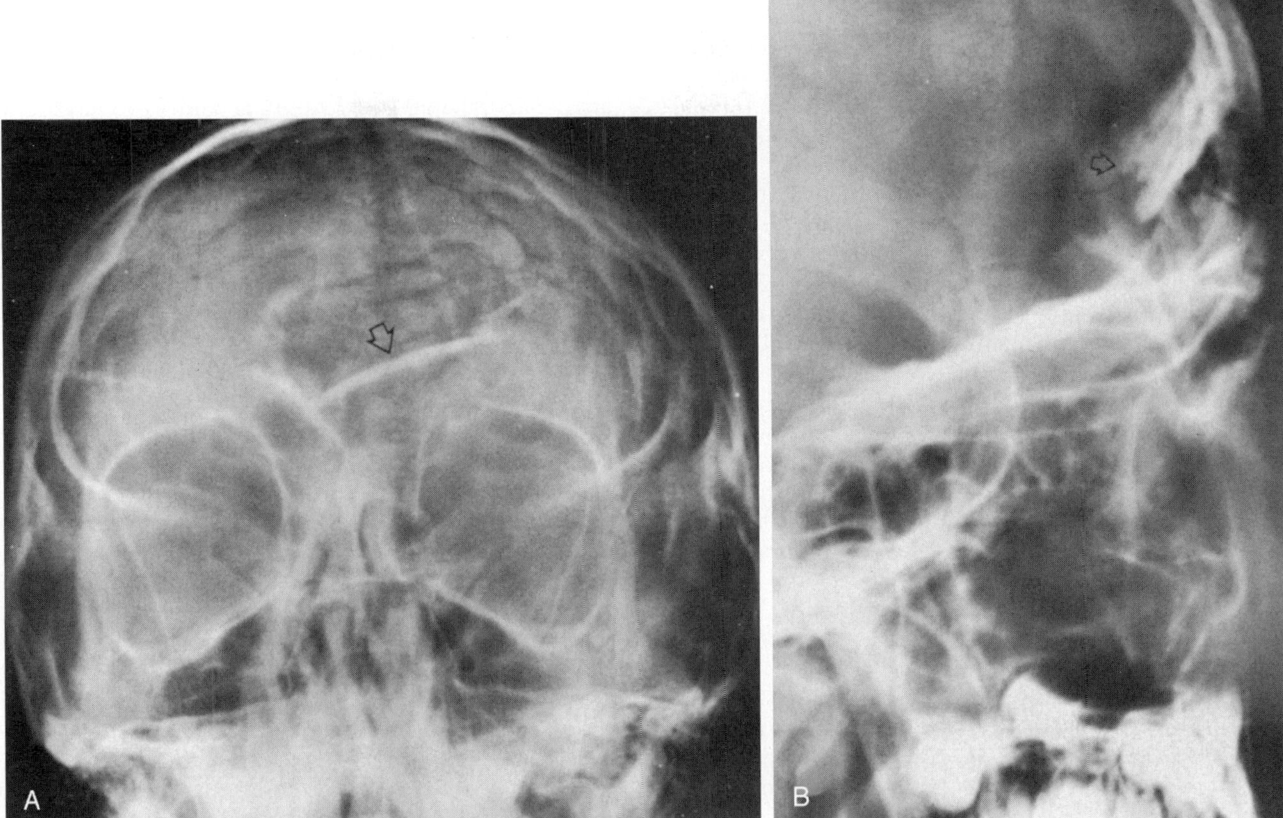

Figure 11–51. Fracture of the anterior and posterior walls of the frontal sinuses: Plain films. *A,* Caldwell's view shows opacification of the frontal and ethmoid sinuses. A large fragment of bone is seen end on within the frontal sinus (*arrow*). *B,* Lateral projection shows depression of the fracture fragments (*arrow*). The posterior wall fracture can be diagnosed only on the lateral view.

it. An occlusal x-ray film of the teeth or a panoramic view should be obtained to allow precise definition of the fracture fragments and associated dental injuries.

When there has been a fracture of the teeth or alveolar process, it is important to examine the chest radiograph closely to exclude the presence of aspirated teeth, which may lead to subsequent atelectasis and pneumonia. Fractures involving the posterior part of the maxilla and pterygoid processes may result in airway compromise secondary to hemorrhage and edema.[229]

LeFort Fractures

René LeFort, a French physician, studied facial fractures in cadavers. His work was published in 1901.[43, 55] By

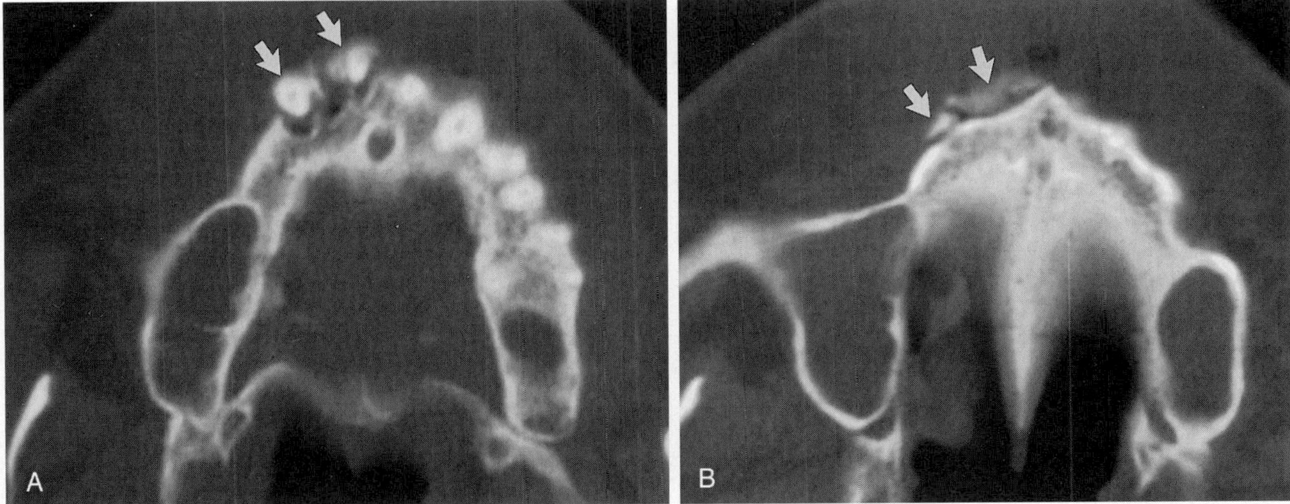

Figure 11–52. Maxillary alveolar fracture: CT findings. *A,* Axial CT image shows displacement of two anterior teeth (*arrows*). *B,* Lower axial image shows fracture fragments (*arrows*) from the alveolar process. Alveolar process fractures were evident clinically because of mobility of the teeth.

varying the strength and direction of blows to various portions of the face, LeFort found that he could create more or less reproducible types of fracture of the facial skeleton. He outlined three principal lines of fracture reflecting relative areas of weakness within the facial skeletal structure. These three lines form the basis of what has become known as LeFort's classification of facial fractures, although he himself did not propose the classification (Figs. 11–53 through 11–58).

The LeFort fractures are easily remembered by thinking of the findings on physical examination. In a *LeFort I fracture* the hard palate is freely movable relative to the remainder of the face. Fracture lines must be seen that free the hard palate and alveolar process of the maxilla (see Fig. 11–54). In a *LeFort II fracture* the maxilla and nose together are movable relative to the remainder of the face. The fracture line follows the border between the nose and maxilla and the remainder of the face (see Fig. 11–55). In a *LeFort III fracture* the maxilla, nose, and zygoma bones are movable relative to the brain case. All of the areas connecting the facial bones to the remainder of the calvaria are fractured (see Fig. 11–56). Mobility may not be present in a LeFort-type fracture if the fracture is incomplete.[210, 225]

By definition, all lines of a LeFort fracture must extend through the posterior face to transect the pterygoid processes. In each type there is partial or complete separation of the maxilla from the remainder of the facial skeleton or calvaria. It is relatively infrequent that these forces are distributed solely along the lines described by LeFort. Combinations of injury[13, 19, 23] are more common than the specific types he originally described. In fact, LeFort stated that comminution and other associated fractures[43, 55] were commonly encountered (see Fig. 11–56). Nevertheless, the forces are more or less focused along these lines of fracture, allowing for easier and more precise identification of the true extent of the injury.

Although LeFort I fractures are frequently encountered in their pure form, pure LeFort II and LeFort III fractures are infrequent. In general, the lines of fracture tend to respect the lines of weakness described. Thus, various combinations of LeFort II and LeFort III fractures are encountered—that is, a LeFort II fracture may be present on one side and a LeFort III on the other. These findings are further complicated by the presence of comminution of the zygoma and maxillary bones and sagittally oriented fractures of the hard palate. LeFort I fractures are occasionally accompanied by unilateral ZMC fractures.

LeFort I Fracture

A LeFort I fracture is a transverse fracture at the base of the maxillary sinuses that separates the alveolar process of the maxilla from the maxillary sinuses and nasal fossa. LeFort noted that such a transverse fracture had been described earlier by Guerin. It is the result of a blow directly under the nose against the alveolar process from either the front or the side.

At CT examination the transverse component of a LeFort I fracture is best visualized on coronal images (see Fig. 11–54). Transverse fractures involve the nasal septum and medial and lateral walls of the maxillary sinus. Coronal images will also show fractures of the pterygoid processes. The axial images will show any associated sagittal fracture of the hard palate.

On plain radiographs, fractures of the anterior maxillary wall, the posterior maxillary wall, and the pterygoid process are seen on the lateral view (see Fig. 11–57). Posterior displacement is frequent, as can be determined on the lateral view by noting the abnormal relationship of the anterior portion of the hard palate to the frontal sinus and the posterior portion to the sphenoid wing. On occasion there may be an associated sagittally oriented

Text continued on page 365

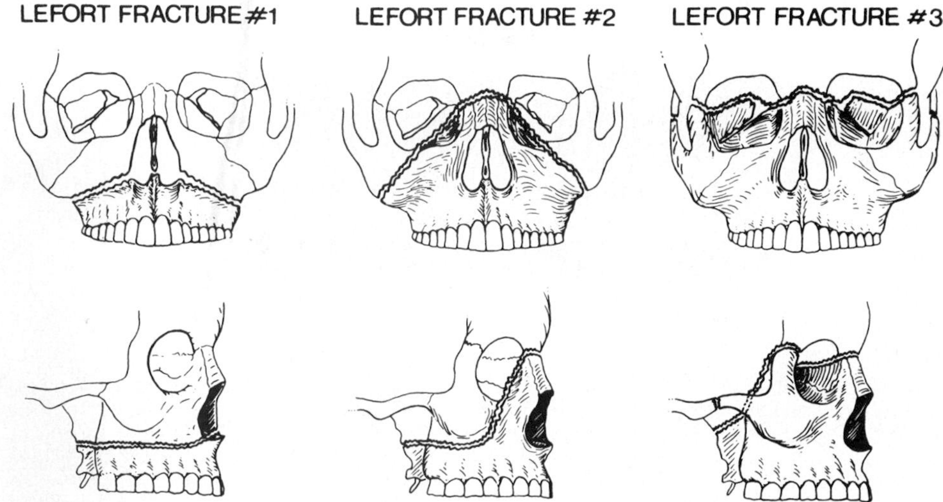

Figure 11–53. LeFort fractures: LeFort I is a transverse fracture in the horizontal plane at the base of the maxillary sinuses separating off the alveolar process of the maxilla; LeFort II, a pyramidal fracture separating off the central portion of the face; and LeFort III, complete separation of the facial skeleton from the skull (craniofacial disjunction). Interpretation of LeFort fractures depends on recognizing not only the location of fractures but also the stronger areas of bone that remain intact. Specifically, the areas to analyze are the pterygoid processes, the zygomatic arches, the zygomaticofrontal suture or frontal process, the nasofrontal suture, the inferior orbital rim, and the lateral walls of the maxillary sinuses. For example, intact inferior orbital rims exclude a LeFort II fracture.

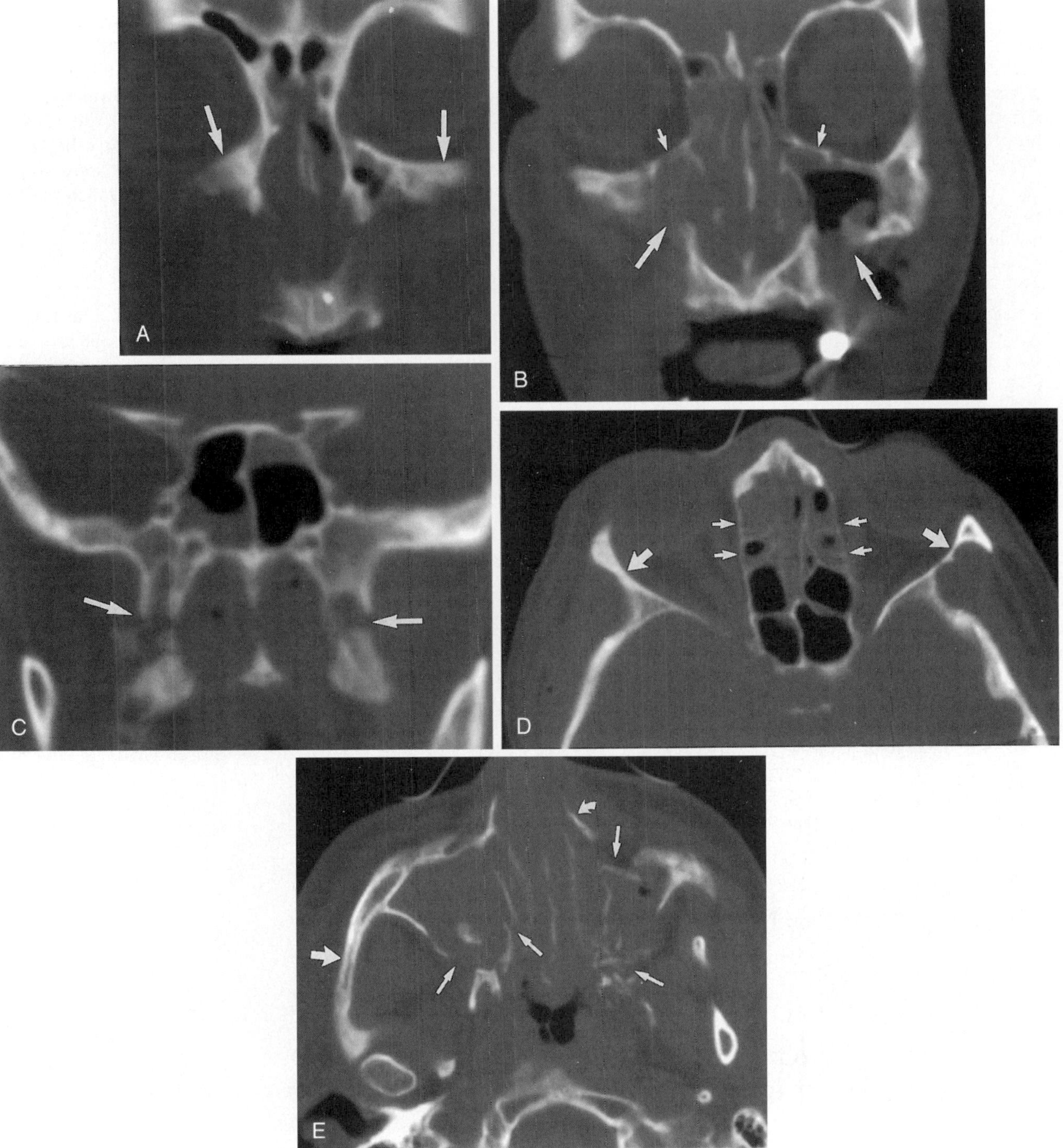

Figure 11–54. LeFort I fracture: CT findings. *A,* Coronal CT image shows the inferior orbital rims to be intact (*arrows*). LeFort II fractures are excluded. *B,* Coronal CT image shows that the lateral walls of the maxillary sinuses are broken (*large arrows*). This finding excludes a LeFort III fracture, in which the lateral walls are intact. Also note the intact orbital floors (*small arrows*). The presence of a LeFort I component remains a possibility. *C,* Coronal CT image shows bilateral fractures of the pterygoid processes (*arrows*). These are broken in all of the LeFort fractures and constitute a clue to the presence of a LeFort fracture. *D,* Axial CT image obtained through the orbits shows intact lateral orbital walls (*large arrows*), which excludes a LeFort III fracture, and intact medial orbital walls (*small arrows*), which excludes a LeFort II or III fracture or an associated naso-orbital-ethmoidal fracture. The density in the anterior ethmoid air cells probably is blood. The presence of blood in a sinus does not necessarily mean that a wall has been fractured. *E,* Axial image shows an intact right zygomatic arch (*large arrow*). The left arch is seen to be intact on other images. This finding also excludes a LeFort III fracture or associated zygomatic complex fracture. All walls of the maxillary sinuses are broken (*small straight arrows*), as seen on this and adjacent axial images. This injury is a very comminuted LeFort I fracture. There is an additional fracture of the left frontal process of the maxilla (*curved arrow*).

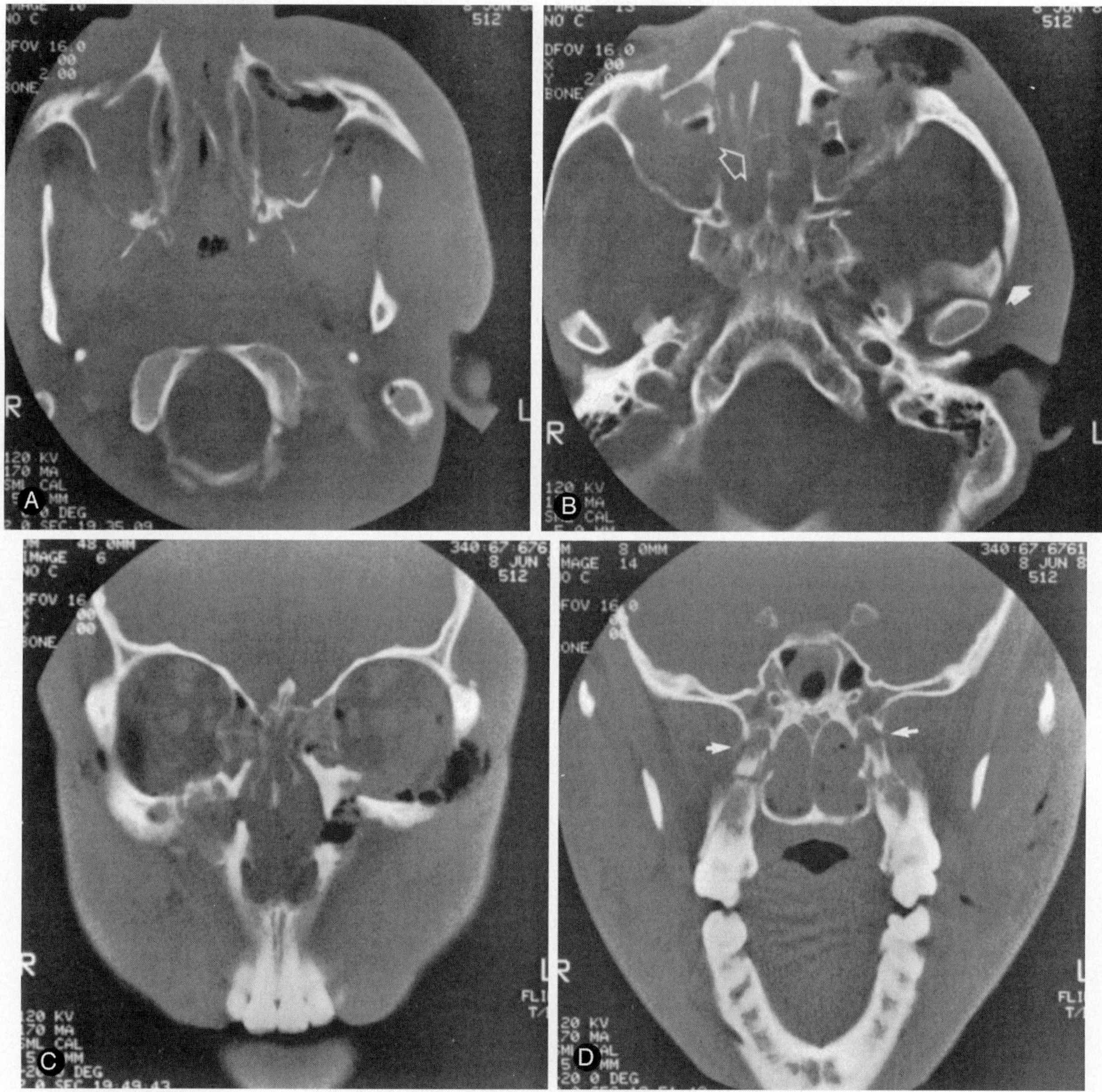

Figure 11–55. LeFort II fracture plus zygomatic arch fracture. *A,* Opacification of the nasal fossa and maxillary sinuses and a large retropharyngeal hematoma are evident. There are comminuted fractures of the anterior and posterolateral maxillary walls and pterygoid processes. A pure LeFort III fracture is excluded because of the anterior maxillary sinus wall fracture. LeFort I and II fractures remain as possibilities. *B,* Axial CT image shows subcutaneous emphysema over the left maxilla. Comminuted fractures of the anterior and posterolateral maxillary walls are identified, as well as fractures and flattening of the nasal bones and a comminuted, folded fracture of the nasal septum (*open arrow*). There is also a fracture of the posterior left zygomatic arch (*white arrow*). *C,* Coronal CT image shows comminuted fractures of the medial walls of the orbits bilaterally, with tilting of the crista galli associated with a fracture of the cribriform plate on the right. Bilateral fractures of the inferior orbital rims and lateral maxillary walls are also present. *D,* Posterior coronal CT image shows comminuted fractures in the pterygoid processes bilaterally (*arrows*). The best diagnosis based on the imaging findings is a LeFort II fracture plus a fracture of the left zygomatic arch.

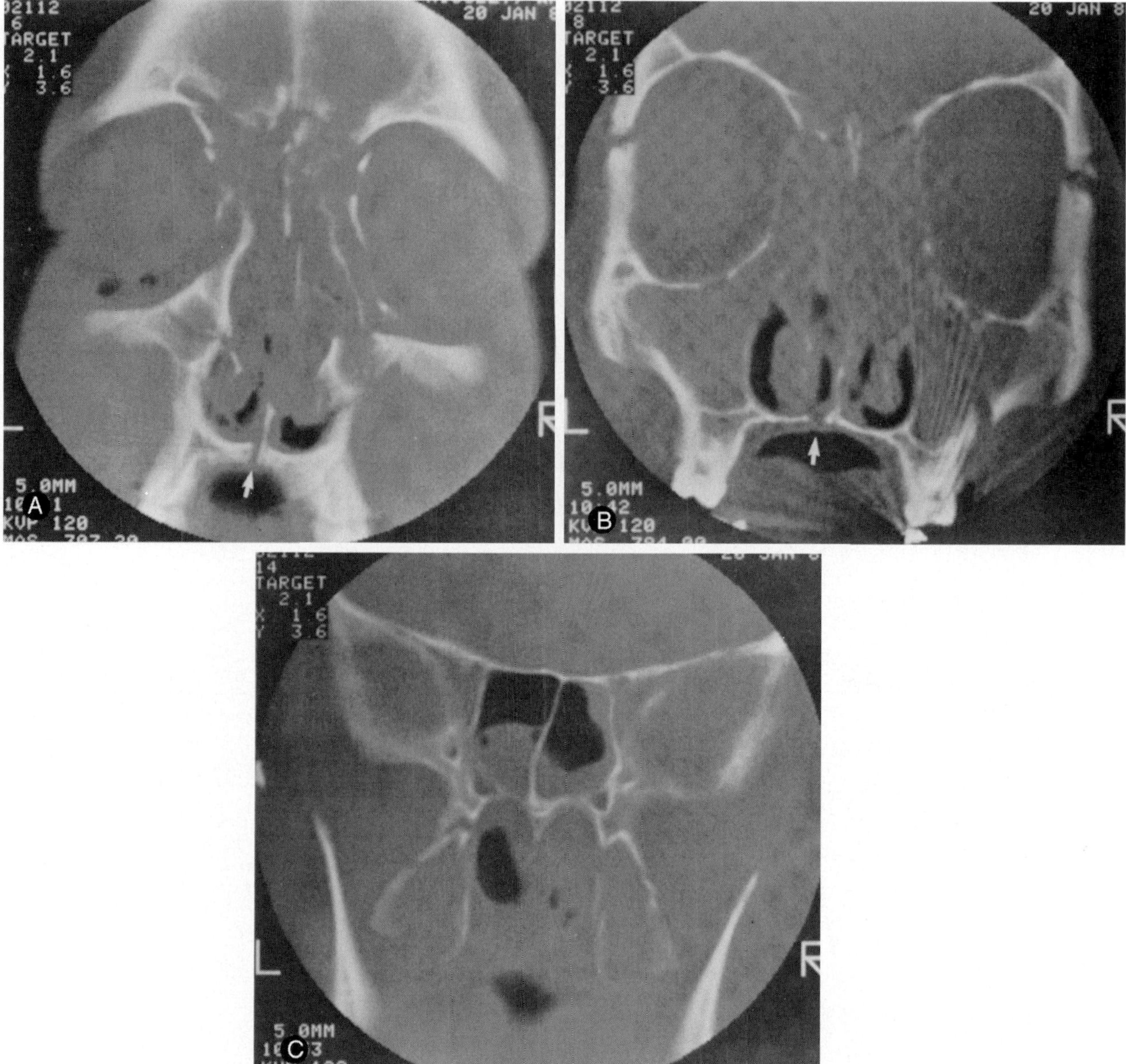

Figure 11–56. Complex LeFort III fracture: CT finding. *A,* LeFort III fractures are seldom found in pure form; usually, other associated fractures are present. Anterior coronal image shows comminuted fractures of the medial orbital walls bilaterally and fractures of the frontal sinuses and nasal septum. These fractures suggest either a LeFort II or LeFort III designation. There are also bilateral fractures of the maxillae at the lateral walls of the nasal fossa inferiorly. These nasal fossa fractures could be seen in a LeFort I fracture or in an extensive naso-orbital-ethmoidal fracture. Note the sagittal fracture of the hard palate (*arrow*). *B,* Coronal CT image through the maxillary sinuses again shows bilateral fractures of the medial orbital walls, as well as fractures within the cribriform plate and bilateral separation of the zygomaticofrontal sutures. If a LeFort designation is appropriate, only with the LeFort III fracture is there bilateral separation of the zygomaticofrontal sutures. The sagittal fracture of the hard palate (*arrow*) and fracture of the lateral wall of the right maxillary antrum are identified. Note the streak artifacts arising from the right alveolar process produced by metallic dental fillings. *C,* Posterior coronal CT image shows bilateral comminuted fractures of the medial and lateral pterygoid plates. Hemorrhage is present within the sphenoid sinuses. These fractures do not fit neatly into a single LeFort classification. The LeFort III designation captures the zygomaticofrontal suture separation, the medial orbital wall fractures, pterygoid plate fractures, and zygomatic arch fractures (not shown). A LeFort II designation would be inappropriate with intact inferior orbital rims. A low naso-orbital-ethmoidal fracture could explain the medial maxillary wall fractures but not the lateral maxillary wall fractures. A LeFort I category would include these maxillary wall fractures and should be described as comminuted because of the sagittal fracture of the hard palate. A summary description that would capture all the fracture components seen in this case would be a LeFort III plus a LeFort I fracture accompanied by a maxillary sagittal fracture.

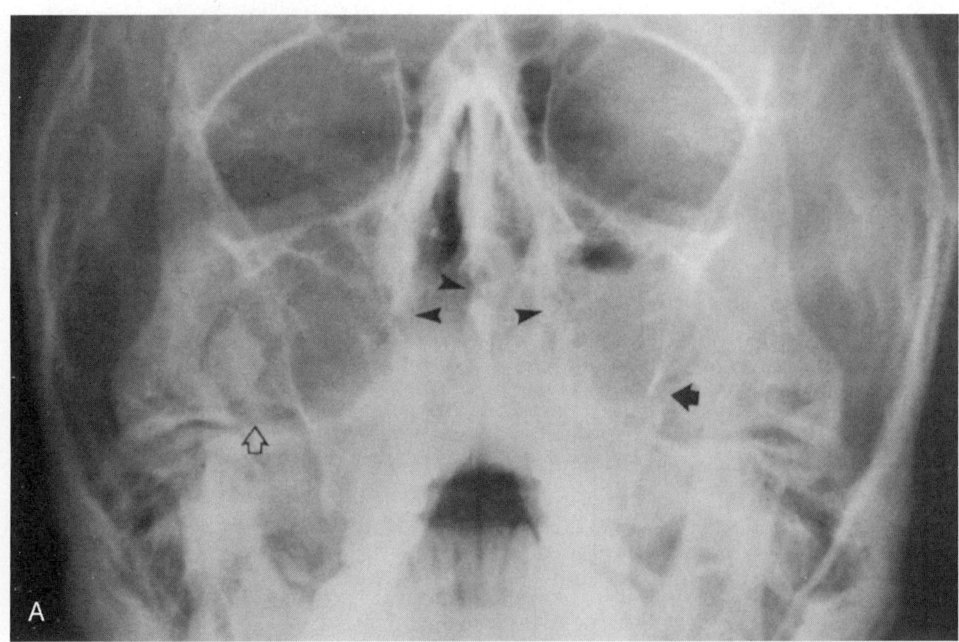

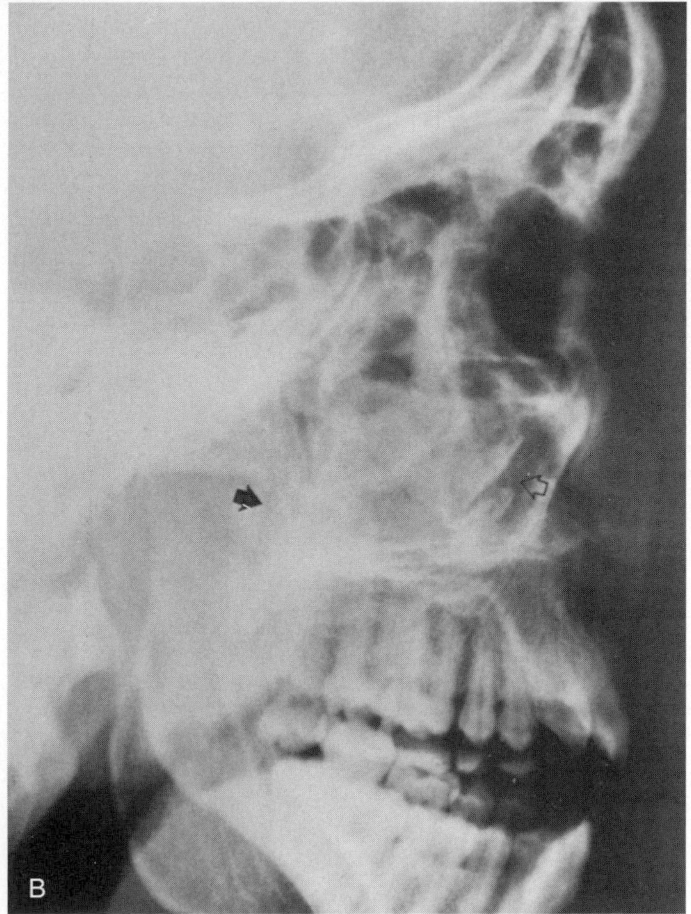

Figure 11–57. LeFort I fracture: Plain radiography findings. *A*, There are fractures of the lateral wall of the left maxillary sinus (*black arrow*) and a comminuted fracture of the lateral wall of the right maxillary sinus (*open arrow*). There is a suggestion of a fracture of the medial wall of both sinuses and of the nasal septum (*arrowheads*). The inferior orbital rims and frontal processes of the zygoma are intact. *B*, Lateral view shows a large retropharyngeal hematoma. The hard palate is displaced posteriorly and tilted, as determined by comparison with Dolan's lines of reference. There are fractures of the posterior walls of the maxillary sinuses and pterygoid processes (*black arrow*) and of the anterior walls of the maxillary sinuses (*open arrow*).

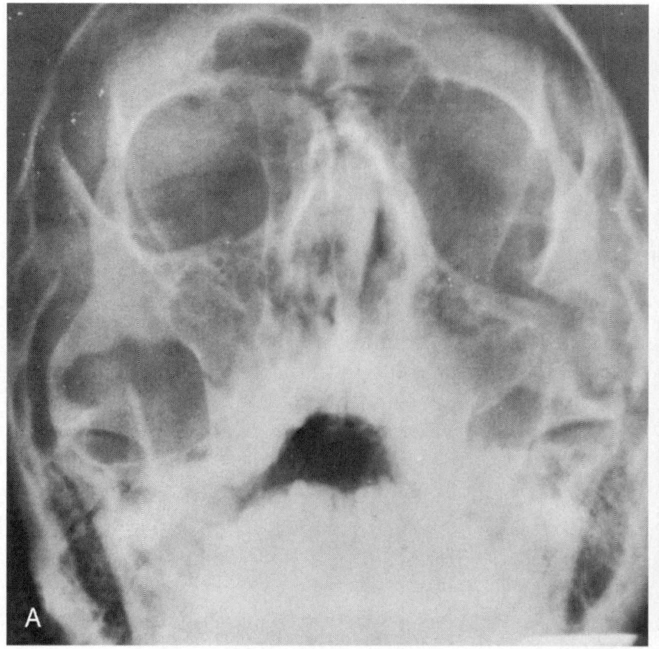

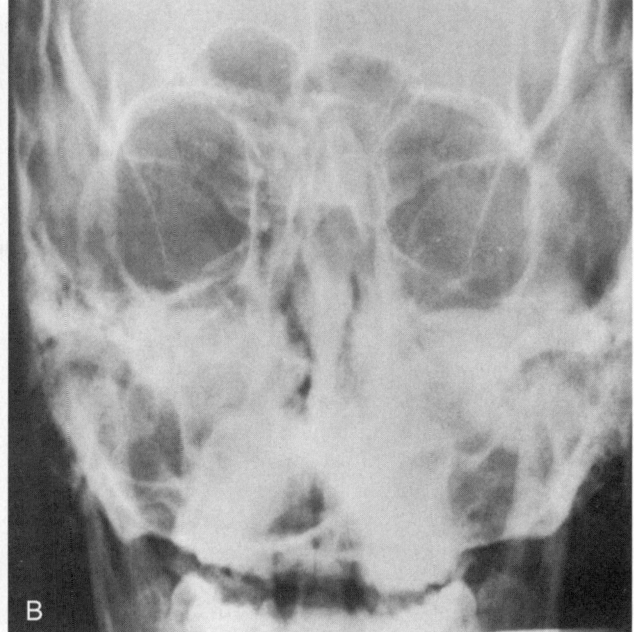

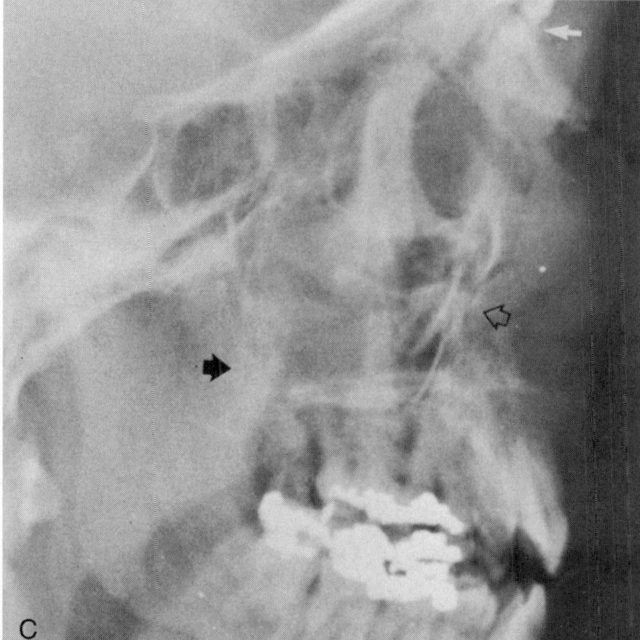

Figure 11–58. Complex LeFort II fracture: Plain radiography findings. *A,* The LeFort II component is on the right, consisting of fracture of the right inferior orbital rim and of the lateral wall of the right maxillary sinus. There is a comminuted fracture in the nasofrontal-ethmoidal region and a comminuted fracture of the left maxilla. There is also a fracture of the lateral wall of the left maxillary sinus and at the junction of the inferior and the lateral orbital rim. Also seen are separation of the left zygomaticofrontal suture and a comminuted fracture of the left zygomatic arch. *B,* Caldwell's projection shows the complex fractures in the nasofrontal-ethmoidal region and the separation of the zygomaticofrontal suture on the left. *C,* Lateral view shows a large retropharyngeal hematoma. Fractures of the pterygoid processes and of the posterior walls (*black arrow*) and the anterior walls of the maxillary sinuses (*open arrow*) are identified. There is a fracture in the region of the nasion (*white arrow*).

Designation of this fracture as LeFort II on the right and LeFort III on the left leaves out the lower left orbital rim and lateral left maxillary sinus fractures. A more complete designation would be a LeFort II fracture on the right and a LeFort III fracture on the left, with additional components of a zygomatic complex fracture on the left. Alternatively, this injury could be called a bilateral LeFort II fracture with atypical lateral position of the left (inferior) orbital rim fracture plus a left zygomatic complex fracture.

fracture through the hard palate, forming two separate fracture fragments. The fracture may be identified by noting an abnormal separation between the teeth.

LeFort II Fracture

A LeFort II fracture is sustained from a blow directed centrally or slightly downward to the central portion of the midface. The force of the blow separates a large, roughly pyramidal fragment consisting of the central portion of the face; thus, the resulting fracture is sometimes called a "pyramidal fracture." The fracture line traverses the nasofrontal region and then extends across the ethmoid bones obliquely on the medial wall of the orbits, across the maxillary surface of the orbit through the inferior orbital rim, obliquely across the maxillary sinuses, and posteriorly through the pterygoid processes. The pyramidal fragment is often displaced posteriorly.

CT in both the coronal and axial planes is recommended for imaging LeFort II fractures (see Fig. 11–55). Major CT findings with a LeFort II fracture include bilateral fractures of the pterygoid processes and inferior orbital rims and fracture or separation across the nasofrontal suture. The zygomatic arches and frontal processes are, by definition, intact. The thinner bones that fracture include the posterior, lateral, and anterior walls of the maxillary sinuses; the floors of the orbits; and the medial walls of the orbits.

At plain radiographic examination, the LeFort II fracture may be suspected on the lateral view when it demonstrates fractures of the pterygoid processes and the nasal area. The Waters view will show the fracture of the lateral wall of the maxillary sinus, and the Caldwell view will show the fractures of the inferior orbital rims (see Fig. 11–58). In the pure form of the LeFort II fracture, the zygomatic bones remain attached to the calvaria through the zygomatic arch and the zygomaticofrontal process.

LeFort III Fracture

The LeFort III fracture entails a complete separation of the facial skeleton from the calvaria or brain case, producing a craniofacial disjunction, or craniofacial separation. The fracture line extends from the nasofrontal area across the ethmoid bones posteriorly to the inferior orbital fissures and pterygoid process and laterally through the lateral wall of the orbits and the zygomatic arches. The face is thus completely separated from the calvaria (see Fig. 11–56).

As with all complex facial injuries, CT in both the coronal and axial planes is the recommended imaging modality. The coronal images are usually more informative. Bilateral fractures of the pterygoid processes, diastasis of the zygomaticofrontal suture or fracture of the frontal process of the zygoma, and fractures across the nasal bones are best shown on coronal images. Fractures of the zygomatic arch, however, are better shown in the axial plane. The inferior orbital rims should be intact in a LeFort III fracture.

On the Waters and Caldwell views, the orbits appear elongated with a LeFort III fracture, with wide separation of the zygomaticofrontal sutures and possibly associated fractures of the frontal process of the zygoma. It may be difficult to appreciate the fractures on the lateral view, although this view may demonstrate the inferior separation of the facial bones from the brain case.

Maxillary Sagittal and Other Hard Palate Fractures

The maxilla may fracture in the sagittal plane (Fig. 11–59), and such fractures are also well shown on CT examination. If the fracture involves the pterygoid plate on the affected side, it may be considered a unilateral LeFort I fracture.

Sagittally oriented fractures of the hard palate may occur in the midline, in a parasagittal location, or in a para-alveolar location.[171] Hard palate fractures may also be transverse or oblique and may be simple or comminuted. Fractures of the hard palate are almost always seen in association with other midfacial fractures, especially the LeFort fractures. In fact, 8% of LeFort fractures are accompanied by a hard palate fracture. The sagittal fracture of the hard palate is more frequent in young patients, whereas the parasagittal and para-alveolar fractures are more common in adults.[171]

Smash and Panfacial Fractures

Severely comminuted fractures of the facial skeleton are often described as *smash fractures* (Figs. 11–60 and 11–61). These complex fractures consist of comminuted pyramidal fractures, with impaction and telescoping of the facial skeleton, particularly of the ethmoid structures, against the base of the skull. The degree of comminution will influence the required surgical approach.[188] Cerebrospinal fluid rhinorrhea and pneumocephalus are potential complications.

Fractures of the Mandible

The prominent position of the mandible exposes this structure to traumatic forces during assaults and motor

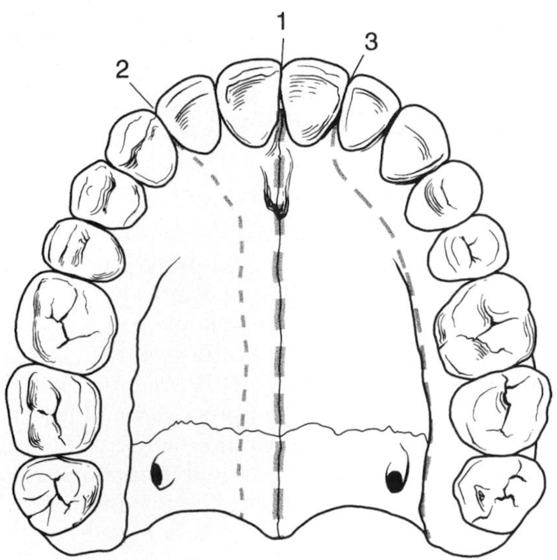

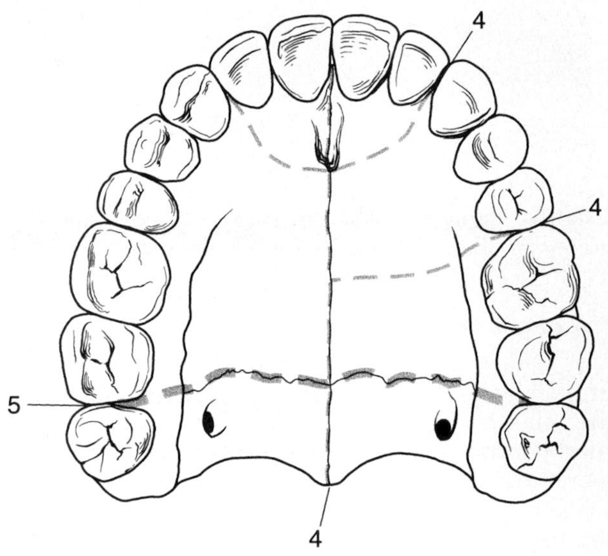

Figure 11–59. Maxillary sagittal and other hard palate fractures. Sagittally oriented fractures may occur in the hard palate in the midline (1), in the parasagittal region (2), and in the paraalveolar region (3). Comminuted fractures (4) and transverse fractures (5) may also be seen.

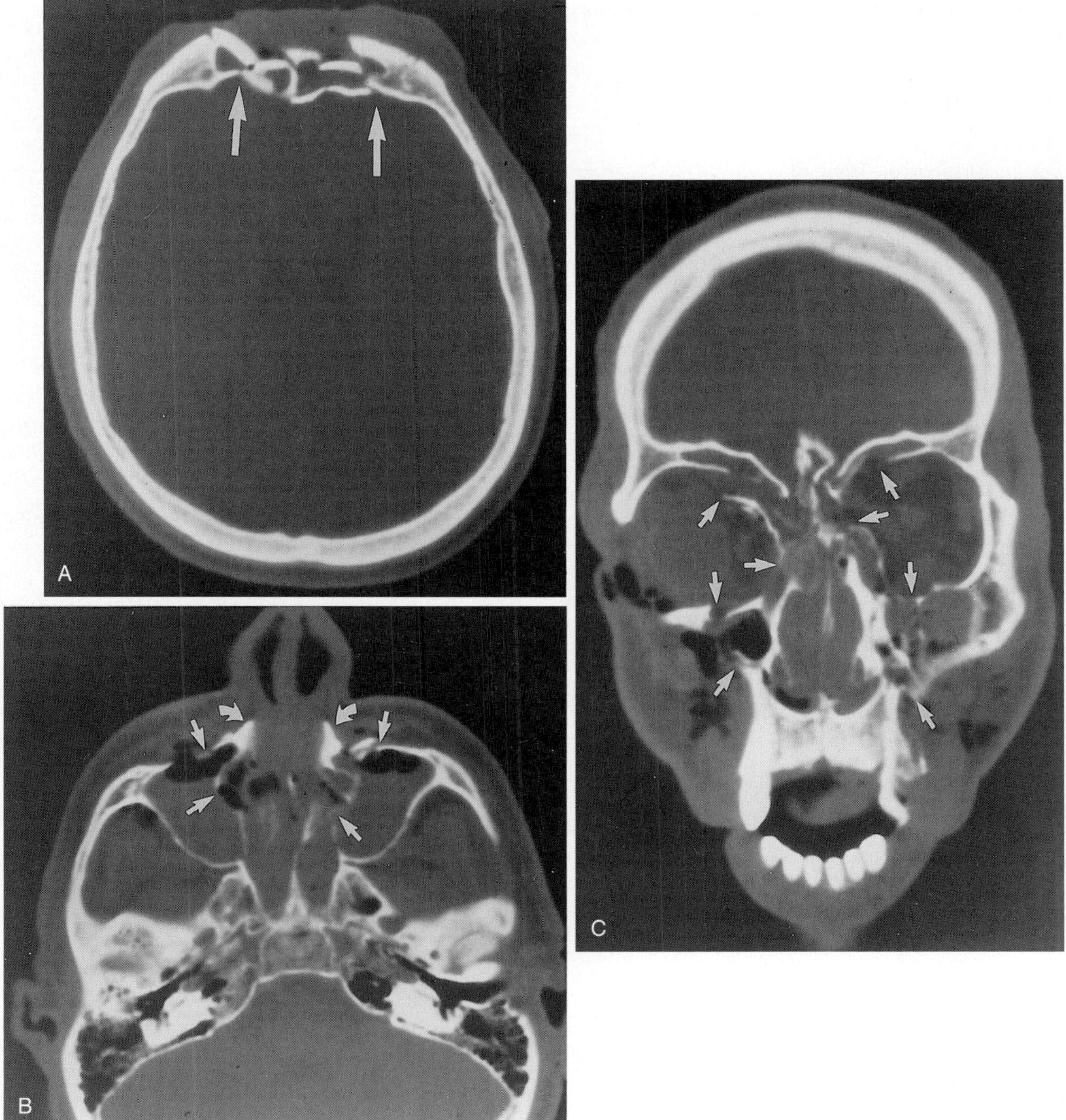

Figure 11–60. Smash fracture: CT findings. The smash fracture is a severely comminuted fracture of the central midface that does not fit into the LeFort classification, primarily because there is no extension posteriorly through the pterygoid processes. *A,* Axial CT image reveals comminution of both walls of the frontal sinuses (*arrows*). *B,* There is comminution of the anterior and medial walls of the maxillary sinuses (*straight arrows*) with posterior displacement of the frontal processes of the maxilla (*curved arrows*). In this patient, the zygomatic arches and pterygoid processes were intact. *C,* Coronal CT image shows fractures of the orbital roofs, ethmoid sinuses, inferior orbital rim on the right, and orbital floor on the left, and medial and lateral walls of the maxillary sinuses (*arrows*).

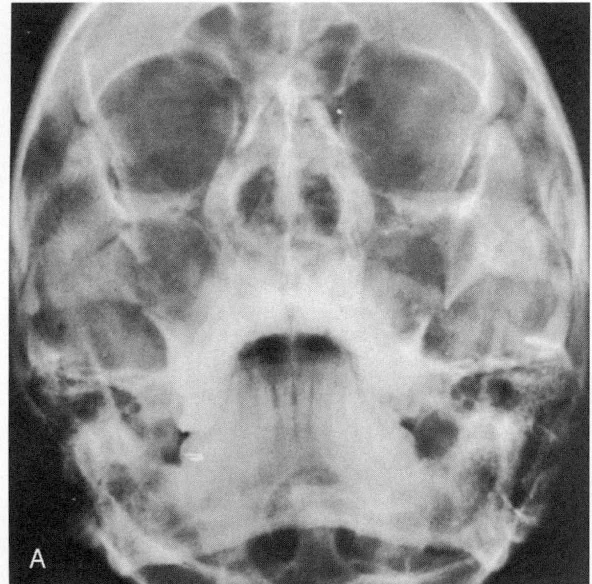

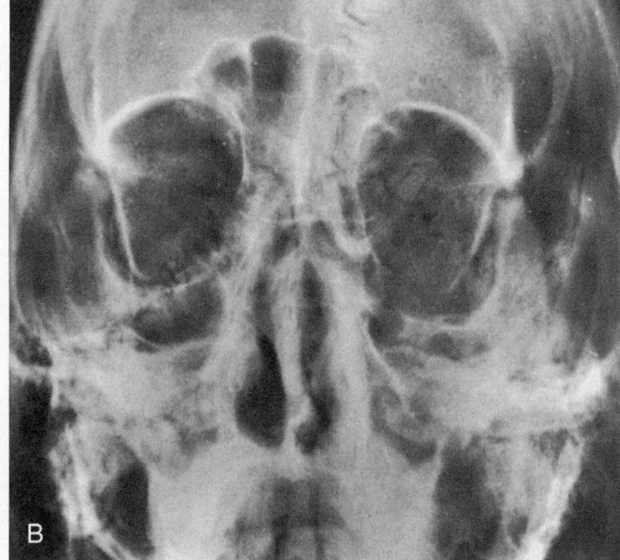

Figure 11–61. Smash fracture: Plain radiography findings. *A*, Waters' projection shows fractures of the lateral walls of the maxillary sinuses, separation of the zygomaticofrontal sutures, and complex fractures in the medial walls of the orbits and nasofrontal-ethmoidal region. *B*, Caldwell's projection shows opacification of the ethmoid and frontal sinuses. The fractures of the medial wall of the orbit are not clearly visualized. Separation of the zygomaticofrontal suture is shown.

vehicle collisions. These two mechanisms account for at least 80% of all mandibular fractures.[116, 117, 122, 129, 134, 136] Traditionally, the ratio of mandibular to facial fractures has been 2:1,[13] with rates of simultaneous occurrence of fractures in the two areas ranging between 6% and 10%.

Fractures of the mandible in children are relatively uncommon, comprising only 5% of all mandibular fractures.[114, 126, 132, 133] If the mandible is fractured in a child, the fracture usually involves the condyle.[156] As many as one third of the reported cases of mandibular fracture in children result from bicycle collisions.[126, 132] Together, automobile and bicycle collisions account for the majority of childhood mandibular fractures[127]; sports activities and falls account for the remainder. Although it usually closes by 1 year of age, the mandibular symphysis may not close until puberty, persisting as a vertical radiolucent line. This finding should not be mistaken for a fracture. Clinical evaluation may be required to make the distinction with certainty.

The mandible is best divided into regions or segments for the purpose of describing the location of fractures[120, 134, 138] (Fig. 11–62). The symphysis extends between the lower canine teeth. The body of the mandible extends between the symphysis and angle. The ramus extends from the angle to the base of the condylar and coronoid processes. The most common site of fracture is in the mandibular body, accounting for 30%[116] to 40%[129, 196] of cases. The next most frequent site is in the mandibular angle, accounting for 25%[116] to 31%[129]; the mandibular condyle accounts for 15%[129] to 35%,[138] and the mandibular symphysis, 7%[129] to 15%.[116] The symphysis fracture line is rarely located exactly in the midline. Fractures of the mandibular ramus account for 3%[129] to 9%[116]; fractures of the coronoid process, 1% to 2%[129]; and those limited to the alveolar process, 2% to 4%.[23, 29]

Rings or arcs of bone are difficult to break in one location because of their relative brittleness. The mandible is protected in this regard because of the presence of the temporomandibular joints, which may absorb some forces by rotation of the condyle within the joint. This protection is far from complete, however, and multiple fractures occur in 50% to 60% of cases.[116, 122, 129] In most reported series, there is an incidence of 1.5 to 1.8 fractures per patient. It is therefore imperative to search for a second fracture after the initial fracture has been identified. The most common combination is fracture of the mandibular angle associated with contralateral fracture of the body. Fractures of the angle and the condylar process on opposite sides are also frequent, but any combination of angle and body, body and condylar process, symphysis and condyle, or the like can be encountered (Figs. 11–63 through 11–66). Only infrequently are these fractures found on the same side of the mandible. Triple fractures occur; the most common combination[122] is a fracture of the symphysis with bilateral fractures of the condylar process. Multiple fractures may allow posterior displacement of the mandible with compromise of the airway.[141]

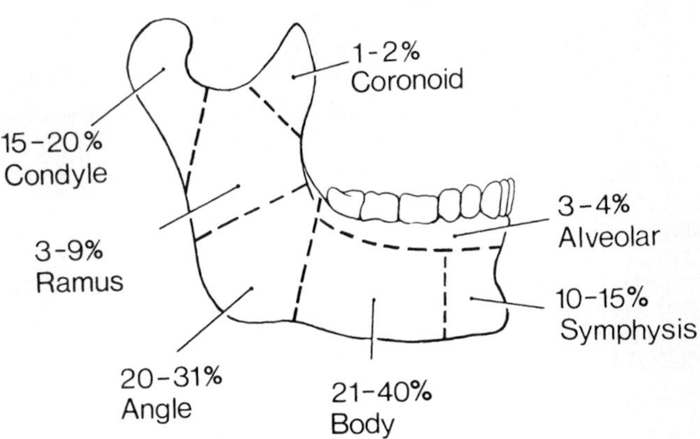

Figure 11–62. Distribution of mandibular fractures. Single fractures of the mandible occur in slightly less than half of patients who sustain mandibular fractures.

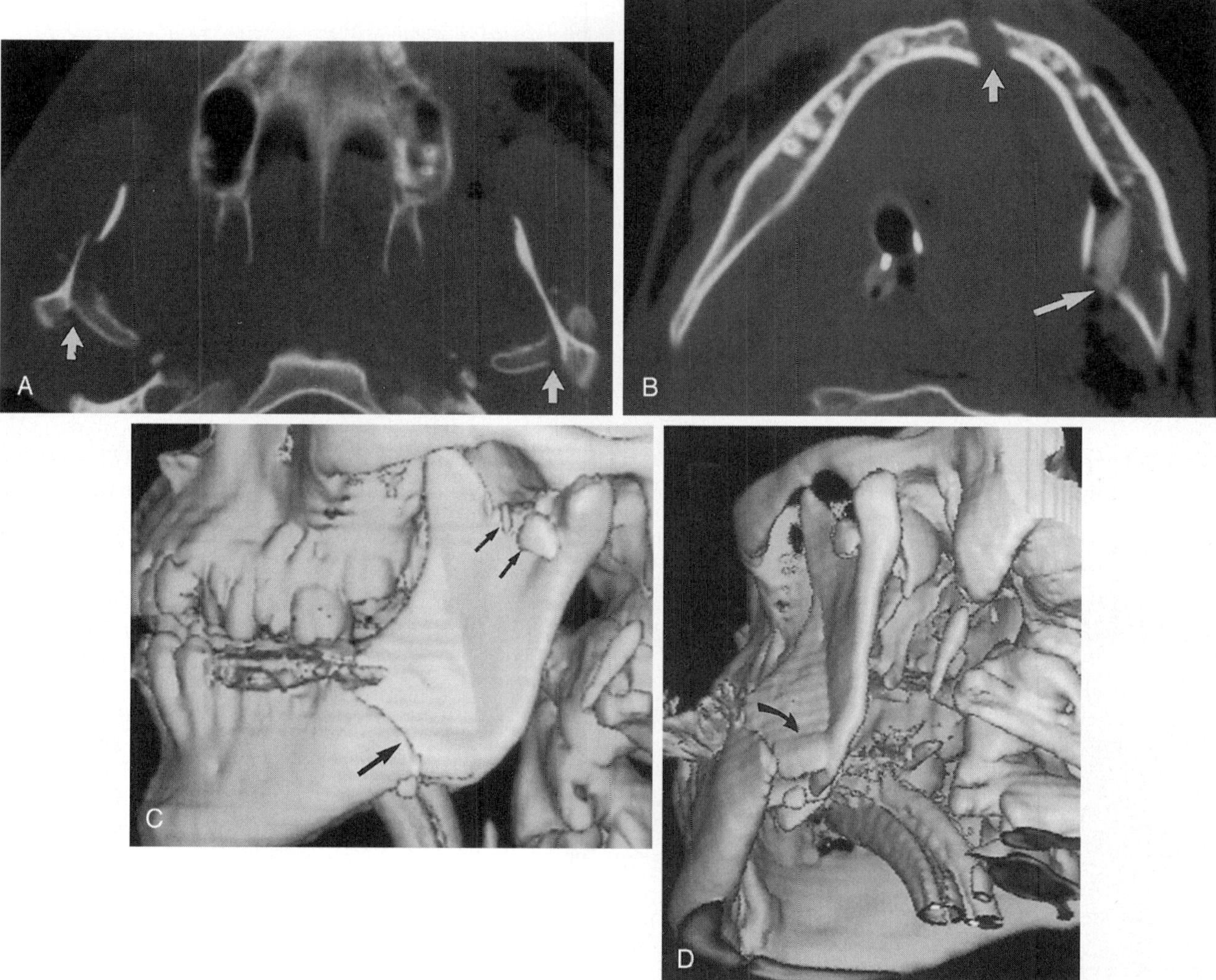

Figure 11–63. Multiple mandibular fractures. *A,* Axial CT image shows bilateral comminuted fractures of the mandibular condyles (*arrows*). There is also a fracture of the right coronoid process (not shown in this image). *B,* There is a fracture at the angle of the mandible on the left that appears comminuted (*long arrow*), and there is a fracture at the symphysis (*short arrow*). *C,* Lateral three-dimensional reformatted image of the left mandible shows mandibular condyle fragments (*small arrows*) and a displaced fracture at the mandibular angle (*large arrow*). *D,* Oblique three-dimensional reformatted image of the left mandible seen from behind was obtained to show better the displacement of the fracture of the left mandibular angle (*arrow*). The degree of medial displacement is more easily appreciated than on the other images.

Dislocation of the temporomandibular joint may occur spontaneously, often during yawning, without an associated fracture. Subsequent dislocations may occur during eating, speaking, or laughing. The mandibular condyle is displaced out of the glenoid fossa and lies anterior to the articular eminence of the temporal bone but remains within the confines of the joint capsule. It should be remembered that with the mouth open, the condyle normally lies below the articular eminence, but in dislocation, the condyle lies anterior to it. A blow on the mandible at the proper angle may drive the condyle upward through the glenoid fossa, dislocating the condyle into the middle cranial fossa. Fewer than 10 such cases[135] have been reported.

CT is an excellent technique for imaging fractures of the mandible (see Figs. 11–63 and 11–64). Fractures of the symphysis and body are well visualized in the axial projection, and those of the ramus and condyle are best seen in the coronal projection.[24, 142] The sagittal splitting fracture of the condyle and fracture of the tympanic plate of the temporomandibular joint may be visualized only with CT[192, 230] (see Fig. 11–64). The position of the condyle relative to the glenoid fossa is more precisely shown with CT than with conventional radiography.[206] The position and morphology of the cartilage of the temporomandibular joint are best assessed with MRI.[200]

The routine radiographic examination of the mandible should include a lateral, posteroanterior, both oblique, and Towne views. Panorex and Orthopantograph views are also helpful if this equipment is available (see Fig. 11–66). The panoramic x-ray film affords a view of the entire mandible, including the condylar and coronoid processes.[118, 119, 123, 131] The symphysis is obscured on the posteroanterior view[123] because of the overlap of the cervical spine and is not visualized in the oblique projection. This problem may be solved by the addition of a Waters view or a base view to the routine radiographic examination of the mandible (see Fig. 11–65). The body and symphysis of the mandible are well visualized on a Waters view and are free of confusing overlap. They are also well

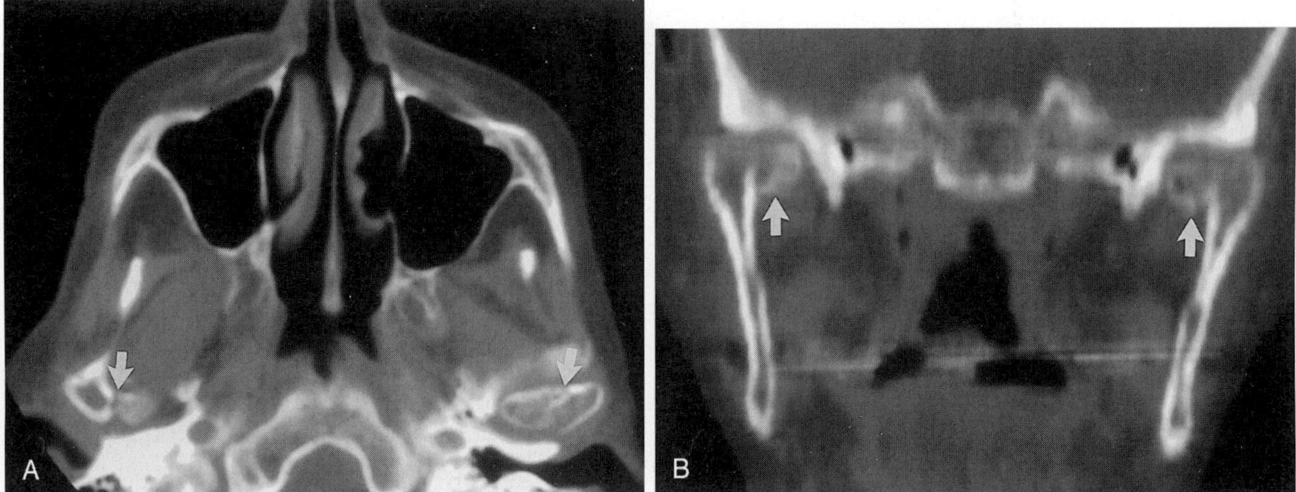

Figure 11–64. Sagittal splitting fracture of the mandibular condyle. *A,* Axial CT image shows sagittally oriented fractures through the condyles bilaterally (*arrows*). *B,* Coronal CT image shows medial displacement of the condylar fragments (*arrows*). Sagittal splitting fractures of the condyles may not be seen on plain films. (*A* and *B,* Reprinted with permission from Rhea, J.T., Rao, P.M., & Novelline, R.N. [1999]. Helical CT and three-dimensional CT of facial and orbital injury. Radiol. Clin. North Am., 37:489.)

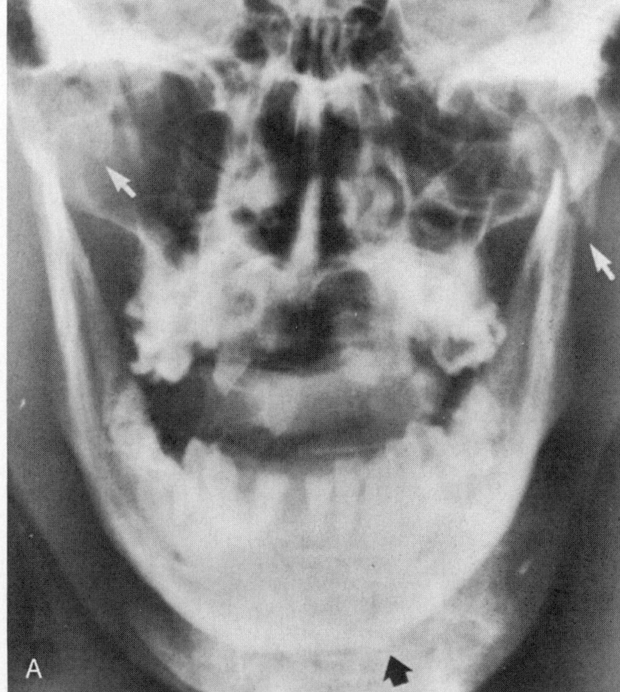

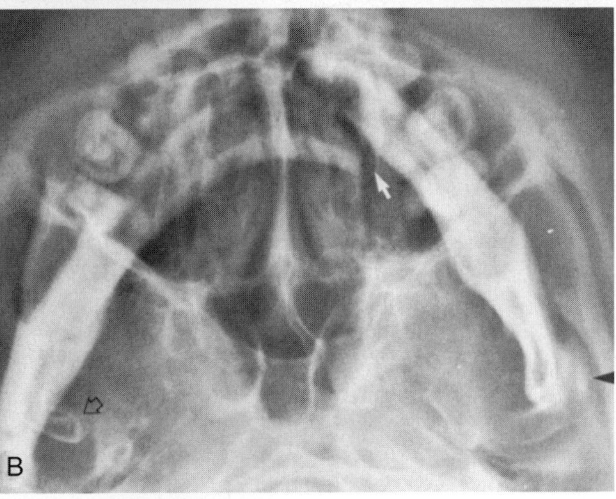

Figure 11–65. Multiple fractures of the mandible: Plain radiography findings. *A,* Posteroanterior view of the mandible shows fractures of both condyles (*white arrows*). The fracture of the symphysis is difficult to see in this projection. There is minimal disruption of the inferior cortex (*black arrow*). *B,* Submentovertex view clearly shows the fracture of the symphysis (*white arrow*). There is anterior and medial displacement of the right condyle (*open arrow*), with lateral displacement of the left condyle (*arrowhead*).

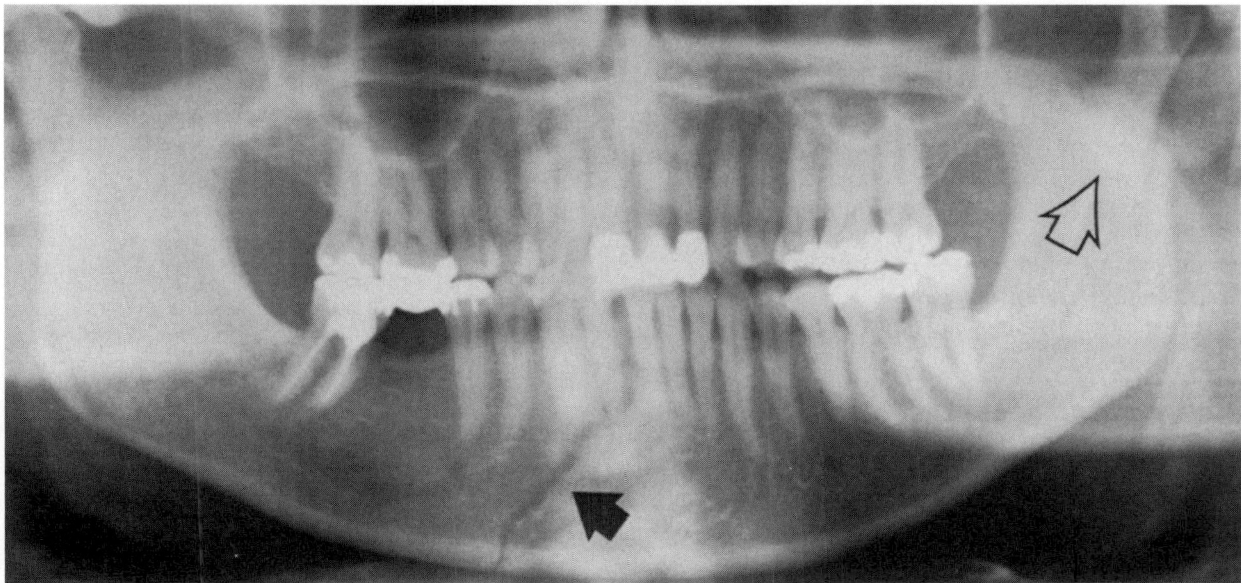

Figure 11–66. Panoramic view of mandibular fractures. An oblique, paramedian fracture of the symphysis (*black arrow*) associated with a fracture of the base of the left condyloid process (*open arrow*) is seen. Overlapping of the fracture fragments results in a zone of increased density at the junction of the neck and ramus.

shown on the base projection. Occlusal films[123] will nicely demonstrate the symphysis and alveolar process.

An indirect sign of a mandibular fracture is malocclusion or displacement of the teeth. Displacement of the fracture fragments is often minimal because the fragments are held in place by their muscular attachments against the opposite teeth of the upper jaw. Because of the frequent lack of displacement it is necessary to trace the inferior cortical margin of the symphysis and body and the cortical margins of the ramus, angle, and coronoid and condyloid processes on all of the views to identify or exclude a fracture. The outlines of the mandibular canal should also be traced. The mandibular canal extends from the mandibular foramen on the inner surface of the ramus to the mental foramen on the outer surface of the mandibular body. It contains the alveolar nerves and vessels and its margin consists of a thin rim of cortical bone, which has the radiographic appearance of fine parallel lines of cortical density. Disruption and offsets in the margins of the canal serve as clues to otherwise obscure fractures.

If the patient is edentulous or lacks opposing teeth in the region of the fracture line, then greater displacement may occur. If there is overlap of fragments, the fracture may be identified by a line or band of increased density. The degree of displacement is also dependent on the angle and position of the fracture line in relation to muscular attachments. The muscles attached anteriorly tend to displace fragments downward and posteriorly, whereas those attached posteriorly pull upward and medially. Mandibular fractures have been classified as favorable or unfavorable. Favorable fracture lines are those held in apposition and alignment by the natural pull exerted by the attached muscles. Unfavorable fracture lines are those displaced by the pull of those muscles.

The mandible is composed of an inner and an outer cortex enclosing the medullary cavity. Accordingly, obliquely oriented vertical fractures may create the false appearance of two separate fracture lines when the mandible is viewed from the side. In fact, these two lines represent a single fracture: one line in the outer cortex and the other in the inner cortex of the same fracture.

Air in the pharynx, particularly on the oblique view, may be mistaken for fracture of the angle, ramus, or condyle. On the posteroanterior view, the lucencies formed by the various portions of the cervical spine and intervertebral disc spaces may be mistaken for fractures of the symphysis. On closer examination, the intact cortex of the mandible can be traced through these lucencies and a fracture safely excluded.

It is also important to identify any pathologic dental condition lying within the fracture line.[115, 116] A fracture that extends through a periapical abscess may result in osteomyelitis and delayed healing if not recognized and treated. Any mandibular fracture involving the teeth must be considered an open fracture.[203]

Fractures of the coronoid and condylar processes frequently occur at their bases.[128] The condyle and condylar processes of the mandible are best shown using the posteroanterior and Towne views. With fractures through the bases of the condylar process, the condyle is characteristically angulated or pulled medially[126, 128] by the lateral pterygoid muscle, resulting in subluxation or dislocation of the temporomandibular joint. The condyle then forms an angle of up to 90 degrees with the ramus. With severe angulation, the condyle is displaced from the glenoid fossa, which then appears vacant. The vacant appearance of the glenoid fossa may lead to recognition of an otherwise obscure displaced fracture of the condyle. Medial dislocation of the condyle may occur rarely without condylar fracture.[143]

Trapnell[137] described a "magnification sign" of triple mandibular fractures. In the presence of a fracture of the symphysis and bilateral fractures of the neck of the condylar process, the mandible appears too wide for the upper jaw because bilateral-lateral displacement of the body, angle, and ramus of the mandible is associated with the fracture. The hinge or fulcrum of this lateral displacement is at the fracture of the symphysis, which allows lateral displacement.

Most mandibular fractures are treated[5, 116, 124, 129] by placement of arch bars and wires about the teeth. The teeth are held in apposition between the upper and lower jaws by additional wires or rubber bands. These appliances reduce the fracture and restore proper occlusion of the teeth. Some fractures are treated with screws, and CT demonstration of stable bicortical bone is of importance before fixation of a comminuted mandibular fracture.[160]

Fractures of the mandible heal slowly, somewhat similarly to skull fractures. The fracture line may remain lucent for prolonged periods[125] despite clinical union. This finding has two implications for the radiographic interpretation. First, it is possible that an old fracture may be mistaken for a new one. Probably, however, the margins of the older fracture will be somewhat blurred. Second, union or healing of mandibular fractures is based on the clinical findings and not on their radiographic appearance.

In children, as healing occurs, the condyles gradually return to their normal position.[126, 130, 132] Apparently, the displaced condylar head undergoes resorption, and a new condyle is gradually formed by appositional bone growth from the growth center on the displaced condylar fragment. Fractures high on the condylar process within the joint capsule may be nondisplaced. They are manifested by persistent pain, and CT is usually required to show them.[121] These fractures are particularly devastating in children because they represent an epiphyseal separation. The condylar ossification center is the only growth center within the mandible, and its destruction results in underdevelopment of the entire mandible.

References

1. Brant-Zawadzki, M.N., Minagi, H., Federle, M.P., & Rowe, L.D. (1982). High resolution CT with image reformation in maxillofacial pathology. A.J.R. Am. J. Roentgenol., *138*:477.
2. Carroll, M.J., Hill, C.M., & Mason, D.A. (1987). Facial fractures in children. Br. Dent. J., *163*:23.
3. Cooper, P.W., Kassel, E.E., & Gruss, J.S. (1983). High-resolution CT scanning of facial trauma. A.J.N.R. Am. J. Neuroradiol., *4*:495.
4. Daffner, R.H., Apple, J.S., & Gehweiler, J.A. (1983). Lateral view of facial fractures: New observations. A.J.R. Am. J. Roentgenol., *141*:587.
5. Dingman, R.O., & Natvig, P. (1964). Surgery of Facial Fractures. W.B. Saunders Co., Philadelphia.
6. Dodd, G.D., & Jing, B.S. (1977). Traumatic lesions involving the paranasal sinuses. p. 146. In Radiology of the Nose, Paranasal Sinuses and Nasopharynx. Williams & Wilkins, Baltimore.
7. Dolan, D.D., & Jacoby, C.G. (1978). Facial fractures. Semin. Roentgenol., *13*:37.
8. Dolan, K., Jacoby, C., & Smoker, W. (1984). The radiology of facial fractures. Radiographics, *4*:577.
9. Frable, M.A., Roman, N.E., Lenis, A., & Lung, J.P. (1974). Hemorrhagic complications of facial fractures. Laryngoscope, *84*:2051.
10. Freimanis, A.K. (1966). Fractures of the facial bones. Radiol. Clin. North Am., *4*:341.
11. Gentry, L.R., Manor, W.F., Turski, P.A., & Strother, C.M. (1983). High-resolution CT analysis of facial struts in trauma: 1. Normal anatomy. A.J.R. Am. J. Roentgenol., *140*:523.
12. Gentry, L.R., Manor, W.F., Turski, P.A., & Strother, C.M. (1983). High-resolution CT analysis of facial struts in trauma: 2. Osseous and soft tissue complications. A.J.R. Am. J. Roentgenol., *140*:533.
13. Gwyn, P.P., Carraway, J.H., Horton, C.E. et al. (1971). Facial fractures—associated injuries and complications. Plast. Reconstr. Surg., *47*:225.
14. Karlson, T.A. (1982). The incidence of hospital-treated facial injuries from vehicles. J. Trauma, *22*:303.
15. Kassel, E.E., & Cooper, P.W. (1983). Radiologic studies of facial trauma associated with a regional trauma centre. Can. Assoc. Radiol. J., *34*:178.
16. Kreipke, D.L., Moss, J.J., Franco, J.M. et al. (1984). Computed tomography and thin-section tomography in facial trauma. A.J.R. Am. J. Roentgenol., *142*:1041.
17. Lewis, V.L. Jr., Manson, P.N., Morgan, R.F. et al. (1985). Facial injuries associated with cervical fractures: Recognition, patterns, and management. J. Trauma, *25*:90.
18. Luce, E.A. (1984). Maxillofacial trauma. Curr. Probl. Surg., *11*:1.
19. Lundin, K., Ridell, A., Sandberg, N., & Ohman, A. (1943). One thousand maxillofacial and related fractures at the ENT clinic in Gothenburg. Acta Otolaryngol., *75*:359.
20. Marsh, J.L., Vannier, M.W., Gado, M., & Stevens, W.G. (1986). In vivo delineation of facial fractures: The application of advanced medical imaging technology. Ann. Plast. Surg., *17*:364.
21. Mayer, J.S., Wainwright, D.J., Yeakley, J.W. et al. (1988). The role of three-dimensional computed tomography in the management of maxillofacial trauma. J. Trauma, *28*:1043.
22. Merrell, R.A., Jr., Yanagisawa, E., Smith, H.W., & Thaler, S. (1968). Radiographic anatomy of the paranasal sinuses. Arch. Otolaryngol., *87*:5.
23. Nakamura, T., & Gross, C.W. (1973). Facial fractures: Analysis of five years of experience. Arch. Otolaryngol., *97*:288.
24. Noyek, A.M., Kassel, E.E., Wortzman, G. et al. (1982). Sophisticated CT in complex maxillofacial trauma. Laryngoscope, *92*:1.
25. Rothman, S.L.G., Allen, W.E., & Kier, E.L. (1973). Stereo roentgenography in craniofacial injuries: A revival of fundamental ideas. Radiol. Clin. North Am., *11*:683.
26. Rowe, L.D., Miller, E., & Brandt-Zawadzki, M. (1981). Computed tomography in maxillofacial trauma. Laryngoscope, *91*:745.
27. Rowe, N.L., & Killey, H.C. (1968). Fractures of the Facial Skeleton. E. & S. Livingstone, Edinburgh.
28. Zilkha, A. (1982). Computed tomography in facial trauma. Radiology, *144*:545.
29. Andreasen, J.O. (1970). Fractures of the alveolar process of the jaw. A clinical and radiographic follow-up study. Scand. J. Dent. Res., *78*:263.
30. Charlton, O.P., Daffner, R.H., Gehweiler, J.A. et al. (1981). Panoramic zonography of fractures of the facial skeleton. A.J.R. Am. J. Roentgenol., *137*:109.
31. Clayton, M.I., & Lesser, T.H.J. (1986). The role of radiography in the management of nasal fractures. J. Laryngol. Otol., *100*:797.
32. deLacey, G.J., Wignall, B.K., Hussain, S., & Reidy, J.R. (1977). The radiology of nasal injuries: Problems of interpretation and clinical relevance. Br. J. Radiol., *50*:412.
33. Dodd, G.D., Collins, L.C., Egan, R.L., & Herrera, J.R. (1959). The systematic use of tomography in the diagnosis of carcinoma of the paranasal sinuses. Radiology, *72*:379.
34. Dolan, K.D., & Hayden, J. (1973). Maxillary "pseudo-fracture" lines. Radiology, *107*:321.
35. El Gammal, T., & Keats, T.E. (1969). The lamina dura (L.D.) of the maxillary antrum: Its value in roentgen diagnosis. A.J.R. Am. J. Roentgenol., *105*:830.
36. Fujii, N., & Yamashiro, M. (1983). Classification of malar complex fractures using computed tomography. J. Oral Maxillofac. Surg., *41*:562.
37. Harris, J.H. Jr., Littleton, J.T., Ray, R.D. et al. (1985). Panoramic zonography ("Zonarc") in the delineation of midface fractures. Radiographics, *5*:653.
38. Johnson, D.H. Jr. (1984). CT of maxillofacial trauma. Radiol. Clin. North Am., *22*:131.
39. Knight, J.S., & North, J.F. (1961). The classification of malar fractures: An analysis of displacement as a guide to treatment. Br. J. Plast. Surg., *13*:325.
40. Kristensen, S., & Tveteras K. (1986). Zygomatic fractures: Classification and complications. Clin. Otolaryngol. *11*:123.
41. Lame, E.L., & Redick, T.J. (1976). A new radiographic technique for fractures of the orbit and maxilla. A.J.R. Am. J. Roentgenol., *127*:473.
42. Larsen, O.D., & Thomsen, M. (1978). Zygomatic fractures. Scand. J. Plast. Reconstr. Surg., *12*:55.
43. LeFort, R. (1901). Étude experimentale sur les fractures de la mâchoire supérieure. Rev. Chir., *23*:208.
44. Mallen, R.W. (1969). Fractures of the nasofrontal complex. Otolaryngol. Clin. North Am., *2*:335.
45. Manson, P.N. (1986). Some thoughts on the classification and treatment of LeFort fractures. Ann. Plast. Surg., *17*:356.
46. McCoy, F.J., Chandler, R.A., Magnan, C.G. et al. (1966). An analysis of facial fractures and their complications. Plast. Reconstr. Surg., *29*:381.
47. Merrell, R.A., & Yanagisawa, E. (1968). Radiographic anatomy of the paranasal sinuses. I. Waters view. Arch. Otolaryngol., *87*:184.
48. Merrell, R.A., Yanagisawa, E., & Smith, H.W. (1969). Abnormal linear density. A useful x-ray sign in the evaluation of maxillofacial fractures. Arch. Otolaryngol., *90*:518.
49. Murray, J.A.M., Maran, A.G.D., Busuttil, A., & Vaughan, G. (1986). A pathological classification of nasal fractures. Injury, *17*:338.
50. Nahum, A.M. (1975). The biomechanics of facial bone fracture. Laryngoscope, *85*:140.
51. Porteder, H., Steinkogler, F.J., & Rausch, E. (1987). 200 fractures of the zygoma. Diagnosis, treatment, complications. Orbit, *6*:223.

52. Robbins, K.T., Harris, J. Jr., Zaluze, D., & Jahrsdoerfer, R. (1986). Radiological evaluation of mid-third facial fractures. J. Otolaryngol., *15*:6.
53. Switzer, P., Pitman, R.G., & Fleming, J.P. (1974). Pneumomediastinum associated with zygomatico-maxillary fractures. Can. Assoc. Radiol. J., *25*:316.
54. Thompson, J.N., Gibson, B., & Kohut, R.I. (1987). Airway obstruction in LeFort fractures. Laryngoscope, *97*:275.
55. Tilson, H.B., McFee, A.S., & Soudah, H.P. (1972). The Maxillo-Facial Works of Rene LeFort. University of Texas, Dental Branch of Houston, Houston.
56. Tofield, J.J. (1977). Pneumomediastinum following fracture of the maxillary antrum. Br. J. Plast. Surg., *30*:179.
57. Valvassori, G.E., & Hord, G.E. (1968). Traumatic sinus disease. Semin. Roentgenol., *3*:160.
58. Whalen, J.P., & Berne, A.S. (1964). The roentgen anatomy of the lateral walls of the orbit (orbital line) and the maxillary antrum (antral line) in the submentovertical view. A.J.R. Am. J. Roentgenol., *91*:1009.
59. Yanagisawa, E., & Greenspan, R.H. (1962). Fractures of zygomatic arch: Unrecognized sign. Arch. Otolaryngol., *75*:424.
60. Yanagisawa, E., Merrell, R.A., & Myerson, M. (1965). X-ray diagnosis of posterior displacement of zygoma. Value of submentovertical base view. Arch. Otolaryngol., *82*:275.
61. Yanagisawa, E., Smith, H.W., & Thaler, S. (1968). Radiographic anatomy of the paranasal sinuses. II. Lateral view. Arch. Otolaryngol., *87*:196.
62. Anda, S., Elsas, T., & Harstad, H.K. (1987). The missing rectus: A CT observation from blow-out fracture of the orbital floor. J. Comput. Assist. Tomogr., *11*:895.
63. Anderson, A.G., Frank, T.W., & Loftus, J.M. (1988). Fractures of the medial infraorbital rim. Arch. Otolaryngol. Head Neck Surg., *114*:1461.
64. Baldwin, L., & Baker, R.S. (1988). Acquired Brown's syndrome in a patient with an orbital roof fracture. J. Clin. Neuro-ophthalmol., *8*:127.
65. Ball, J.B. Jr. (1987). Direct oblique sagittal CT of orbital wall fractures. A.J.R. Am J. Roentgenol., *148*:601.
66. Ball, J.B. Jr., Towbin, R.B., Staton, R.E., & Cowdrey, K.E. (1985). Direct sagittal computed tomography of the head. Radiology, *155*:822.
67. Carothers, A. (1978). Orbitofacial wounds and cerebral artery injuries caused by umbrella tips. J.A.M.A., *239*:1151.
68. Catone, G.A., Morrissette, M.P., & Carlson, E.R. (1988). A retrospective study of untreated orbital blow-out fractures. J. Oral Maxillofac. Surg., *46*:1022.
69. Crikelair, G.F., Rein, J.M., Potter, G.D., & Cosman, B. (1972). A critical look at the "blowout" fracture. Plast. Reconstr. Surg., *49*:375.
70. Crumley, R.L., Leibsohn, J., Krause, C.J., & Burton, T.C. (1977). Fractures of the orbital floor. Laryngoscope, *87*:934.
71. Curtin, H.D., Wolfe, P., & Schramm, V. (1982). Orbital roof blow-out fractures. A.J.N.R. Am. J. Neuroradiol., *3*:531.
72. Dallow, R.L. (1974). Ultrasonography in ocular and orbital trauma. Int. Ophthalmol. Clin., *14*:23.
73. de Visscher, J.G.A.M., & van der Wal, K.G.H. (1988). Medial orbital wall fracture with enophthalmos. J. Craniomaxillofac. Surg., *16*:55.
74. Dodick, J.M., Galin, M.A., Littleton, J.T., & Sod, L.M. (1971). Concomitant medial wall fracture and blowout fracture of the orbit. Arch. Ophthalmol., *85*:273.
75. Dufresne, C.R., Manson, P.N., & Iliff, N.T. (1988). Early and late complications of orbital fractures. Clin. Plast. Surg., *15*:239.
76. Emery, J.M., & von Noorden, G.D. (1975). Traumatic "pseudoprolapse" of orbital tissues into the maxillary antrum: A diagnostic pitfall. Trans. Am. Acad. Ophthalmol. Otolaryngol., *79*:873.
77. Fueger, G.F., Milauskas, A.T., & Britton, W. (1966). The roentgenological evaluation of orbital blow-out injuries. A. J. R. Am. J. Roentgenol., *97*:614.
78. Fujino, T., & Makino, K. (1980). Entrapment mechanism and ocular injury in orbital blowout fracture. Plast. Reconstr. Surg., *65*:571.
79. Gilbard, S.M., Mafee, M.F., Lagouros, P.A., & Langer, B.G. (1985). Orbital blowout fractures. The prognostic significance of computed tomography. Ophthalmology, *92*:1523.
80. Gould, H.R., & Titus, C.O. (1966). Internal orbital fractures: The value of laminagraphy in diagnosis. A.J.R. Am. J. Roentgenol., *97*:618.
81. Guyon, J.J., Brant-Zawadzki, M., & Seiff, S.R. (1984). CT demonstration of optic canal fractures. A.J.N.R. Am. J. Neuroradiol, *5*:575.
82. Habal, M.B., Beart, R., & Murray, J.E. (1977). Mediastinal emphysema secondary to fracture of orbital floor. Am. J. Surg., *123*:606.
83. Hammerschlag, S.B., Hughes, S., O'Reilly, G.V. et al. (1982). Blow-out fractures of the orbit: A comparison of computed tomography and conventional radiography with anatomical correlation. Radiology, *143*:487.
84. Haverling, M. (1972). Diagnosis of blow-out fractures of the orbit by tomography. Acta Radiol., *12*:347.
85. Kersten, R.C. (1987). Blowout fracture of the orbital floor with entrapment caused by isolated trauma to the orbital rim. Am. J. Ophthalmol., *103*:215.
86. Kulwin, D.R., & Leadbetter, M.G. (1984). Orbital rim trauma causing a blowout fracture. Plast. Reconstr. Surg., *74*:969.
87. Leibsohn, J., Burton, T.C., & Scott, W.E. (1976). Orbital floor fractures: A retrospective study. Ann. Ophthalmol., *8*:1057.
88. Lloyd, G.A.S. (1966). Orbital emphysema. Br. J. Radiol., *39*:933.
89. Lloyd, G.A.S. (1975). Fractures of the orbit. p. 180. In Radiology of the Orbit. W.B. Saunders Co., Philadelphia.
90. McArdle, C.B., Amparo, E.G., & Mirfakhraee, M. (1986). MR imaging of orbital blow-out fractures. J. Comput. Assist. Tomogr., *10*:116.
91. Milauskas, A.T., & Fueger, G.F. (1966). Serious ocular complications associated with blowout fractures of the orbit. Am. J. Ophthalmol., *62*:670.
92. Potter, G.D. (1977). Maxillofacial trauma. Syllabus for the Categorical Course on Trauma presented at the Annual Meeting of the American College of Radiology, Houston, 1971.
93. Sanderov, B., & Viccellio, P. (1988). Fractures of the medial orbital wall. Ann. Emerg. Med., *17*:973.
94. Smathers, R.L. (1981). Traumatic intraocular air-fluid level. Can. Assoc. Radiol. J., *32*:180.
95. Smith, B., & Regan, W.F. Jr. (1957). Blow-out fracture of the orbit. Am. J. Ophthalmol., *44*:733.
96. Tonami, H., Nakagawa, T., Ohguchi, M. et al. (1987). Surface coil MR imaging of orbital blowout fractures: A comparison with reformatted CT. A.J.N.R. Am. J. Neuroradiol., *8*:445.
97. Trokel, S.L., & Potter, G.D. (1969). Radiographic diagnosis of fracture of the medial wall of the orbit. Am. J. Ophthalmol., *67*:772.
98. Unger, J.M. (1984). Orbital apex fractures: The contribution of computed tomography. Radiology, *150*:713.
99. Wagle, W.A., Eames, F.A., & Wood, G.W. (1987). Orbital roof blow-in fractures: CT demonstration. J. Comput. Assist. Tomogr., *11*:918.
100. Waring, G.O., & Flanagan, J.C. (1975). Pneumocephalus. A sign of intracranial involvement in orbital fracture. Arch. Ophthalmol., *93*:847.
101. Wojno, T.H. (1987). The incidence of extraocular muscle and cranial nerve palsy in orbital floor blow-out fractures. Ophthalmology, *94*:682.
102. Zilkha, A. (1981). Computed tomography of blow-out fracture of the medial orbital wall. A.J.N.R. Am. J. Neuroradiol., *2*:427.
103. Zizmor, J., Smith, B., Fasano, C., & Converse, J.M. (1962). Roentgen diagnosis of blow-out fractures of the orbit. A.J.R. Am. J. Roentgenol., *87*:1009.
104. Adkins, W.Y., Cassone, R.D., & Putney, F.J. (1979). Solitary frontal sinus fracture. Laryngoscope, *89*:1099.
105. Hybels, R.L., & Weimert, T.A. (1979). Evaluation of frontal sinus fractures. Arch. Otolaryngol., *105*:275.
106. Levine, S.B., Rowe, L.D., Keane, W.M., & Atkins, J.P. Jr. (1986). Evaluation and treatment of frontal sinus fractures. Otolaryngol. Head Neck Surg., *95*:19.
107. Noyek, A.M., & Kassel, E.E. (1982). Computed tomography in frontal sinus fractures. Arch. Otolaryngol., *108*:378.
108. Stanley, R.B. Jr. (1989). Fractures of the frontal sinus. Clin. Plast. Surg., *16*:115.
109. Wallis, A., & Donald, P.J. (1988). Frontal sinus fractures: A review of 72 cases. Laryngoscope, *98*:593.
110. Gruss, J.S. (1982). Fronto-naso-orbital trauma. Clin. Plast. Surg., *9*:577.
111. Gruss, J.S. (1986). Complex nasoethmoid-orbital and midfacial fractures: Role of craniofacial surgical techniques and immediate bone grafting. Ann. Plast. Surg., *17*:377.
112. Gruss, J.S., Mackinnon, S.E., Kassell, E.E., & Cooper, P.W. (1985). The role of primary bone grafting in complex craniomaxillofacial trauma. Plast. Reconstr. Surg., *75*:17.
113. Paskert, J.P., Manson, P.N., & Iliff, N.T. (1988). Nasoethmoidal and orbital fractures. Clin. Plast. Surg., *15*:209.
114. Amaratunga, N.A.S. (1986). Mandibular fractures in children—a study of clinical aspects, treatment needs, and complications. J. Oral Maxillofac. Surg., *46*:637.
115. Amaratunga, N.A.S. (1987). The effect of teeth in the line of mandibular fractures on healing. J. Oral Maxillofac. Surg., *45*:312.
116. Bernstein, L., & McClurg, F.L. (1977). Mandibular fractures: A review of 156 consecutive cases. Laryngoscope, *87*:957.
117. Busuito, M.J., Smith, D.J. Jr., & Robson, M.C. (1986). Mandibular fractures in an urban trauma center. J. Trauma, *26*:826.
118. Chayra, G.A., Meador, L.R., & Laskin, D.M. (1986). Comparison of panoramic and standard radiographs for the diagnosis of mandibular fractures. J. Oral Maxillofac. Surg., *44*:677.
119. Ching, M., & Hase, M.P. (1987). Comparison of panoramic and standard radiographic radiation exposures in the diagnosis of mandibular fractures. Med. J. Aust., *147*:226.
120. Chuong, R., Donoff, R.B., & Guralnick, W.C. (1983). A retrospective analysis of 327 mandibular fractures. J. Oral Maxillofac. Surg., *41*:305.
121. Davis, W.M. Jr. (1989). An interesting condylar fracture revealed by use of computed tomography. Oral Surg. Oral Med. Oral Pathol., *67*:31.
122. Goldberg, M.G., & Williams, A.C. (1969). The location and occurrence of mandibular fractures. Oral Surg., *28*:336.
123. Henny, F.A. (1971). Fractures of the jaws. Semin. Roentgenol., *6*:397.
124. Howard, P., & Wolfe, S.A. (1986). Fractures of the mandible. Ann. Plast. Surg., *17*:391.
125. Kappael, D.A., Craft, P.D., Robinson, D.W., & Masters, F.W. (1974). The significance of persistent radiolucency of mandibular fractures. Plast. Reconstr. Surg., *53*:38.
126. Keniry, A.J., & Orth, D. (1971). A survey of jaw fractures in children. Br. J. Oral Surg., *8*:231.
127. Lehman, J.A., & Sadawi, N.D. (1976). Fractures of the mandible in children. J. Trauma, *16*:773.
128. Lindahl, L. (1977). Condylar fractures of the mandible. Int. J. Oral Surg., *6*:12.
129. Melmed, E.P., & Koonin, A.J. (1975). Fractures of the mandible: A review of 909 cases. Plast. Reconstr. Surg., *56*:323.

130. Miller, R.I., & McDonald, D.K. (1986). Remodeling of bilateral condylar fractures in a child. J. Oral Maxillofac. Surg., *44*:1008.
131. Moilanen, A. (1982). Primary radiographic diagnosis of fractures in the mandible. Int. J. Oral Surg., *11*:299.
132. Morgan, W.C. (1975). Pediatric mandibular fractures. Oral Surg., *40*:320.
133. Myall, R.W.T., Sandor, G.K.B., & Gregory, C.E.B. (1987). Are you overlooking fractures of the mandibular condyle? Pediatrics, *79*:639.
134. Olson, R.A., Fonseca, R.J., Zeitler, D.L., & Osbon, D.B. (1982). Fractures of the mandible: A review of 580 cases. J. Oral Maxillofac. Surg., *40*:23.
135. Seymour, R.L., & Irby, W.B. (1976). Dislocation of the condyle into the middle cranial fossa. J. Oral Surg., *34*:180.
136. Tinder, L.E. (1973). The relationship of mid-face fractures to mandibular fractures in various forms of trauma: Study of 4,015 cases. Mil. Med., *138*:487.
137. Trapnell, D.H. (1977). The "magnification sign" of triple mandibular fracture. Br. J. Radiol., *50*:97.
138. Watts, P.G. (1988). An unusual type of mandibular fracture. Br. J. Oral Maxillofac. Surg., *26*:157.
139. Antonyshyn, O., Gruss, J.S., & Kassel, E.E. (1989). Blow-in fractures of the orbit. Plast. Reconstr. Surg., *84*:10.
140. Ashley, M., & Jones, C. (1997). Pneumomediastinum: An unusual radiographic finding following mid-facial trauma injury. Injury, *28*:229.
141. Assael, L.A. (1993). Clinical aspects of imaging in maxillofacial trauma. Radiol. Clin. North Am., *31*:209.
142. Avrahami, E., Frishman, E., & Katz, R. (1994). CT evaluation of otorrhagia associated with condylar fractures. Clin. Radiol., *49*:877.
143. Avrahami, E., Rabin, A., & Mejdan M. (1997). Unilateral medial dislocation of the temporomandibular joint. Neuroradiology, *39*:602.
144. Bains, R.A., & Rubin, P.A. (1995). Blunt orbital trauma. Int. Ophthalmol. Clin., *35*:37.
145. Beirne, J.C., Butler, P.E., & Brady, F.A. (1995). Cervical spine injuries in patients with facial fractures: A 1-year prospective study. Int. J. Oral Maxillofac. Surg., *24*:26.
146. Boorstein, J.M., Titelbaum, D.S., Patel, Y. et al. (1995). CT diagnosis of unsuspected traumatic cataracts in patients with complicated eye injuries: Significance of attenuation value of the lens. A.J.R. Am. J. Roentgenol., *164*:181.
147. Burm, J.S., Chung, C.H., & Oh, S.J. (1999). Pure orbital blowout fracture: New concepts and importance of medial orbital blowout fracture. Plast. Reconstr. Surg., *103*:1839.
148. Burns, J.A., & Park, S.S. (1997). The zygomatic-sphenoid fracture line in malar reduction. A cadaver study. Arch. Otolaryngol. Head Neck Surg., *123*:1308.
149. Burstein, F., Cohen, S., Hudgins, R., & Boydston, W. (1997). Frontal basilar trauma: Classification and treatment. Plast. Reconstr. Surg., *99*:1314.
150. Cahan, M.A., Fischer, B., Iliff, N.T. et al. (1996). Less common orbital fracture patterns: The role of computed tomography in the management of depression of the inferior oblique origin and lateral rectus involvement in blow-in fractures. J. Craniofac. Surg., *7*:449.
151. Carr, R.M., & Mathog, R.H. (1997). Early and delayed repair of orbitozygomatic complex fractures. J. Oral Maxillofac. Surg., *55*:253.
152. Chacko, J.G., Figueroa, R.E., Johnson, M.H. et al. (1997). Detection and localization of steel intraocular foreign bodies using computed tomography. A comparison of helical and conventional axial scanning. Ophthalmology, *104*:319.
153. Chirico, P.A., Mirvis, S.E., Kelman, S.E., & Karesh, J.W. (1989). Orbital "blow-in" fractures: Clinical and CT features. J. Comput. Assist. Tomogr., *13*:1017.
154. Creasman, C.N., Markowitz, B.L., Kawamoto, H.K. Jr. et al. (1992). Computerized tomography versus standard radiography in the assessment of fractures of the mandible. Ann. Plast. Surg., *29*:109.
155. Daly, B.D., Russell, J.L., Davidson, M.J., & Lamb, J.T. (1990). Thin section computed tomography in the evaluation of naso-ethmoidal trauma. Clin. Radiol., *41*:272.
156. Demianczuk, A.N., Verchere, C., & Phillips, J.H. (1999). The effect on facial growth of pediatric mandibular fractures. J. Craniofac. Surg., *10*:323.
157. Dingman, R.O., & Natvig, P. Eds. (1964). Surgery of Facial Trauma. pp. 230–235. W. B. Saunders Co., Philadelphia.
158. Donat, T.L., Endress, C., & Mathog, R.H. (1998) Facial fracture classification according to skeletal support mechanisms. Arch. Otolaryngol. Head Neck Surg., *124*:1306.
159. Dunya, I.M., Rubin, P.A., & Shore, J.W. (1995). Penetrating orbital trauma. Int. Ophthalmol. Clin., *35*:25.
160. Evans, G.R., Clark, N., Manson, P.N. et al. (1995). Role of mini- and microplate fixation in fractures of the midface and mandible. Ann. Plast. Surg., *34*:453.
161. Fox, L.A., Vannier, M.W., West, O.C. et al. (1995). Diagnostic Performance of CT, MPR and 3DCT imaging in maxillofacial trauma. Comput. Med. Imaging Graph., *19*:385.
162. Freeman, L.N., Selff, S.R., Aguilar, G.L. et al. (1991). Self-compression plates for orbital rim fractures. Ophthal. Plast. Reconstr. Surg., *7*:198.
163. Gabrielli, M.A., Vieira, E.H., Gabrielli, M.F., & Barbeiro, R.H. (1997). Orbital roof blow-in fracture: Report of a case. J. Oral Maxillofac. Surg., *55*:1475.
164. Garri, J.I., Perlyn, C.A., Johnson, M.J. et al. (1999). Patterns of maxillofacial injuries in powered watercraft collisions. Plast. Reconstr. Surg., *104*:922.
165. Gassner, R., Tuli, T., Emshoff, R., & Waldhart, E. (1999). Mountainbiking—a dangerous sport: Comparison with bicycling on oral and maxillofacial trauma. Int. J. Oral Maxillofac. Surg., *28*:188.
166. Gassner, R., Hackl, W., Tuli, T., & Emshoff, R. (1999). Facial injuries in skiing. A retrospective study of 549 cases. Sports Med., *27*:127.
167. Gillespie, J.E., Isherwood, I., Barker, G.R. et al. (1987). Three-dimensional reformation of computed tomography in the assessment of facial trauma. Clin. Radiol., *38*:523.
168. Grant, M.P., Iliff, N.T., & Manson, P.N. (1997). Strategies for the treatment of enophthalmos. Clin. Plast. Surg., *24*:539.
169. Gruss, J.S., & Hurwitz, J.J. (1990). Isolated blow-in fracture of the lateral orbit causing globe rupture. Ophthal. Plast. Reconstr. Surg., *6*:221.
170. Heine, R.D., Catone, G.A., Bavitz, J.B., & Grenadier, M.R. (1990). Naso-orbital-ethmoid injury: Report of a case and review of the literature. Oral Surg. Oral Med. Oral Pathol., *69*:542.
171. Hendrickson, M., Clark, N., Manson, P.N. et al. (1998). Palatal fractures: Classification, patterns, and treatment with rigid internal fixation. Plast. Reconstr. Surg., *101*:319.
172. Hunts, J.H., Patrinely, J.R., Holds, J.B. et al. (1994). Orbital emphysema. Staging and acute management. Ophthalmology, *101*:960.
173. Iinume, T., Hirota, Y., & Ishio, K. (1994). Orbital wall fractures. Conventional views and CT. Rhinology, *32*:81.
174. Johnson, D.H. Jr., Colman, M., Larsson, S. et al. (1984). Computed tomography in medial maxillo-orbital fractures. J. Comput. Assist. Tomogr., *8*:416.
175. Karesh, J.W., Kelman, S.E., Chirico, P.A., & Mirvis, S.E. (1991). Orbital roof "blow-in" fractures. Ophthal. Plast. Reconstr. Surg., *7*:77.
176. Kirath, H., Tumer, B., & Bilgic, S. (1999). Management of traumatic luxation of the globe. A case report. Acta Ophthalmol. Scand., *77*:340.
177. Koltai, P.J., & Rabkin, D. (1996). Management of facial trauma in children. Pediatr. Clin. North Am., *43*:1253.
178. Kuhn, F., Hulda, T., Witherspoon, C.D. et al. (1996). Intraocular foreign bodies: Myths and truths. Eur. J. Ophthalmol., *6*:464.
179. Laine, F.J., Conway, W.F., & Laskin, D.M. (1993). Radiology of maxillofacial trauma. Curr. Probl. Diagn. Radiol., *22*:145.
180. Lambert, D.M., Mirvis, S.E., Shanmuganathan, K. et al. (1997). Computed tomography exclusion of osseous paranasal sinus injury in blunt trauma patients: The "clear sinus" sign. J. Oral Maxillofac. Surg., *55*:1207.
181. Larsen, M., & Wieslander, S. (1999). Acute orbital compartment syndrome after lateral blow-out fracture effectively relieved by lateral cantholysis. Acta Ophthalmol. Scand., *77*:232.
182. Li, K.K., Caradonna, D., Lauretano, A.M., & Iwamoto, M.A. (1997). Delayed blindness after facial fracture repair. Otolaryngol. Head Neck Surg., *116*:251.
183. Linberg, J.V. (1987). Orbital compartment syndrome following trauma. Ophthal. Plast. Reconstr. Surg., *6*:51.
184. Lombardi, S., Sheller, B., & Williams, B.J. (1998). Diagnosis and treatment of dental trauma in a children's hospital. Pediatr. Dent., *20*:112.
185. Longaker, M.T., & Kawamoto, H.K. Jr. (1998). Evolving thoughts on correcting posttraumatic enophthalmos. Plast. Reconstr. Surg., *101*:899.
186. Lustrin, E.S., Brown, J.H., & Novelline, R. (1996). Radiologic assessment of trauma and foreign bodies. Neuroimaging Clin. N. Am., *6*:219.
187. Manfre, L., Nicoletti, G., Lombardo, M. et al. (1993). Orbital "blow-in" fracture: MRI. Neuroradiology, *35*:612.
188. Manson, P.N., Markowitz, B., Mirvis, S. et al. (1990). Toward CT-based facial fracture treatment. Plast. Reconstr. Surg., *85*:202.
189. Martello, J.Y., & Vasconez, H.C. (1997). Supraorbital roof fractures: A formidable entity with which to contend. Ann. Plast. Surg., *38*:223.
190. Mason, P.N., Hoopes, J.E., & Su, C.T. (1980). Structural pillars of the facial skeleton: An approach to the management of LeFort fractures. Plast. Reconstr. Surg., *66*:54.
191. Mayer, J.S., Wainwright, D.J., Yeakley, J.W. et al. (1988). The role of three-dimensional computed tomography in the management of maxillofacial trauma. J. Trauma, *28*:1043.
192. McGrath, C.J., Egbert, M.A., Tong, D.C. et al. (1996). Unusual presentations of injuries associated with the mandibular condyle in children. Br. J. Oral Maxillofac. Surg., *34*:311.
193. McLoughlin, P., Gilhooly, M., & Wood, G. (1996). The management of zygomatic complex fractures—results of a survey. Br. J. Oral Maxillofac. Surg., *32*:284.
194. Moon, M., Pietris, G., & Shapter, M. (1997). Dislocation of the globe into the ethmoid sinuses. Aust. N. Z. J. Ophthalmol., *25*:175.
195. Moore, M.H., David, D.J. & Cooter, R.D. (1990). Oblique craniofacial fractures in children. J. Craniofac. Surg., *1*:4.
196. Moreno, J.C., Fernandez, A., Ortiz, J.A., & Montalvo, J.J. (2000). Complication rates associated with different treatments for mandibular fractures. J. Oral Maxillofac. Surg., *58*:273.
197. Myllyla, V., Pyhtinen, J., Paivansalo, M. et al. (1987). CT detection and location of intraorbital foreign bodies. Fortschr. Rontgenstr., *146*:639.
198. Nolasco, F.P., & Mathog, R.H., (1995). Medial orbital wall fractures: Classification and clinical profile. Otolaryngol. Head Neck Surg., *112*:549.
199. Novelline, R.A. (1993) Three-dimensional CT of facial trauma. p. 323. In Thrall, J.H. Ed.: Current Practice of Radiology. Mosby–Year Book, St. Louis.
200. Oezmen, Y., Mischkowski, R.A., Lenzen, J., & Fischbach, R. (1998). MRI examination of the TMJ and functional results after conservative and surgical treatment of mandibular condyle fractures. Int. J. Oral Maxillofac. Surg., *27*:33.

201. Paoli, J.R., Lauwers, F., Kany, M., & Babayan, G. (2000). Traumatic intracranial impaction of the zygoma: Case report. J. Oral Maxillofac. Surg., *58*:238.
202. Patel, B.C., & Hoffmann, J. (1998). Management of complex orbital fractures. Facial Plast. Surg., *14*:83.
203. Pathria, M.N., & Blaser, S.I. (1989). Diagnostic imaging of craniofacial fractures. Radiol. Clin. North. Am., *27*:839.
204. Perry, M., Banks, P., Richards, R. et al. (1998). The use of computer-generated three-dimensional models in orbital reconstruction. Br. J. Oral Maxillofac. Surg., *36*:275.
205. Rashid, M.A., Wikstrom, T., & Ortenwall, P. (1999). Pneumomediastinum after nasal fracture. Eur. J. Surg., *165*:903.
206. Raustia, A.M., Pyhtinen, J., Oikarinen, K.S. et al. (1990). Conventional radiographic and computed tomographic findings in cases of fracture of the mandibular condylar process. J. Oral Maxillofac. Surg., *48*:1258.
207. Rehm, C.G., & Ross, S.E. (1995). Diagnosis of unsuspected facial fractures on routine head computerized tomographic scans in the unconscious multiply injured patient. J. Oral Maxillofac. Surg., *53*:522.
208. Rhea, J.T., Rao, P.M., Novelline, R.A. (1999). Helical CT and three-dimensional CT of facial and orbital injury. Radiol. Clin. North Am., *37*:489.
209. Rohrich, R.J., Hollier, L.H., & Watumuli, D. (1992). Optimizing the management of orbitozygomatic fractures. Clin. Plast. Surg., *19*:149.
210. Romano, J.J., Manson, P.N., Mirvis, S.E. et al. (1990). Le Fort fractures without mobility. Plast. Reconstr. Surg., *85*:355.
211. Rose, E.H., Norris, M.S., & Rosen, J.M. (1993). Application of high-tech three-dimensional imaging and computer-generated models in complex facial reconstructions with vascularized bone grafts. Plast. Reconstr. Surg., *91*:252.
212. Saleh, T., & Leatherbarrow, B. (1999). Traumatic prolapse of the globe into the maxillary sinus diagnosed as traumatic enucleation of the globe. Eye, *13*:678.
213. Schuknecht, B., Carls, F., Valavanis, A. et al. (1996). CT assessment of orbital volume in late post-traumatic enophthalmos. Neuroradiology, *38*:470.
214. Segev, Y., Goldstein, M., Lazar, M. et al. (1995). CT appearance of a traumatic cataract. A.J.N.R. Am. J. Neuroradiol., *16*:1174.
215. Seiff, S.R., Good, W.V. (1996). Hypertropia and the posterior blowout fracture. Ophthalmology, *103*:152.
216. Seno, H., Mizunuma, M., Nishida, M. et al. (1999). 3D-CT stereoscopic imaging in maxillofacial surgery. J. Comput. Assist. Tomogr., *23*:276.
217. Sevel, D., Krausz, H., Ponder, T. et al. (1983). Value of computed tomography for the diagnosis of a ruptured eye. J. Comput. Assist. Tomogr, *7*:870.
218. Shumrick, K.A., & Campbell, A.C. (1998). Management of the orbital rim and floor in zygoma and midface fractures: Criteria for selective exploration. Facial Plast. Surg., *14*:77.
219. Stamper, R.L. (1995). Intraocular pressure: Measurement, regulation, and flow relationships. pp. 1–31. In Tasman, W., & Jaeger, E.A. Eds.: Duane's Foundations of Clinical Ophthalmology. Vol. 2. Lippincott-Raven Publishers, Philadelphia.
220. Stanley, R.B. Jr., Sires, B.S., Funk, G.F., & Nerad, J.A. (1998). Management of displaced lateral orbital wall fractures associated with visual and ocular motility disturbances. Plast. Reconstr. Surg., *102*:972.
221. Storrs, B.B., & Byrd, S.E. (1988). Radiation exposure to the ocular lens during CT scanning. Pediatr. Neurosci., *14*:254.
222. Strong, E.B., & Sykes, J.M. (1998). Zygoma complex fractures. Facial Plast. Surg., *14*:105.
223. Szachowicz, E.H. (1995). Facial bone wound healing. Otolaryngol. Clin. North Am., *28*:865.
224. Tello, R., Suojanen, J., Costello, P. et al. (1994). Comparison of spiral CT and conventional CT in 3D visualization of facial trauma: Work in progress. Comput. Med. Imaging Graph., *18*:423.
225. Thompson, R., Myer, C.M. 3rd. (1988). Sagittal palate fracture. Ann. Otol. Rhinol. Laryngol., *97*:432.
226. Villarreal, P.M., de Vicente, J.C., & Junquera, L.M. (2000). Traumatic optic neuropathy. A case report. Int. J. Oral Maxillofac. Surg., *29*:29.
227. Weissman, J.L., Beatty, R.L., Hirsch, W.L. et al. (1995). Enlarged anterior chamber: CT finding of a ruptured globe. A.J.N.R. Am. J. Neuroradiol. *16*(4 Suppl.):936.
228. Wesley, R.E., & McCord, C.D. (1982). Tension pneumocephalus from orbital roof fracture. Ann. Ophthalmol., *14*:184.
229. Wittram, C. (1997). Nasopharyngeal cavity narrowing associated with posterior maxilla and pterygoid plate fracture: Report of three cases. Eur. J. Radiol., *24*:222.
230. Yamaoka, M., Furusawa, K., & Iguchi, K. (1994). The assessment of fracture of the mandibular condyle by use of computerized tomography. Incidence of sagittal split fracture. Br. J. Oral Maxillofac. Surg., *32*:77.
231. Yoshioka, N., Tominaga, Y., Motomura, H., & Muraoka, M. (1999). Surgical treatment for greater sphenoid wing fracture (orbital blow-in fracture). Ann. Plast. Surg., *42*:87.

Chapter 12

THE CERVICAL SPINE

with Diego Nuñez Jr., MD, MPH

Formerly, most spinal fractures and spinal cord injuries were due to industrial accidents, particularly in mining,[313, 315, 321, 322] but these types of accidents have decreased because safety precautions have been instituted. However, there has been a definite increase in the number of spinal fractures and associated spinal cord injuries[69] attributable to an increase in auto traffic and traffic accidents.

The pattern, frequency, and distribution of spinal injury vary with the age of the patient, with the nature of the patient population served by the reporting institution, and to some extent with the inclusive dates of the injuries reported.[13, 15, 20, 34] It is generally recognized that the distribution of spinal fractures and dislocations varies throughout the length of the spine, indicating a variance in susceptibility to injury from segment to segment.[1, 11] There are three peaks[11, 324] of incidence (Fig. 12–1): C1-C2, C5-C7, and T12–L2. These peaks were first recognized by Jefferson.[11] In children, fractures of the cervical spine are less frequent, and an appreciable incidence is found in the midthoracic spine and in the upper lumbar spine.[26, 31] In children younger than 12 years of age, injuries commonly involve C1, C2, and the atlanto-occipital articulation.[21, 23, 28] In children older than 12, injuries are distributed throughout the cervical spine similarly to adults.

Fractures involving adjacent vertebrae are also relatively common in children,[24, 26, 27, 29] but fractures of widely dispersed segments of the spinal column are generally rare and a manifestation of severe trauma, and they are often accompanied by spinal cord injury.[324–326] Approximately 20% of spinal fractures are associated with fractures elsewhere.[18, 126]

Spinal cord injuries occur in 10% to 14% of spinal fractures and dislocations.[75] The distribution of spinal fractures in patients who sustain cord injury varies to some extent from the general distribution of spinal fractures noted earlier. The three peaks of incidence (see Fig. 12–1) are in the lower cervical spine, the thoracolumbar junction, and the midthoracic spine.[324] Injuries of the cervical spine produce neurologic damage in approximately 40% of cases,[84, 102] whereas injuries of the thoracolumbar junction produce an incidence rate of 4%, and injuries of the thoracic spine produce an incidence rate of approximately 10%. However, in patients sustaining fractures of the vertebral bodies and posterior elements with some degree of malalignment of the spine, the incidence rate of neurologic deficit is approximately 60%.[22] In 85% of cases spinal cord injury occurs immediately (i.e., at the time of trauma); 5% to 10% of injuries are late complications,[132] and, alarmingly, 5% to 10% of injuries occur[84, 129] in the immediate postinjury period.[17, 84, 319] Late complications are quite likely due to mishandling of the

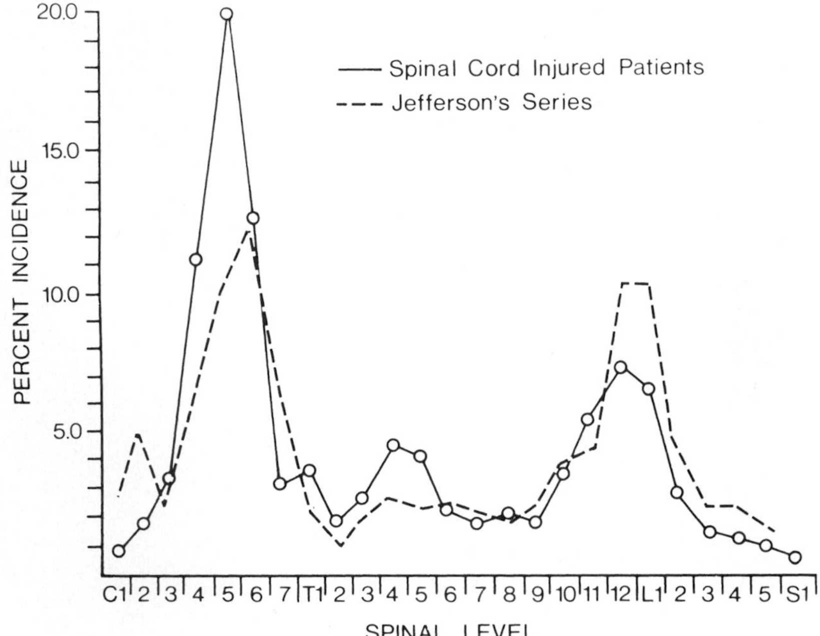

Figure 12–1. Comparison of the distribution of 2006 cases of nonselected injuries of the spine in Jefferson's series[11] with 710 patients of Calenoff and associates[324] with spinal cord injury.

patient, a very important consideration for all concerned in the care of patients with suspected or proven spinal injury. In 10% of cases of traumatic cord injury there is no overt radiographic evidence of vertebral injury.[68, 75, 78, 80, 131, 135] Generally, these cases are in older patients with degenerative arthritic changes of the spine who have sustained hyperextension injuries.[73, 74, 316] The spinal cord becomes compressed between the osteophytic spurs on the posterior margin of the vertebral bodies and the hypertrophied ligamentum flavum, resulting in hematomyelia and an associated neurologic deficit (see Fig. 12–50). On occasion a young individual may sustain a hyperextension injury that results in a spinal cord injury without an associated fracture or dislocation, even in the absence of degenerative changes of the spine.[22, 36]

Anatomy

A vertebra is made up of two components, the *vertebral body* and the *neural arch* (Fig. 12–2). The entire spine can be similarly subdivided into anterior and posterior components. The principal anterior structures are the vertebral bodies, intervertebral discs, and anterior and posterior longitudinal ligaments. The intervertebral disc consists of two portions: the gelatinous, central nucleus pulposus and the surrounding concentric, peripheral layers of the annulus fibrosis. The anterior longitudinal ligament is a taut structure, closely applied to the anterior aspects of the vertebral body and the annulus of the intervertebral discs. The posterior longitudinal ligament, applied to the posterior surface of the vertebral bodies and intervertebral discs, is considerably weaker and less important. The posterior component, the neural arch, is formed by the pedicles, facets, apophyseal joints, laminae, spinous processes, and all intervening ligaments. The ligamentum flavum lines the dorsal surface of the canal, and it is tightly applied to the laminae. The interspinous ligaments interconnect the spinous processes and are overlain by the supraspinous ligament, which connects the dorsal tip of the spinous processes contiguously from the sacrum to the occiput. The capsules of the apophyseal joints complete the principal ligamentous and soft tissue support of the spine.

Biomechanics

Sir Frank Holdsworth[10] subdivided the spine conceptually into two columns: the anterior and the posterior.[16, 19] The anterior column consisted of the vertebral bodies and surrounding and intervening soft tissue structures, whereas the posterior column consisted of the neural arch and intervening soft tissue structures. Holdsworth's basic concept of stability stated that if one of the two columns remained intact, the injury was considered stable. If both columns were disrupted, the injury was unstable. It has since been demonstrated that an isolated disruption of

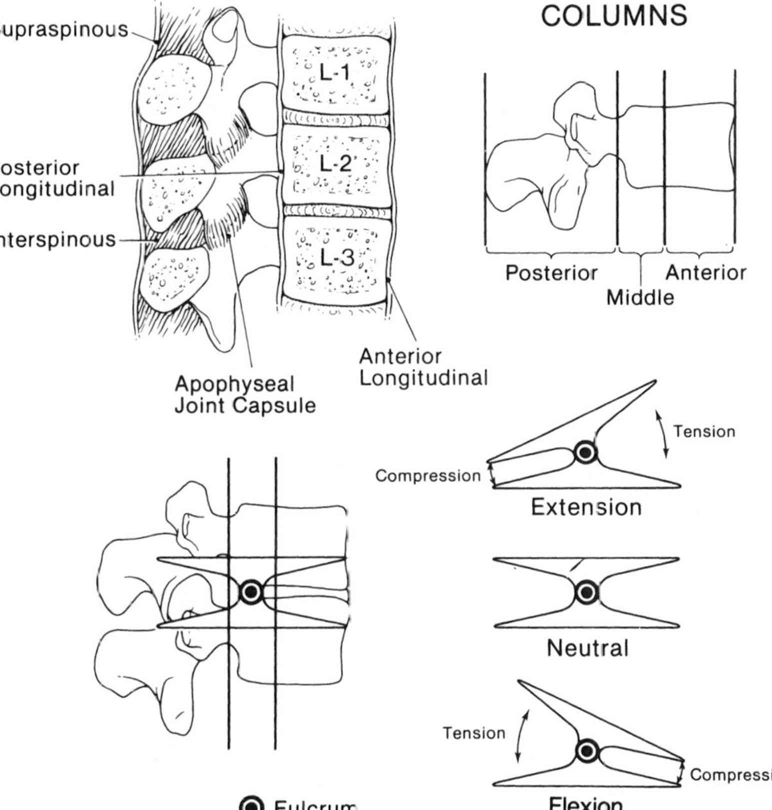

Figure 12–2. Anatomy and biomechanics of the spine. Biomechanically the spine is divided into three columns *(upper right)*. The middle column functions as a fulcrum between two adjacent vertebrae *(lower left)*. In flexion the anterior column is placed in compression and the posterior column in tension, whereas in extension the reverse occurs.

the posterior column associated with an injury of the anterior column does not, in fact, necessarily create instability.

Denis[6, 312] modified Holdsworth's concepts and proposed a three-column theory of spinal stability that better accommodates clinical observations (see Fig. 12–2). The Denis concept is helpful in understanding the biomechanics of injury, and it is useful in the diagnosis and treatment of spinal fractures and dislocations.

The three-column concept proposes that the spine consists of *anterior, middle*, and *posterior* columns. The posterior column is the same as what was proposed by Holdsworth. The Denis anterior column subdivides Holdsworth's anterior column into anterior and middle columns. The Denis anterior column consists of the anterior longitudinal ligament, anterior annulus fibrosis, and anterior part of the vertebral body. The middle or third column consists of the posterior longitudinal ligament, posterior annulus fibrosis, and posterior part of the vertebral body. Conceptually, the third column binds the posterior to the anterior column and functions as a hinge between the two during flexion and extension. It serves as a pivot, like the fulcrum of a teeter-totter, between the anterior and posterior columns. Usually, spinal injuries in which the middle column remains intact are stable, and those in which the middle column is disrupted are unstable.[14]

Pathomechanics of Injury

Injuries to the spine are the result of indirect forces generated by movement of the head and trunk and are only rarely the result of direct blows to the vertebrae. An appreciation of the forces involved[66, 67, 318] in the creation of spinal fractures aids in the assessment of injury. The forces involved are frequently multiple and therefore complex. The combination of flexion, compression, rotation, and shearing is particularly common.[314, 318, 321, 322] However, it is of value to consider the potential forces separately, because each is associated with a relatively specific pattern of injury[4, 5, 7, 8] (Fig. 12–3). In general, compression forces create fractures and rotational and shearing forces disrupt ligaments.

Flexion

Flexion is the most common force operative in spinal injury.[321, 322] In *flexion* the spine is arched anteriorly, pivot-

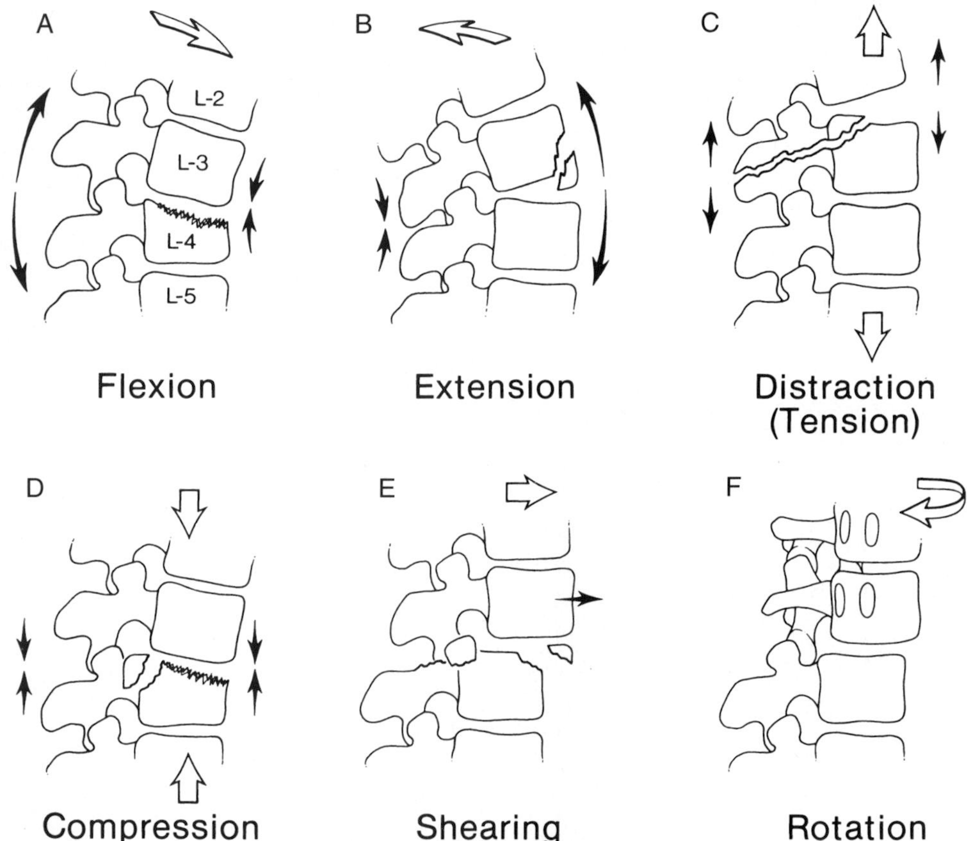

Figure 12–3. Pathomechanics of spinal injury. Each force produces a characteristic injury as visualized on the lateral radiograph. *A*, Flexion creates an anterior, wedged deformity of the vertebral body. *B*, Extension results in a small, triangular fragment separating from the anterior inferior margin of the vertebral body. *C*, Distraction creates horizontal fractures in the posterior elements, and there is little or no wedging of the vertebral body. *D*, Axial compression (as in burst fractures) is characterized by anterior wedging of the vertebral body and retropulsion of the posterior superior margin of the vertebral body. *E*, Shearing is the dominant force in fracture-dislocations, manifested by anterior displacement of the vertebra above the level of dislocation, carrying with it a triangular avulsion fracture from the anterior superior margin of the vertebral body below. Fractures of the laminae and superior facets are commonly encountered. *F*, Rotational forces are combined with shearing to produce an anterior lateral dislocation of the spine.

ing about the fulcrum of the middle column, which results in the generation of compression in the vertebral body and tension within the neural arch posterior to the fulcrum. The maximum forces are focused at the anterior portion of the vertebral bodies, which results in anterior wedging of the vertebral body. As the vertebral bodies are compressed anteriorly, the posterior elements, particularly the spinous processes, laminae, and intervening ligaments, are placed in tension. These tensile forces may produce ligamentous injuries and fractures of the posterior elements. As the head is flexed on the trunk, the maximum force is focused in the cervical spine on the bodies of C4 through C7. As the trunk is flexed on itself the force is focused at the thoracolumbar junction and accounts for the high percentage of fractures occurring between T12 and L2. The force may be directed either anteriorly or laterally. The anterior flexion forces are directed toward the anterior superior margin, and the lateral flexion forces are directed toward the lateral superior margin of the vertebral bodies.

Compression

Compressive forces are difficult to separate from flexion forces. It is helpful to think of the vertebrae in a neutral position, sustaining a vertical or axial load without angulation of the spine. This position results in compression in all three columns, particularly in the anterior and middle columns. The middle column does not function as a fulcrum, as it does in flexion; instead it is subjected to compressive forces. The intact vertebrae and intervertebral discs serve as a shock-absorbing mechanism. As the spine is compressed, the major distortion is a bulge of the vertebral end plate. This bulging causes blood to be squeezed out of the cancellous bone of the vertebral body. As the pressure increases, the end plate bulges more. If the resilience of the end plate is exceeded, a concave fracture of the end plate results. If the compressive forces are even greater, the disc virtually explodes into the vertebral body, creating a comminuted fracture, displacing the fragments centripetally and often resulting in a sagittally oriented fracture within the vertebral body. These fractures have been designated *explosion* or *bursting fractures*.[321, 322] In the lumbar spine this type is known as a burst fracture characterized by retropulsion (posterior displacement) of a fragment from the posterior superior margin of the vertebral body into the spinal canal. In the cervical spine a special variety of this type has been termed a *teardrop fracture* because of the characteristic appearance of the anterior inferior fragment of the vertebral body.[76]

Extension

Extension is the opposite of flexion; the spine is arched posteriorly, pivoting about the fulcrum of the middle column and placing the anterior column in tension and the posterior column in compression. Extension of the head on the trunk creates tension in the anterior longitudinal ligament, which may tear either at the intervertebral disc space or at the margin of a cervical vertebral body and avulse a small fragment from the anterior superior or anterior inferior margin of the vertebral body.[111, 122, 323] The posterior elements of the cervical spine are simultaneously compressed, which may result in fractures of the spinous processes, laminae, and facets. Extension plays a very minor role in thoracolumbar fractures.[25] It probably accounts for the fractures of the pars interarticularis and articular processes of the lower lumbar spine that are occasionally encountered.

Rotation

Rotational forces disrupt the interspinous ligaments and fracture the posterior elements, particularly the articular facets, and laminae. The spinal ligaments withstand tensile and compression forces rather well, but they are very susceptible to disruption by rotation and shearing forces. Rotational forces play a major role in fracture-dislocations of the spine.[321, 322] If you want to dispatch a chicken, you do not flex or extend its neck; you wring it.

Shearing

Shearing refers to a horizontal force applied to one portion of the spine relative to another. The horizontal force may be directed in any direction—anterior, posterior, lateral, or in between. Shearing forces tend to disrupt ligaments and are frequently operative in fracture-dislocation of the thoracic or lumbar spine. Shearing and rotational forces are frequently combined.

Distraction

Distraction refers to forces that are pulling in opposite directions (the opposite of compression). These tensile forces are operative in cervical injuries. The head weighs 10 pounds and is therefore capable of creating a significant degree of inertia and moments of force. The momentum of the head is translated into tensile forces within the cervical spine. The direction of the tensile force is directly dependent on the direction of the movement of the head. If the head is moving away from the trunk, the severity of the compression generated by other simultaneously operating forces, such as flexion or extension, is countered or lessened, and injury of the interspinous ligaments and displacement of the vertebral body elements occur without significant degrees of bony injury.

Pathomechanical Classification

Using the three-column concept of Denis[6, 312] and the forces of injury described earlier, a simplistic classification of spinal cord injuries can be developed (Table 12–1), which is not meant to be comprehensive. Occasional injuries will be encountered that do not readily fit the classification. Some degree of overlap is inevitable; however, the most common injuries are accommodated. The

Table 12–1. Pathomechanical Classification of Spinal Injury

Flexion
Atlantoaxial
Fracture of odontoid
Fracture of lateral mass of C1 or C2 (lateral flexion)
C spine
Compression fracture
T-L spine
Compression fracture
Extension
Atlantoaxial
Atlas (C1)
Neural arch fracture
Avulsion fracture of anterior arch
Axis
Hangman's fracture
Fracture of odontoid
Teardrop fracture of C2
C spine
Hyperextension strain
Spondylytic injury
Spinous process fracture
T-L spine
Pedicle or laminar fracture
Burst
Atlantoaxial
Jefferson's fracture of C1
C spine
Classic teardrop fracture
Classic burst fracture (C6, C7)
Sagittal fracture, vertebral body
T-L spine
Classic burst fracture
Distraction
Atlantoaxial
Atlantoaxial subluxation
C spine
Hyperflexion strain
T-L spine
Classic seat belt fracture (Chance fracture)
Fulcrum fracture
Hyperflexion strain
Translation (Dislocation)
Atlantoaxial
Atlanto-occipital dislocation
Atlantoaxial dislocation
C spine
Unilateral facet lock
Bilateral facet lock
T-L spine
Fracture-dislocation
Dislocation without fracture

mobility and mechanical characteristics warrant dividing the spine into three separate sections: the atlantoaxial spine, consisting of the occipital condyles, atlas (C1), and axis (C2); the cervical (C) spine, consisting of the third through the seventh cervical vertebrae; and the thoracolumbar (T-L) spine, consisting of all the thoracic and lumbar vertebrae. The principal categories in this classification are flexion, extension, burst, distraction, and translation or dislocation. From the standpoint of stability, the middle column remains intact in both pure flexion and extension injuries, whereas it is always disrupted and therefore inherently unstable in burst, distraction, and translation or dislocation injuries. The injury under study can usually be readily classified on the basis of a characteristic appearance of the vertebral body as seen on anteroposterior and lateral radiographs (see Fig. 12–3). Flexion is characterized by an anterior wedge compression of the vertebral body; in extension the vertebral body is either intact or a minimally displaced small avulsion fracture occurs at the anterior superior or anterior inferior margin of the vertebral body. Burst fractures are characterized by retropulsion of a vertebral body fragment into the spinal canal. In distraction injuries the normal anterior height of the vertebral body is maintained, and there is often a horizontally oriented fracture in the neural arch and posterior aspect of the vertebral body. Translation or dislocation refers to either subluxation or frank dislocation as evidenced by malalignment of adjacent vertebral bodies in the axial plane. In flexion, burst, and distraction injuries, there may be angulation of the spine, either anteriorly or laterally, but there is no displacement between the adjacent vertebral segments in the horizontal or axial plane. Using these observations, the principal injuries of the spine can be placed into this pathomechanical classification.

Imaging Techniques

Radiography

With a spinal injury there are two prime questions to be asked: (1) Is a fracture or dislocation present? and (2) Is the injury stable or unstable? The stability of the spinal column is maintained by a combination of bony elements (the vertebrae) and the ligaments, apophyseal joint capsules, and intervertebral discs.[320] The degree of instability depends on the extent of the disruption and the relative strength of the structures that remain intact.[3, 321, 322]

Disruption through bone or soft tissue is equally important in this determination. Because there is no direct radiographic evidence of soft tissue injury, the presence of such injuries must be implied by variations in the alignment of or distance between the bony elements joined by the soft tissue structures[107, 127, 133, 317] in question (Fig. 12–4). Thus, an important clue to the presence of a significant injury is a variation in the distance, either widening or narrowing, between vertebral elements (see Fig. 12–57), particularly the intervertebral disc spaces, the apophyseal joints, and the spinous processes. Similarly, anterior, lateral, or posterior offsetting of adjacent vertebral structures is equally important. Such changes indicate disruption of the intervening soft tissue structures, the intervertebral disc, the apophyseal joint, and the interspinous ligament. It is as important to determine the presence or absence of alignment and the distances between the various portions of the vertebral bodies as it is to identify fractures of the vertebrae themselves. At the time of the radiographic examination, only the residual displacement between vertebral elements is visualized. At the time of injury, there may have been gross displacements that have spontaneously reduced partially or completely, leaving minimal deformities.

Radiographic examination of a possible spinal injury must be tailored to the patient's clinical signs and symptoms.[8, 12] The patient who has an obvious neurologic deficit may require only anteroposterior and lateral views

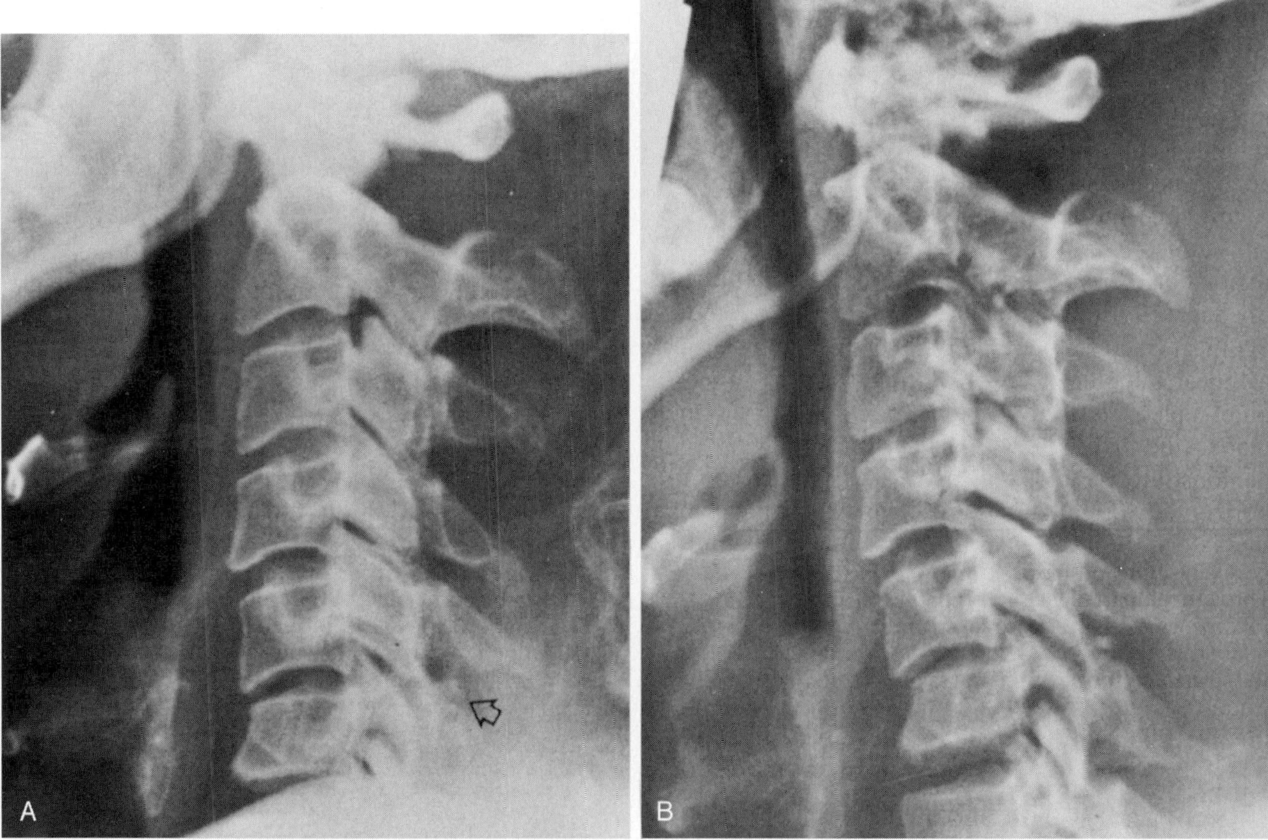

Figure 12–4. Hyperflexion strain at C5-C6 in a 42-year-old man. *A*, The findings on the initial radiographic examination are subtle. The C5-C6 interspace is more narrowed anteriorly than posteriorly. The apophyseal joints at this level are not parallel. A small fracture of the lamina is apparent (*arrow*). *B*, Eleven days later the subluxation is much more obvious. C5 is now offset anteriorly 3 mm.

of the area in question to sufficiently define a fracture or fracture-dislocation, before undergoing computed tomography (CT) or magnetic resonance imaging (MRI). A patient with an acute injury without localizing signs or symptoms will probably require a more complete examination, including oblique projections, to identify or exclude a fracture or dislocation. If these examinations suggest the presence of an injury, either additional special projections or CT might be necessary to clarify or substantiate the lesion in question. The patient whose symptoms persist for some time following injury, even though previous radiographic examination showed no abnormalities, may require all of the special projections, including angled anteroposterior views of the cervical spine and angled oblique views of the facet joints, to exclude or identify an occult fracture. Such an extended examination does not have to be obtained initially in every patient who sustains spinal trauma; this would not be either medically or economically justifiable. On occasion, particularly in the cervical spine, stress views may be required. Stress views are lateral views of the cervical spine obtained in flexion and extension (see Fig. 12–58). They should never be obtained as a matter of routine. When deemed necessary in an acutely injured patient, they should be obtained under the immediate supervision of a physician to avoid creation or extension of a neurologic injury. The patient with multiple organ injuries and suspected cervical spine trauma may benefit from a limited radiographic examination followed by screening CT of the cervical spine.

Computed Tomography

There is some danger of creating or extending an existing neurologic deficit by movement of a patient with an unstable injury of the spine. CT is advantageous because the patient is examined in the supine position, and it can be performed while cervical immobilization or traction is maintained.[62]

The integrity of the spinal canal is easily assessed by CT[2, 49, 60] (Fig. 12–5). The axial projection gives a unique and excellent view that allows precise localization of fracture fragments in relation to the spinal canal[42] and reveals otherwise obscure fractures of the posterior elements.[39, 47, 53, 61, 64] However, horizontal or axially oriented fractures, often only 1 to 2 mm in width, can be overlooked or missed because of partial volume averaging (see Fig. 12–5).

Disruptions of the middle column, particularly those occasioned by burst fractures, are readily assessed and, of equal importance, the distinction is easily made between burst and standard compression fractures.[65] Likewise, CT is useful in assessing fractures that are elusive to radiography, such as those involving the C1-C2 complex, the posterior elements, and the transverse processes.

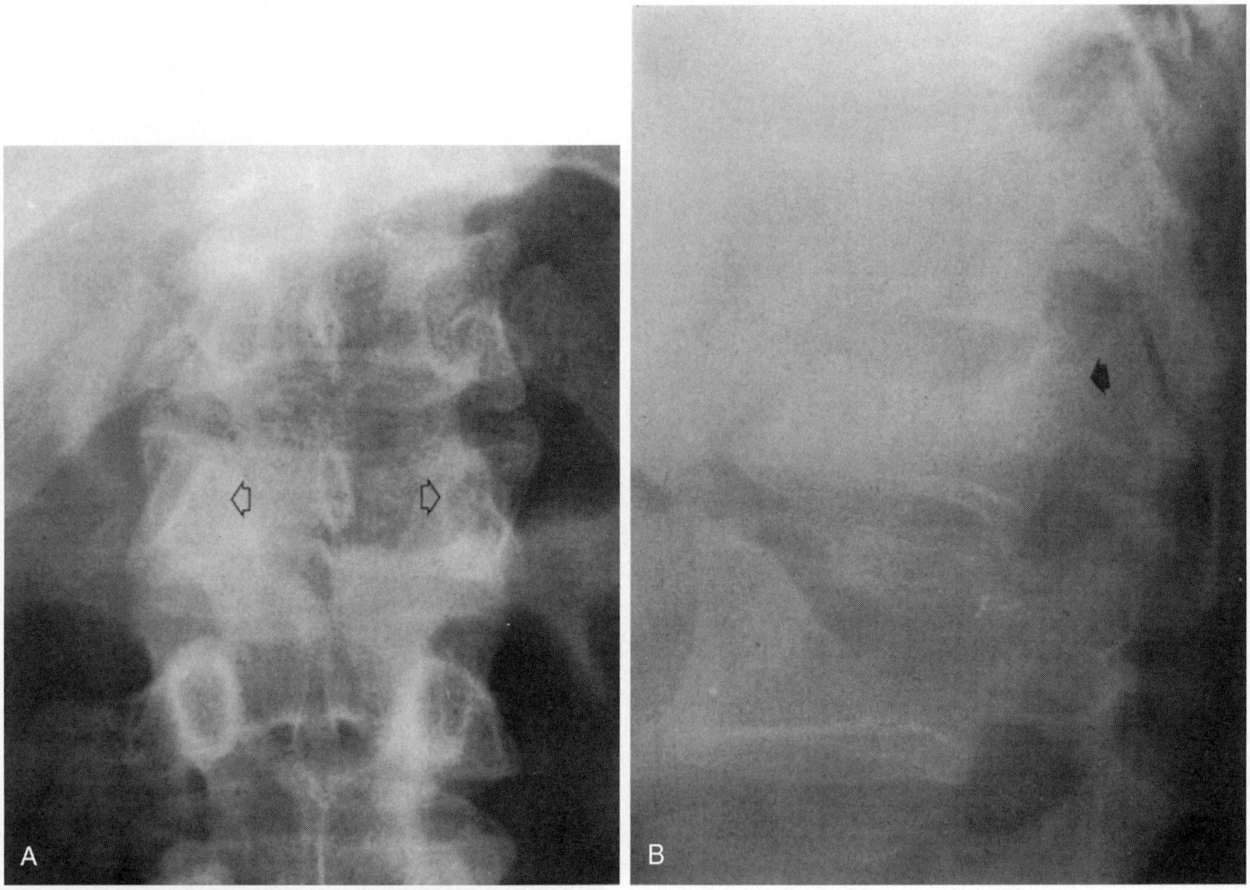

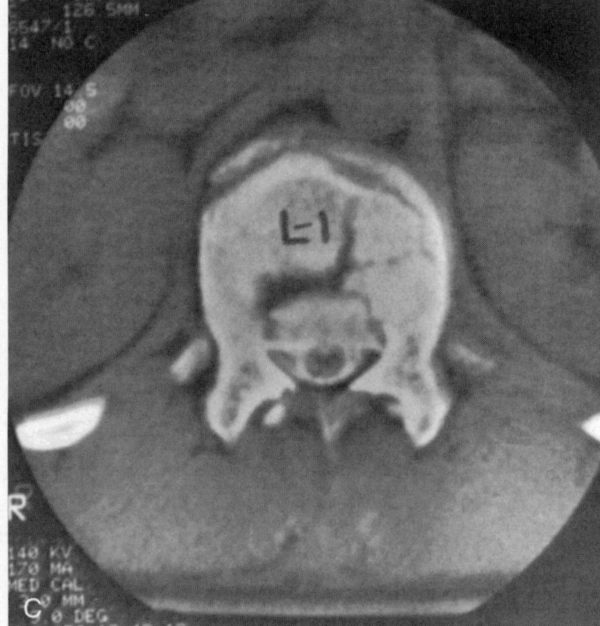

Figure 12–5. Burst fracture of L1 in a 24-year-old man. *A*, Anteroposterior projection demonstrates widening of the interpediculate distance (*arrows*), characteristic of a burst fracture. The vertebral body is flattened. *B*, Lateral radiograph reveals anterior wedging of L1 and retropulsion of a fragment from the posterior superior aspect of the vertebral body (*arrow*), compromising the spinal canal. *C*, CT scan with metrizamide shows retropulsed fragment from the posterior superior margin of the vertebral body compressing the cauda equina. The superior end plate is fragmented. The retropulsed fragment characteristically extends from the medial cortex of one pedicle to that of the other.

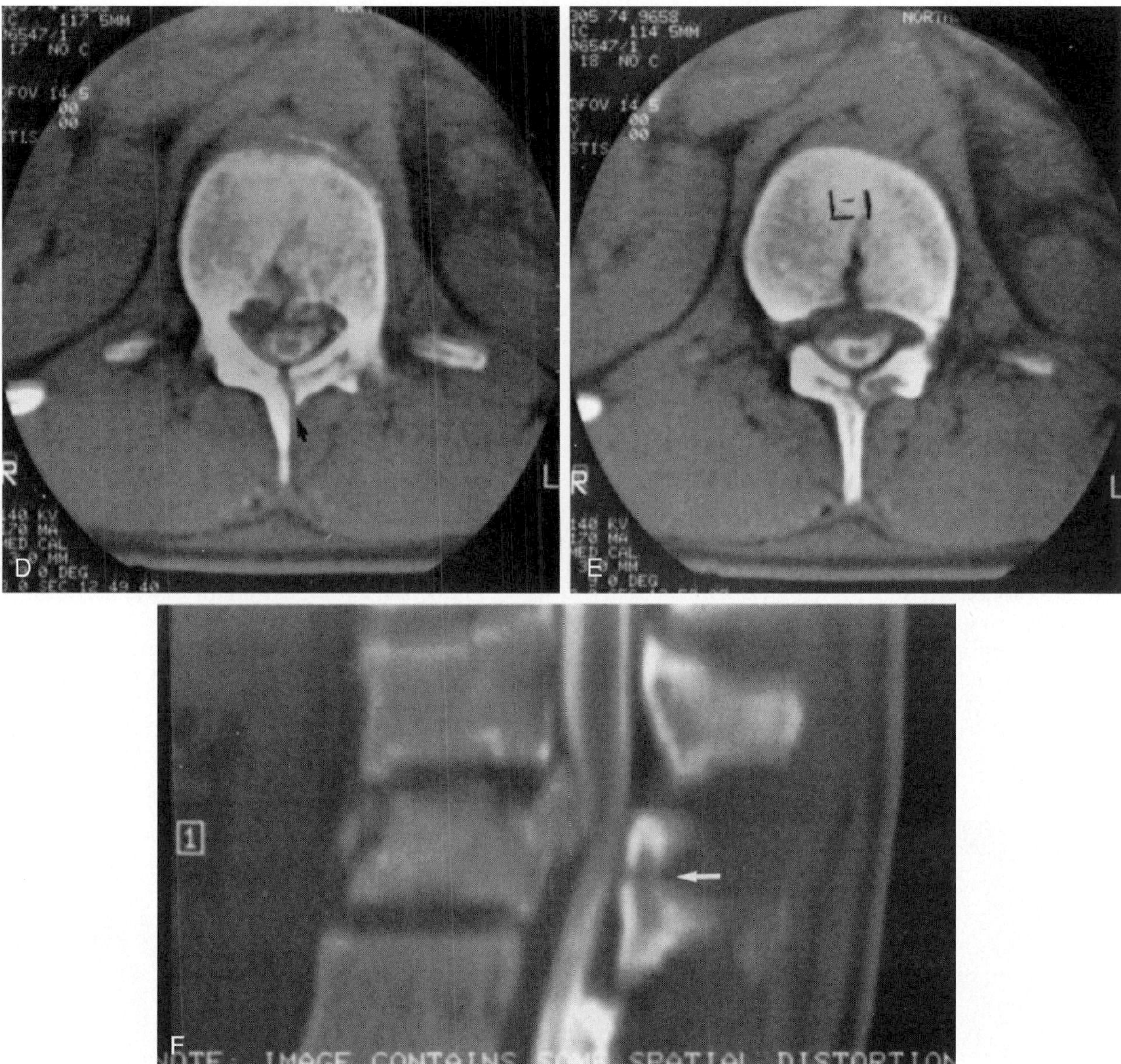

Figure 12–5 *(Continued). D,* A section 5 mm inferior to *C* demonstrates the characteristic fracture of the lamina at its junction with the spinous process *(arrow)*. A hematoma below the level of the burst fragment displaces the subarachnoid space and cauda equina posteriorly. *E,* Characteristic sagittal fracture through the inferior portion of the L1 vertebral body is identified. *F,* Sagittal reconstruction demonstrates the features of a burst fracture to excellent advantage. Note that the reconstruction discloses a horizontally oriented fracture involving the lamina and spinous process *(arrow)* not evident on the axial images.

Although CT affords an exceptional and, in many ways, better view of any given vertebra, the important relationship between adjacent vertebrae is not as easily demonstrated in the axial plane. However, sagittal and coronal reconstructions of CT images do afford an adequate visualization of the relationship between adjacent vertebrae. This is particularly true when using helical (or spiral) CT imaging. Helical CT scanning has expanded the clinical applications of CT and produced a significant impact on how CT examinations are performed. The advantages of helical CT compared with single-section CT include a faster acquisition of a volumetric data set, resulting in a shorter overall examination time. Motion and misregistration artifacts are minimized, and high-quality multiplanar and three-dimensional reconstructions can be obtained. Images obtained with a slice thickness of 3 mm, reconstructed at 1- or 1.5-mm intervals, are typically used for spine imaging and to generate coronal and sagittal reformations.

These advantages are particularly relevant in acutely ill patients and multitrauma victims who require rapid and accurate imaging assessment. In addition, the number of segments that can be examined at any time is no longer limited, as is the case with single-section CT. Longer segments of the spine can now be included in a single acquisition and the recent introduction of multidetector technology will further reduce the time of examination of helical scanning and improve the quality of multiplanar imaging. CT has been used increasingly as a screening modality for patients with high suspicion of cervical spine injury. Thoracic and lumbar spine injuries also can be detected on chest and abdominal CT scans of trauma patients. Such injuries can be assessed by means of reconstructed images, using smaller overlapping intervals from the original data set of images. Ultimately, more detailed information about the extent of injury can be obtained with dedicated spine examinations, using thinner collimation. Thoracolumbar injuries are covered in detail in Chapter 13.

CT myelography (see Fig. 12–5) improves evaluation of the spinal canal, demonstrates dural tears (see Fig. 12–62),[51, 56] and eliminates the need for standard myelography, with the added advantage of not requiring manipulation of the patient.[40, 58] Tomography has been largely replaced by CT, and it is no longer available in most radiology departments.

Magnetic Resonance Imaging

MRI affords a unique and very desirable view of the spine and spinal canal differentiating cerebrospinal fluid and the spinal cord without necessitating the use of contrast media.[46, 55] Furthermore, images may be obtained in any plane without necessitating reconstruction. T_1-weighted, proton density, and T_2-weighted sequences are typically performed for evaluation of spine and cord injuries. The sagittal and axial planes are particularly helpful. Myelomalacia, cord contusion, and transections can be visualized[41, 45, 48, 50, 52, 272] (Fig. 12–6). Unfortunately, the acutely injured patient may not be able to tolerate the examination, and most life-support systems cannot be used in the immediate environment of the MRI system. This notwithstanding, it is possible to demonstrate acute herniations of discs (Fig. 12–7), cord edema, hemorrhage and ligamentous disruptions.[44] When a spinal cord injury is encountered in the absence of fracture or dislocation (or any abnormality) on the plain films and the patient does not require life support, an MRI scan will very likely demonstrate the intrinsic lesion of the cord accounting for the neurologic symptoms.[54] MRI is particularly helpful in the subsequent demonstration of post-traumatic spinal cord atrophy and syringomyelia.[59, 63] MRI has eliminated the need for myelography in the evaluation of spinal cord injury.

Fractures of the Cervical Spine

When there is a strong suspicion of injury to the cervical spine, the initial radiograph should be a horizontal beam lateral view[86, 93, 97, 98, 100, 101, 267]; *this must include all seven cervical vertebrae*[9, 17, 82, 87, 88, 110, 274] (Figs. 12–8 through 12–10). Injuries of C6 and C7 are quite common, but they are easily overlooked if these vertebrae are not included on the lateral radiograph. They are frequently obscured by the overlying shoulders. Pulling down on the arms (see Fig. 12–9) by holding the wrists improves the visualization. If this technique should fail, the swimmer's projection (see Fig. 12–10) should be ob-

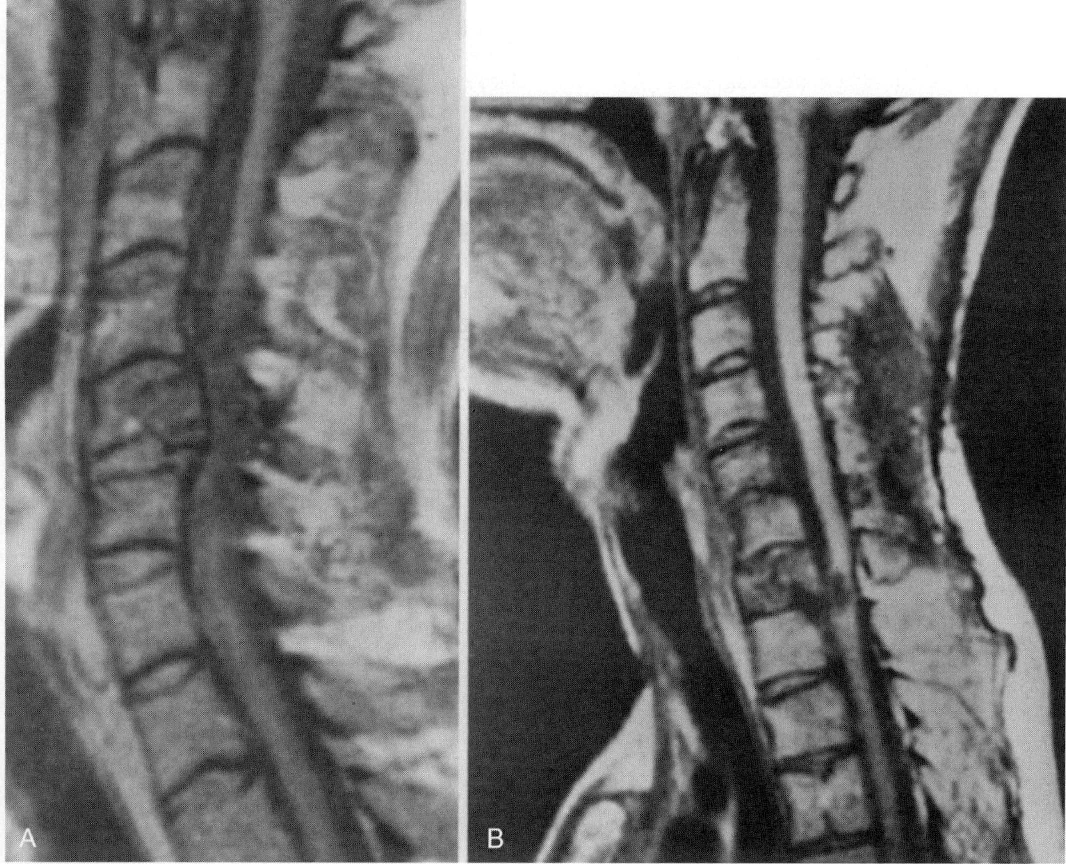

Figure 12–6. Magnetic resonance imaging of spinal cord injuries. *A*, Teardrop fracture of C4 in a 40-year-old man. Sagittal T_1-weighted image demonstrates retropulsion of the vertebral body of C4 with complete transection of the spinal cord. *B*, T_1-weighted image demonstrates focal area of myelomalacia in the spinal cord at the level of a C7 fracture-dislocation in a 25-year-old man.

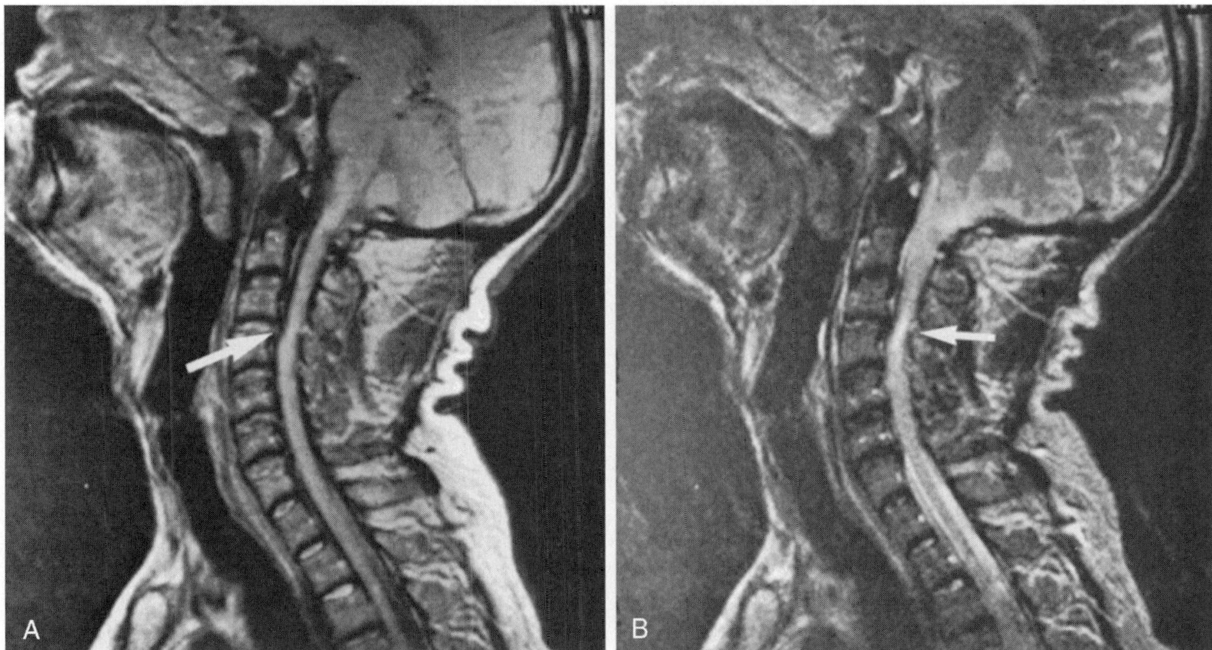

Figure 12–7. Acute herniation of intervertebral disc and spinal cord hematoma without associated fracture or dislocation in a 54-year-old man injured in an auto accident. *A*, T_1-weighted image demonstrates the presence of discal herniation at C3-C4 (*arrow*) compressing the spinal cord. *B*, T_2-weighted image reveals hematoma within the spinal cord at this level (*arrow*).

tained, in which one arm of the patient is extended over the head while the other arm remains by the side. This position places the upper torso in a slightly oblique projection and allows visualization of the cervicothoracic junction. Ultimately, it may prove necessary to resort to CT to demonstrate the lower cervical vertebral bodies. Next, an anteroposterior view of the spine and an open-

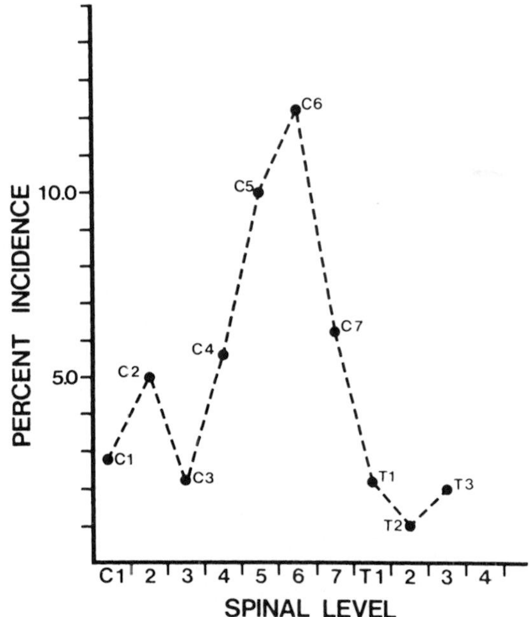

Figure 12–8. Fracture incidence in the cervical and upper thoracic spine. Note the high frequency at C7 and the low frequency at T1 and T2, confirming the importance of including C7 on a lateral radiograph when evaluating cervical trauma.

mouth view of the atlas and axis (C1 and C2) should be obtained. All of these radiographs must be reviewed in sequence to exclude an overt injury (Fig. 12–11) before the decision is made to move the patient to obtain oblique projections or other additional radiographs.[83] It is possible to obtain oblique radiographs while the patient is in the supine position.[1, 88] The tube is angled 30 degrees from the horizontal, and a nongrid cassette is placed flat on the table adjacent to the patient's neck on the side opposite the tube. In the acutely injured patient, flexion and extension views should be obtained only under direct supervision of the physician. The standard cervical spine series consists of five projections: lateral, anteroposterior, anteroposterior open-mouth, and right and left oblique. A basic three-projection trauma series comprising lateral, anteroposterior and open-mouth radiographs is also accepted and performed in many trauma centers.[344, 345] The examination must be tailored to the patient's clinical signs and symptoms and to clarification of abnormalities found on the more routine projections.[90, 104] Special pillar projections, angled views, and flexion and extension views are not obtained unless there is some question of an abnormality on the initial views or in the event of persistent pain following an injury in which the routine views were thought to be normal. We are quite likely to perform CT in the last circumstance.[83]

Radiographic Evidence of Injury

Retropharyngeal Soft Tissue Swelling

An increase in the retropharyngeal soft tissue caused by hemorrhage or edema would seem an obvious clue to the presence of underlying fracture or dislocation of the

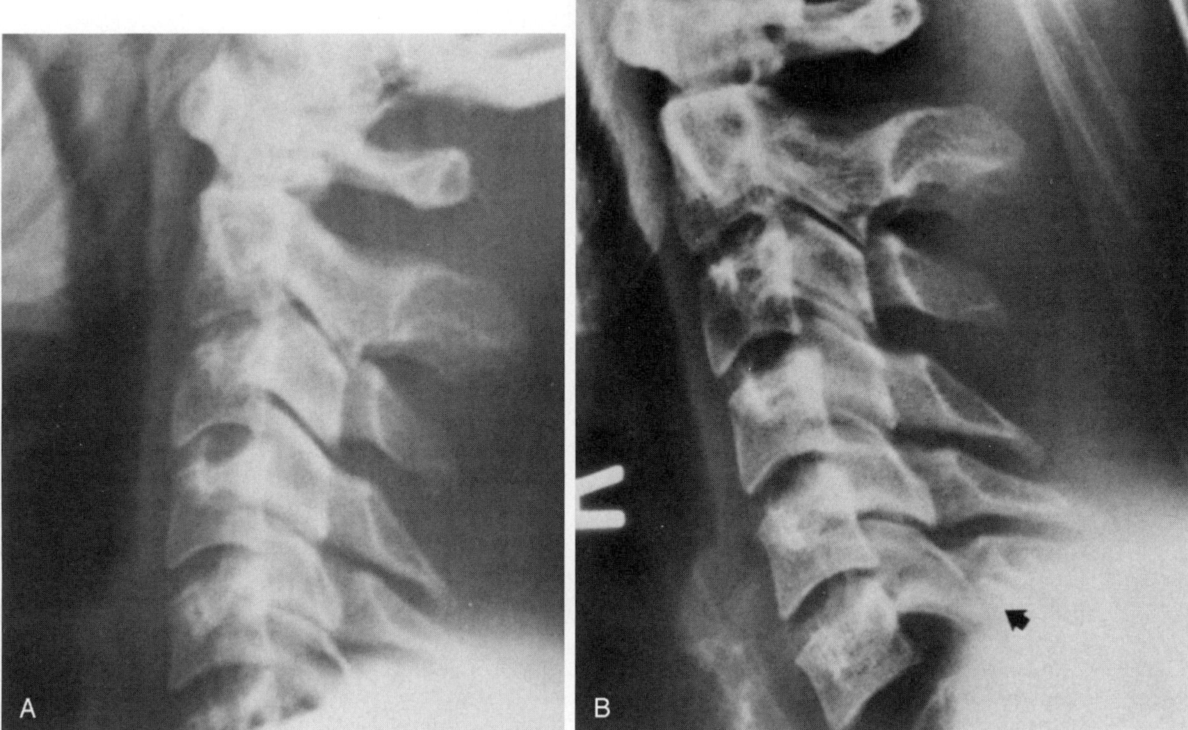

Figure 12–9. Injury to the cervical spine sustained in an auto accident by a 22-year-old man. *A*, At the initial radiographic examination only the first six cervical vertebrae are visualized, and no abnormalities are evident. *B*, Repeat examination obtained while the shoulders were pulled down demonstrates anterior dislocation of C6 upon C7. The anterior displacement of C6 is greater than 50% of the width of the vertebral bodies and is accompanied by bilateral facet locking. Note that the inferior facet of C6 lies anterior to the superior facet of C7 (*arrow*).

cervical spine. Unfortunately, this is only partially true.[92, 95, 103] Because of the broad range of measurements and considerable overlap, it is impossible to establish absolute values that consistently discriminate between normal and abnormal. Penning[95] has suggested the following measurements for retropharyngeal soft tissue as the upper limits of the normal range in adults: 10 mm anterior to the arch of C1, 5 mm anterior to the base of C2, 7 mm anterior to C3 and the upper margin of C4, and 20 mm anterior to C6 and C7. Others have suggested lower values, but lower values are used at the risk of making the measurement too sensitive and the false-positive rate extremely high, as evidenced by the work of Templeton and coworkers[103] (Fig. 12–12). As a rule of thumb, with measurements of 5 mm or less anterior to C3 and C4, underlying injuries are unlikely; with measurements between 5 and 7 mm, injuries are possible but relatively infrequent; with those between 7 and 10 mm, injuries are likely; and with those over 10 mm, injuries are quite probable. Measurements between 5 and 7 mm require close review for underlying injury, but they could be dismissed with no further evaluation beyond a standard five-film series examination. Measurements greater than 7 mm may require further evaluation (i.e., flexion or extension views, pillar views, or CT) to exclude underlying injury, and measurements over 10 mm require stabilization of the spine before any further evaluation, because an injury is almost certainly present whether or not it is immediately obvious on the initial radiographs.

Measurements below C4 are rarely increased even in the presence of extensive injuries of the lower cervical spine; however, increases in these measurements should occasion a closer look at the underlying spine. In particular, make certain that all seven cervical vertebrae are included on the radiograph, and then exclude a C7–T1 dislocation or injury of the upper thoracic spine.

Swelling of the nasopharyngeal soft tissues may be a clue to injuries of C1 and C2, as well as fractures of the facial skeleton. Penning[95] suggested the soft tissues should measure no more than 10 mm anterior to the anterior arch of C1. The presence of adenoidal tissue in children makes this determination more difficult in the younger population than in adults.

In emergency rooms, most lateral radiographs of the spine are obtained with a 40-inch focal spot–film distance. Focal spot–film distance and relative degree of flexion and extension have no appreciable effect on these measurements. As in children, it seems that the thickness of the retropharyngeal soft tissues of adults is increased to some extent in expiration and decreased in inspiration, but this is difficult to control in the traumatized patient.

Although the exact temporal relationship between injury and the appearance of retropharyngeal soft tissue swelling is unknown, hematomas may not be evident on immediate postinjury examinations performed within 2 hours of injury, but they may appear subsequently. Most hematomas clear and the measurements return to normal within 5 to 14 days of injury. Injuries involving anterior structures are more likely to cause an increase in the retropharyngeal soft tissues than those limited to the posterior elements, but this occurrence also is not absolute.

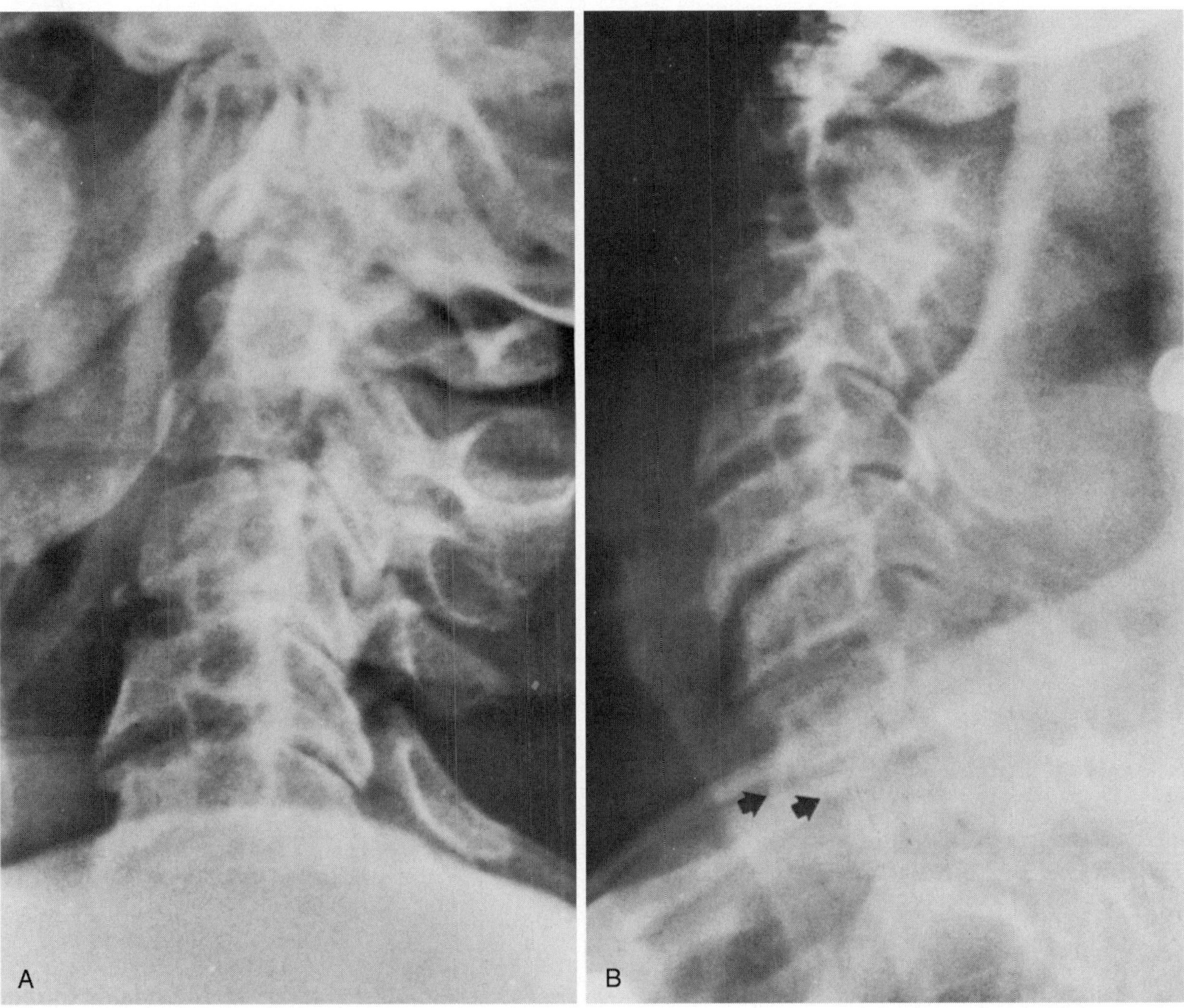

Figure 12–10. Fracture-dislocation in which C7–T1 was not visualized on the initial examination of a 67-year-old man. *A*, Initial radiographic examination visualizes only the first five cervical vertebrae. The patient is heavyset, and it was impossible to visualize the lower cervical spine by pulling down on the arms. *B*, Swimmer's view demonstrates the dislocation at C7 upon T1 (*arrows*).

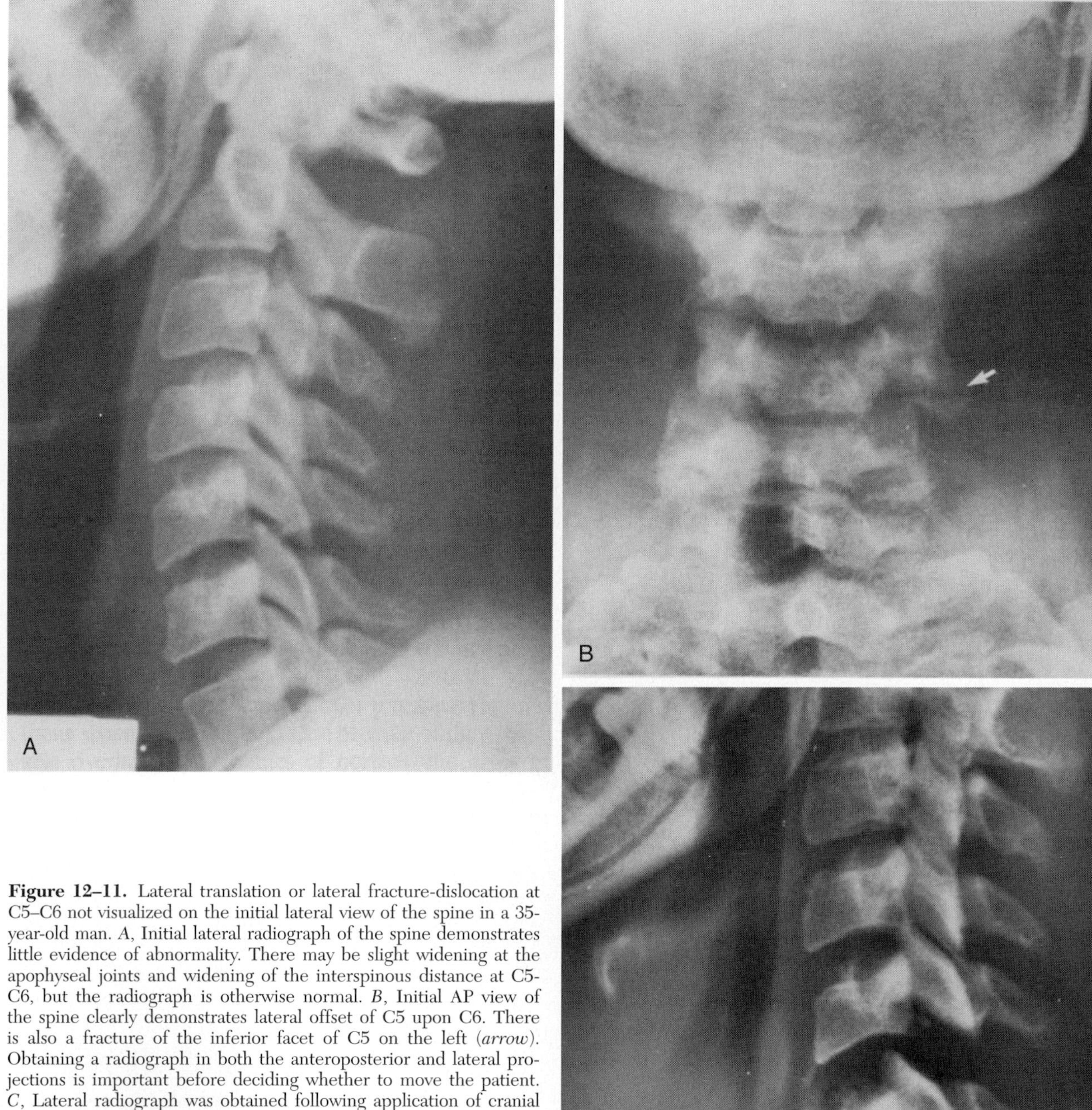

Figure 12–11. Lateral translation or lateral fracture-dislocation at C5–C6 not visualized on the initial lateral view of the spine in a 35-year-old man. *A*, Initial lateral radiograph of the spine demonstrates little evidence of abnormality. There may be slight widening at the apophyseal joints and widening of the interspinous distance at C5-C6, but the radiograph is otherwise normal. *B*, Initial AP view of the spine clearly demonstrates lateral offset of C5 upon C6. There is also a fracture of the inferior facet of C5 on the left (*arrow*). Obtaining a radiograph in both the anteroposterior and lateral projections is important before deciding whether to move the patient. *C*, Lateral radiograph was obtained following application of cranial tongs and 20 pounds of traction. The traction is obviously excessive. There is wide separation of C5 from C6, indicating complete disruption of the intervertebral disc, facet joints, and all intervening ligamentous structures. The extent of the injury is not obvious on the initial radiographic examinations.

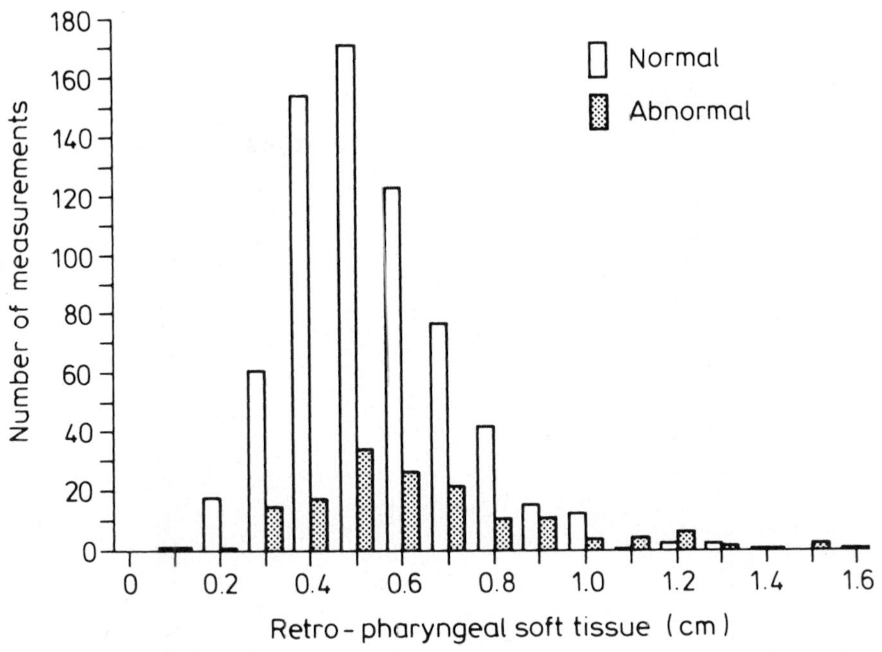

Figure 12–12. Retropharyngeal soft tissue measurements. Histogram of measurements of the retropharyngeal soft tissues at C2, C3, and C4 in 318 patients, including 260 normal subjects and 58 with cervical fractures and/or dislocations. At 7 mm the probability of abnormality increases relative to normality. At 9 mm and greater there is a strong probability of a fracture of dislocation. (From Templeton, P. A., Young, J. W. R., Mirvis, S. E., & Buddemeyer, E. U. [1987]. The value of retropharyngeal soft tissue measurements in trauma of the adult cervical spine. Skeletal Radiol., *16*:98.)

The prevertebral fat stripe,[105] a lucent stripe just anterior to the anterior longitudinal ligament, is identified with insufficient frequency for changes or displacements to be of value in the diagnosis of underlying spinal injury. In most cases, the cervical fat stripe is not demonstrated.

In general, measurements of the retropharyngeal soft tissue space are of limited value because of the considerable overlap of the ranges of normal and abnormal. Many patients with fractures do not demonstrate an increase in the width of the retropharyngeal soft tissues.

Malalignment

Very serious injuries may be manifested by seemingly minor degrees of malalignment (Fig. 12–13; see also Figs. 12–4 and 12–61). They are often subtle and easily overlooked unless specifically sought by employing disciplined search patterns.[115] By visually joining component parts of the vertebral column, lines and curves can be formed that are useful in determining the presence or absence of correct alignment. On the lateral view, four separate gently anterior convex lines are formed (Figs. 12–14 and 12–15) by joining the anterior and posterior margins of the vertebral bodies, the anterior margins of the spinous processes at their junction with the laminae, and finally the posterior tips of the spinous processes.[9, 87, 88, 161] In actuality, only the first three of these lines are of any value. The anterior vertebral line is the most obvious and useful, but as patients get older and spur formation and other changes of spondylosis occur, it becomes increasingly difficult to draw the curve accurately. In older patients, the alignment of the vertebral bodies is better determined by the posterior vertebral body line. Subtle malalignments are often more readily appreciated when the spine is viewed horizontally rather than vertically (see Fig. 12–61). Similarly, on the frontal view (see Fig. 12–15), lines joining the lateral margins of the vertebrae on each side and another joining the spinous processes in the midline should form a straight line or at best three parallel gentle curves in the presence of muscle spasm of the neck or angulation of the head on the neck. Any abrupt reversal in angulation or disruption of these lines should alert the observer to the possibility of an underlying injury. The lateral cortex or lateral margin of the lateral masses should form a smooth, undulating, uninterrupted line. The line is disrupted by fractures of the lateral mass and dislocations of the facet joints. The normal lordotic curvature of the cervical spine depends on the status of contraction of the paravertebral muscles and the relative position of the head. In the presence of muscle spasm the curve is straightened. When the head is flexed on the neck in the military position with the chin tucked in, the lordotic curve is actually slightly reversed. One should be aware of these positional variations. The fulcrum of flexion in adults is at C5-C6, whereas in children it is at C2-C3. In the young child a physiologic anterior offset of C2 upon C3 may be visualized (Fig. 12–16).[45] Occasionally, there is a similar offset of C3 upon C4. The latter may occur either in isolation or in association with a similar offset at C2-C3. These may be seen or encountered even up to age 30 and should not be mistaken for subluxation.

It is easy to overlook the soft tissue manifestations of significant underlying spinal trauma. It is particularly important to evaluate the width of the intervertebral disc spaces. Trauma to the intervertebral disc is manifested by a decrease in height of the disc space[115] (see Fig. 12–4). This may be subtle. Recognition depends on the observation that the involved disc space is narrower than the adjacent intervertebral disc spaces above and below the space in question. Minimal narrowings may be very difficult to visualize at first glance. Pure lateral translocation of the spine without anterior-posterior offset may be manifest on the lateral view only by apparent narrowing of the intervertebral disc space. Thus, it is important to obtain an anteroposterior and lateral view of the spinal area in question before manipulating the patient.

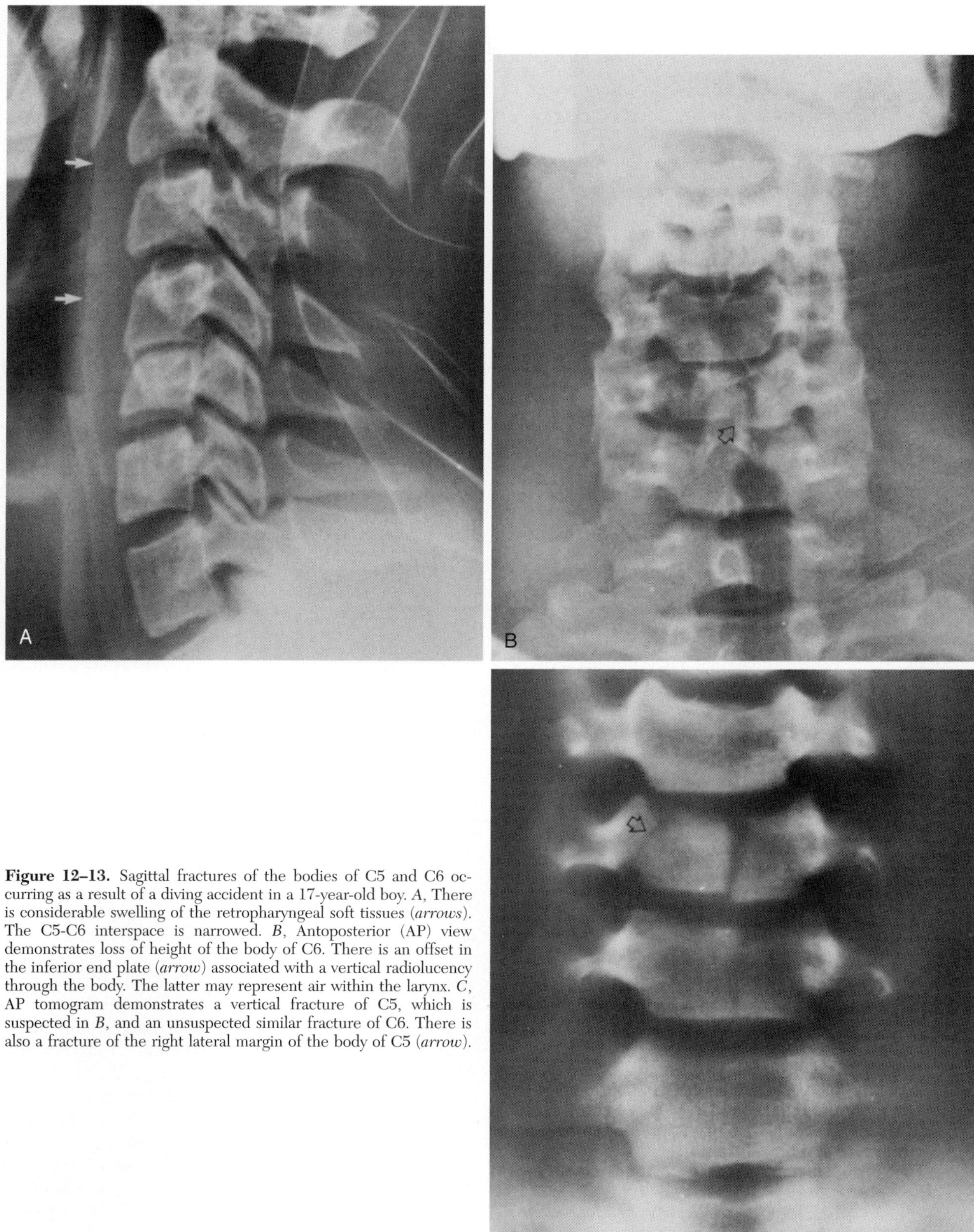

Figure 12–13. Sagittal fractures of the bodies of C5 and C6 occurring as a result of a diving accident in a 17-year-old boy. *A*, There is considerable swelling of the retropharyngeal soft tissues (*arrows*). The C5-C6 interspace is narrowed. *B*, Antoposterior (AP) view demonstrates loss of height of the body of C6. There is an offset in the inferior end plate (*arrow*) associated with a vertical radiolucency through the body. The latter may represent air within the larynx. *C*, AP tomogram demonstrates a vertical fracture of C5, which is suspected in *B*, and an unsuspected similar fracture of C6. There is also a fracture of the right lateral margin of the body of C5 (*arrow*).

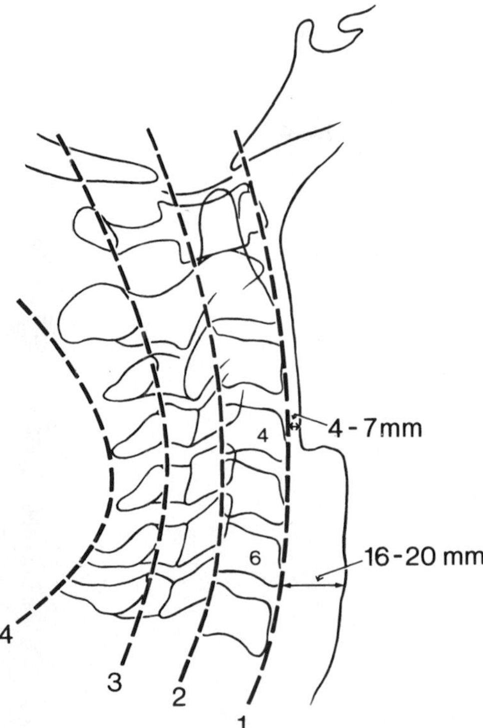

Figure 12–14. Convex lines of the cervical spine. The first line is formed by joining the anterior margin of all vertebral bodies, the second by joining the cortical margins of the vertebral bodies, the third by joining the anterior margins of the junctions of the spinous processes and laminae, and the fourth by joining the posterior tips of the spinous processes. The fourth line is useless. The retropharyngeal soft tissue measurements given here must be considered relative, as explained in the text. (From Rogers, L. F., & Lee, C. (1984). Cervical spine trauma. Clin. Emerg. Med., 3:275.)

The distance between the spinous processes[88, 125] (the interspinous distance) of the cervical spine is an important clue to injuries of the interspinous ligaments and therefore the posterior column (see Fig. 12–11). Widening of the interspinous distance can be demonstrated on either the lateral or frontal view.[125] At times the spinous processes are not well visualized on the initial lateral radiograph. Rotational displacement is demonstrated by lateral displacements of the spinal processes to the affected side as visualized on the anteroposterior projection (see Fig. 12–55*A*).

Abnormalities of Height of the Vertebral Body

Variations in height of the vertebral body consist of varying degrees of anterior wedging with or without comminution of the vertebral body.[103] The height of the fourth or fifth vertebral or both may be less than that of the adjacent third and sixth vertebral bodies. This decrease is generalized without associated wedging and is a normal variant. If the anterior height of a vertebral body measures 3 mm or more less than the posterior height, a fracture of the vertebral body can be assumed. Anterior wedging of the vertebra is due to varying combinations of flexion and axial compression. The wedge is formed predominantly by a depression of the superior end plate (see Fig. 12–46). If a pure flexion force is operative, a simple wedge fracture occurs. At times this may be accompanied by a small triangular fragment from the anterior superior surface of the vertebral body (see Fig. 12–46*B*).

The Value of Computed Tomography and Magnetic Resonance Imaging

Radiography remains accepted as the technique of choice for initial evaluation of an injured cervical spine. This practice is supported by the fact that if the results of an adequately exposed and properly positioned radiographic series of the spine are normal, it is unlikely that CT will reveal a fracture. However, there is sufficient evidence that a significant number of fractures can be missed if the evaluation of the cervical spine relies exclusively on radiography.* These claims are particularly valid for the subset of patients who meet multiple trauma criteria for whom radiography has a limited value. Woodring and Lee[347] reported the limitations of radiography in detecting fractures, using a retrospective review of radiographs and CT scans in 216 patients with cervical spine fractures. They determined prospectively that radiography did not detect fractures in 23% of their patients and that the cervical injuries were unstable in 50%. Our own experience[337, 339] indicates that radiography can miss up to 57% of fractures. In a series by Acheson and colleagues,[38] only 47% of fractures were seen or suspected on initial screening radiographs when compared with those ultimately detected by CT. A frequent limitation of radiography is the inadequate visualization of the cervical thoracic junction in unconscious and uncooperative multiple trauma victims. In addition, overlying nasogastric and endotracheal tubes, dental pieces, and motion can affect optimal demonstration of the C1-C2 complex. Thus, significant delays can occur when largely relying on radiography to determine that the spine is not injured. Repeated exposures are frequently necessary before adequate radiographs are obtained in this subset of obtunded and uncooperative patients. To overcome these shortcomings of radiography, other imaging protocols have been proposed with the goal of improving sensitivity while avoiding unnecessary delays.[337, 338]

CT has been proposed as an adjunct to radiography in the setting of cervical spine trauma.[327, 329, 334, 336–338, 340] The use of section-limited CT to image the portions of the spine that are inadequately shown by radiography has been proposed. Specifically, the routine evaluation of the C1-C2 complex in patients undergoing CT of the brain has been recommended, based on the high frequency of undetected fractures of the cranial cervical junctions by radiography.[329, 334] From the standpoint of efficient patient care in a busy trauma center, a significant delay of clearance of the cervical spine is still found with this approach. One can be frequently confronted with a problem of having to obtain multiple radiographs to clear the proximal or distal cervical spine, and even after obtaining those films, this ability of those areas may still be unsatisfactory. Nuñez and associates[337] describe the routine CT examina-

---

*See references 329, 330, 334, 337, 339, 341–343, 346, 347.

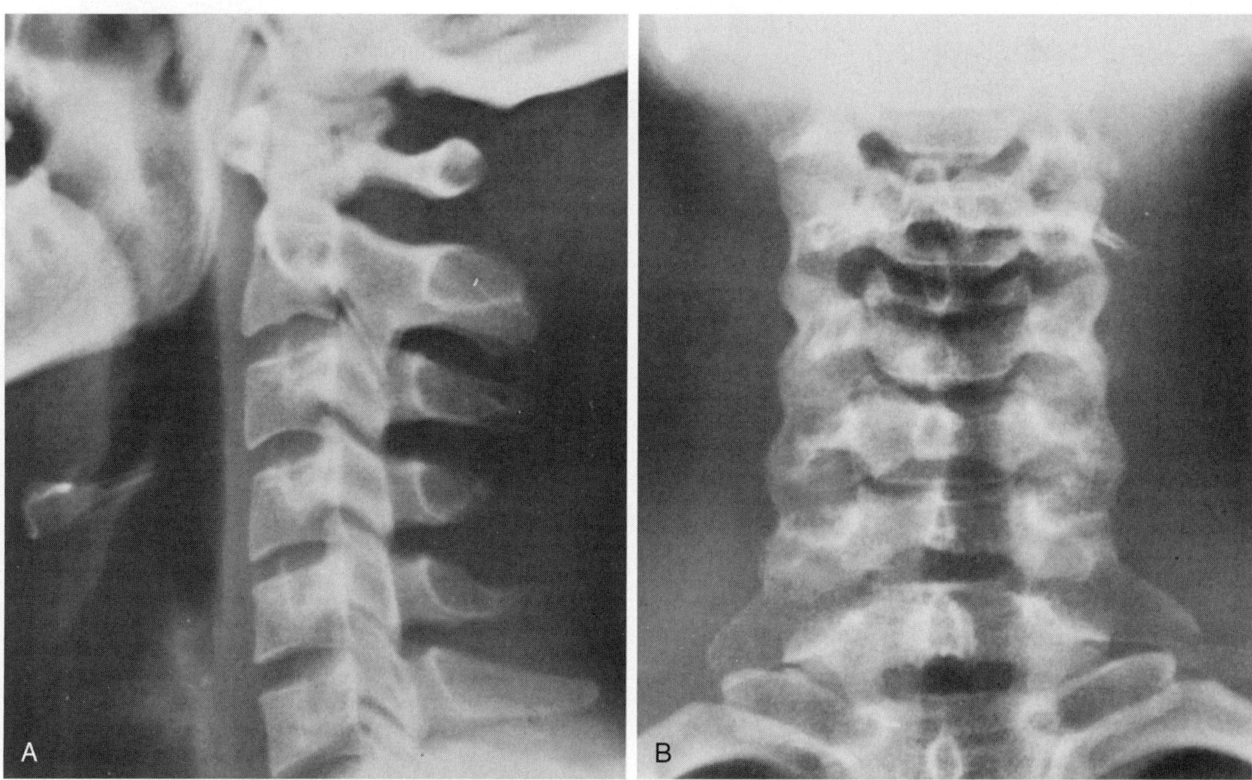

Figure 12–15. Normal cervical spine. *A*, Alignment of the cervical spine is evaluated on the lateral view by means of four separate anteriorly convex lines (see text for explanation). The degree of convexity of these lines is reduced by muscle spasm and the position of the chin. The curves are increased when the head is extended on the neck and reduced when the head is flexed. Note also the prevertebral fat stripe. *B*, The alignment of the cervical spine is evaluated on the anteroposterior view by means of lines. Note that the vertebral bodies are equal in height and that the apposing cortical margin of the intervertebral disc and the apophyseal joints are roughly parallel.

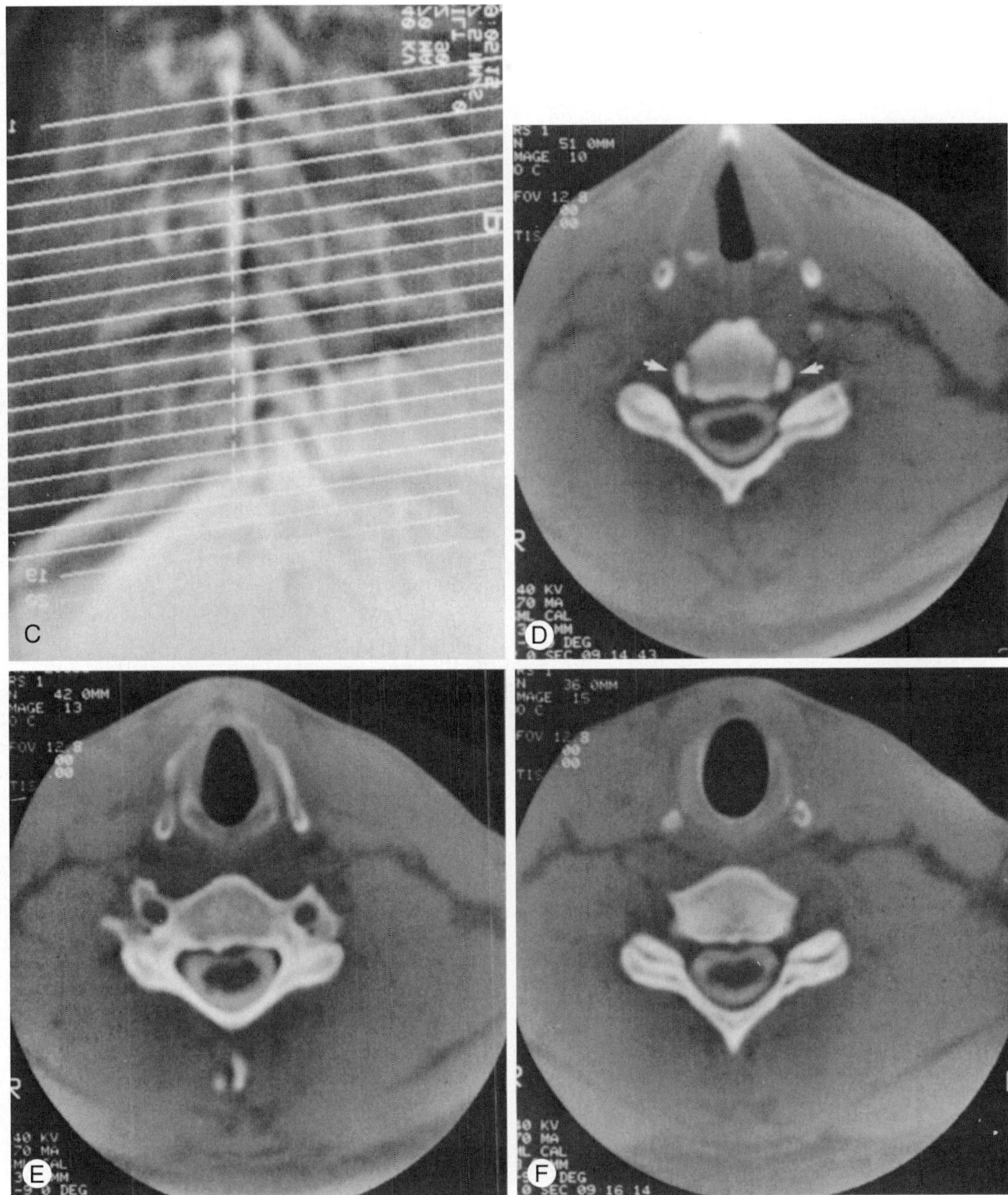

Figure 12–15 *Continued. C*, Lateral digital radiograph demonstrating plane of 3-mm slices. *D*, Slice 10 through the inferior end plate of C5 demonstrates uncinate processes of C4 (*arrows*). Metrizamide outlines the subarachnoid space and spinal cord. The superior facet of C6 is convex anteriorly and lies anterior to the inferior facet of C6, which is convex posteriorly and contiguous with the laminae. *E*, Slice 13 through the upper portion of the sixth cervical vertebra at the level of the pedicles demonstrates the lateral processes and foramen for the vertebral artery. *F*, Slice 15 through the lower aspect of the sixth vertebral body demonstrates the characteristic silhouette of the facets at this level. Note the biconvexity of the superior facets anteriorly and the clawlike appearance of the inferior facets posteriorly.

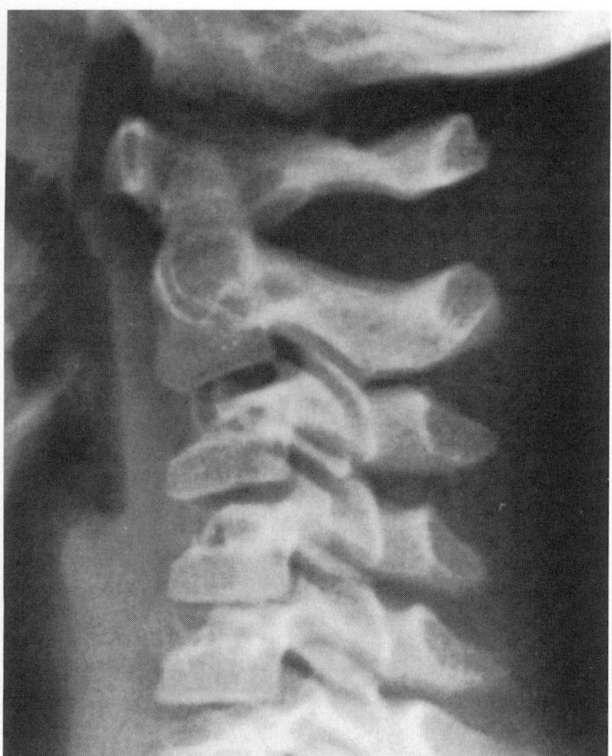

Figure 12–16. Pseudosubluxation of C2 upon C3 in a 5-year-old boy. Lateral radiograph demonstrates characteristic angulation occurring in youngsters at the level of C2-C3. This is normal, but it can be misconstrued as a dislocation by the unwary. Note also the V-shaped predens space.

tion, not only for documented spine trauma but also for patients who were undergoing CT of the brain and/or abdomen to evaluate other possible injuries. Using CT in this manner avoided double use of the scanner, and with this practice they also demonstrated that an important number of fractures are not shown by radiography. A recent publication by Blackmore and colleagues[328] has supported this practice from a cost-effectiveness point of view. In addition, Hanson and coworkers[333] have reported on the validity of a clinical decision rule that can distinguish between patients at high and low risk for cervical spine injury. Patients who are stratified as being at high risk for injury are selected to undergo helical CT screening of the cervical spine. The current trend is to rely on radiography for patients at a lower risk for cervical spine injury in whom an adequate examination can be easily obtained. For patients at higher risk, who are obtunded and clinically unevaluable, there appears to be a role for screening CT. In general, patients with suspected acute cervical spine injury are initially evaluated by radiography (lateral radiograph and/or complete trauma series), and depending on the clinical scenario, cervical CT may be used as a screening or as a complementary modality to radiography. MRI is indicated in all patients with partial or progressive neurologic deficit after cervical spine injury,[331, 332] as well as in patients with potential mechanical instability owing to ligament injury or associated intervertebral disc injury. Emergency MRI is indicated in these cases, because surgical decisions may be based in part on MRI findings.[340] The presence of hemorrhagic versus nonhemorrhagic cord contusion and how that relates to neurologic recovery have been reported. In addition, the presence or absence of cord compression by bone, disc, or hematoma allows one to answer the basic question of whether immediate decompressive surgery should be performed.[340]

Specific Cervical Spine Injuries

Craniovertebral Junction (Atlanto-occipital Articulation) and Junction of C1 and C2

The atlas and axis are structurally and functionally distinct from the remaining cervical vertebrae.[155, 169] The atlas, or C1, is a ring structure consisting of two lateral articular masses joined by thin anterior and posterior arches. The lateral articular masses contain the superior and inferior facets. A thin transverse process extends from each lateral articular mass and contains a foramen through which passes the vertebral artery. The superior facets of the atlas articulate with the occipital condyles, and the inferior articular facets articulate with the superior articular facets of the axis. The axis, or C2 (Fig. 12–17), consists of a vertebral body on which is situated a bony protrusion, the dens. The dens articulates with the anterior arch of the axis. The superior articular facets of the axis are broad, sloping surfaces on the superior surface of the pedicles and vertebral body just lateral to the dens. They are sloped laterally. At their medial margin a notch is formed with the base of the dens. This notch is variable in appearance and may be mistaken for a cortical disruption, suggesting a fracture. The pedicles of the axis are pierced by the foramina transversaria transversing superiorly and posterolaterally. The foramina divide the pedicles into two short segments, one thin and more variable, located anteriorly and inferiorly, and one more substantial, located posteriorly and superiorly. The posterior segments form broad bases with the laminae. The laminae are broadened on their inferior margins to form the inferior articular facets.

The peculiar bony structure at the craniovertebral junction is associated with its own unique ligamentous structure.[87, 88] Broad ligamentous structures extend from the anteroposterior surfaces of the spinal canal to the margins of the foramen magnum. The dens is attached to the anterior margin of the foramen magnum by three separate ligaments, one apical and two alar, each extending from the right and left lateral surfaces of the dens. A tough ligament extends between the lateral articular masses of C1: the transverse ligament or ligamentum transversum. The dens lies between this ligament and the anterior arch of the atlas. A true joint is formed between the dens and the anterior arch of the atlas, and a synovial-lined pouch is present between the posterior surface of the dens and the ligamentum transversum to form a true joint on the posterior surface.

These peculiar structural arrangements confer a great range of rotation, flexion, and extension upon the cranium relative to the cervical spine. The fulcrum of flexion and extension of the cranium on the neck lies at C2.[150] The

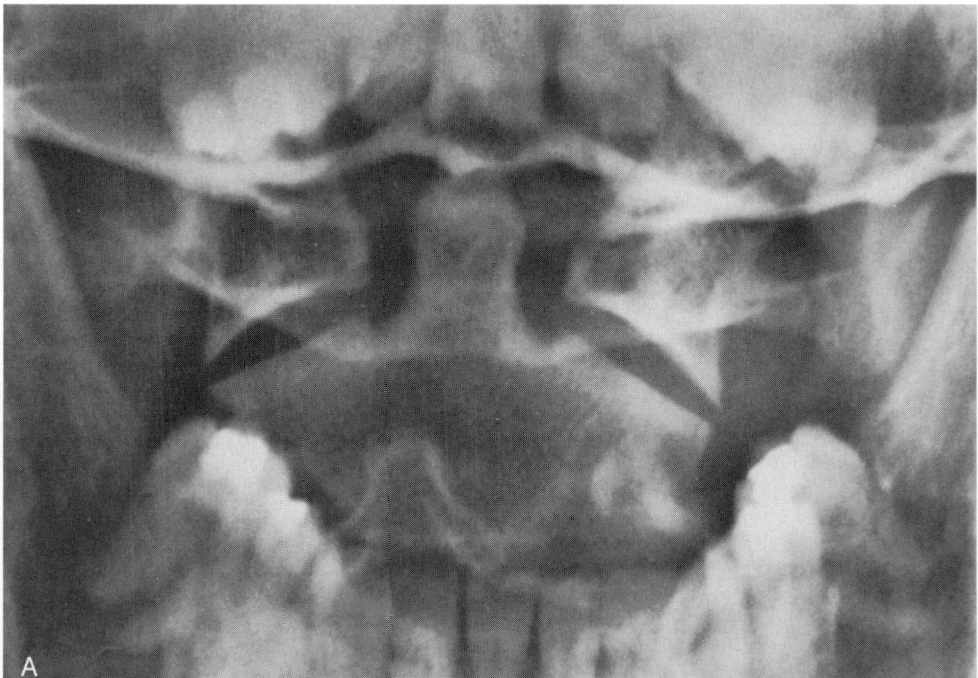

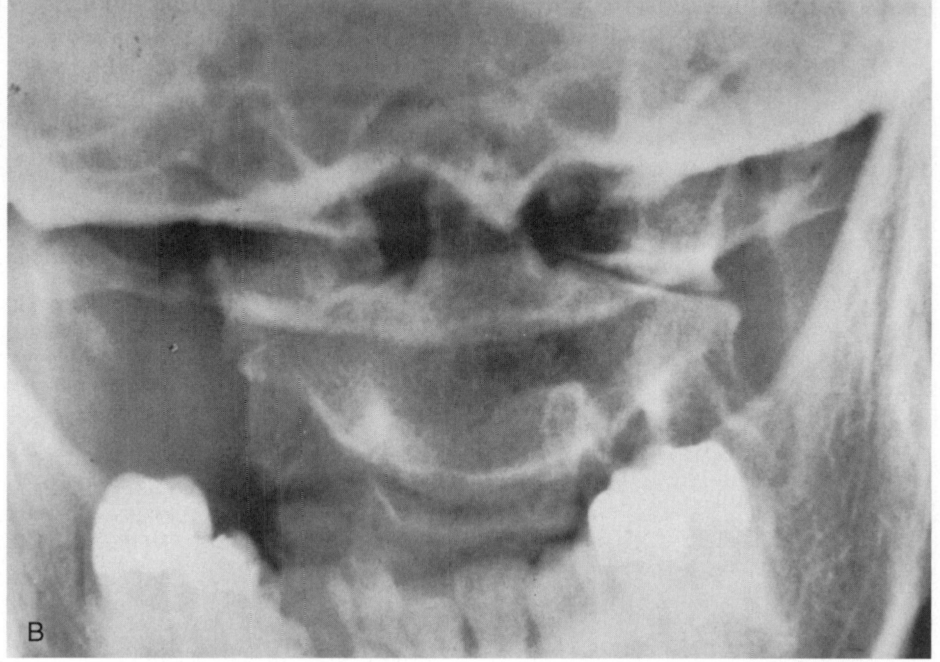

Figure 12–17. Open-mouth anteroposterior view of C1 and C2. *A*, This radiograph was obtained with the head in the neutral position. Note the normal notches at the base of the dens. *B*, In this radiograph with the head tilted to the right, the right lateral mass of C1 is offset laterally from the lateral margin of C2, whereas the left lateral mass of C1 is medially offset in comparison with the apposing margin of C2. Furthermore, the distance between the medial margin of the right lateral mass and the dens is now increased, whereas the same distance on the left is correspondingly decreased.

weight of the cranium is transmitted through the occipital condyles and atlas to the superior articular facets of the axis. It is then divided into three portions and transmitted inferiorly and anteriorly through the vertebral bodies and intervertebral discs and posteriorly through the pedicles onto the inferior articular facet and from there to the other apophyseal joints.

In a properly positioned radiograph, in the neutral position C1 sits squarely upon C2 without offset (see Fig. 12–17*A*); that is, the lateral margin of the lateral articular mass of C1 lies exactly opposite the apposing lateral margin of C2.[87, 88, 156, 157, 170] The distance between the medial margin of the lateral articular mass of C1 and the dens is symmetric. With rotation or tilting of the head, C1 moves as a unit toward the side to which the head is rotated or abducted (see Figs. 12–17*B* and 12–15). The lateral articular mass of C1 is then offset laterally toward the side of this motion, and the distance between the medial margin and the lateral mass and the dens increases on this side. On the opposite side there is a corresponding medial offset of the lateral articular mass of C1 and abbreviation of the distance between the medial borders of the lateral mass of the dens, which produces a unilateral offset, usually of a magnitude of 1 to 2 mm, and rarely up to 4 mm.

Fracture of the craniovertebral junction is rarely the result of direct trauma. These fractures usually result from forces transmitted through the cranium and its contents. The nature of the resultant injury depends on the extent and direction of the force and the relative position of the head and neck. From the clinical standpoint, fractures and dislocations at the craniovertebral junction are rarely associated with permanent neurologic deficits, although transient paresis may occur, but examination of individuals who died in automobile and other traffic accidents has demonstrated an appreciable incidence of craniovertebral junction injuries.[110, 137, 138] There is no discrepancy between these statements because a neurologic deficit at this level in most situations leads to immediate death. With immediate resuscitation it is possible that an occasional patient with a high spinal cord transection may survive.

The important radiographs in the evaluation of craniovertebral injuries are the anteroposterior open-mouth projection and the lateral view of the cervical spine. CT is frequently required for full clarification of all abnormalities.[142] Many injuries at the craniovertebral junction are only minimally displaced or simply overlooked if CT is

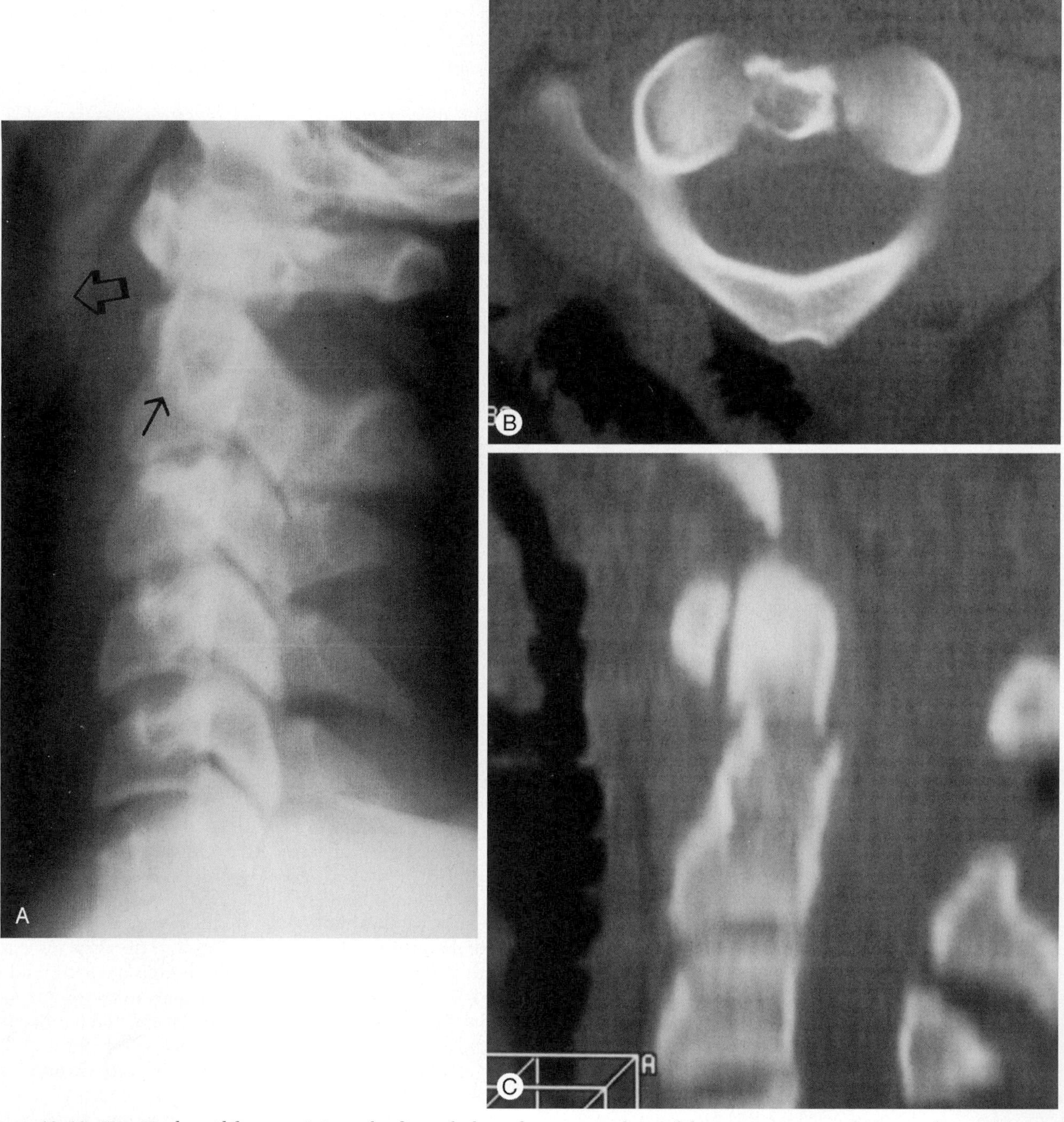

Figure 12–18. Type II odontoid fracture. *A*, Lateral radiograph shows discrete irregularity of the anterior contour of C2 ring of cortical bone (*solid arrow*) and evidence of soft tissue swelling (*open arrow*). *B*, Axial CT image reveals focal irregularity of the anterior contour of C2, at the level of the base of the odontoid. *C*, Sagittal CT reformation shows a moderately displaced, transversely oriented fracture of the base of the odontoid.

not performed (see Fig. 12–34). Similarly, axially oriented, minimally displaced fractures may be overlooked on CT because of partial volume averaging if reconstructed images are not obtained. Therefore, before all injuries can be safely excluded, it is necessary to obtain reconstructed CT in both projections (Fig. 12–18). In difficult cases, CT may ultimately have to be performed before all questions are satisfactorily resolved. Craniovertebral injuries are frequently associated with soft tissue swelling in the retropharynx and nasopharynx (see Fig. 12–28). The important bony relationships to determine are of the dens to the anterior arch of the atlas, the lateral masses of C1 to the superior facets of C2, the dens to the body of C2, and the body of C2 to the body of C3. If all these relationships are normal, the majority of significant injuries can be excluded.

Approximately 25% of fractures of C1 and C2 are associated with other fractures of the spine.[147, 164, 178, 235] The most common combination is fracture of the atlas associated with a second fracture of the axis[209] (see Fig. 12–21A); however, associated fractures and fracture-dislocations of the lower cervical spine and cervicothoracic junction are not unusual, occurring in approximately 8%[164] (Fig. 12–19). Less commonly, the second injury is located in the midthoracic spine or thoracolumbar junction. The combination of injuries may be due to sequential flexion and extension, but simultaneous forces acting at two or more levels of the spine seems more likely. For instance, the head could be extended on the neck, creating hyperextension fractures of the craniovertebral junction, at the same time the neck is flexed on the body, resulting in flexion injuries at the cervicothoracic junction (Fig. 12–20). On occasion, fractures are identified at three levels; for example, craniovertebral junction, lower cervical spine, and upper thoracic spine.

Injuries of the craniovertebral junction infrequently result in spinal injury at this level. When a neurologic deficit is encountered and a fracture of C1 or C2 is

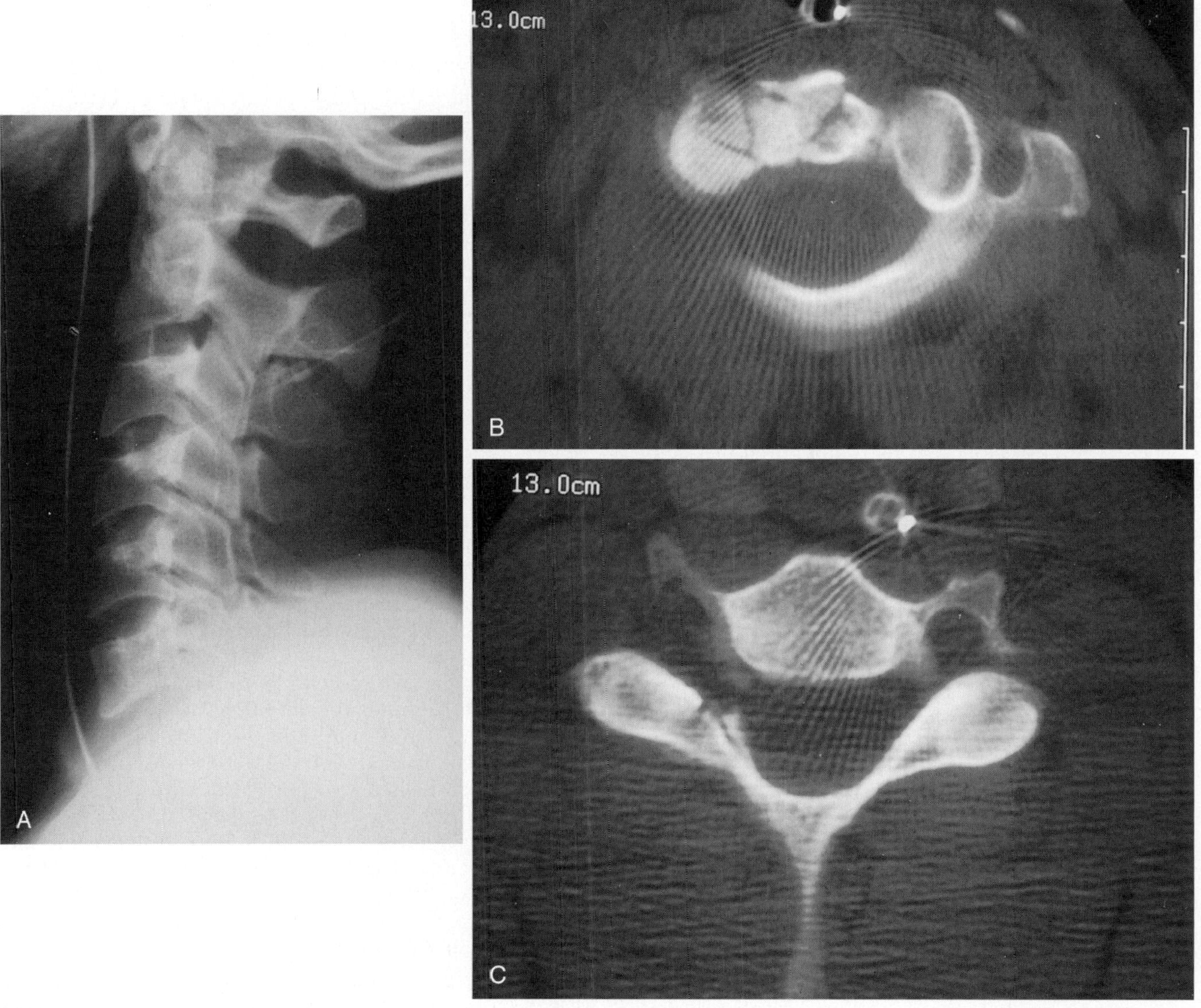

Figure 12–19. Type III odontoid fracture, and associated right laminar fracture of C6. *A*, Lateral radiograph shows indistinctness of the C2 ring anteriorly. *B*, Axial CT image at the level of C2 reveals comminuted type III odontoid fracture with extension to the lateral aspect of the vertebral body. *C*, Axial CT image obtained at the level of C6 reveals fracture of the right lamina with displaced bony fragment into the spinal canal.

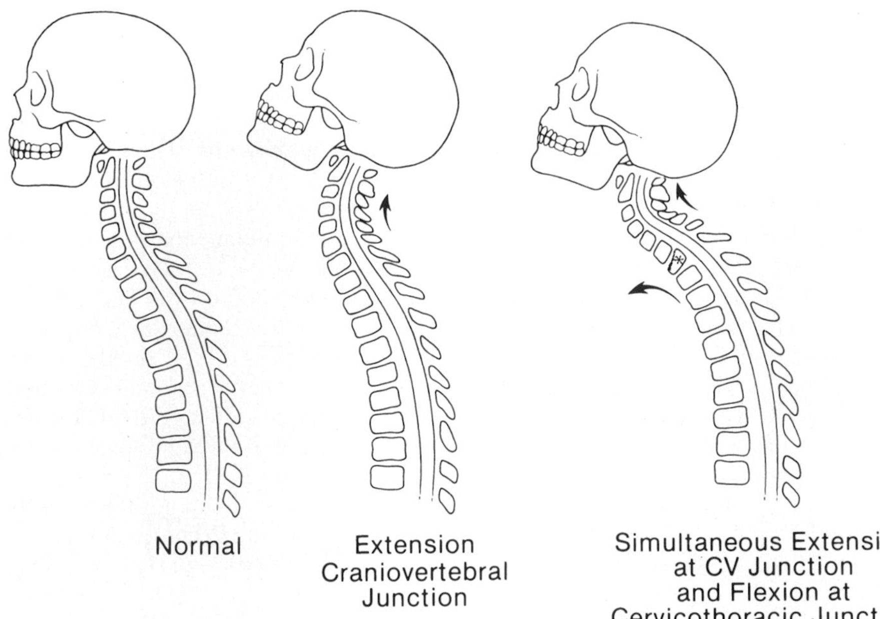

Figure 12–20. Simultaneous injuries of the craniovertebral and cervicothoracic junction are most likely the result of simultaneous extension of the head on the neck and flexion of the neck on the thorax (*right*).

identified, it is quite likely that a second lower level injury resulted in the neurologic deficit. Whenever a fracture of C1 or C2 is identified, one must still visualize the seventh cervical vertebra, and if a neurologic deficit is present, the entire spine should be examined in the anteroposterior and lateral projections.[242]

Atlas

Fracture of the Neural Arch

The most common fracture of C1 is a bilateral vertical fracture through the neural arch[177, 179, 209, 212] (Fig. 12–21*A*). This type of fracture is caused by hyperextension of the head on the neck, which compresses the neural arch of C1 between the occiput and the neural arch of C2. It is best demonstrated on the lateral view. Characteristically, because of the ligamentous attachments, there is minimal displacement, but there may be some angulation at the fracture site. It carries no risk of neurologic deficit. This fracture must be distinguished from developmental defects (see Fig. 12–21*B*). These vary from complete absence of the posterior neural arch to short segmental defects located laterally that might be mistaken for fractures. The margins of these defects are rounded and consist of cortical bone. In addition, the apposing portions of the neural arch at the defect are often slightly tapered. Lateral views of the cervical spine obtained with the head tilted result in an oblique projection of the arch of C1 that may give the false impression of one or more fractures or developmental defects of the arch. A repeat examination in the true lateral position will demonstrate that the arches are intact (Fig. 12–22). Fractures of the neural arch also occur as a component of Jefferson's fractures of C1 and may be evident on the lateral projection. Before concluding that a fracture identified in the neural arch represents an isolated injury, examine the anteroposterior open-mouth view to determine if there is spreading of the lateral masses as is characteristic of Jefferson's fracture.

Unilateral fractures of the neural arch are occasionally encountered, as are unilateral ossification defects.[215, 218]

Small ossicles of congenital origin may be found between the inferior tip of the clivus and the anterior arch of the atlas. These are readily distinguished from fractures by their completely intact cortical margins and the fact that avulsion fractures are rarely encountered in this region.

Isolated fracture of the medial portion of the lateral mass of the atlas has been reported.[141] These fractures are difficult to identify on plain film but may be visualized by CT (see Fig. 12–34). They represent an avulsion at the site of origin of the transverse ligament. Isolated unilateral or bilateral fractures of the transverse process of C1 have also been described.[205] These fractures are best visualized on basal views of the skull or by CT.

Horizontal fractures of the anterior arch of the atlas have been described.[181, 182, 211, 216] These fractures are characteristically minimally displaced, best visualized on the lateral view, and often associated with fractures of the dens. Horizontal fractures result from an avulsion mediated through the tendinous ligamentous insertion on the anterior tubercle by the anterior longitudinal ligament and the longus colli muscle. Horizontal fractures may be missed by CT examination, but they are readily visualized on the lateral radiograph or in reconstructed CT images.

Segmental fractures of the anterior arch of C1 and disruption of the apophyses or synchondroses of the anterior arch of C1 have been described[214, 215] and are likely caused by hyperextension. Such fractures in adults are sometimes associated with transverse fractures of the dens.[254]

Jefferson's Fracture

Jefferson's fracture[168, 177, 212] is a comminuted fracture of the ring involving both the anterior and posterior arches (Figs. 12–23 and 12–24). This allows centripetal displacement of the fragments. Bursting fractures of the

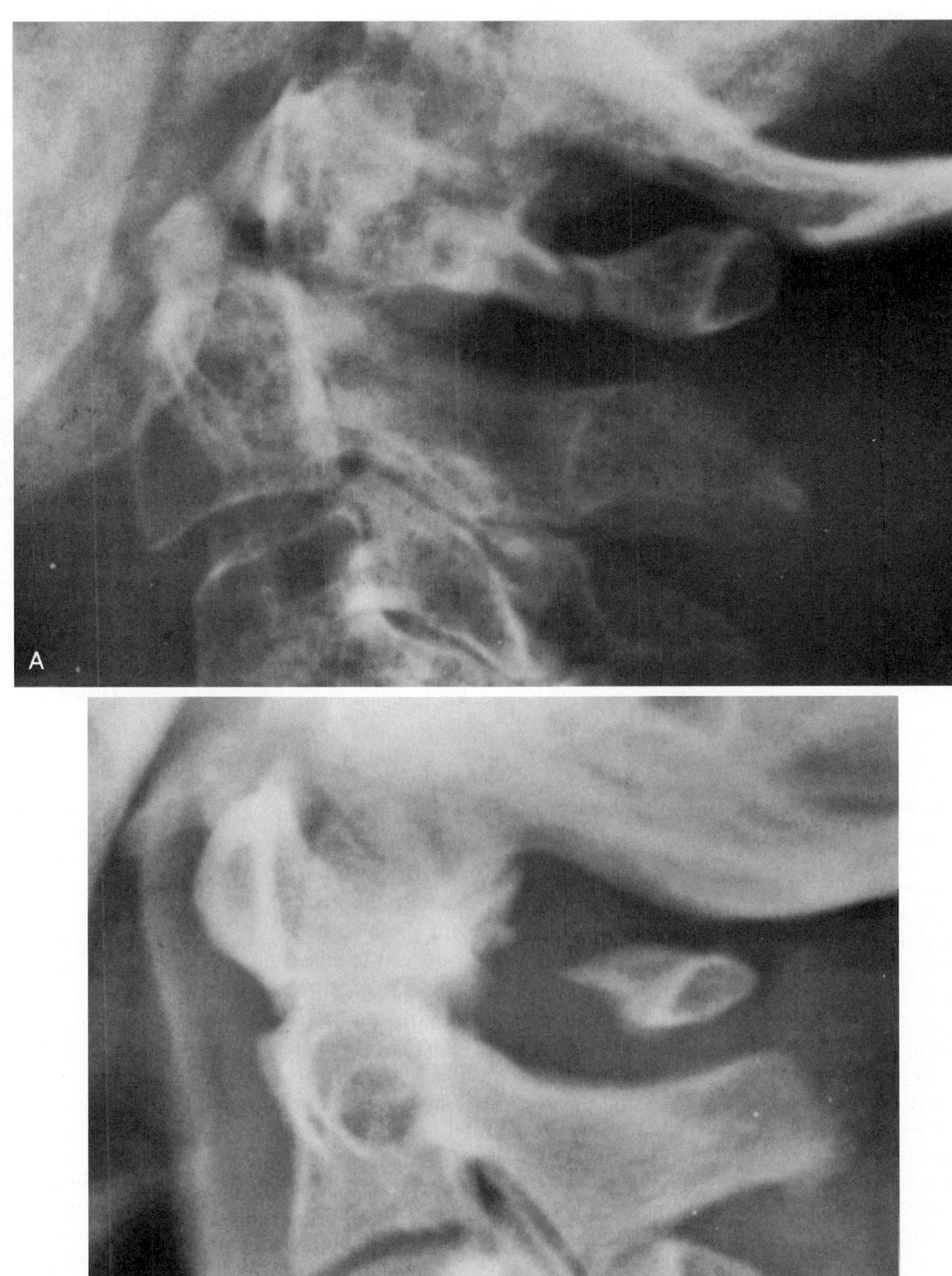

Figure 12–21. Abnormalities of the neural arch of C1. *A*, Simultaneous fractures of the neural arch of C1 and the dens of C2 in an 89-year-old woman. This is a hyperextension injury with marked posterior displacement of the dens. Note the vertical fracture in the neural arch of C1. *B*, Bilateral congenital absence of a segment of the neural arch of C1 is seen in a 12-year-old girl. Note the smooth tapered cortical surface on the anterior aspect of the posterior segment. The posterior segment is in normal position. The neural arch is completed by a band of fibrous tissue, which, of course, is radiolucent. Note also the V-shaped predens space.

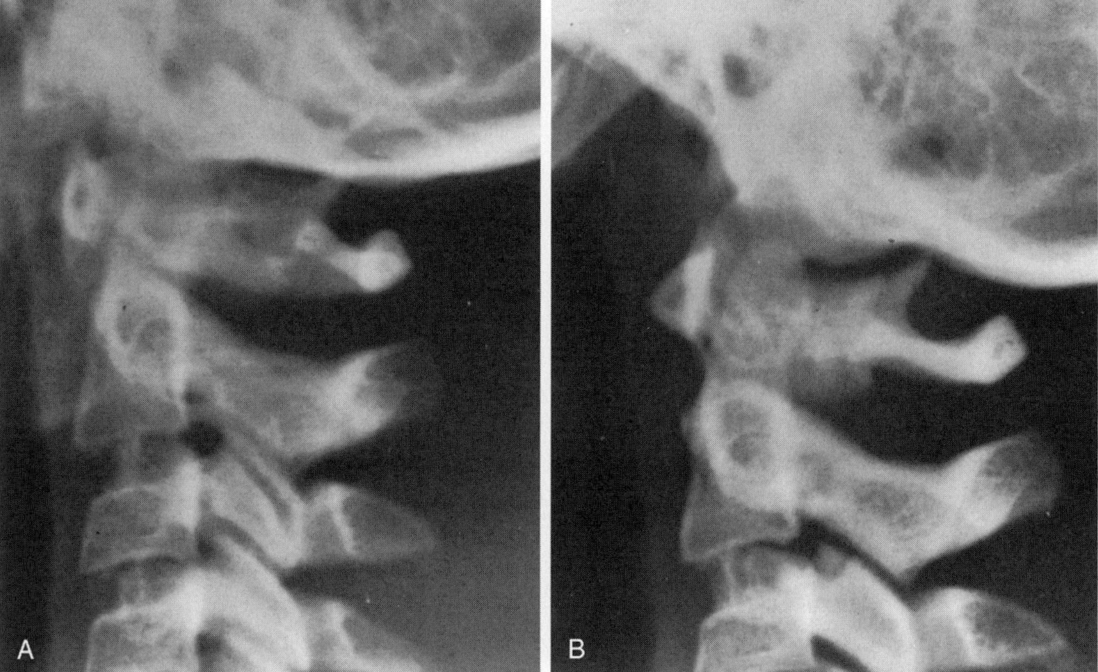

Figure 12–22. Oblique projection of C1 giving false impression of fracture of the neural arch in an 11-year-old girl. *A*, The head is rotated upon the cervical spine, which gives an oblique and somewhat tilted projection of T1. This easily could be misconstrued as a fracture of the neural arch. *B*, A true lateral projection shows the neural arch is intact.

ring of the atlas have been designated Jefferson's fractures in recognition of Sir Geoffrey Jefferson, a British neurosurgeon who in 1919[158] first described the mechanism of injury. A Jefferson's fracture is created by blows on the vertex. The force is transmitted from the cranium to the cervical spine through the occipital condyles. The lateral articular masses of the atlas become compressed between the occipital condyles and the superior articular facets of the axis. The lateral articular masses of C1 are wedge shaped. The superior articular facets of the atlas slope inward, and the inferior articular facets slope outward. Therefore, as the occipital condyles are driven toward the axis, the lateral articular masses of the atlas are displaced laterally. The weaker segments of the atlas—the anterior and posterior arches—are stressed and finally broken, disrupting the ring and forcing the lateral articular masses of the atlas to spread apart. Most commonly there are two fractures in the posterior arch, one on each side, and a single fracture in the anterior arch off the midline[212] (see Fig. 12–24). At times there is a single fracture in both arches.[210] Occasionally, there are two fractures in both arches.

Jefferson's fractures mostly are the result of automobile accidents. Blows to the vertex and falls in which the head is struck account for the remainder. The symptoms and physical findings are nonspecific. Diagnosis depends on proper interpretation of radiographs of the cervical spine. The most significant findings are on the frontal projections of the atlas and axis. The crucial observation is the bilateral offset or spreading of the lateral articular masses of C1[87, 88] in relation to the apposing articular surfaces of C2 (see Fig. 12–23). It is often difficult to visualize the lines of fracture per se,[206, 207] but the presence of the fracture may be implied from lateral displacement of the lateral masses of C1 relative to the peripheral margins of the superior facet of C2. Occasionally, the fractures are demonstrated on the lateral projection. Demonstration of these fractures is not an absolute necessity. Bilateral offset or spreading of the lateral articular masses is sufficient for diagnosis.

It has been suggested that the degree of offset distinguishes between stable and unstable Jefferson's fractures.[217, 248] A stable Jefferson's fracture, defined as one in which the transverse ligament is intact, is implied by total offset of the two sides of less than 7 mm. An unstable fracture is one in which the transverse ligament is disrupted, as evidenced by lateral displacement in excess of 7 mm, often in association with an increase in the atlantoaxial distance on the lateral view. On occasion, the lateral masses of C1 and C2 are aligned on one side but offset on the other. This carries the same implications as a bilateral offset. CT confirms the presence of the comminuted fracture (see Fig. 12–24).

Bilateral offset of the lateral articular masses of C1 upon C2 is also seen under two other circumstances. In children younger than age 5, the ossification of the lateral mass of C1 often exceeds that of the ossification of C2, giving rise to what has been termed "pseudospread" of C1 upon C2[219, 220] (Fig. 12–25). Such offsets are normal findings in young children, and fortunately Jefferson's fractures are very rare. Developmental defects in the arch of C1 are also associated with bilateral offset, particularly spondyloschisis, which consists of a developmental cleft in both the anterior and the posterior arches[208, 213] (Fig. 12–26). Under these circumstances, the bilateral offset usually amounts to no more than 2 mm, whereas offset

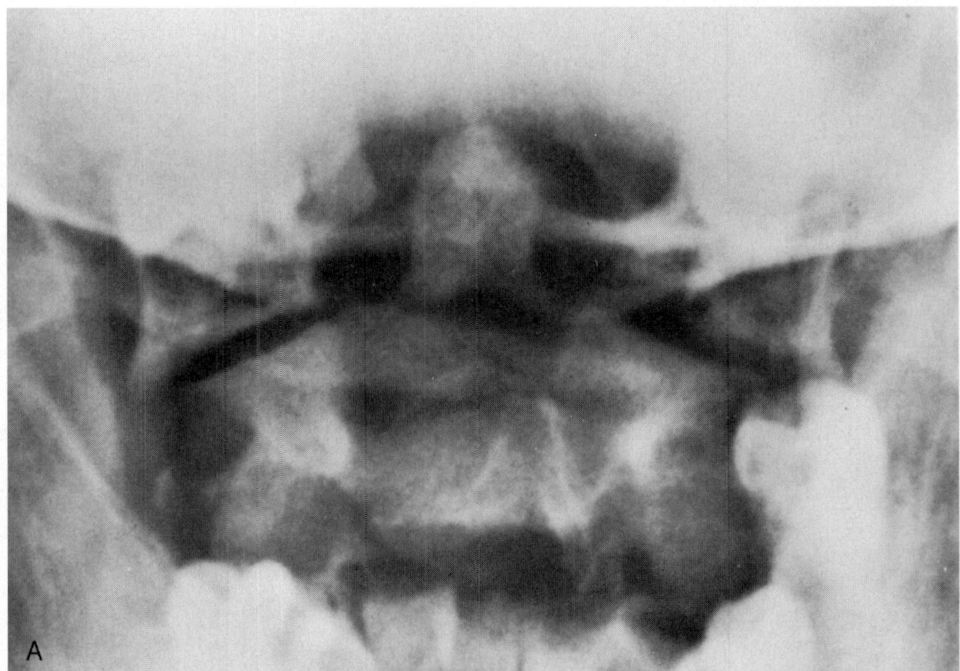

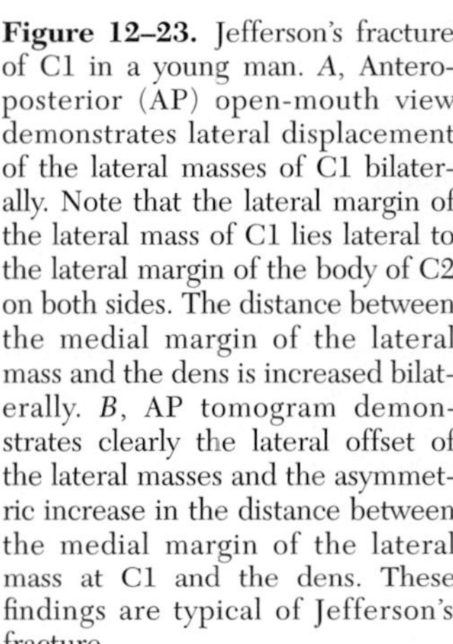

Figure 12–23. Jefferson's fracture of C1 in a young man. *A*, Anteroposterior (AP) open-mouth view demonstrates lateral displacement of the lateral masses of C1 bilaterally. Note that the lateral margin of the lateral mass of C1 lies lateral to the lateral margin of the body of C2 on both sides. The distance between the medial margin of the lateral mass and the dens is increased bilaterally. *B*, AP tomogram demonstrates clearly the lateral offset of the lateral masses and the asymmetric increase in the distance between the medial margin of the lateral mass at C1 and the dens. These findings are typical of Jefferson's fracture.

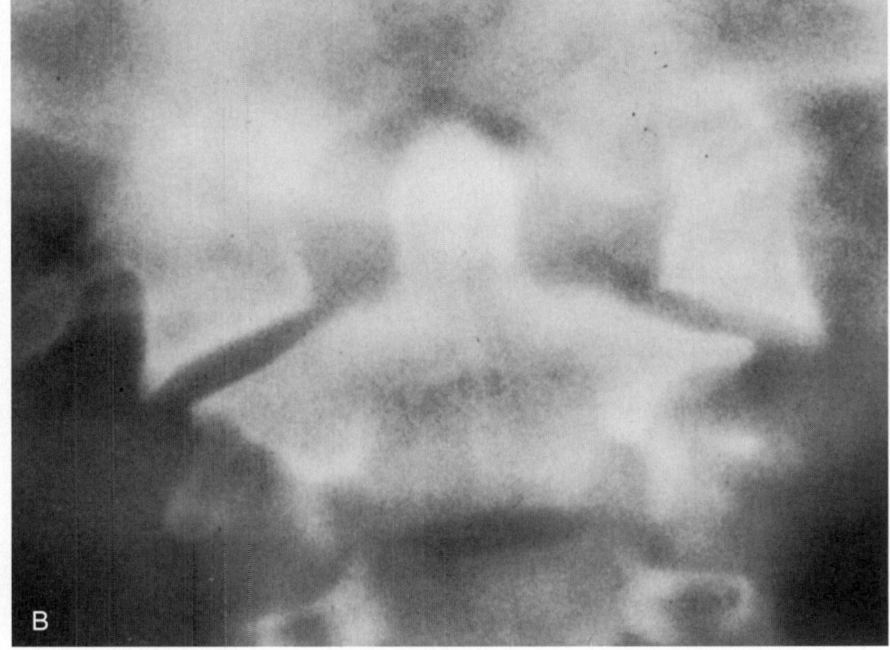

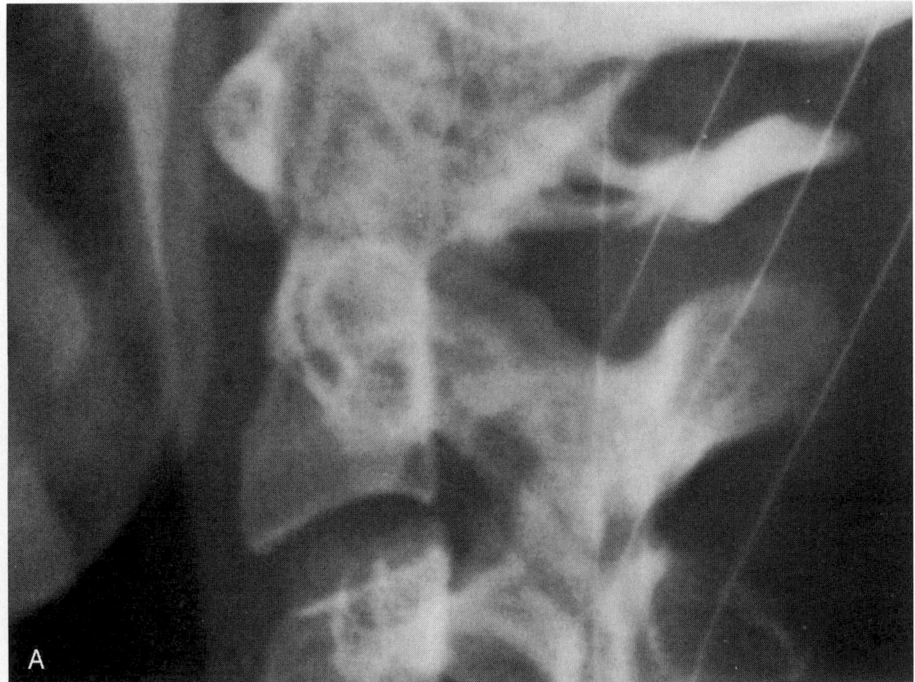

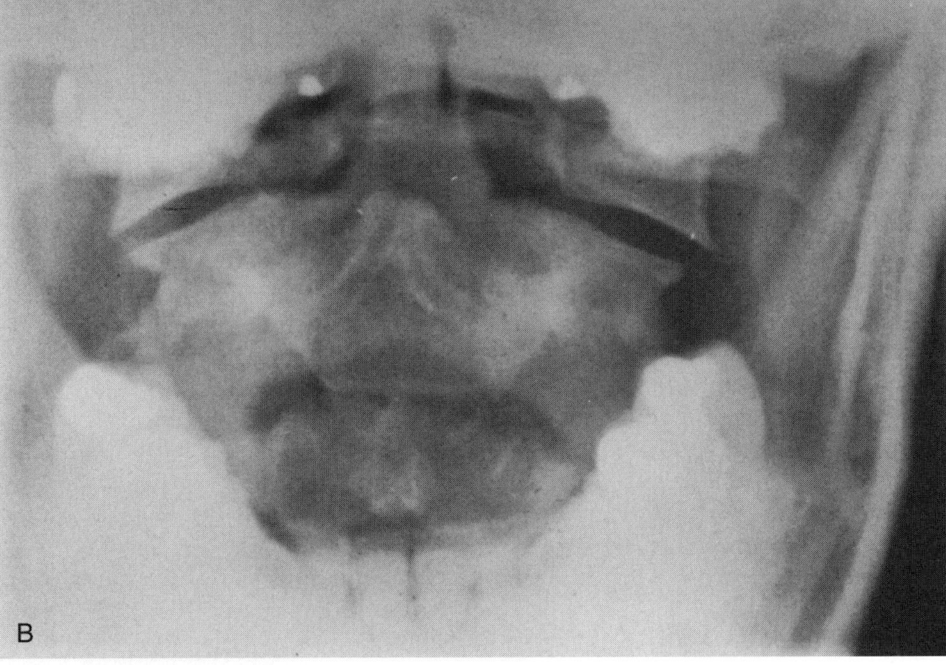

Figure 12–24. Jefferson's fracture of C1 in a 28-year-old woman. *A*, Lateral radiograph is marred by several linear artifacts, but there is no definite fracture. Soft tissue swelling is present anterior to C1 and the upper margin of C2. *B*, Anteroposterior open-mouth view demonstrates minimal lateral offset of C1 upon C2 bilaterally.

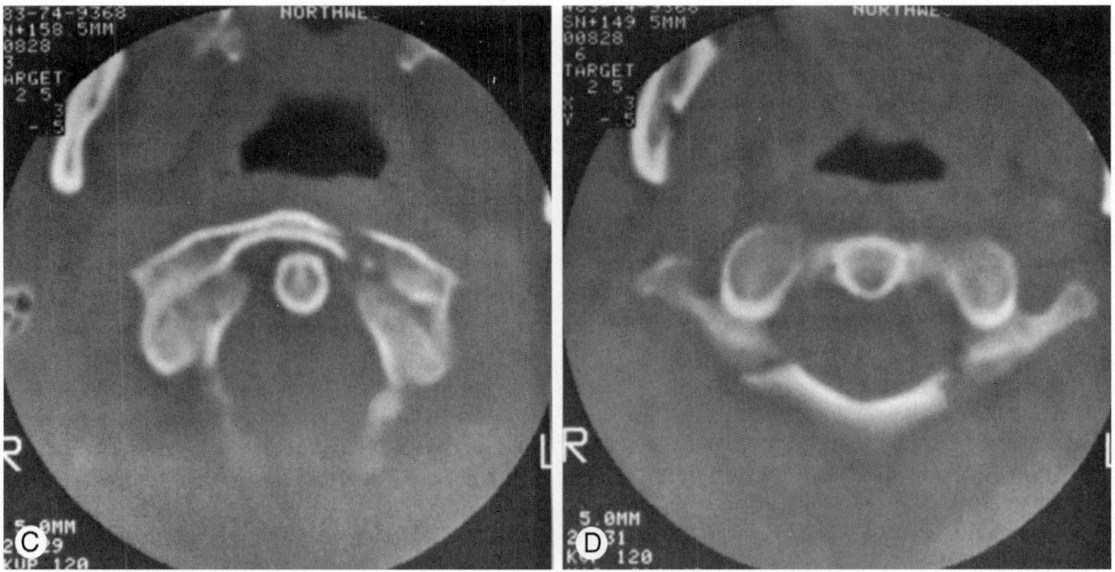

Figure 12–24 *(Continued). C,* CT scan reveals fracture through the anterior arch of C1. *D,* A second scan obtained more inferiorly shows bilateral fractures of the posterior neural arch of C1.

associated with Jefferson's fracture usually, but not always, exceeds 3 mm on each side. CT makes the distinction readily in questionable cases.

Axis (C2)

About 15% of cervical fractures involve the axis, 40% of which are associated with head injuries and 18% with other cervical spine injuries.[242, 263, 288, 289] Approximately 25% are hangman's fractures, over half (55%) are odontoid fractures, and the remainder are miscellaneous fractures involving the body, lateral mass, or spinous process or single fractures of the neural arch.[151, 229, 230]

Hangman's Fracture

Hangman's fractures are variously known as traumatic spondylolisthesis of the axis, fractures of the neural arch of the axis, or fractures of the ring of the axis. Schneider and associates[174] noted that this injury is identical to that created by judicial hanging,[163, 183] thus the designation hangman's fracture.[150, 174, 236] Hangman's fractures are usually the result of acute hyperextension of the head on the neck, in keeping with this designation, but some of these fractures may be due to hyperflexion and axial compression.

Fracture of the neural arch of the axis is one of the most common injuries of the cervical spine.[117, 145, 167, 171] The full force of acute hyperextension of the head on the neck is transmitted through the pedicles of C2 onto the apophyseal joints.[150] The weakest points in this chain are the interarticular segments of the pedicle.[150] Thus, the arch of C2 is fractured anterior to the inferior facet (Fig. 12–27). The anterior longitudinal ligament is placed under tension and is disrupted. These injuries are commonly sustained in automobile accidents as the chin or forehead encounters the steering wheel or dashboard, forcing the head into hyperextension.

It is difficult to visualize the fracture on the anteroposterior view; it is best demonstrated on the lateral view. The atlantoaxial joint and dens are intact. Fractures of the neural arch of the axis are often anterior to the inferior facets. They are oblique, extending from superior posterior to inferior anterior. The fractures may be symmetric, but they usually vary slightly in obliquity and relative anteroposterior position. When bilateral fractures of the neural arch are symmetric, they are easily visualized (see Fig. 12–27), but they may be difficult to see when they are in different portions of the arch on each side (Fig. 12–28) because of the resultant overlap. Oblique views may demonstrate the fracture. CT is of definite value in questionable cases (Fig. 12–29). CT has demonstrated quite clearly that fractures of the arch commonly extend into the posterior aspect of the vertebral body.[227, 235] Such extension also may be evident on the plain films. Widely separated fractures may be associated with disruption and dislocation of the C2-C3 facet joints or even locking of the facets (see Fig. 12–27), with the facets of C2 coming to rest anterior to the facets of C3. An avulsion fracture of the anterior inferior margin of the axis (see Fig. 12–28A) or anterior superior margin at C3 is often present and identifies the site of rupture of the anterior longitudinal ligament. It may serve as an important clue to obscure hangman's fracture. Whenever a fracture is identified at the anterior inferior margin of the body at C2 the neural arch should be examined closely for evidence of fracture. The ligament may rupture at the level of the C2-C3 interspace; therefore, avulsion fracture does not occur. At times there may be an associated fracture of the neural arch of C1.

Effendi and associates[225] have proposed a classification of hangman's fractures[234] (Fig. 12–30). Type I fractures are isolated hairline fractures of the neural arch with minimal displacement of the body of C2. In types II and III the fracture is widely separated. In type II the anterior fragment is displaced with obvious disruption of the C2-C3 disc. The body of the axis may be tilted, as in extension or flexion, or displaced anteriorly. In type III there is obvious displacement of the body of the axis forward in

Text continued on page 408

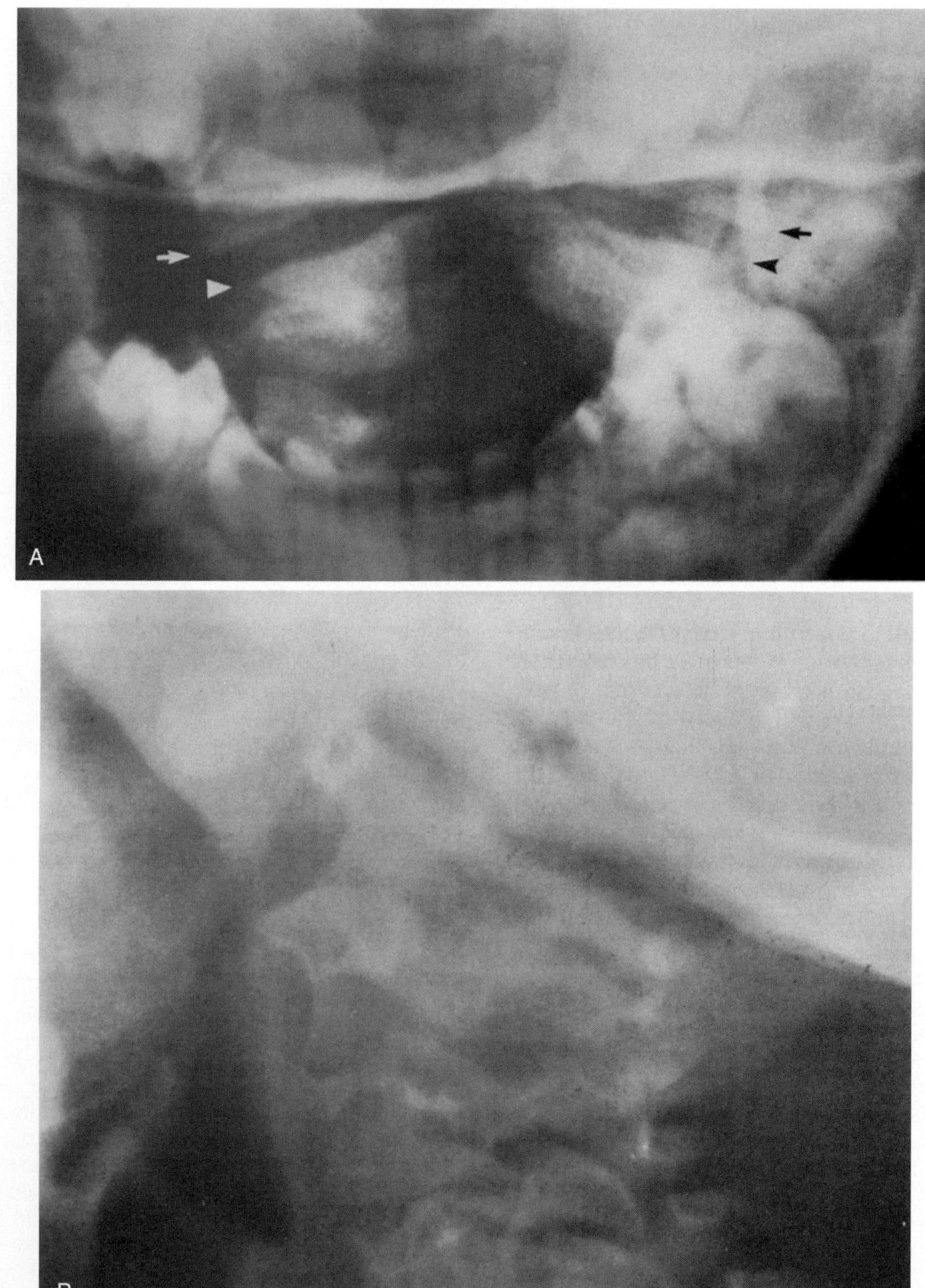

Figure 12–25. Pseudospread of C1 upon C2 in a 3-year-old girl with a normal cervical spine. *A*, The lateral border of C1 (*arrows*) lies well beyond the lateral margins of C2 (*arrowheads*) bilaterally. *B*, Lateral radiograph obtained in a slightly oblique projection reveals no abnormality. Pseudospreading of C1 is a normal finding in patients younger than 5 years of age.

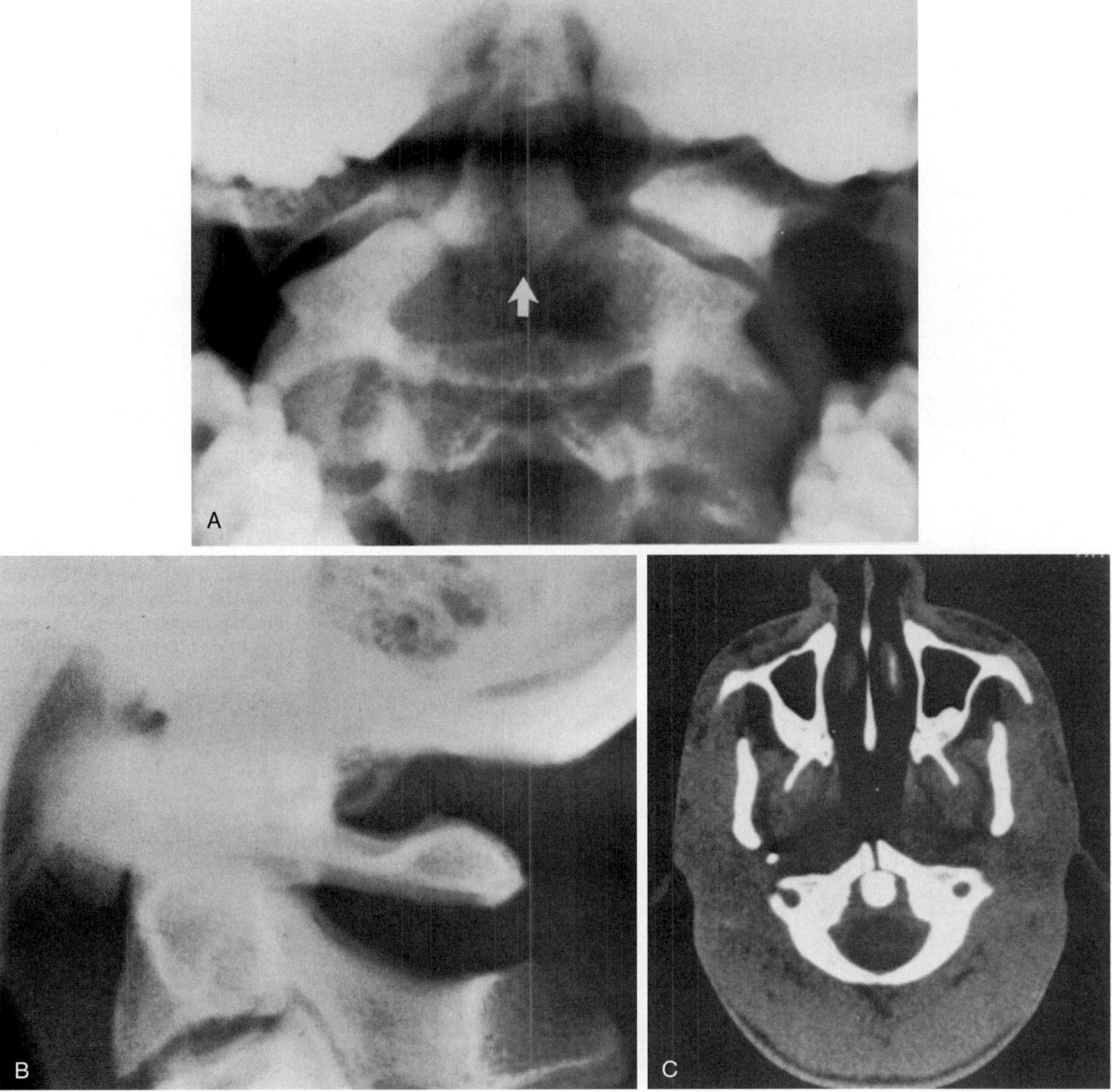

Figure 12–26. Developmental defects in the anterior and posterior arches of C1 in an 18-year-old man giving rise to a pseudospread of C1 upon C2. *A*, The lateral margin of C1 lies slightly lateral to that of C2 bilaterally. There is a peculiar vertical lucency overlying the dens (*arrow*) caused by the defect in the anterior arch of C1. *B*, Lateral radiograph demonstrates enlarged anterior arch of C1 without other obvious abnormalities. *C*, CT scan demonstrates the absence of fusion of the anterior and posterior arches of C1. The anterior arch of C1 is hypertrophied, accounting for its appearance of the lateral radiograph. (Case courtesy of Kendrick C. Davidson, MD, Kansas City, Mo.)

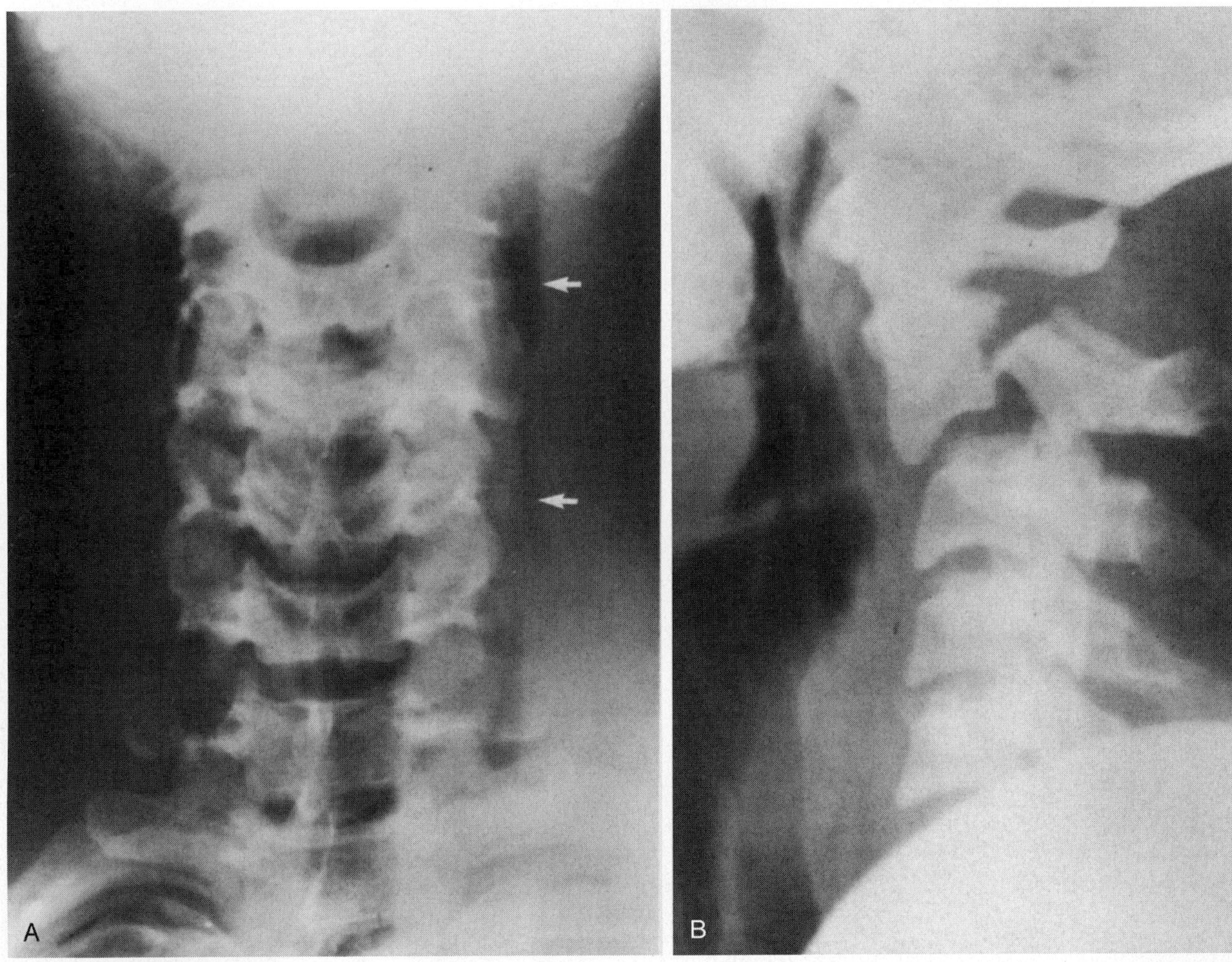

Figure 12–27. Hangman's fracture associated with fracture of the larynx in a young man injured in an auto accident. *A*, Anteroposterior view of the spine reveals no evidence of bony injury. C2 is not visualized; there is air within the soft tissue lying outside of the larynx (*arrows*). *B*, Lateral view of the cervical spine clearly demonstrates bilateral fracture of the neural arch of C2 with anterior dislocation of C2 upon C3. The findings are typical of a hangman's fracture. In addition, there is abnormal air within the soft tissues and anterior to the larynx and trachea. Note that the air column within the larynx is distorted. These findings are typical of fracture of the larynx. (Case courtesy of Lincoln Russin, MD, Amherst, Mass.)

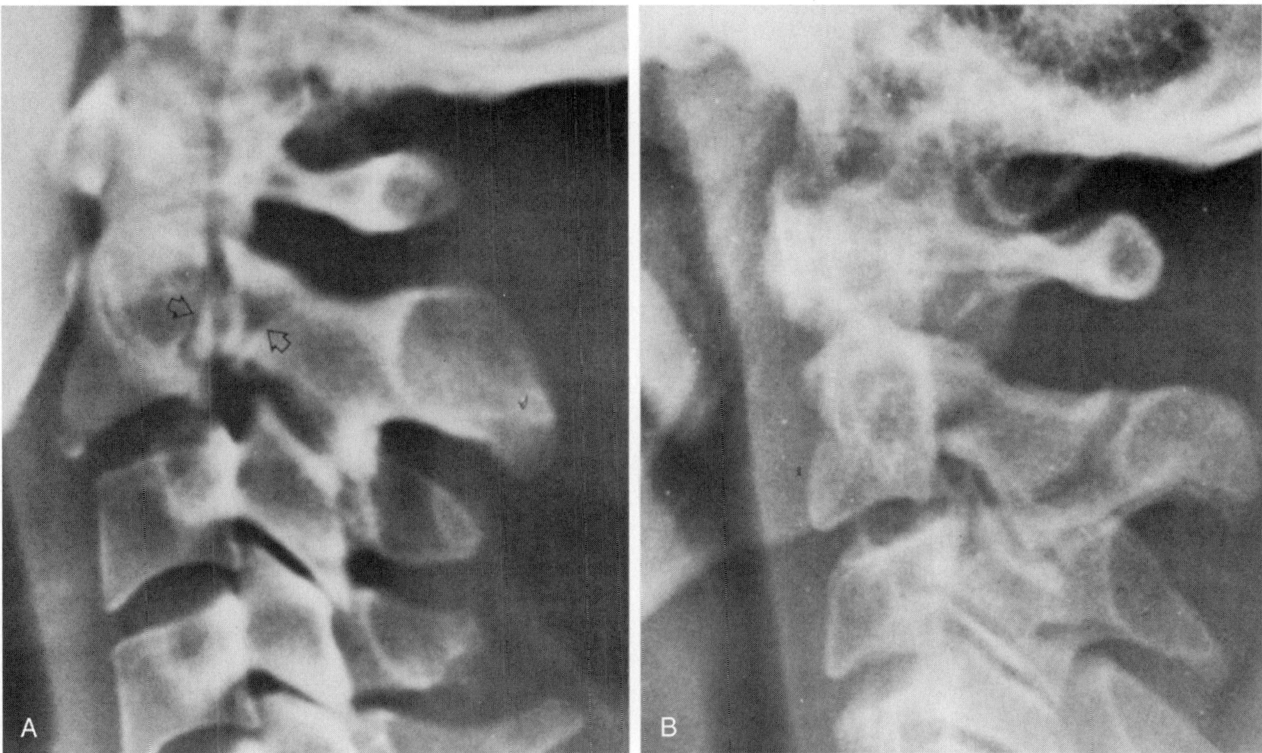

Figure 12–28. Two cases of hangman's fracture. *A*, Soft tissue swelling is present in the retropharynx. There is a small avulsion fracture from the anterior inferior surface of the body of C2. Close examination revealed that this is associated with fractures of the neural arch (*arrows*). *B*, In this case there is minimal anterior subluxation of C2 upon C3 with soft tissue swelling in the retropharynx. Fractures are present in the neural arch bilaterally. When the fractures of the neural arch are asymmetric, they are often obscure.

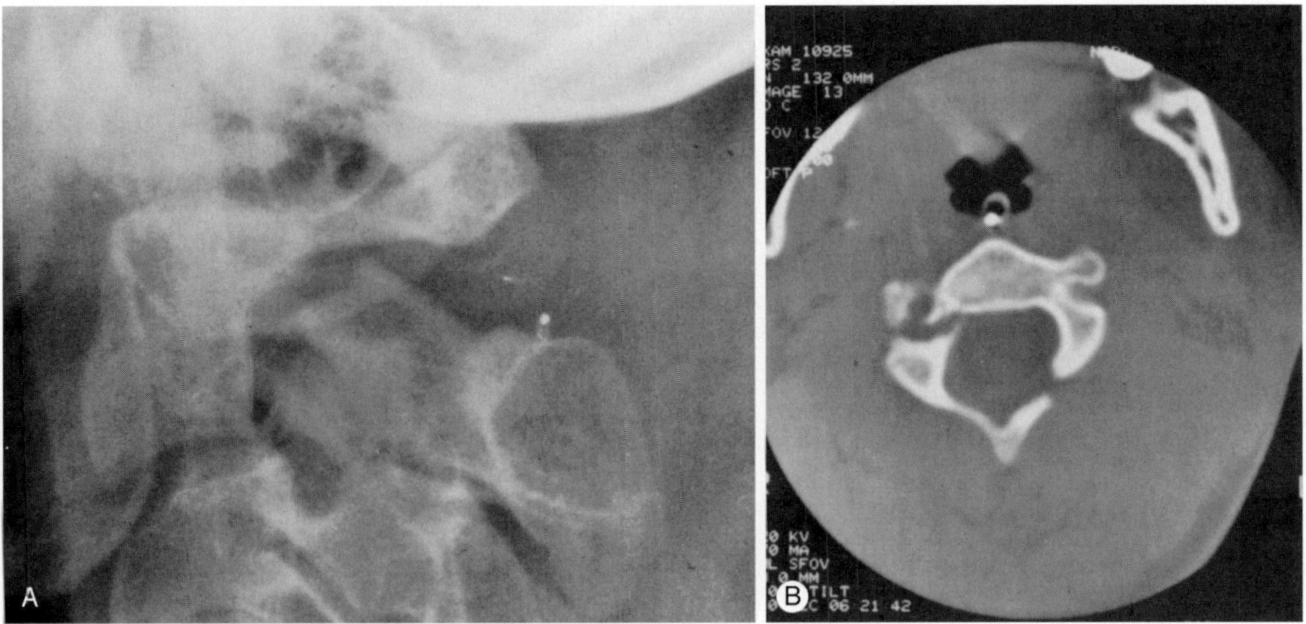

Figure 12–29. Hangman's fracture in a 26-year-old man. *A*, Lateral radiograph reveals fractures of the neural arch of C2 with anterior subluxation of C2 upon C3 and disruption of the facet joints. *B*, CT scan demonstrates fractures through the pedicle on the right and through the neural arch on the left.

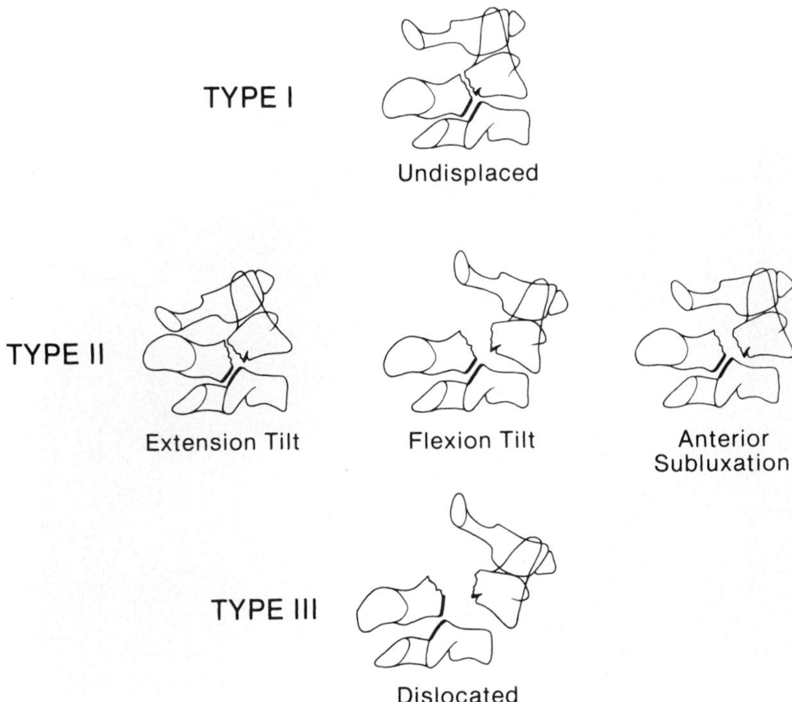

Figure 12–30. Effendi and associates'[225] classification of hangman's fractures.

the flexion position associated with disruption of the facet joints of C2-C3, which are either simply dislocated or locked.[224, 245] In Effendi's series,[225] 65% of hangman's fractures were type I, 28% were type II, and 7% were type III. Atypical hangman's fractures, occurring through the posterior aspect of the vertebral body have been described.[349] Because of the fracture pattern, this injury can produce canal compression and neurologic dysfunction, rather than expansion without deficits.

Hangman's fractures or fractures of the neural arch of the axis have been described in which the mechanism of injury appears to have been hyperflexion, as evidenced by an intact anterior longitudinal ligament at postmortem examination.[249] Occasionally, hangman's fractures are found associated with compression fractures of the C3 vertebral body. These fractures and those associated with the locking of the facets are more easily explained by some element of flexion, as opposed to pure extension.

"Unilateral" hangman's fractures, in which a fracture of the neural arch is found on one side without a corresponding fracture on the opposite side, rarely occur. CT should be obtained in order to exclude a fracture on the opposite side before this diagnosis is accepted[227] (Fig. 12–31).

Synchondroses between the neural arch and body of C2 or within the neural arch have been described in children,[169] occasionally resulting in defects that may be associated with spondylolisthesis.[33, 226, 233, 239] Hangman's fractures are rare in children,[35, 37, 246] and care must be taken to distinguish between these infrequent ossification defects and a fracture. The opposing margins of the ossification defects are usually smooth and sharply defined.

There is a surprising paucity of neurologic findings in fractures of the neural arch of C2 when encountered in the clinical situation.[244] Alker and associates,[138] in postmortem study of head and neck injuries in fatal traffic accidents, did find that this was the most frequent fracture of the cervical spine in their series, however. Transient hyperextension may result in fracture without neurologic deficit.[150] If the force is sustained following creation of the fracture, the cord is susceptible to transection, as is seen in judicial hanging.[222, 254]

Fractures of the Odontoid Process

Fractures of the odontoid process are often difficult to visualize because of minimal displacement. They are rare in children but are relatively common in the aged.[253] Most fractures of this type are transverse, in the axial plane, and located at the base of the dens.[140, 173, 175] Oblique fractures limited to the odontoid process occur but are infrequent. Oblique fractures beginning at the base of the dens and extending into the body of the axis anteriorly or posteriorly are relatively common. The dens may be displaced anteriorly or posteriorly depending on the principal mechanism of injury: anteriorly with flexion and posteriorly with extension. The degree of lateral offset is variable.[221] Fragments are rarely distracted more than 2 or 3 mm.

Anderson and d'Alonzo[139] proposed a classification of dens fracture (Fig. 12–32) consisting of three types[223, 247, 252]: type I, an oblique fracture limited to the dens, accounting for only 4%; type II, a transverse fracture at the base of the dens and by far the most common, accounting for 66%; and type III, an oblique fracture at the base of the dens and extending into the body, accounting for the remaining 30%. In type III flexion injuries, the oblique line of fracture extends from the posterior aspect of the base of the dens obliquely into the anterior

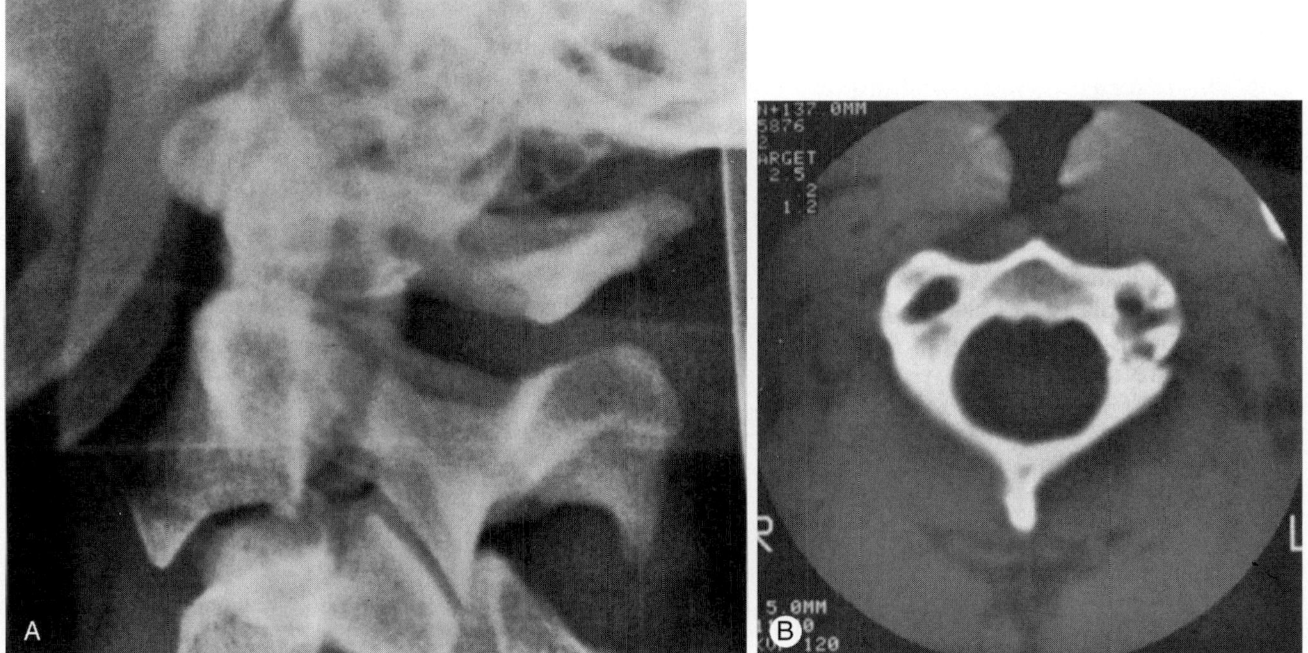

Figure 12–31. Unilateral neural arch fracture of C2 in an 18-year-old man. *A*, Lateral radiograph demonstrates fractures of the neural arch and anterioinferior margin of the body of C2 with subluxation of C2 upon C3. *B*, CT demonstrates only a single fracture through the neural arch on the left without an accompanying fracture on the right. Strict definition of hangman's fractures requires bilateral fractures of the neural arch.

aspect of the body of the axis, and the dens is displaced anteriorly. When fracture is caused by extension, it begins at the anterior base of the dens and extends to the posterior cortex of the body, and the dens is displaced posteriorly. The latter fractures appear to be more common in the elderly.[245, 254]

In types I and II dens fractures the diagnosis depends primarily on radiographic findings in the anteroposterior open-mouth projection (Fig. 12–33). On lateral projections soft tissue swelling is seen anterior to the nasopharynx and within the retropharyngeal tissues, but minimal displacement often precludes demonstration of the fracture line. The anterior and posterior cortical margins of the dens and body of C2 should be examined closely on

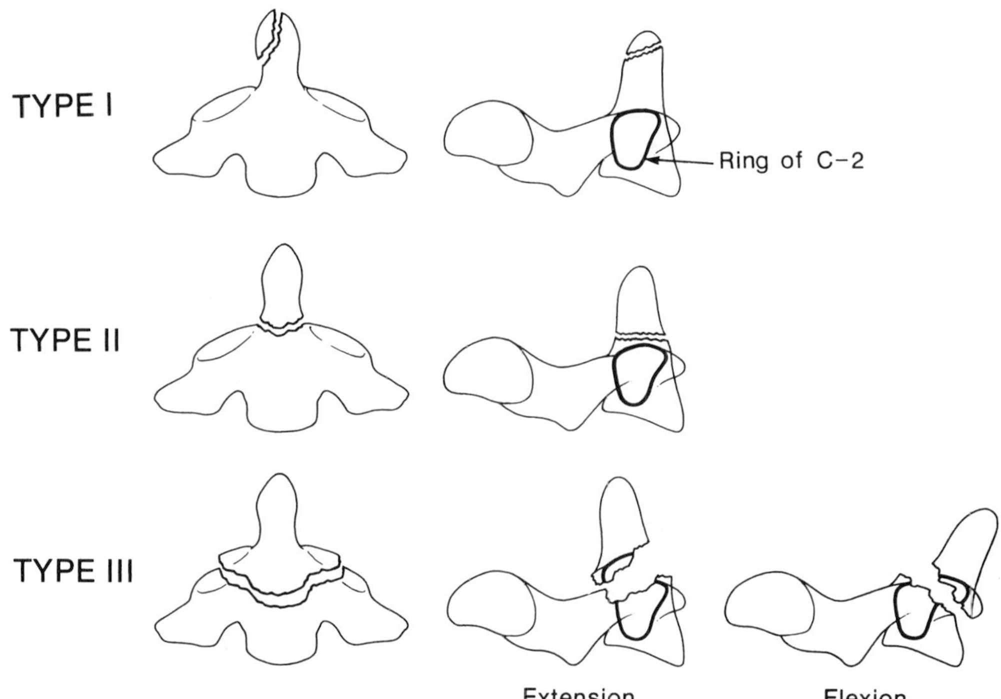

Figure 12–32. Anderson and d'Alonzo's classification of dens fractures.[139] Note the "ring" of C2 is disrupted in type III, but it remains intact in types I and II.

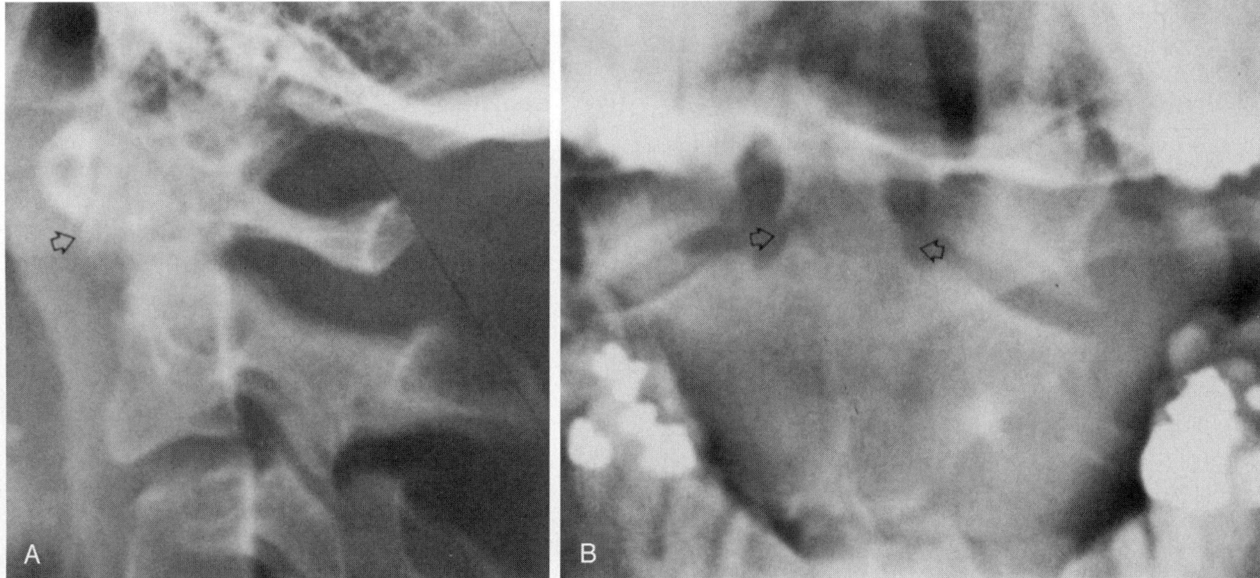

Figure 12–33. Fracture of the odontoid process in a 21-year-old man. *A*, Lateral view demonstrates soft tissue swelling in the nasopharynx and posterior displacement of the body of C2 in relation to the odontoid process (*arrow*). The anterior cortex of the dens is clearly visualized and is in normal relationship to the anterior arch of C1. *B*, Open-mouth view demonstrates transverse fracture at the base of the dens. Note the cortical disruption (*arrows*).

the lateral projection for evidence of cortical disruption. Type III fractures are almost always better visualized on the lateral projection and, in fact, may not be evident on the anteroposterior plain film. CT is better suited for depiction of this type of injury (see Fig. 12–19*B*).

On the anteroposterior view, a notch is commonly present at the base of the dens at its junction with the superior articular facet. This notch should not be mistaken for a fracture. In a small percentage of cases the dens joins the body of C2 at a slightly oblique angle with the long axis of the dens tilted posteriorly. This is a normal variant. The cortex of the dens is best studied on the lateral view by noting the anterior and posterior cortex of both the dens and body. The anterior cortical margin is sometimes difficult to visualize with certainty because of its slightly undulant and sloping character. The posterior cortical margin is straight and more vertically oriented; therefore, it is more easily identified. Disruptions in either the anterior or posterior cortex are, of course, indicative of fracture.

Fractures of the body of the axis, including type III fractures of the odontoid process, are often difficult to visualize because of the combination of minimal displacement and complex anatomy. On the lateral view a ring of cortical bone is projected over the body of the axis, representing a composite of several structures[232, 238] (see Figs. 12–32 and 12–40). Fractures of the body of the axis disrupt the cortical margins of the ring (see Fig. 12–37), which is a clue to otherwise inapparent fractures. The upper margin of the ring at the approximate level of the junction of the dens and body is formed by the joint surface of the superior articular facet. The anterior margin represents the anterior cortex of the axis at the junction of the body and neural arch; the posterior vertically oriented component is produced by the posterior cortex of the body. The ring may be incomplete inferiorly. At times there is a circular component within the ring, representing the foramen transversarium, a distinct, completely or partially corticated lucency at the inferior portion of the ring through which passes the vertebral artery.

CT may be of value in some cases (see Fig. 12–37*H*),[228, 237] but the axial orientation of the fractures may result in obscuration as a consequence of partial volume averaging, and reconstructed images are needed for adequate evaluation (see Fig. 12–18).

The transverse fracture at the base of the dens must be differentiated from a developmental abnormality termed *os odontoideum*,[153] which is rounded, has a cortical margin around its entire surface, and is usually more widely separated from the base of the odontoid than a fracture. Admittedly, at times this distinction may be difficult. A further problem is that nonunion of this type of fracture is rather frequent in adults, and when the ossicle is closely approximated with the base of the odontoid, is normal in shape, and has a smooth inferior cortical margin, it may be impossible to distinguish an os odontoideum from an old ununited fracture.

Dens fractures are infrequent in children, but occasionally apophyseal separations are encountered that involve the dentocentral synchondrosis between the ossification centers of the dens and body[23, 169, 240] (Fig. 12–35). This synchondrosis begins to close at age 5 and is essentially closed by age 7; however, small horizontally oriented remnants of the synchondrosis persist until about age 14. Most apophyseal separations through the synchondrosis occur in children younger than age 6. The synchondrosis and its remnants should not be misconstrued as fractures.

Diagnosis of fracture of the dens is complicated by the combination of the minimal displacement of the fracture fragment and the complexity of the overlying structures as demonstrated radiographically. A Mach effect (Fig. 12–36) is frequently seen at the base of the dens on the anteroposterior view and is caused by either the inferior cortex of the posterior neural arch of the atlas or the

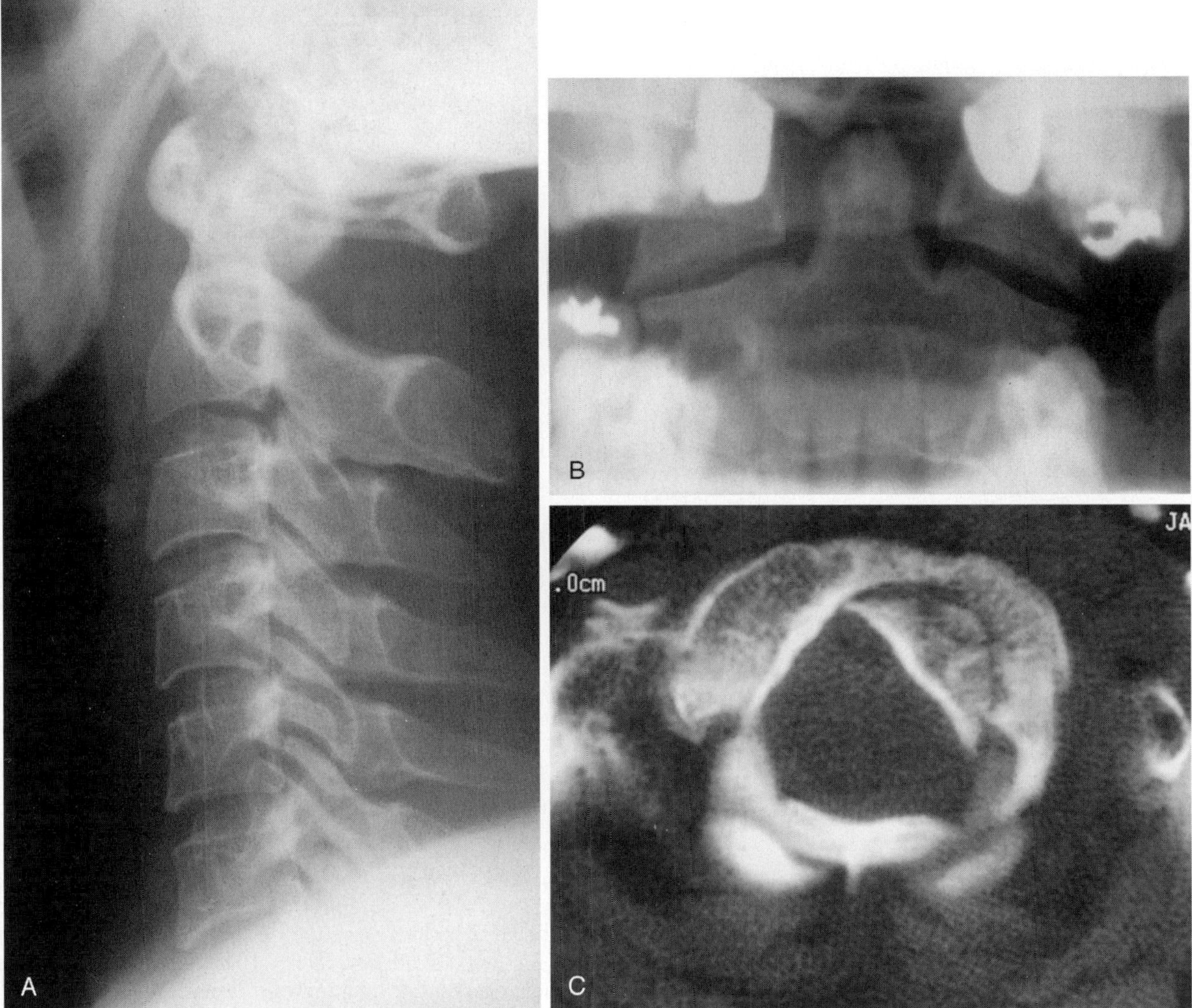

Figure 12–34. Fracture of the craniovertebral junction. *A*, Lateral radiograph shows discrete prevertebral soft tissue swelling adjacent to C1. *B*, Open-mouth odontoid view shows no abnormalities. *C*, Axial CT image reveals displaced fracture of the left occipital condyle that extended to the lateral mass of C1. The displaced bone fragment reduces the size of the spinal canal.

superior cortex of the neural arch of the axis. There are several normal variants that might be mistaken for fractures. In children the synchondrosis between the ossification center of the body and dens may be confused with a fracture. The os terminale is a small accessory ossification center found at the tip of the dens. The upper central incisors frequently overlap the dens, and a lucency is seen between them. This situation might be mistaken for a vertical fracture of the dens. Similarly, a vertical cleft in the anterior arch of the atlas has been described that also overlaps the dens[172] (see Fig. 12–26*A*). This distinction is simplified by awareness that vertical fractures of the dens are virtually impossible to create, and none has been reported.

Fractures of the dens are occasionally associated with atlantoaxial dislocations[148] and fractures of C1[165, 250] (see Fig. 12–21*A*), usually of the posterior neural arch but also of the anterior arch and Jefferson's fractures. Because fractures of the dens often are not readily apparent, it is important to specifically look for an associated fracture of the dens when there is fracture of C1 or an atlantoaxial dislocation.

Nonunion is a troublesome complication of type II fractures at the base of the dens.[223, 231, 243, 247] Types I and III fractures usually heal without difficulty. A vacuum phenomenon within an ununited dens fracture has been described.

Fractures of the Body

Fractures are limited to the body of C2 without involving the odontoid process in less than 10% of all axis fractures. When in the coronal plane, these fractures are readily identified on the lateral radiograph, but when oriented obliquely, they may be inapparent on both anteroposterior and lateral projections. The fragments often separate so as to broaden the anteroposterior diameter of the body of C2. Normally, lines drawn tangential to the anterior and posterior surfaces of C3 align with the anterior and posterior surfaces of C2. In the presence of a fracture of the body with displacement of the fragments,

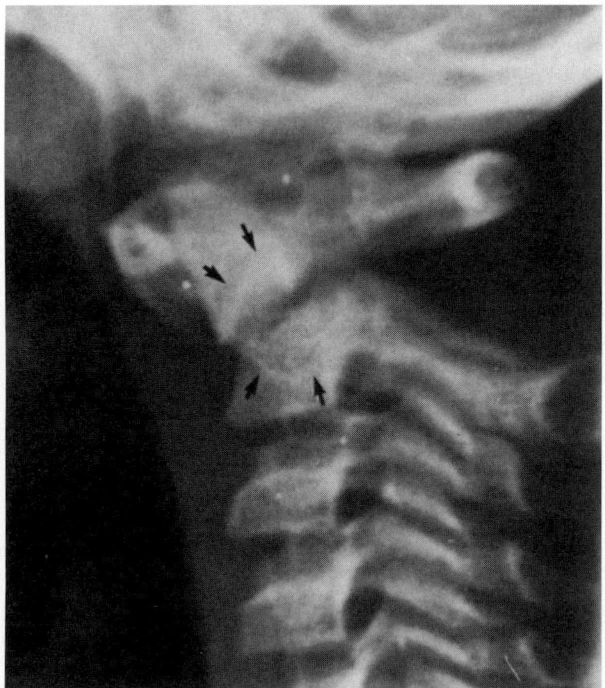

Figure 12–35. Fracture through the synchondrosis of the dens in a 4-year-old girl. Note the anterior displacement and tilting of the dens and upper portion of the body of C2. Also note that the "ring" of C2 is disrupted. *Arrows* point to the top and bottom half of the ring. This type of fracture occurs in children younger than 5 years of age.

the body of C2 becomes wider than that of C3 (Fig. 12–37), which was designated by Smoker and Dolan[251] as the "fat" C2 sign. On a lateral radiograph the anteroposterior diameter of the C2 vertebral body will be larger than the anteroposterior diameter of the subjacent normal C3 vertebral body, hence the term *fat C2*. Such fractures are often better visualized by pluridirectional tomography than by CT even with reconstruction.

Isolated Fractures of the Anterior Inferior Margin

Isolated fractures of the anterior inferior margin of C2 occur (Fig. 12–38). The avulsion is mediated through tension in the anterior longitudinal ligament. At times a similar lesion occurs at C3 or in any of the other cervical vertebral bodies. The injury is due to hyperextension, and the resultant fracture has been termed the *hyperextension teardrop*. Because this fracture is frequently a component of a hangman's fracture,[150] it is important to determine that the neural arch of C2 is intact before making the definitive diagnosis of a hyperextension teardrop fracture.

Isolated fractures of the articular facet or spinous process are occasionally encountered.

Fractures of the Occipital Condyle

Fractures of the occipital condyle are rarely encountered, but they may be demonstrated by CT (see Fig. 12–34), especially when reformatted in the coronal plane. The fractures are usually avulsions mediated by the alar ligaments[184, 187, 190] or extensions or fractures of the occiput.[184, 190, 194]

Dislocations and Subluxations Involving the Craniovertebral Junction[197]

Atlantoaxial Dislocation

Atlantoaxial dislocation is the most common dislocation involving the craniovertebral junction and is usually associated with rheumatoid arthritis[152] or its variants or with Down's syndrome.[30, 43, 57] It is also a transient occurrence caused by ligamentous laxity in association with severe infections of the head and neck.[143, 146, 166] It is rarely

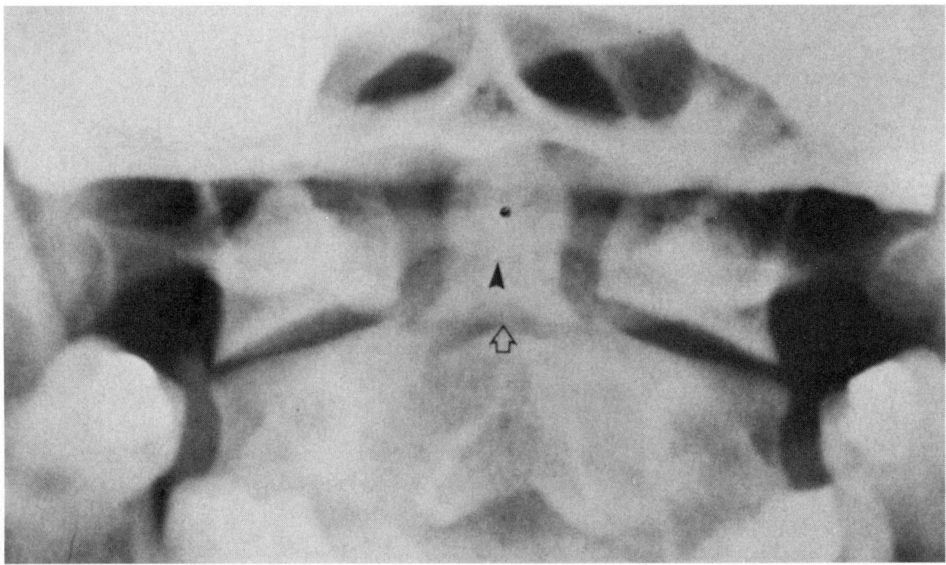

Figure 12–36. The Mach effect simulating fracture at the base of the dens. The horizontal lucent area at the base of the dens (*arrow*) is a Mach effect caused by the underlying posterior arch of C1. There is a similar lucent area caused by the anterior arch of C1 across the midportion of the dens (*arrowhead*). These may easily be mistaken for fracture. The Mach effect is particularly common at the base of the dens. The misinterpretation is aided by mistaking the normal notches between the base of the dens and the articular surface of C2 as evidence of cortical disruption.

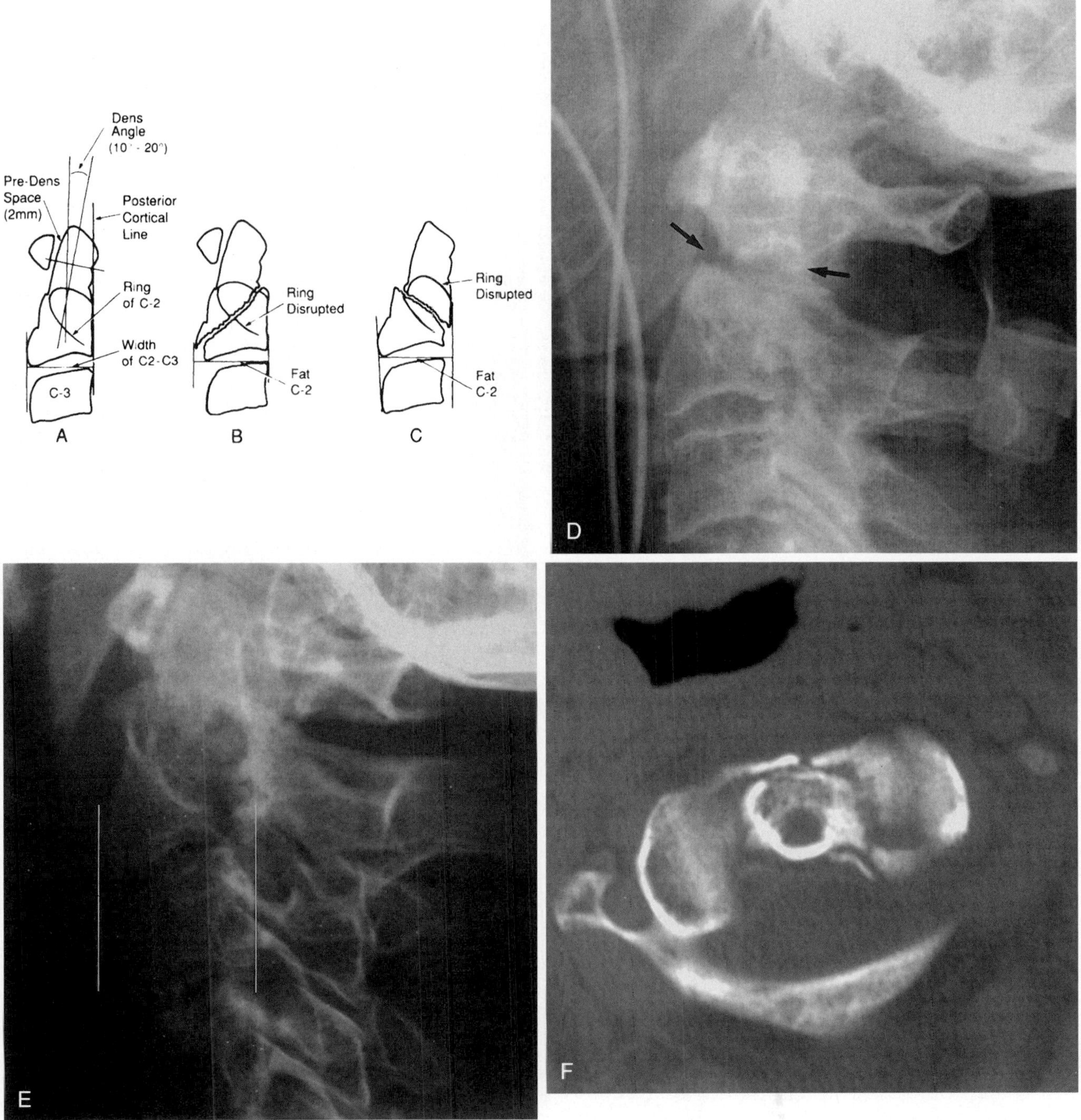

Figure 12–37. Fractures of the body of C2 (type 3 fractures of the odontoid) emphasizing the value of the "ring of C2" and "fat C2." *A* to *C*, Diagram of C2 and C3. *A*, Normal relationship of C2 to C3. The anteroposterior width of C2 equals that of C3. Note the "ring of C2," the posterior cortical line, and normal 10- to 20-degree posterior angulation of the dens. *B* and *C*, Type 3 fracture of the dens caused by flexion (*B*) and extension (*C*). Note typical course of fracture lines, disruption of "ring of C2," and "fat C2." (*A to C*, From Rogers, L.F. (1993). Injuries of the axis vertebra (C2). Contemporary Diagnostic Radiology, 16:1, with permission.) *D*, A 56-year-old man with extension, type 3 fracture. Note also the disruption of the "ring of C2" (*arrows*). *E* to *H*, A 57-year-old woman with extension, type 3 fracture (*E*). Note particularly the "fat C2"; the width of C2 exceeds that of C3. The "ring of C2" is also disrupted. *F* and *G*, CT confirms the presence of a fracture. *F*, CT of dens and upper body of C2.

Illustration continued on following page

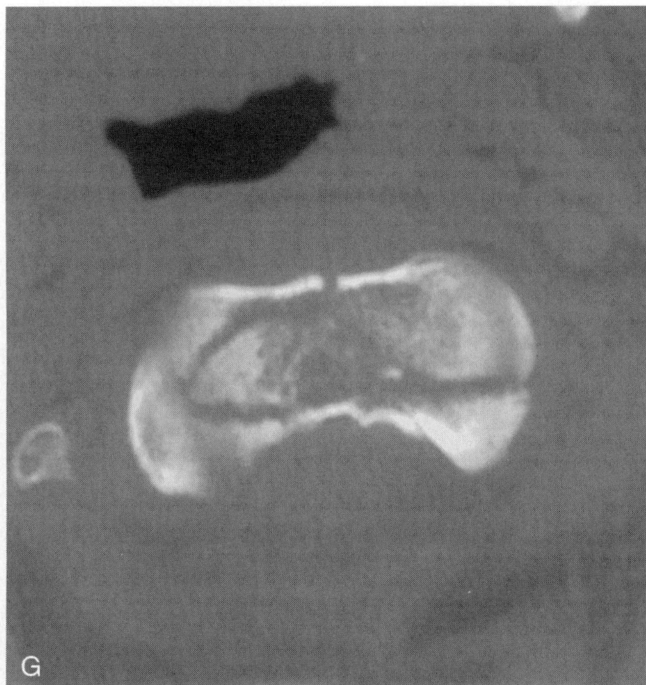

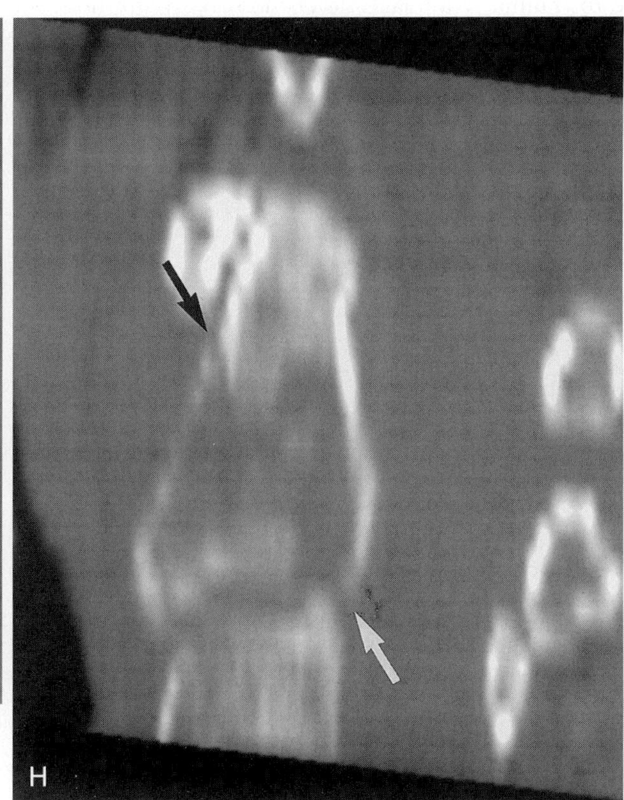

Figure 12–37 *Continued. G,* CT of lower body of C2. *H,* Sagittal reconstruction depicts the line of fracture (*arrows*).

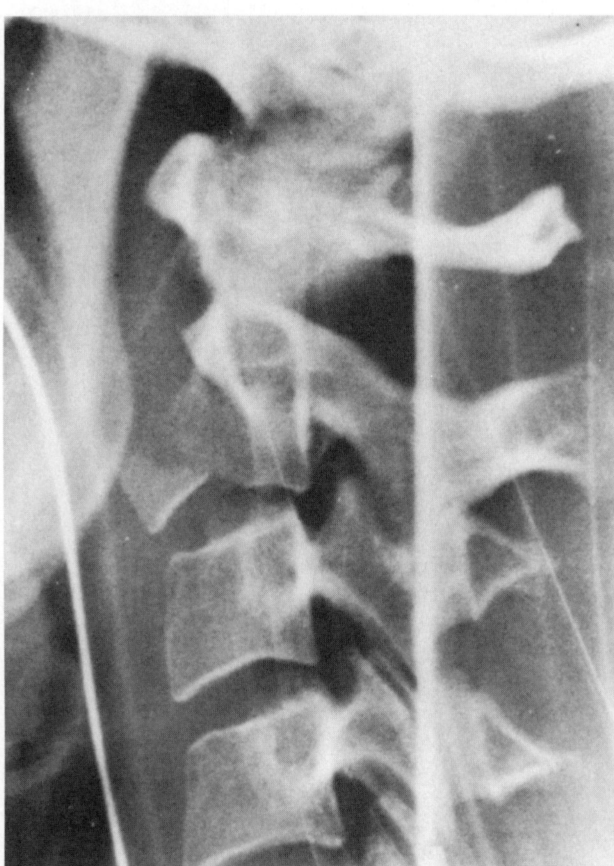

Figure 12–38. Hyperextension teardrop fracture of C2 in a 19-year-old woman. There is a large triangular fragment arising from the anterior inferior margin of C2 with minimal posterior subluxation of C2 upon C3. The neural arch is intact.

due to trauma. Traumatic dislocations do occur, however (Fig. 12–39). In the arthritides the dislocation or subluxation is due to laxity of the transverse ligament of the atlas. In traumatic subluxation or dislocation the ligament is disrupted, which is presumed to be caused by a combination of hyperflexion and shearing. The injury is demonstrated on the lateral projection and may not be evident with the spine in neutral position or in extension. Flexion may be necessary to disclose the subluxation. The normal measurement between the anterior cortex of the dens and posterior cortex of the anterior arch of the atlas is 2.5 mm in adults and 5 mm in children.[169] Measurements in excess of these dimensions are indicative of an atlantoaxial subluxation. Traumatic subluxation is the result of a rupture of the transverse ligament either as an isolated injury or as a component of Jefferson's fracture of C1. Whenever the atlantoaxial distance is increased, the possibility of an associated Jefferson's fracture should be considered.

In less than 10% of cases the predens space is V-shaped; that is, the posterior cortex of the arch of C1 and the anterior cortex of the dens are not parallel.[144, 169] The space is widened with the open end oriented cranially (Fig. 12–40). In such cases, the space between C1 and the dens usually measures 4 mm or less at the cranial end of the V. On occasion it may measure up to 7 mm and still be within normal range. The V-shaped predens space is usually identified in flexion and occasionally is seen in the neutral position, but it is practically always eliminated in extension. The V-shaped predens space is a normal finding and should not be misconstrued as evidence of a partial rupture of the transverse ligament,

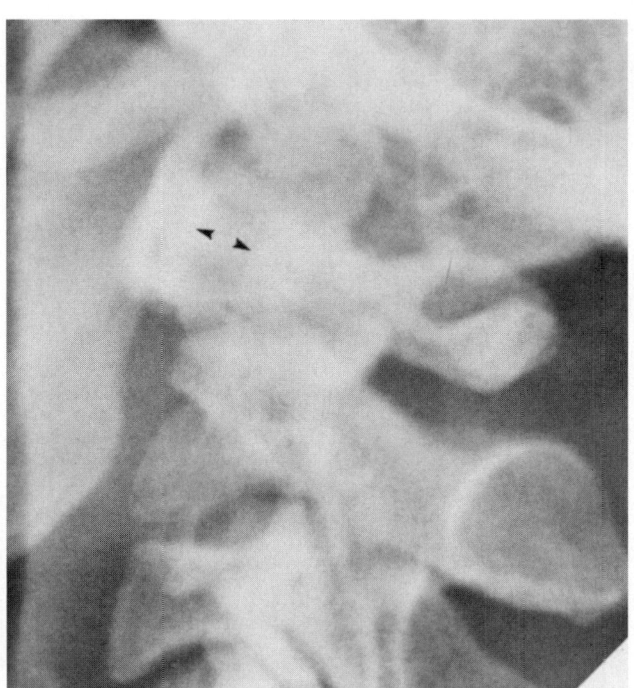

Figure 12–39. Traumatic atlantoaxial dislocation in a 27-year-old man as a result of an auto accident. There is soft tissue swelling in the nasopharynx and retropharynx. C2 is displaced posteriorly in relation to C1 without evidence of fracture. The distance between the dens and anterior arch of C1 (*arrowheads*) measures 7 mm.

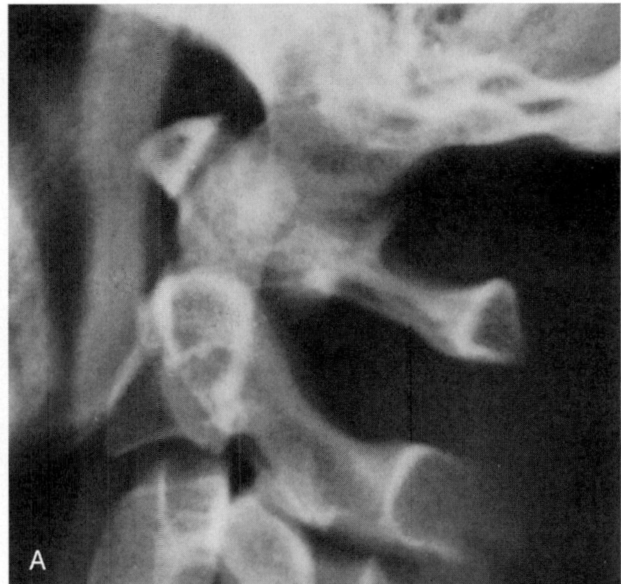

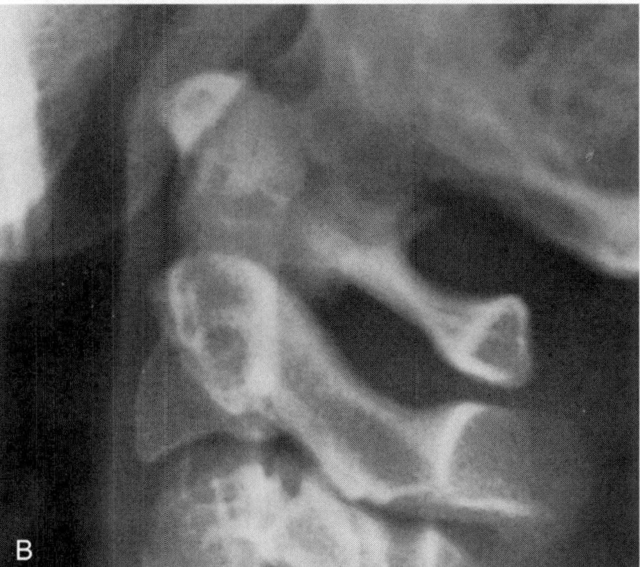

Figure 12–40. V-shaped predens space in a 23-year-old woman. *A*, Lateral view with the head flexed on the neck demonstrates a V-shaped predens space, characteristically wide superiorly and narrow inferiorly. Measurements of the predens space in such cases should be made in the middle of the V. The measurement is normal in this case. *B*, Repeat lateral view with the head in slight extension. (Note the change in position of the angle of the mandible between *A* and *B*.) Extension of the head causes the anterior arch of C1 to become parallel to the upper surface of the dens.

which has been alleged to occur but never with pathologic proof.

Craniovertebral instabilities owing to ligamentous laxity are encountered in patients with Down's syndrome.[176, 180] Atlantoaxial subluxation occurs in approximately 20% of persons with Down's syndrome, and atlanto-occipital instability has also been described.[201] Many cases have been brought to light because of screening for participation in the Special Olympics. Atlantoaxial subluxation is disclosed by lateral radiographs obtained in flexion, whereas atlanto-occipital instability, manifested by posterior displacement of the occiput relative to C1, is identified on extension films.

Posterior dislocation of the atlas on the axis (C1 upon C2) has been reported.[154, 155] In this injury the anterior arch of the atlas comes to rest against the posterior surface of the dens (Fig. 12–41). These abnormalities are easily demonstrated on the lateral view of the spine.

Atlanto-occipital Dislocation

Atlanto-occipital dislocations are usually fatal, but survivals have been reported with increasing frequency, attributable in great measure to better immediate postinjury care.[185, 186, 188, 191, 200, 204] Significant displacement is usually accompanied by disruption of the medulla oblongata and immediate death.[203] Survivals are reported in children with three times the frequency of those in adults.[202] The diagnosis is established by observations on the lateral radiograph, but it is difficult to identify the various important landmarks with certainty—in particular, the basion, or tip of the clivus at the anterior margin of the foramen magnum; the opisthion, or posterior margin of the foramen magnum; the occipital condyles; and the atlanto-occipital joint. Marked soft tissue swelling is an important clue to the possibility of this injury, particularly without any obvious accompanying fracture or dislocation[193] (Fig. 12–42). However, injuries have been described without significant soft tissue swelling. A bare or naked appearance of the occipital condyles and condylar fossa caused by longitudinal distraction of the atlanto-occipital joint is helpful in some cases; with the common anterior dislocation the upper cervical spine is well removed and free of the ramus of the mandible. The clarity with which it is seen should serve as a clue.

There are three principal forms of traumatic atlanto-occipital dislocation[186, 202] (Fig. 12–43). The first is an anterior dislocation of the head displaced anterior to the cervical spine; the second and less common is a longitudinal distraction injury resulting in a separation of the occiput from the atlas;[195] and the third, and least frequent, is a posterior dislocation of the cranium in relation to the spine. It is presumed that the injury requires a complete disruption of the ligamentous structures at the atlanto-occipital articulation.

On the lateral cervical radiograph the relationship of the dens and clivus and related structures can be established in several ways. The middle half of the upper end of the odontoid process normally lies 5 mm directly beneath the basion. In infants and young children, this distance may measure up to 1 cm. Evarts[191] stated that the tip of the odontoid process should point to the anterior tip of the foramen magnum in the middle sagittal plane. The correct alignment of the cervical spine in the skull is confirmed when a line extended from the surface of the clivus intersects the odontoid process somewhere in its posterior third and when the curved spinolaminar line of C1 extended posteriorly and superiorly meets the region of the posterior margin of the foramen magnum or opisthion. The width of the atlanto-occipital joint may be measured directly on a radiograph or more easily by reformatted CT. In children the joint averages 5 mm in width; however, some normal joints measure up to 10 mm. The joint is difficult to measure. When it exceeds 5 mm, the diagnosis of atlanto-occipital dislocation should be considered.

Because direct observations and measurements are difficult, observers have turned to the construction of various lines to determine the proper relationship between anatomic structures at the craniovertebral junction. The most suggested method is the Powers ratio.[199] Powers and col-

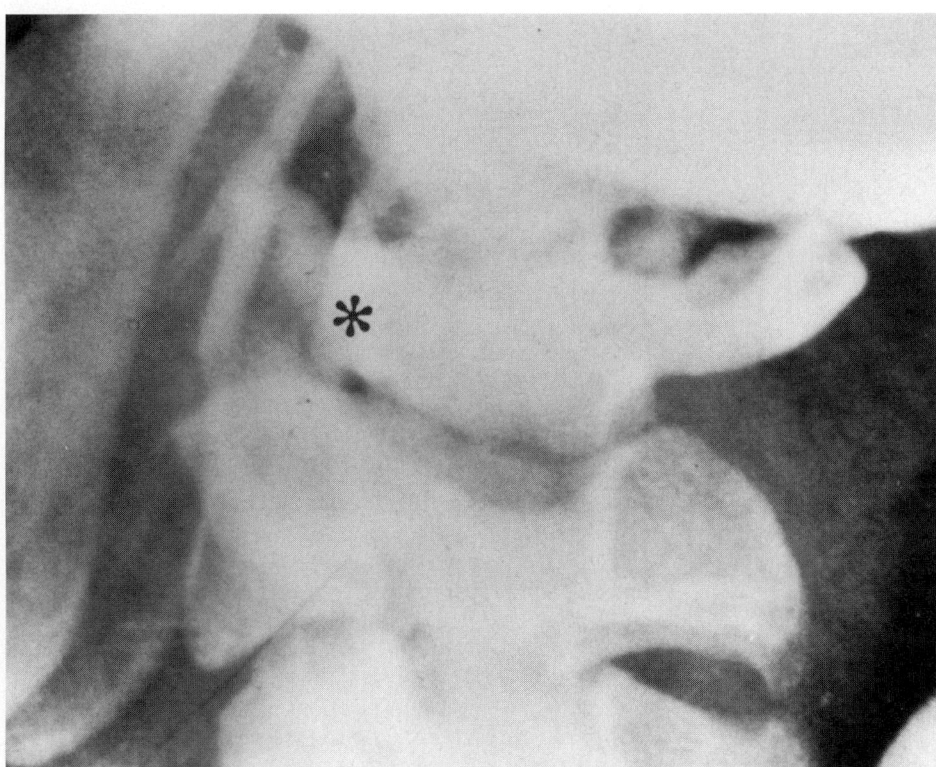

Figure 12–41. Atlantoaxial dislocation in a 21-year-old man without a neurologic deficit. The dens rests anterior to the anterior arch of C1 (*). (Case courtesy of Charles Resnick, MD, Baltimore.)

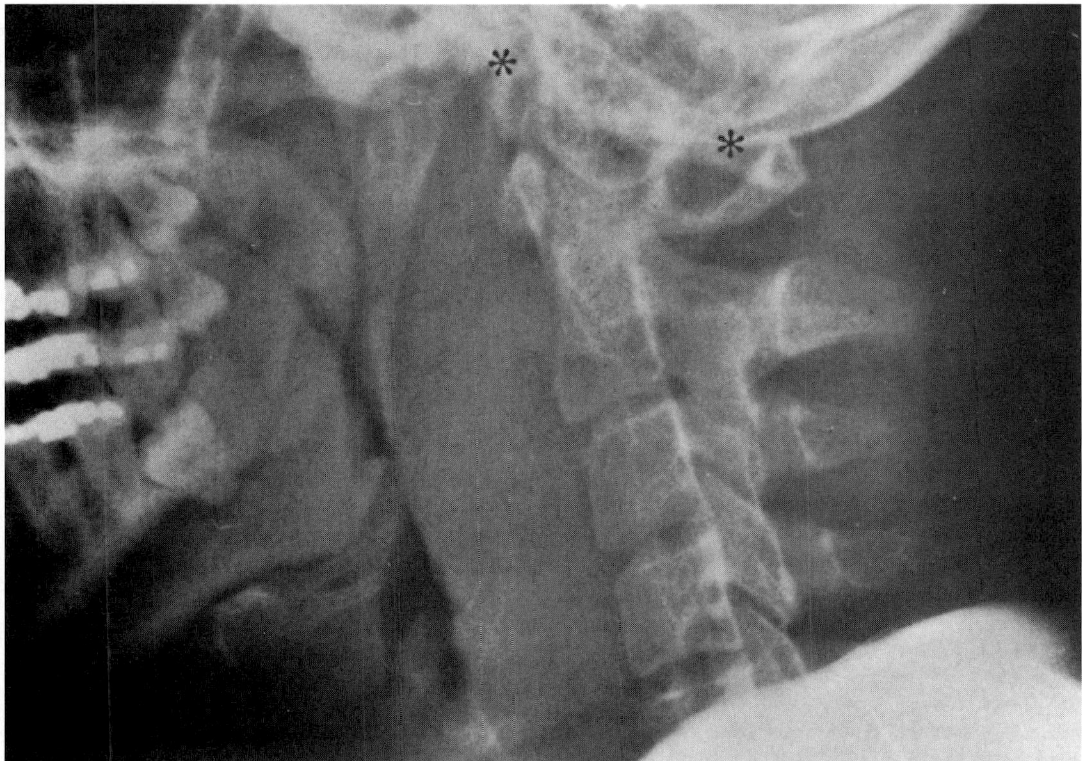

Figure 12–42. Posterior atlanto-occipital dislocation in a 27-year-old man. Note the massive retropharangeal soft tissue swelling and the relative clarity of the upper cervical spine. It is seen so clearly because the spine lies well posterior to its normal position. The tip of the clivus and the opisthion are seen (*). By constructing the X line as in Figure 12–43, it can be seen that the line from the opisthion to the third vertebral body lies well anterior to the spinolaminar junction of C1 and the line from the clivus to the spinolaminar junction of C2 passes through the dens. This clearly demonstrates that the spine lies posterior to its normal position. (Case courtesy of Charles Lee, MD, Lexington, Ky.)

leagues[198] proposed the ratio of the length of two lines as an indicator of atlanto-occipital dislocation: one line is the distance between the basion (B) and the posterior arch of C1 (C), and the other line is the distance from the opisthion (O) to the anterior arch of the atlas (A). The mean BC/OA value in a normal population is 0.77. Any value greater than 1 is considered indicative of atlanto-occipital dislocation. Unfortunately, the Powers ratio is only abnormal in approximately one third of cases.[196] The ratio may be less than 1 in cases of posterior atlanto-occipital dislocation as well as with pure longitudinal distraction. Lee and associates[196] have proposed an X line method of evaluation (see Fig. 12–43). On a normal lateral radiograph a line is drawn from the tip of the basion to the midpoint of the C2 spinolaminar line. This line just intersects with the posterior superior margin of the dens in most cases. A second line is drawn from the posterior inferior corner of the body to the tip of the opisthion. This line intersects with the highest point of the C1 spinolaminar line. With an anterior dislocation both limbs of the X are displaced forward from their reference points, and with posterior dislocation both limbs are displaced posteriorly. With longitudinal distraction, the basion-C2 spinolaminar line is displaced posteriorly from the dens and the C2-opisthion line is displaced anteriorly from its intersection with the posterior arch of C1. In the series by Lee and associates, the X line was the most accurate means of establishing a diagnosis and was positive in 77% of cases.

The diagnosis of atlanto-occipital dislocation may not be easy. It must first be suspected on the basis of soft tissue swelling or questionable relationships at the atlanto-occipital junction; then various measurements and linear relationships can be determined to either exclude or confirm the diagnosis. Reformatted CT may be required.[187, 189, 192, 193]

Rotatory Atlantoaxial Dislocation

Rotatory atlantoaxial dislocation occurs in two principal forms.[24] *Torticollis*, or *wryneck*, is an atlantoaxial rotatory displacement frequently encountered in childhood and early adolescence (Fig. 12–44). This type of dislocation may occur spontaneously or in association with acute infectious diseases of the upper respiratory tract or following minor trauma to the head and neck. The second form of rotatory atlantoaxial dislocation is caused by acute trauma (Fig. 12–45). Both types are characterized by a tilting of the head in one direction and simultaneous rotation of the head in the opposite direction. This positioning has been likened to that of a robin listening for a worm, the so-called cock-robin appearance.[159] Lesser degrees of injury are due to laxity of the supporting atlantoaxial ligaments. The principal atlantoaxial ligaments are the transverse and the paired alar ligaments. The alar ligaments prevent excessive rotation. With severe displacement it is likely that one or more of the ligaments are disrupted. With severe rotational displacement, as is occasionally encountered following trauma, the radiographs reveal an obvious malalignment of the atlas and

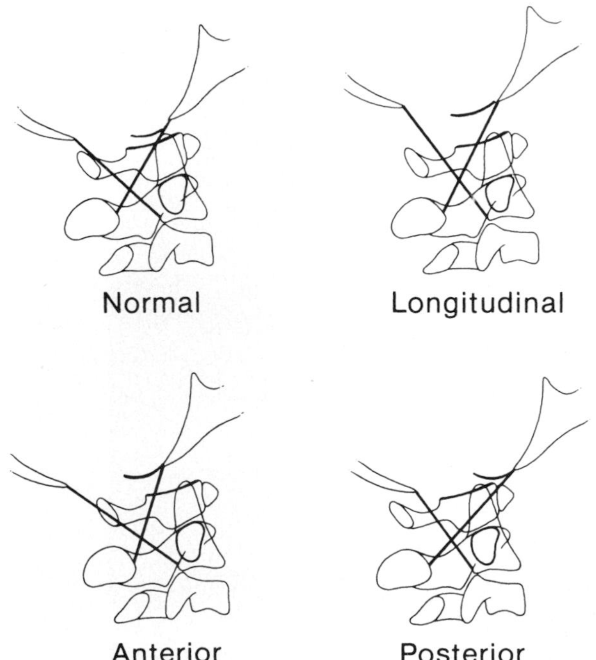

Figure 12–43. The X line method of identifying and classifying atlanto-occipital dislocations. See text for explanation. (Adapted from Lee, C., Woodring, J. H., Goldstein, S. J. et al. [1987]. Evaluation of atlantooccipital dislocation. A.J.N.R., 8:19.)

axis; with lesser degrees of injury, the findings are much more subtle.

The radiographic findings (see Figs. 12–44 and 12–45) include asymmetry of the space between the dens and the articular masses of the axis, asymmetry of the lateral margins of the lateral atlantoaxial joints, increase in the transverse diameter of the anteriorly rotated articular mass of the atlas, decrease in the width of the posteriorly rotated articular mass, and displacement of the spinous process of the axis from the midline in the direction opposite that toward which the head is rotated. There is narrowing of the joint space at C1-C2 or overlap on the side on which the articular mass is widened, whereas the contralateral narrowed articular mass is associated with widening of the C1-C2 joint space. On the lateral projection the rotation and lateral tilt of the atlas and axis result in loss of definition of normal anatomy. The complex distortion is very difficult to describe, but it is characteristic and should pose no difficulty in the proper clinical setting.

CT demonstrates the abnormality quite nicely. Contiguous slices demonstrate the obvious rotary displacement of C1 upon C2[162] (see Fig. 12–45). In most cases there is disruption of one of the facet joints pivoting about the opposite intact facet joint. Displacement may be sufficient to result in locking of the facets. Occasionally, both facet joints are dislocated.[149, 160] With greater displacement, the anterior arch of the atlas may be displaced anteriorly 5 mm or more relative to the dens. Displacements of this or greater magnitude imply ligamentous disruption. The acute traumatic form may often be reduced by traction and rotation of the head.[24] At times the joint remains unstable because of ligamentous disruption, often manifested by recurrent dislocations, which ultimately require surgical stabilization (usually some form of fusion).[159] Torticollis and other lesser forms usually resolve spontaneously.

Associated Neurologic Injury

It is reasonable to ask how anyone could sustain any of the various fractures and dislocations of the craniovertebral junction without sustaining neurologic injury. The spinal cord occupies only 50% of the spinal canal at this level, which in itself affords some margin of safety. It is possible to reduce the dimensions of the spinal canal by 50% without necessarily injuring the spinal cord. At C1 approximately one third of the ring is occupied by the dens and its associated ligaments, one third by the spinal cord, and the remaining third by the subarachnoid space, meninges, and epidural fat. In spite of the presence of the dens, there still is a 50% margin of safety at C1; therefore, when dislocation occurs, provided there is no more than a 50% reduction in the dimension of the spinal canal, neurologic injury need not occur. Fracture of the ring of the atlas, either the posterior arch or Jefferson's fracture, or hangman's fracture of C2 actually increases the width of the spinal canal by displacement of the fragments. In Jefferson's fracture (see Fig. 12–23), the fragments are centrifugally displaced; in fractures of the posterior arch of C1 and of the neural arch of C2 (see Figs. 12–27 and 12–28), the fragments are posteriorly displaced to some extent; these in effect increase the dimensions of the spinal canal, and neurologic injury is avoided.

Lower Cervical Spine

The usual way to present injuries of the cervical spine is by classification according to the nature of the force that created the injury.[255] Each particular force or combination of forces tends to result in a relatively specific pattern of injury. These classifications are valuable in their explanation of how the injury is produced and in their implications regarding the type of treatment that is best for the patient. Before the injury can be classified, however, it must be recognized. A pattern should be developed for searching radiographs. After the injury is recognized, it can be classified according to the forces involved, and then the appropriate treatment plan can be outlined.

The initial radiograph is a horizontal lateral view of the cervical spine. It is essential that all seven cervical vertebrae are included on the radiograph (see Fig. 12–9) so that significant injuries of the cervicothoracic junction are not missed.[9, 87, 88, 274] It is easy to erroneously assume that all seven vertebrae are present. It is best to simply count the vertebrae to confirm their presence; this will avoid error. Interpretation of the radiograph of the lower cervical spine should include analysis of the retropharyngeal soft tissues and the height and continuity of the vertebral body, determination of the alignment of the vertebral elements,[87, 88, 90, 115] and exclusion of fractures of the articular pillars and posterior elements of the vertebral bodies.[167] In this manner one can be reasonably assured that no significant injury has been overlooked.

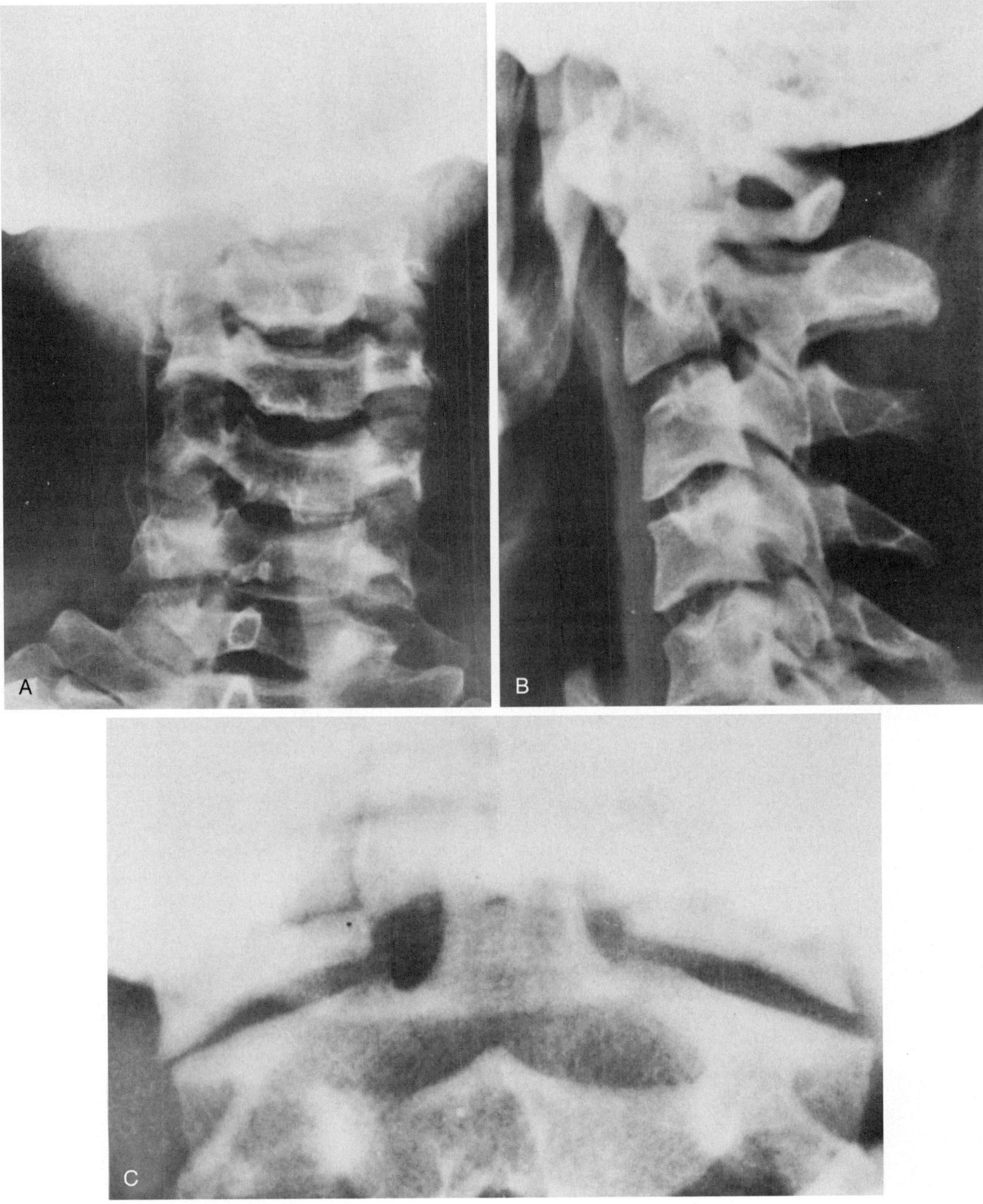

Figure 12–44. Torticollis in a 28-year-old man. *A*, Anteroposterior view demonstrates scoliosis of the cervical spine. The head is tilted and rotated to the right in relation to the spine. *B*, Lateral view of the cervical spine demonstrates rotation and tilting of C1 in relation to C2. *C*, Open-mouth view of C1 to C2 demonstrates that C1 is tilted and offset to the right with asymmetry of the space between the dens and the articular masses of C1. There is also asymmetry of the joint space at C1-C2. The findings are typical of torticollis. There was no history of trauma in this case.

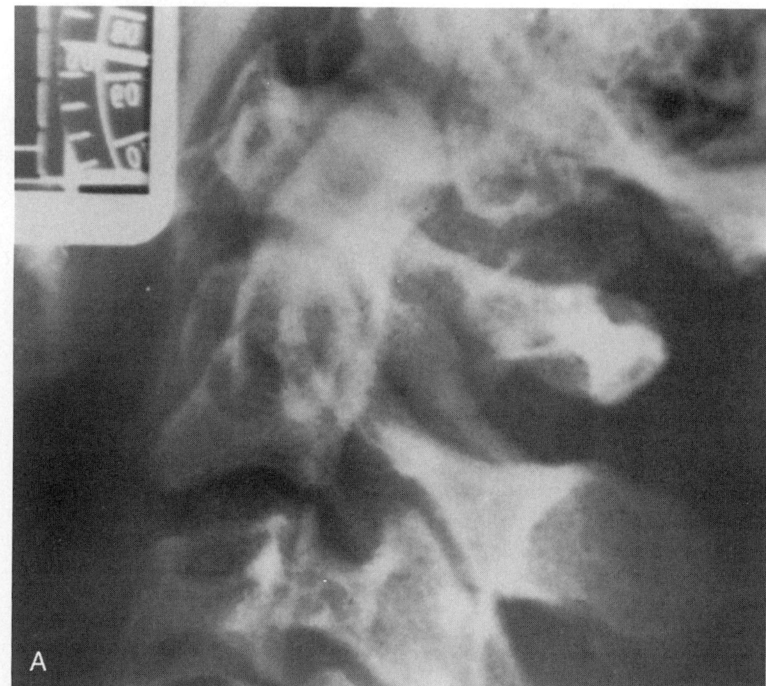

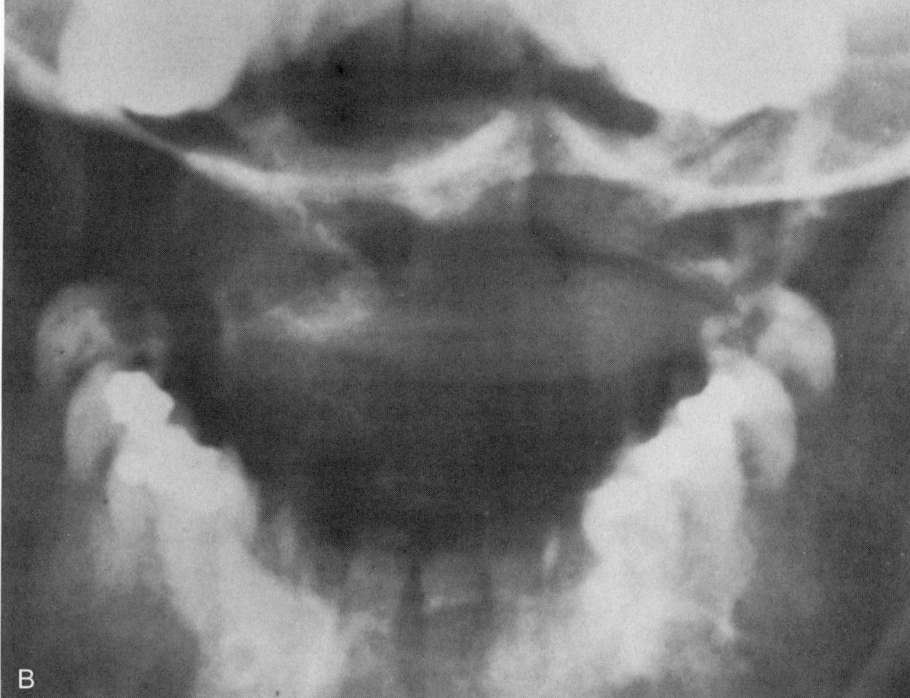

Figure 12–45. Rotatory atlantoaxial subluxation with facet lock in a 23-year-old woman. *A*, Lateral radiograph of the craniovertebral junction demonstrates marked rotation of the lateral masses of C1 with foreshortening of the neural arch. *B*, Open-mouth view of the craniovertebral junction reveals rotation of C1 as evidenced by variation in the distance between the medial margin of the lateral masses of C1 and the dens. Note that the C1-C2 facet joint is not clearly visualized on the right and appears narrowed on the left.

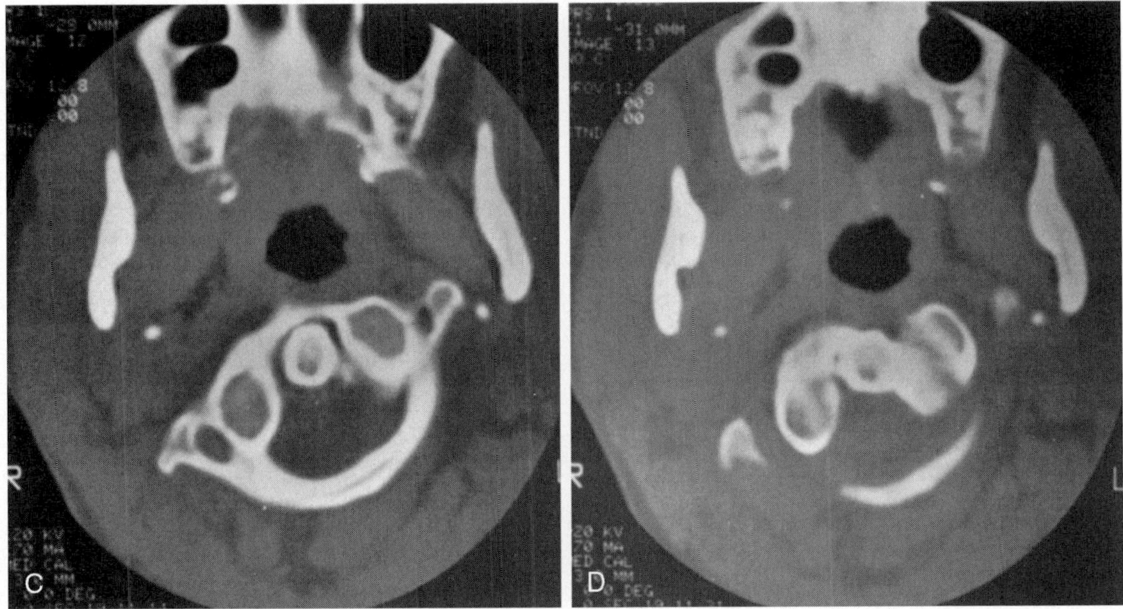

Figure 12–45 *Continued.* *C*, CT scan demonstrates rotation of C1 in relation to the dens and facial skeleton. *D*, CT scan at a slightly inferior level shows anterior subluxation of the left lateral mass of C1 and a complete posterior dislocation of the lateral mass on the right.

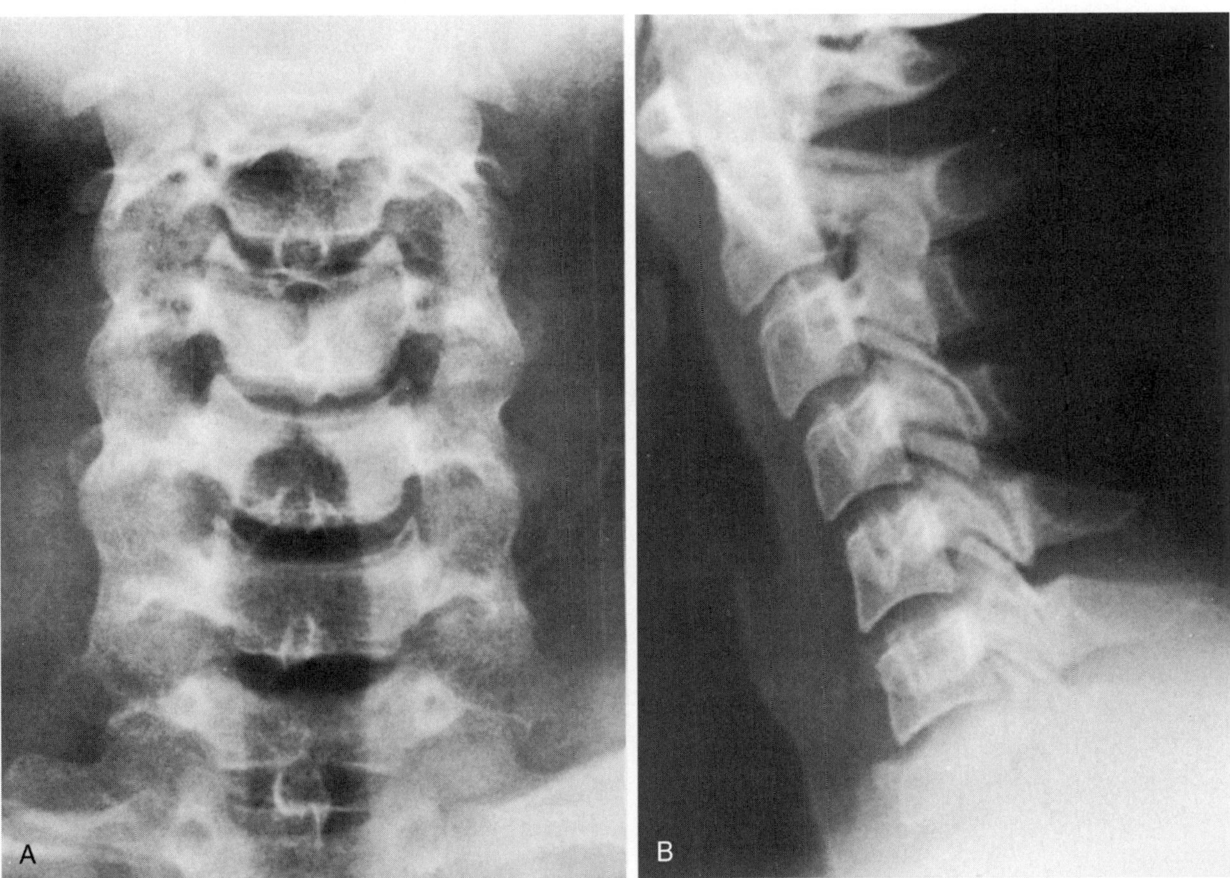

Figure 12–46. Compression fracture of C7 in a 21-year-old man who dove into a shallow pool. *A*, Anteroposterior view demonstrates the loss of height of the body of C7. The superior end plate of the vertebral body is poorly defined. *B*, Lateral view demonstrates anterior wedge compression of the body of C7. There is a small triangular fragment separated from the anterior superior portion of the vertebral body.

Burst Fracture

When axial compression forces predominate, the intervertebral disc is driven into the vertebral body below, and the vertebral body is exploded into several fragments. This is termed a *burst fracture* (Fig. 12–47). The fragments are driven centrifugally, and a fragment from the posterior superior surface of the involved vertebra is driven into the spinal canal (see Fig. 12–47), which frequently results in spinal cord injury. It may be difficult, if not impossible, to visualize this posteriorly displaced fragment on the plain radiograph. The posterior cortex of the vertebral body is normally visible on the lateral radiograph, projecting as a thin line of cortical bone that is referred to as the posterior cortical line. In a burst fracture this line is disrupted and the posteriorly displaced fragment can be identified within the spinal canal, or, alternatively, the superior segment of the line is not visualized. When the posterior superior margin of the vertebra is not visualized or in the presence of a severe comminuted or markedly compressed vertebral body, CT should be performed to exclude or identify a posteriorly displaced fragment in the spinal canal (see Fig. 12–47*C* and *D*). Such injuries are more common in the thoracolumbar spine and are more fully described in Chapter 13.

Teardrop Fracture

The *teardrop fracture*[271] is a specific form of the burst fracture described by Schneider and Kahn.[132] The injury is a fracture-dislocation consisting of a comminuted fracture of a vertebral body with a characteristic triangular or quadrilateral fragment (Fig. 12–48) from the anterior inferior margin of the vertebral body (the teardrop). The teardrop fracture is usually accompanied by a spinal cord injury. Indeed, it was the frequency of spinal cord injury as much as the configuration at the anterior fragment that led Schneider and Khan[132] to designate this as a teardrop fracture.[268, 270, 275, 278] With more severe injuries, the fracture is accompanied by a posterior dislocation, widening of the interspinous distance, and disruption of the facet joints. With lesser degrees of injury, there may be just a slight posterior offset of the affected vertebra and the facet joints may remain intact. In just less than 50% of cases a vertical, sagittal split is identifiable in the vertebral body, either on the anteroposterior plain film or subsequently by CT (Fig. 12–49); similar complete or incomplete fractures may be found in adjacent vertebral bodies.[275] The teardrop fragment may also be a split sagittally. As in Jefferson's fracture, it is impossible to disrupt a ring of bone in only one position; thus, a sagittally oriented fracture anteriorly is accompanied by fractures of the neural arch posteriorly. These commonly occur at the junction of the laminae and lateral masses and are often bilateral.

Vertical Split of Vertebral Body

On occasion a vertical split of the vertebral body[124, 128, 134, 277] may be seen without other associated abnormalities (see Fig. 12–13). This injury is created by predominantly compressive forces in the sagittal plane. It is thought to be created by acute herniation of the intervertebral disc into the vertebral body below. The fracture line is apparent only on the frontal projection and may easily be mistaken for air in the larynx. The vertebra is split in the sagittal plane into almost equal parts. The obscure vertical fracture may be evident on the plain film if the end plates of the vertebral bodies are closely observed.[277] Disruption in the end plate may indicate the presence of sagittal fractures. In the majority of fractures, two or, less commonly, three contiguous vertebral bodies will be so affected. Lateral radiographs may demonstrate very slight anterior, wedged compression, but often there is no obvious deformity of the vertebral body. Most cases will have associated fractures in the posterior arch involving either the lamina or the pedicle. Posterior fractures are rarely evident on the plain film but will be disclosed by CT.

Despite its relatively innocuous appearance, this fracture is commonly accompanied by spinal cord injury.

Facet Locking

When a vertebral body is displaced anteriorly so that 50% or more overrides the vertebral body below there is practically always associated bilateral locking of the facets[109, 118] (Figs. 12–52 and 12–53). Flexion[127] combined with distraction forces results in ligamentous disruption. The apophyseal joints at the affected level are completely disrupted, allowing the superiorly located vertebra to displace anteriorly to such a degree that the facets become locked in a position anterior to the facets of the vertebral body below. This situation requires at least 50% displacement of one vertebral body on the other. The spinal canal is, of course, severely compromised by this displacement, and spinal cord injuries are frequent.

Lesser degrees of displacement, usually in the range of 25% and measuring approximately 4 to 5 mm of one vertebra on the other, are usually due to unilateral locking of the facets[109, 118, 259] (Figs. 12–52, 12–53*B*, 12–54, and 12–55).

Unilateral facet dislocation occurs most frequently at C5-C6 or C6-C7 and less commonly at C3-C4, C4-C5, and C7–T1.[262, 283]

A combination of flexion, distraction, and rotation results in unilateral displacement and locking of the facet joints.[106] The radiographic clue to this injury on the lateral view rests with recognition that the articular pillars are visualized in the true lateral profile above the injury but are in the oblique profile below the injury, or vice versa.[9, 156] The obliquity of the spine causes the articular pillar on the side of rotation to project anterior to the unrotated articular pillar on the opposite side. When the rotated articular pillar is projected at the anterior margin of the unrotated pillar, the rhomboid outline of the pillars creates a characteristic "bow tie" or "butterfly" appearance (see Fig. 12–53*B*). In some cases rotation is not immediately obvious. The first clue is often the presence of a minimal dislocation or subluxation. Rotation may then be recognized by noting the rounded pedicle in the anterior superior margin of the rotated vertebral bodies above the level of injury. A search for evidence of the "bow tie" configuration of the pillars confirms rotation. This configuration may not be evident at the level of injury, but it may be seen two or three segments proximally. Young and colleagues[298] noted a reduction in the

Text continued on page 432

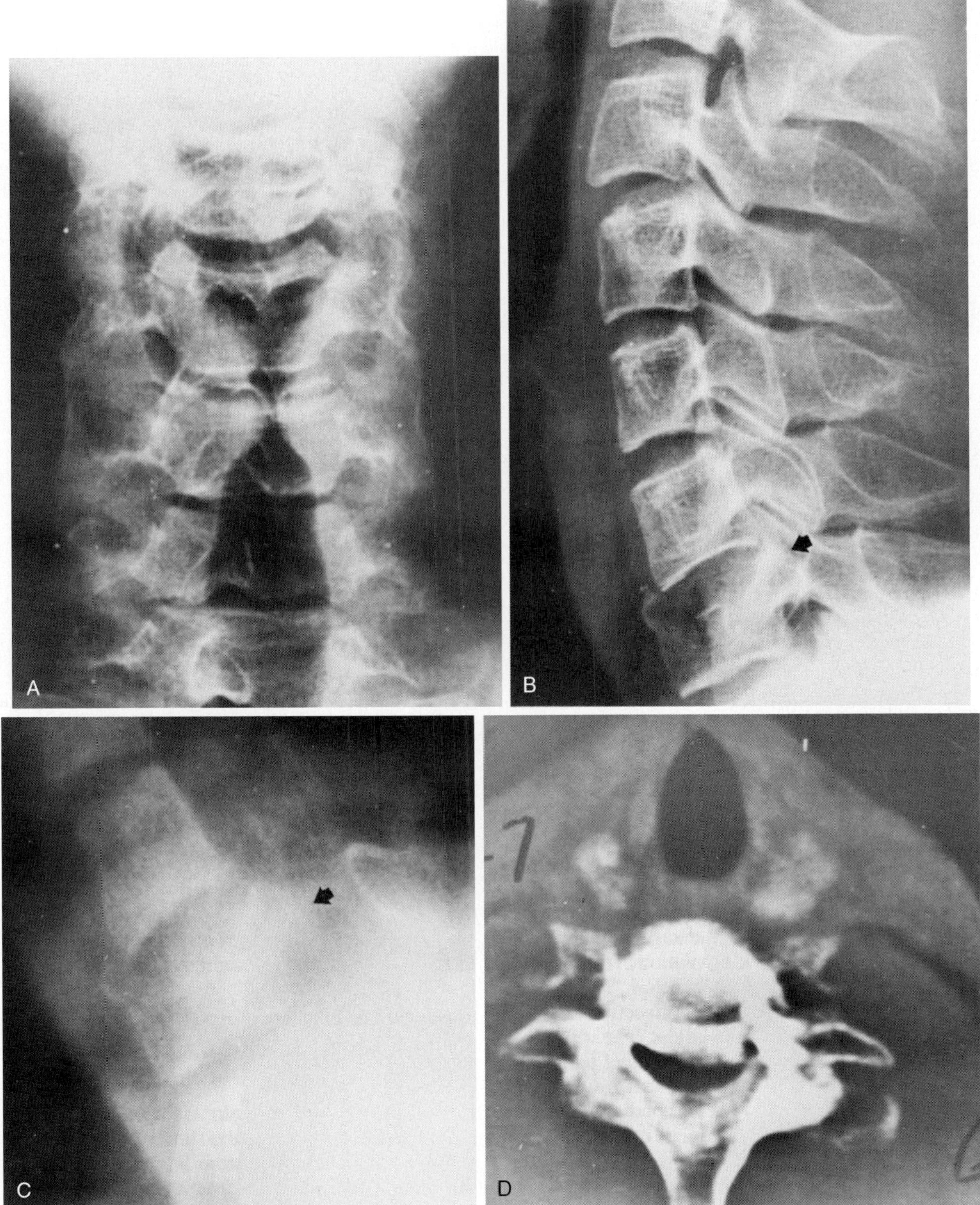

Figure 12–47. Burst fracture of C7 in a 17-year-old boy. *A*, Anteroposterior view fails to demonstrate any evidence of abnormality. Neither the body of C6 nor the body of C7 is well visualized. *B*, Lateral view demonstrates severe depression of the superior end plate of C7. There is a suggestion that a fragment from the posterior superior surface of the vertebral body is displaced into the spinal canal (*arrow*). *C*, Lateral tomogram confirms the presence of a posteriorly displaced fragment (*arrow*) from the posterior superior portion of the vertebral body. *D*, CT scan clearly demonstrates the posteriorly displaced fragment that severely compromises the spinal canal. (Case courtesy of Michael Mikhael, MD, Evanston, Ill.)

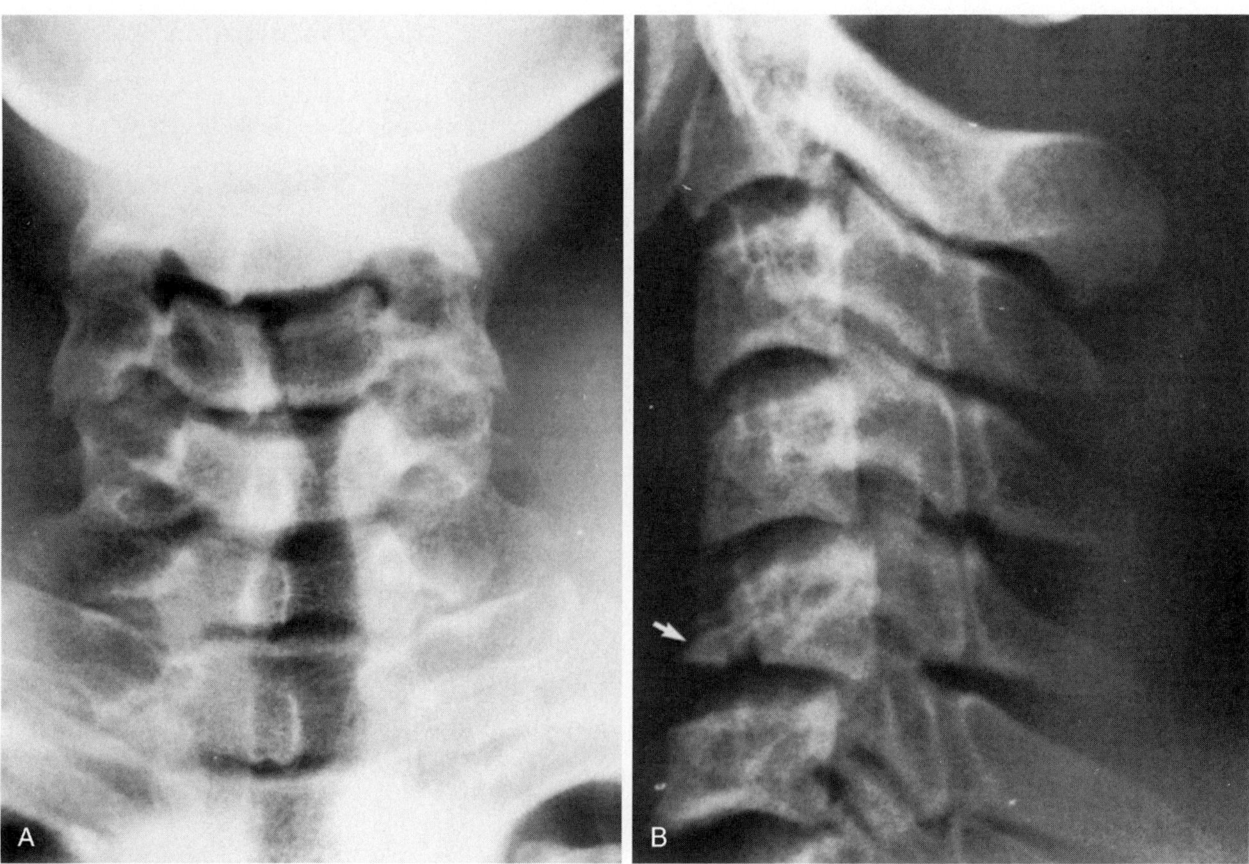

Figure 12–48. Teardrop fracture of C5 in an 18-year-old boy. *A*, Anteroposterior view demonstrates a lucency in the sagittal plane of C5. Close examination reveals that this is cortical disruption of both the superior and inferior end plates. *B*, Lateral view demonstrates compression of the body of C5 associated with a posterior dislocation of C5 upon C6. The fragment from the anterior inferior surface of C5 (*arrow*) is the teardrop.

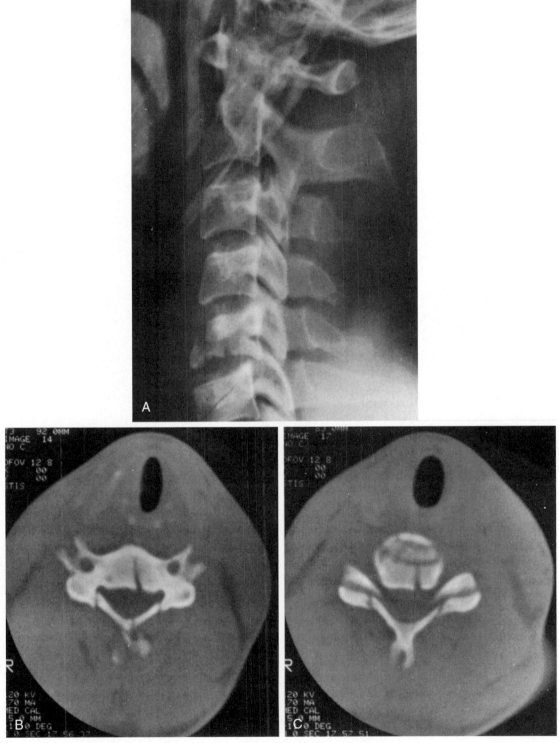

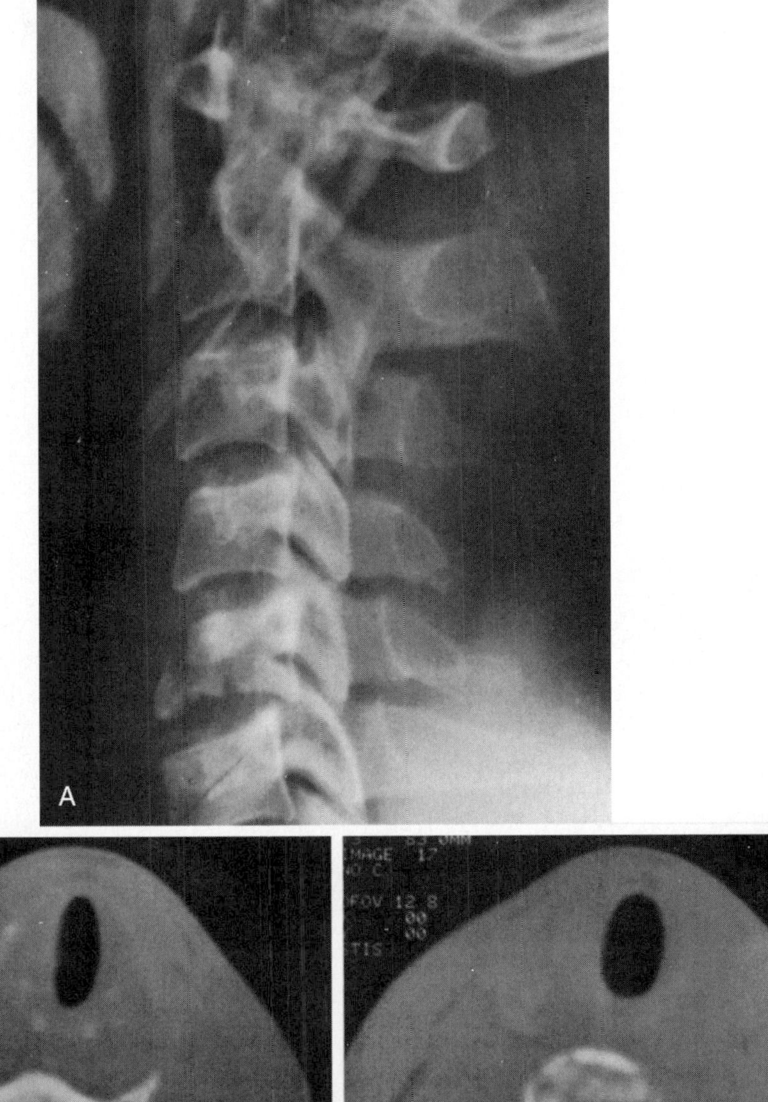

Figure 12–49. Teardrop fracture of C5 in a 22-year-old man. *A*, Characteristic teardrop fracture manifested by posterior dislocation at C5-C6 with a triangular fragment arising from the anterior inferior margin of C5. The facet joints and interspinous distance are within normal limits. *B*, CT scan through the top half of C5 demonstrates a sagittal fracture of the vertebral body and bilateral fractures of the laminae at their junctions with the lateral masses. *C*, CT scan through the lower half of C5 demonstrates slight widening of the facet joints bilaterally. The sagittal fracture of the vertebral body and comminuted fracture of the anterior inferior end plate of the vertebra are identified. The laminar fractures are again shown.

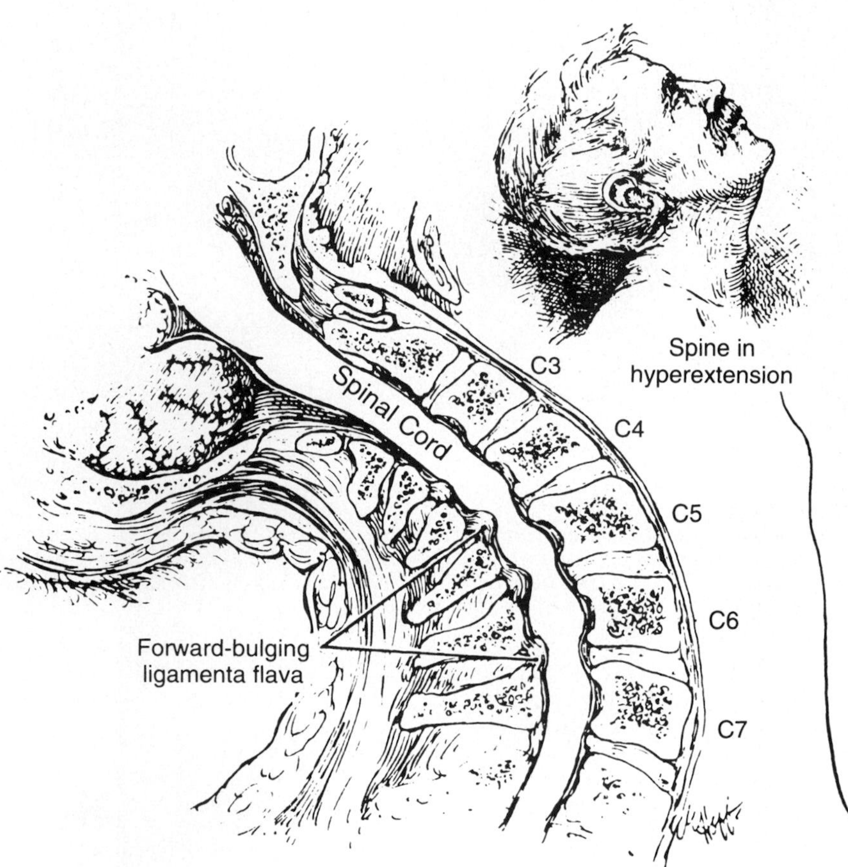

Figure 12–50. Mechanism of injury of the spinal cord in spondylosis. Hyperextension causes the spinal cord to be pinched by posterior spur formation at the margins of the intervertebral space anteriorly and enfolding of hypertrophied ligamentum flavum posteriorly. (From Schneider, R. C., Cherry, G., & Pantek, H. [1954]. The syndrome of acute central cervical spinal cord injury. J. Neurosurg., *11*:546, with permission.)

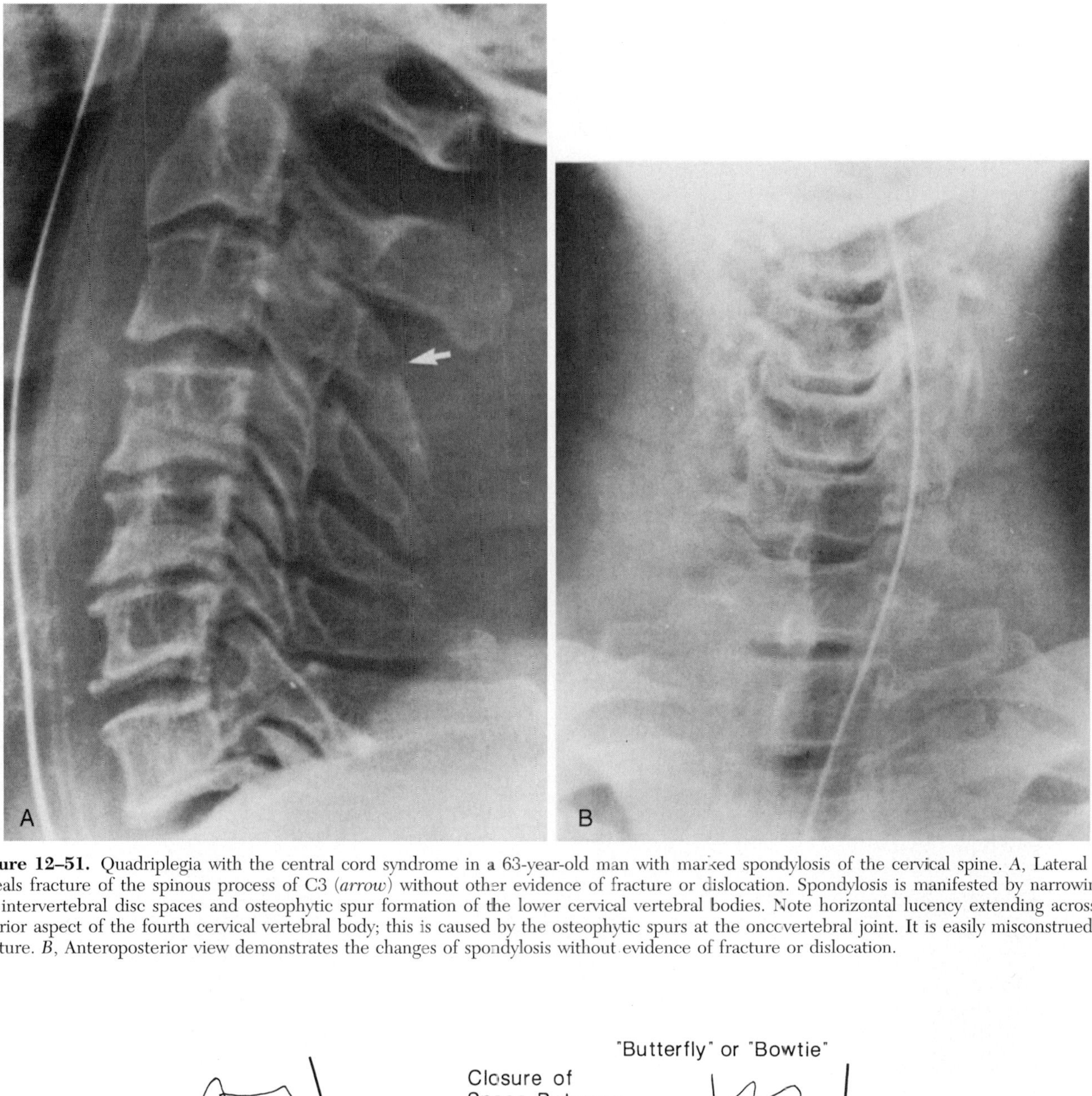

Figure 12–51. Quadriplegia with the central cord syndrome in a 63-year-old man with marked spondylosis of the cervical spine. *A*, Lateral view reveals fracture of the spinous process of C3 (*arrow*) without other evidence of fracture or dislocation. Spondylosis is manifested by narrowing of the intervertebral disc spaces and osteophytic spur formation of the lower cervical vertebral bodies. Note horizontal lucency extending across the inferior aspect of the fourth cervical vertebral body; this is caused by the osteophytic spurs at the oncovertebral joint. It is easily misconstrued as a fracture. *B*, Anteroposterior view demonstrates the changes of spondylosis without evidence of fracture or dislocation.

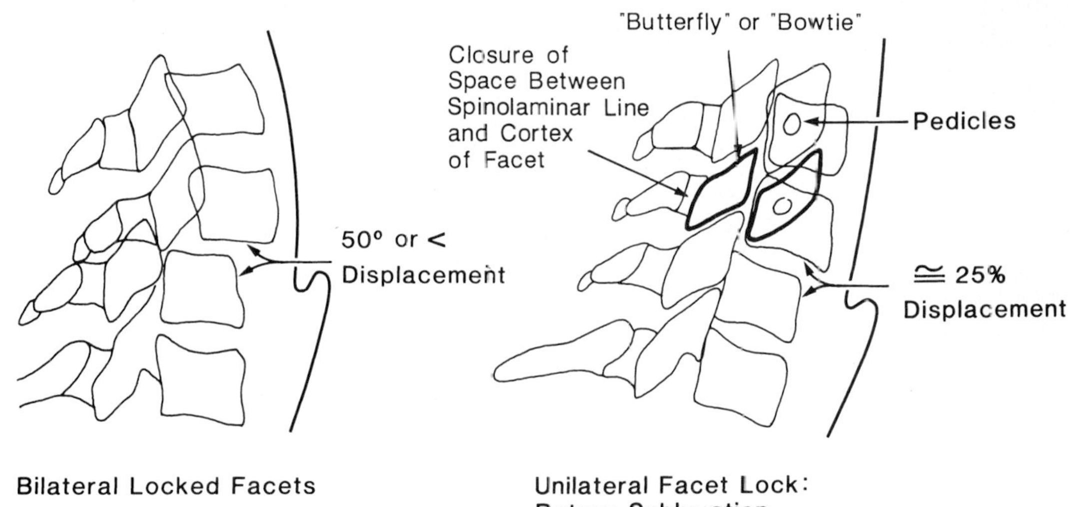

Figure 12–52. Facet locking. In bilateral facet lock, the vertebra above is displaced 50% or more of the anteroposterior diameter of the vertebral body and the inferior facets of the anteriorly displaced vertebra lie anterior to the superior facets of the vertebra below. In unilateral facet lock, the vertebra is characteristic displaced anteriorly approximately 25%. The vertebrae above are seen in oblique profile and vertebrae below this level in true lateral profile. The facets are locked only on one side. Note the locking depicted by the "butterfly" or "bow tie" appearance of the facets. Also, the distance between the posterior surface of the lateral masses and spinolaminar junction is reduced at the level of the dislocation.

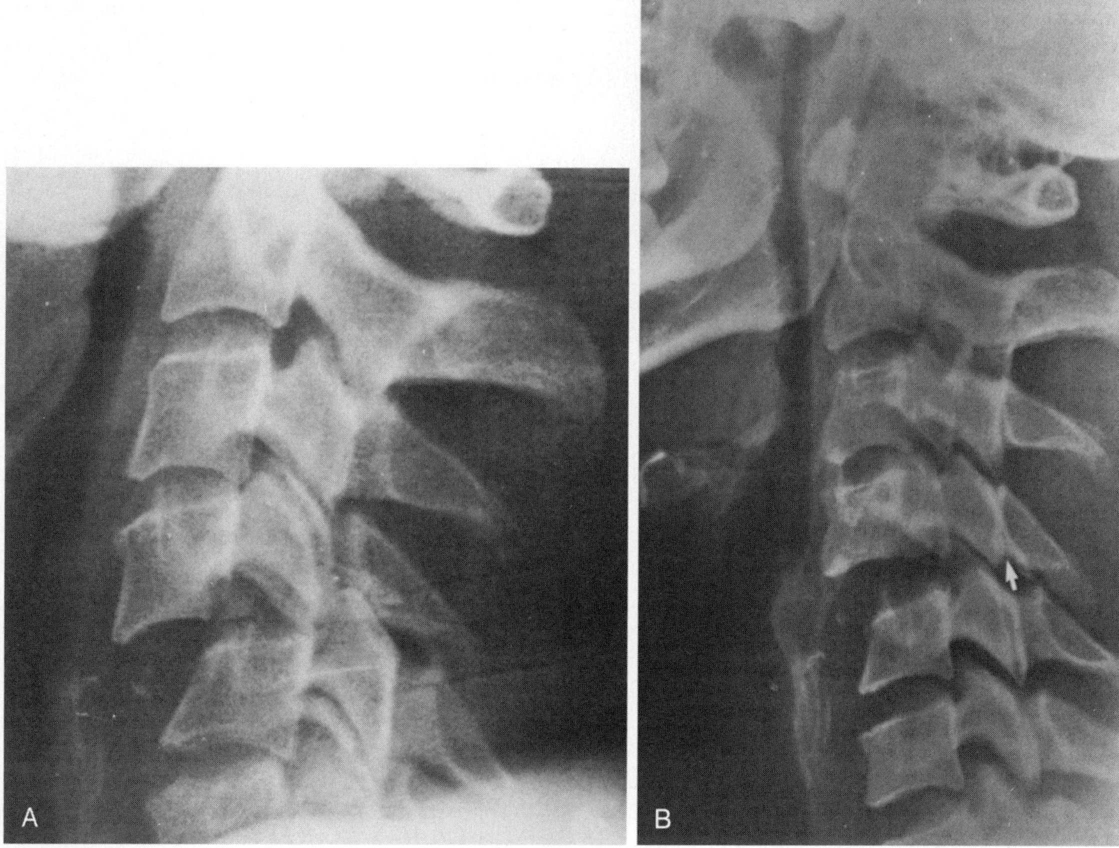

Figure 12–53. Fracture-dislocation with locking of the facets at C4-C5 as a result of an auto accident in a 31-year-old man. *A*, Initial lateral view demonstrates anterior dislocation of C4 upon C5. The displacement is greater than 50% of the width of the vertebral bodies. There is an associated fracture from the posterior inferior margin of the vertebral body and bilateral locking of the facets. The inferior facet of C4 lies anterior to the superior facet of C5. *B*, Following application of cranial traction, bilateral locking of the facets was converted to unilateral. The body of C4 remains anteriorly dislocated approximately 25% of the width of the body, as is characteristic of unilateral locking of the facets. Note that the bodies of vertebrae C5 and below are in true lateral profile, whereas those of C4 and above are seen in oblique profile. The rotated facets at C4 and above assume the characteristic "bow tie" or "butterfly" appearance. Note also that the distance between the posterior margin of the facets and the spinolaminar junction decreases and actually is obliterated at the level of the rotated facets (*arrow*). Narrowing or obliteration of this space is characteristic and helpful when the "bow tie" appearance is not so obvious.

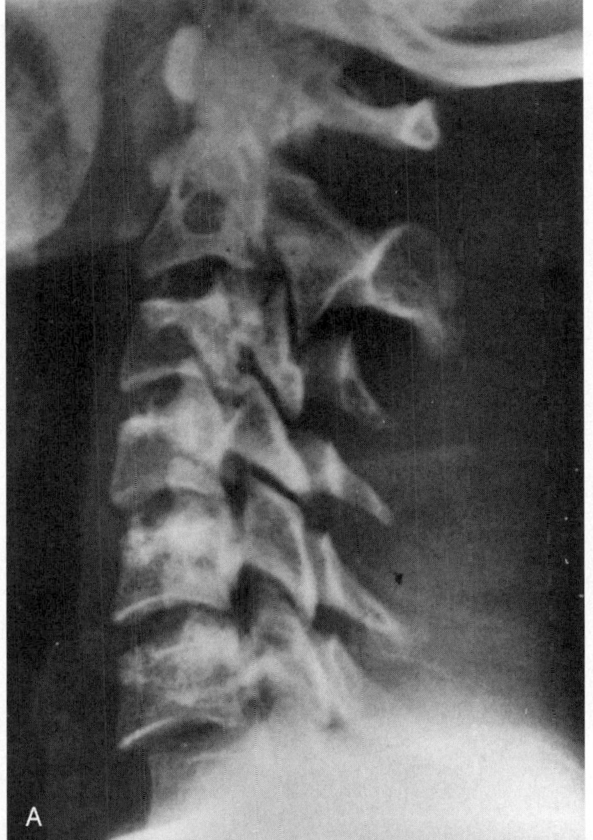

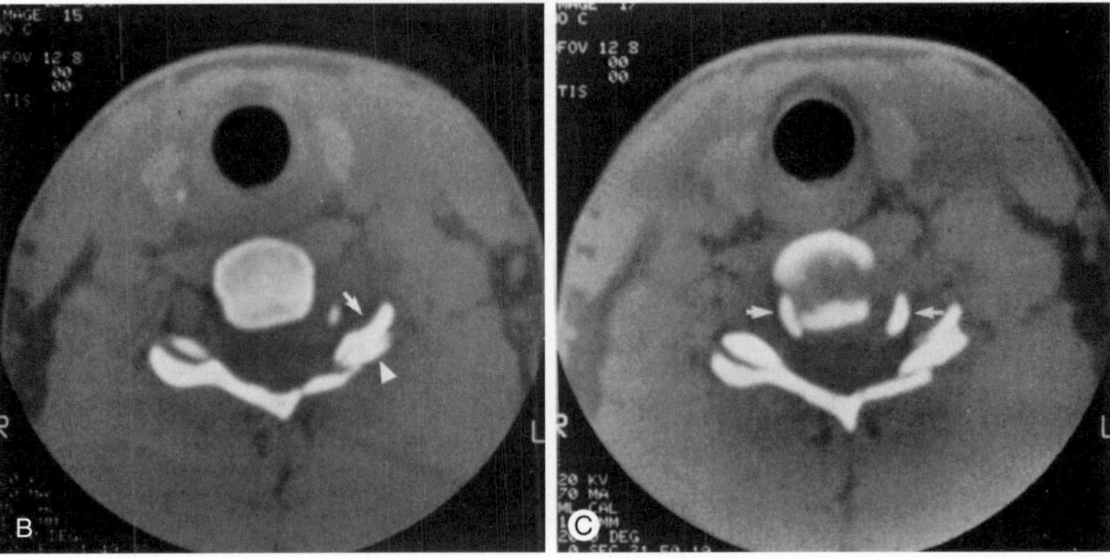

Figure 12–54. Unilateral facet lock at C6-C7 in a 27-year-old man. *A*, Lateral radiograph shows anterior displacement of C6 upon C7 approximating 25%. Other plain film features of locking of the facets are not clearly identified. *B*, Axial CT scan at the midportion of the sixth cervical vertebral body demonstrates slight widening of the facet joint on the right. There is a fracture of the lamina on the left at its junction with the lateral mass. The left inferior facet of C6 is identified by the characteristic concave anterior surface (*arrow*) and lies anterior to the superior facet (*arrowhead*) of C7. *C*, CT scan at the inferior end plate of C6 demonstrates rotation of the vertebral body in relation to the uncinate processes (*arrows*) of C7. The displacement and locking of the left inferior facet of C6 anterior to the superior facet of C7 is again identified. These are characteristic CT findings of a unilateral facet lock.

Illustration continued on following page

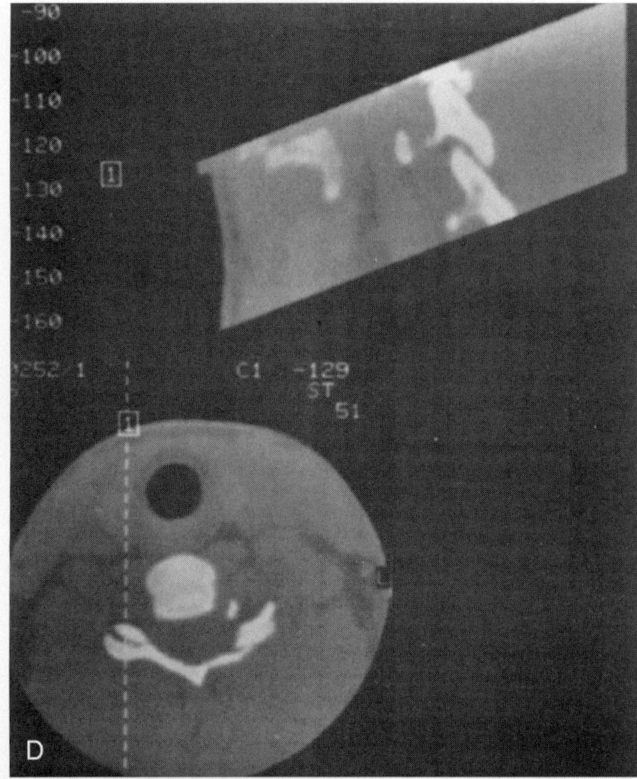

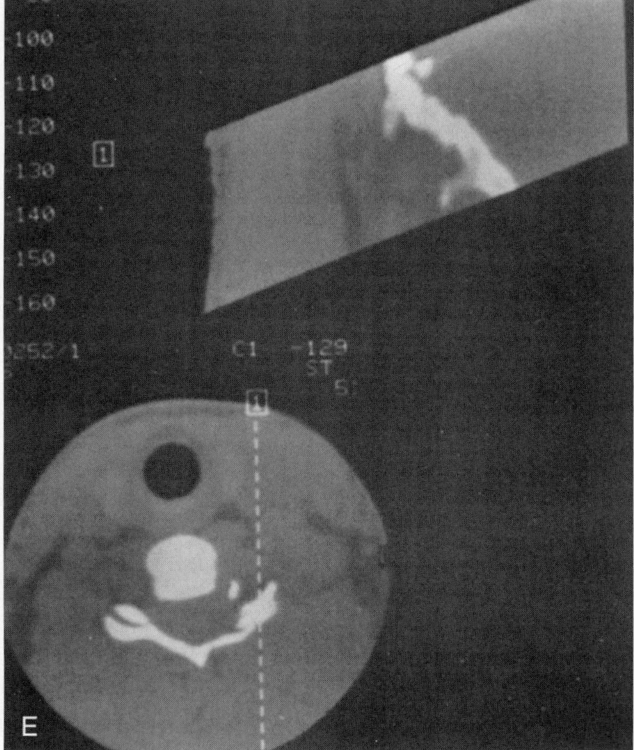

Figure 12–54 *Continued. D*, Reconstruction in the sagittal plane through the right facets at C6-C7 demonstrates slight subluxation of the facet joint. *E*, Reconstruction through the left facet joint clearly demonstrates locking of the inferior facet of C6 anterior to the superior facet of C7.

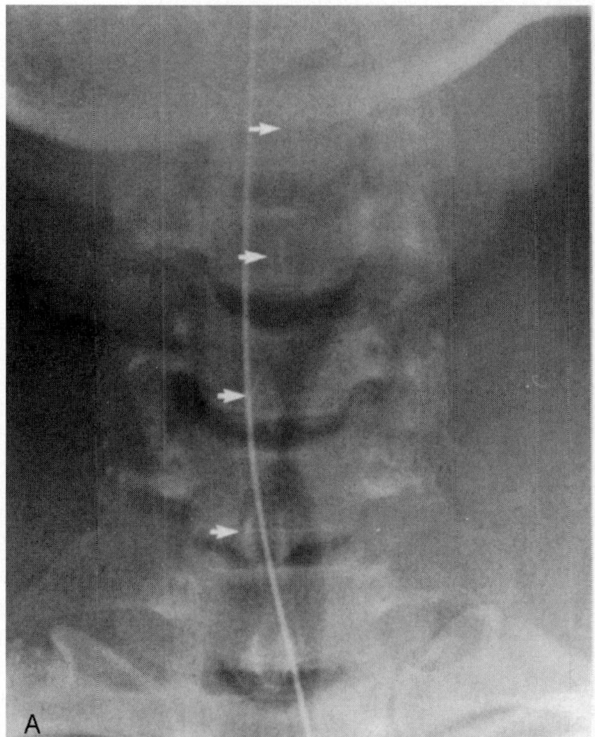

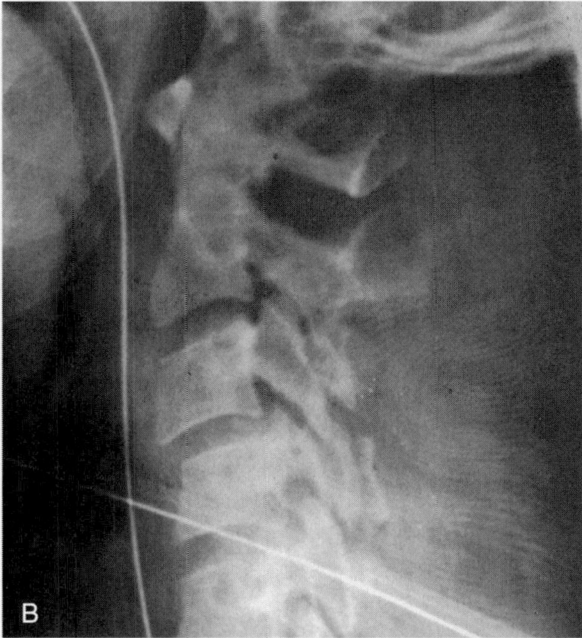

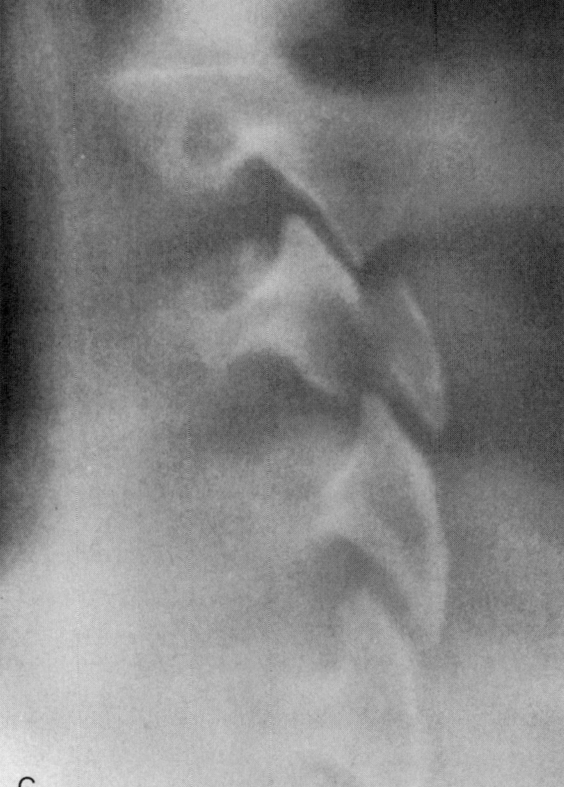

Figure 12–55. Unilateral facet fracture with minimal subluxation and facet locking in a 35-year-old man. *A*, Anteroposterior view shows the spinous processes (*arrows*) rotated to the left and the smooth undulating lateral margin of the facets disrupted on the left at the level of C3. *B*, Lateral view demonstrates anterior displacement of C3 upon C4 of less than 25%. *C*, Lateral polytomogram through the left lateral masses demonstrates anterior displacement of the third facet relative to the fourth. Note vertical fracture through the lateral mass of the third facet. The fractured facet of C3 appears locked anterior to the superior facet of C4.

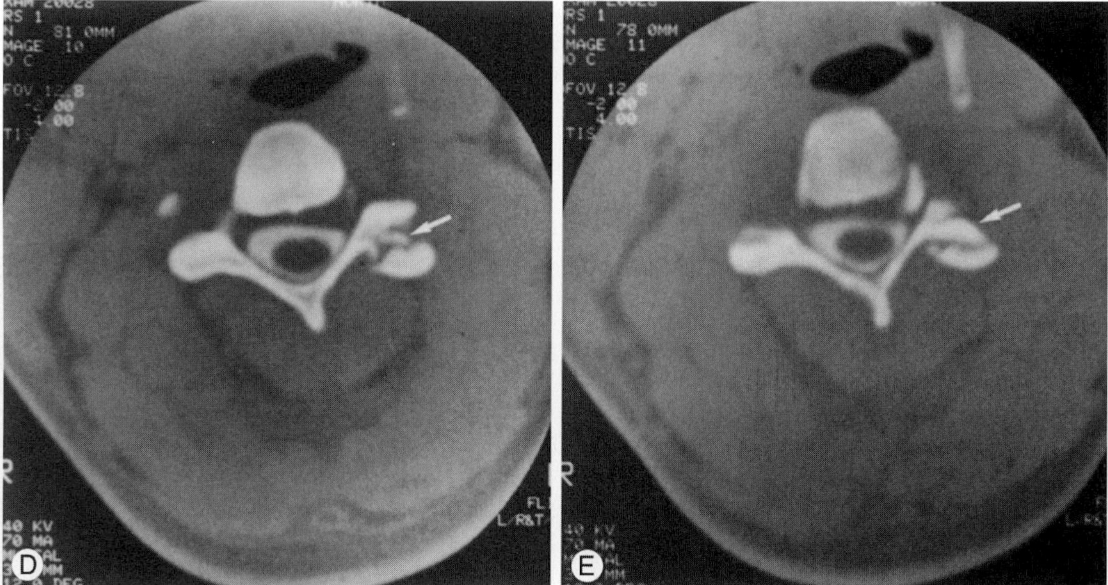

Figure 12–55 *Continued. D*, CT scan through the inferior portion of the body of C3 demonstrates a fractured facet that is displaced anterior to the tip of the superior facet of C4 (*arrow*). *E*, At a slightly lower level rotation of the third vertebral body relative to the uncinate processes of C4 is identified. Note the superior facet of C4 (*arrow*) projecting between two separate fragments of the inferior facets of C3. Compare CT scan with tomogram in *C*.

distance between the spinolaminar line and the posterior cortex of the articular pillars at the level of a unilateral locked facet. An abrupt reduction in the distance at two adjacent levels is an excellent clue to the presence of an otherwise obscure unilateral facet lock (see Fig. 12–53*B*). On the anterior posterior view the spinous processes are displaced toward the affected side at the level of injury (see Fig. 12–55). Oblique views demonstrate the facet locking to good advantage. The anteriorly displaced articular pillar is readily visualized. The intervertebral foramen on the affected side is reduced in size and partially obliterated by the rotated articular pillar. Because the spinal canal is much less compromised by unilateral rotational displacement, spinal cord injuries are less frequent. The degree of anterior displacement may be decreased by an associated fracture of the affected facet (see Fig. 12–55). Such fractures usually involve the posterior margin of the anteriorly displaced facet. Less commonly, fractures occur in the superior margin of the opposing undisplaced facet. The fragment does not displace with the remainder of the articular pillar; therefore, there is less rotational displacement.

CT will demonstrate both facet locking and facet fractures (see Figs. 12–54 and 12–55). The locking of the facets in the cervical spine is manifested by an oblique rotation of one vertebra anterior to the other with disruption of the facet joint on the affected side, and the recognition that the inferior facet lies anterior to the superior facet (see Fig. 12–54). The superior facet is rounded anteriorly and straight posteriorly at the joint surface, whereas the opposite is true of the inferior facet—it is flat anteriorly at the joint surface and rounded posteriorly. When the joints are normal, the flattened joint surfaces face each other (see Fig. 12–15*D* and *F*); when they are locked, the rounded or half-moon surfaces face each other (so-called back-to-back half-moons). Perching of the facets is demonstrated by the half-moon–shaped superior articular facet with a flat posterior surface being seen on a more inferior slice than an unapposed inferior articular facet, identified by a flat anterior surface, on the more superior slice. This is referred to as the "bare" or "naked facet" sign. Facet locking and associated fractures are sometimes more evident on lateral tomograms (see Fig. 12–55). If there is any question on the CT findings, a lateral tomogram should be obtained for clarification.

Unilateral Facet Fracture

Unilateral facet fractures, or *horizontal facet fractures*, may also result in a unilateral rotation and displacement similar to that encountered in unilateral facet lock.[269] The fractured articular pillar is rotated into the horizontal plane and its articular surfaces are readily visualized on standard frontal radiographs (Fig. 12–56). On CT the tilted articular mass appears as a broad, flat surface with fractures both anteriorly in the pedicle and posteriorly within the adjacent lamina.

Hyperflexion Strain

Hyperflexion strain refers to an injury caused by a combination of distraction and flexion that disrupts the ligamentous structures between two adjacent vertebrae—the interspinous ligament, apophyseal joint capsule, posterior longitudinal ligament, and intervertebral disc—without disruption of the anterior longitudinal ligament. The apophyseal joints are disrupted and sublux with minimal displacement.[258, 286, 292] On the lateral view the articular pillars are not properly seated, but the displacement is insufficient for facet locking (Fig. 12–57; see also Fig. 12–4). This injury is usually accompanied by anterior angulation of the spine at the involved interspace

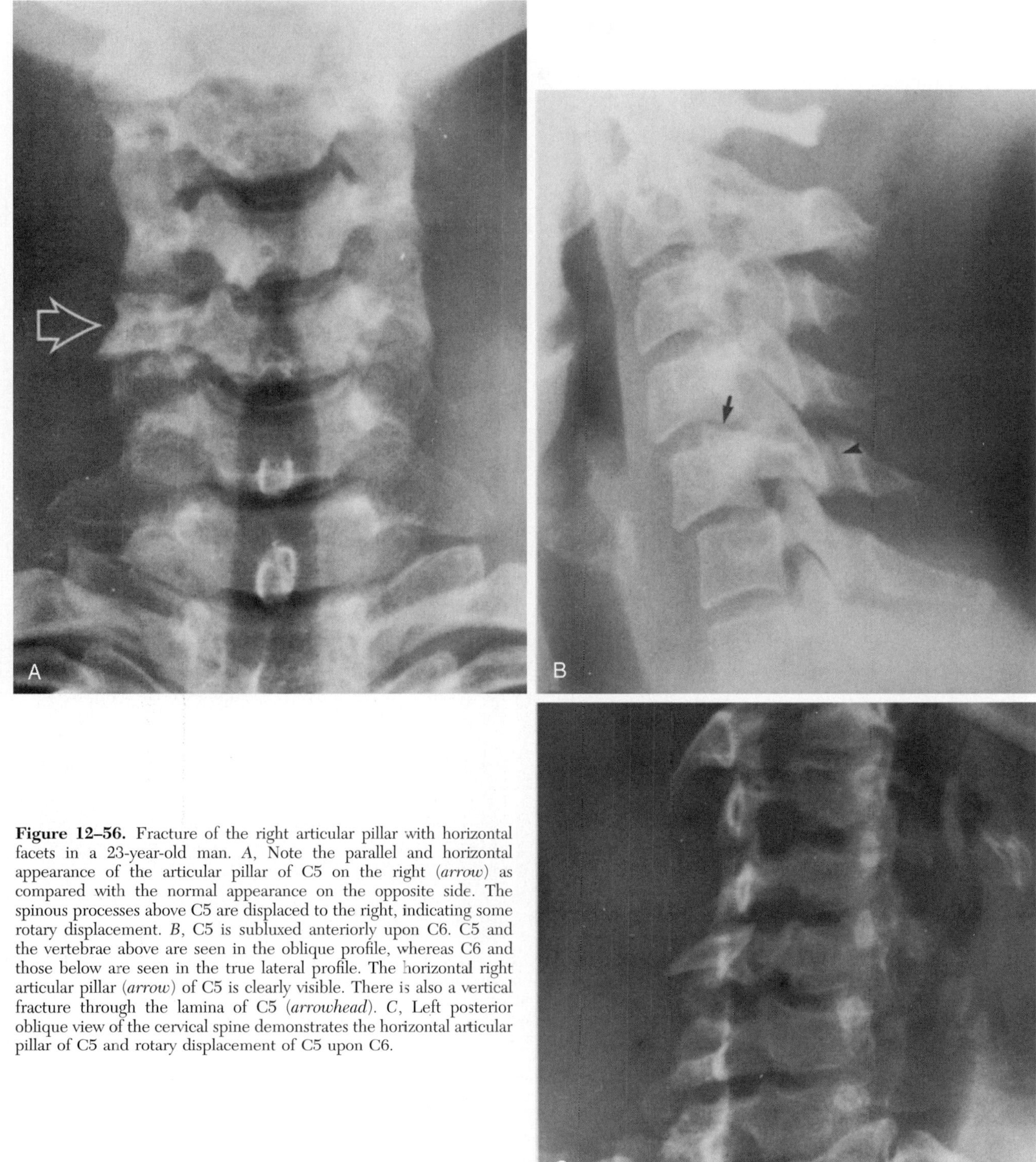

Figure 12–56. Fracture of the right articular pillar with horizontal facets in a 23-year-old man. *A*, Note the parallel and horizontal appearance of the articular pillar of C5 on the right (*arrow*) as compared with the normal appearance on the opposite side. The spinous processes above C5 are displaced to the right, indicating some rotary displacement. *B*, C5 is subluxed anteriorly upon C6. C5 and the vertebrae above are seen in the oblique profile, whereas C6 and those below are seen in the true lateral profile. The horizontal right articular pillar (*arrow*) of C5 is clearly visible. There is also a vertical fracture through the lamina of C5 (*arrowhead*). *C*, Left posterior oblique view of the cervical spine demonstrates the horizontal articular pillar of C5 and rotary displacement of C5 upon C6.

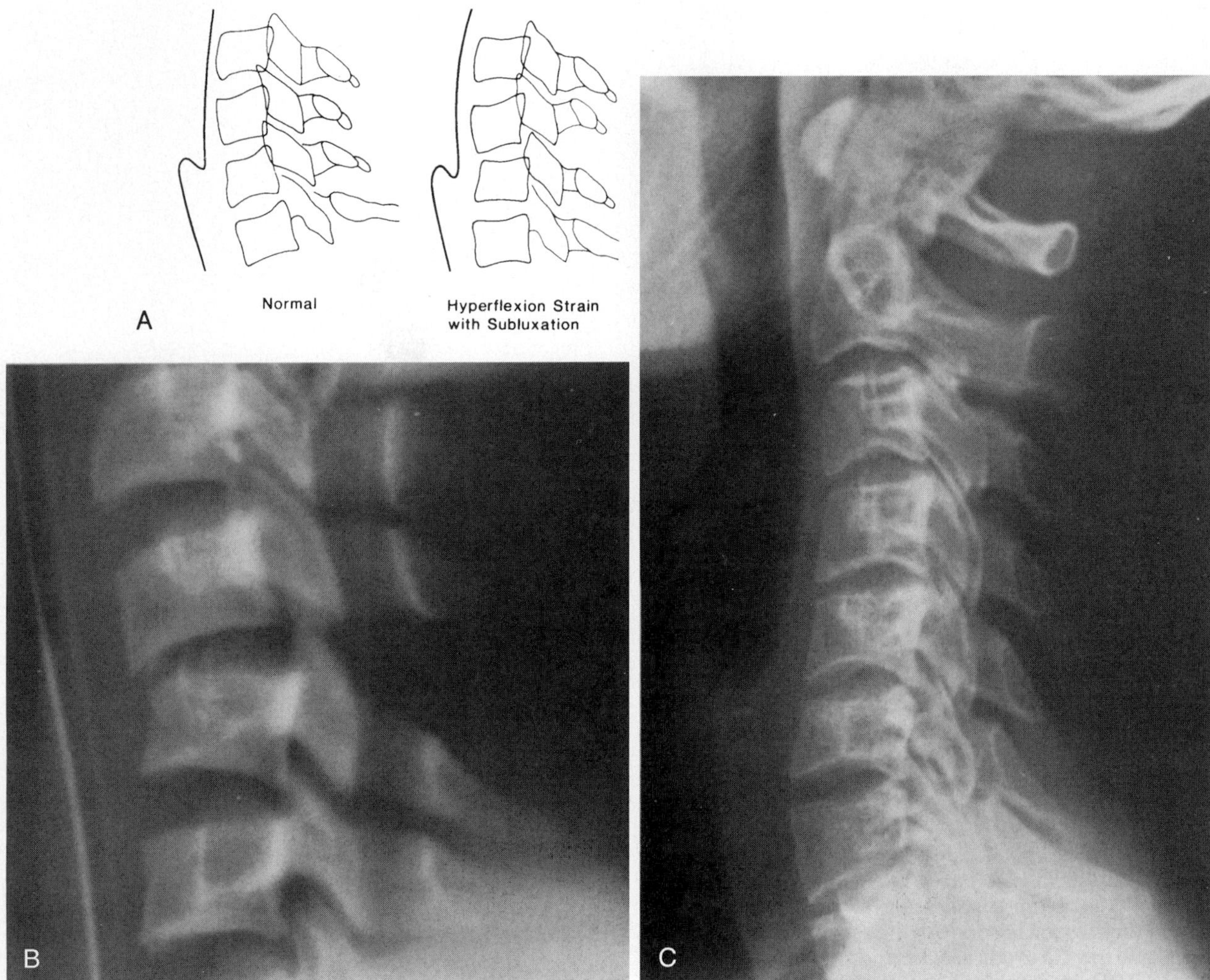

Figure 12–57. Hyperflexion strain. *A*, Characteristic features of hyperflexion strain are an abrupt change in the normal convexity of the spine focused at one interspace—the anterior height of the interspace is narrowed and the posterior height is widened; the facet joints at this level are disrupted, and the opposing cortical margins are no longer parallel—the interspinous distance is increased. *B* and *C*, Hyperflexion strain compared with reversal of the cervical curve owing to muscle spasm. *B*, Hyperflexion strain in a 16-year-old boy. Note the abrupt change in the alignment of the spine at the C4-C5 interspace, with narrowing of the disc space anteriorly and widening posteriorly. The facet joints at this level are disrupted and the interspinous distance is widened. *C*, Reversal of cervical curve resulting from muscle spasm in a 30-year-old man. Note change in alignment at C3-C4 interspace without corresponding changes in the intervertebral disc space or facet joints or widening of the interspinous distance.

and widening of the interspinous distance between the affected vertebrae (Fig. 12–58). The affected intervertebral disc is often wedge shaped, being decreased in height anteriorly and increased in height posteriorly. Hyperflexion strain is usually evident or at least suggested on lateral radiographs in the neutral position, but it can be accentuated or confirmed by flexion and often completely reduced in extension (Fig. 12–59). There may be minimal anterior subluxation of the vertebral body at the affected interspace. Abel[1] has referred to this displacement as *sagging* and has found it to be highly suggestive of instability of the posterior elements. Minimal subluxations or changes in alignment are sometimes better appreciated by viewing the spine horizontally instead of vertically on the lateral view. The phrase "delayed dislocation of the cervical spine"[120] has been used to describe cases in which the initial radiographs are normal but some degree of subluxation is identified on a subsequent examination

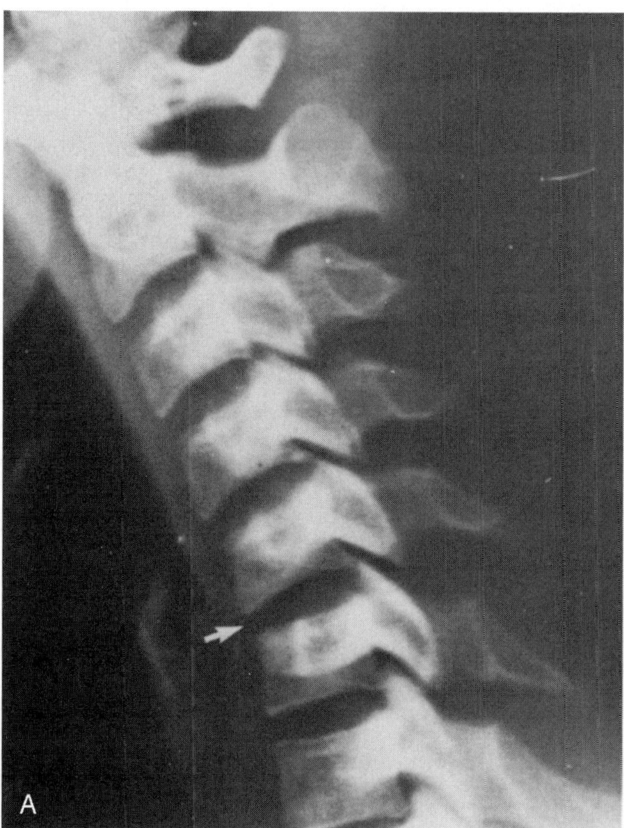

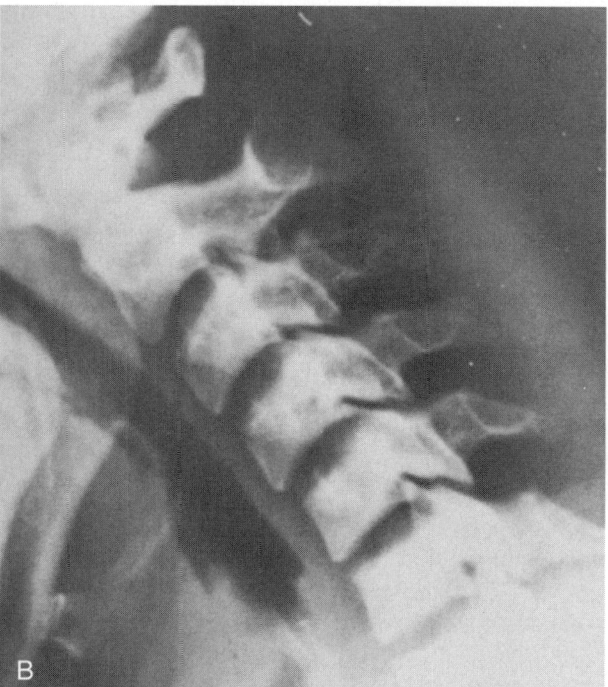

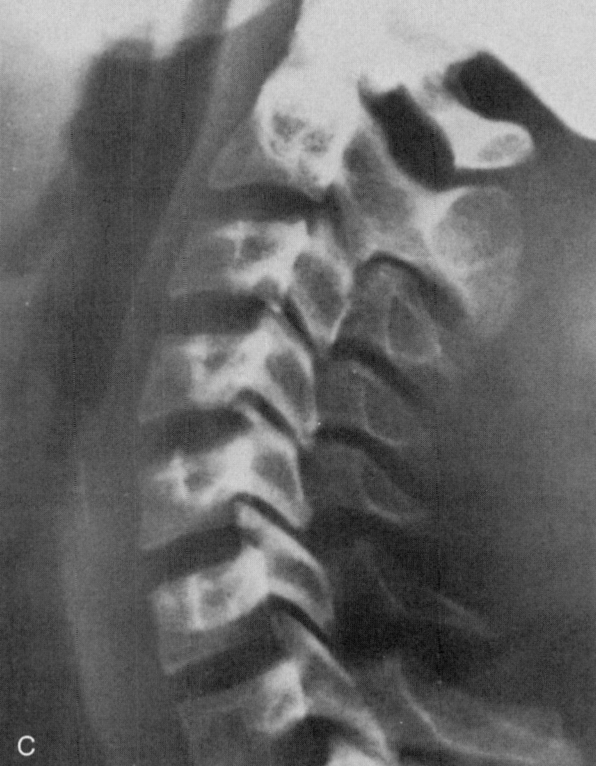

Figure 12–58. Hyperflexion strain at C5-C6 in a 25-year-old woman. *A*, Initial lateral radiographic examination was obtained with a slight degree of flexion and demonstrates narrowing of the C5-C6 interspace anteriorly (*arrow*) and loss of parallelism of the apposing joint surfaces of the apophyseal joint at C5-C6. *B*, Lateral view in flexion accentuates the findings suspected on the initial lateral view. Note the forward displacement of the facet joints and widening of the interspinous distances at C5-C6. *C*, Lateral view in extension reveals no evidence of abnormality. The subluxation at C5-C6 has been reduced. (Case courtesy of William Daniel, MD, Birmingham, Ala.)

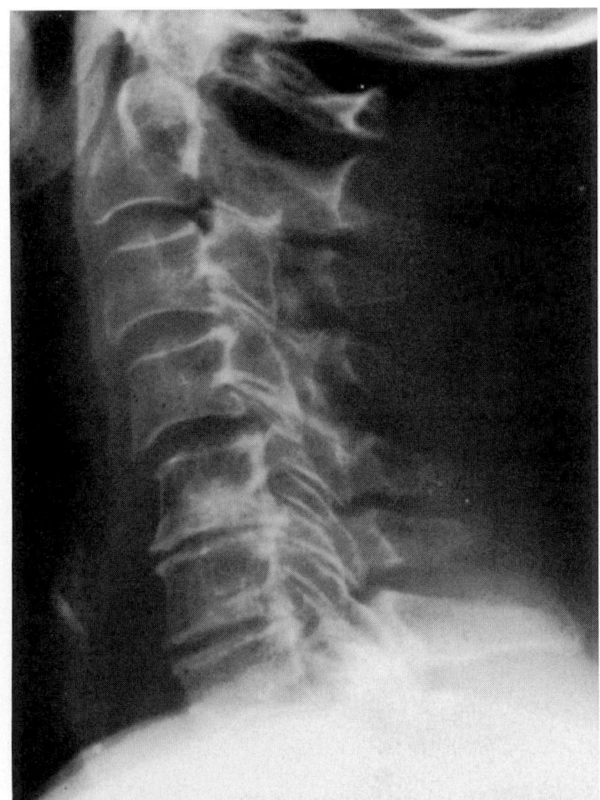

Figure 12–59. Spondylosis of the cervical spine with anterolisthesis at the C4-C5 interspace in an 87-year-old woman. Note the narrowing of the intervertebral disc spaces at C6-C7 and C7–T1. There is a slight retrolisthesis at the C5-C6 interspace. Anterolisthesis at C4-C5 is due to the degenerative disease of the facets at this level. These findings are characteristic of spondylosis. At times the degree of anterior subluxation is greater than in this case.

(see Fig. 12–4). These are actually nothing more than ligamentous disruptions of the cervical spine that either are not demonstrated or are not recognized on the initial radiographs but later are accentuated when the spine is either intentionally or inadvertently placed in some degree of flexion.[285] Despite subtle radiographic findings, these injuries prove to be highly unstable because, if untreated, they may ultimately progress to complete dislocation. When a hyperflexion strain is identified, some form of posterior fusion or stabilization is usually advised to prevent subsequent complications.[292]

All of the ligamentous structures between two adjacent vertebrae may be disrupted without associated bony injury. The radiographic manifestation of these severe injuries may be alarmingly subtle and easily overlooked, despite the severity of the injury and its resultant instability. Gross instability is often first demonstrated after the patient is placed in cranial tongs and the vertebrae become widely separated despite the use of only 10 to 15 pounds of traction (see Fig. 12–11*C*). The only way to avoid error is to be suspicious of seemingly minor variations in alignment. Flexion stress views obtained under direct supervision of a physician may be required for confirmation.

Although most of the comments have been directed to displacements of the anteroposterior plane, it is equally important to determine the presence or absence of displacements in the lateral plane (see Fig. 12–11*A*), but these are less frequent.

Lateral dislocation, also called lateral translation, may occur without significant anterior or posterior displacement. Under this circumstance the spine appears normally aligned on the lateral view (see Fig. 12–11). Apparent narrowing of an intervertebral disc space, particularly narrowing in the absence of other signs of degenerative disc disease (i.e., subchondral sclerosis or osteophytic spur formation), may be the only clue to the underlying injury. The possibility of lateral translocation is good reason to insist on both anteroposterior and lateral views of the spine before allowing movement of the patient in the emergency room.

Retrolisthesis and anterolisthesis occur in association with spondylosis or degenerative arthritis of the cervical spine[276, 279] (see Fig. 12–59). Retrolisthesis is usually minimal, measuring 1 to 2 mm, and found at the level of a narrowed, degenerated disc, usually accompanied by spur formation and changes typical of degenerative disc disease. Degenerative disc disease is most commonly encountered at the C5-C6 and C6-C7 levels. Anterolisthesis occurs as a result of degenerative disease in the facets, usually either one level above or one level below a narrowed intervertebral disc space; therefore it is commonly located at C4-C5 or C7–T1.[279] Usually the anterolisthesis is minimal, but it may measure 3 to 5 mm. The intervertebral disc at this level is characteristically normal. The degenerative nature of the process can be confirmed by an examination of the facet joints. The articular masses are usually thinned and the facet joint is often more horizontal. Subchondral sclerosis and osteophytic spur formation are also identified, particularly a spur at the posterior margin of the inferior facet.[276] The absence of soft tissue swelling, the minimal nature or absence of symptoms, and the characteristic location and changes of spondylosis should allow the distinction between degenerative listhesis and acute traumatic dislocation.

Whiplash Injury

Whiplash refers to the flexion and extension reverberatory movements of the cervical spine[1, 89, 119, 130, 261] caused by sudden deceleration of the trunk and continued oscillatory movements of the unrestrained head. This type of injury is usually associated with automobile accidents. The term has been popularized by the lay press and lawyers. Usually, the injury results in sprain or intervertebral disc injury[96] without associated fracture or dislocation.[119] The spine is usually straightened because of associated muscle spasm. At times there are fractures,[1] however. These commonly involve the posterior elements, particularly the articular pillars and laminae; special views of the cervical spine or CT scan probably will be required to demonstrate or to exclude with certainty the presence of a fracture under these circumstances.

MRI does not have a role in the routine evaluation of patients with acute whiplash injury who have normal radiography and no neurologic deficit.[350]

Hyperextension Injuries

The cervical spine can be hyperextended by blows to the head. There are three principal forms of hyperexten-

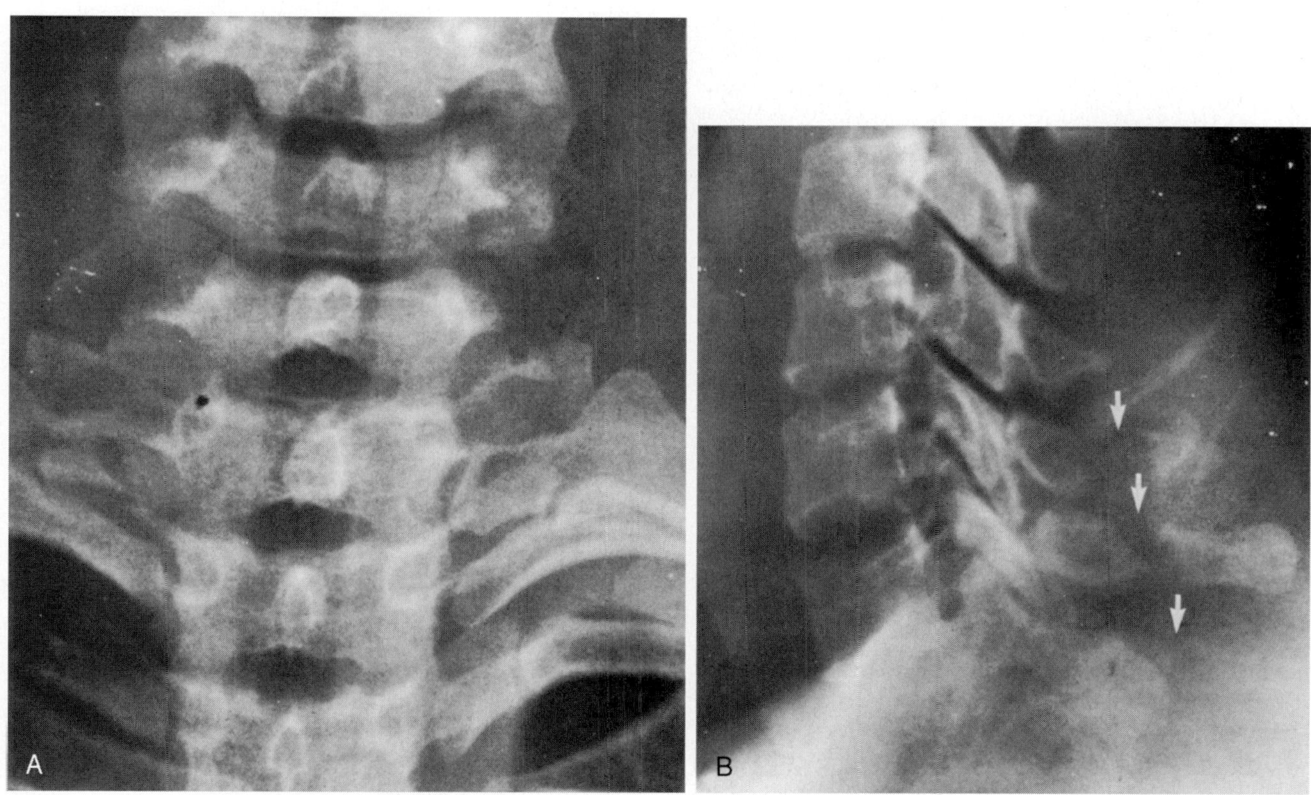

Figure 12–60. Hyperextension injury with fractures of the spinous processes of C6, C7, and T1 in a 24-year-old woman. *A*, Anteroposterior view demonstrates double cortical margins of the spinous processes at C6, C7, and T1. *B*, In lateral view note fractures of the spinous processes of C6, C7, and T1 (*arrows*). The double cortical outline on the frontal view is better appreciated when comparing the appearance of the fractured spinous processes with that of the intact spinous process of T3.

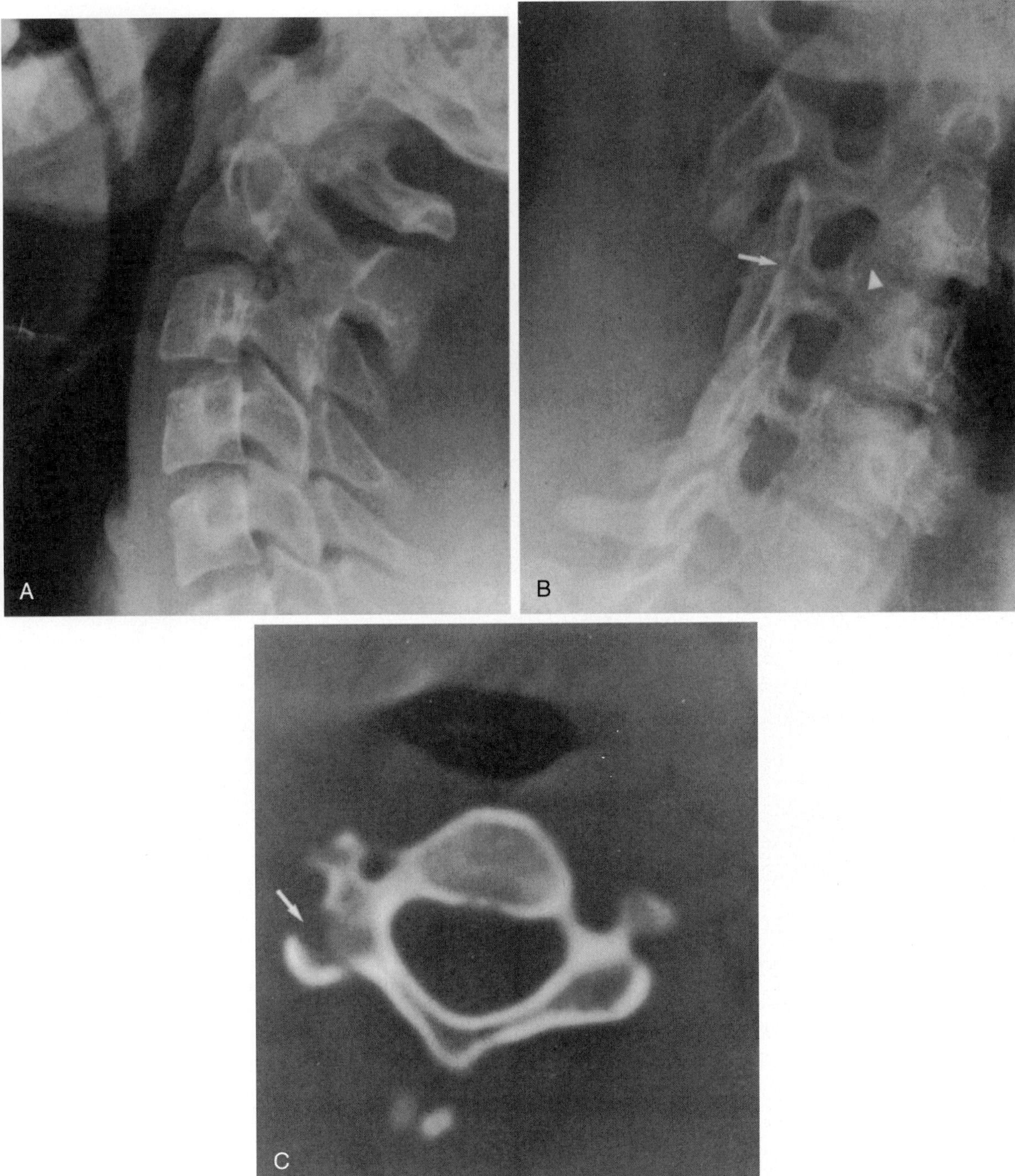

Figure 12–61. Fracture of facet of C3 in a 17-year-old boy. *A*, There is no obvious abnormality when viewed in the usual vertical position. If the reader turns the page 90 degrees and views the spine horizontally, the subluxation at C3-C4 becomes evident. *B*, Right oblique view also demonstrates subluxation of C3 upon C4. Note disruption of the oncovertebral joint (*arrowhead*). Compare with other oncovertebral joints. Also note loss of imbrication of the laminae at this level (*arrow*). Compare with laminae at other levels. *C*, CT scan at C3 demonstrates fracture of the posterior margin of the lateral mass on the right (*arrow*). (Case courtesy of W. Michael Hensley, MD, Parkersburg, WVa.)

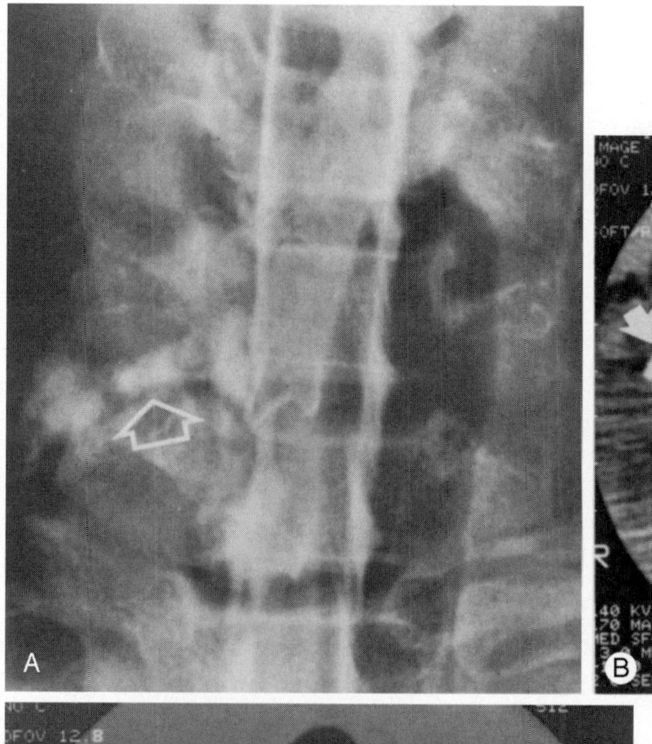

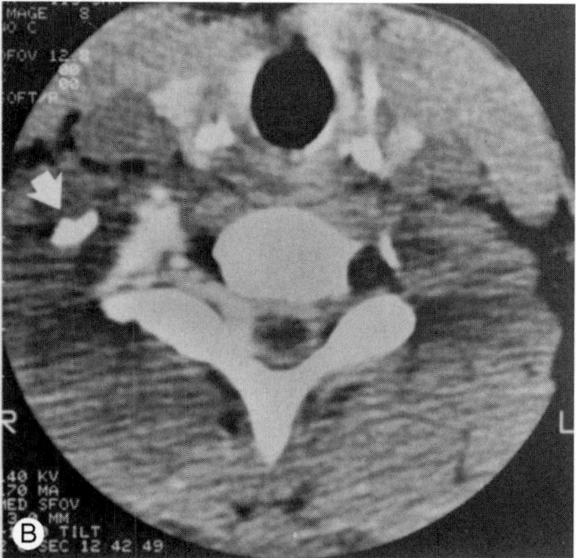

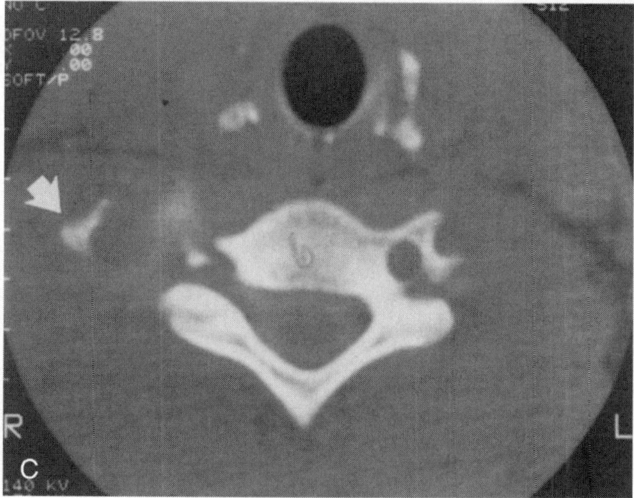

Figure 12–62. Brachial plexus injury in a 26-year-old man. *A*, Myelogram demonstrates extravasation (*arrow*) along the nerve root at the level of C6-C7 indicative of an avulsion injury. *B*, CT scan (soft tissue window) also demonstrates extravasation of metrizamide as well as a fracture of the transverse process (*arrow*). *C*, In bone window image obtained 3 mm higher than *B*, extravasation is less evident but bony injury is seen with greater clarity. There was no injury of the vertebral artery despite the fracture of the surrounding bone.

sion injury of the lower cervical spine (Fig. 12–63). The distinguishing features are the age of the patient, the presence or absence of spondylosis or degenerative arthritis, and the degree of force necessary to create the injury.

Hyperextension Strain

Hyperextension strain, also known as hyperextension dislocation,[257, 266] generally occurs in younger individuals as a result of high-impact trauma, and most instances show evidence of facial injury and have signs and symptoms of acute central spinal cord syndrome. Severe hyperextension leads to an acute angulation of the spine that disrupts the anterior longitudinal ligament and avulses the intervertebral disc from the superior vertebral body at the level of injury, frequently accompanied by a small avulsion fracture at the insertion of Sharpey's fibers in the anulus fibrosis of the intervertebral disc. Posterior displacement strips the posterior longitudinal ligament from the dorsal surface of the inferiorly situated vertebrae. Impact of the displaced vertebral body against the anterior surface of the cord and the pinching action of the infolded ligamentum flavum posteriorly leads to a central hematomyelia and gives rise to the central cord syndrome. The dislocation is momentary and reduces spontaneously.

The radiographic signs are subtle, the hallmarks being normal vertebral alignment with extensive prevertebral soft tissue swelling. In two thirds of cases a thin, transversely oriented avulsion fracture arises from the anterior aspect of the inferior end plate of one of the cervical vertebrae.[266] Vacuum defects in the intervertebral discs are sometimes identified, and occasionally the affected intervertebral disc is noted to be widened anteriorly with a loss of parallelism of the opposing end plates (Fig. 12–64). Less commonly, fractures of posterior elements, particularly spinous processes, are encountered (see Fig. 12–60). The small, thin avulsion fracture must be distinguished from the larger triangular fragment referred to as the "hyperextension teardrop" of C2, which carries no

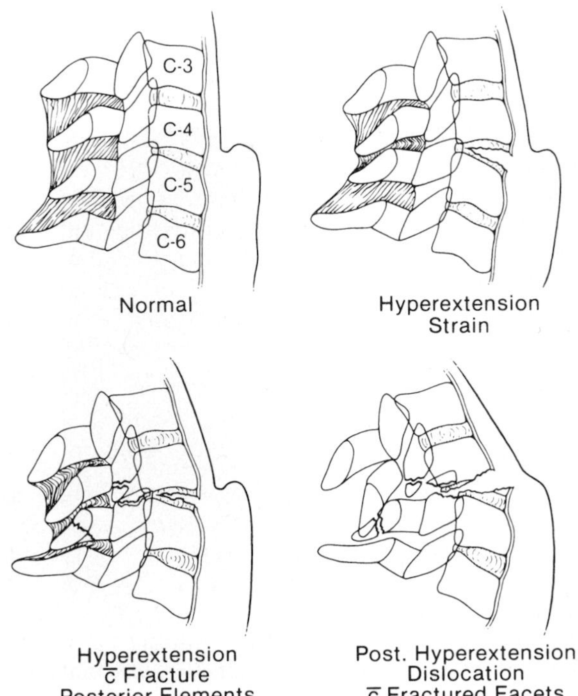

Figure 12–63. Hyperextension injuries of the cervical spine. Hyperextension strain is evidenced by widening of the intervertebral disc space anteriorly and narrowing posteriorly. The facet joints are disrupted and the interspinous distance is narrowed. Hyperextension is essentially the opposite of hyperflexion strain (compare with Figure 12–57A). More severe hyperextension may result in fractures of the posterior elements with or without associated dislocation. (From Rogers, L. F., & Lee, C. [1984]. Cervical spine trauma. Clin. Emerg. Med., 3:275, with permission.)

connotation or actuality of spinal cord injury. The avulsion fragment is smaller, thinner, and broader in its anterior-posterior dimension than in its height, whereas the height and width of the hyperextension teardrop fragment are approximately equal. Extension stress films may demonstrate minimal displacement and widening of the anterior intervertebral disc space at this level. Inadvertent hyperextension during the course of a myelogram or lateral tomogram may demonstrate posterior displacement and widening of the disc space anteriorly. Hyperextension strain, as described by Edeiken-Monroe and associates[266] is generally seen in younger individuals, with a mean age of 31, as opposed to the hyperextension injuries seen in distinctly older (mean age of 61 years) patients with spondylosis, as reported by Regenbogen and coworkers.[282]

Avulsion Fractures of Vertebral Body Margins

Isolated avulsion fractures of the anterior inferior margins of the vertebral bodies may occur. These fractures are due to hyperextension and most commonly affect C2 (see Fig. 12–38).[278] Small avulsion fractures of the anterior inferior surface of the vertebral body or of an osteophytic spur often accompany spinal cord injuries resulting from hyperextension. Indeed, such fractures may be the only radiographic evidence of injury in these patients.[111, 116, 123, 278]

An isolated avulsion of the inferior ring apophysis of the cervical vertebral body is occasionally encountered, and less commonly a fracture-dislocation occurs through the apophysis.[27]

Cervical spine injuries in patients older than 40 years of age with spondylosis or degenerative arthritis are often due to hyperextension resulting from lower impact forces, such as a fall from a standing height.[261, 273, 282, 284, 287, 295] As a consequence, the cord is compressed between the hypertrophied ligamentum flavum and osteophytic spur formation on the posterior margin of the vertebral body (see Fig. 12–50). This pinching of the cord leads to hematomyelia, manifested clinically as a central cord syndrome. In half of those patients so afflicted, there is no evidence of fracture or dislocation but simply the changes of spondylosis, at times associated with swelling of the retropharyngeal soft tissue accompanying disruption of the anterior longitudinal ligament.[282] In the other half, there are small or minor fractures of the anterior margins of the vertebral bodies, the osteophytic spurs, or the spinous process and laminae.

Avulsion fractures of the uncinate process may occur.[167] These fractures are the result of either rotation and shearing or lateral flexion. The uncinate process is the perpendicular projection on the lateral edge of the cervical vertebra in which sits the intervertebral disc and the inferior vertebral end plate of the adjacent vertebra. De-

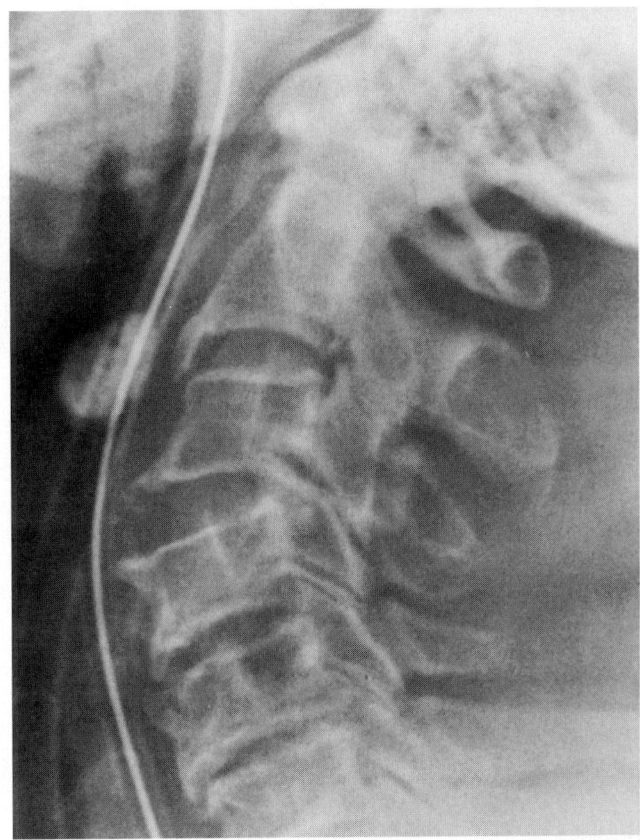

Figure 12–64. Hyperextension strain in an 82-year-old man who fell, striking his chin. The disc space is widened anteriorly and narrowed posteriorly at the level of the injury. The interspinous distance is narrowed, but there is no frank dislocation. (From Rogers, L. F., & Lee, C. [1984]. Cervical spine trauma. Clin. Emerg. Med., 3:275, with permission.)

generative changes in the uncovertebral joint between the uncinate process and the lateral margin of the apposing vertebral body give rise to osteophytic spur formation. On the lateral radiograph this results in a linear, horizontal lucency between the spurs that traverses the inferior aspect of the cervical vertebral body, which can be misinterpreted by the unwary as a fracture[264, 276] (see Fig. 12–51). The proper interpretation is made easy by the characteristic location and the presence of obvious appropriately situated spur formation on the frontal view.

Hyperextension Injury with Spondylosis

Hyperextension injuries are more common in older individuals in association with spondylosis or degenerative arthritis of the cervical spine[282, 284, 287] (see Fig. 12–51). In contradistinction to hyperextension sprain, as described earlier, these injuries occur as a result of low-impact trauma, often just a simple fall from a standing height. Three fourths of patients sustain an incomplete cervical cord lesion, often the central cord syndrome, and one fourth of the patients have complete lesions. Approximately half of the injuries occur at the C5 level, followed in frequency by C4, C6, and C7. Fifty percent of patients demonstrate little or no evidence of fracture or dislocation. In the series of Regenbogen and coworkers,[282] 28% of patients had no demonstrable bony abnormalities and 20% had only minimal evidence of bony injury, consisting principally of small avulsions from the anterior inferior or, less commonly, from the anterior superior aspect of the vertebral body. Isolated spinous process fractures may also occur (see Fig. 12–51). Prevertebral soft tissue swelling was present in 60% of patients. Widening of the anterior disc space is occasionally identified (see Fig. 12–64), and may be disclosed or accentuated by inadvertent hyperextension during the course of a myelogram or tomogram. Cervical spondylosis is practically universal, and osteophytic spur formation is commonly identified, both anteriorly and posteriorly, at the level of injury. The neurologic injury is due to pinching of the spinal cord between osteophytic spurs on the posterior margin of the vertebral body and the enfolded hypertrophied ligamentum flavum lining the posterior surface of the spinal canal[273] (see Fig. 12–50).

Hyperextension Fracture-Dislocation

Hyperextension fracture-dislocation is an unusual injury most often encountered in the elderly with severe spondylosis or in the spine ankylosed from whatever etiology. It occasionally occurs in younger individuals as the result of a severe hyperextension strain.[294] Characteristically, the spine above the level of involvement is retrolisthesed or posteriorly displaced, the intervertebral disc space is widened anteriorly and narrowed posteriorly, and the facet joints are disrupted, often in association with fractures of the spinous processes, laminae, and articular masses.

Fractures of the Posterior Elements[88, 90]

Fractures of the Spinous Processes

Isolated fracture of the spinous processes (see Fig. 12–60) of the lower cervical and upper thoracic spine occurs as a result of rotation of the trunk relative to the head and neck. This type of injury is known as a *clay shoveler's fracture,* having been first described in these workers. The spinous processes in this area are often not visualized on the lateral view; however, the fracture may be seen on an anteroposterior view by recognizing the double cortical profile of the spinous processes[112, 113, 260] caused by the slightly displaced fracture fragment overlying the base (see Fig. 12–60*A*). Fractures of the spinous processes may also occur as a result of extension[108, 116] (see Fig. 12–51*A*). In extension the neural arches of the spinous processes are compressed against each other and may fracture.

Fractures of the Articular Pillars and Facets

Fractures of the articular pillars and facets occur as a result of the compressive forces associated with hyperextension[108] or shearing and compression forces associated with hyperflexion. Unilateral fractures may result from lateral bending. These fractures are frequently difficult to visualize.[1, 167, 296] On both the anteroposterior and oblique projections the lateral margins of the articular pillars present a smooth, undulating surface. Any cortical disruption or break in this line may indicate a fracture. The articular pillars normally lie at a 25- to 30-degree angle with the horizontal; therefore, when normally situated, the articular surfaces of the facets cannot be visualized in profile on any radiograph using a perpendicular central ray. The fractured articular pillar or facet is frequently rotated so that it becomes horizontal (see Fig. 12–56), and its articular surface is readily visualized on the standard frontal projection (the *horizontal facet*). The articular pillars and facets of C3 through C7 are best demonstrated by anteroposterior views obtained with 20 to 30 degrees of caudad angulation of the central ray, which are known as pillar views.[1, 136] They allow a profile view of the articular pillars and laminae, and fractures involving these structures can be more easily visualized. However, facet fractures usually are undisplaced or involve either the superior margin or the posterior inferior margin of the facet. Most fractures of the articular pillars or facets are not visualized on plain films, but they are subsequently identified by CT (see Fig. 12–61). In Woodring and Goldstein's series,[296] fractures of the articular masses were quite common, occurring in 20% of all patients with cervical spine fractures, but only 12.5% were apparent on plain films.

Fractures in the articular pillar are difficult to detect by CT in some cases, or to distinguish from facet joints in others.[297] CT demonstration of a distracted facet joint or an uncovertebral joint is a sign of subluxation or dislocation that may be more readily recognized and precisely defined on plain radiographs.

The fractures are variable in appearance. There may be a vertical or horizontal fracture line, compression with flattening or wedging of the articular pillar (see Fig. 12–56), or even circular or elliptical lucencies[1] within the cancellous portion of the pillar. These lucencies are the result of compression or crushing of the pillar with subsequent re-expansion or distraction of the fracture by opposing forces. A combination of such forces—a crush or compression of the pillar by hyperextension and distraction by hyperflexion—is operative in whiplash injuries. Horizontal shearing and rotational forces with significant compression create horizontal fractures through the articular pillar. One of the articular surfaces or facets may then become displaced anteriorly or posteriorly, depending on the direction of the forces involved. Fractures of the articular pillar may extend into the adjacent pedicle or lamina. Articular pillar isolation can occur with simultaneous fracture through the lamina and ipsilateral pedicle. The recognition of the isolated pillar has important implications for surgical management, because patients may have two-level instability that requires fixation of three contiguous vertebrae.[351]

Acute cervical radiculopathy is an important clue to the presence of a fracture of the articular pillar.[296] If plain film results are negative, but this symptom is present, tomography or CT should be considered to search for an occult fracture in the region of the neural foramen (see Fig. 12–62).

Fractures of the Laminae

Fractures of the laminae may be either vertical or horizontal. Occasionally, they occur in isolation,[114, 290] but usually they are components of a more complex fracture involving the vertebral body and other posterior elements.[167]

Fractures of the Transverse Processes

Transverse process fractures of cervical vertebrae are considered to be rare and insignificant, but they accounted for 13% of all cervical fractures in Woodring and coworkers'[352] review of 216 patients. Of note, cervical radiculopathy and brachial plexus lesions were present in 10% of patients. In addition, CT revealed that the fractures extended to the vertebral foramen in 78% of the patients. However, the researchers also pointed out that although vertebral artery lesions may be common secondary to these fractures, symptomatic vertebral-basilar stroke is rare, owing to the dual blood supply. They reserved vertebral artery assessment with angiography for patients who had clinical signs and symptoms of vertebral-basilar stroke. Friedman and colleagues[348] also found vertebral artery injuries to be common in patients with cervical spine fractures and recognized that most cases remain clinically occult. However, these researchers proposed noninvasive assessment of the vertebral arteries by means of magnetic resonance angiography in all patients with an acutely injured cervical spine without discrimination for the type of fracture. This approach may not be practical with regard to logistics and cost-effectiveness. LeBlang and Nuñez[335] have suggested the performance of CT angiography in patients with fractures that involve the vertebral canal, because this procedure can be obtained at the time of the standard cervical spine helical CT scan, performed routinely for injury assessment.

Transverse process fractures appear to be more common than previously recognized, perhaps because of the increasing use of CT. Although most remain clinically silent, nerve root injuries and vertebral artery injuries are definitely possible. Only occasionally, vertebral artery injury may evolve into a devastating vertebral-basilar stroke.

Spinal Cord Injury without Obvious Fracture

Approximately 10% of spinal cord injuries have no evidence of fracture or dislocation.[73, 74, 75, 135] This is usually the case in older individuals with spondylosis (see Figs. 12–50 and 12–51) as described earlier, but it may also occur in individuals with relative narrowing of the spinal canal (Fig. 12–65*A*) and is sometimes encountered in children in both the cervical and upper dorsal spine without any obvious congenital abnormality or relative narrowing of the canal[36, 85, 91, 290] (Fig. 12–65*B*). The normal anteroposterior diameter of the cervical spinal canal is stated to be 12 to 21 mm. Canals measuring less than 12 mm in the midcervical spine have a relative stenosis. There are some difficulties in making accurate measurements on the radiograph and accounting for differences in magnification, occasioned by differences in focal spot–film distance. This problem can be overcome by comparing the anteroposterior width of the canal with that of the vertebral body[94] (see Fig. 12–65). Generally, these widths are approximately equal. When the canal measures less than 80% of the width of the vertebral body, it can be safely stated that a relative stenosis exists. Individuals who incur a spinal cord injury in association with narrowed or stenotic canals generally have a spinal canal–to–vertebral body ratio of 0.8 or less.

Vertical, sagittal fractures are often accompanied by spinal cord injury (see Fig. 12–13).[277] Occasionally, an acute ruptured disc causes a spinal cord injury, and of course the results of plain films will be normal. The injury can be disclosed by myelography, metrizamide-aided CT, or MRI (see Fig. 12–7). Acute ruptured discs are sometimes encountered in association with fractures or fracture-dislocations.

Associated Neurologic Injury

Spinal cord injuries are usually associated with fracture-dislocation of the spine[18, 70, 72, 75, 121]; 85% of cases of bilateral locking of facets, 75% of teardrop and severe crush fractures, and 30% of unilateral locking of facets are accompanied by spinal cord injury. In approximately 4% of fracture-dislocations of the cervical spine with spinal cord injury there will be a second fracture at the thoracolumbar junction.[324]

The likelihood of a neurologic injury depends on two principal factors: the energy level of the force of injury and the sagittal diameter of the spinal canal. The greater the force and the narrower the canal, the greater the chance of neurologic damage.[85, 91, 94]

To some extent it is possible to predict the type of bony injury of the spine from the neurologic deficit.[72, 79, 121] Total motor and sensory loss below the level of injury is usually associated with bilateral locking of the facets or severe burst fracture of the vertebral body. Central spinal cord injury syndrome[71, 76, 78, 99] consists of disproportionately more motor impairment of the upper than lower extremity, bladder dysfunction, urinary retention, and varying degrees of sensory loss below the level of the lesion.

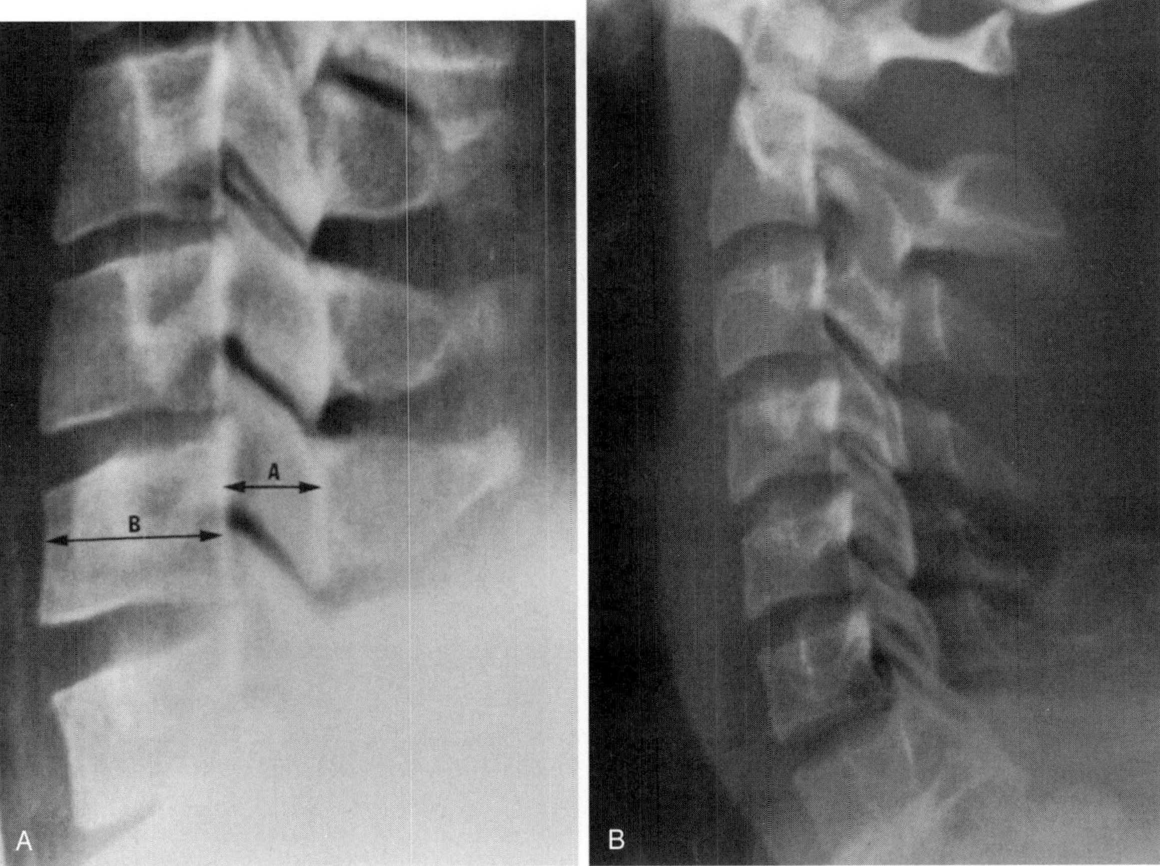

Figure 12–65. Diameter of spinal canal. *A*, Congenital spinal stenosis with central cord injury in a 23-year-old man. Lateral view of the mid and lower cervical spine demonstrates narrowing of the anteroposterior diameter of the spinal canal. The ratio of the width of the spinal canal (A) to the width of the vertebral bodies (B) is approximately 0.5 (50%), well below the lower limits of normal of 0.8 (80%). *B*, A 15-year-old boy sustained a C5 quadriparesis in an auto accident without obvious fracture or dislocation and with normal width of the spinal canal. The ratio of the spinal canal to the vertebral body at C4 is 1.0. Rarely, neurologic injury may occur even in the presence of a normal spinal canal without a fracture or dislocation, which is much less common than the occurrence of the spinal injury in patients with congenital spinal stenosis.

This syndrome is associated with hyperextension injuries, including those without obvious fractures. Anterior spinal cord injury syndrome[77, 79, 99] is characterized by immediate, complete paralysis, with hypesthesia and hypalgesia to the level of the lesion and with preservation of motion, position, and vibratory sense. This syndrome is usually associated with burst and teardrop fractures of the vertebral body. Motor weakness or paresis in all four limbs or limited to the upper extremity without sensory loss is frequently associated with fracture of the axis, either a hangman's fracture[153] or fracture of the dens, or with unilateral locking of facets of the lower cervical spine. The deficit is usually transient. Brown-Séquard syndrome[79, 81] consists of unilateral motor paralysis and contralateral loss of pain and temperature sensation. This is commonly associated with unilateral locking of the facets or burst fractures, and occasionally it may be seen as the result of a hyperextension injury.

MRI may directly visualize cord injuries (see Figs. 12–6 and 12–7). With extensive injury the cord may be completely disrupted, but in those situations wherein there is no obvious fracture or dislocation, one may demonstrate acute herniated disc or parenchymal hemorrhage and/or edema within the cord. The latter is manifested by an increased signal on T_2-weighted images. MRI also may demonstrate cord impingement by spondylosis.

Fracture of the Larynx

The soft tissues of the neck must be examined closely on every radiograph for evaluation of cervical spinal trauma to exclude laryngeal trauma. The immediate diagnosis of fracture of the larynx is very important. Delays result in scarring, fibrosis, and contraction of the airway and larynx, thereby compromising respiration and speech.[299, 305, 306, 311] The greater the delay, the less functional the end result of treatment. The diagnosis is frequently overlooked either because of lack of awareness of the possibility of this injury or because of distraction by other seemingly or actually more severe associated injuries.[305, 306] If a fracture of the larynx is suspected, anteroposterior and lateral examinations of the soft tissues of the neck[300, 309] should be ordered. Quite frequently, however, the difficulty in respiration is attributed to facial or chest injuries, and views of the cervical spine are obtained only for evaluation of possible spinal injury.

Laryngeal fractures are often the result of a head-on

collision.[309] Usually, either the driver or front-seat passenger not wearing a seat belt is involved. As the vehicle decelerates, the body continues forward because of its inertia. Normally, the head becomes flexed on the chest, protecting the neck, but on occasion the neck becomes extended, exposing it to injury. The hyperextended neck is then thrust forward against either the dashboard or steering wheel, pinning and crushing the larynx against the cervical spine. The resultant injuries vary[303, 305, 306] from simple hematoma to cartilage dislocation to fracture of the cartilages, usually accompanied by mucosal lacerations. Frequently, they are found in varying combinations. In addition, the hypopharynx or cervical esophagus may be lacerated from being pinned between the thyroid or cricoid cartilages and the spine.

The injuries are classified[305, 306] as glottic, supraglottic, and subglottic. Supraglottic injuries include fractures of the thyroid cartilage and mucosal laceration of vocal cords or supraglottic tissues, including avulsion of the epiglottis. Subglottic injuries include fractures of the cricoid cartilage and upper tracheal rings. Glottic and supraglottic injuries are more common in women; subglottic, in males. Presumably the more slender, longer female neck exposes the thyroid cartilage to injury.

The symptoms[32, 303, 309] are pain, difficulty in breathing and swallowing, and change in quality or loss of speech. Physical examination reveals flattening of the contour of the anterior portion of the neck and crepitus to palpation, signs that are subtle and easily overlooked.

The radiographic signs of laryngeal fracture (Figs. 12–66 and 12–67) are cervical emphysema and distortion of the laryngeal air column. Cervical emphysema is secondary to mucosal laceration and resultant seepage of air into the soft tissues of the neck, frequently extending into the mediastinum. Distortion of the laryngeal air column is due to cartilage displacement, hematoma, edema, and blood clots. On rare occasion, in an older individual, the thyroid and cricoid cartilages may be sufficiently calcified to delineate a fracture. Transection of the cervical trachea may be revealed by recognizing elevation of the hyoid bone.[307] Normally, the hyoid bone lies at the level of the upper border of the third cervical vertebra and approximately 2 cm distal to the body of the mandible. When the trachea is transected, the larynx is retracted upward, with the result that the hyoid lies closer to the mandible and above the third cervical vertebra. CT is the examination of choice for the delineation of injuries of the larynx.[302, 304, 310] Laryngography has been performed in the acute phase, but it is poorly tolerated and unnecessary. Examination after the patient swallows contrast material is of value in delineation of pharyngeal and esophageal tears. A water-soluble contrast medium or propyliodone (Dionosil) should be used because aspiration is likely to occur, and if lacerations of the hypopharynx or esophagus exist, there will be extravasation into the soft tissues.

CT is warranted in every case of suspected laryngeal trauma.[310] The larynx can be examined easily by CT at the same time as the brain, skull, and facial skeleton even in the presence of severe injuries. The amount of calcium is always sufficient to allow the distinction of cartilage from surrounding soft tissues. The unique cross-sectional display clearly depicts the presence of cartilage fractures

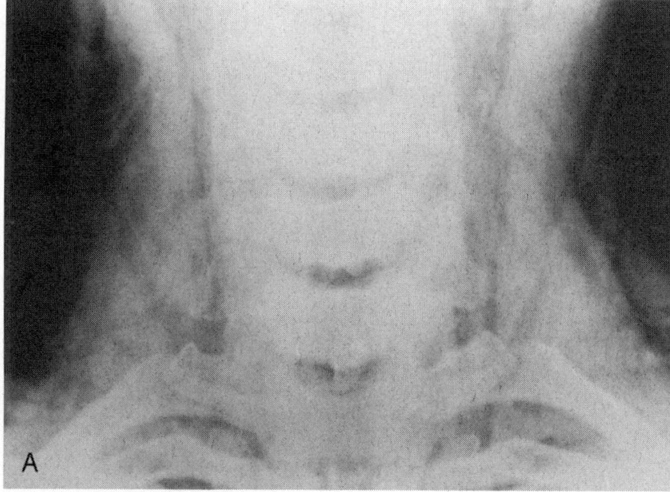

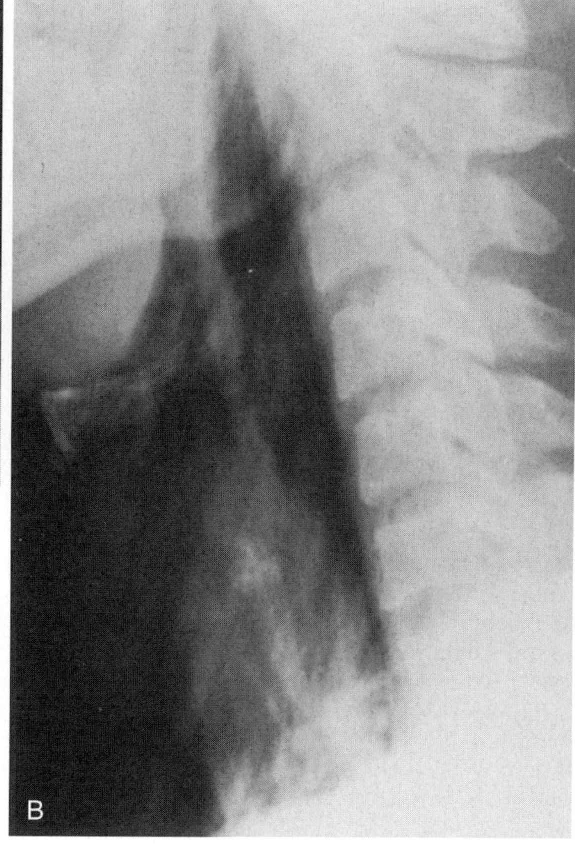

Figure 12–66. Fracture of the larynx sustained in an auto accident by a 33-year-old man. *A*, Anteroposterior view of the neck demonstrates considerable interstitial emphysema. *B*, Lateral view of the neck demonstrates interstitial and retropharyngeal emphysema and obliteration of the normal laryngeal airway. Tracheostomy was performed. A stellate fracture of the thyroid cartilage was reduced and laceration of the right true cord was closed at operation.

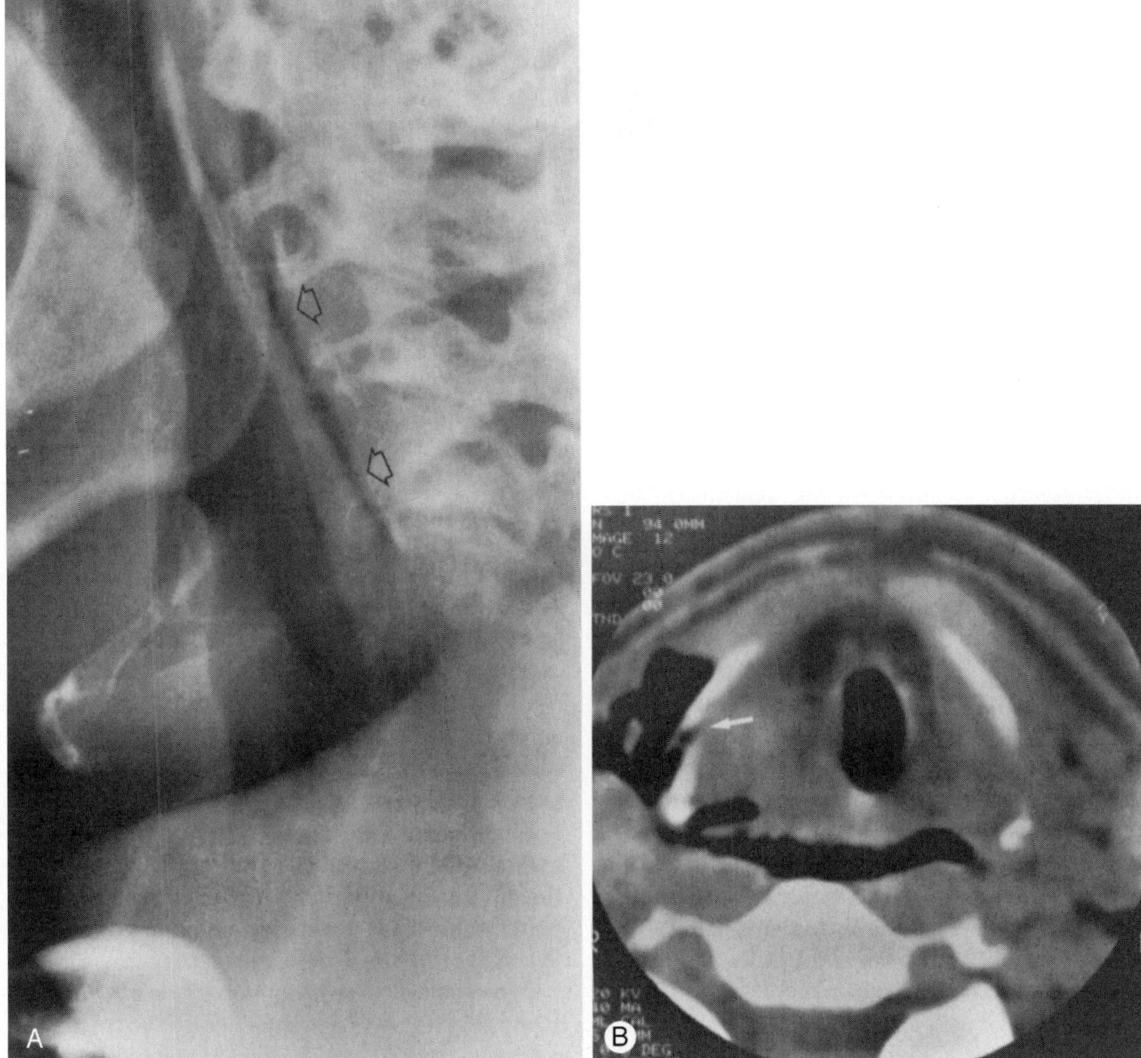

Figure 12–67. Fracture of thyroid cartilage in a 26-year-old man. *A*, An oblique lateral radiograph of the cervical spine demonstrates retropharyngeal air (*arrows*) lying adjacent to the vertebral bodies. The laryngeal air column is distorted and not well visualized. *B*, CT scan demonstrates retropharyngeal air just anterior to the vertebral body. There is soft tissue swelling in the right larynx with flattening of the air column. Fracture of the right thyroid cartilage is visualized (*arrow*). Air has dissected outside the larynx and overlies the lateral surface of the thyroid cartilage.

and their displacement, the extent of related soft tissue injury, and the degree of compromise of the airway (see Fig. 12–67). In supraglottic injuries there is usually a vertical fracture of the thyroid cartilage about the midline and a dislocation of the arytenoids. Similarly, in glottic injuries the thyroid cartilage is also fractured vertically in the parasymphyseal region, and the arytenoid cartilages are often dislocated. In addition, the cricoid is fractured. In subglottic injuries there is a fracture of the ring of the cricoid, both anteriorly and posteriorly. Typically the posterior cricoid fragments are sprung apart and widely separated. Injuries may be limited to the soft tissues without fracture of cartilages. In these cases CT demonstrates the presence of a hematoma and compromise of the airway. When confirmed by laryngoscopy such injuries may be treated conservatively and may not even require a tracheostomy.

Fracture of the hyoid bone[301, 308] may occur as a result of a direct blow to the neck or by compression, as in strangulation (Fig. 12–68) or hanging. A rare cause is contraction of the attached suprahyoid and infrahyoid musculature during the act of swallowing or from sudden hyperextension of the neck.[308] The fracture results in pain in the neck and throat that is increased by swallowing. There may also be some change in the quality of the voice or hoarseness. The hyoid bone is composed of a centrally located body from which extend two linear ossicles called the greater cornua. In their normal position the cornua are roughly parallel to the mandible as visualized in the lateral projection. The greater cornua do not fuse with the body until the age of 35 to 45 years; occasionally they do not fuse at all. Prior to this there is a fibrous junction. Fractures of the hyoid bone usually involve the cornua and are best visualized on the lateral projection. The cornual fragment is frequently displaced, resulting in malalignment of the two cornua. At times there may be perforation to the pharynx resulting in emphysema in the soft tissues of the neck. This is not common. Fractures of the cornua are often associated with fractures of the mandible[308]; therefore, when a frac-

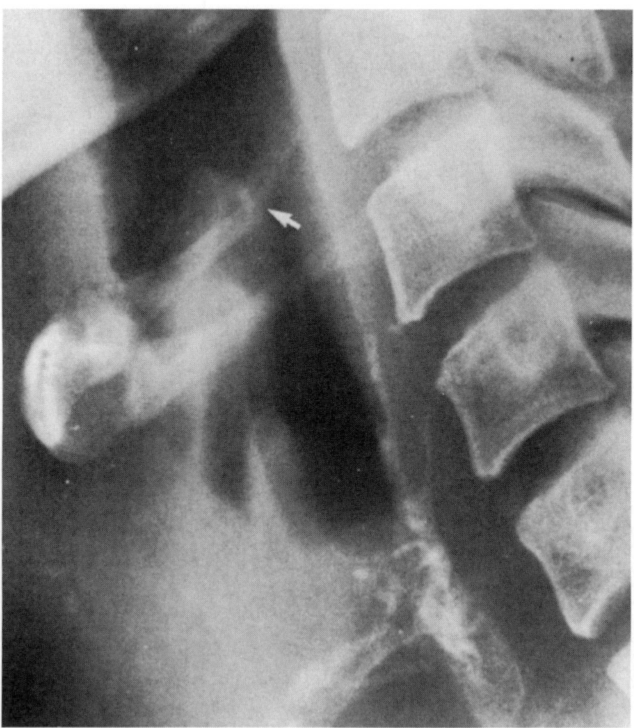

Figure 12–68. Fracture of the cornu of the hyoid bone (*arrow*) owing to attempted strangulation of this 25-year-old man.

ture of the mandible is encountered, it is important that cornual fracture be excluded. There are a few pitfalls in the diagnosis. The normal line of radiolucency between the ununited body and greater cornua should not be mistaken for a fracture. On occasion there are ununited small lesser cornua that might be mistaken for fractures of the body. These are located superiorly. Irregular ossification of the thyrohyoid ligament or radiolucent lines owing to air in the air passages of the neck might be also mistaken for a fracture.

Esophageal Laceration

Lacerations of the esophagus have been reported in association with hyperextension injuries of the cervical spine, presumably as a result of lacerations by adjacent spurs or entrapment and pinching by the underlying opened intervertebral disc space at the time of injury.[256, 280, 281, 291, 293] Delays in diagnosis are common. Retropharyngeal and mediastinal air suggest this possibility. Endoscopy and esophagrams are often required to establish the diagnosis.

References

General

1. Abel, M. S. (1983). Occult Traumatic Lesions of the Cervical and Thoracolumbar Vertebrae. 2nd Ed. Warren Green, St. Louis.
2. Banna, M. (1985). Clinical Radiology of the Spine and Spinal Cord. Aspen Systems Corp., Rockville, Md.
3. Bedbrook, G. M. (1971). Stability of spinal fractures and fracture dislocations. Paraplegia, *9*:23.
4. Daffner, R. H. (1988). Imaging of Vertebral Trauma. Aspen Publishers, Rockville, Md.
5. Daffner, R. H., Deeb, Z. L., & Rothfus, W. E. (1986). "Fingerprints" of vertebral trauma—A unifying concept based on mechanisms. Skeletal Radiol., *15*:518.
6. Denis, F. (1984). Spinal instability as defined by the three-column spine concept in acute spinal trauma. Clin. Orthop., *189*:65.
7. Dorr, L. D., & Harvey, J. P. Jr. (1981). The traumatic lesions in fatal acute spinal column injuries. Clin. Orthop., *157*:178.
8. Gehweiler, J. A. Jr., Osborne, R. L. J., & Becker, R. F. (1980). The Radiology of Vertebral Trauma. Vol. 16. In Saunders Monographs in Clinical Radiology. W. B. Saunders Co., Philadelphia.
9. Harris, J. H. Jr. (1978). Acute injuries of the spine. Semin. Roentgenol., *13*:53.
10. Holdsworth, F. W. (1954). Traumatic paraplegia. Ann. R. Coll. Surg., *15*:281.
11. Jefferson, G. (1927–28). Discussion on spinal injuries. Proc. R. Soc. Med., *21*:625.
12. Kassel, E. E., Cooper, P. W., & Rubenstin, J. D. (1983). Radiology of spinal trauma—Practical experience in a trauma unit. J. Can. Assoc. Radiol., *34*:189.
13. Kraus, J. F. (1980). A comparison of recent studies on the extent of the head and spinal cord injury problem in the United States. J. Neurosurg., *53*:35.
14. Louis, R. (1977). Unstable fractures of the spine. III. Instability. A. Theories concerning instability. Rev. Chir. Orthop., *63*(5):423.
15. Odeku, E. L., & Richard, D. R. (1971). Peculiarities of spinal trauma in Nigeria. West Afr. Med. J., *20*:211.
16. Panjabi, M. M., & White, A. A. III. (1980). Basic biomechanics of the spine. Neurosurgery, *7*:76.
17. Reid, D. C., Henderson, R., Saboe, L., & Miller, J. D. R. (1987). Etiology and clinical course of missed spine fractures. J. Trauma, *27*:980.
18. Stauffer, E. S., & Kaufer, H. (1975). Fractures and dislocations of the spine. p. 817. In Rockwood, C. A. Jr., & Green, D. P. Eds.: Fractures. Vol. 2. J. B. Lippincott Co., Philadelphia.
19. White, A. A. III, & Panjabi, M. M. (1978). Clinical Biomechanics of the Spine. J. B. Lippincott Co., Philadelphia.

Spinal Fractures in Children

20. Anderson, J. M., & Schutt, A. H. (1980). Spinal injury in children. A review of 156 cases seen from 1950 through 1978. Mayo Clin. Proc., *55*:499.
21. Apple, J. S., Kirks, D. R., Merten, D. F., & Martinez, S. (1987). Cervical spine fractures and dislocations in children. Pediatr. Radiol., *17*:45.
22. Burke, D. C. (1971). Spinal cord trauma in children. Paraplegia, *9*:1.
23. Ehara, S., El-Khoury, G. Y., & Sato, Y. (1988). Cervical spine injury in children: Radiologic manifestations. A.J.R., *151*:1175.
24. El-Khoury, G. Y., Clark, C. R., & Gravett, A. W. (1984). Acute traumatic rotatory atlanto-axial dislocation in children. J. Bone Joint Surg. [Am.], *66*:774.
25. Ferrandez, L., Usabiaga, J., Curto, J. M. et al. (1989). Atypical multivertebral fracture due to hyperextension in an adolescent girl. Spine, *14*:645.
26. Hegenbarth, R., & Ebel, K. D. (1976). Roentgen findings in fractures of the vertebral column in childhood: Examination of 35 patients and its results. Pediatr. Radiol., *5*:34.
27. Henrys, P., Lyne, E. D., Lifton, C., & Salciccioli, G. (1977). Clinical review of cervical spine injuries in children. Clin. Orthop., *129*:172.
28. Hill, S. A., Miller, C. A., Kosnik, E. J., & Hunt, W. E. (1984). Pediatric neck injuries. A clinical study. J. Neurosurg., *60*:700.
29. Horal, J., Nachemson, A., & Scjeller, S. (1972). Clinical and radiological long term follow-up of vertebral fractures in children. Orthop. Scand., *43*:491.
30. Hubbard, D. D. (1974). Injuries of the spine in children and adolescents. Clin. Orthop., *100*:56.
31. Hubbard, D. D. (1976). Fractures of the dorsal and lumbar spine. Orthop. Clin. North Am., *7*:605.
32. Lusk, R. P. (1986). The evaluation of minor cervical blunt trauma in the pediatric patient. Clin. Pediatr., *25*:445.
33. Matthews, L. S., Vetter, W. L., & Tolo, V. T. (1982). Cervical anomaly simulating hangman's fracture in a child. Case report. J. Bone Joint Surg. [Am.], *64*:299.
34. McPhee, I. B. (1981). Spinal fractures and dislocations in children and adolescents. Spine, *6*:533.
35. Pizzurillo, P. D., Rocha, E. F., D'Astous, J. et al. (1986). Bilateral fracture of the pedicle of the second cervical vertebra in the young child. J. Bone Joint Surg. [Am.], *68*:892.
36. Pollack, I. F., Pang, D., & Sclabassi, R. (1988). Recurrent spinal cord injury without radiographic abnormalities in children. J. Neurosurg., *69*:177.
37. Ruff, S. J., & Taylor, T. K. F. (1986). Hangman's fracture in an infant. J. Bone Joint Surg. [Br.], *68*:702.

Computed Tomography, Magnetic Resonance Imaging

38. Acheson, M. B., Livingston, R. R., Richardson, M. L., & Stimac, G. K. (1987). High-resolution CT scanning in the evaluation of cervical spine fractures: Comparison with plain film examinations. A.J.R., *148*:1179.
39. Brant-Zawadzki, M., Jeffrey, R. B. Jr., Minagi, H., & Pitts, L. H. (1982). High resolution CT of thoracolumbar fractures. A.J.N.R., *3*:69.
40. Brown, B. M., Brant-Zawadzki, M., & Cann, C. E. (1982). Dynamic CT scanning of spinal column trauma. A.J.R., *139*:1177.
41. Chakeres, D. W., Flickinger, F., Bresnahan, J. C. et al. (1987). MR imaging of acute spinal cord trauma. A.J.N.R., *8*:5.

42. Colley, D. P., & Dunsker, S. B. (1978). Traumatic narrowing of the dorsolumbar spinal canal demonstrated by computed tomography. Radiology, *129*:95.
43. Dershner, M. S., Goodman, G. A., & Perlmutter, G. S. (1977). Computed tomography in the diagnosis of an atlas fracture. A.J.R., *128*:688.
44. Goldberg, A. L., Rothfus, W. E., Deeb, Z. L. et al. (1988). The impact of magnetic resonance on the diagnostic evaluation of acute cervicothoracic spinal trauma. Skeletal Radiol., *17*:89.
45. Hackney, D. B., Asato, R., Joseph, P. M. et al. (1986). Hemorrhage and edema in acute spinal cord compression: Demonstration by MR imaging. Radiology, *161*:387.
46. Haughton, V. M. (1988). MR imaging of the spine. Radiology, *166*:297.
47. Imhof, H., Hajek, P., Kumpan, W. et al. (1986). CT in der akutdiagnostic von wirbelsaulentraumen. Radiologe, *26*:242.
48. Kadoya, S., Nakamura, T., Kobayashi, S., & Yamamoto, I. (1987). Magnetic resonance imaging of acute spinal cord injury. Report of three cases. Neuroradiology, *29*:252.
49. Keene, J. S., Goletz, T. H., Lilleas, F. et al. (1982). Diagnosis of vertebral fractures. J. Bone Joint Surg. [Am.], *64*:586.
50. Kulkarni, M. V., Bondurant, F. J., Rose, S. L., & Narayana, P. A. (1988). 1.5 tesla magnetic resonance imaging of acute spinal trauma. RadioGraphics, *8*:1059.
51. Marshall, R. W., & DeSilva, R. D. D. (1986). Computerised axial tomography in traction injuries of the brachial plexus. J. Bone Joint Surg. [Br.], *68*:734.
52. Mathis, J. M., Wilson, J. T., Barnard, J. W., & Zelenik, M. E. (1988). MR imaging of spinal cord avulsion. A.J.N.R., *9*:1232.
53. McAfee, P. C., Yuan, H. A., Fredrickson, B. E., & Lubicky, J. P. (1983). The value of computed tomography in thoracolumbar fractures. J. Bone Joint Surg. [Am.], *65*:461.
54. Mirvis, S. E., Geisler, F. H., Jelinek, J. J. et al. (1988). Acute cervical spine trauma: Evaluation with 1.5 T MR imaging. Radiology, *166*:807.
55. Modic, M. T., Masaryk, T. J., Mulopulos, G. P. et al. (1986). Cervical radiculopathy: Prospective evaluation with surface coil MR imaging, CT with metrizamide, and metrizamide myelography. Radiology, *161*:753.
56. Morris, R. E., Hasso, A. N., Thompson, J. R. et al. (1984). Traumatic dural tears: CT diagnosis using metrizamide. Radiology, *152*:443.
57. O'Callaghan, J. P., Ullrich, C. G., Yuan, B. A., & Kieffer, S. A. (1980). CT of facet distraction in flexion injuries of the thoracolumbar spine: The "naked facet." Am. J. Neuroradiol., *1*:97.
58. Quencer, R. M., Green, B. A., & Eismont, F. J. (1983). Posttraumatic spinal cord cysts: Clinical features and characterization with metrizamide computed tomography. Radiology, *146*:415.
59. Quencer, R. M., Sheldon, J. J., Post, M. J. D. et al. (1986). Magnetic resonance imaging of the chronically injured cervical spinal cord. A.J.N.R., *7*:457.
60. Sheldon, J. J., Sersland, T., & Leborgne, J. (1977). Computed tomography of the lower lumbar vertebral column. Radiology, *124*:113.
61. Shetty, A. K., Deeb, Z. L., & Hryshko, F. G. (1984). Computed tomography of spine trauma. CT, *8*:105.
62. Stimac, G. K., Burch, D., Livingston, R. R. et al. (1987). A device for maintaining cervical spine stabilization and traction during CT scanning. A.J.R. *149*:345.
63. Tracy, P. T., Wright, R. M., & Hanigan, W. C. (1989). Magnetic resonance imaging of spinal injury. Spine, *14*:292.
64. Trafton, P. G., & Boyd, C. A. Jr. (1984). Computed tomography of thoracic and lumbar spine injuries. J. Trauma, *24*:506.
65. White, R. R., Newberg, A., & Seligson, D. (1980). Computerized tomographic assessment of the traumatized dorsolumbar spine before and after Harrington instrumentation. Clin. Orthop., *146*:150.

Spinal Cord Injury

66. Black, P. (1973). Injuries of the vertebral column and spinal cord: Mechanism and management in the acute phase. p. 198. In Ballinger, W. F., Rutherford, R. B., & Zuidema, G. D. Eds.: The Management of Trauma. W. B. Saunders Co., Philadelphia.
67. Braakman, R., & Penning, L. (1973). Mechanisms of injury to the cervical cord. Paraplegia, *10*:314.
68. Del Bigio, M. R., & Johnson, G. E. (1989). Clinical presentation of spinal cord concussion. Spine, *14*:37.
69. Gehrig, R., & Michaelis, L. S. (1968). Statistics of acute paraplegia and tetraplegia on a national scale: Switzerland 1960–77. Paraplegia, *6*:93.
70. Gosch, H. H., Gooking, E., & Schneider, R. C. (1972). An experimental study of cervical spine and cord injuries. J. Trauma, *12*:570.
71. Marar, B. C. (1974). Hyperextension injuries of the cervical spine. The pathogenesis of damage to the spinal cord. J. Bone Joint Surg. [Am.], *56*:1665.
72. Marar, B. C. (1974). The pattern of neurological damage as an aid to the diagnosis of the mechanism in cervical spine injuries. J. Bone Joint Surg. [Am.], *56*:1648.
73. Maxted, M. J., & Dowd, G. S. E. (1982). Acute central cord syndrome without bony injury. Injury, *14*:103.
74. Merriam, W. F., Taylor, T. K. F., Ruff, S. J., & McPhail, M. J. (1986). A reappraisal of acute traumatic central cord syndrome. J. Bone Joint Surg. [Br.], *68*:708.
75. Riggins, R. S., & Kraus, J. F. (1977). The risk of neurologic damage with fractures of the vertebrae. J. Trauma, *17*:126.
76. Schneider, R. C. (1955). The syndrome of acute anterior spinal cord injury. J. Neurosurg., *12*:95.
77. Schneider, R. C. (1970). Concomitant craniocerebral and spinal trauma with special reference to the cervicomedullary region. Clin. Neurosurg., *17*:266.
78. Schneider, R. C., Cherry, G., & Pantek, H. (1954). The syndrome of acute central cervical spinal cord injury. J. Neurosurg., *11*:546.
79. Schneider, R. C., Crosby, E. C., Russo, R. H., & Gosch, H. H. (1973). Traumatic spinal cord syndromes and their management. Clin. Neurosurg., *20*:424.
80. Selecki, B. R. (1970). Cervical spine and cord injuries: mechanisms and surgical implications. Med. J. Aust., *1*:838.
81. Taylor, R. G., & Gleave, J. R. W. (1957). Incomplete spinal cord injuries with Brown-Sequard phenomena. J. Bone Joint Surg. [Br.], *39*:438.

Cervical Spine, General

82. Annis, J. A. D., Finlay, D. B. L., Allen, M. J., & Barnes, M. R. (1987). A review of cervical-spine radiographs in casualty patients. Br. J. Radiol., *60*:1059.
83. Berquist, T. H. (1988). Imaging of adult cervical spine trauma. RadioGraphics, *8*:667.
84. Castellano, V., & Bocconi, F. L. (1970). Injuries of the cervical spine with spinal cord involvement (myelic fractures): Statistical considerations. Bull. Hosp. Joint Dis., *31*:188.
85. Ersmark, H., & Loewenhielm, P. (1988). Factors influencing the outcome of cervical spine injuries. J. Trauma, *28*:407.
86. Fischer, R. P. (1984). Cervical radiographic evaluation of alert patients following blunt trauma. Ann. Emerg. Med., *13*:905.
87. Gerlock, A. J., Kischner, S. G., Heller, R. M., & Kay, J. J. (1978). The Cervical Spine in Trauma. W. B. Saunders Co., Philadelphia.
88. Harris, J. H. Jr., & Mirvis, S. E. (1994). The Radiology of Acute Cervical Spine Trauma. 3rd Ed. Williams & Wilkins, Baltimore.
89. Hohl, M. (1974). Soft-tissue injuries of the neck in automobile accidents. J. Bone Joint Surg. [Am.], *56*:1675.
90. Kattan, K. R. Ed. (1975). "Trauma" and "No-Trauma" of the Cervical Spine. Charles C Thomas, Springfield, Ill.
91. Matsuura, P., Waters, R. L., Adkins, R. H. et al. (1989). Comparison of computerized tomography parameters of the cervical spine in normal control subjects and spinal cord-injured patients. J. Bone Joint Surg. [Am.], *71*:183.
92. Miles, K. A., & Finlay, D. (1988). Is prevertebral soft tissue swelling a useful sign in injury of the cervical spine? Injury, *19*:177.
93. Mirvis, S. E., Diaconis, J. N., Chirrico, P. A. et al. (1989). Protocol-driven radiologic evaluation of suspected cervical spine injury: Efficacy study. Radiology, *170*:831.
94. Pavlov, H., Torg, J. S., Robie, B., & Jahre, C. (1987). Cervical spinal stenosis: Determination with vertebral body ratio method. Radiology, *164*:771.
95. Penning, L. (1980). Prevertebral hematoma in cervical spine injury: Incidence and etiologic significance. A.J.N.R., *1*:557.
96. Reymond, R. D., Wheeler, P. S., Perovic, M., & Block, B. (1972). The lucent cleft, a new radiographic sign of cervical disc injury or disease. Clin. Radiol., *23*:188.
97. Roberge, R. J., Wears, R. C., Kelly, M. et al. (1988). Selective application of cervical spine radiography in alert victims of blunt trauma: A prospective study. J. Trauma, *28*:784.
98. Ross, S. E., Schwab, C. W., David, E. T. et al. (1987). Clearing the cervical spine: Initial radiologic evaluation. J. Trauma, *27*:1055.
99. Schneider, R. C. (1951). A syndrome in acute cervical spine injuries for which early operation is indicated. J. Neurosurg., *8*:360.
100. Shaffer, M. A., & Doris, P. E. (1981). Limitation of the cross table lateral view in detecting cervical spine injuries: A retrospective analysis. Ann. Emerg. Med., *10*:508.
101. Streitwieser, D. R., Knopp, R., Wales, L. R. et al. (1983). Accuracy of standard radiographic views in detecting cervical spine fractures. Ann. Emerg. Med., *12*:538.
102. Taylor, R. G., & Gleave, J. R. W. (1962). Injuries to the cervical spine. Proc. R. Soc. Med., *55*:33.
103. Templeton, P. A., Young, J. W. R., Mirvis, S. E., & Buddemeyer, E. U. (1987). The value of retropharyngeal soft tissue measurements in trauma of the adult cervical spine. Skeletal Radiol., *16*:98.
104. Wales, L. R., Knopp, R. K., & Morishima, M. S. (1980). Recommendations for evaluation of the acutely injured cervical spine: A clinical radiologic algorithm. Ann. Emerg. Med., *9*:422.
105. Whalen, J. P., & Woodruff, C. L. (1970). The cervical prevertebral fat stripe: A new aid in evaluating the cervical prevertebral soft tissue space. A.J.R., *109*:445.
106. Whitley, J. E., & Forsyth, H. F. (1960). The classification of cervical spine injuries. A.J.R., *83*:633.
107. Zatzkin, H. R., & Kveton, F. W. (1960). Evaluation of the cervical spine in whiplash injuries. Radiology, *75*:577.

Fracture of the Cervical Spine

108. Babcock, J. L. (1976). Cervical spine injuries: Diagnosis and classification. Arch. Surg., *3*:646.

109. Beatson, T. R. (1963). Fractures and dislocations of the cervical spine. J. Bone Joint Surg. [Br.], *45*:21.
110. Bucholz, R. W. (1984). Fracture-dislocations of the cervical spine. p. 179. In The Multiple Injured Patient with Complex Fracture. Lea & Febiger, Philadelphia.
111. Burke, D. C. (1971). Hyperextension injuries of the spine. J. Bone Joint Surg. [Br.], *53*:3.
112. Cancelmo, J. J. Jr. (1972). Clay shoveler's fracture: A helpful diagnostic sign. A.J.R. *115*:540.
113. Chiroff, R. T., & Sachs, B. L. (1976). Discontinuity of the spinous process on standard roentgenographs as an aid in the diagnosis of unstable fractures of the spine. J. Trauma, *16*:313.
114. Cimmino, C. V., & Scott, D. W. (1977). Laminar avulsion in a cervical vertebra. A.J.R., *129*:57.
115. Clark, W. M., Gehweiler, J. A., & Laib, R. H. (1977). The twelve significant indirect signs of cervical spine trauma. Exhibit, 61st Annual Meeting, Radiological Society of North America, Chicago.
116. Forsyth, H. F. (1964). Extension injuries of the cervical spine. J. Bone Joint Surg. [Am.], *46*:1792.
117. Gehweiler, J. A. Jr., Clark, W. M., Schaaf, R. E. et al. (1979). Cervical spine trauma: The common combined conditions. Radiology, *130*:77.
118. Harviainen, S., Lahti, P., & Davidsson, L. (1972). On cervical spine injuries. Acta Chir. Scand., *138*:349.
119. Hohl, M. (1974). Soft-tissue injuries of the neck in automobile accidents. J. Bone Joint Surg. [Am.], *56*:1675.
120. Kessler, L. A. (1973). Delayed, traumatic dislocation of the cervical spine. J.A.M.A., *224*:124.
121. King, D. M. (1967). Fractures and dislocations of the cervical part of the spine. Aust. N.Z. J. Surg., *37*:57.
122. Macnab, I. (1964). Acceleration injuries of the cervical spine. J. Bone Joint Surg. [Am.], *46*:1797.
123. Marar, B. C. (1974). Hyperextension injuries of the cervical spine. J. Bone Joint Surg. [Am.], *56*:1655.
124. McCoy, S. H., & Johnson, K. A. (1976). Sagittal fracture of the cervical spine. J. Trauma, *16*:310.
125. Naidich, J. B., Naidich, T. P., Garfein, C. et al. (1977). The widened interspinous distance: A useful sign of anterior cervical dislocation in the supine frontal projection. Radiology, *123*:113.
126. O'Malley, K. F., & Ross, S. E. (1988). The incidence of injury to the cervical spine in patients with craniocerebral injury. J. Trauma, *28*:1476.
127. Penning, L. (1970). Diagnostic clues by x-ray injuries of the lower cervical spine. Acta Neurochir., *22*:234.
128. Richman, S., & Friedman, R. L. (1954). Vertical fracture of cervical vertebral bodies. Radiology, *62*:536.
129. Rogers, W. A. (1957). Fractures and dislocations of the cervical spine: An end-result study. J. Bone Joint Surg. [Am.], *39*:341.
130. Sampson, P. (1977). Will the real whiplash patient tip back his head? J.A.M.A., *238*:2341.
131. Scher, A. T. (1976). Cervical spinal cord injury without evidence of fracture or dislocation: An assessment of the radiological features. S. Afr. Med. J., *50*:962.
132. Schneider, R. C., & Kahn, E. A. (1956). Chronic neurological sequelae of acute trauma to the spine and spinal cord. J. Bone Joint Surg. [Am.], *38*:985.
133. Selecki, B. R. (1970). Cervical spine and cord injuries: Mechanisms and surgical implications. Med. J. Aust., *1*:838.
134. Skold, G. (1978). Sagittal fractures of the cervical spine. Injury, *9*:294.
135. Taylor, A. R., & Blackwood, W. (1948). Paraplegia in hyperextension cervical injuries with normal radiographic appearances. J. Bone Joint Surg. [Br.], *30*:245.
136. Vines, F. S. (1969). The significance of "occult" fractures of the cervical spine. A.J.R., *107*:493.

Fracture of the Atlantoaxial Spine

137. Alker, G. J., Oh, Y. S., & Leslie, E. V. (1978). High cervical spine and craniovertebral junction injuries in fatal traffic accidents. Orthop. Clin. North Am., *9*:1003.
138. Alker, G. J., Young, S. O., Leslie, E. V. et al. (1975). Postmortem radiology of head and neck injuries in fatal traffic accidents. Radiology, *114*:611.
139. Anderson, L. D., & d'Alonzo, R. T. (1974). Fractures of the odontoid process of the axis. J. Bone Joint Surg. [Am.], *56*:1663.
140. Apuzzo, M. L. J., Heiden, J. S., Weiss, M. H. et al. (1978). Acute fractures of the odontoid process. J. Neurosurg., *48*:85.
141. Barker, E. G., Krumpelman, J., & Long, J. M. (1976). Isolated fracture of the medial portion of the lateral mass of the atlas: A previously undescribed entity. A.J.R., *126*:1053.
142. Baumgarten, M., Mouradian, W., Boger, D., & Watkins, R. (1985). Computed axial tomography in C1-C2 trauma. Spine, *10*:187.
143. Bicknell, J. M., Kirsch, W. M., Seigel, R., & Orrison, W. (1987). Atlanto-axial dislocation in acute rheumatic fever. Case report. J. Neurosurg., *66*:286.
144. Bohrer, S. P., Klein, A., & Martin, W. III. (1985). "V" shaped predens space. Skeletal Radiol., *14*:111.
145. Brashear, H. R., Venters, G. C., & Preston, E. T. (1975). Fractures of the neural arch of the axis. J. Bone Joint Surg. [Am.], *57*:879.
146. Clark, W. C., Coscia, M., Acker, J. D. et al. (1988). Infection-related spontaneous atlantoaxial discloation in an adult. J. Neurosurg., *69*:455.
147. Dickman, C. A., Hadley, M. N., Browner, C., & Sonntag, V. K. H. (1989). Neurosurgical management of acute atlas-axis combination fractures. J. Neurosurg., *70*:45.
148. Eismont, F. J., & Bohlman, H. H. (1978). Posterior atlanto-occipital dislocation with fractures of the atlas and odontoid process. J. Bone Joint Surg. [Am.], *60*:397.
149. El-Khoury, G. Y., Clark, C. R., & Wroble, R. R. (1985). Fixed atlantoaxial rotary deformity with bilateral facet dislocation. Skeletal Radiol., *13*:217.
150. Elliott, J. M., Rogers, L. F., Wissinger, J. P., & Lee, J. F. (1972). The hangman's fracture. Radiology, *104*:303.
151. Ersmark, H., & Kalen, R. (1987). Injuries of the atlas and axis. A follow-up study of 85 axis and 10 atlas fractures. Clin. Orthop., *217*:257.
152. Fehring, T. K., & Brooks, A. L. (1987). Upper cervical instability in rheumatoid arthritis. Clin. Orthop., *221*:137.
153. Fielding, W. J., Hensinger, R. N., & Hawkins, R. J. (1980). Os odontoideum. J. Bone Joint Surg. [Am.], *62*:376.
154. Fox, J. L., & Jerez, A. (1977). An unusual atlanto-axial dislocation. Case report. J. Neurosurg., *47*:115.
155. Haralson, R. H. III., & Boyd, H. B. (1969). Posterior dislocation of the atlas on the axis without fracture. J. Bone Joint Surg. [Am.], *51*:561.
156. Jacobson, G., & Adler, D. C. (1953). An evaluation of lateral atlanto-axial displacement in injuries of the cervical spine. Radiology, *61*:355.
157. Jacobson, G., & Adler, D. C. (1956). Examination of the atlanto-axial joint following injury. A.J.R., *76*:1081.
158. Jefferson, G. (1919–20). Fracture of the atlas vertebra. Report of four cases, and a review of those previously recorded. Br. J. Surg., *7*:407.
159. Johnson, D. P., & Fergusson, C. M. (1986). Early diagnosis of atlanto-axial rotatory fixation. J. Bone Joint Surg. [Br.], *68*:698.
160. Jones, R. N. (1984). Rotatory dislocation of both atlanto-axial joints. J. Bone Joint Surg. [Br.], *66*:6.
161. Kattan, K. R. (1977). Backward "displacement" of the spinolaminal line at C2: A normal variation. A.J.R., *129*:289.
162. Kowalski, H. M., Cohen, W. A., Cooper, P., & Wisoff, J. H. (1987). Pitfalls in the CT diagnosis of atlantoaxial rotary subluxation. A.J.N.R., *8*:697.
163. Lachman, E. (1972). Anatomy of judicial hanging. Resident Staff Phys., *46*:54.
164. Lee, C., Rogers, L. F., Woodring, J. H. et al. (1984). Fractures of the craniovertebral junction associated with other fractures of the spine: Overlooked entity? A.J.N.R., *5*:775.
165. Lipson, S. J. (1977). Fractures of the atlas associated with fractures of the odontoid process and transverse ligament ruptures. J. Bone Joint Surg. [Am.], *59*:940.
166. Mathern, G. W., & Batzdorf, U. (1989). Grisel's syndrome. Clin. Orthop., *244*:131.
167. Miller, M. D., Gehweiler, J. A., Martinez, S. et al. (1978). Significant new observations on cervical spine trauma. A.J.R., *130*:659.
168. O'Brien, J. J., Butterfield, W. L., & Gossling, H. R. (1977). Jefferson fracture with disruption of the transverse ligament. Clin. Orthop., *126*:135.
169. Ogden, J. A., Murphy, M. J., Southwick, W. O., & Ogden, D. A. (1986). Radiology of postnatal skeletal development. Skeletal Radiol., *15*:433.
170. Paul, L. W., & Moir, W. W. (1949). Non-pathologic variations in relationship of the upper cervical vertebrae. A.J.R., *62*:519.
171. Plaut, H. F. (1938). Fractures of the atlas resulting from automobile accidents: A survey of the literature and report of six cases. A.J.R., *40*:867.
172. Polga, J. P., & Cramer, G. G. (1974). Cleft anterior arch of atlas simulating odontoid fracture. Radiology, *113*:341.
173. Schatzker, J. (1971). Fractures of the dens (odontoid process): An analysis of thirty-seven cases. J. Bone Joint Surg. [Br.], *53*:392.
174. Schneider, R. D., Livingstone, K. E., Cove, A. J. E., & Hamilton, G. (1965). "Hangman's fracture" of the cervical spine. J. Neurosurg., *22*:141.
175. Seimon, L. P. (1977). Fracture of the odontoid process in young children. J. Bone Joint Surg. [Am.], *59*:943.
176. Shaffer, T. E., Dyment, P. G., Luckstead, E. F. et al. (1984). Atlantoaxial instability in Down syndrome. Pediatrics, *74*:152.
177. Shapiro, R., Youngberg, A. S., & Rothman, S. L. (1973). The differential diagnosis of traumatic lesions of the occipito-atlanto-axial segment. Radiol. Clin. North Am., *11*:505.
178. Shear, P., Hugenholtz, H., Richard, M. T. et al. (1987). Non-contiguous fractures of the cervical spine. Can. J. Neurol. Sci., *14*:212.
179. Sherk, H. H., & Nicholson, J. T. (1970). Fractures of the atlas. J. Bone Joint Surg. [Am.], *52*:1017.
180. Shikata, J., Mikawa, Y., Ikeda, T., & Yamamuro, T. (1985). Atlanto-axial subluxation with spondyloschisis in Down syndrome. Case report. J. Bone Joint Surg. [Am.], *67*:1414.
181. Stewart, G. C. Jr., Gehweiler, J. A. Jr., Laib, R. H., & Martinez, S. (1977). Horizontal fracture of the anterior arch of the atlas. Radiology, *122*:349.
182. von Torklus, D., & Gehle, W. (1972). The Upper Cervical Spine. Grune & Stratton, New York.
183. Wood-Jones, F. (1913). The ideal lesion produced by judicial hanging. Lancet, *1*:53.

Fracture of the Atlanto-occipital Joint

184. Anderson, P. A., & Montesano, P. X. (1988). Morphology and treatment of occipital condyle fractures. Spine, *13*:731.

185. Banna, M., Stevenson, G. W., & Tumiel, A. (1983). Unilateral atlanto-occipital dislocation complicating an anomaly of the atlas. J. Bone Joint Surg. [Am.], *65*:685.
186. Bucholz, R. W., & Burkhead, W. Z. (1978). The pathological anatomy of fatal atlanto-occipital dislocations. J. Bone Joint Surg. [Am.], *61*:248.
187. Burguet, J. L., Sick, H., Dirheimer, Y., & Wackenheim, A. (1985). CT of the main ligaments of the cervico-occipital hinge. Neuroradiology, *27*:112.
188. Collalto, P. M., DeMuth, W. W., Schwentker, E. P., & Boal, D. K. (1986). Traumatic atlanto-occipital dislocation. J. Bone Joint Surg. [Am.], *68*:1106.
189. Daniels, D. L., Williams, A. L., & Haughton, V. M. (1983). Computed tomography of the articulations and ligaments at the occipito-atlantoaxial region. Radiology, *146*:709.
190. Deeb, Z. L., Rothfus, W. E., Goldberg, A. L., & Daffner, R. H. (1988). Occult occipital condyle fractures presenting as tumors. J. Comput. Tomogr., *12*:261.
191. Evarts, C. M. (1970). Traumatic occipito-atlantal dislocation. J. Bone Joint Surg. [Am.], *52*:1653.
192. Gerlock, A. J. Jr., Mirfakhraee, M., & Benzel, E. C. (1983). Computed tomography of traumatic atlantooccipital dislocation. Neurosurgery, *13*:316.
193. Grobovschek, M., & Scheibelbrandner, W. (1983). Atlanto-occipital dislocation. Neuroradiology, *25*:173.
194. Harding-Smith, J., MacIntosh, P. K., & Sherbon, K. J. (1981). Fracture of the occipital condyle. J. Bone Joint Surg. [Am.], *63*:1170.
195. Kaufman, R. A., Dunbar, J. S., Botsford, J. A., & McLaurin, R. L. (1982). Traumatic longitudinal atlanto-occipital distraction injuries in children. A.J.N.R., *3*:415.
196. Lee, C., Woodring, J. H., Goldstein, S. J. et al. (1987). Evaluation of traumatic atlantooccipital dislocation. A.J.N.R., *8*:19.
197. Levine, A. M., & Edwards, C. C. (1989). Traumatic lesions of the occipitoatlantoaxial complex. Clin. Orthop., *239*:53.
198. Powers, B., Miller, M. D., Kramer, R. S. et al. (1979). Traumatic anterior atlanto-occipital dislocation. Neurosurgery, *4*:17.
199. Putnam, W. E., Stratton, F. T., Rohr, R. J. et al. (1986). Traumatic atlanto-occipital dislocations: Value of the Powers ratio in diagnosis. J. Am. Osteopath. Assoc., *86*:798.
200. Ramsay, A. H., Waxman, B. P., & O'Brien, J. F. (1986). A case of traumatic atlanto-occipital dislocation with survival. Injury, *17*:412.
201. Rosenbaum, D. M., Blumhagen, J. D., & King, H. A. (1986). Atlantooccipital instability in Down syndrome. A.J.R., *146*:1269.
202. Traynelis, V. C., Marano, G. D., Dunker, R. O., & Kaufman, H. H. (1986). Traumatic atlanto-occipital dislocation. Case report. J. Neurosurg., *65*:863.
203. Van Den Bout, A., & Dommisse, G. F. (1986). Traumatic atlantooccipital dislocation. Spine, *11*:174.
204. Woodring, J. H., Selke, A. C. Jr., & Duff, D. E. (1981). Traumatic atlantooccipital dislocation with survival. A.J.N.R., *2*:251.

Fractures of the Atlas (C1)

205. Clyburn, T. A., Lionberger, D. R., & Tullos, H. S. (1982). Bilateral fracture of the transverse process of the atlas. J. Bone Joint Surg. [Am.], *64*:948.
206. England, A. C. III, Shippel, A. H., & Ray, M. J. (1985). A simple view for demonstration of fractures of the anterior arch of C1. A.J.R., *144*:763.
207. Flournoy, J. G., Cone, R. O., Saldana, J. A., & Jones, M. D. (1980). Jefferson fracture Presentation of a new diagnostic sign. Radiology, *134*:88.
208. Gehweiler, J. A. Jr., Daffner, R. H., & Roberts, L. Jr. (1983). Malformations of the atlas vertebra simulating the Jefferson fracture. A.J.N.R., *4*:187.
209. Hadley, M. N., Dickman, C. A., Browner, C. M., & Sonntag, V. K. H. (1988). Acute traumatic atlas fractures: Management and long term outcome. Neurosurgery, *23*:31.
210. Hays, M. B., & Alker, G. J. Jr. (1988). Fractures of the atlas vertebra. The two-part burst fracture of Jefferson. Spine, *13*:601.
211. Jevtich, V. (1986). Horizontal fracture of the anterior arch of the atlas. J. Bone Joint Surg. [Am.], *68*:1094.
212. Landells, C. D., & Van Peteghem, P. K. (1988). Fractures of the atlas: Classification, treatment and morbidity. Spine, *13*:450.
213. Lipson, S. J., & Mazur, J. (1978). Anteroposterior spondyloschisis of the atlas revealed by computerized tomography scanning. J. Bone Joint Surg. [Am.], *60*:1104.
214. Mikawa, Y., Watanabe, R., Yamano, Y., & Ishii, K. (1987). Fracture through a synchondrosis of the anterior arch of the atlas. J. Bone Joint Surg. [Br.], *69*:483.
215. Ogden, J. A. (1984). Radiology of postnatal skeletal development. XI. The first cervical vertebra. Skeletal Radiol., *12*:12.
216. Roush, R. D., & Salciccioli, G. G. (1982). Fracture of the anterior tubercle of the atlas. Case report. J. Bone Joint Surg. [Am.], *64*:626.
217. Schlicke, L. H., & Callahan, R. A. (1981). A rational approach to burst fractures of the atlas. Clin. Orthop., *154*:18.
218. Suss, R. A., & Bundy, K. J. (1984). Unilateral posterior arch fractures of the atlas. A.J.N.R., *5*:783.
219. Suss, R. A., Zimmerman, R. D., & Leeds, N. E. (1983). Pseudospread of the atlas: False sign of Jefferson fracture in young children. A.J.N.R., *4*:183.
220. Wirth, R. L., Zatz, L. M., & Parker, B. R. (1987). CT detection of a Jefferson fracture in a child. A.J.R., *149*:1001.

Fractures of the Axis (C2)

221. Autricque, A., Lesoin, F., Villette, L. et al. (1986). Fracture de l'odontoide et lucation laterale C1-C2. Ann Chir., *40*:397.
222. Bucholz, R. W. (1981). Unstable hangman's fractures. Clin. Orthop., *154*:119.
223. Clark, C. R., & White, A. A. III. (1985). Fractures of the dens. J. Bone Joint Surg. [Am.], *67*:1340.
224. Dussault, R. G. Effendi, B., Roy, D. et al. (1983). Locked facets with fracture of the neural arch of the axis. Spine, *8*:365.
225. Effendi, B., Roy, D., Cornish, B. et al. (1981). Fractures of the ring of the axis. A classification based on the analysis of 131 cases. J. Bone Joint Surg. [Br.], *63*:319.
226. Fardon, D. F., & Fielding, J. W. (1981). Defects of the pedicle and spondylolisthesis of the second cervical vertebra. J. Bone Joint Surg. [Br.], *63*:526.
227. Gerlock, A. J. Jr., & Mirfakhraee, M. (1983). Computed tomography and hangman's fractures. South Med. J., *76*:727.
228. Hadley, M. N., Browner, C. M., Liu, S. S., & Sonntag, V. K. H. (1988). New subtype of acute odontoid fractures (type IIA). Neurosurgery, *22*:67.
229. Hadley, M. N., Browner, C., & Sonntag, V. K. H. (1985). Axis fractures: A comprehensive review of management and treatment in 107 cases. Neurosurgery, *17*:281.
230. Hadley, M. N., Sonntag, V. K. H., Grahm, T. W. et al. (1986). Axis fractures resulting from motor vehicle accidents. The need for occupant restraints. Spine, *11*:861.
231. Hanssen, A. D., & Cabanela, M. E. (1987). Fractures of the dens in adult patients. J. Trauma, *27*:928.
232. Harris, J. H., Burke, J. T., Ray, R. D. et al. (1984). Low (type III) odontoid fracture: A new radiographic sign. Radiology, *153*:353.
233. Kish, K. K., & Wilner, H. I. (1983). Spondylolysis of C2: CT and plain film findings. J. Comput. Assist. Tomogr., *7*:517.
234. Levine, A. M., & Edwards, C. C. (1985). The management of traumatic spondylolisthesis of the axis. J. Bone Joint Surg. [Am.], *67*:217.
235. Mirvis, S. E., Young, J. W. R., Lim, C., & Greenberg, J. (1987). Hangman's fracture: Radiologic assessment in 27 cases. Radiology, *163*:713.
236. Mollan, R. A. B., & Watt, P. C. H. (1982). Hangman's fracture. Injury, *14*:265.
237. Nepper-Rasmussen, J. (1989). CT of dens axis fractures. Neuroradiology, *31*:104.
238. Nicolet, V., Chalaoui, J., Vezina, J. V., & Dussault, R. G. (1984). C2 "target": Composite shadow. A.J.N.R., *5*:331.
239. Nordstrom, R. E. A., Lahdenranta, T. V., Kaitila, I. I., & Laasonen, E. M. I. (1986). Familial spondylolisthesis of the axis vertebra. J. Bone Joint Surg. [Br.], *68*:704.
240. Ogden, J. A. (1984). Radiology of postnatal skeletal development. XII. The second cervical vertebra. Skeletal Radiol., *12*:169.
241. Pepin, J. W., Bourne, R. B., & Hawkins, R. J. (1985). Odontoid fractures, with special reference to the elderly patient. Clin. Orthop., *193*:178.
242. Pepin, J. W., & Hawkins, R. J. (1981). Traumatic spondylolisthesis of the axis: Hangman's fracture. Clin. Orthop., *157*:133.
243. Roberts, W. A., & Wickstrom, J. (1973). Prognosis of odontoid fractures. Acta Orthop. Scand., *44*:21.
244. Robertson, W. G. A. (1935). Recovery after judicial hanging. Br. Med. J., *1*:121.
245. Roda, J. M., Castro, A., & Blazquez, M. G. (1984). Hangman's fracture with complete dislocation of C2 on C3. J. Neurosurg., *60*:633.
246. Rush, G. A., & Burke, S. W. (1984). Hangman's fracture in a patient with osteogenesis imperfecta. Case report. J. Bone Joint Surg. [Am.], *66*:778.
247. Ryan, M. D., & Taylor, T. K. F. (1982). Odontoid fractures. A rational approach to treatment. J. Bone Joint Surg. [Br.], *64*:416.
248. Segal, L. S., Grimm, J. O., & Stauffer, E. S. (1987). Nonunion of fractures of the atlas. J. Bone Joint Surg. [Am.], *69*:1423.
249. Sherk, H. H., & Howard, T. (1983). Clinical and pathologic correlations in traumatic spondylolisthesis of the axis. Clin. Orthop., *174*:122.
250. Signoret, F., Bonfait, H., Feron, J. M., & Patel, A. (1986). Fractured odontoid with fractured superior articular process of the axis. J. Bone Joint Surg. [Br.], *68*:182.
251. Smoker, W. R. K., & Dolan, K. D. (1987). The "fat" C2: A sign of fracture. A.J.R., *148*:609.
252. Southwick, W. O. (1980). Current Concept Review. Management of fractures of the dens (odontoid process). J. Bone Joint Surg. [Am.], *62*:482.
253. Wisoff, H. S. (1984). Fracture of the dens in the aged. Surg. Neurol., *22*:547.
254. Wozasek, G. E., Strassegger, H., & Rizzi, C. (1989). Fatal hanged man's fracture. Unfallchirurg, *92*:32.

Lower Cervical Spine (C3–C7)

255. Aebi, M., & Nazarian, S. (1987). Klassification der halswirbelsaulenverletzungen. Orthopade, *16*:27.
256. Agha, F. P., & Raji, M. R. (1982). Case reports. Oesophageal perforation with fracture dislocation of cervical spine due to hyperextension injury. Br. J. Radiol., *55*:369.
257. Barquet, A., & Pereyra, D. (1988). An unusual extension injury to the cervical spine. J. Bone Joint Surg. [Am.], *70*:1393.
258. Braakman, M., & Braakman, R. (1987). Hyperflexion sprain of the cervical spine. Follow-up of 45 cases. Acta Orthop. Scand., *58*:388.
259. Braakman, R., & Vinken, P. J. (1967). Unilateral facet interlocking in the lower cervical spine. J. Bone Joint Surg. [Br.], *49*:249.

260. Cancelmo, J. J. Jr. (1972). Clay shoveler's fracture: A helpful diagnostic sign. A.J.R., *115*:540.
261. Cloward, R. B. (1980). Acute cervical spine injuries. Ciba Clin. Symp., *32*:2.
262. Cotler, H. B., Miller, L. S., DeLucia, F. A. et al. (1987). Closed reduction of cervical spine dislocations. Clin. Orthop., *214*:185.
263. Cybulski, G. R., Stone, J. L., Arnold, P. M. et al. (1989). Multiple fractures of the cervical and upper thoracic spine without neurological deficit: Case report. Neurosurgery, *24*:768.
264. Daffner, R. H., Deeb, Z. L., & Rothfus, W. E. (1986). Pseudofractures of the cervical vertebral body. Skeletal Radiol., *15*:295.
265. Dolan, K. D. (1977). Cervical spine injuries below the axis. Radiol. Clin. North Am., *15*:247.
266. Edeiken-Monroe, B., Wagner, L. K., & Harris, J. H. Jr. (1986). Hyperextension dislocation of the cervical spine. A.J.N.R., *7*:135.
267. Evans, D. K. (1983). Dislocations at the cervicothoracic junction. J. Bone Joint Surg. [Br.], *65*:124.
268. Favero, K. J., & VanPeteghem, P. K. (1989). The quadrangular fragment fracture. Roentgenographic features and treatment protocol. Clin. Orthop., *239*:40.
269. Fuentes, J. M., Benezech, J., Lusszie, B., & Bloncourt, J. (1987). Fracture separation of the articular process of the inferior cervical vertebra: A comprehensive review of 13 cases. p. 227. In Cervical Spine I. Springer-Verlag, Berlin, Germany.
270. Fuentes, J. M., Bloncourt, J., & Vlahovitch, B. (1983). La tear drop fracture. Contribution a l'etude de mecanisme et des lesions osteo-disco-ligamentaires. Neurochirurgie, *29*:129.
271. Garger, W. N., Fisher, R. G., & Halfmann, H. W. (1969). Vertebrectomy and fusion for "tear drop fracture" of the cervical spine: Case report. J. Trauma, *9*:887.
272. Goldberg, A. L., Rothfus, W. E., Deeb, Z. L. et al. (1989). Hyperextension injuries of the cervical spine. Skeletal Radiol., *18*:283.
273. Hayashi, H., Okada, K., Hamada, M. et al. (1987). Etiologic factors of myelopathy. A radiographic evaluation of the aging changes in the cervical spine. Clin. Orthop., *214*:200.
274. Jacobs, B. (1975). Cervical fractures and dislocations (C3-7). Clin. Orthop., *109*:18.
275. Kim, K. W., Chen, H. H., Russell, E. J., & Rogers, L. F. (1988). Flexion teardrop fracture of the cervical spine: Radiographic characteristics. A.J.N.R., *9*:1221.
276. Kim, K. S., Rogers, L. F., & Regenbogen, V. (1986). Pitfalls in plain films diagnosis of cervical spine injuries: False positive interpretation. Surg. Neurol., *25*:381.
277. Lee, C., Kim, K. S., & Rogers, L. F. (1982). Sagittal fracture of the cervical vertebral body. A.J.R., *139*:55.
278. Lee, C., Kim, K. S., & Rogers, L. F. (1982). Triangular cervical vertebral body fractures: Diagnostic significance. A.J.R., *138*:1123.
279. Lee, C., Woodring, J. H., Rogers, L. F., & Kim, K. S. (1986). The radiographic distinction of degenerative slippage (spondylolisthesis and retrolisthesis) from traumatic slippage of the cervical spine. Skeletal Radiol., *15*:439.
280. Makoyo, P. Z. (1979). Rupture of cervical esophagus from blunt trauma with concomitant fracture dislocation of C4-C5 vertebra. J. Natl. Med. Assoc., *71*:473.
281. Reddin, A., Mirvis, S. E., & Diaconis, J. N. (1987). Rupture of the cervical esophagus and trachea associated with cervical spine fracture. J. Trauma, *27*:564.
282. Regenbogen, V. S., Rogers, L. F., Atlas, S. W., & Kim, K. W. (1986). Cervical spinal cord injuries in patients with cervical spondylosis. A.J.R., *146*:277.
283. Rorabeck, C. H., Rock, M. G., Hawksin, R. J., & Bourne, R. B. (1987). Unilateral facet dislocation of the cervical spine. An analysis of the results of treatment in 26 patients. Spine, *12*:23.
284. Rowed, D. W., & Tator, C. H. (1982). Cervical spondylosis in acute cervical cord injuries. p. 335. In Tator, C. H. Ed.: Early Management of Acute Spinal Cord Injury. Raven Press, New York.
285. Salomone, J. A. III, & Steele, M. T. (1987). An unusual presentation of bilateral facet dislocation of the cervical spine. Ann. Emerg. Med., *16*:1390.
286. Scher, A. T. (1979). Anterior cervical subluxation: An unstable position. A.J.R., *133*:275.
287. Scher, A. T. (1983). Hyperextension trauma in the elderly: An easily overlooked spinal injury. J. Trauma, 23:1066.
288. Shacked, I., Rappaport, Z. H., Barzilay, Z., & Ohri, A. (1983). Two-level fracture of the cervical spine in a young child. J. Bone Joint Surg. [Am.], *65*:119.
289. Shear, P., Hugenholtz, H., Tichard, M. T. et al. (1988). Multiple noncontiguous fractures of the cervical spine. J. Trauma, *28*:655.
290. Snyder, L. A. (1976). The lower cervical spine in trauma: A study of false-negative and false-positive findings. South Med. J., *69*:764.
291. Spenler, C. W., & Benfield, J. R. (1976). Esophageal disruption from blunt and penetrating external trauma. Arch. Surg., *111*:663.
292. Stauffer, E. S. (1989). Subaxial injuries. Clin. Orthop., *239*:30.
293. Stringer, W. L., Kelly, D. L., Johnston, F. R., & Holliday, R. H. (1980). Hyperextension injury of the cervical spine with esophageal perforation. Case report. J. Neurosurg., *53*:541.
294. Sumchai, A., Eliastam, M., & Werner, P. (1988). Seatbelt cervical injury in an intersection type vehicular collision. J. Trauma, *28*:1384.
295. Torg, J. S., Pavlov, H., Genuario, S. E. et al. (1986). Neurapraxia of the cervical spinal cord with transient quadriplegia. J. Bone Joint Surg. [Am.], *68*:1354.
296. Woodring, J. H., & Goldstein, S. J. (1982). Fractures of the articular processes of the cervical spine. A.J.R., *139*:341.
297. Yetkin, Z., Osborn, A. G., Giles, D. S., & Haughton, V. M. (1985). Uncovertebral and facet joint dislocations in cervical articular pillar fractures: CT evaluation. A.J.N.R., *6*:633.
298. Young, J. W. R., Resnik, C. S., DeCandido, P., & Mirvis, S. E. (1989). The laminar space in the diagnosis of rotational flexion injuries of the cervical spine. A.J.R., *152*:103.

Fracture of the Larynx

299. Angood, P. D., Attia, E. L., Brown, R. A., & Mulder, D. S. (1986). Extrinsic civilian trauma to the larynx and cervical trachea—Important predictors of long-term morbidity. J. Trauma, *26*:869.
300. Ballenger, J. J. (1969). Trauma of the larynx. In Ballenger, J. J. Ed.: Diseases of the Nose, Throat, and Ear. 11th Ed. Lea & Febiger, Philadelphia.
301. Guernsey, L. H. (1954). Fractures of the hyoid bone. J. Oral Surg., *12*:241.
302. Gussack, G. S., & Jurkovich, G. J. (1988). Treatment dilemmas in laryngotracheal trauma. J. Trauma, *28*:1439.
303. Harris, H. H., & Tobin, H. A. (1970). Acute injuries of the larynx and trachea in 49 patients (observations over a 15-year period.) Laryngoscope, *80*:1376.
304. Myers, E. M., & Iko, B. O. (1987). The management of acute laryngeal trauma. J. Trauma, *27*:448.
305. Nahum, A. M. (1969). Immediate care of acute blunt laryngeal trauma. J. Trauma, *9*:112.
306. Ogura, J. H., & Powers, W. E. (1964). Functional restitution of traumatic stenosis of the larynx and pharynx. Laryngoscope, *74*:1081.
307. Polanski, A., Resnick, D., Sofferman, R. A., & Davidson, T. M. (1984). Hyoid bone elevation: A sign of tracheal transection. Radiology, *150*:117.
308. Porrath, S. (1969). Roentgenologic considerations of the hyoid apparatus. Am. J. Roentgenol. Radium Ther. Nucl. Med., *105*:63.
309. Shumrick, D. A. (1967). Trauma of the larynx. Arch. Otolaryngol., *86*:109.
310. Stanley, R. B. Jr. (1984). Value of computed tomography in the management of acute laryngeal injury. J. Trauma, *24*:359.
311. Stanley, R. B. Jr., Cooper, D. S., & Florman, S. H. (1987). Phonatory effects of thyroid cartilage fractures. Ann. Otol. Rhinol. Laryngol., *96*:493.

Thoracolumbar Spine

312. Denis, F. (1983). The three column spine and its significance in the classification of acute thoracolumbar spinal injuries. Spine, *8*:817.
313. Griffith, H. B., Gleave, J. R. W., & Taylor, R. G. (1966). Changing patterns of fracture in the dorsal and lumbar spine. Br. Med. J., *1*:891.
314. Howorth, M. B. (1956). Fracture of the spine. Am. J. Surg., *92*:573.
315. Nicoll, E. A. (1949). Fractures of the dorso-lumbar spine. J. Bone Joint Surg. [Br.], *31*:376.
316. Olsson, O. (1951). Fractures of the upper thoracic and cervical vertebral bodies. Acta Chir. Scand., *102*:87.
317. Quesada, R. S., Greenbaum, E. I., Hertl, A., & Zoda, F. (1975). Widened interpedicular distance secondary to trauma. J. Trauma, *15*:167.
318. Roaf, R. (1960). A study of the mechanics of spinal injuries. J. Bone Joint Surg. [Br.], *42*:810.
319. Rogers, W. A. (1938). Cord injury during reduction of thoracic and lumbar vertebral body fracture and dislocation. J. Bone Joint Surg., *20*:689.
320. White, A. A., & Hirsch, C. (1971). The significance of the vertebral posterior elements in the mechanics of the thoracic spine. Clin. Orthop., *81*:2.
321. Holdsworth, F. W. (1963). Fractures, dislocations and fracture-dislocations of the spine. J. Bone Joint Surg. [Br.], *45*:6.
322. Holdsworth, F. W. (1970). Fractures, dislocations and fracture-dislocations of the spine. J. Bone Joint Surg. [Am.], *52*:1534.
323. Jonas, J. G. (1976). Fracture-dislocation of the dorsal spine. South. Med. J., *69*:1502.

Multiple-Level Spinal Injuries

324. Calenoff, L., Chessare, J. W., Rogers, L. F. et al. (1978). Multiple level spinal injuries: Importance of early recognition. A.J.R., *130*:665.
325. Kewalramani, L. S., & Taylor, R. G. (1976). Multiple non-contiguous injuries to the spine. Acta Orthop. Scand., *47*:52.
326. Scher, A. T. (1978). Double fractures of the spine—an indication for routine radiographic examination of the entire spine after injury. S. Afr. Med. J., *53*:411.

Additional References

Computed Tomography, Magnetic Resonance Imaging

327. Berne, J. D., Velmahos, G. C., El-Tawil, Q. et al. (1999). Value of complete cervical helical computed tomographic scanning in identifying cervical spine injury in the unevaluable blunt trauma patient with multiple injuries: A prospective study. J. Trauma, *47*:896.

328. Blackmore, C. C., Ramsey, S. D., Mann, F. A., & Deyo, R. A. (1999). Cervical spine screening with CT in trauma patients: A cost-effectiveness analysis. Radiology, *212*:117.
329. Blacksin, M. F., & Lee, H. J. (1995). Frequency and significance of fractures of the upper cervical spine detected by CT in patients with severe neck trauma. A.J.R., *165*:1201.
330. Borock, E. C., Gabram, S. G. A., Jacobs, L. M., & Murphy, M. A. (1991). A prospective analysis of a two-year experience using computed tomography as an adjunct for cervical spine clearance. J. Trauma, *31*:1001.
331. Flanders, A. E., Schaefer, D. M., Doan, H. T. et al. (1997). Acute cervical spine trauma: Correlation of MR imaging findings with degree of neurologic deficit. Radiology, *177*:25.
332. Hall, A. J., Wagle, V. G., Raycroft, J. et al. (1993). Magnetic resonance imaging in cervical spine trauma. J. Trauma, *34*:21.
333. Hanson, J. A., Blackmore, C., Mann, F. A., & Wilson, A. J. (2000). Cervical spine injury: A clinical decision rule to identify high-risk patients for helical CT screening. A.J.R., *174*:713.
334. Link, T. M., Schuierer, G., Hufendiek, A. et al. (1995). Substantial head trauma: Value of routine CT examination of the cervicocranium. Radiology, *196*:741.
335. LeBlang, S. D., & Nuñez, D. B. (1999). Helical CT of cervical spine and soft tissue injuries of the neck. Radiol. Clin. North Am., *37*:515.
336. Nuñez, D. B. (1998). Helical CT for the evaluation of cervical vertebral injuries. Semin. Musculoskelet. Radiol. 2:19.
337. Nuñez, D. B., Ahmad, A. A., Coin, C. G. et al. (1994). Clearing the cervical spine in multiple trauma victims: A time-effective protocol using helical computed tomography. Emergency Radiology, *1*:273.
338. Nuñez, D. B., & Quencer, R. (1998). The role of helical CT in the assessment of cervical spine injuries. A.J.R., *171*:951.
339. Nuñez, D. B., Zuluaga, A., Fuentes-Bernardo, D. A. et al. (1996). Cervical spine trauma: How much more do we learn by routinely using helical CT? RadioGraphics, *16*:1307.
340. Quencer, R. M., Nuñez, D. B., & Green, B. A. (1997). Controversies in imaging acute cervical spine trauma. A.J.N.R., *18*:1866.
341. Woodring, J. H., & Lee, C. (1992). The role and limitations of computed tomographic scanning in the evaluation of cervical trauma. J. Trauma, *33*:698.

Cervical Spine, General

342. Blackmore, C. C., & Deyo, R. A. (1997). Specificity of cervical spine radiography: Importance of clinical scenario. Emergency Radiology, *4*:283.
343. Davis, J. W., Phreaner, D. L., Hoyt, D. B., & Mackersie, R. C. (1993). The etiology of missed cervical spine injuries. J. Trauma, *34*:342.
344. Freemyer, B., Knopp, R., Piche, J. W. et al. (1989). Comparison of five-view and three-view cervical spine series in the evaluation of patients with cervical trauma. Ann. Emerg. Med. *18*:818.
345. MacDonald, R. L., Schwartz, M. L., Mirich, D. et al. (1990). Diagnosis of cervical spine injury in motor vehicle crash victims: How many x-rays are enough? J. Trauma, *30*:392.
346. Vandemark, R. M. (1990). Radiology of the cervical spine in trauma patients: Practice pitfalls and recommendations for improving efficiency and communication. A.J.R., *155*:465.
347. Woodring, J. H., & Lee, C. (1993). Limitations of cervical radiography in the evaluation of acute cervical trauma. J. Trauma, *34*:32.

Fracture of the Cervical Spine

348. Friedman, D., Flanders, A., Thomas, C., & Millar, W. (1995). Vertebral artery injury after acute cervical spine trauma: Rate of occurrence as detected by MR angiography and assessment of clinical consequences. A.J.R., *164*:443.

Fractures of the Axis (C2)

349. Starr, J. K., & Eismont, F. J. (1993). Atypical hangman's fractures. Spine, *18*:1954.

Lower Cervical Spine (C3–C7)

350. Ronnen, H. R., de Korte, P. J., Brink, P. R. G. et al. (1996). Acute whiplash injury: Is there a role for MR imaging? A prospective study of 100 patients. Radiology, *201*:93.
351. Shanmuganathan, K., Mirvis, S. E., Dowe, M., & Levine, A. L. (1996). Traumatic isolation of the cervical articular pillar: Imaging observations in 21 patients. A.J.R., *166*:897.
352. Woodring, J. H., Lee, C., & Duncan, V. (1993). Transverse process fractures of the cervical vertebrae: Are they insignificant? J. Trauma, *34*:797.

Chapter 13

THE THORACIC AND LUMBAR SPINE

with Richard H. Daffner, MD, FACR

Injuries to the thoracic and lumbar regions of the spine occur less commonly than those to the cervical region. Although the majority of cervical injuries are the result of flexion or extension mechanisms, thoracic and lumbar injuries are virtually all due either to primary flexion or to a mechanism in which flexion also plays a major role. Other differences between cervical injuries and thoracic and lumbar injuries are related to the stabilizing effect of the ribs and sternum, with moderation of the degree of injury and any resulting instability.[35, 36] Nevertheless, injuries to the thoracic and lumbar regions of the spine, like cervical injuries, produce a well-recognized spectrum of abnormalities on imaging studies, the findings being dependent on the incident mechanism.

This chapter describes the key anatomic, biomechanical, and pathomechanical aspects of injuries to the thoracic and lumbar regions of the spine. The pertinent imaging features are also covered. In addition, the radiographic signs that constitute the "footprints" and the "fingerprints" of these injuries are reviewed.

Incidence, Distribution, and Biomechanics

Two thirds of all fractures involving the thoracic and lumbar spine occur at T11–L2;[26, 104, 145] 90% occur between T11 and L4[145] (Fig. 13–1). In a review of 1908 vertebral injuries seen at Allegheny General Hospital in Pittsburgh, a Level I Trauma Center, 472 (25%) were found to be thoracic, and 490 (26%), lumbar. Of these, 509 (56%) occurred between T11 and L2 (T11: 60 injuries; T12: 121; L1: 236; and L2: 90).[36] The majority of fractures between T2 and T8 occurred in motorcyclists.[40] Fractures of the mid- and upper dorsal spine are otherwise relatively uncommon in adults except for those resulting from convulsions caused by either electroshock therapy[101, 143] or tetany.[16] There is, however, in my experience and that of others an incidence of approximately 20% of noncontiguous fractures (either within the same anatomic segment or in the cervical-thoracic, thoracic-lumbar, or cervical-lumbar regions) throughout the vertebral column.[26, 36] Thus, it is imperative that the thoracic and lumbar regions be evaluated in any patient who has sustained a cervical fracture.

Although there are 12 separate thoracic and 5 separate lumbar vertebrae, from a biomechanical and clinical standpoint there are only 4 distinct functional segments, derived from the incidence patterns of injury. These segments and their vertebral components are as follows: T1, part of the cervicothoracic junction; T2 through T9, the mid-thoracic region; T10 through L2, the thoracolumbar region; and L3 through S1, the lower lumbar and lumbosacral regions.

As noted, most injuries occur at the thoracolumbar junction; this preponderance is related to the unique anatomy and biomechanics of the area. The thoracic spine from T1 through T8 is relatively immobile, allowing only minimal degrees of flexion and extension because of the stabilizing and restrictive effect of the ribs.[36, 191] However, beginning at T9 and T10 the ribs no longer have this effect, so that a greater degree of flexion as well as limited motion in extension, lateral bending, and rotation is permitted. The T10–L2 segment is the most mobile portion of the thoracic and lumbar regions. The arrangement of the facet joints (at an angle of nearly 90 degrees) at the thoracolumbar level permits only flexion and extension and almost no rotation. Unfortunately, with traumatic injury the lower torso may be fixed in one position while the upper torso is twisted, placing undue stress on severely restricted motion segments. This mechanism of injury frequently results in disruptive fractures and dislocations at the junction point of the more mobile lumbar region and the markedly less mobile thoracic region.[191]

In contrast, the highest incidence of thoracic and lumbar fractures in children is at T4, T5, and L2.[89, 95, 98] Fractures involving adjacent vertebrae are relatively common, particularly in children, in whom multiple contiguous fractures are the rule rather than the exception.[60, 89, 95] In the Allegheny General Hospital series, 18% of patients (of all ages) had multilevel contiguous or noncontiguous vertebral injuries.[36]

Approximately 20% of thoracolumbar fractures are associated with other skeletal injuries.[93, 94, 145] The frequent association of compression fractures of the thoracolumbar junction with fractures of the calcaneus is particularly noteworthy.[93] Wedge compression fractures of the upper thoracic spine are at times associated with fractures of the sternum. This entity is described in detail in Chapter 14.

The clinical and historical indications for evaluation of the thoracic and lumbar spinal segments for possible injury are the same as for evaluation of the cervical spine:

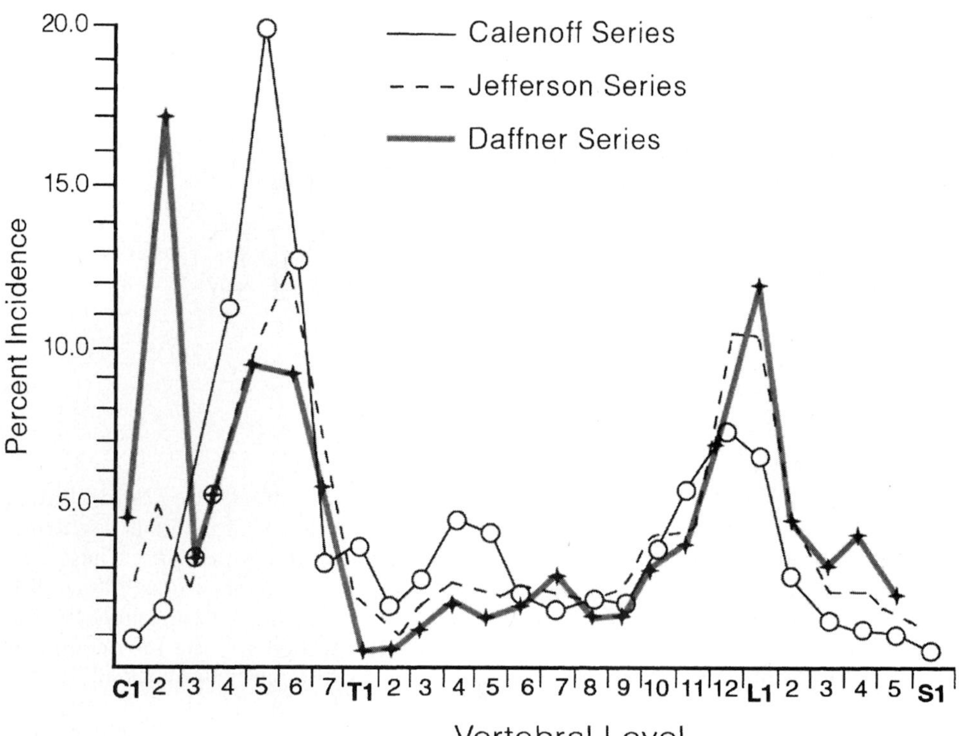

Figure 13–1. Distribution of vertebral injuries in three large reported series. The Calenoff series comprised 710 patients; the Jefferson series, 2006 cases; and the Daffner series, 1908 injuries. The C2 peak for the Daffner series (the author's) reflects the large elderly population in the geographic region served. (Data from references 26, 36, and 104.)

high-velocity blunt trauma, multiple peripheral fractures, presence of a cervical fracture, altered mental status following trauma (unconsciousness, alcohol or drug use), fall from a height of greater than 10 feet, rigid vertebral disease (ankylosing spondylitis, diffuse idiopathic skeletal hyperostosis [DISH]), and paresthesias or burning in the (lower) extremities.[35, 36, 52, 187]

Imaging of Suspected Fracture

Radiography

Radiography of the thoracic and lumbar spine is the single most important study for diagnosing injuries to these regions. Unlike fractures of the cervical spine, with its unique anatomy, thoracic and lumbar fractures are rarely occult. In addition to being easy to perform, radiographic studies of these regions allow (1) determination of the primary mechanism of injury, (2) delineation of the extent of injury, and (3) identification of the areas on which to focus more definitive studies such as computed tomography (CT) or magnetic resonance imaging (MRI).

At Allegheny General Hospital, all examinations are performed with the patient supine. The examination begins with properly exposed and positioned anteroposterior and cross-table lateral views of the thoracic and lumbar regions (Fig. 13–2). Because of the preponderance of spinal fractures at the thoracolumbar junction, it is very important that the lower thoracic vertebrae be included in examinations for suspected lumbar spine trauma and likewise that the upper lumbar vertebrae be included in examinations of the thoracic spine. A swimmer's view is required to adequately demonstrate the upper thoracic column. Oblique views of the thoracic and lumbar spine are rarely informative and can be safely omitted; in any case, because of the patient's condition it may not be possible to obtain oblique views of the lumbar spine.[36] Also included is an anteroposterior view of the pelvis in all trauma patients because of the high incidence of pelvic fractures concomitant with vertebral injuries.[35] Finally, it should be remembered that thoracic spine fractures can often be detected on portable chest radiographs obtained initially.[122]

General Approach

Fractures and dislocations in the thoracic and lumbar regions may be recognized by direct or indirect signs. The use of a systematic approach to viewing radiographs is recommended. For this purpose I have devised a system termed the *ABCS system,* wherein *A* denotes abnormalities of *a*natomy or *a*lignment, *B* denotes abnormalities of *b*one integrity (frank fracture), *C* denotes abnormalities of the *c*artilage or joint spaces, and *S* denotes *s*oft tissue abnormalities.[35, 36] Unlike injuries in the cervical region, as previously mentioned, thoracic and lumbar injuries tend to be less subtle but are nonetheless diagnostically challenging.

Abnormalities of Anatomy or Alignment

Abnormalities of anatomy and alignment include disruption of the anterior or posterior vertebral body line, disruption of the spinolaminar line, rotation of spinous processes, widening of the interspinous distance, and widening of the interpedicle distance. The posterior vertebral body line should be oriented with the long axis of the vertebra and should be interrupted only in the center by nutrient vessels. Any displacement, angulation, rotation, duplication, or absence of this line is abnormal[36, 39, 136]

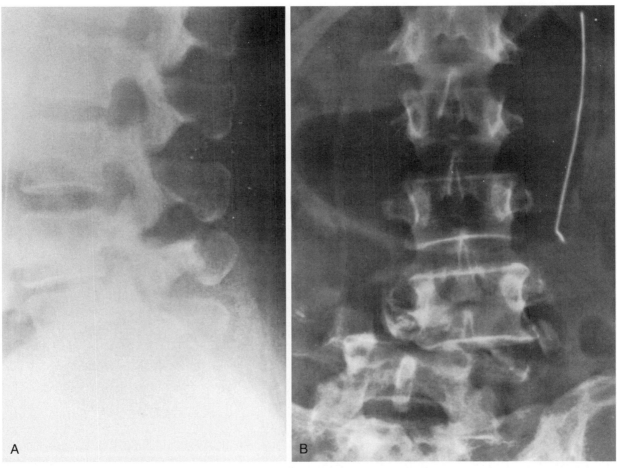

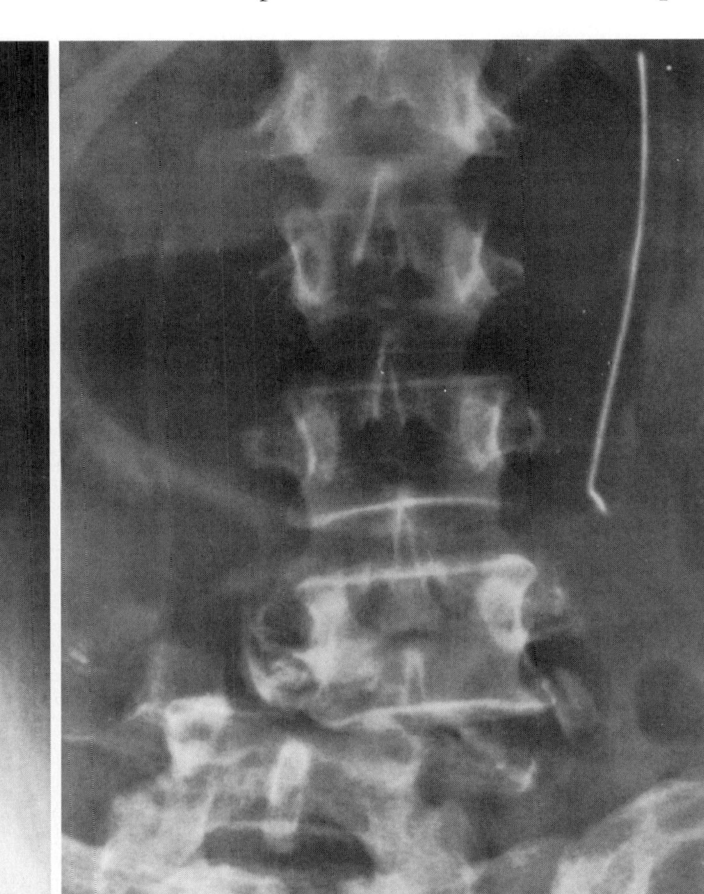

Figure 13–2. Lateral fracture-dislocation of L4-L5. *A*, Lateral radiograph reveals narrowing of the L4-L5 interspace, giving no hint of the severity of the injury. *B*, Frontal (anteroposterior) view demonstrates marked left lateral translation (dislocation) of L4 on L5. *Both* views should be examined before the patient is moved.

(Fig. 13–3). The interspinous space is measured from the bottom of one spinous process to the top of the one below on frontal radiographs. This distance should not vary by more than 2 mm from level to level[36] (Fig. 13–4). The interpedicle distance—the space between the inner margins of the pedicles—likewise should not vary by more than 2 mm from level to level (Fig. 13–5). Widening of the interpedicle distance indicates that a burst fracture has occurred, with involvement of not only the vertebral body but also the lamina.[35, 36] Other, nonspecific findings are kyphotic angulation, loss of lordosis, scoliosis, and loss of the psoas stripe.

Abnormalities of Bone Integrity

Abnormalities of bone integrity include any overt evidence of fracture. Such evidence may include any of the aforementioned signs. A careful search for fractures of ribs or transverse processes should also be made because the presence of such fractures is useful for differentiating shearing and rotary injuries from the more common burst fractures.[35, 36]

Cartilage or Joint Space Abnormalities

The most common joint space abnormality encountered in the thoracic or lumbar region is narrowing of an intervertebral disc space with or without facet narrowing. Traumatic joint abnormalities are much less common in the thoracic and lumbar spine than in the cervical region. However, widening or distraction of facet joints or even the presence of so-called naked facets indicates that a severe posterior ligamentous injury has occurred (Fig. 13–6). This sign is almost always associated with widening of the interspinous distance. A wide disc space should always be viewed with suspicion because this finding is usually an indication of an extension injury[35, 36] (Fig. 13–7).

Soft Tissue Abnormalities

There are only two important soft tissue abnormalities that accompany thoracic or lumbar injuries: the presence of a paraspinous soft tissue mass and loss of the psoas stripe.[35, 36] Of these two signs, the presence of paraspinous changes is the more useful for identifying thoracic injuries because such changes can be identified on a chest radiograph (Fig. 13–8). Paraspinous masses in these cases represent hematomas accumulated beneath and dissecting along the paraspinous ligaments. They are bilateral but usually asymmetrical, and may extend considerably beyond the site of fracture. The paraspinous hematoma associated with fracture of the upper thoracic spine may dissect over the apex of the lung, forming a

Text continued on page 460

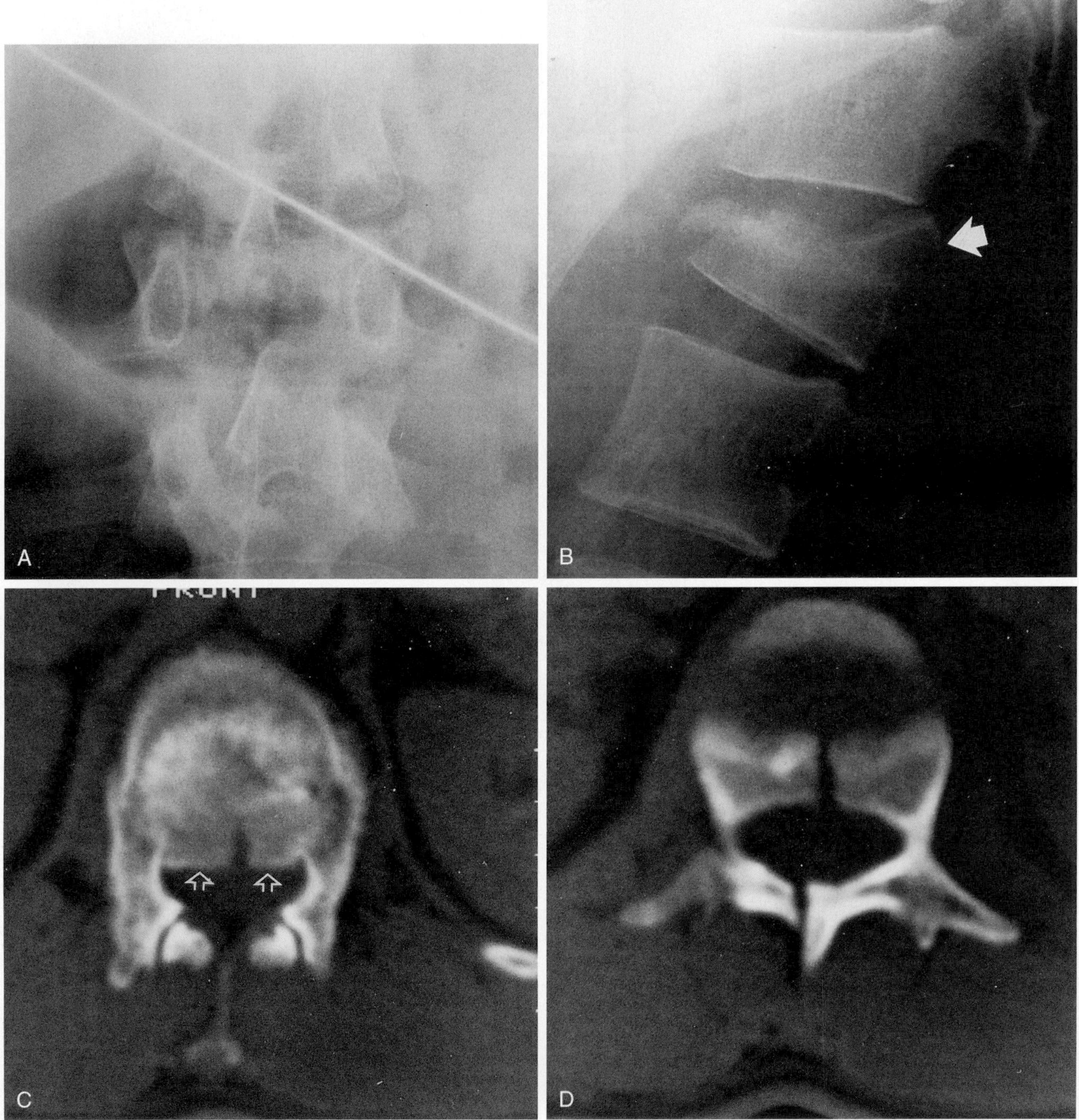

Figure 13–3. Burst fracture of L1, with an abnormal posterior vertebral body line. *A*, Anteroposterior view shows loss of height of the body of L1 and widening of the interpedicle distance. *B*, Lateral view shows body compression anteriorly and retropulsion and bowing of the upper part of the posterior vertebral body line *(arrow)*. *C*, CT image through the upper portion of L1 shows encroachment of the vertebral canal by the retropulsed fragments *(arrows)*. *D*, CT image through the lower portion of L1 demonstrates sagittal fractures through the body as well as through the lamina. This finding accounts for the wide interpedicle distance.

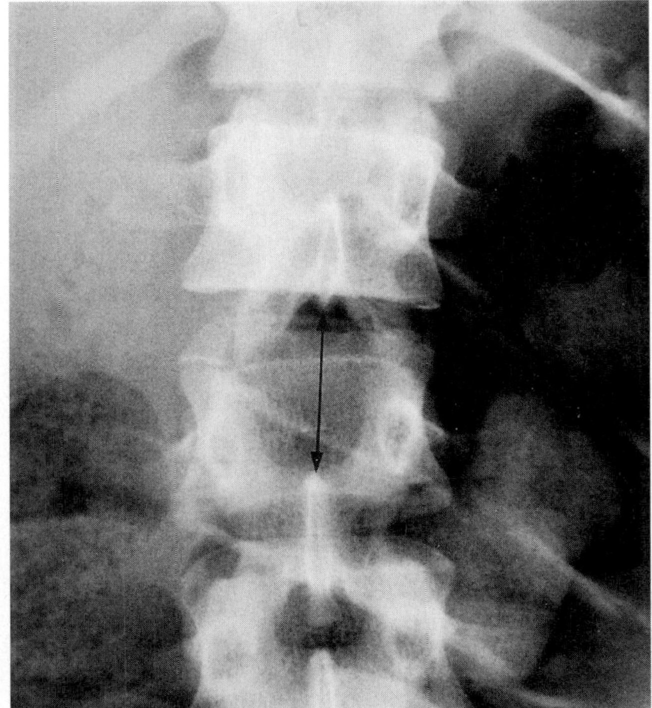

Figure 13–4. Wide interspinous space *(double arrow)* in a distraction injury of L1–L2. Note the naked facets resulting from the distraction.

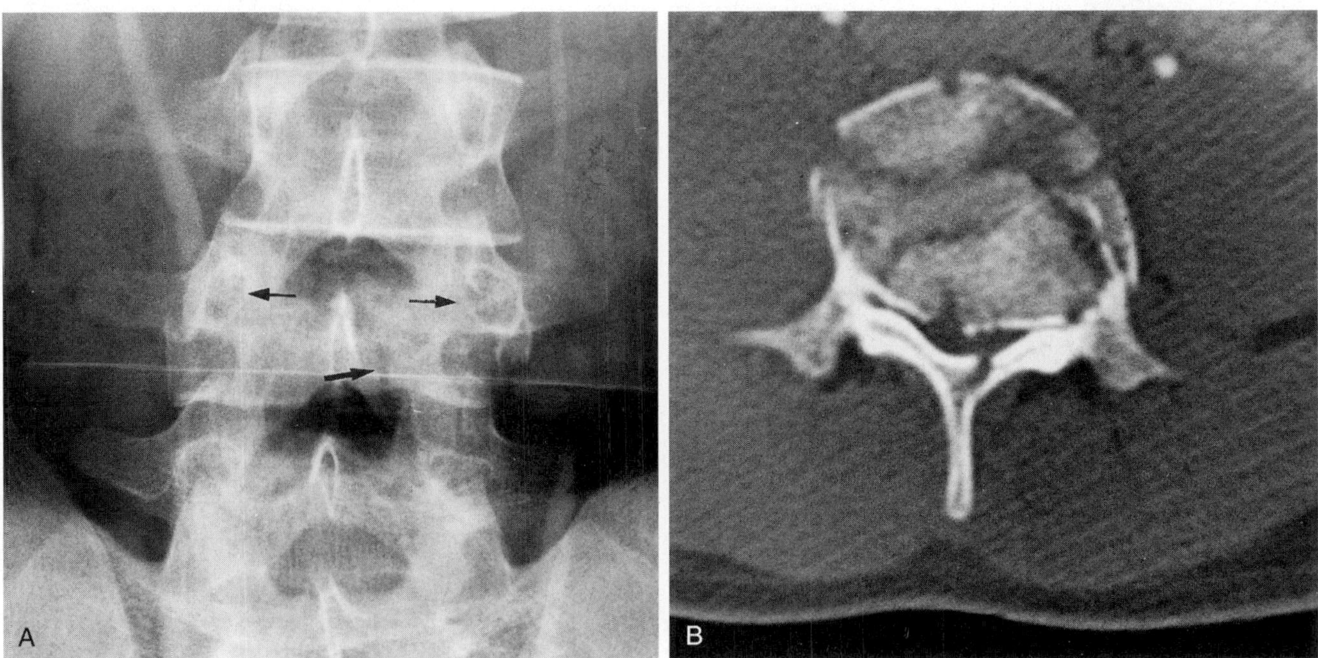

Figure 13–5. Wide interpedicle distance in L4 resulting from a burst fracture. *A*, Anteroposterior view shows an increase in the interpedicle distance *(upper thin arrows)*. The laminar fracture can also be seen on the left *(lower arrow)*. *B*, CT image shows the vertebral canal nearly completely occluded by retropulsed bone fragments. Note the laminar fracture on the left. (See also Fig. 13–3.)

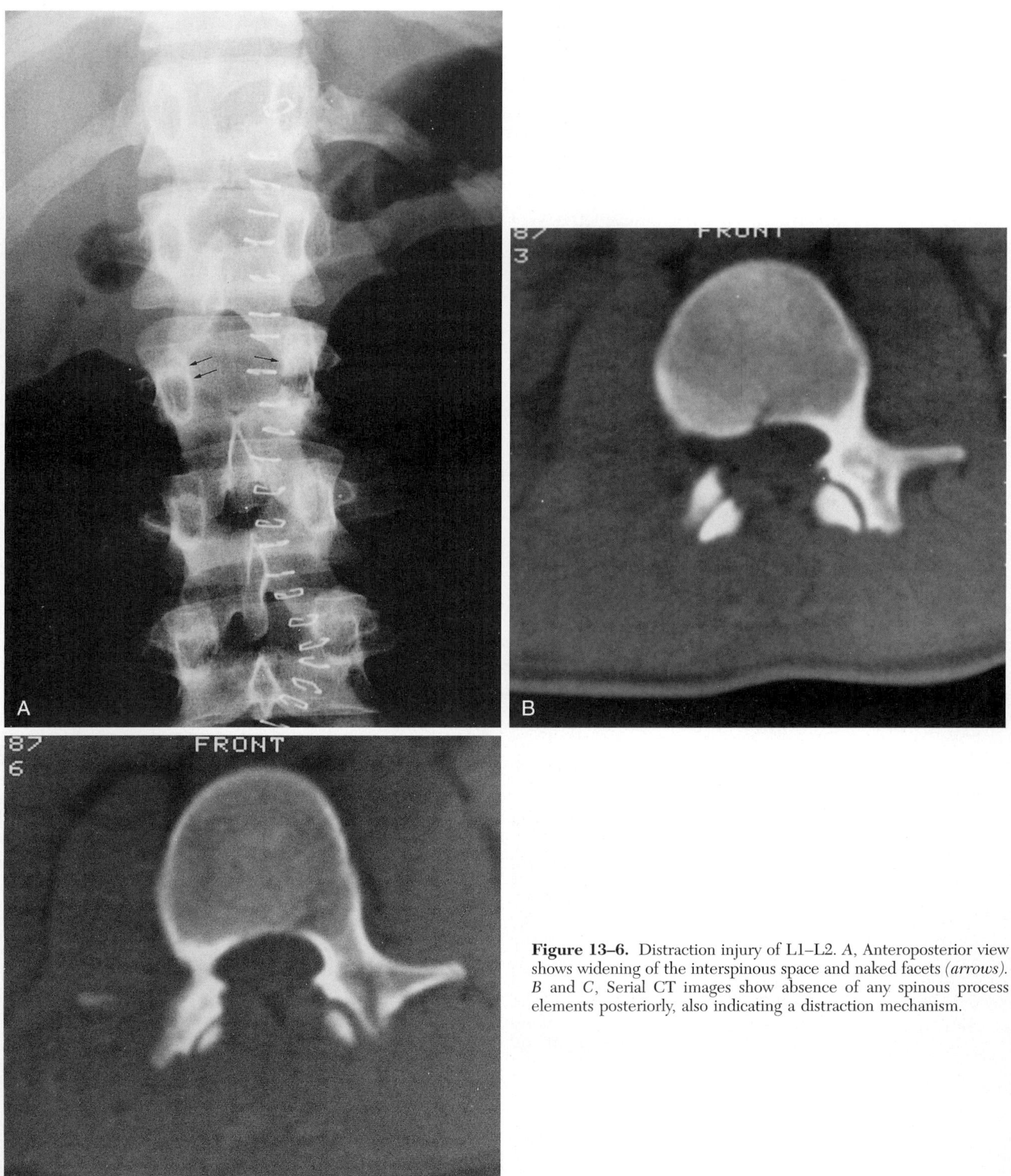

Figure 13–6. Distraction injury of L1–L2. *A*, Anteroposterior view shows widening of the interspinous space and naked facets *(arrows)*. *B* and *C*, Serial CT images show absence of any spinous process elements posteriorly, also indicating a distraction mechanism.

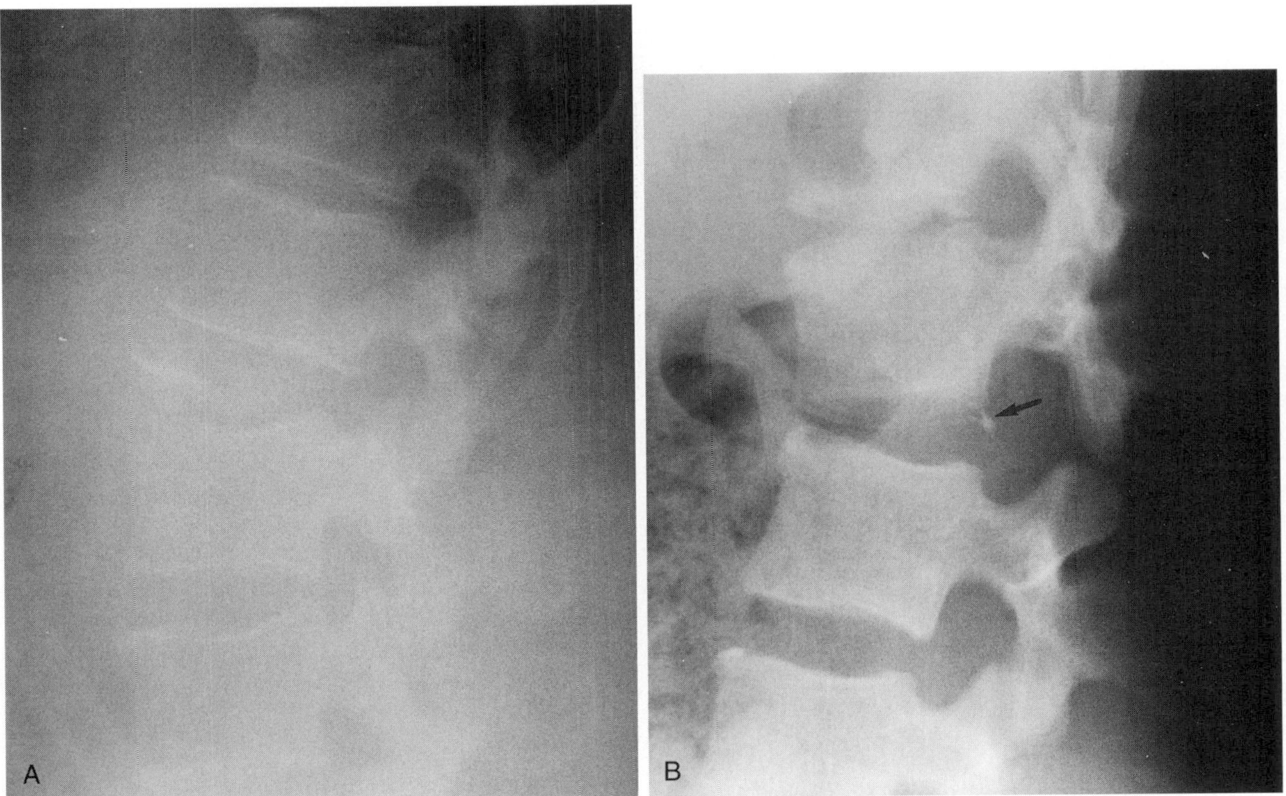

Figure 13–7. Wide disc spaces. *A*, Extension injury of L1–L2. Lateral view shows anterior widening of the L1 disc space. Note the avulsed fragment of bone from L2. *B*, Flexion-distraction injury of L1–L2. Lateral view shows posterior widening of the L1 disc space. Note the small avulsed fragment of bone from the posterior inferior margin of L1 *(arrow)*, as well as perching of the facets.

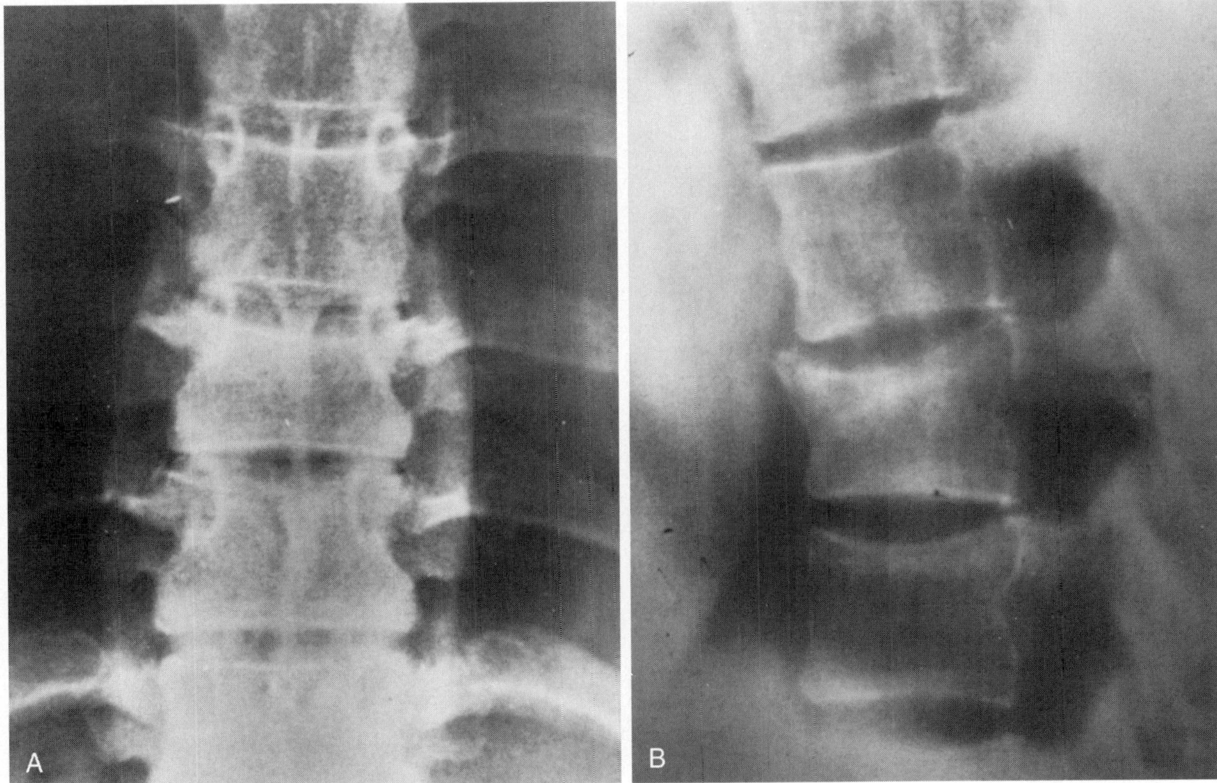

Figure 13–8. Paraspinous hematoma associated with compression fractures of T8 and T9. *A*, Anteroposterior view demonstrates bilateral paraspinous soft tissue swelling. Note the decreased height of T8 and T9. The superior end plates of these two vertebrae are not as well defined as those of the other vertebrae. *B*, Lateral tomogram demonstrates depression of the superior end plates of T8 and T9, with a small triangular fragment at the superior margin of each vertebra. A line of sclerosis beneath each depressed end plate indicates impaction.

pleural cap (Fig. 13–9). This configuration is precisely the same as for the hematoma associated with traumatic disruption of the aorta. When such a posterior mediastinal hematoma is encountered, both possibilities must be considered and the spine examined closely for evidence of fracture before the patient is unnecessarily submitted to aortography. As a rule, a chest CT study is sufficient to make this distinction (Fig. 13–10).

Other Considerations

The importance of identifying a dislocation or loss of height of a vertebral body, indicating the presence of a compression fracture, is universally appreciated. However, it is also important to determine the status of the posterior elements. Their disruption represents an important clue to the possibility of an unstable fracture.[30] It is particularly important to be aware of the appearance of the posterior elements on the anteroposterior view of the spine,[164] for two reasons: First, because of the critical status of many patients in the immediate postinjury period, only an anteroposterior view may be obtained. Second, the posterior elements of the spine are insufficiently visualized for evaluation on many lateral views obtained under these circumstances.

On the anteroposterior view of the thoracolumbar spine, the cortical margins of the spinous processes are tear-shaped and the pedicles are ovoid. The laminae are solid plates of bone. The inferior articular facets are well seated within the superior articular facet of the adjacent inferior vertebral body. The majority of the vertebral body is overlain by the posterior elements. The whole unit has the appearance of an owl's face, with the pedicles representing the eyes and the spinous process the beak. Any posterior distractive injury will result in widening of the posterior elements, making the beak of the owl disappear.

On the frontal view there are two clues to the recognition of disruption of the posterior elements.[30, 159, 164] With either a transverse fracture of the posterior elements or disruption of the ligaments, there may be sufficient angulation of the superior fragment or vertebra that a portion of the vertebral body is no longer overlain by the posterior elements. This separation plus elevation of the posterior elements gives rise to an empty or vacant appearance of the involved vertebral body (Fig. 13–11). Closer examination will demonstrate a widening of the interspinous distance or, if there is a transverse fracture through the spinous process, a distinct separation of the fragments. Another key is recognition of a break in the continuity (Fig. 13–12) of the oval cortex of the pedicles or the tear-shaped cortex of the spinous process, or both. A fracture line may be visualized within the laminae or articular processes. Confirmation rests with an adequately exposed lateral view of the spine.

In the thoracic spine it is more difficult to identify fractures of the posterior elements[163] and in some cases even fractures of the vertebral bodies (see Fig. 13–9)

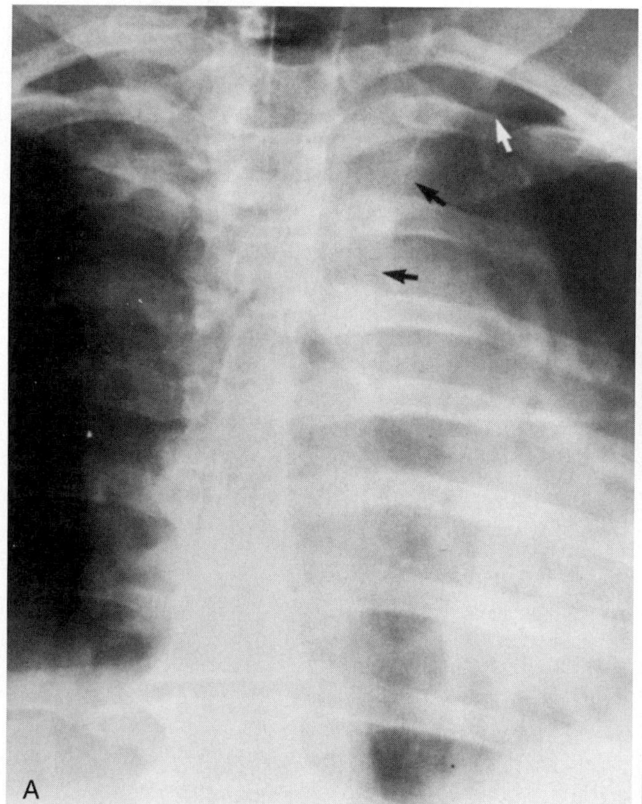

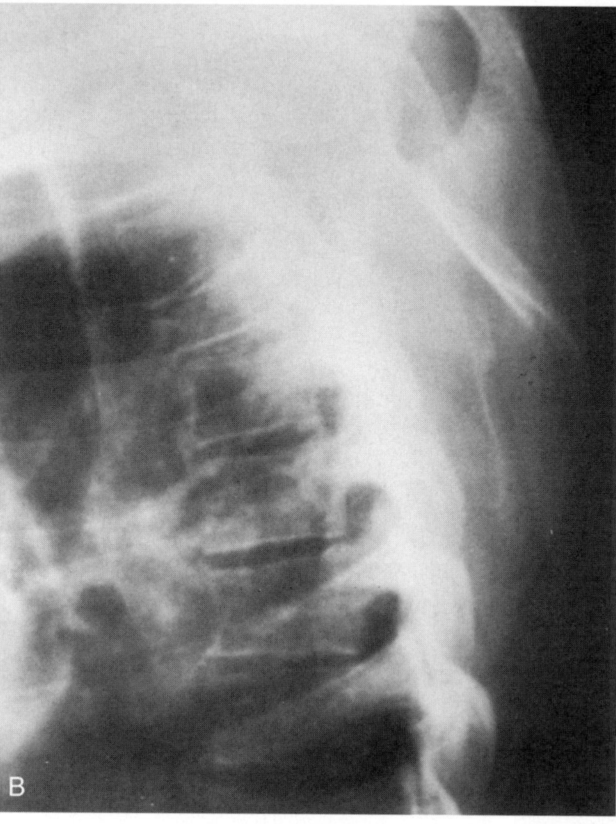

Figure 13–9. Fracture-dislocation of T4–T5. *A*, Anteroposterior view demonstrates narrowing of T4 without significant lateral offset. A paraspinous hematoma is present and extends over the left apex *(arrows)*. *B*, Lateral view reveals compression of T5. The posterior elements are not demonstrated in this image. (From Rogers, L.F., Thayer, C., Weinberg, P.E., & Kim, K.S. [1980]. Acute injuries of the upper thoracic spine associated with paraplegia. A.J.R. Am. J. Roentgerol., *134*:67.)

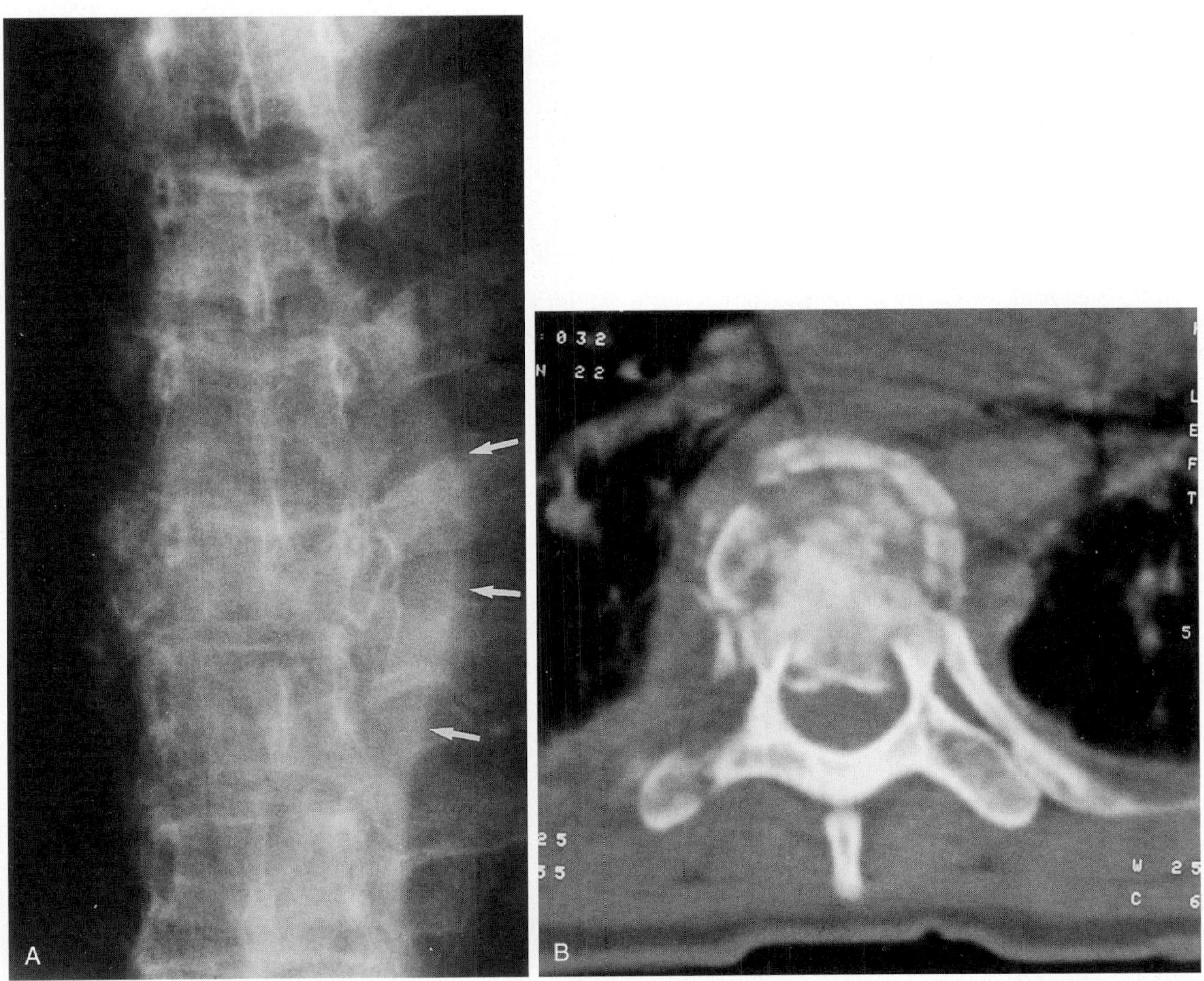

Figure 13–10. Burst fracture of T8 with paraspinal hematoma. *A*, Anteroposterior radiograph shows loss of height of T8 as well as paraspinal widening centered on T8 *(arrows)*. *B*, CT image shows the retropulsed bone fragment in the vertebral canal, as well as bilateral paraspinal soft tissue hematoma.

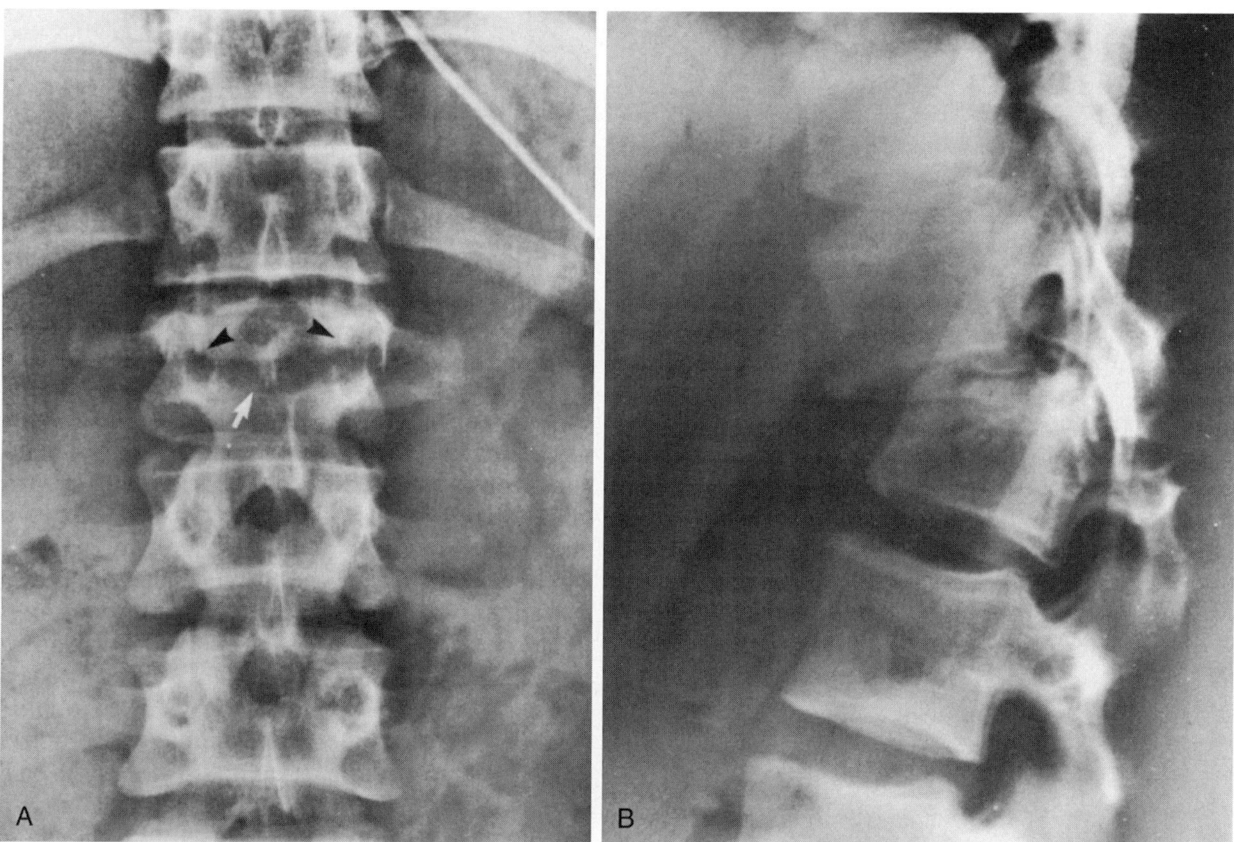

Figure 13–11. T12–L1 fracture-dislocation. *A*, Anteroposterior view demonstrates disruption of the cortical margins of the pedicles of L1 *(arrowheads)* and a horizontal fracture of the lamina and spinous process *(white arrow)*, as well as the transverse process on the left. The end plates of L1 are indistinct. *B*, Lateral view demonstrates anterior dislocation of T12 on L1 and anterior wedge compression of the body of L1.

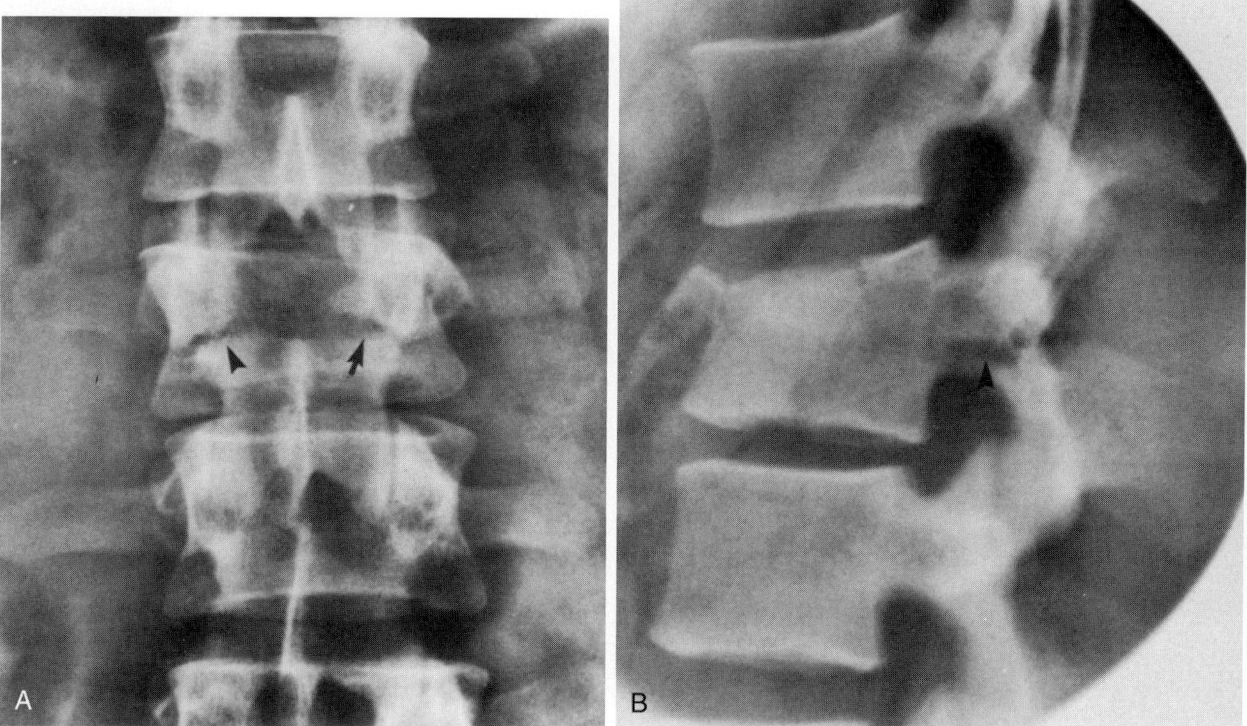

Figure 13–12. Flexion-distraction (Smith-type) fracture of L2 associated with posterior element fractures. *A*, Anteroposterior view demonstrates compression of the left side of the body of L2. There is a horizontal fracture through the inferior margin of the pedicle on the right *(arrowhead)* and through the lamina on the left *(arrow)*. *B*, There is an anterior wedge compression fracture as well as a horizontal fracture through the pedicle *(arrowhead)*.

themselves. Fracture lines are partially obscured by the overlying cardiac and mediastinal structures, and the laminae, spinous processes, and articular facets are more vertically oriented and overlap in a shingle-like fashion. Fractures of the upper dorsal spine are infrequently angulated in the lateral plane and are characteristically minimally displaced when viewed in the frontal projection. Minimal lateral offsets may be difficult to determine. Alignment is evaluated by closely observing the alignment of the spinous processes and lateral margins of the vertebral bodies. In the mid- and lower dorsal spine, injuries are manifested on the anteroposterior view by paraspinous hematomas or as abrupt angulations in the alignment of the vertebrae (Fig. 13–13). The identification of questionable malalignment or angulation of the spine on a chest radiograph following trauma is an indication for obtaining anteroposterior and lateral views of the dorsal spine. On the lateral view the vertebral bodies and particularly the posterior elements are obscured by the overlying pectoral girdle. A modified swimmer's view or, better, a CT scan is helpful.

Diagnostic Pitfalls

Pitfalls in radiographic evaluation relate to patient size and adequate visualization of the cervicothoracic and the lumbosacral junctions. Patients who are obese are extremely difficult to radiograph, particularly in the lateral projection. For these patients, use of CT may be necessary. In addition, imaging the cervicothoracic and the lumbosacral junctions always present a diagnostic and technical challenge because of the overlying shoulder girdle and pelvis and buttock, respectively, particularly in large patients. Again, it may be necessary to resort to CT as an alternative examination.

Computed Tomography

CT is simple to perform in patients with suspected or known vertebral trauma. The advent of helical CT has significantly reduced the scanning time to a matter of seconds. Newer refinements in CT technology such as multislice scanning have further reduced the time needed for study in critically injured patients. In addition, with helical CT of the thorax or abdomen, the data acquired at the time of examination can be processed later to produce diagnostic images of the thoracic and lumbar spinal regions. This capability eliminates the need for a separate vertebral CT examination.

At Allegheny General Hospital, each thoracic and lumbar CT examination is tailored to the specific area(s) of (suspected) injury for each patient. Unlike with cervical helical CT, which often includes the entire cervical spine, the levels for study are selected by review of the radiographs of the area. The CT scout film may also be used for this purpose. The helical technique of choice uses contiguous 4-mm slices, reviewed at 3 mm, with a pitch of 1. The area of study is overlapped from at least one full level above to one full level below for all suspected injured vertebrae.[35, 36] If several levels are in question, separate studies are performed, unless the distance between the involved vertebrae is only one or two vertebrae. In that instance, a contiguous study is performed. It is important to examine the levels above and below all suspected injuries because additional fractures may be present at contiguous levels that are not apparent on the radiographs (Fig. 13–14). As previously stated, approximately 20% of patients may have noncontiguous injuries.[26, 36] It is important for the spine surgeon to know whether or not contiguous injuries are present in planning spinal stabilization.

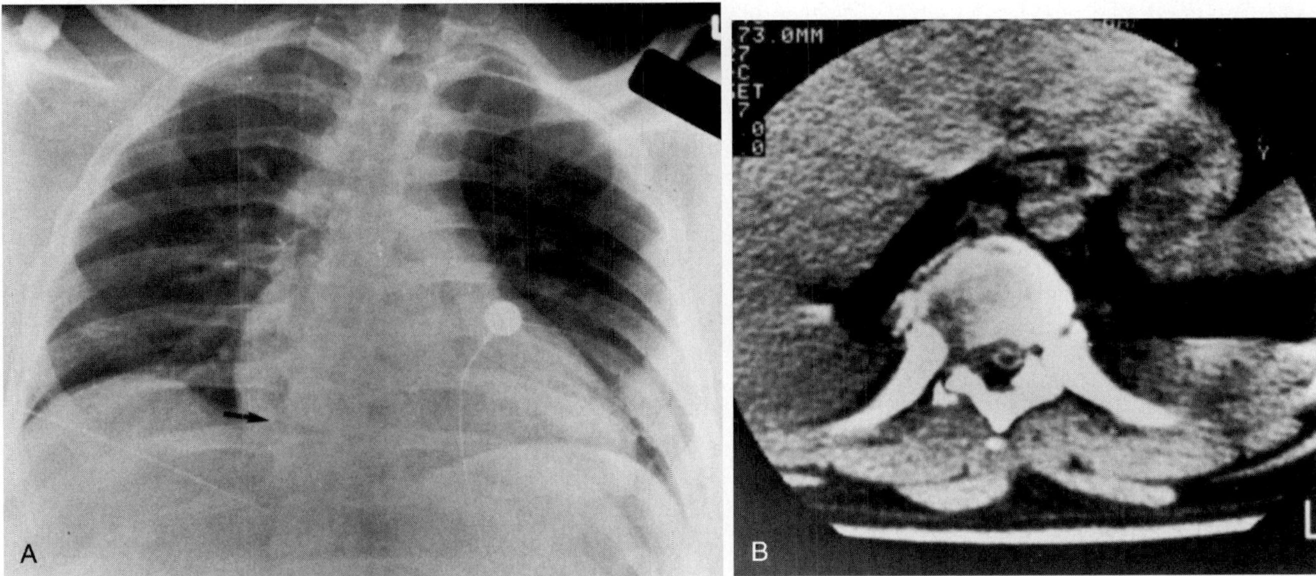

Figure 13–13. Fracture-dislocation at T9–T10. *A*, Initial chest radiograph demonstrates angulation of the vertebral column with widening of the right lateral aspect of the T9 disc space *(arrow)*. *B*, CT myelographic image obtained at the level of the inferior end plate of T9 demonstrates a fracture of the vertebral body and displacement of the subarachnoid space to the left by a soft tissue density projecting posteriorly and medially into the vertebral canal. This finding was proved to represent a herniated intervertebral disc, which was associated with partial paraplegia. (Case courtesy of Fred M.H. Ziter, Jr., MD, Hartford, Conn.)

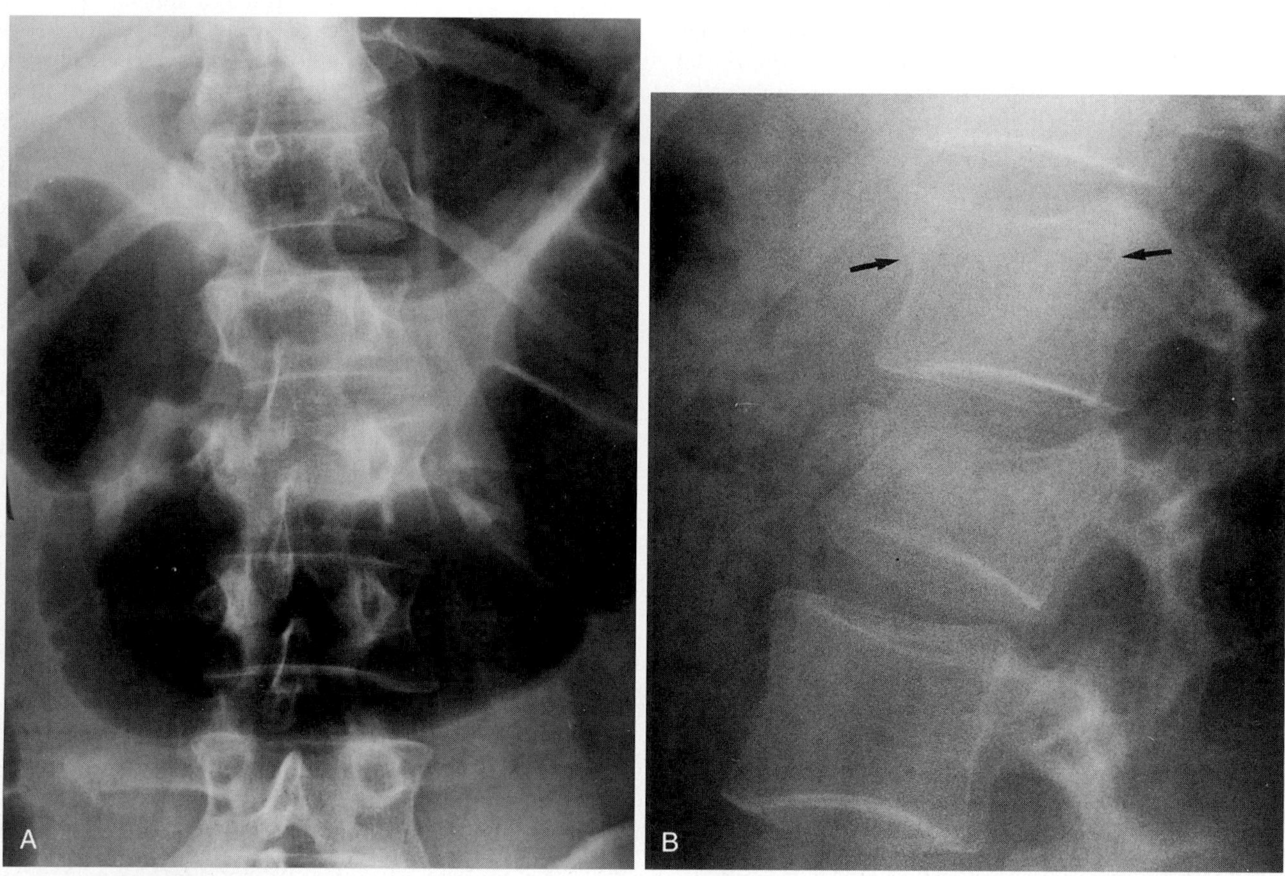

Figure 13–14. Contiguous fractures of L1 and L2. *A*, Anteroposterior radiograph shows an obvious burst fracture of L2. The L1 fracture is not as obvious. *B*, Lateral radiograph shows the characteristic findings with a burst fracture of L2. Note the buckling of the anterior and posterior vertebral body lines of L1 *(arrows)*.

The survey (scout) view is an important portion of the examination and allows accurate correlation of the axial images with the proper levels. It should therefore be obtained in such a way that allows delineation of the anatomic levels. If the suspected injury is between C6 through T8, the anteroposterior survey view is selected. For injuries at T8 and below, anteroposterior or lateral survey views are obtained; I prefer the lateral view. In addition, the CT technologists may be directed to print the scout views in a 2-on-1 format using widely spaced reference lines on one image and all reference lines on the other (Fig. 13–15).

All studies are filmed using bone and soft tissue windows. This technique permits evaluation for not only the fracture but also any disc herniation (Fig. 13–16); different window settings should be used in obtaining digital images as well. In addition, reconstruction in sagittal or coronal planes is performed for an additional imaging perspective on the area of injury; on occasion, three-dimensional (3-D) reformatting is also performed. An intravenous contrast agent is not given, although the patient may have already received such an agent for an associated body scan.

Unlike in the cervical region, in which CT is being used more and more as a screening study (see Chapter 12), in the thoracic and lumbar regions CT is used to delineate the extent of injury. It is the best method for determining the presence and degree of vertebral canal compromise (Fig. 13–17) and pedicle and laminar injuries (Fig. 13–18), as well as the integrity of facet joints (Fig. 13–19).[35, 36, 81, 136, 155] The ability to quickly perform multiplanar or 3-D reconstruction also aids in diagnosing

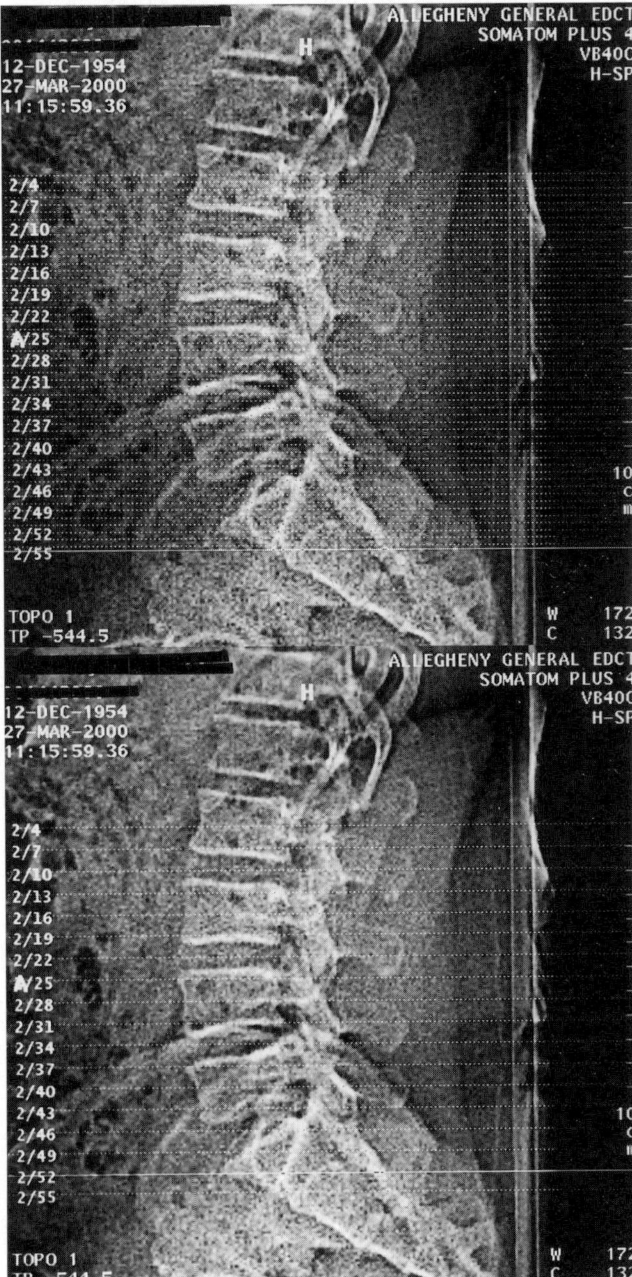

Figure 13–15. Dual scout views. The *upper* image shows the exact level of each image; the *lower* image is for overall orientation.

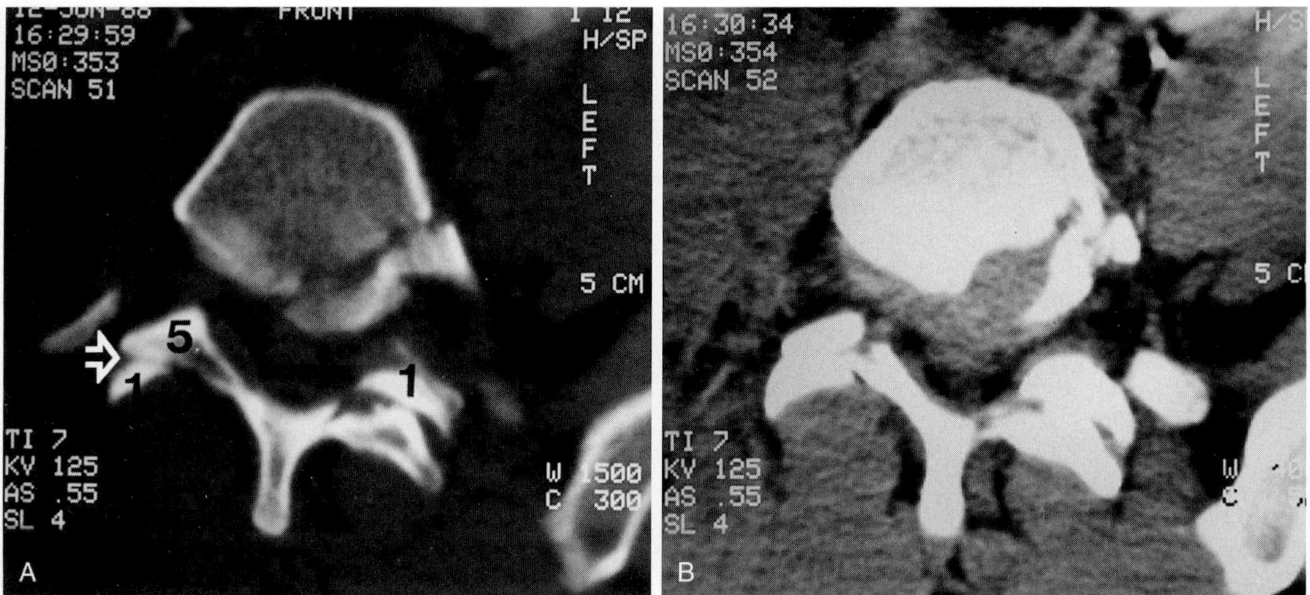

Figure 13–16. Fracture of L5 with disc herniation and unilateral facet lock of L5 on S1 on the right. *A*, CT image obtained at bone window setting shows the unilateral locked facets on the right *(arrow)*. In addition, there is a fracture of the posterior body of L5. *B*, Same image obtained at soft tissue window setting shows a herniated intervertebral disc, which was responsible for the patient's neurologic abnormalities. (From Daffner, R.H. [1989]. Dislocation at L-5–S-1 with unilateral facet lock. Skeletal Radiol., *18*:489. Copyright: © 1989 Springer-Verlag.)

the injuries. Rapid 3-D imaging is particularly useful in evaluation of a severely comminuted and disrupted fracture because it allows determination of the spatial relationships of the bone fragments that will be encountered at the time of surgery.

CT may be combined with myelography whenever MRI is not feasible. The addition of a water-soluble contrast agent to the subarachnoid space will allow demonstration of the status of the spinal cord, conus medullaris, and nerve roots and the integrity of the meninges (Fig. 13–20). In most centers, however, MRI is the procedure of choice when the integrity of the spinal cord is questionable or when blockage of flow of cerebrospinal fluid is suspected.

Pitfalls in CT examination include partial volume-averaging effect and fractures within the plane of the scan. Partial volume averaging occurs when structures from contiguous levels are projected into the main field, producing lucent lines that may be misinterpreted as fractures. This phenomenon most often occurs because of facet joints or adjacent spinous processes and is more commonly encountered in the cervical region. Angular deformities of the spine (scoliosis or kyphosis) may produce an axial CT image that suggests a fracture of the vertebral body. Acute angulation places the end plates of adjacent vertebral bodies and the intervening intervertebral disc on the same axial plane. Scoliosis usually creates a pseudofracture in the sagittal plane of the vertebral body, whereas kyphosis usually creates a pseudofracture in the coronal plane. The pseudofractures lack associated soft tissue swelling and have poorly defined, irregular borders that are widely separated by disc material. The characteristic appearance and correlation with radiographs or digital images should allow ready distinction between such findings and true fractures.

Horizontal fractures that are oriented in the plane of the scan, such as the Chance-type injury, may not always be demonstrated by CT. However, helical CT has been useful in overcoming this diagnostic problem because of overlapping imaging of contiguous segments. Furthermore, these injuries are more likely to be demonstrated on sagittal and coronal reconstructions (Fig. 13–21). Once again, correlation with radiographs is of paramount importance in the diagnosis.

CT should be performed in any patient suspected of having anything more than a simple wedge compression fracture. In older patients with a history of minimal trauma, CT may aid in distinguishing between an osteoporotic compression fracture and a pathologic fracture by demonstrating areas of cortical destruction and a surrounding soft tissue mass in pathologic fractures. However, MRI is better suited for this purpose. In more severe trauma, CT demonstrates the status of the middle and posterior spinal columns, which in great measure determines the stability or instability of the injury; this aspect of spinal trauma is discussed in detail later in the chapter. CT readily distinguishes between simple wedge compression and burst fractures by clearly defining the status of the posterior wall of the vertebral body and precisely localizing fracture fragments in relation to the vertebral canal (see Fig. 13–17).[*]

Magnetic Resonance Imaging

Although radiography and CT scanning are the first-line imaging studies for diagnosing acute vertebral injuries, they are unable to demonstrate changes within or injury to the spinal cord. MRI, however, fills the void by its ability not only to image the spinal cord but also to

*See references 30, 35, 36, 39, 81, 136, 155, 159, 163, 164.

Text continued on page 471

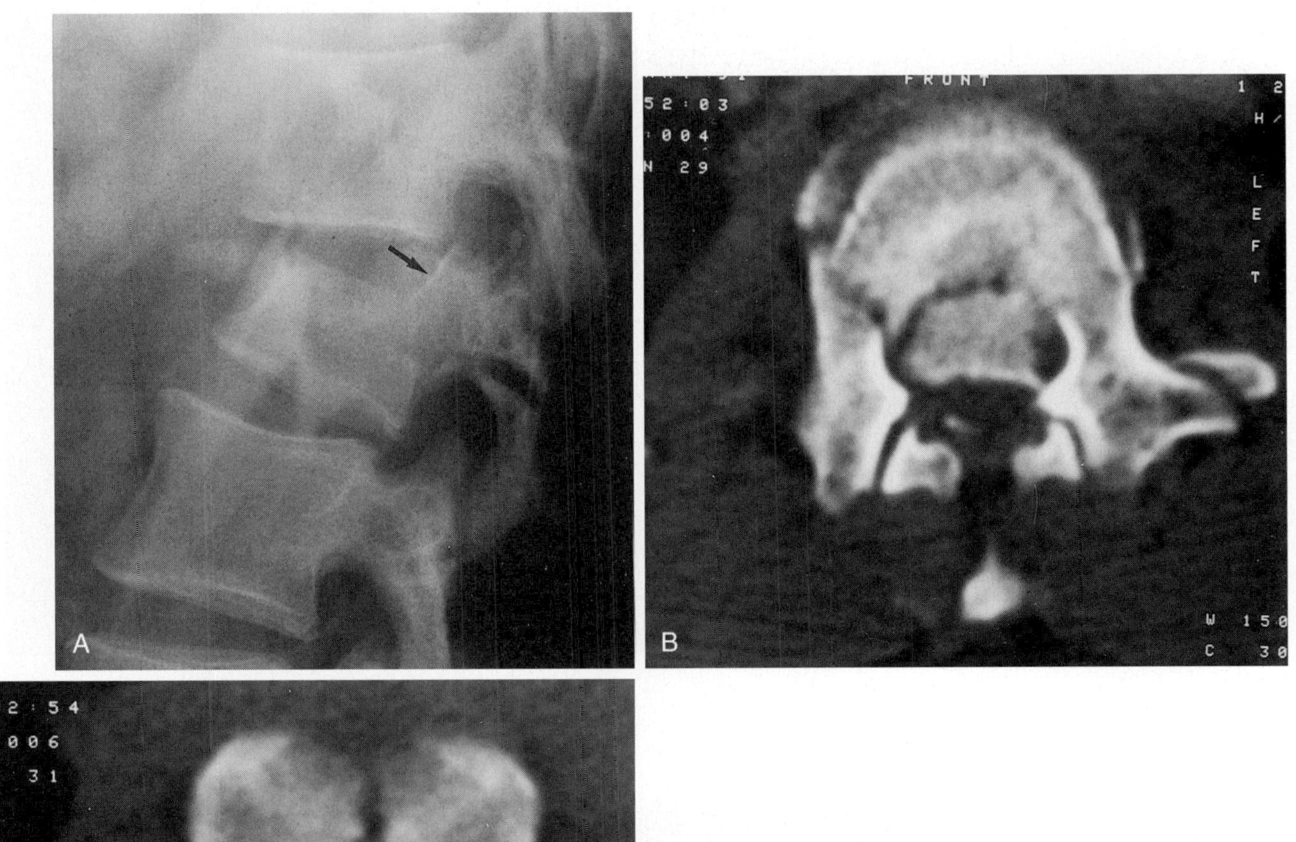

Figure 13–17. Burst fracture of L1 with canal compromise. *A*, Lateral radiograph shows a burst fracture of L1 with rotation of a fragment from the posterior vertebral body line *(arrow)*. *B*, CT image obtained through the upper portion of L1 shows the large fragment displaced into the vertebral canal. *C*, CT image obtained at a slightly lower level shows sagittal fractures through the vertebral body and lamina of L1. Note the pedicle fracture on the right.

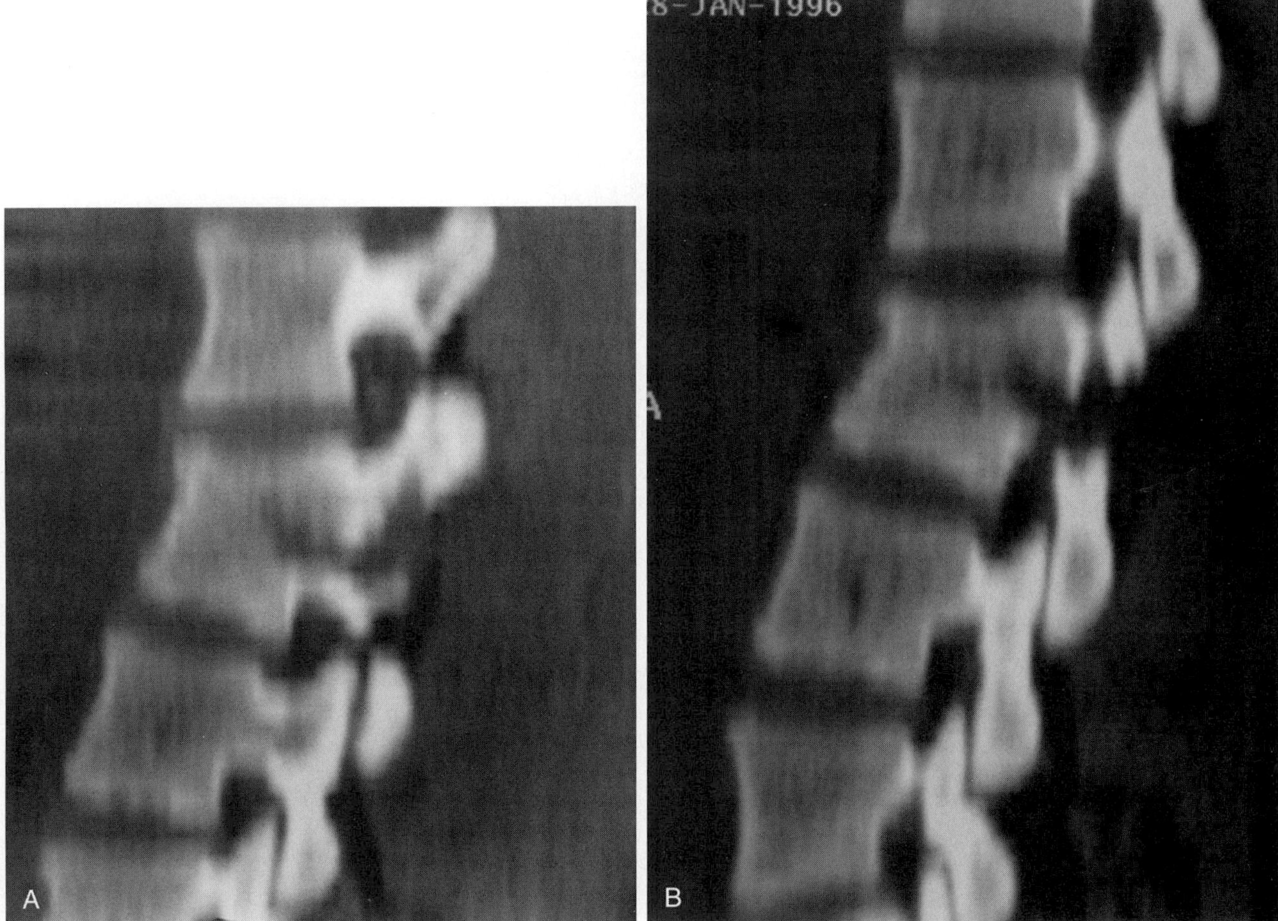

Figure 13–18. Utility of CT for visualizing pedicle fractures. *A* and *B*, Sagittal tomographic reconstructions show bilateral pedicle fractures in a patient with a Smith fracture of L2.

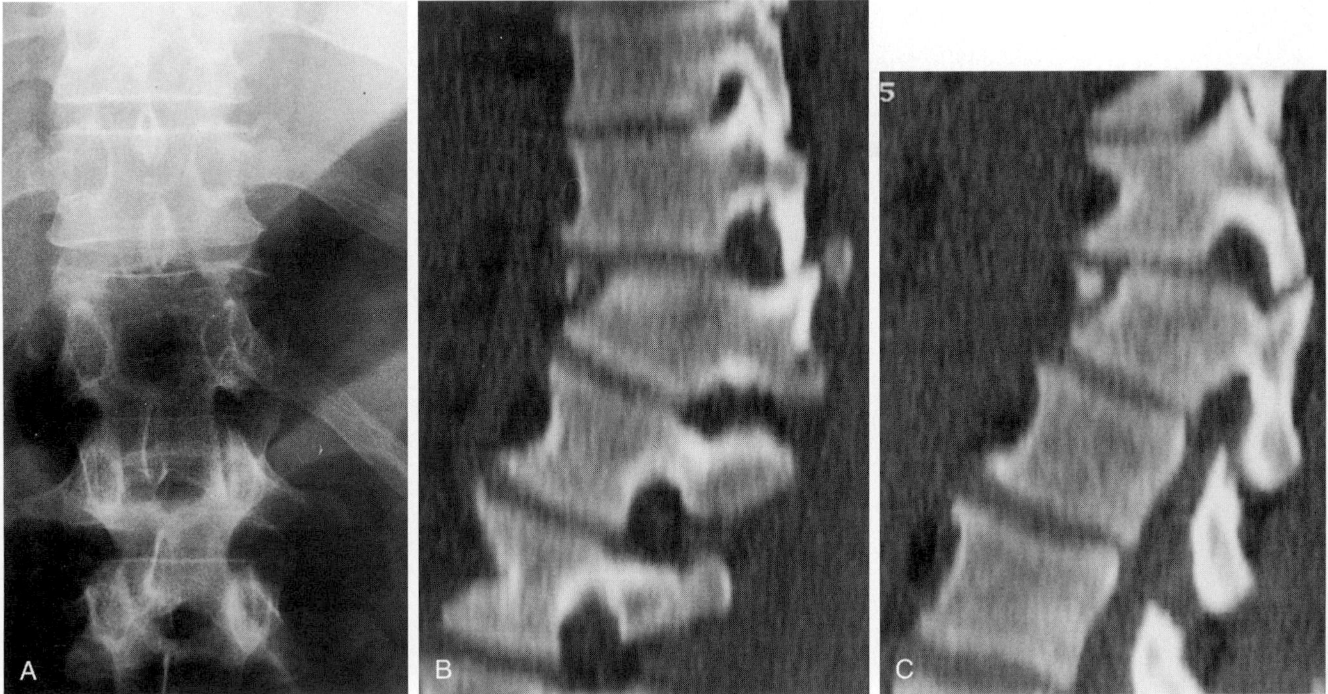

Figure 13–19. T11–T12 dislocation with facet lock. *A*, Anteroposterior radiograph shows widening of the interspinous space between T11 and T12. Note the naked facets. *B* and *C*, Sagittal tomographic reconstructions show bilateral facet lock.

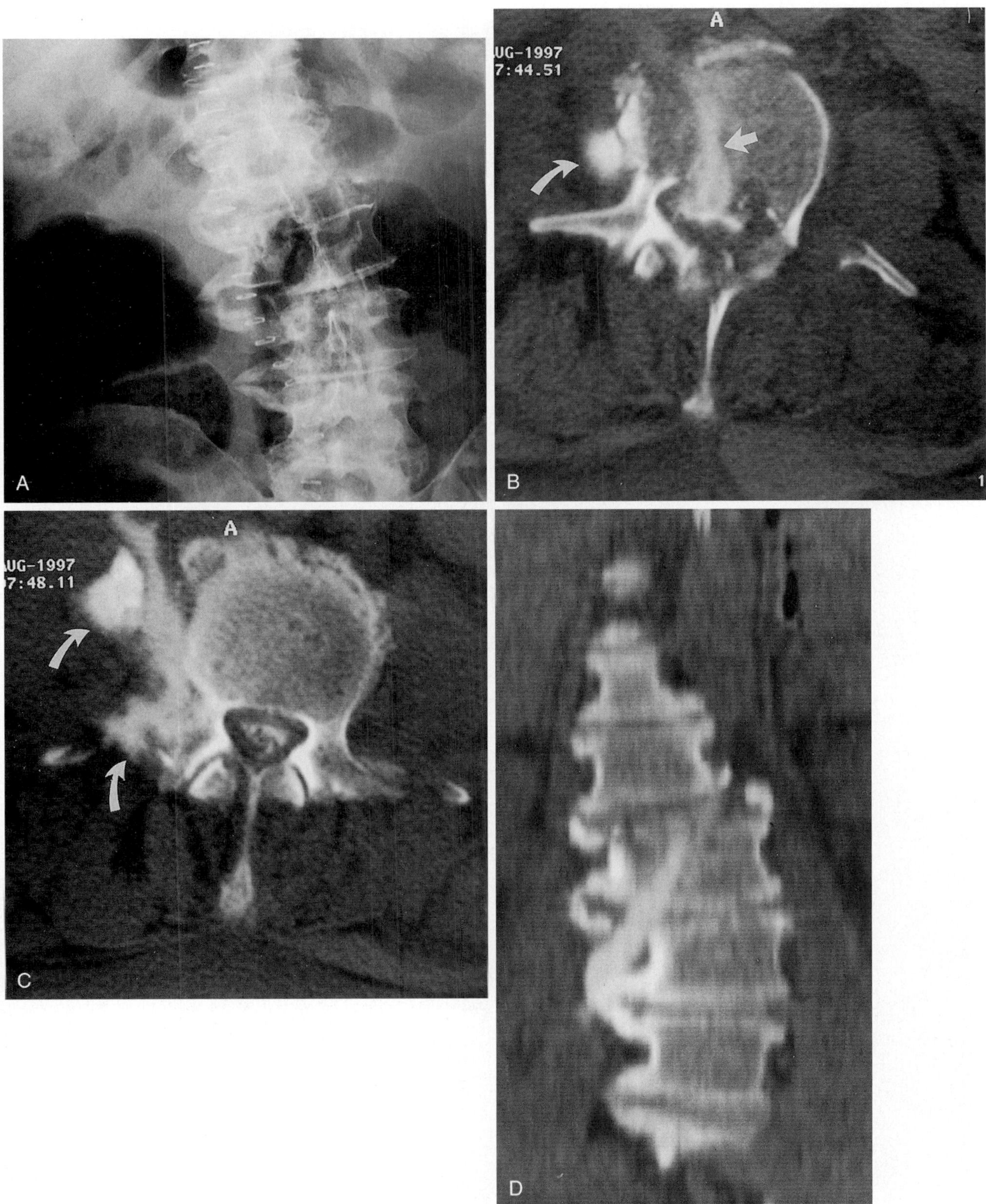

Figure 13–20. L1–L2 fracture dislocation with torn thecal sac. *A*, Anteroposterior radiograph shows a "windswept" appearance to the spine, with laterolisthesis of L1 on L2 on the right. The right side of the body of L2 is fractured. *B*, Image from a CT myelogram shows contrast extravasating through the fracture of the body of L2 *(straight arrow)* as well as contrast in the paraspinal soft tissues *(curved arrow)*. *C* Image from the CT obtained at a slightly lower level shows gross extravasation of contrast material into the paraspinal soft tissues *(curved arrows)*. A, Anterior. *D*, CT reconstruction shows the extent of injury, with the contrast extravasating through the fracture into the paraspinous soft tissues on the right side.

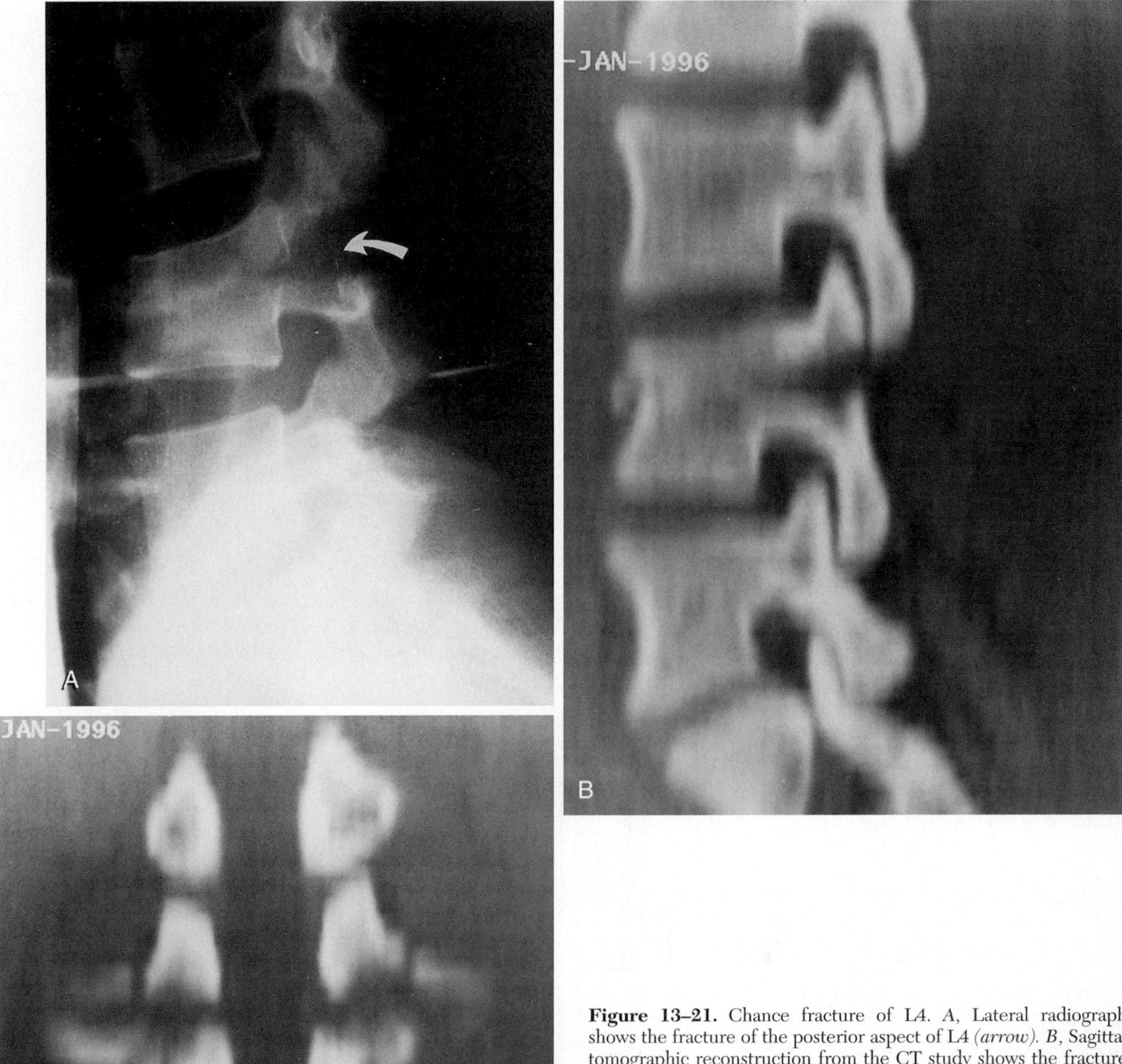

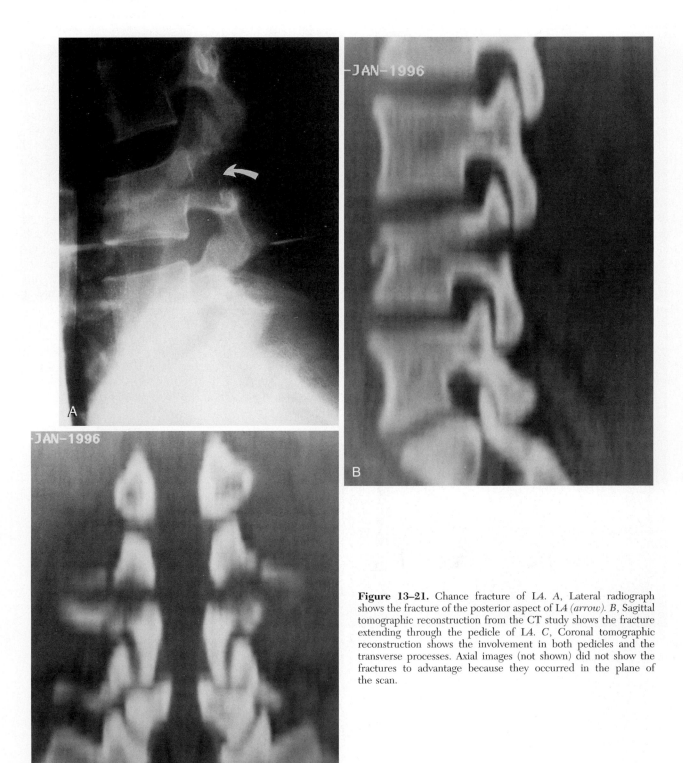

Figure 13–21. Chance fracture of L4. *A*, Lateral radiograph shows the fracture of the posterior aspect of L4 *(arrow)*. *B*, Sagittal tomographic reconstruction from the CT study shows the fracture extending through the pedicle of L4. *C*, Coronal tomographic reconstruction shows the involvement in both pedicles and the transverse processes. Axial images (not shown) did not show the fractures to advantage because they occurred in the plane of the scan.

define its internal anatomy. In addition, this modality has the capability of imaging supine patients directly in sagittal, coronal, or, as occasionally required, oblique planes, as well as in the traditional axial plane. Thus, MRI is useful for demonstrating areas of direct spinal cord injury (Figs. 13–22 and 13–23), epidural hematomas (Figs. 13–24 and 13–25), and herniation of intervertebral discs (Fig. 13–26), as well as alignment abnormalities (Fig. 13–27).[28, 35, 36, 62, 74, 120, 154] MRI is also useful for definitively differentiating osteoporotic collapse from that due to a pathologic fracture.[6] The typical osteoporotic compression fracture is of low signal intensity on T_1-weighted images, with orientation of signal changes in a *linear* fashion along the lines of collapse (Fig. 13–28*A* and *B*). Pathologic fractures, on the other hand, demonstrate *rounded* areas of low signal intensity on T_1-weighted images (see Fig. 13–28*C*).

In dealing with acutely traumatized patients, time is of the essence. At Allegheny General Hospital, we have therefore tailored the MRI examination to four sequences designed to optimally demonstrate all aspects of the injury in as short a time period as possible: (1) a T_1-weighted sagittal spin-echo sequence, (2) a sagittal turbo (T2*) spin echo sequence, (3) an axial T_1-weighted sequence, and (4) an axial gradient echo sequence. Because there is a low risk of vascular injury in the thoracic or lumbar region, we do not perform MR angiography unless there is a suspected aortic injury. If only one set of images can be obtained for a patient, the long spin echo sequence is preferred because it clearly differentiates the spinal cord from the cerebrospinal fluid.[36, 104] Because of the nature of MRI, its use in the trauma setting demands that the patient be hemodynamically stable. In addition to frequently observing the vital signs of these patients, the electrical leads of all monitoring equipment must be kept off the skin surface to prevent a thermal burn in unconscious or neurologically compromised patients.[36]

MRI surpasses other imaging modalities for evaluating vertebral injuries in several ways. MRI is useful in determining the relationship of bone fragments that may have been displaced into the vertebral canal to impinge upon the spinal cord (Fig. 13–29). It can also show the full extent of the damage in acute spinal injury. In addition to demonstrating transection of the spinal cord (see Fig. 13–22), MRI can now differentiate between spinal cord edema (contusion) (Fig. 13–30) and hemorrhage (see Fig. 13–23).[36, 62, 74, 82, 120] This capability has prognostic significance in that patients with edema may recover full function, whereas those with hemorrhage usually do not.[173] In acute spinal cord injury, the cord is expanded to fill the vertebral canal. The epidural fat is usually obliterated because of hemorrhage or edema. Acute spinal cord hemorrhage typically produces isointense signal on T_1-weighted images and low signal intensity on T_2-weighted images over the first 24 hours. Typically the low signal intensity on the T_2-weighted sequences is surrounded by a high-intensity zone of edema (Fig. 13–31). Between 24 hours and 3 weeks the signal intensity is

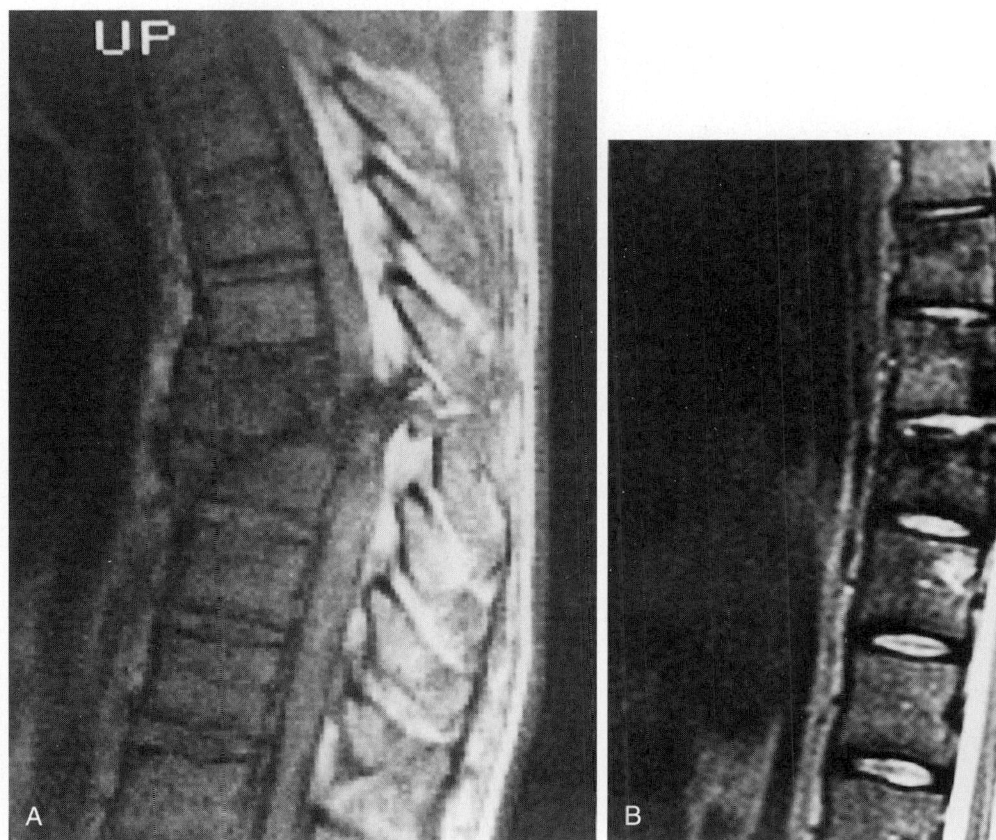

Figure 13–22. Spinal cord transections. *A*, T_1-weighted sagittal image shows complete transection of the spinal cord and its linings as a result of a T9–T10 dislocation. *B*, T_2-weighted sagittal image from another patient shows complete transection of the spinal cord, with retraction of the severed ends to produce a gap *(arrow)*.

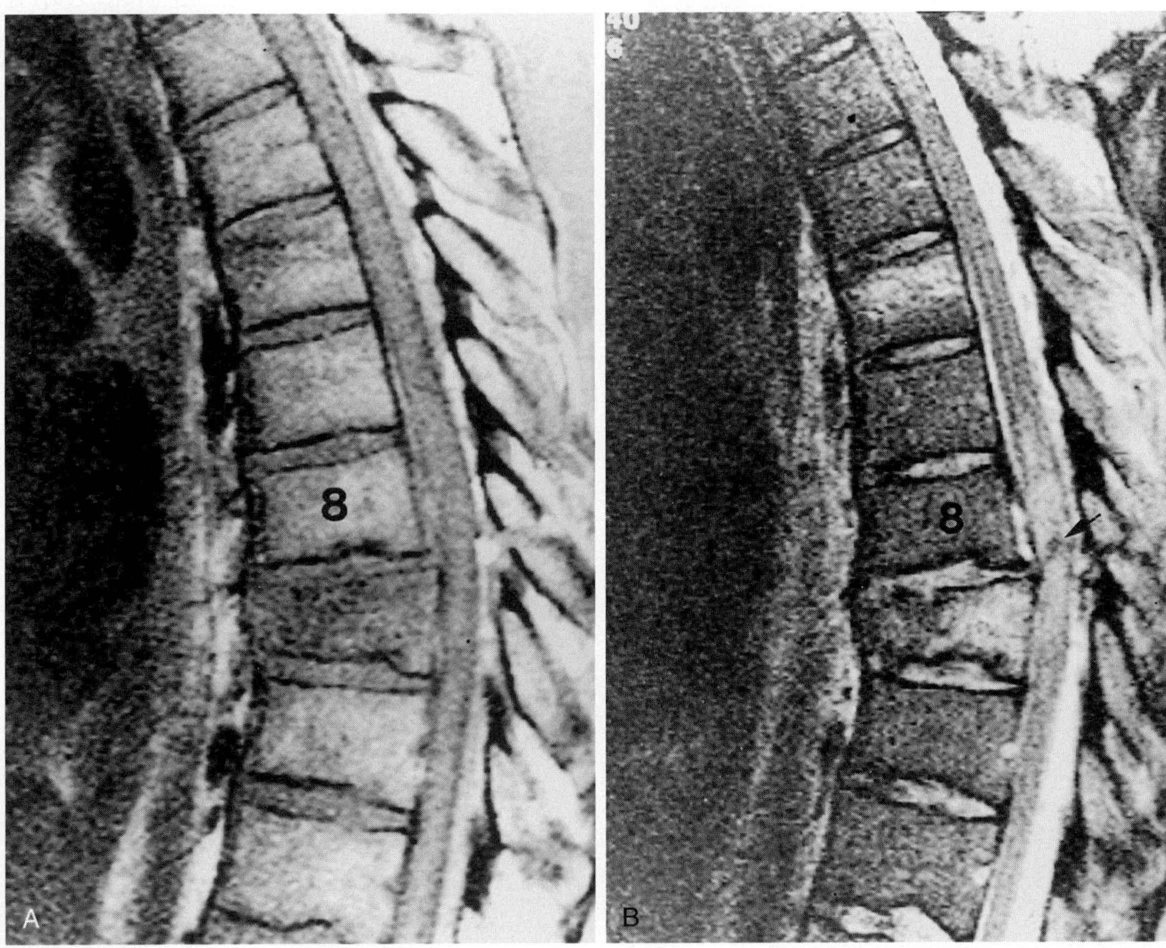

Figure 13–23. Spinal cord hemorrhage in a patient with a T8–T9 injury. *A*, T_1-weighted sagittal image shows low signal intensity in the compressed body of T9. Note the rupture of the posterior longitudinal ligament at the T8 disc space. The spinal cord is swollen and demonstrates isointense signal. *B*, Gradient echo sagittal image shows the low-signal-intensity hematoma in the substance of the spinal cord *(arrow)*, with a surrounding zone of edema. Note the high signal intensity in the bodies of T9 and T6, representing a noncontiguous and unsuspected injury.

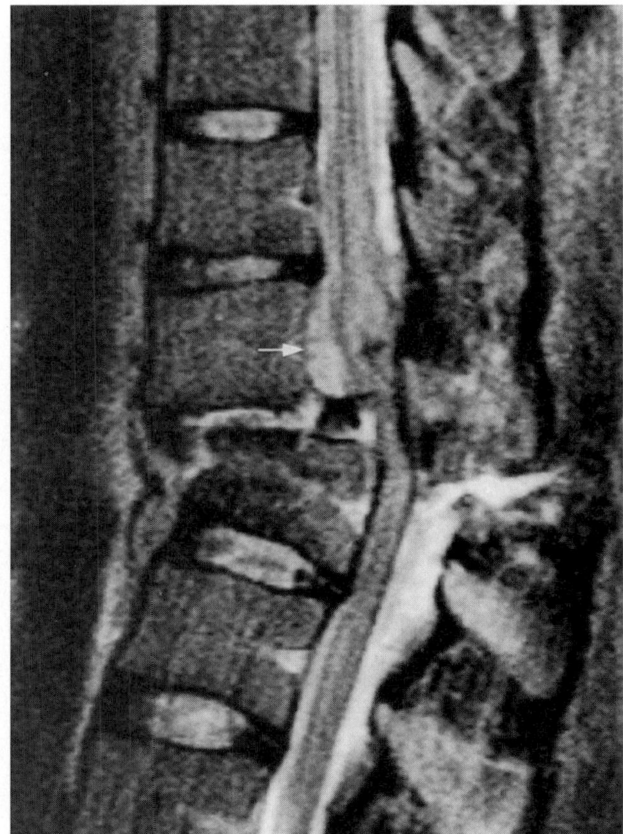

Figure 13–24. Epidural hematoma *(arrow)* in a patient with diffuse idiopathic skeletal hyperostosis (DISH) and a T9–T10 fracture-dislocation. Note the low-signal-intensity cord hemorrhage at T9 on this T_2-weighted image. Also note the high-signal-intensity hematoma in the posterior soft tissues from T10 downward.

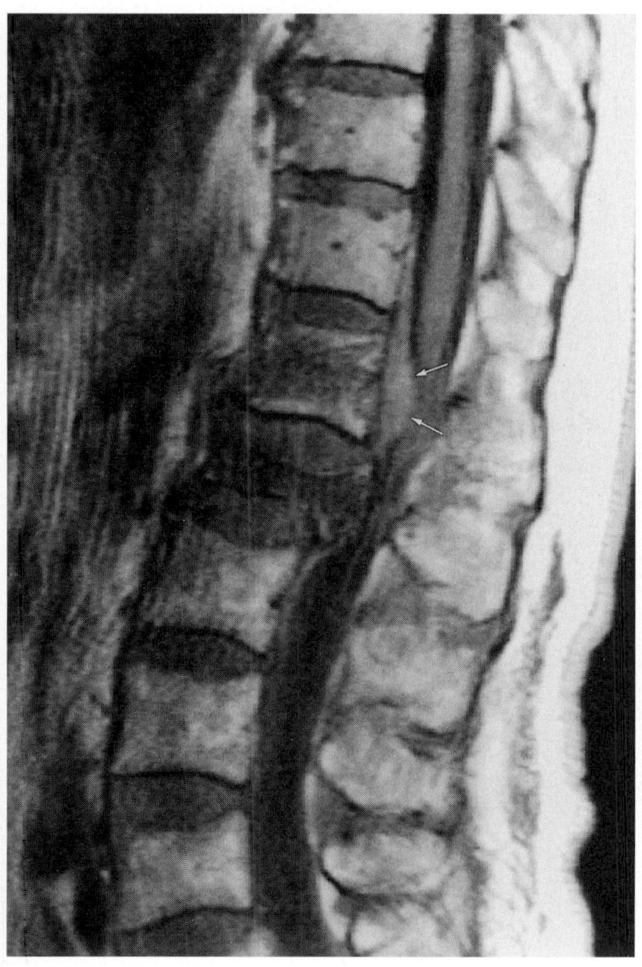

Figure 13–25. Epidural hematoma in a patient with a burst fracture of L1. T_1-weighted image shows the epidural hematoma posterior to T12 compressing the thecal sac *(arrows)*. Note an occult fracture in T12, manifested as low-signal-intensity marrow edema.

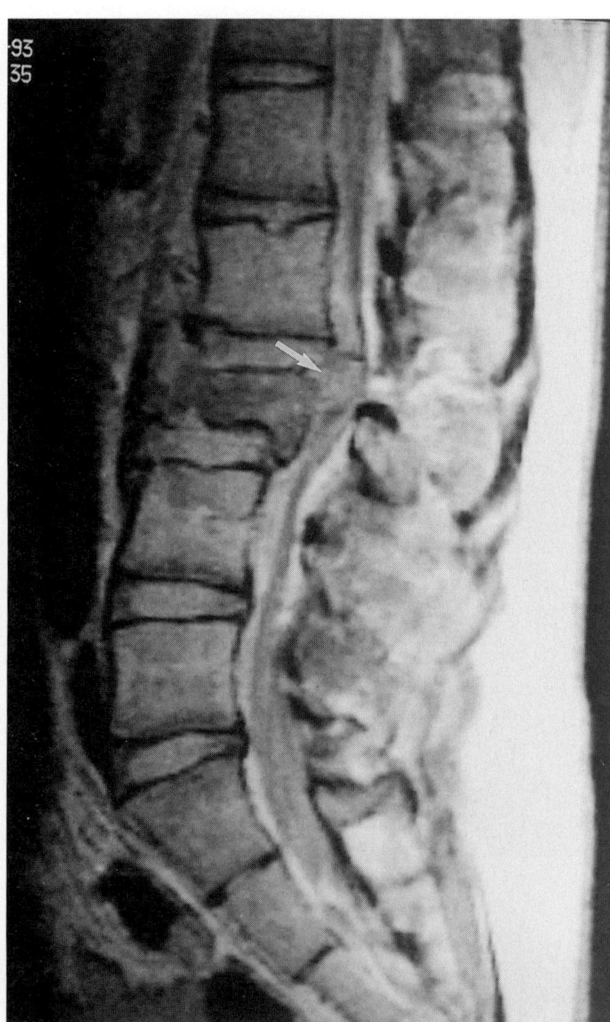

Figure 13–26. Herniation of the L2 intervertebral disc incurred as a result of an L3 fracture. Proton density image shows the herniated disc material *(arrow)* posterior to L3.

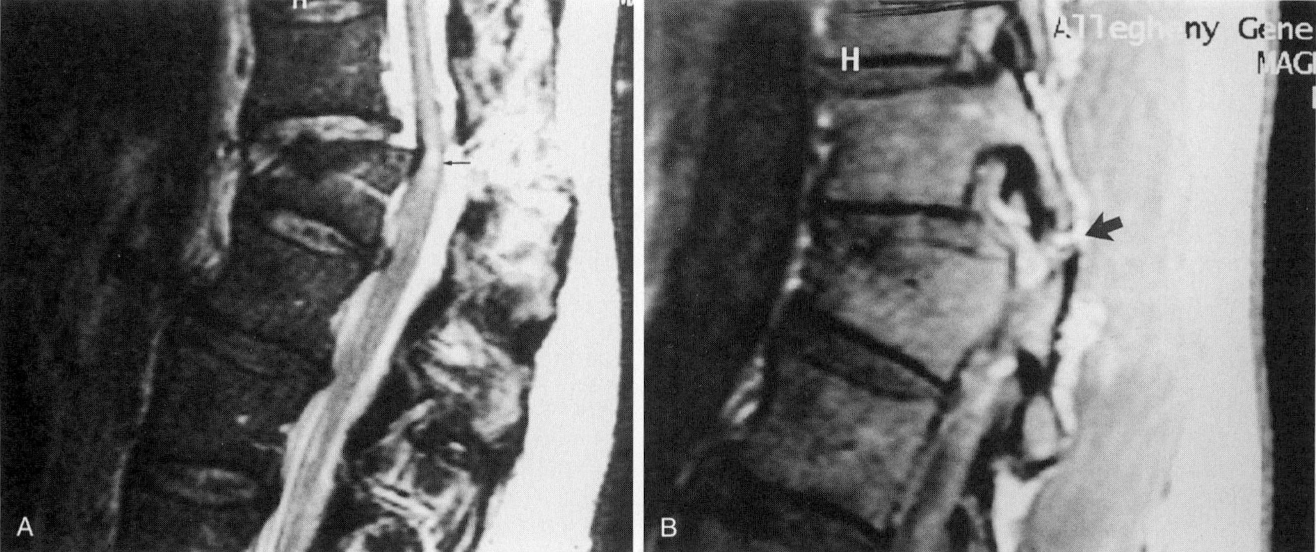

Figure 13–27. Alignment abnormalities from a T10–T11 fracture-dislocation demonstrated by MRI. *A*, T_2-weighted sagittal image shows anterolisthesis of T10 on T11. Note rupture of the posterior longitudinal ligament and cord edema at the level of injury *(arrow)*. *B*, Paraspinal sagittal T_1-weighted section shows perched facets *(arrow)*. The contralateral side (not shown) looked similar.

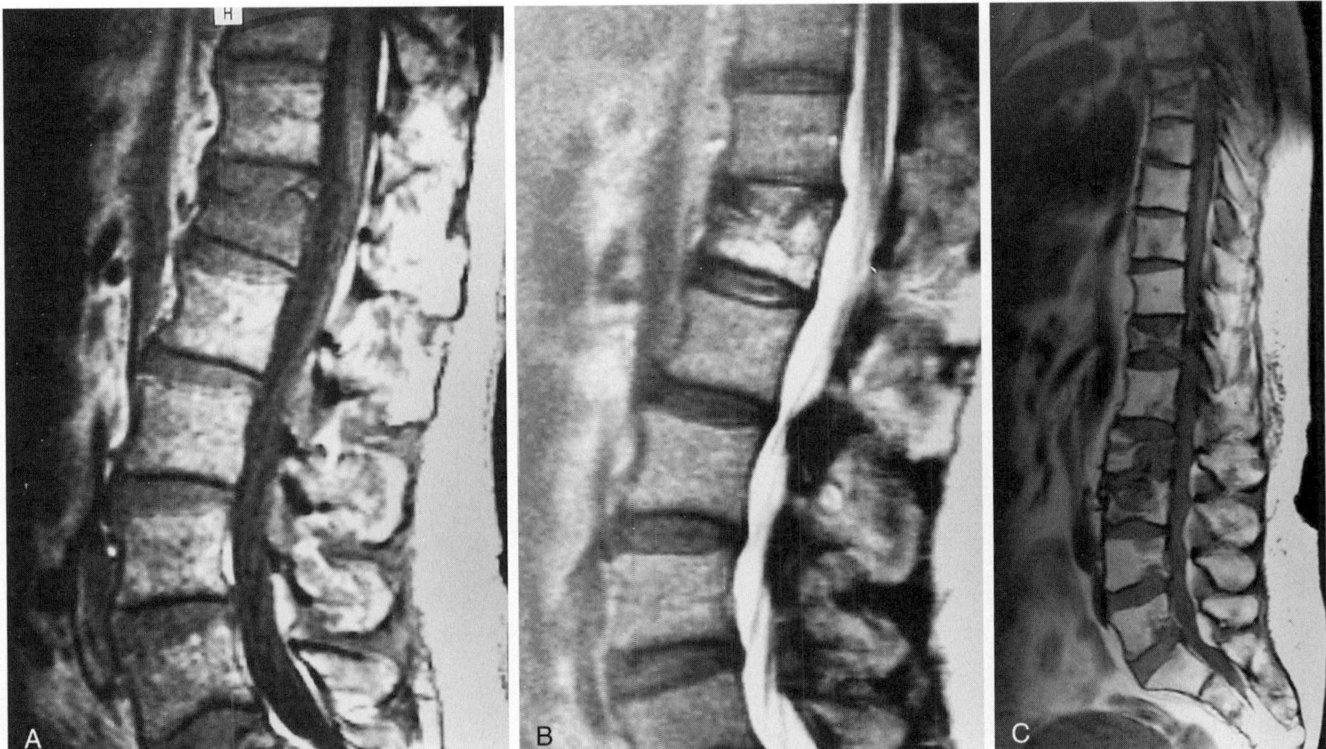

Figure 13–28. Differentiation of osteoporotic compression fracture from pathologic compression fracture by magnetic resonance imaging. *A*, T_1-weighted sagittal image in an osteoporotic patient shows compression of L1. Note the low signal intensity in the body. *B*, T_2-weighted sagittal image from the same patient shows increased signal at the same level. In both of these images, the signal changes are *linear*. *C*, Sagittal T_1-weighted image from a patient with diffuse metastatic disease and multiple compression fractures shows multiple compressed vertebrae of low signal intensity. The pattern is more *globular*. Compare with *A*.

increased on both T_1-weighted and T_2-weighted sequences. After 3 weeks there is low signal intensity in the cord on T_1-weighted images and high signal intensity on T_2-weighted sequences. Spinal cord edema behaves like edema elsewhere in the body, with low signal intensity on T_1-weighted images and high signal intensity on T_2-weighted images (see Fig. 13–30).

MRI is also useful for identifying extradural compressive lesions such as intervertebral disc herniation (see Fig. 13–26) and epidural hematoma (see Figs. 13–24 and 13–25). The sagittal imaging capability of MRI is especially useful for delineating abnormalities at the cervicothoracic junction.[75] This area is particularly difficult to evaluate radiographically, and sometimes to a lesser extent by CT, because of the overlap of the patient's shoulders. MRI is also useful for identifying the integrity of the vertebral ligaments (Fig. 13–32). This distinction is paramount in determining the stability of the spine[19] (see later on). Finally, MRI is the procedure of choice for identifying areas of post-traumatic syringomyelia or myelomalacia in the follow-up evaluation of patients with vertebral trauma[54] (Fig. 13–33). The signal changes produced by these abnormalities are identical to those produced by edema.

Classification: Mechanisms of Injury and Characteristic Radiographic Features

The injuries depicted in this book are illustrative of the principle that fractures and dislocations produced by a specific mechanism result in distinctive radiographic findings. These findings are characteristic of the mechanism of injury and are termed "fingerprints," because the radiographic changes are similar in appearance no matter where the location. In the vertebral column, therefore, the findings due to a particular mechanism will be identical whether the injury is in the cervical, thoracic, or lumbar region. There are four basic mechanisms of injury based upon the major force vectors: flexion, rotation, shear, and extension.[35, 36, 41, 52, 162, 191] In each of the first three mechanisms, some degree of flexion and axial loading are common denominators. The importance of recognizing these radiographic fingerprints lies in the ability to define the extent of the injury—a factor of importance in treatment.

Flexion injuries are the most common type encountered throughout the entire vertebral column.[35, 36, 40, 41, 52, 162] These injuries occur when compressive forces are applied anteriorly and are combined to a greater or lesser degree with posterior distractive forces (Fig. 13–34). In the thoracic and lumbar regions, vertebral injury results most commonly when unrestrained front seat occupants of motor vehicles involved in crashes forcibly flex on the steering wheel or dashboard, or are ejected from the vehicle. Most injuries incurred by this mechanism occur between T10 and L2. Motorcyclists who are ejected over the handlebars after striking a solid object are more prone to suffer thoracic injuries between T2 and T8[35, 36, 40] (Fig. 13–35). Rear seat occupants of motor vehicles wearing lap-type seat belts only may suffer a severe distractive flexion injury in the thoracolumbar region (see Fig. 13–21).[29, 35, 36, 164, 176] In this

Text continued on page 480

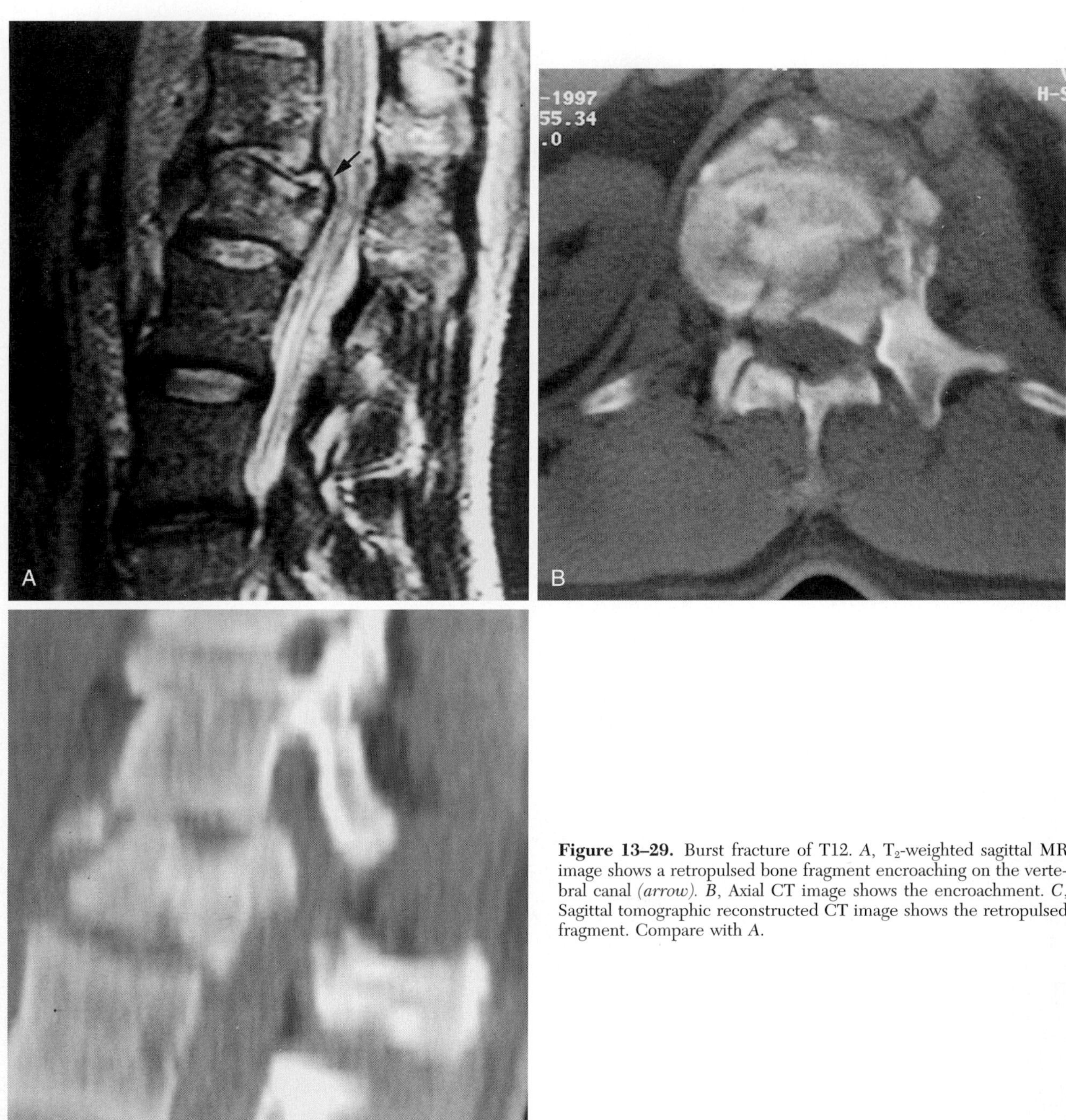

Figure 13–29. Burst fracture of T12. *A*, T_2-weighted sagittal MR image shows a retropulsed bone fragment encroaching on the vertebral canal *(arrow)*. *B*, Axial CT image shows the encroachment. *C*, Sagittal tomographic reconstructed CT image shows the retropulsed fragment. Compare with *A*.

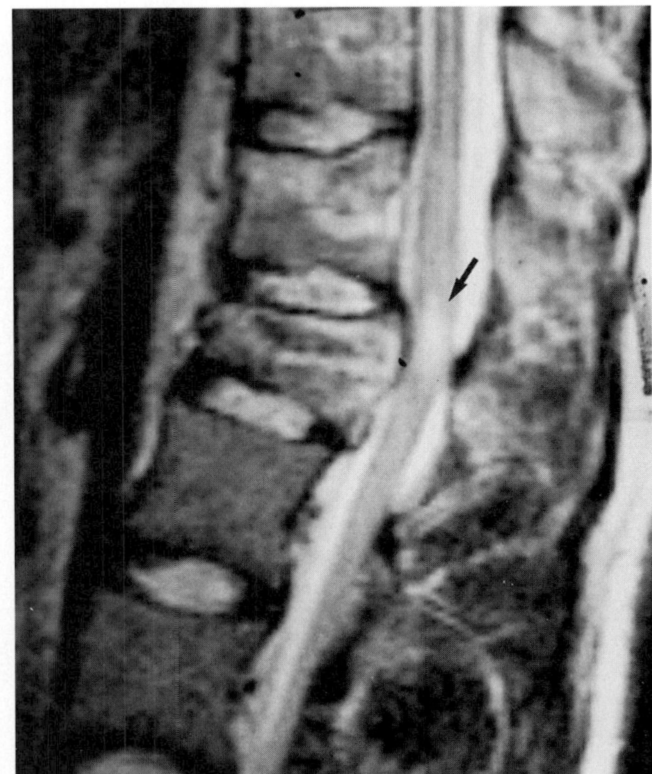

Figure 13–30. Spinal cord contusion. Sagittal T_2-weighted image shows increased signal intensity representing cord edema *(arrow)* at the level of the T12 burst fracture. On the T_1-weighted images (not shown), the abnormal area was of diminished signal intensity.

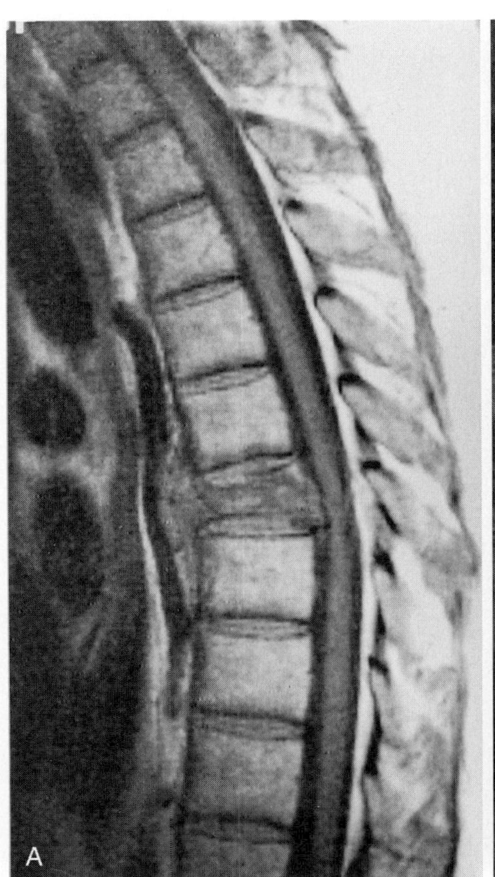

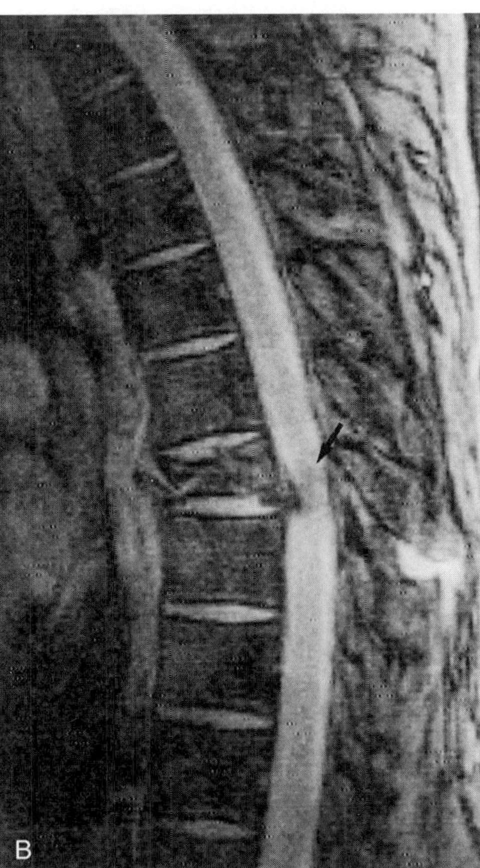

Figure 13–31. Spinal cord hemorrhage due to burst fracture of T8. *A*, T_1-weighted sagittal image shows bone fragments retropulsed into the vertebral canal. The spinal cord is of isointense signal. *B*, T_2-weighted sagittal image shows an area of low signal intensity within the spinal cord representing hemorrhage *(arrow)*. Compare with Figure 13–30.

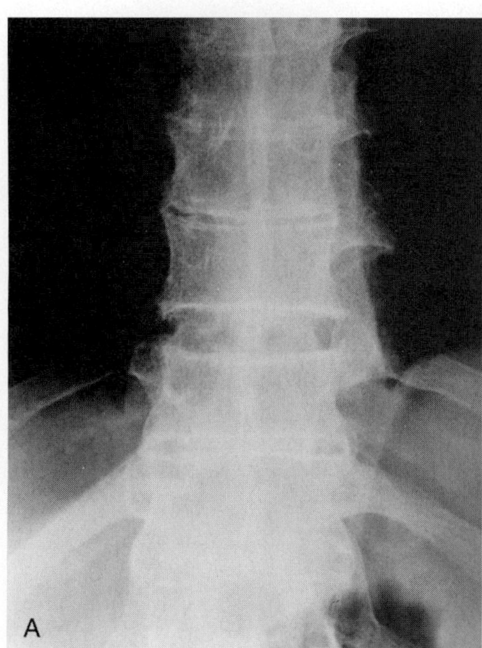

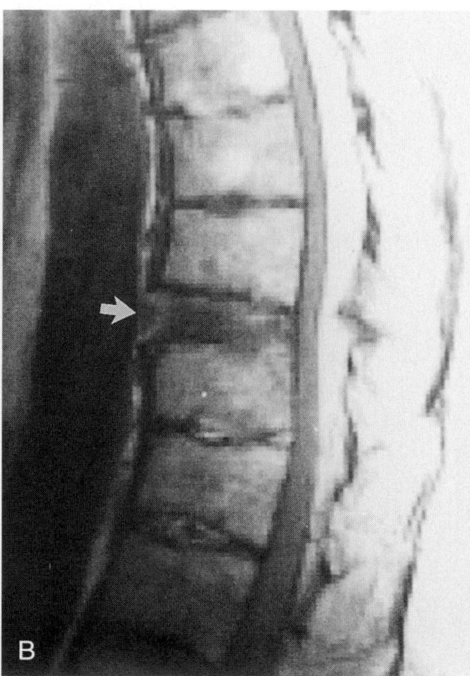

Figure 13–32. Extension injury at T9–T10 disc space. *A*, Anteroposterior radiograph shows widening of the T9 disc space. *B*, Sagittal T_1-weighted magnetic resonance image shows the ruptured anterior longitudinal ligament *(arrow)* and the wide disc space, with low signal intensity representing hemorrhage at the disc.

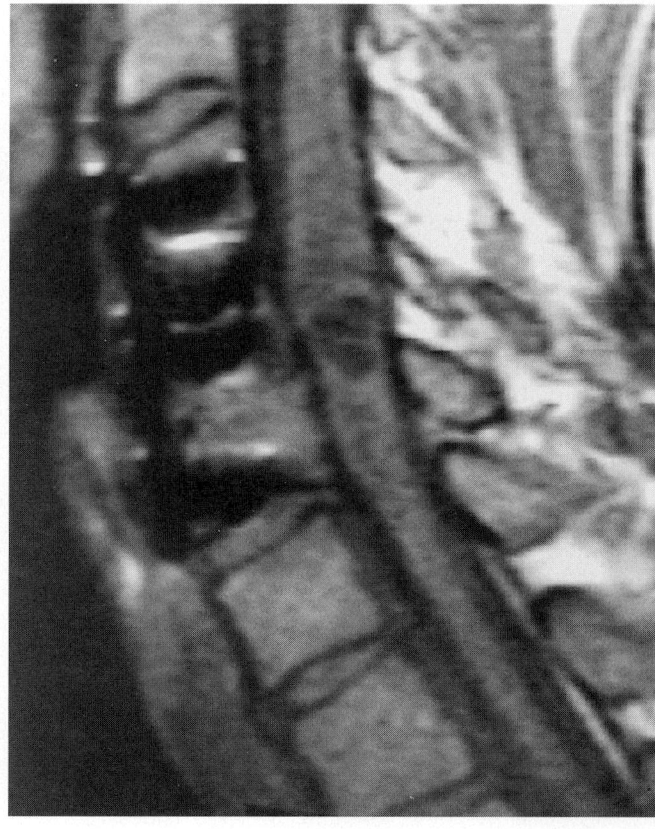

Figure 13–33. Syringomyelia. Sagittal T_1-weighted magnetic resonance image of the cervical region shows the characteristic areas of low signal intensity within a swollen spinal cord. The artifacts over the vertebrae are from a surgical plate and screws. Thoracic syringomyelia is unusual.

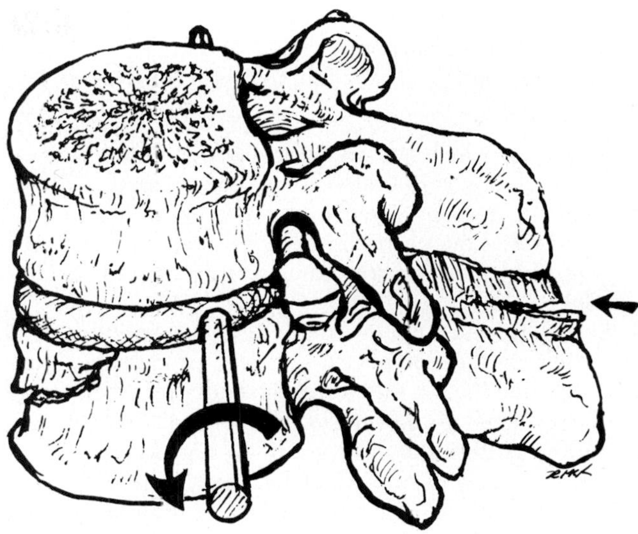

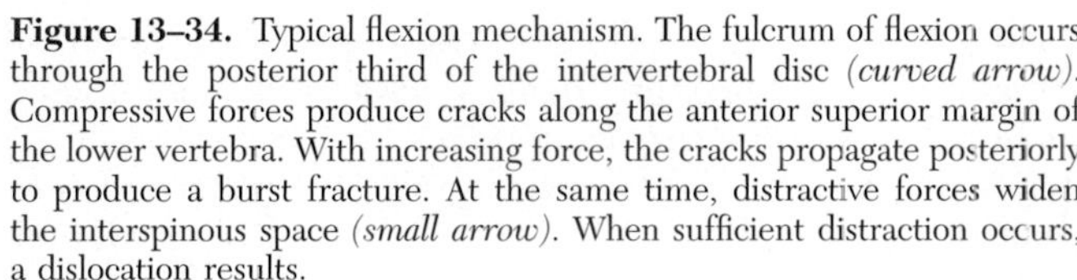

Figure 13–34. Typical flexion mechanism. The fulcrum of flexion occurs through the posterior third of the intervertebral disc *(curved arrow)*. Compressive forces produce cracks along the anterior superior margin of the lower vertebra. With increasing force, the cracks propagate posteriorly to produce a burst fracture. At the same time, distractive forces widen the interspinous space *(small arrow)*. When sufficient distraction occurs, a dislocation results.

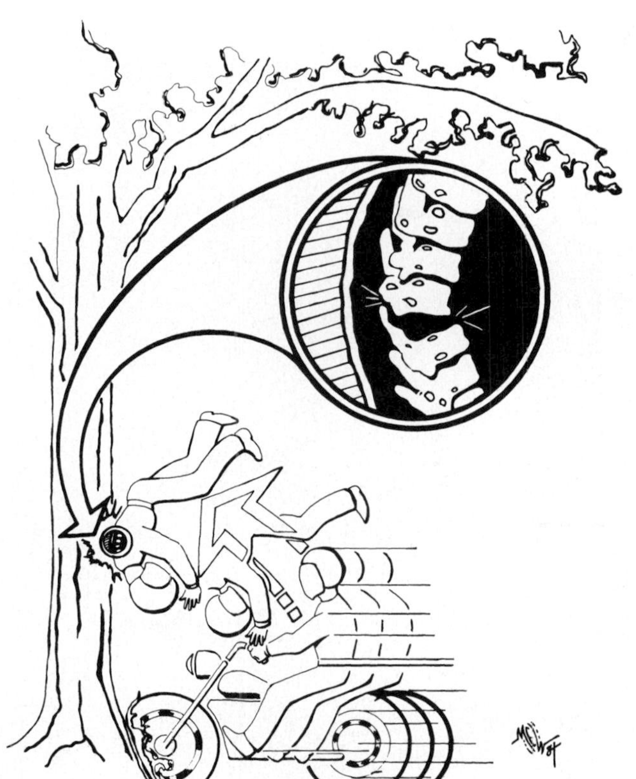

Figure 13–35. Mechanism of flexion injury in a motorcycle accident. This mechanism typically produces flexion injuries from T2 to T8. (From Daffner, R. H., Deeb, Z. L., & Rothfus, W. E. [1987]. Thoracic fractures and dislocations in motorcyclists. Skeletal Radiol., *16*:280. Copyright © 1987 Springer-Verlag.)

type of injury, the seat belt is responsible for shifting the fulcrum of flexion from the posterior third of the intervertebral disc to the abdominal wall. Identical injuries may be encountered in skiers who have struck their midsection on a fence or other solid object. These injuries are discussed in detail later on.

Radiographically, flexion injuries may be divided into four subtypes:

Simple, in which the anterior superior or inferior aspect of the vertebral body is compressed, with or without disc space narrowing above the level of injury, while the posterior vertebral body line and posterior ligamentous structures remain intact (Fig. 13–36)

Burst, in which the vertebra literally explodes as a result of the compressive forces, producing severe comminution of the vertebral body, retropulsion of bone fragments into the vertebral canal, and cleavage of the posterior arch (Figs. 13–37 and 13–38)

Distraction, with or without fracture, in which there is widening of the interspinous (interlaminar) and interfacet distances without dislocation (Fig. 13–39). A variant of this injury is the Chance-type injury, in which there are accompanying horizontal fractures (Fig. 13–40)

Dislocation, in which there is complete loss of continuity of the articular surfaces (Fig. 13–41)

The radiographic fingerprints of flexion injuries, therefore, are (1) compression, fragmentation, and burst of vertebral bodies; (2) wide interspinous or interlaminar space; (3) wide facet joints; (4) anterolisthesis; (5) disruption of the posterior vertebral body line; (6) naked facets; and (7) narrowing of the disc space *above* the level of injury. These findings are identical with those from similar mechanisms in the cervical region.

Rotary or *grinding injuries* result from rotary or torsional forces applied about the long axis of the vertebral column. In nearly every instance there is an associated flexion vector. These injuries are the most disruptive of all vertebral injuries and tend to occur almost exclusively at the thoracolumbar junction, owing to the restrictions the facet alignment places on any degree of rotary motion.[36, 191] Disruption occurs not only in the vertebral body but also in the posterior elements and the ligaments.

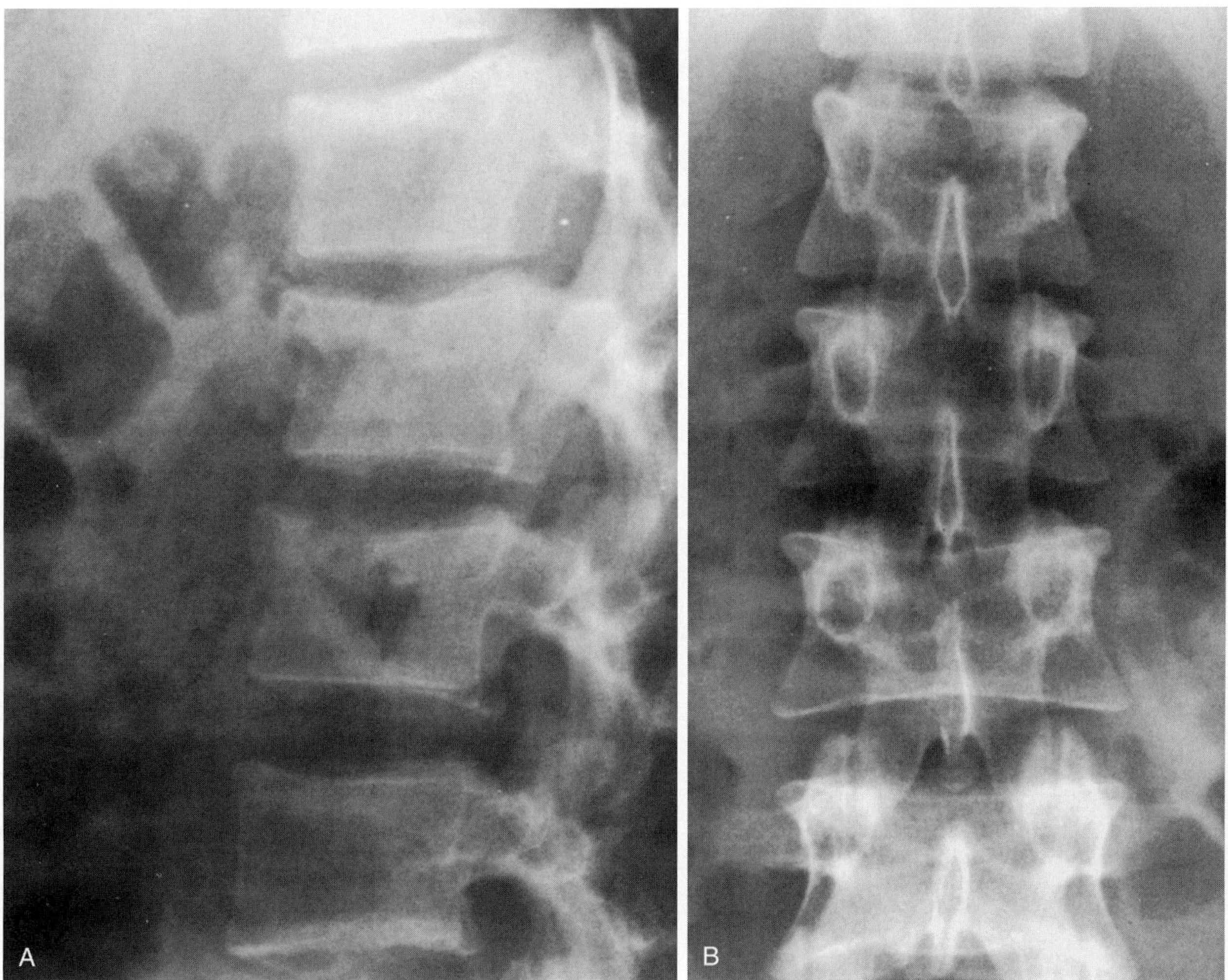

Figure 13–36. Simple compression fractures of L1 to L3. *A,* Lateral view demonstrates compression deformities of the superior end plates of L1 to L3. Note the characteristic beak at the anterior superior margin of each of the involved vertebrae. *B,* Anteroposterior view demonstrates poorly defined superior end plates of L1 and L2 and a mild compression deformity of the superior end plate of L3.

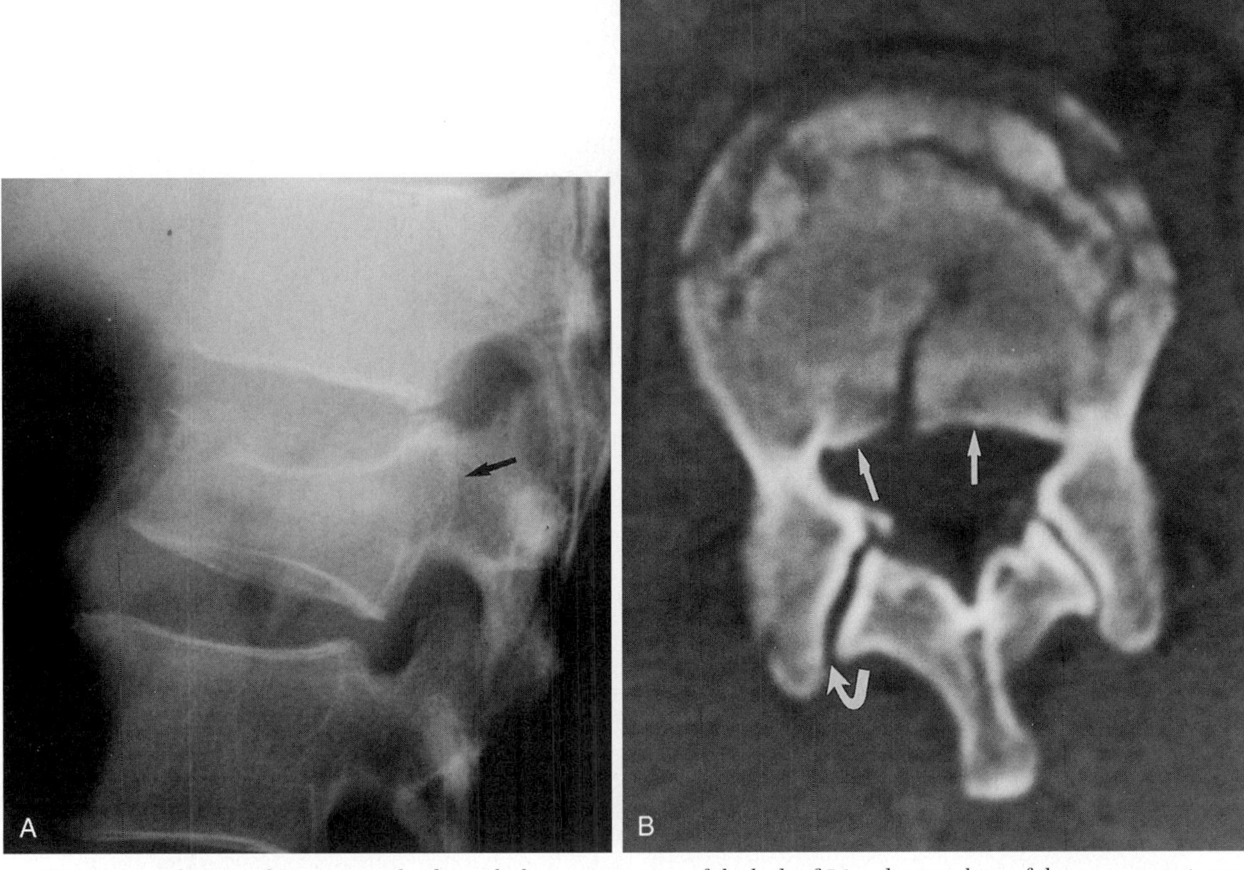

Figure 13–37. Burst fracture of L1. *A*, Lateral radiograph shows compression of the body of L1 and retropulsion of the upper posterior vertebral body line *(arrow)*. *B*, CT image demonstrates comminution of the retropulsed fragments *(straight arrows)* and widening of the facet joint on the right *(curved arrow)*.

In the process, the vertebral body is literally pulverized—hence the epithet "grinding injury." Not surprisingly, patients with these injuries have a high incidence of neurologic deficit. Rotary injuries are the result of a heavy blow to the upper torso that compresses the vertebrae and flexes and twists the torso laterally. In my practice, these injuries occur most commonly as the result of ejection of the victim from a motor vehicle (Fig. 13–42).

The radiographic fingerprints of a rotary or grinding injury are (1) severe distortion of vertebral anatomy with a "ripped can top" appearance of the vertebral body; (2) rotation; (3) dislocation; (4) facet and pillar fractures; (5) transverse process or rib fractures; and (6) a circular array of bone fragments with unilateral widening of the facet joints on the antirotational side on a CT scan. These features can be seen in Figure 13–43. It is important to distinguish this injury from a burst fracture because the treatment is significantly different for each. A key feature for making that differentiation is the linear (horizontal) distribution of bone fragments in a burst fracture, as depicted on both radiographs and CT images, as opposed to the rotary distribution of fragments and facet joint disruption on rotary injuries. In addition, the presence of transverse process or rib fractures indicates that the injury is more severe than a burst fracture. Compare Figures 13–43 and 13–37.

Shearing injuries are produced by force vectors that are horizontal or obliquely directed on the thoracic or lumbar spine. Forward or lateral flexion contributes to the injury. On rare occasions, shearing injuries may result from hyperextension.[47] Shearing injuries typically occur when the lower portion of the body is fixed and the more mobile vertebral column and upper torso receive a severe blow and move in response to it (Fig. 13–44). As with rotary injuries, and for the same reasons, shearing injuries are most common at the thoracolumbar junction. They are typically found in trauma victims who have been ejected from motor vehicles. Shearing injuries are also extremely disruptive and frequently result in severe neurologic compromise.

The radiographic fingerprints of shearing injuries are (1) distortion of vertebral anatomy in a "windswept" appearance (Fig. 13–45); (2) lateral distraction; (3) lateral dislocation; (4) transverse process or rib fractures; and (5) a linear oblique windswept array of bone fragments on a CT scan. As with rotary injuries, it is important to distinguish shearing injuries from burst fractures, again because of treatment considerations. Key features for differentiating these injuries include the linear horizontal distribution of bone fragments on both radiographs and CT in burst injuries and the windswept, linear oblique array of bone fragments in a shearing injury. Furthermore, the presence of transverse process or rib fractures should alert the

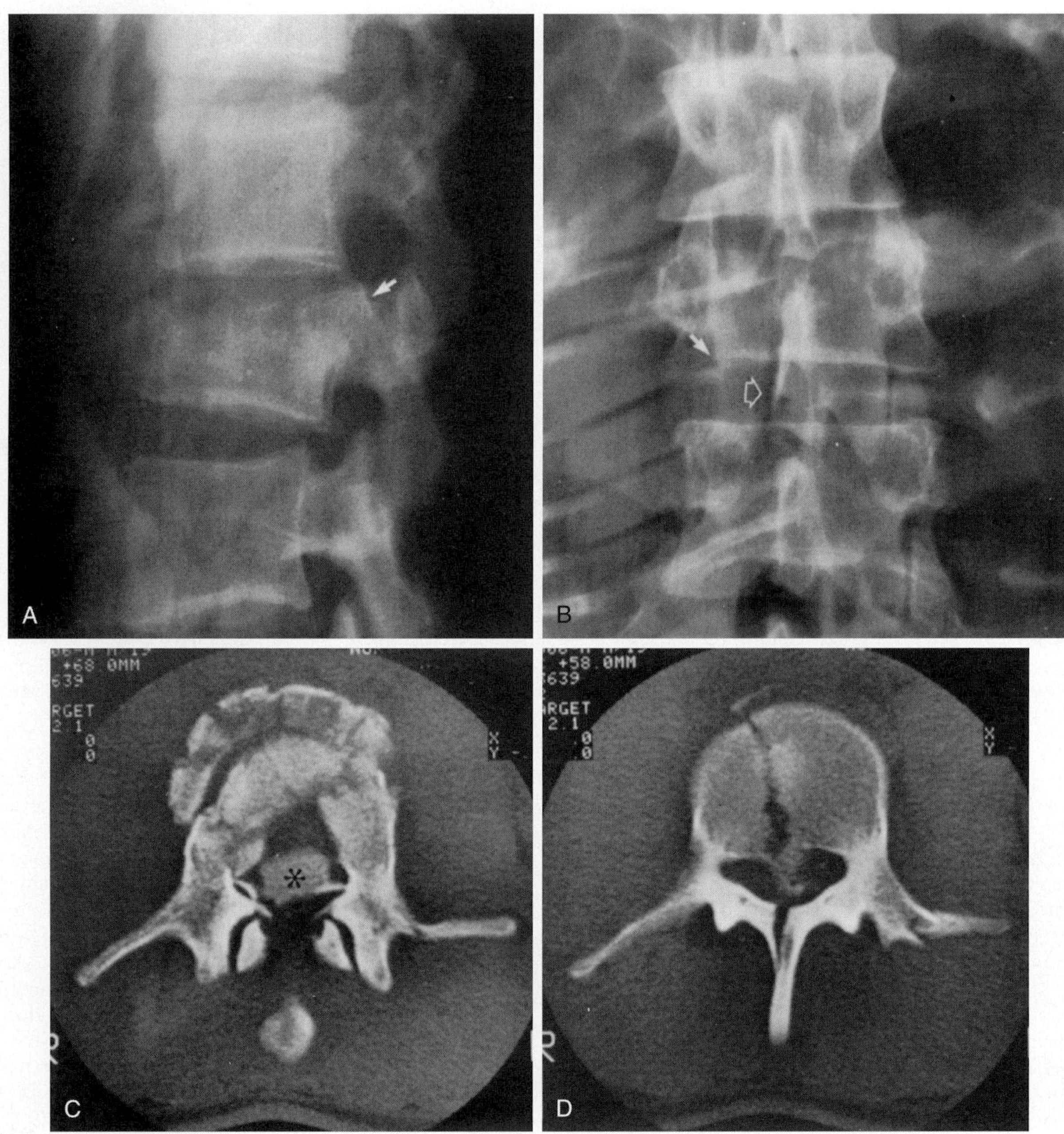

Figure 33–38. Burst fracture of L3. *A*, Lateral view shows wedging of the vertebral body anteriorly and a fragment displaced from the posterior vertebral body line *(arrow)*. *B*, Anteroposterior view demonstrates flattening of the body of L3. The superior vertebral end plate is not seen. Note the wide interpedicle distance. In this patient, a break in the inferior end plate *(solid arrow)* and a fracture of the lamina *(open arrow)* are also present just to the right of the spinous process. *C*, CT image obtained through the upper portion of L3 demonstrates comminution of the superior end plate and the retropulsed fragment *(asterisk)* with resultant significant narrowing of the vertebral canal. The transverse process is also fractured on the left. *D*, CT image obtained through the lower portion of L3 demonstrates sagittal fractures of both the vertebral body and the lamina just to the right of the spinous process.

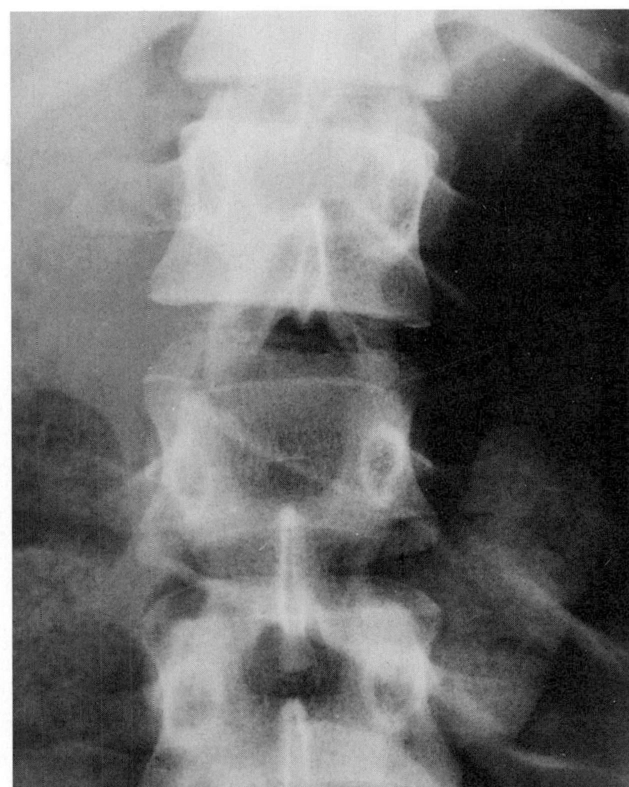

Figure 13–39. Distraction injury of L1–L2. Note the wide interspinous space and naked facets.

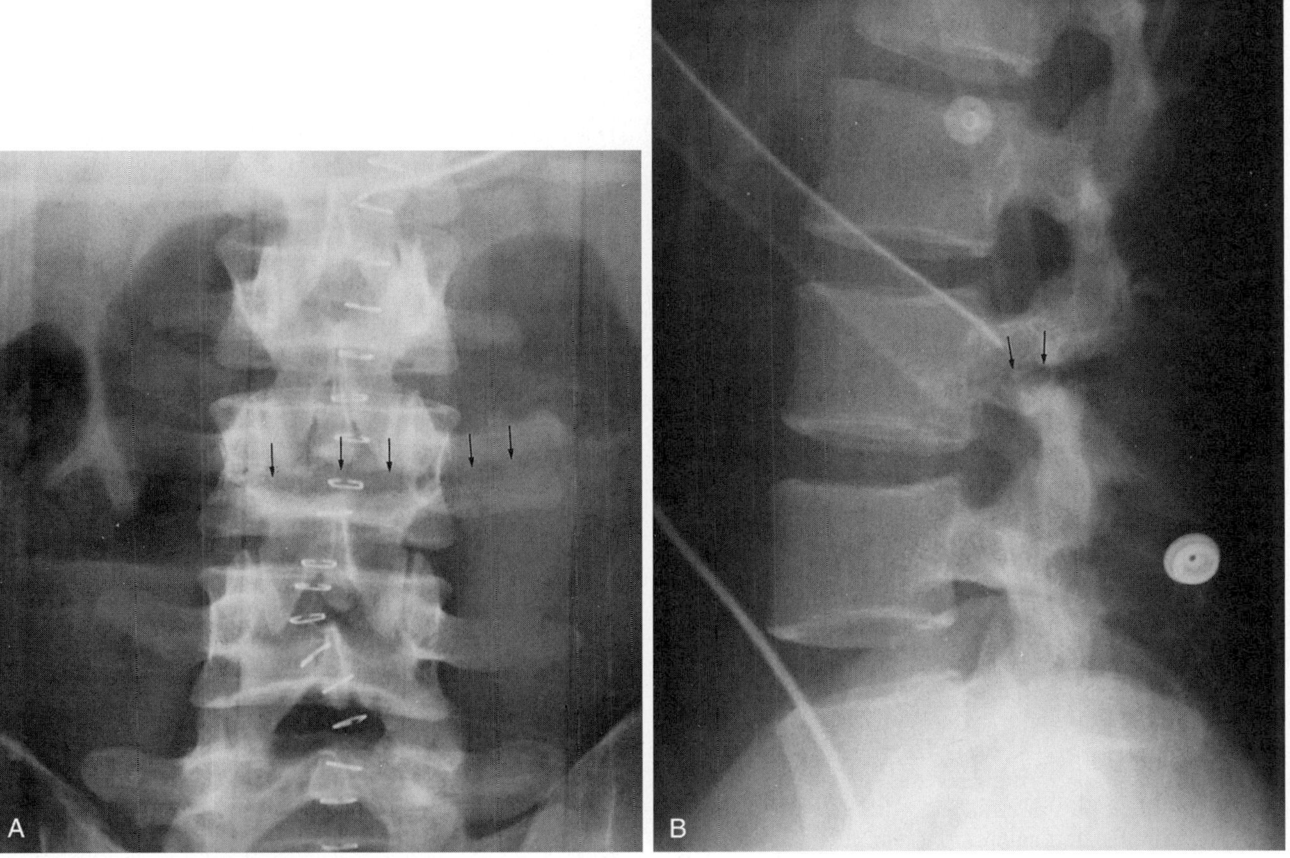

Figure 13–40. Chance-type fracture. *A*, Anteroposterior radiograph shows a horizontal fracture line that extends across the pedicles, lamina, and transverse process on the left *(arrows)*. The staples are from a laparotomy to repair a mesenteric injury caused by the patient's seat belt. *B*, Lateral radiograph shows involvement of the pedicles and lamina *(arrows)*.

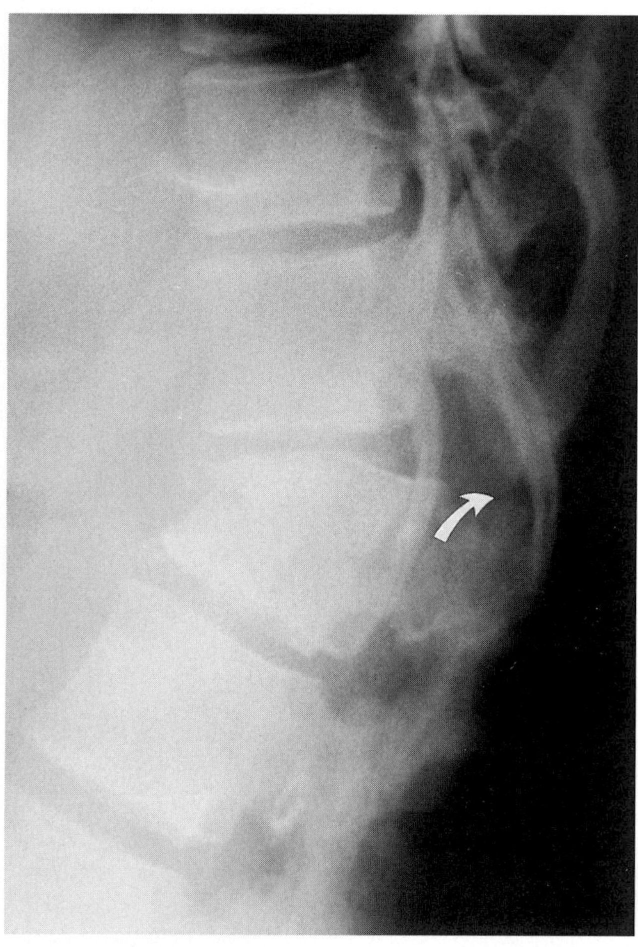

Figure 13–41. Flexion dislocation of T12–L1. Lateral radiograph demonstrates anterolisthesis of T12 on L1, anterior compression of L1, and perching of facets *(arrow)*.

examiner to the fact that the injury is not a burst fracture. Compare Figures 13–45 and 13–37.

Extension injuries are uncommon in the thoracic and lumbar spine. They are the result, in almost every instance, of falling backwards and hyperextending over a solid object. Patients with rigid spine disease such as ankylosing spondylitis and DISH are predisposed to suffer this type of injury.[70, 80, 90] The radiographic fingerprints of an extension injury in the thoracic and lumbar regions are (1) wide disc space and (2) retrolisthesis (Fig. 13–46).

Most other classifications are also based largely on the radiographic appearance of the fractures and the forces presumed to have created the injury.[46, 59, 105, 135] These classifications have been modified and refined by a greater understanding of spinal biomechanics and the improved visualization provided by CT. McAfee and colleagues[135] proposed a classification system based on the three principal forces that injure the middle column: axial compression, axial distraction, and translation within the transverse plane. Consideration of these forces and their resultant injuries allows reasonable prediction of the stability of involved segment(s). These investigators believed that axial compression and axial distraction forces cannot coexist in the same segment of the spine, and that if either one occurs in combination with translation, then translation usually determines the amount of instability. (A notable exception to this concept is found in the Chance-type injury.) These considerations led McAfee and coworkers to propose six kinds of injury: wedge compression fracture, stable burst fracture, unstable burst fracture, Chance fracture, flexion-distraction injuries, and translational injuries.[135] Their classification considers rotary and shearing injuries as subsets of flexion mechanisms and does not include extension injuries. For this reason, I feel that this classification is seriously flawed. However, a review of these injury types is useful here because the orthopedic literature still follows its modifications.

By far the majority of thoracolumbar fractures are simple wedge compression fractures of the vertebral bodies, the posterior elements remaining intact; by comparison, fractures limited to the posterior elements without involving the vertebral body are quite unusual.[46, 59, 105] In the McAfee classification a wedge compression fracture is an injury causing an isolated failure of the anterior column (see Fig. 13–36). The fracture results from forward flexion and is rarely associated with neurologic deficit. The vertebral body or bodies are wedge shaped. This injury is also known as a simple compression fracture.[36, 41]

A “stable” burst fracture is one in which the anterior and middle columns fail because of the compressive load, with no loss of integrity of the posterior elements. This type of injury is uncommon and is usually found in the thoracic region, in the presence of intact ribs. If the same fracture occurs in the presence of rib or sternal fractures, the stabilizing effect of these structures is lost.

An unstable or classic burst fracture is one in which the anterior and middle columns fail in compression and

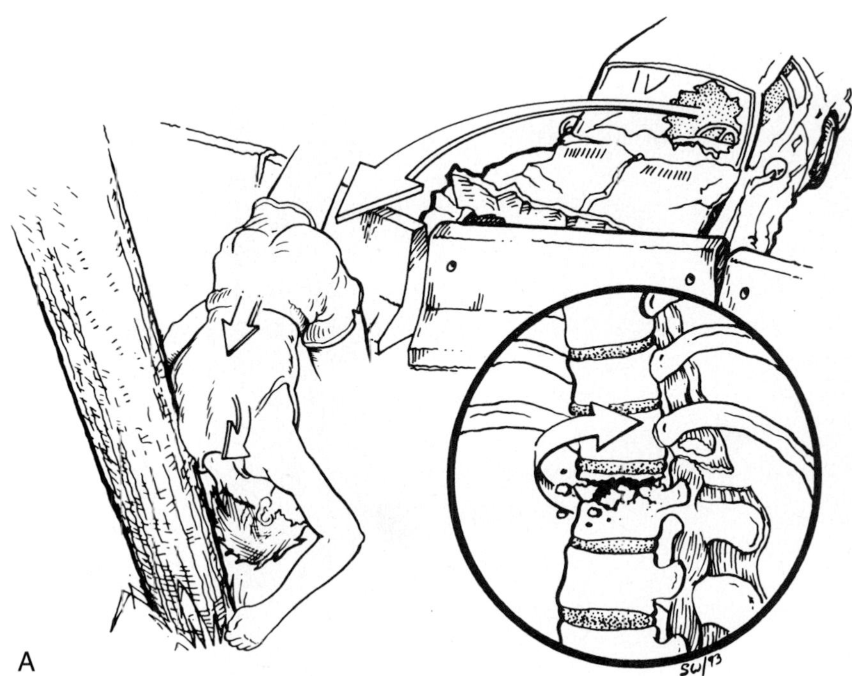

A

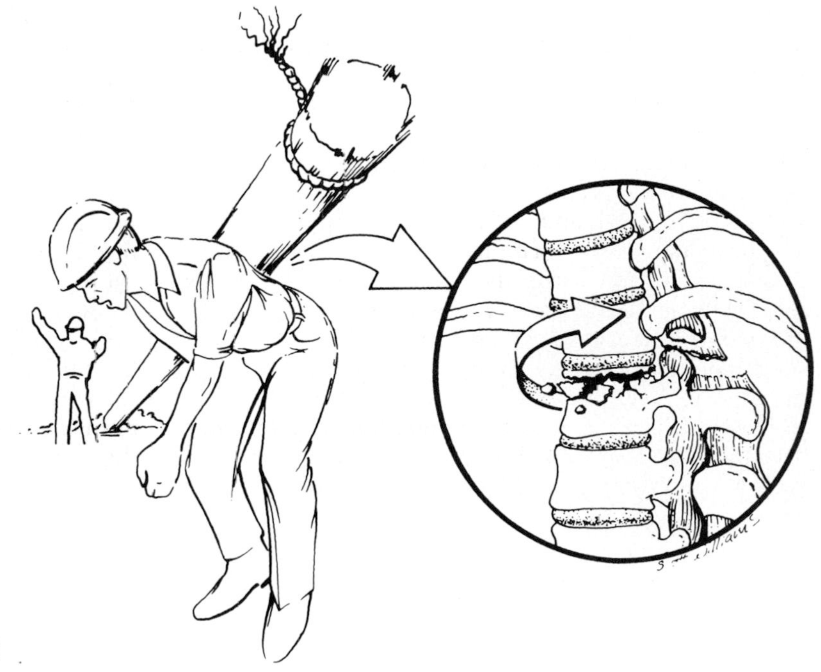

B

Figure 13–42. Mechanisms of rotary or grinding thoracolumbar injuries. *A*, The most common mechanism, due to a traumatic defenestration from a motor vehicle. *B*, Less common mechanism, due to a blow from a solid object. In each instance, one portion of the torso is fixed and the other is forcibly flexed and turned. (From Daffner, R.H. [1996]. Imaging of Vertebral Trauma. 2nd Ed. Lippincott Raven Publishers, Philadelphia. Illustrated by Scott Williams.)

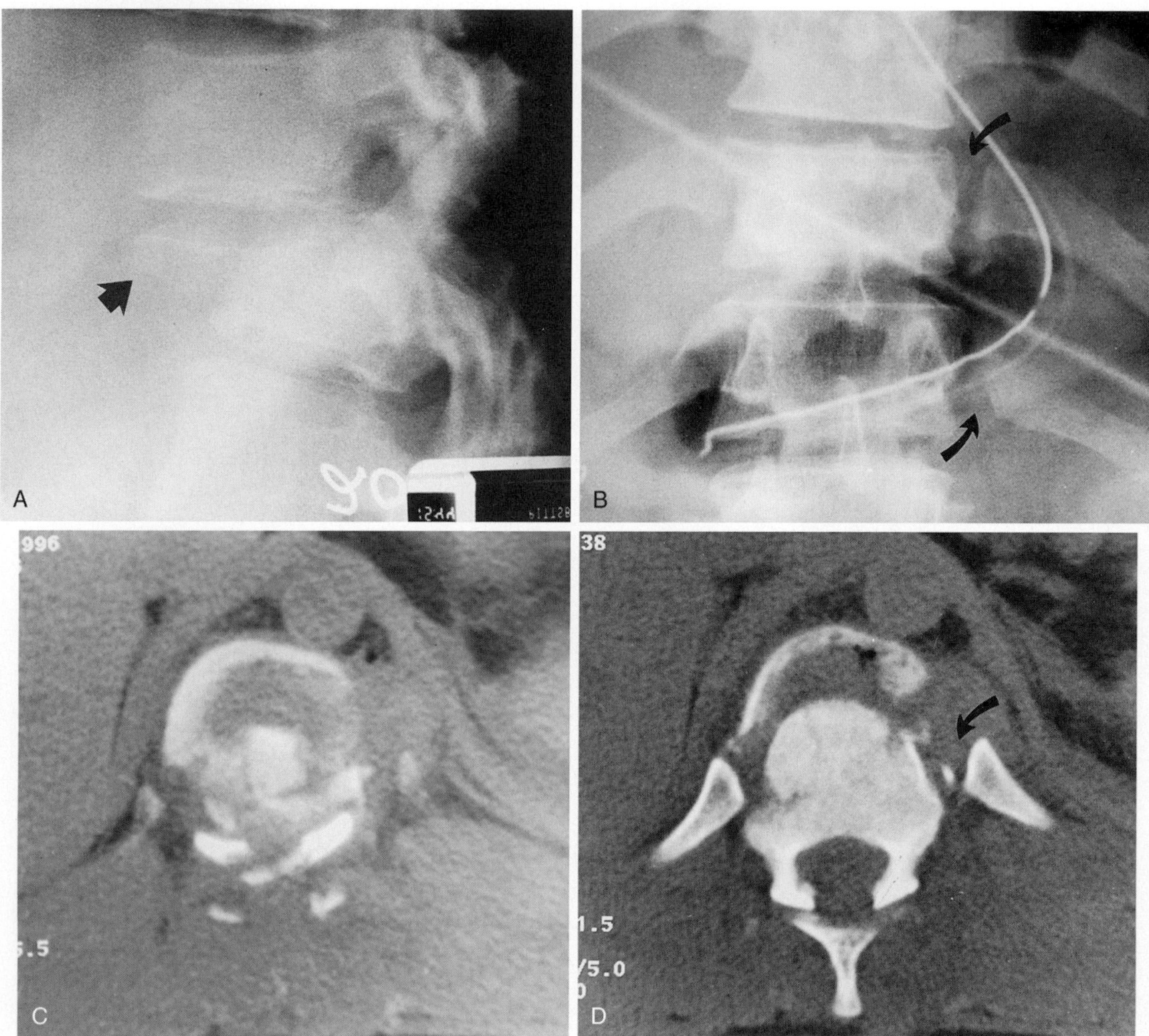

Figure 13–43. Rotary fracture-dislocation of T11 on T12. *A*, Lateral radiograph shows anterior dislocation of T11 on T12. A fragment of the superior portion of T12 has been avulsed, giving the vertebra the appearance of a "ripped can top" *(arrow)*. *B*, Anteroposterior radiograph shows transverse process fractures of T11 and T12 on the left *(arrows)*. *C*, CT image shows pulverization of T12. Note the circular array of bone fragments. *D*, Higher-level CT image shows the avulsed fragment anteriorly and avulsion of the eleventh rib on the left *(arrow)*.

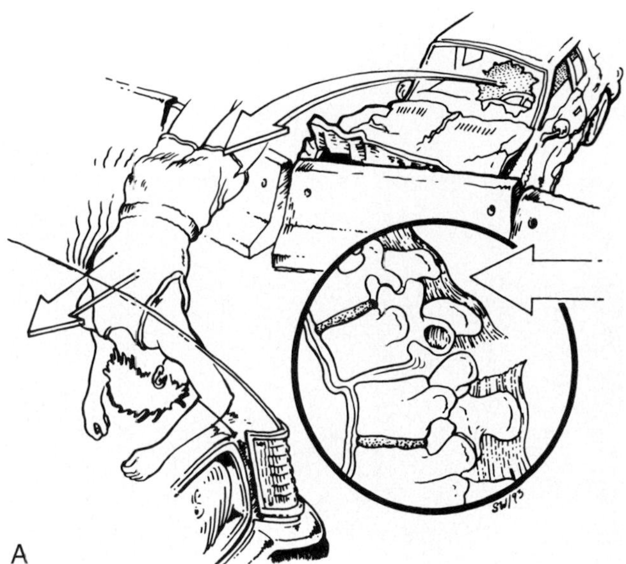

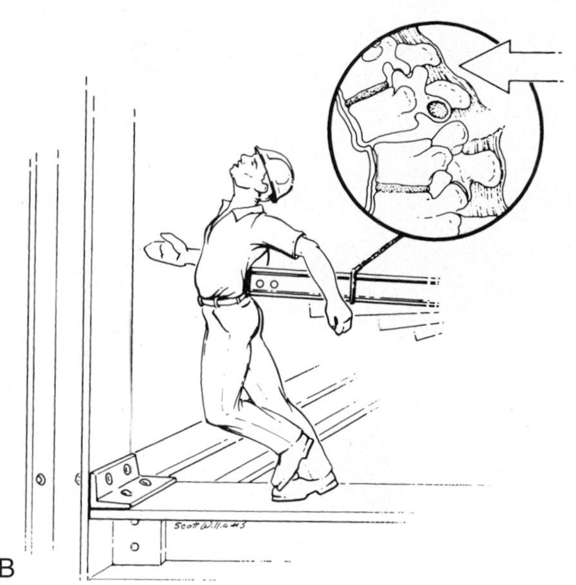

Figure 13–44. Mechanism of shearing injuries. *A*, The most common mechanism, due to a traumatic defenestration from a motor vehicle. *B*, Less common mechanism, due to a blow from a solid object. In each instance, one portion of the torso is fixed and the other is struck a glancing, angled blow. (From Daffner, R.H. [1996]. Imaging of Vertebral Trauma. 2nd Ed. Lippincott Raven Publishers, Philadelphia. Illustrated by Scott Williams.)

the posterior column is disrupted (see Fig. 13–38). According to McAfee and colleagues, disruption of the posterior column leads to instability.[135] As discussed later, stability is most dependent on the integrity of the *middle* column, not the posterior. Hence, by radiologic criteria, all burst fractures are unstable.

A Chance-type fracture is a transverse fracture of the vertebra resulting from distraction about the horizontal plane, with the fulcrum anterior to the anterior longitudinal ligament, so that the entire vertebra is pulled apart by tensile forces (see Fig. 13–40).[29, 164, 176]

In a flexion-distraction injury the axis of flexion is in the middle column (Fig. 13–47). The anterior column fails in compression, while the posterior and middle columns fail through distraction. Failure in the middle column results in a tear or attenuation of the posterior longitudinal ligament. All such injuries are potentially unstable because not only are the ligamentum flavum and interspinous and supraspinous ligaments torn, but the posterior longitudinal ligament and posterior third of the disc may be torn as well.

Translation (dislocation) injuries are those in which the alignment of the neural canal has been disrupted by displacement of the spinal column in the transverse plane in any direction (see Figs. 13–2 and 13–11). Usually, all three columns have failed as a result of rotary or shearing forces.

More recently, Magerl and associates[129] proposed the sophisticated AO classification as an aid to surgical planning for vertebral injuries. This scheme is defined by common morphologic and injury-producing characteristics, particularly to the soft tissues, and comprises three main types of injury, each of which has several variants.[129] Type A injuries are due to compression from axial loading without soft tissue disruption in the transverse plane. Type B injuries are due to anterior or posterior distraction with soft tissue disruption in the horizontal plane. Type C injuries are rotary disruptions.

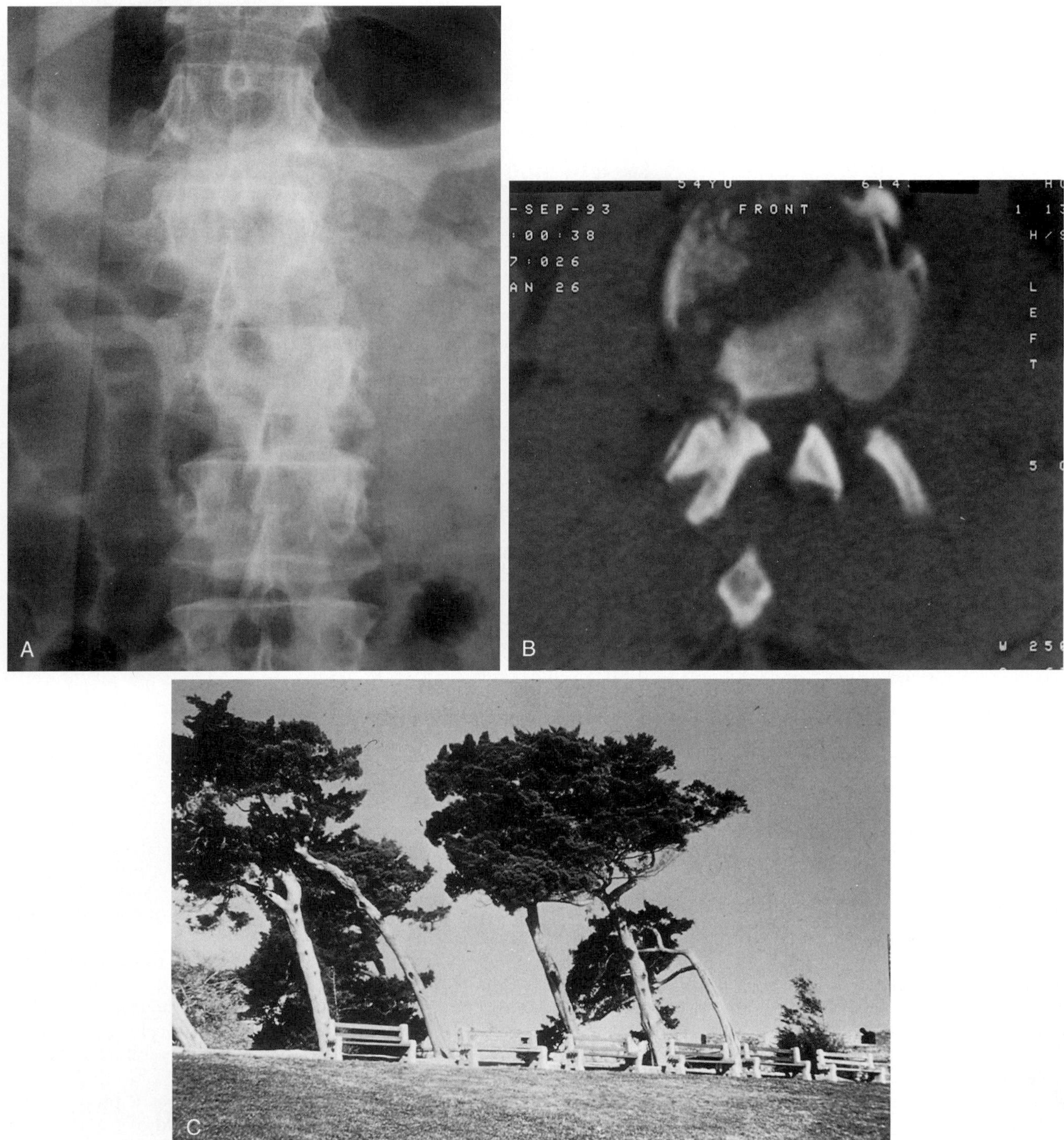

Figure 13–45. Shearing injury involving L1 and L2. *A*, Anteroposterior radiograph shows right laterolisthesis of L1 on L2. Note the "windswept" appearance of L1 and L2 and fracture of the transverse process of L1 on the left. *B*, CT image shows severe comminution of the upper portion of L2. Note the wide facet joint on the left. *C*, Windswept trees. Note the similarities in appearance to the vertebrae in *A*. (*C*, From Daffner, R.H. [1996]. Imaging of Vertebral Trauma. 2nd Ed. Lippincott Raven Publishers, Philadelphia.)

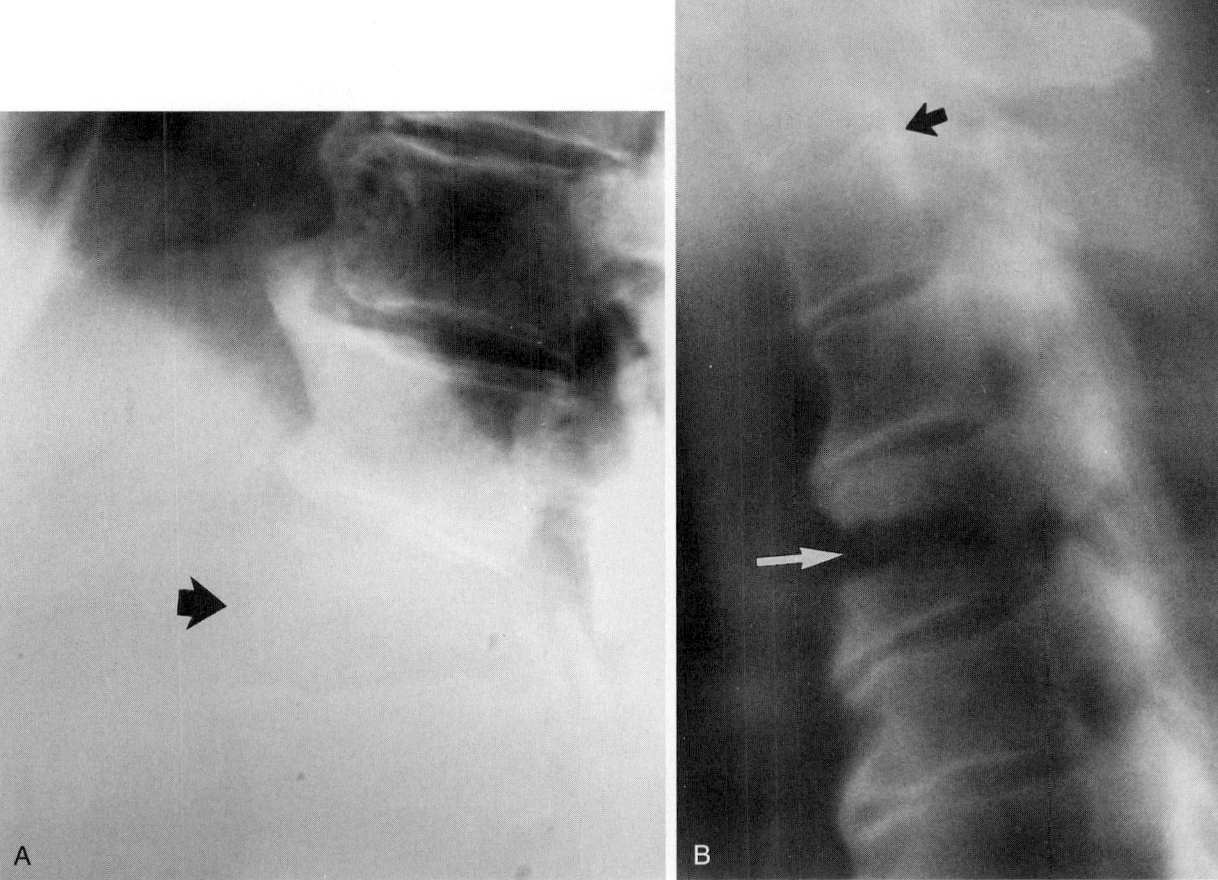

Figure 13–46. Extension injuries in a patient with diffuse idiopathic skeletal hyperostosis (DISH). *A*, Lateral radiograph of the thoracolumbar junction shows widening of the disc space of T11–T12 *(arrow)*. *B*, Lateral tomogram of the upper thoracic region shows a horizontal fracture through the body of T1 *(long white arrow)* and ossification of the posterior longitudinal ligament of C6 *(black arrow)*.

The mechanistic classification based on the *principal* pattern of injury is helpful for both diagnosis and therapy.[36, 41] The radiographic findings in each type of injury are described in detail later on.

Compression Fractures

Simple compression fractures are best identified in the lateral projection. The vertebral body is seen to be wedge-shaped, with most of the compression focused anteriorly.[36, 162] The superior end plate is depressed and forms a concavity in the superior portion of the vertebra (Figs. 13–48 and 13–49). Beneath the concave depression there is a band of poorly marginated sclerosis indicative of impaction of bony trabeculae (see Fig. 13–49*A*). The anterosuperior margin of the wedged vertebra usually forms an irregular beak projecting beyond the anterior border of the vertebral body (see Figs. 13–48 and 13–49*A*). This beak has a sharp point projecting inferiorly. In some cases, the anterosuperior margin of the vertebral body may be displaced anteriorly as a separate small triangular fragment. If so, the possibility of an unstable rotary injury should be considered and the articular facets, laminae, and transverse processes or ribs at this level should be closely examined. CT may be necessary to carefully check the posterior elements. If the inferior end plate is affected, the findings are the same, except that the beak points superiorly (see Fig. 13–49*B*). In children, vertebral compression is more like a torus fracture; therefore, the beak that is formed is contiguous with the wedged vertebra (see Fig. 13–48).[89, 98] Characteristically, the intervertebral disc at the level(s) above the compressed vertebra(e) will be narrowed. This sign is not as reliable in older persons, who often have degenerative disc disease. However, in younger patients, it is a valid and valuable sign.

CT demonstrates comminution of the end plate, with fragments displaced in an arclike fashion, laterally and anterior to the normal confines of the vertebral body. The posterior cortex of the vertebral body should be intact and undisplaced. This finding is the principal distinguishing feature between a simple wedge compression and a burst fracture. CT also demonstrates the cortical disruption, areas of bone destruction, and associated soft tissue mass in wedge compression deformities due to pathologic fractures.

The *limbus vertebra,* or *vertebral edge separation,* is considered by some investigators to be a normal variant and should not be confused with an acute fracture (Fig. 13–50). There are two schools of thought regarding its origin. The first holds that the limbus fragment is an

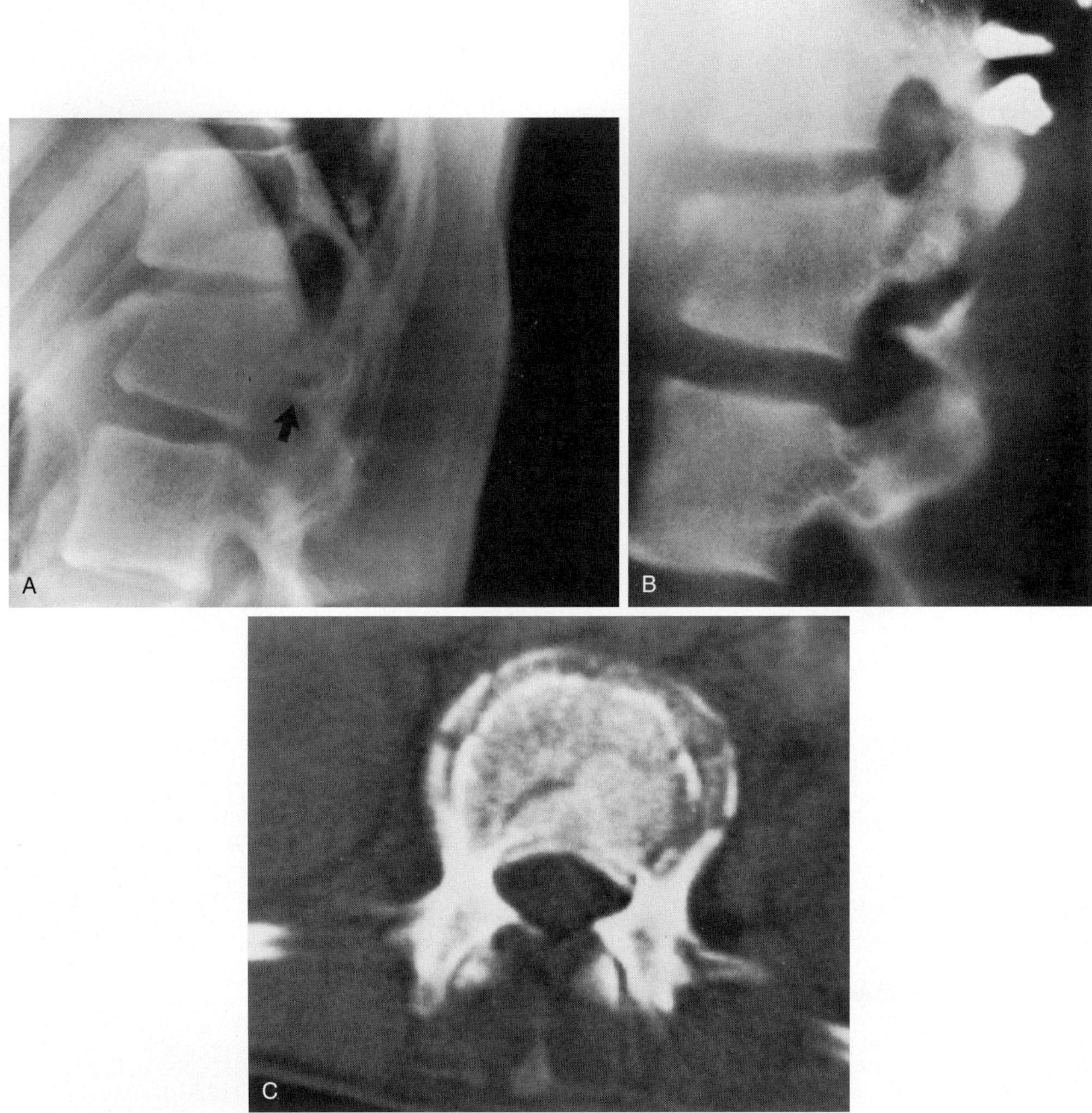

Figure 13–47. Flexion-distraction fracture of L1. *A*, Lateral view demonstrates anterior wedge compression of the body of L1 with a small triangular fragment arising from the anterior superior surface of the vertebra. There is also a horizontal fracture through the pedicle *(arrow)*. *B*, Lateral tomogram demonstrates the pedicle fracture to advantage. *C*, CT image clearly demonstrates the comminuted fractures. The fractured pedicle was not visualized by CT.

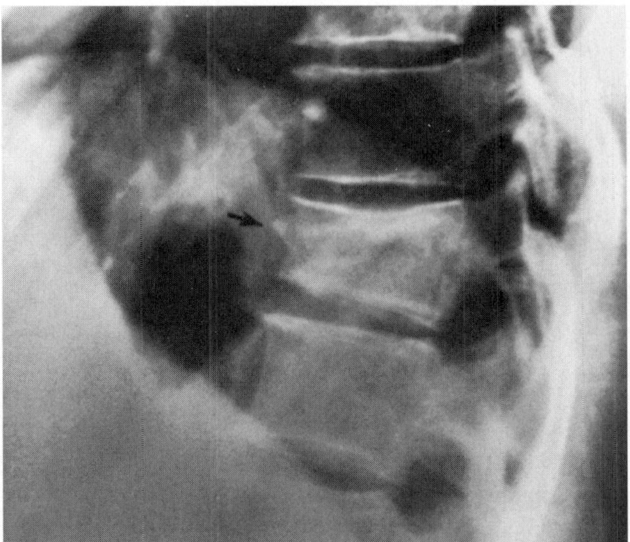

Figure 13–48. Simple compression fracture of T11. Angular distortion of the anterior cortex of the vertebral body can be seen *(arrow)*. Note the increased density beneath the superior end plate, representing impaction. Distortion of the anterior margin of the end plate is more common in children than in adults. (Case courtesy of John Tampas, MD, and Bradley Soule, MD, Burlington, Vt.)

accessory center of ossification at the anterior superior margin of the vertebra. The anterior superior and anterior inferior apophyseal rings are frequently visualized in adolescents at the margins of the vertebral bodies on lateral views. Before the apophyseal rings ossify, there is a small indentation of the vertebra in this location. Neither the ring nor the indentation should be mistaken for a fracture of the vertebral body. The second and prevailing opinion considers all limbus deformities to be the result

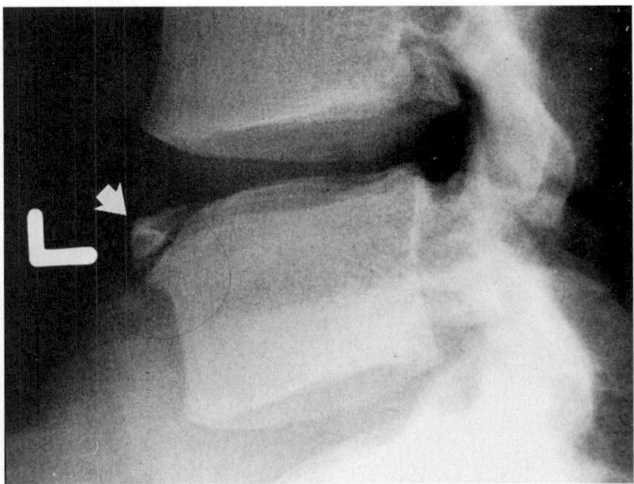

Figure 13–50. Vertebral edge separation (limbus deformity). Lateral radiograph shows a bone fragment off the anterior superior margin of L2 *(arrow)*. Note the narrowed L1 disc space.

of discovertebral trauma—so-called anterior Schmorl nodes[97, 132] (Fig. 13–51). Posterior limbus deformities also occur, frequently producing signs and symptoms of disc herniation. The limbus fragment and the subjacent vertebral body have well-defined margins with sclerotic cortical borders. These findings serve to distinguish this entity from an acute cortical fracture. As a rule, the disc *above* the limbus fragment is narrowed.

The presence of a severe wedge deformity should suggest the possibility of either flexion-distraction or burst injury. It is therefore prudent to perform a CT examination when the patient has a moderate or severe wedge compression deformity of the vertebral body, either to demonstrate associated fractures of the posterior ele-

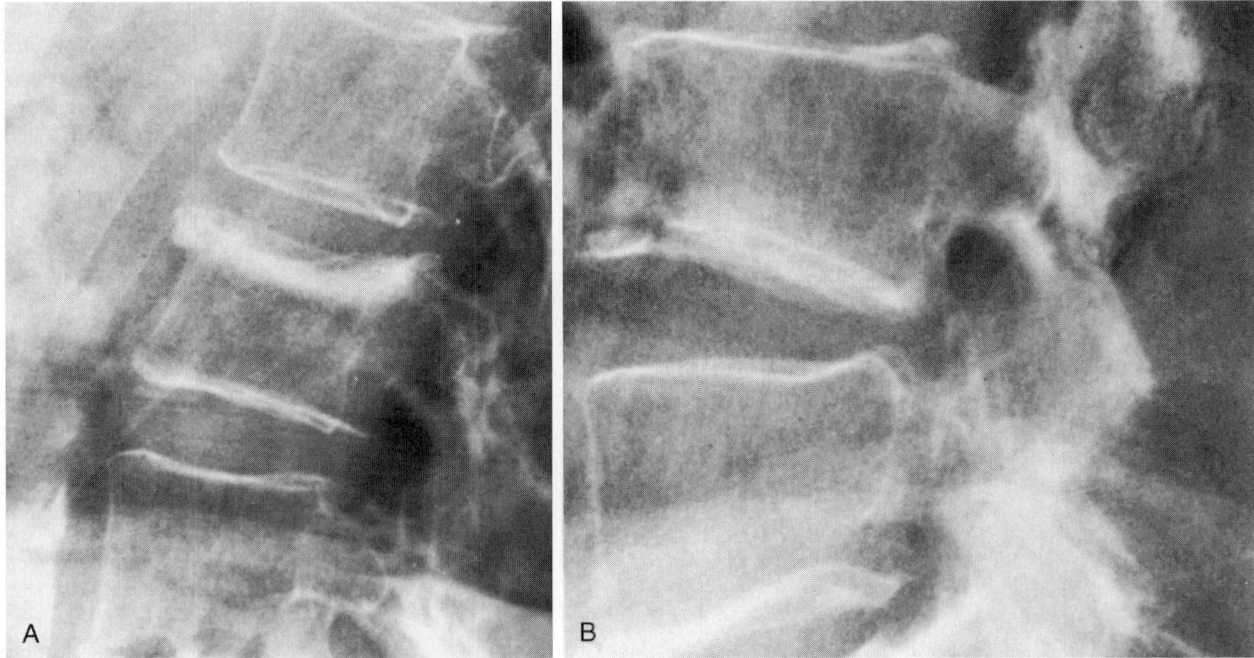

Figure 13–49. Osteopenic compression. *A*, L3 compression deformity. The superior end plate is compressed, with considerable impaction, evidenced by the increased density of the superior aspect of the vertebral body. *B*, L4 compression fracture in another patient. There is anterior wedging due to the compression of the inferior end plate. The vague increase in density is due to impaction.

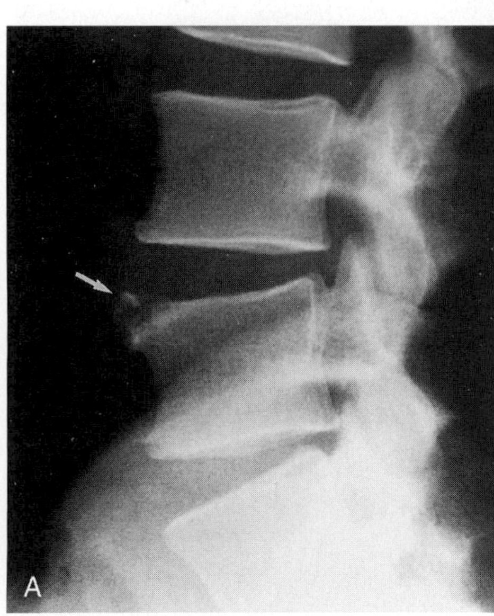

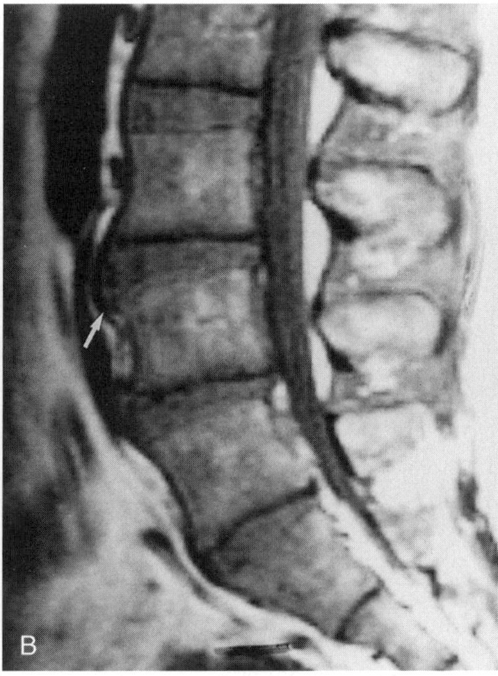

Figure 13–51. Subacute limbus deformity of L5. *A,* Lateral radiograph shows a bone fragment off the anterior superior margin of L5 *(arrow). B,* Sagittal gradient echo MR image shows herniation of disc material into the gap between the fragment and the vertebral body *(arrow),* under the anterior longitudinal ligament.

ments or to disclose the posteriorly displaced fragment indicative of a burst fracture.

Osteoporotic Compression

The diagnosis of acute spinal fracture in older persons is complicated by the frequency of vertebral compression associated with osteoporosis.[17, 65, 87, 88, 138, 146, 185] Osteoporotic fractures are more common after the age of 50 years and increase in prevalence with each succeeding decade. They are particularly common and appear earlier in females than in males and are much more frequent in whites than in blacks.[20, 65] The risk of compression fractures in postmenopausal women increases as vertebral trabecular bone density decreases.[24, 49] The highest incidence of osteoporotic vertebral compression is in the mid-dorsal spine and thoracolumbar junction,[188] resulting in a classic kyphotic deformity of the mid- and upper dorsal spine commonly referred to as a "dowager's hump" (Fig. 13–52). Vertebral compression is rarely, if ever, encountered in the cervical spine. In osteoporosis, selective deficiency or removal of horizontal trabeculae has been histologically associated with microfractures[111] of the vertically oriented trabeculae beneath the superior and inferior vertebral end plates. It is thought that the loss of the horizontally oriented trabeculae increases the stresses placed upon the vertical trabeculae, which in turn results in trabecular fracture. Microscopic callus of woven bone forms about these trabecular microfractures, confirming that these lesions are true fractures.

What criteria can be used to distinguish between compression of a vertebra due to osteoporosis and that due to acute trauma?[17, 88, 138, 188] Evidence of cortical disruption and the presence of a paraspinous soft tissue mass are obvious indications of acute trauma. An ill-defined increase in density beneath the end plate of an involved vertebra indicates impaction of bone due to acute fracture (see Fig. 13–49). The deformed vertebral body that has undergone osteoporotic compression or sustained a previous fracture is similar in density to adjacent vertebrae (Fig. 13–53). Furthermore, these vertebral bodies frequently show evidence of osteophytic spurs with the apposing margins of the adjacent vertebral body. A radioisotope bone scan is of little use in making this distinction because the findings may well be abnormal for a variety of reasons—osteoporotic compression, old fracture, recent fracture, or degenerative changes.

The end stage of an osteoporotic collapse may result in a "vacuum vertebra." With this pathologic entity, the vertebral body contains gas, which can be identified on the radiograph[18] but is more readily apparent on CT images.[22, 121, 133, 181] In extreme cases, the vertebral body is seen to be a gas-containing, wafer-thin, hollow bony shell (Fig. 13–54). Similar changes have also been described in patients on long-term steroid therapy. The gas is presumed to be nitrogen, as is more commonly found in dessicated intervertebral discs. Unless care is taken in the interpretation of the CT findings, gas within the collapsed vertebral body may be dismissed as gas within a disc space.

Severe osteoporotic compression fractures may result in neurologic deficits due to spinal cord or cauda equina encroachment created by retropulsion of a fragment from the posterior surface of the vertebral body.[133] This injury is analogous to a burst fracture.

Vertebral osteomyelitis may present as a wedge compression fracture in patients with osteoporosis.[137] The diagnosis should be considered in osteoporotic patients with severe back pain, wedge compression fractures, and unexplained fever or elevated erythrocyte sedimentation rate. Key to the diagnosis is the presence of vertebral end plate destruction and disc space involvement, features not present in osteoporotic collapse.

Spontaneous fractures of the sternum also occur in association with severe osteoporotic kyphosis.[31, 102] The fracture usually occurs in or about the manubriosternal joint, with characteristic posterior displacement of the superior fragments.

Multiple osteoporotic vertebral compressions are often contiguous. When noncontiguous vertebral fractures are encountered, the possibility of metastatic disease or multiple myeloma must be considered. An MRI examination may be necessary to demonstrate cortical destruction, surrounding soft tissue mass, and focal deposits in other vertebrae. Unfortunately, MRI may not be able to distinguish an osteoporotic compression fracture from pathologic collapse due to metastatic disease when the findings consist of only decreased signal intensity within the vertebral body.[7, 63] If, however, the area of low signal intensity has a linear horizontal pattern (Fig. 13–55) instead of a globular pattern, the findings are more suggestive of osteoporotic collapse. With neoplastic collapse, there is typically low signal intensity in the entire marrow space of the vertebral body or in a globular pattern, usually in the center of the body (Fig. 13–56). Diffusion-weighted MRI shows promise in distinguishing benign from malignant collapse.[7] In addition, gadolinium-enhanced MRI examination has been reported to be effective in making the differentiation.[34]

Pathologic Fracture of the Spine

Metastatic disease to the spine commonly produces pathologic compression fractures of vertebral bodies.

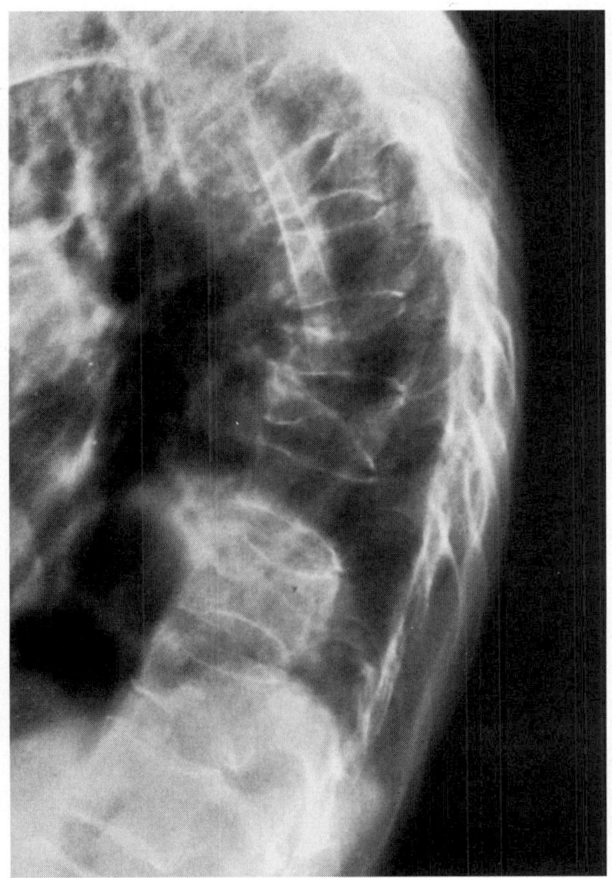

Figure 13–52. Osteopenic collapse. "Dowager's hump" deformity due to multiple anterior wedge compression fractures in an elderly woman. The hump is characteristically located in the middle and upper thoracic regions.

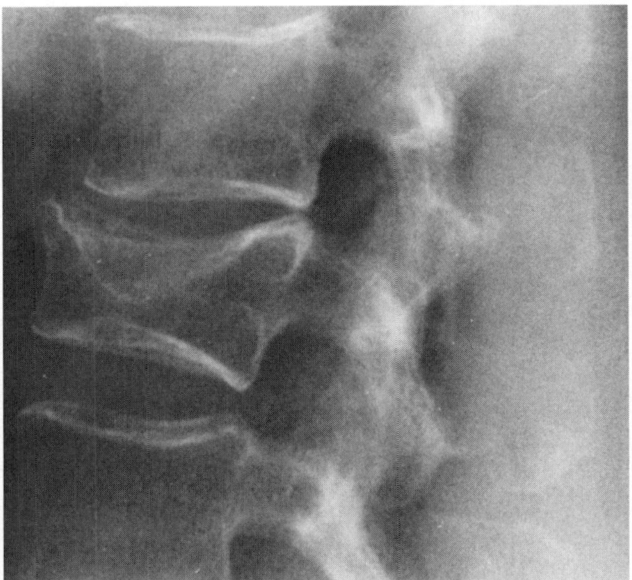

Figure 13–53. Old compression fracture of L2 in an elderly osteoporotic woman. There is anterior wedging of the vertebral body, with considerable depression of the end plate. However, there is no increase in bone density within the vertebral body, and a small spur is present on the anterior superior margin of the body. These findings indicate that the fracture is old.

Other forms of pathologic fracture occur but are rare. The distinctive radiographic feature of a pathologic fracture is the presence of bone destruction, particularly involving the cortex (Fig. 13–57; see also Fig. 13–56). Although the cortex of the pedicle always comes to mind in this context, recognition of cortical destruction of any component of the vertebra is equally important and diagnostic. The pedicles may not be involved by the malignant process and, furthermore, are often spared in multiple myeloma. It is a good habit to search for areas of cortical destruction in any compression fracture of the vertebral body in older persons and particularly when the fractures are multiple or noncontiguous, or both. The history, of course, may be helpful in that the injury or inciting episode may have been trivial, but this feature does not allow discrimination between an insufficiency fracture of osteoporosis and a pathologic fracture associated with metastatic disease. The presence of a surrounding soft tissue mass is further evidence suggesting metastatic disease, but it could be due to a hematoma alone, particularly if the mass is small.

Whenever there is any question of a pathologic fracture, an MRI examination should be performed because of its greater sensitivity in detecting metastatic deposits in the marrow and the extended view of the spine that can be obtained in both the sagittal and coronal planes (see Fig. 13–57).[141, 198] MRI not only will demonstrate or exclude lesions at the level in question but may simultaneously demonstrate lesions at other levels often not previously suspected to be involved. Furthermore, any spinal cord compression due to extension from the focus of metastatic disease will be clearly shown.

The Kümmell Phenomenon: Post-traumatic Collapse

In 1891 Kümmell described delayed post-traumatic collapse of the vertebral body leading to a gibbus defor-

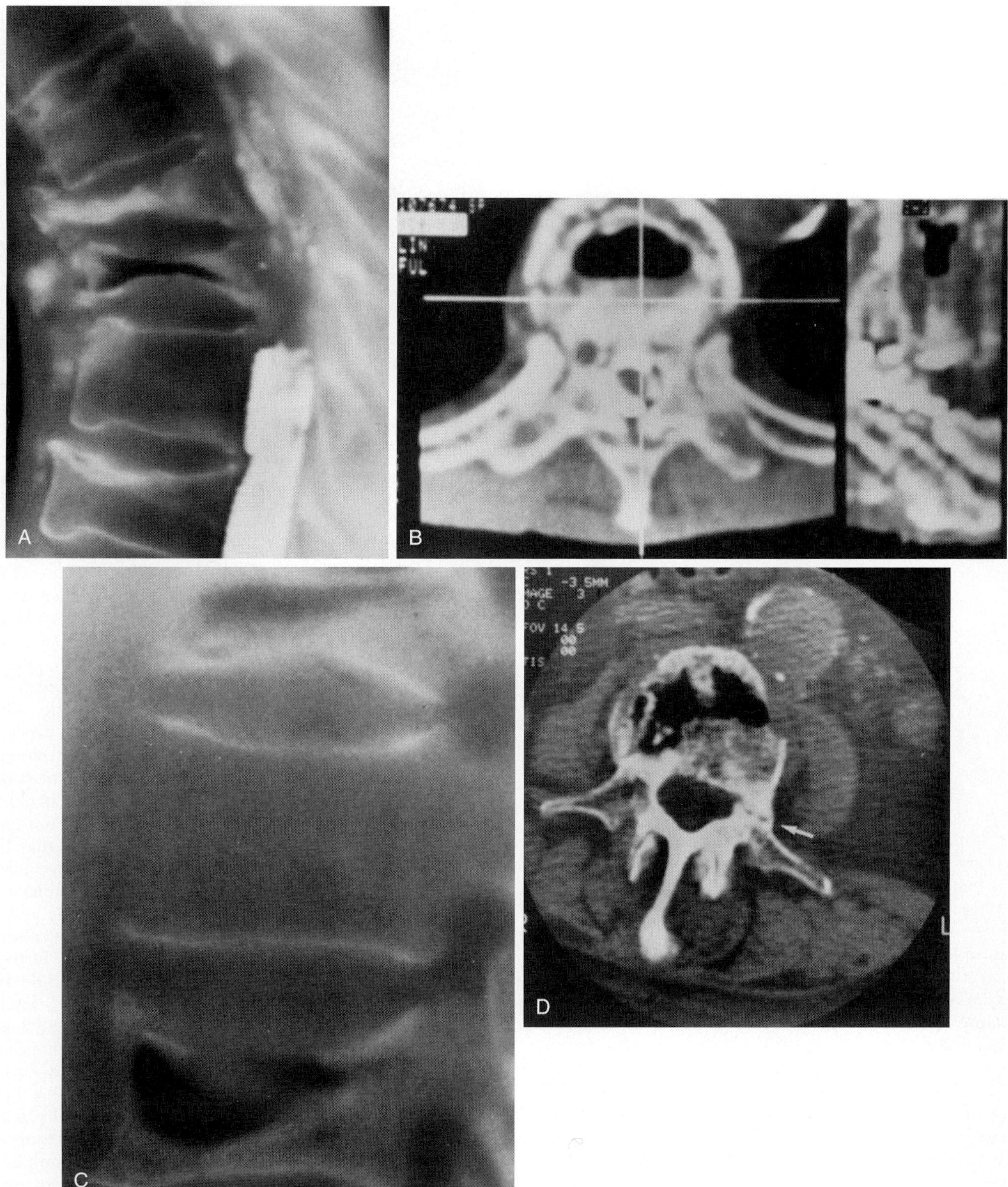

Figure 13–54. Far-advanced osteoporotic vertebral collapse, with gas within affected structures. *A*, Lateral conventional tomogram demonstrates a complete, wafer-thin collapse of two contiguous vertebral bodies in the midthoracic region. The more inferior body is almost completely filled with gas. There is residual contrast material from a previous myelogram, and a partial block at the apex of the kyphosis is present. *B*, CT image demonstrates a gas-fluid level within the vertebral body on both the axial *(left)* and sagittal *(right)* reconstructed images. *C*, Lateral tomogram of the upper lumbar region demonstrates wedge compression deformities of L1 and L3, both of which contain gas. *D*, CT image obtained through L3 demonstrates gas within the vertebral body and an insufficiency fracture of the left pedicle *(arrow)*.

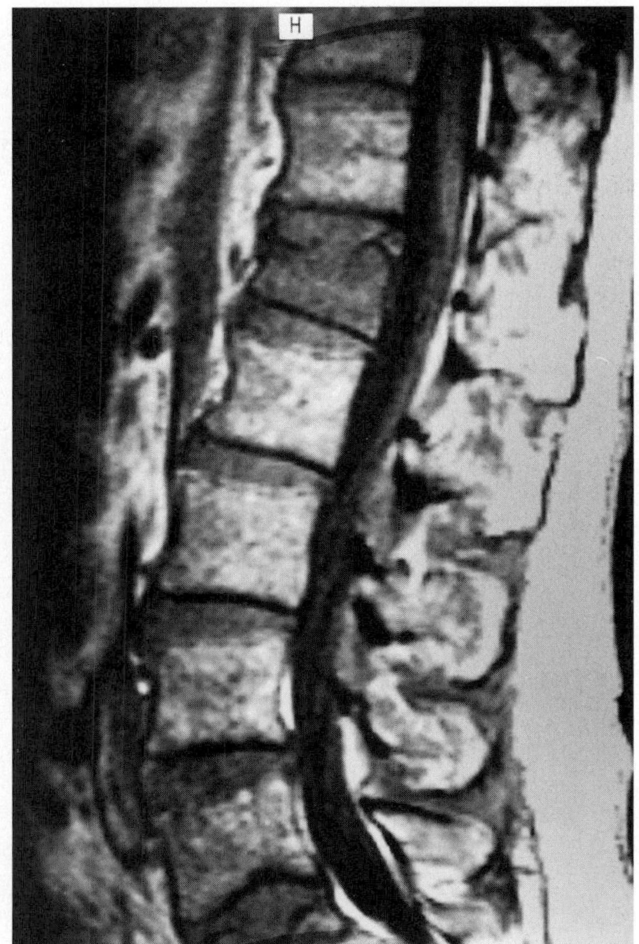

Figure 13–55. Osteopenic collapse: MRI appearance. T_1-weighted sagittal image shows a uniform loss of signal in the body of L1. The distribution is more linear and fills the vertebra, as opposed to a more globular appearance characteristic of metastatic disease (see Fig. 13–56).

mity. Since then, other investigators have noted the occurrence of a delayed, progressive, angular deformity following either radiographically inapparent or minimal fractures[130, 161] (Fig. 13–58). Such progression is occasionally encountered after an otherwise routine compression fracture.[86] The collapse is more likely to occur in the thoracolumbar region. It should not be construed as a manifestation of pathologic fracture. The etiologic factor is presumed to be weakness secondary to vascular damage, although this association has not been proved. The collapse generally occurs within 8 weeks of the initial injury. Abel described a similar phenomenon involving the articular pillars of the lower cervical spine.[1]

The Kümmell phenomenon is to be distinguished from post-traumatic spinal neuroarthropathy—the development of a Charcot joint in the spine after spinal cord injury. Associated changes include juxta-articular bone destruction and the formation of dense appositional new bone, large osteophytes, and bony debris in the surrounding soft tissues.[33, 175, 177, 194] These changes may occur at or below the level of the initial injury. The Kümmell phenomenon should also be distinguished from infectious spondylitis, in which there is involvement of the disc space and the two adjacent vertebral bodies—findings typical of infection.

Flexion-Distraction Injury

Fractures of the posterior elements often accompany more severe compression fractures of the vertebral bodies and therefore should be considered separately and distinguished from simple wedge compression fractures.[5, 83, 140] The greater the degree of compression, the more likely the presence of posterior element fractures. The majority are horizontal fractures involving the laminae, spinous processes, pedicles, and margins of the facets (Fig. 13–59; see also Fig. 13–12). The best explanation for these injuries lies in the three-column concept of Denis.[46] If the middle column is considered as a midpoint or fulcrum, then with flexion the anterior column is compressed and simultaneously the posterior column is placed in tension (distraction), as in the motion of a teeter-totter or seesaw. The compression forces anteriorly cause wedge deformities of the vertebral bodies, and the tensile (distractive) forces posteriorly create horizontal fractures and ligamentous disruptions in the posterior column. This injury might therefore be referred to as a "teeter-totter" fracture.

In some injuries, the tensile component may extend into the posterior aspect of the vertebral body within the middle column. The ultimate in flexion-distraction

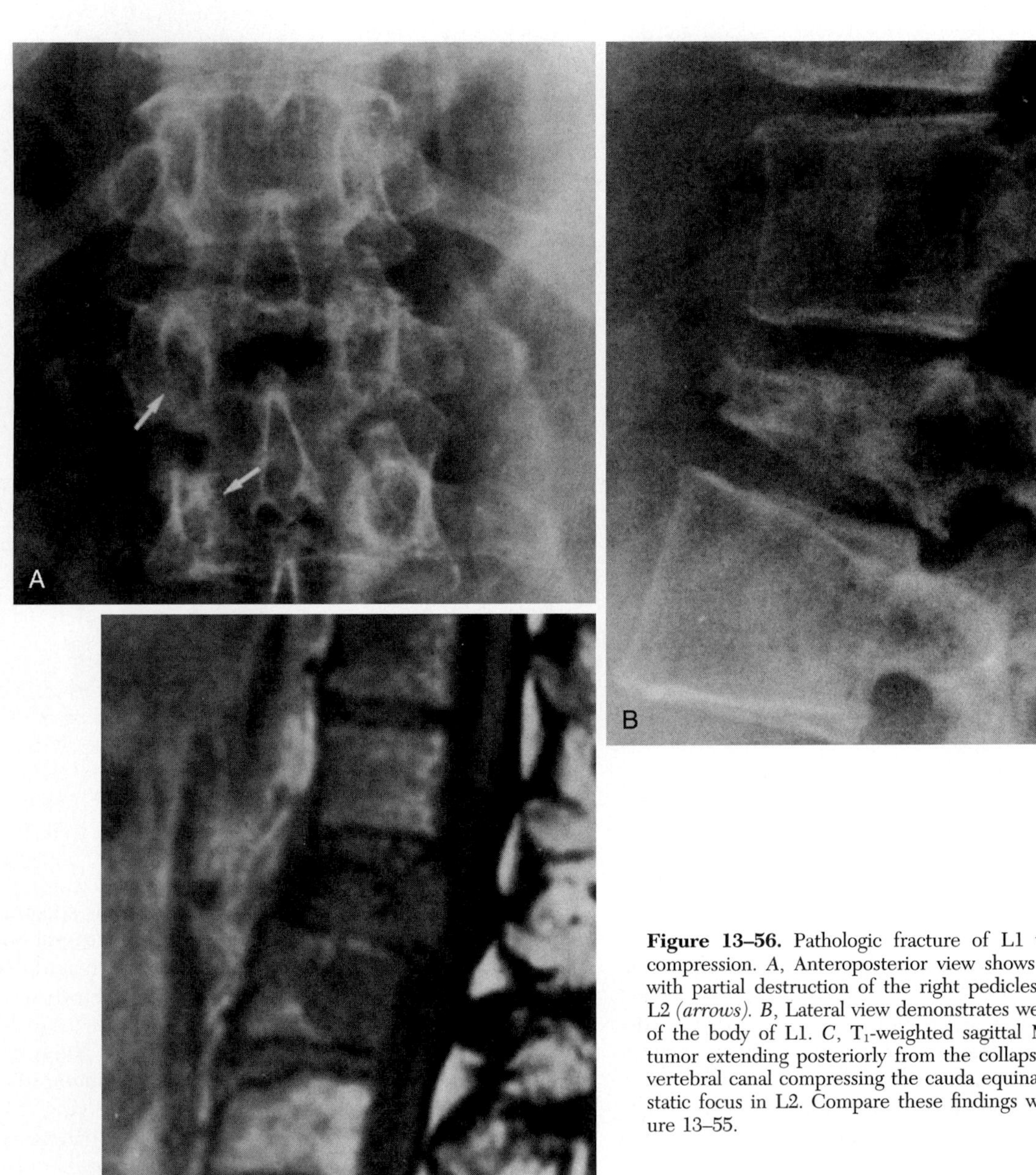

Figure 13–56. Pathologic fracture of L1 with spinal cord compression. *A*, Anteroposterior view shows flattening of L1 with partial destruction of the right pedicles of both L1 and L2 *(arrows)*. *B*, Lateral view demonstrates wedge compression of the body of L1. *C*, T_1-weighted sagittal MR image shows tumor extending posteriorly from the collapsed body into the vertebral canal compressing the cauda equina. Note the metastatic focus in L2. Compare these findings with those in Figure 13–55.

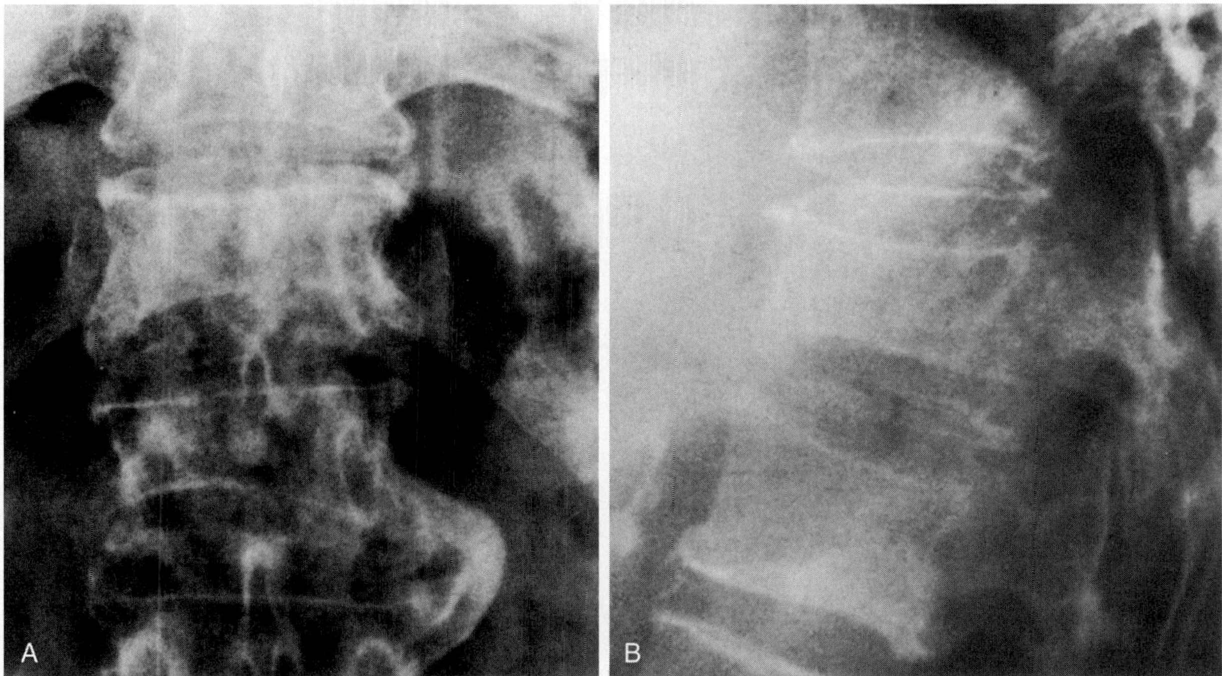

Figure 13–57. Pathologic fractures of T12 and L1 in a patient with metastatic breast carcinoma. *A*, Anteroposterior view shows obvious compression of the bodies of T12 and L1. The pedicles of T12 and L1 are absent on the right, and there is an area of cortical destruction along the anterior inferior margins of the bodies of both vertebrae, manifested as loss of the inferior end plates. *B*, Lateral view demonstrates anterior wedging of the body of T12. Note the indistinct posterior vertebral body lines of each vertebra. In older osteopenic individuals, the cortical margins of the vertebra, including the pedicles, should be closely examined for evidence of destruction to exclude the possibility of a pathologic fracture.

fracture at the thoracolumbar junction was described by Hall and Robertson:[83] a vertebral body fracture with a 50% loss in anterior height associated with posterior ligamentous and bony disruption. This injury included a horizontal fracture through the body and pedicles exiting through the laminae and interspinous ligament and avulsing the inferior spinous process of the adjacent cephalic vertebra. The facet joints remained intact, and there was no anterior or lateral displacement. Flexion-distraction fractures are also to be differentiated from Chance-type fractures (see Figs. 13–21 and 13–40), wherein a distraction force is placed across the entire vertebra, including all three columns.[29, 71, 140, 164, 170] In the Chance-type injury, the tensile forces pull the vertebra apart, resulting in little or no compression of the vertebral body. The absence of compression of the vertebral body distinguishes the Chance-type fracture or pure distraction injury from the flexion-distraction injury described here.

Burst Fractures

The burst fracture is a specific form of compression fracture caused by axial compression forces whereby one or more fragments from the posterior (usually superior) margin of the vertebral body are displaced into the vertebral canal[5, 9, 36, 39, 118, 190, 192] (Figs. 13–60 through 13–62). Although in most cases there is a severe wedge deformity, occasionally burst fractures are encountered with no measurable loss of height at the anterior margin of the involved vertebral body (Fig. 13–63). The severe compressive forces drive the nucleus pulposus into the vertebral body, resulting in a virtual explosion that displaces bony fragments centrifugally. The posterior superior fragment originating between the pedicles is characteristically driven into the spinal canal. The lateral component of the fracture extends from the pedicle walls to the basivertebral foramen, giving the fragment a roughly triangular shape. A single fragment is retropulsed in approximately half of the cases; in 40%, the fragment is split in the sagittal plane (see Fig. 13–61); and in the remaining 10% to 20%, the injuries are due to lateral flexion and compression, resulting in a unilateral retropulsed fragment that commonly extends toward the intervertebral neural foramen on the side of injury[5, 36] (Fig. 13–64). The retropulsed fragment results in neurologic injury to the spinal cord, conus medullaris, or cauda equina in approximately two thirds of the cases. By far the majority of burst fractures occur at the thoracolumbar junction, with 50% occurring at L1.[5, 36]

A second characteristic feature of burst fractures is a sagittal fracture of the vertebral body, occurring in approximately 90% of cases (see Figs. 13–63 and 13–64).[9, 117] This fracture involves the inferior half of the vertebra, extending to the region of the basivertebral foramen. In 85% of cases the posterior elements are involved, characteristically with a sagittal fracture at the junction of the laminae and spinous process (see Fig. 13–38). The combination of sagittal fractures both anteriorly and posteriorly leads to widening of the interpedicle distance in the majority of cases (see Fig. 13–62).

To distinguish between the simple wedge compression fracture and a burst fracture, the posterior vertebral body cortex, or posterior vertebral line, should be identified on lateral radiographs[36, 39] (Fig. 13–65). This radiographic feature is the fine line of cortex outlining the posterior

Text continued on page 504

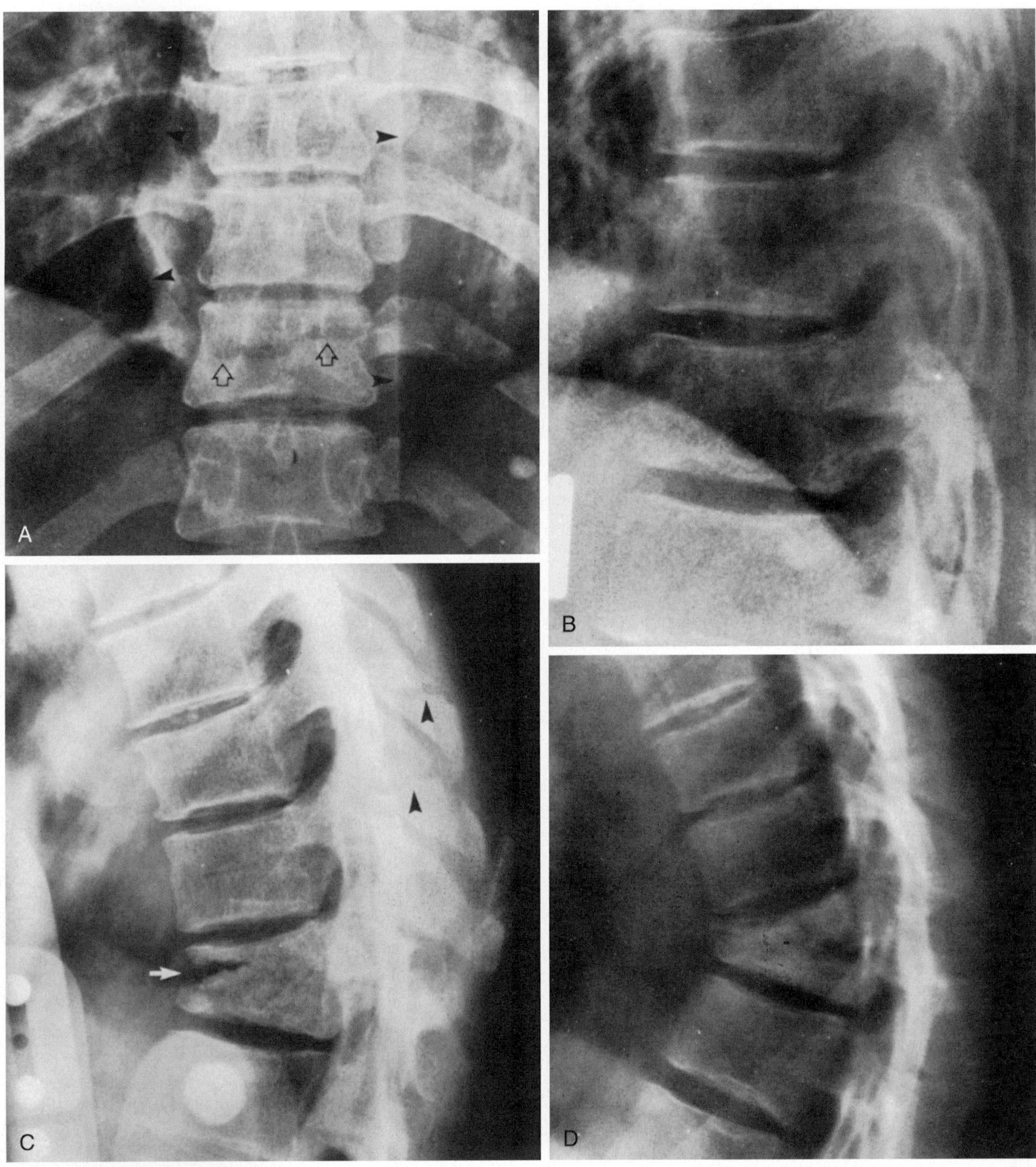

Figure 13–58. Kümmell's phenomenon. *A*, Anteroposterior view shows a transverse fracture involving the pedicles and lamina of T11 *(arrows)*. A paraspinous hematoma is present bilaterally *(arrowheads)*. *B*, Lateral radiograph demonstrates minimal anterior wedging of T11. *C*, Lateral view 9 weeks later demonstrates anterior compression of T11, with a peculiar lucency extending into the vertebral body *(arrow)*. Fractures of the laminae of T9 and T10 are also seen *(arrowheads)*, and the body of T11 is slightly increased in density. *D*, Lateral view 5 months post-injury demonstrates further collapse and increased density in the body of T11. The collapse has led to a kyphotic deformity, requiring surgical stabilization. The progressive collapse and increased density are indicative of the Kümmell phenomenon, probably representing a form of avascular necrosis.

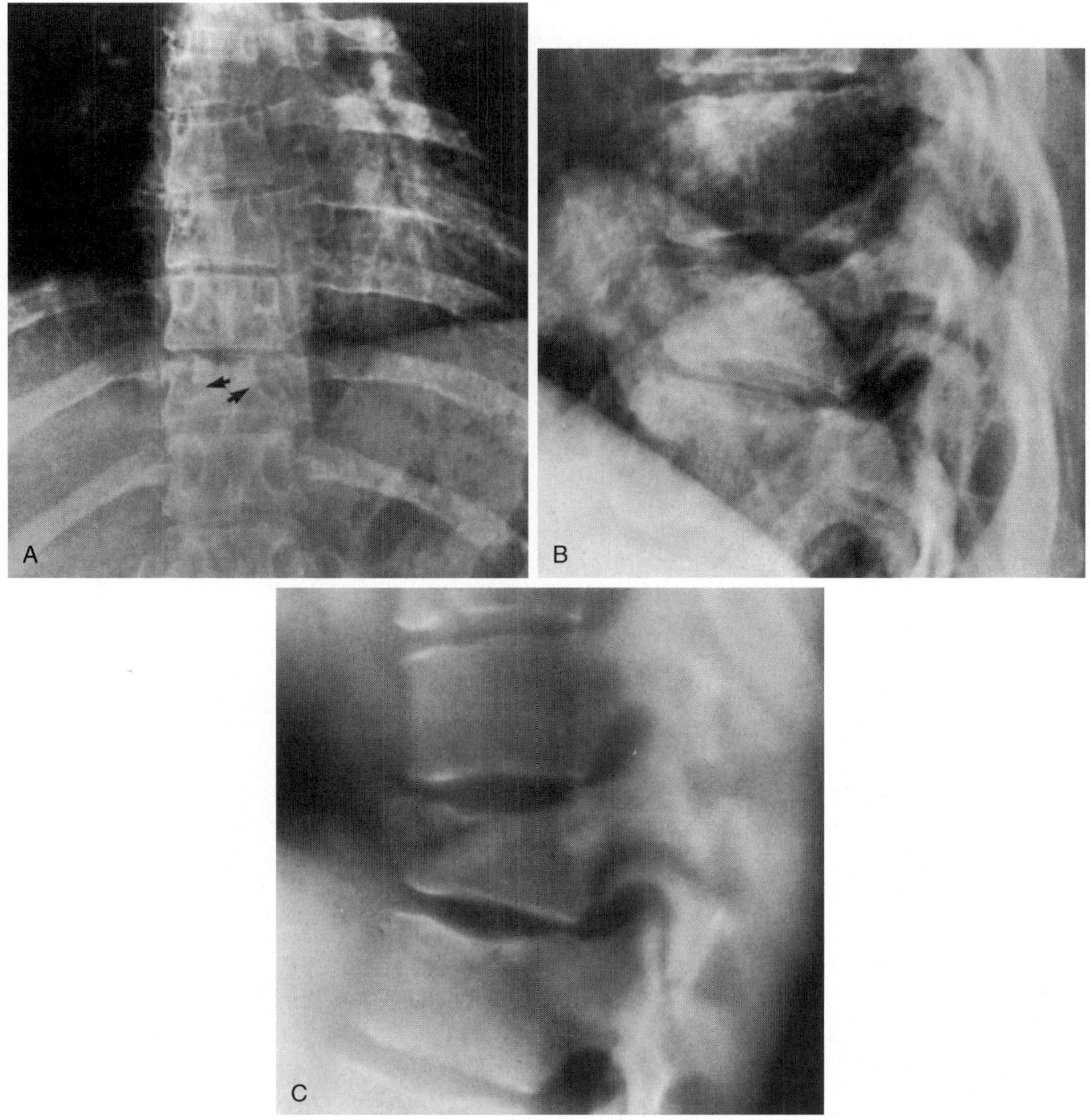

Figure 13–59. Flexion-distraction fracture of T10. *A*, Anteroposterior radiograph demonstrates a compression fracture of T10 with subtle disruption of the outline of the pedicles *(arrows)* and surrounding paraspinous hematoma. There are also compression fractures of T6 and T8. *B*, Lateral radiograph demonstrates an edge compression fracture of T10. *C*, Lateral tomogram reveals a horizontal fracture of the pedicle extending posteriorly through the lamina. Anteriorly, there is a vertical component of the fracture.

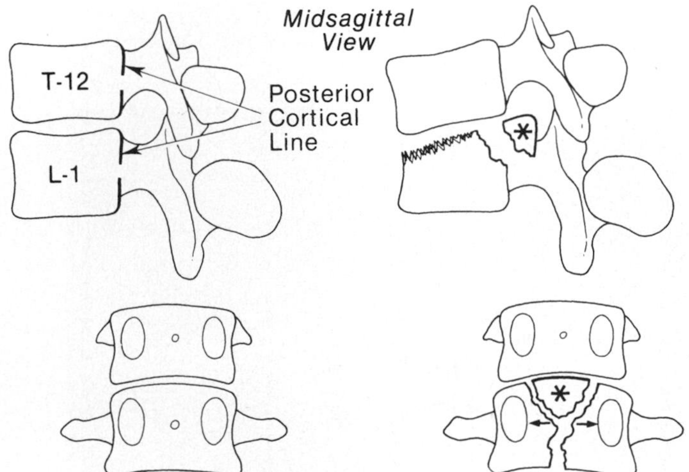

Figure 13–60. Features of burst fractures. On the lateral projection, the injury is characterized by an anterior wedge deformity of the vertebral body and retropulsion of a fragment from the posterior margin of the vertebral body. On frontal views, the injury is characterized by widening of the interpedicle distance and sagittal fractures of the inferior half of the vertebral body and lamina.

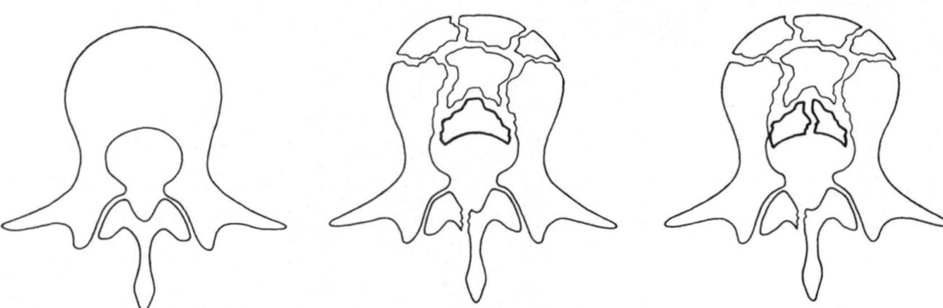

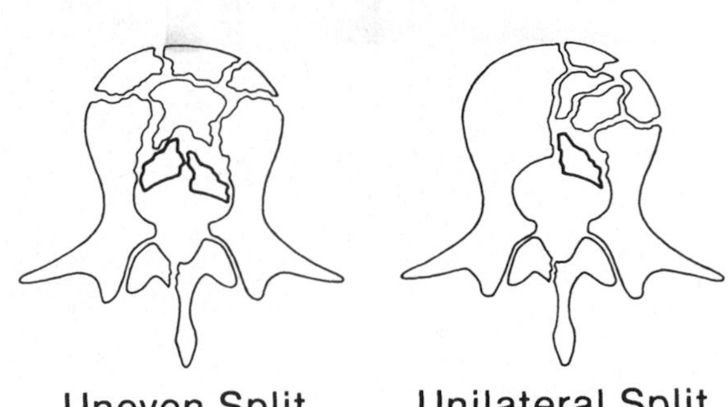

Figure 13–61. Variations in the configurations of burst fragments on CT. Most commonly, there is a single fragment, but often this fragment is separated into two or more components. On occasion, there is a single, unilateral fragment.

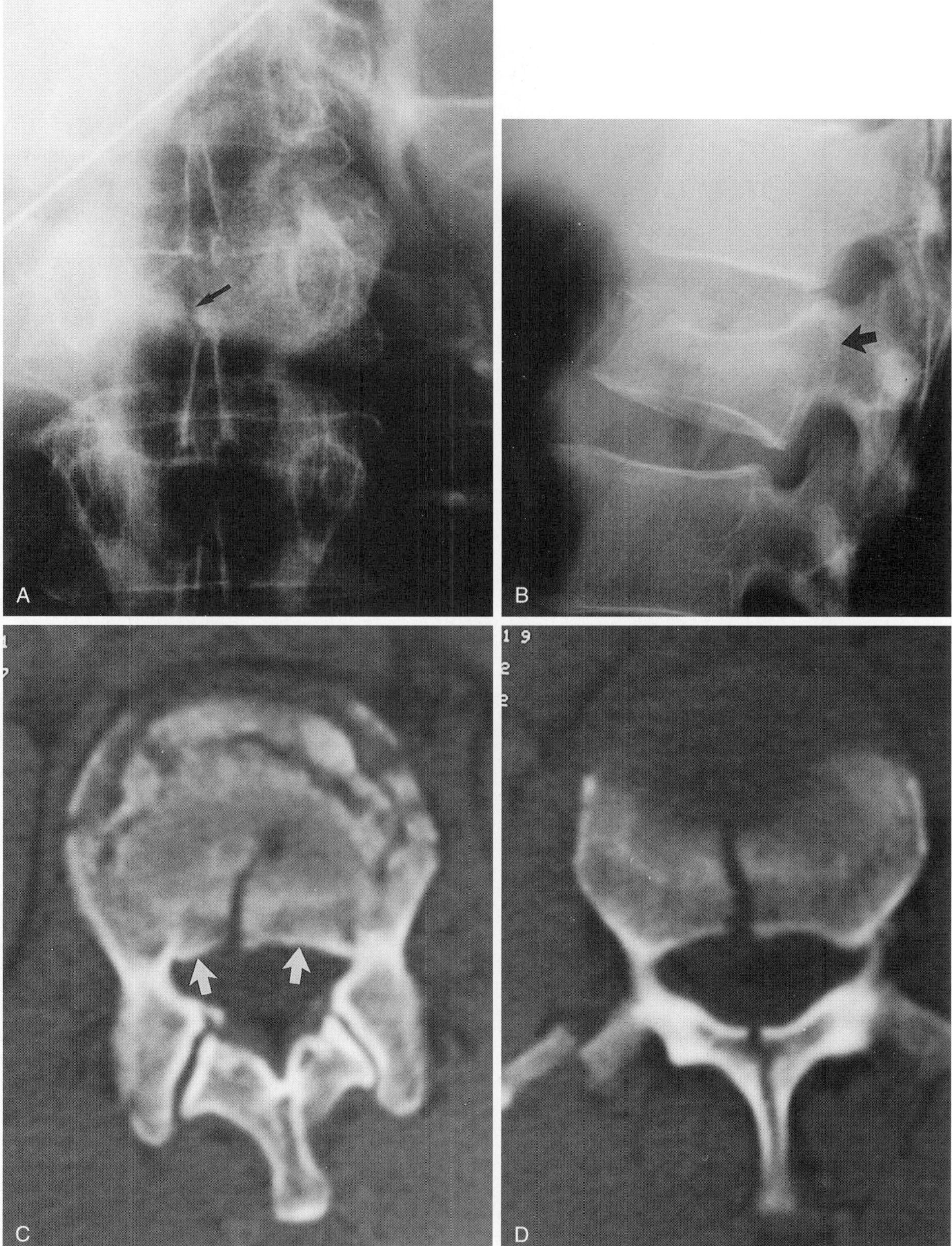

Figure 13–62. Classic radiographic appearance of a burst fracture. *A*, Anteroposterior view shows loss of height of the body of L1. The interpedicle distance is slightly widened. Note the sagittal fracture through the lamina *(arrow)*. *B*, Lateral radiograph shows anterior wedging, a small anterior superior bone fragment, and posterior displacement of the upper portion of the posterior vertebral body line *(arrow)*. *C*, CT image obtained through the upper portion of L1 shows two fragments of the posterior body displaced into the canal *(arrows)*. Note the anterior fragmentation and widening of the right facet joint. *D*, CT image obtained through the lower portion of L1 shows sagittal fractures of the vertebral body and the lamina. There is also a fracture of the right transverse process.

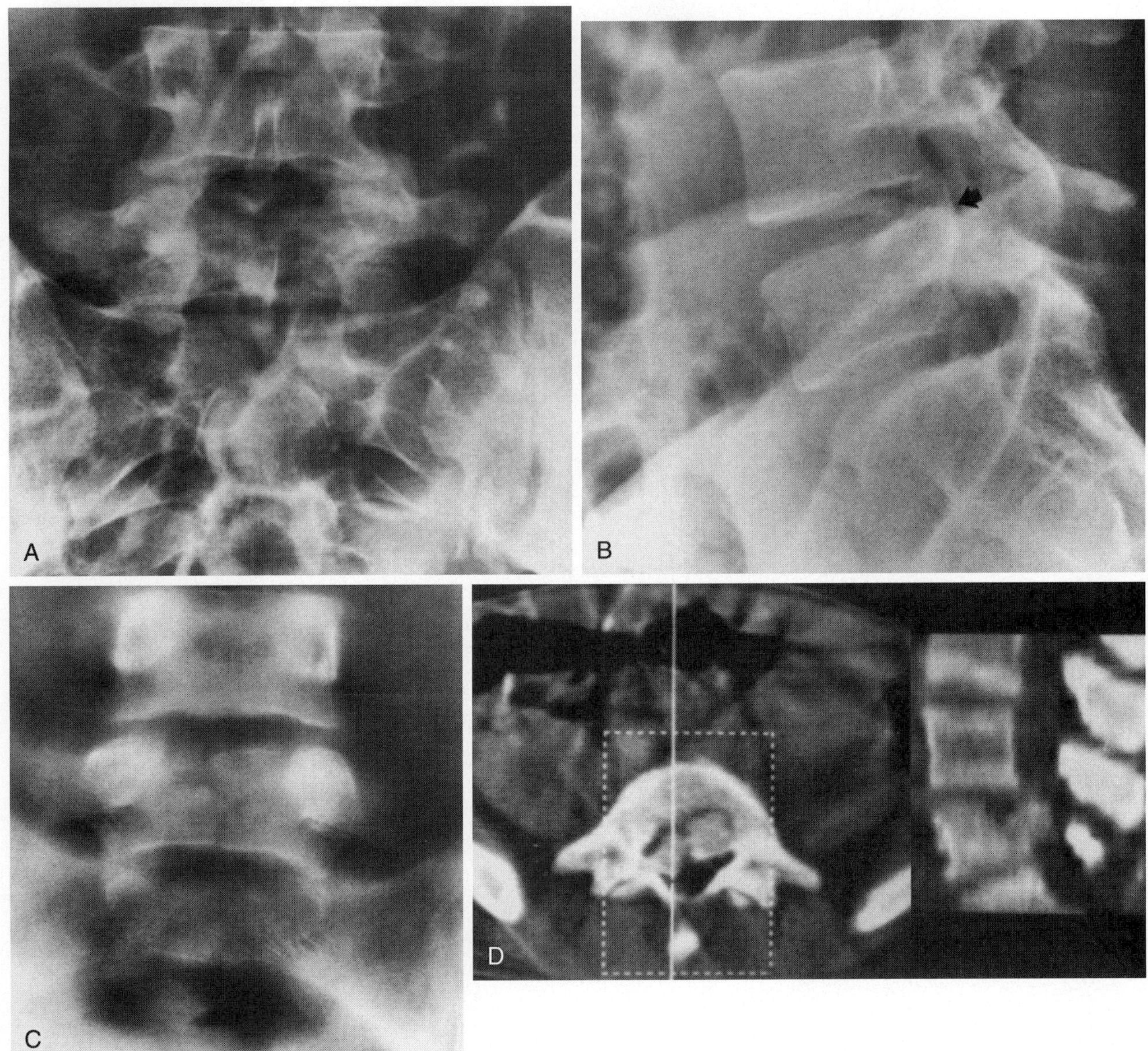

Figure 13–63. L5 burst fracture without significant loss of height. *A*, Anteroposterior view demonstrates a vague vertical lucency in L5. The superior end plate is poorly defined. *B*, Lateral radiograph shows minimal anterior wedging of L5, with posterior bowing of the posterior vertebral body line. A small fragment is displaced anteriorly *(arrow)*. *C*, Anteroposterior tomogram demonstrates a comminuted sagittal fracture of the vertebral body. *D*, CT image with sagittal reconstruction demonstrates the comminuted fracture of L5 with displacement of fragments into the vertebral canal. (Case courtesy of the late George Alker, MD, Buffalo, N.Y.)

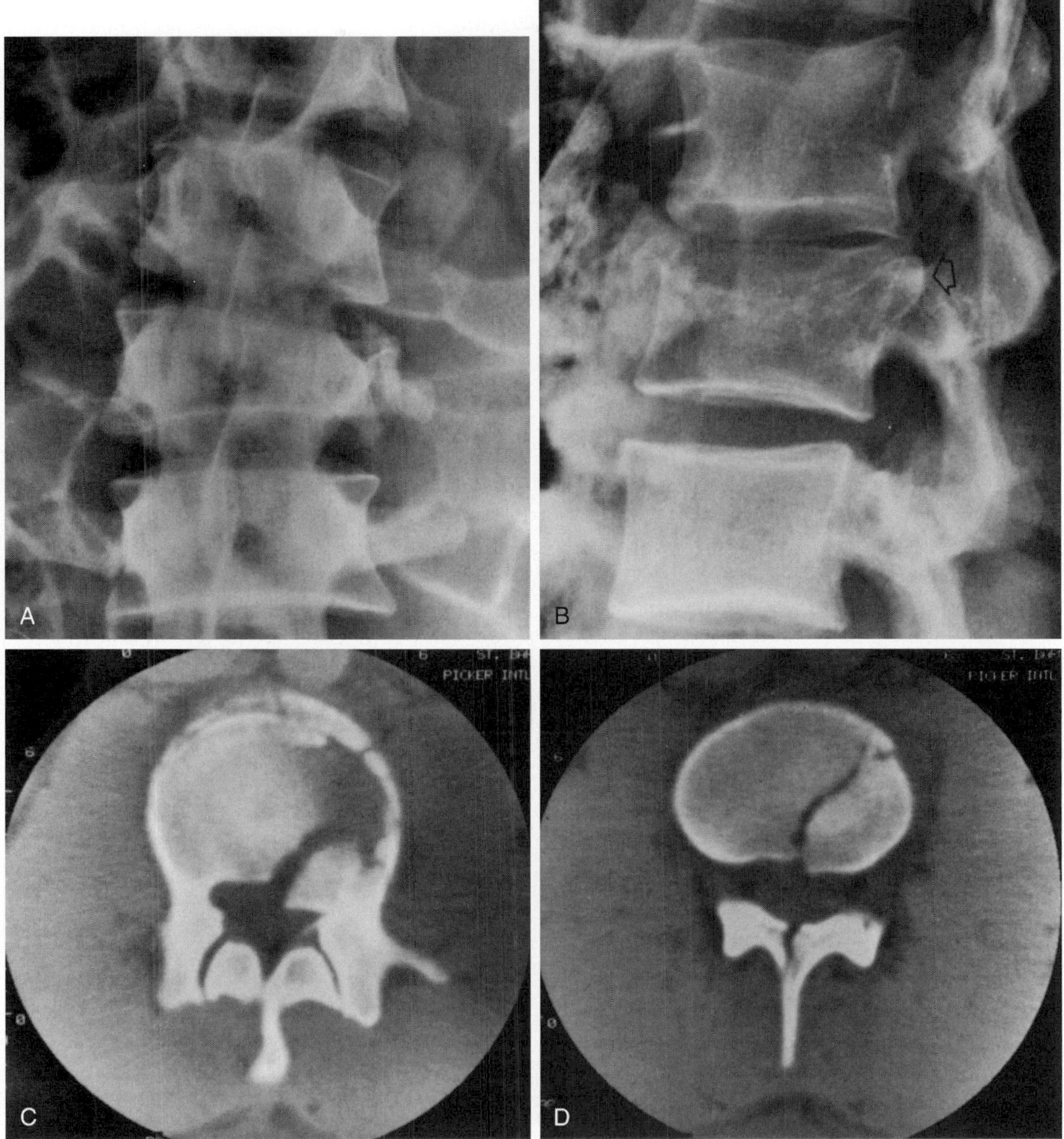

Figure 13–64. Unilateral burst fracture of L2. *A*, Anteroposterior view shows lateral wedge compression of L2 on the left. The interpedicle distance is widened. *B*, Lateral view demonstrates retropulsion of a fragment of the posterior vertebral body line with canal compromise *(arrow)*. *C*, CT image of the upper portion of L2 shows a comminuted fracture of the margins of the vertebral body and retropulsion of a unilateral bone fragment into the vertebral canal on the left. Note the wide facet joints. *D*, CT image of the lower portion of L2 reveals an obliquely oriented fracture of the inferior aspect of the vertebral body, as well as a laminar fracture. (Case courtesy of Mark Mishkin, MD, Philadelphia, Pa.)

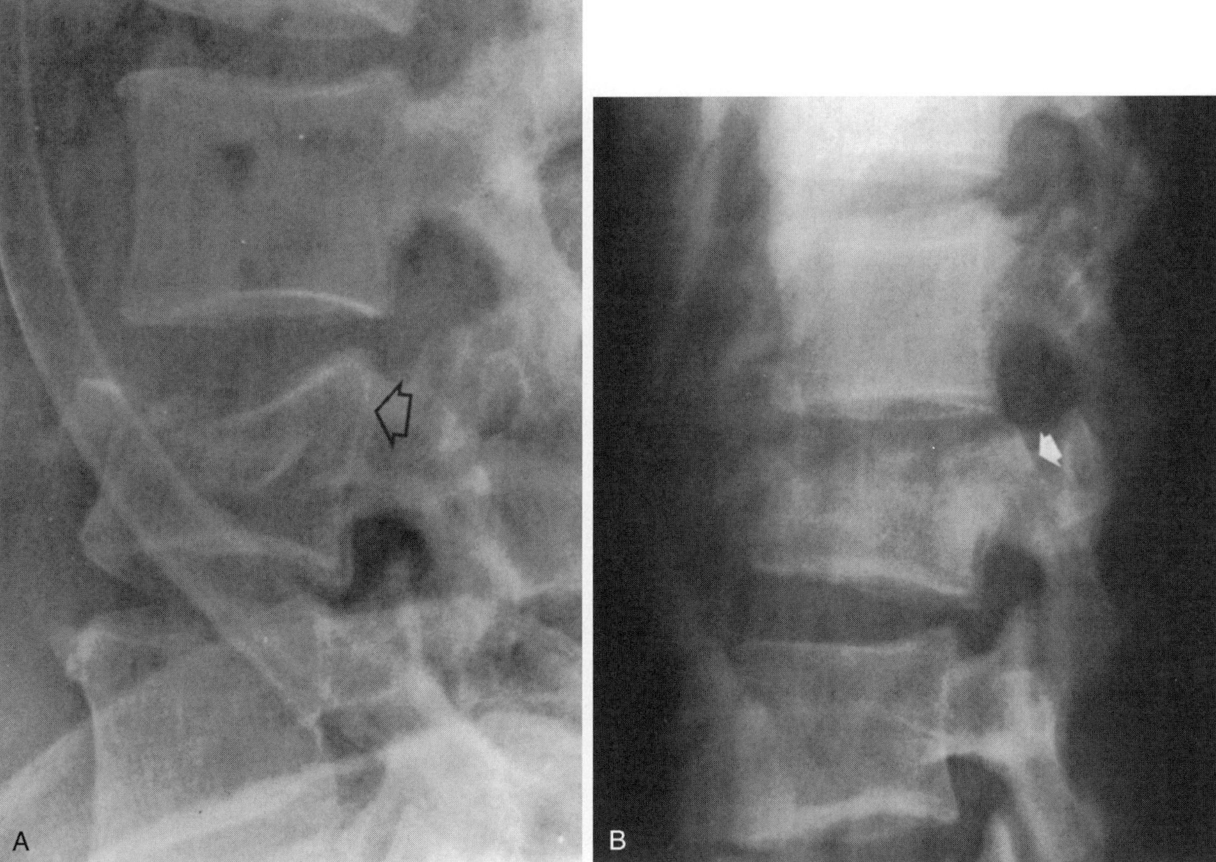

Figure 13–65. Differentiation of simple wedge fracture from a burst fracture. *A*, Lateral radiograph of a simple wedge compression fracture of L4 shows anterior compression and fragmentation. The posterior vertebral body line *(arrow)* of L4 remains aligned with that of adjacent vertebrae. *B*, Lateral radiograph of a burst fracture of L3 shows absence of the upper portion of the posterior vertebral body line, due to displacement into the vertebral canal *(arrow)*. The posterior vertebral body line is a reliable landmark to use in differentiating these two injuries.

wall of the vertebral body from the posterior superior corner and extending inferiorly to the midportion of the vertebral body, where it may not be as sharply defined in the region of the basivertebral foramen. The line then resumes again inferiorly, outlining the posterior inferior margin of the vertebral body. Any displacement, angulation, rotation, duplication, or absence of this line is abnormal and constitutes an indication for a CT examination. With a burst fracture, the superior or inferior portion of this line is displaced posteriorly or retropulsed into the vertebral canal (see Figs. 13–62 through 13–64). With a simple wedge compression fracture, this line may bulge slightly but is not retropulsed. On the frontal view the injury is occasionally suggested by the presence of a sagittal fracture in the inferior aspect of the vertebral body (see Figs. 13–38 and 13–63*A* and *C*). This finding is often obscured but is occasionally manifested by a distinct disruption of the inferior end plate in the midsagittal plane. Another more common and more easily identified sign is widening of the interpedicle distance of the involved vertebra. In 80% of cases this distance will be at least 2 mm greater than that for the vertebra above or below the level of injury.[5, 36] This widening is a sign of instability and is due to the combination of the sagittal fracture of the vertebra and simultaneous fractures in the laminae posteriorly.

CT will confirm the presence of the retropulsed fragment(s) and demonstrate fractures in the posterior elements, particularly the laminae, and the sagittal component in the vertebral body (see Figs. 13–38, 13–63, and 13–64).[81] The neurologic injury cannot be predicted by measuring the degree of displacement of the retropulsed fragment.[61, 158, 172] This limitation is logical when it is realized that the image demonstrates only the position in which the fragment came to rest. The fragment may have been retropulsed to a greater extent during the injury. The retropulsed fragment is rotated anteriorly to some extent.[81] In most cases, cortical bone will be seen on the posterior margin of the fragment, but with moderate to severe anterior tilting, the anterior margin of the fragment may consist of cortical bone, representing the tilted or rotated superior end plate.

If a burst fracture appears to have an anterior or lateral translational component, the injury is probably a rotary or shearing injury. These highly unstable injuries must be distinguished from burst fractures because their treatment requires stabilizing the rotary or oblique translational components in addition to the sagittal linear components. Features that indicate a rotary or shearing injury include anterior or lateral displacement, "windswept" appearance to the vertebrae, facet joint disruption, and rib or transverse process fractures. On CT images there is disruption of the facet joints with a circular array of bone fragments in rotary injuries (Fig. 13–66) and an oblique

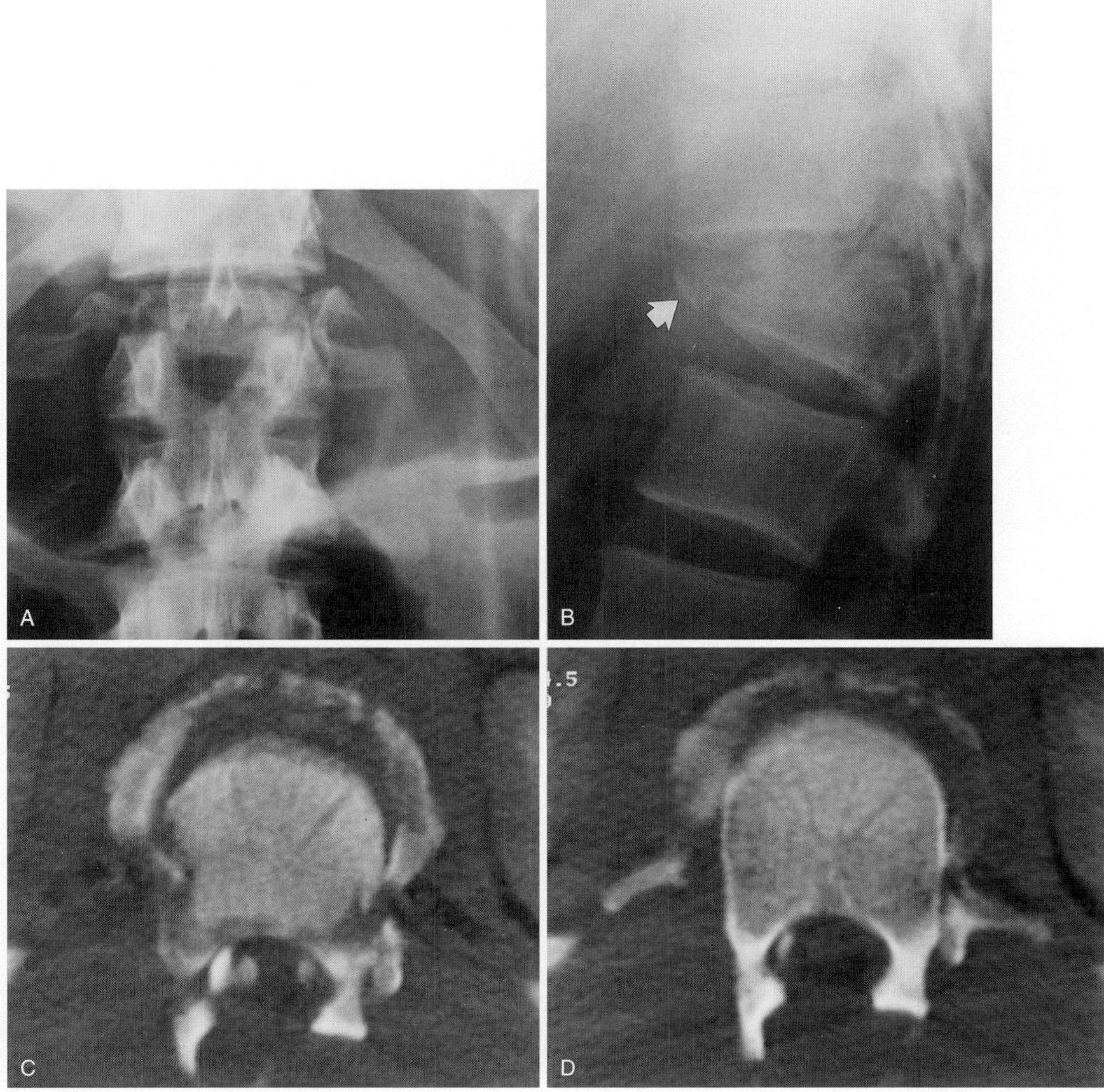

Figure 13–66. Classic radiographic appearance of a rotary ("grinding") injury. *A*, Anteroposterior radiograph shows comminution of the body of L1. The upper portion of the vertebral body is torn off, however. Note the transverse process fracture of L1 on the right. *B*, Lateral radiograph shows anterior dislocation of T12 on L1. An avulsed fragment of the anterior superior portion of L1 is displaced forward, maintaining its normal anatomic relationship to T12 *(arrow)*. This appearance is termed the "ripped can top sign." *C*, CT image obtained through the upper portion of L1 shows the avulsed, fractured segments arrayed in circular fashion anteriorly, fractures of the pedicles, bone fragments in the vertebral canal, and naked facets. *D*, CT image obtained at a slightly higher level reveals the naked facets posteriorly and fractures of both transverse processes.

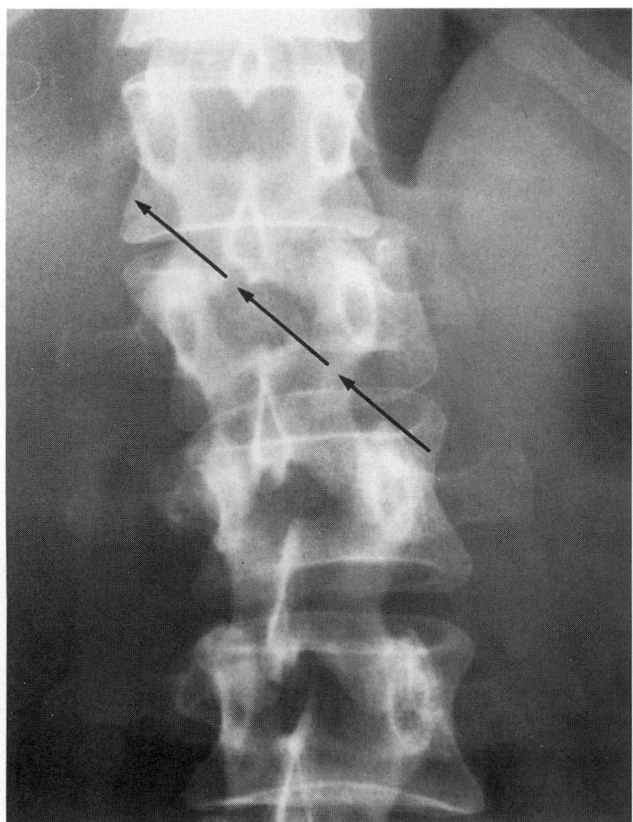

Figure 13–67. Classic radiographic appearance of a shearing injury. This anteroposterior radiograph shows a "windswept" appearance of the spine. The *arrows* indicate the direction of the injury forces. Note the transverse process fracture of L2 on the left.

linear array of fragments (windswept appearance) in shearing injuries[36] (Fig. 13–67).

Burst fractures are, by definition, unstable because they involve all three of Denis' columns.[36, 39, 46] Nonetheless, some burst fractures considered "stable" can be treated conservatively if the posterior longitudinal ligament, although stretched by the retropulsed fragment, is otherwise intact. The determination of the integrity of this ligament can be made by MRI. Other factors that will aid the surgeon in the decision between conservative and operative treatment include the distance of the retropulsed fragment (over 2 mm), the presence of a sagittal split component to the injury, and the presence of posterior element fractures. It is important for the radiologist to accurately describe all of the findings in the report and to communicate verbally any opinions regarding instability.

Surgical stabilization of fractures and fracture-dislocations is performed to prevent subsequent deformities, the development of neurologic abnormalities, or the worsening of such existing abnormalities.[107, 114, 126, 139] These deformities arise from instability due to a combination of disruptions in each of the three columns—the anterior, middle, and posterior—with post-traumatic collapse of the vertebral body. This is discussed in greater detail later.

Fracture-Dislocations: Translation, Rotary, and Shearing Injuries

Fracture-dislocation is the result of a combination of flexion, axial compression, rotational, and shearing forces.[162] The characteristic features are anterior or lateral displacement of the vertebrae above the level of injury with a variable degree of anterior wedging of the vertebra below, with a characteristic triangular fragment torn from the anterior superior margin.[36, 113] The appearance is that of a ripped top of an aluminum can (see Fig. 13–66). Less commonly, there is lateral displacement or translation and, rarely, posterior displacement.[144, 160] In rotary injuries, the posterior vertebral body line is disrupted. It may or may not be involved in shearing injuries. Posterior column injuries consist of tears of the supraspinous, interspinous, and yellow (ligamentum flavum) ligaments and disruption of the facet joints, with accompanying fractures of the superior facets and laminae (Fig. 13–68). Perching or locking of the facets is common.[69, 125, 131, 144, 160] Fractures of the transverse processes or lower ribs (see Fig. 13–66) are common features, reflecting the rotary or shearing forces that produced the injury.[36] When rotatory and shearing forces are added to or superimposed on axial compression, flexion-distraction, or distraction mechanisms, a dislocation occurs in association with fractures consistent with these underlying forces. The injuries are all grossly unstable because the disruption involves all

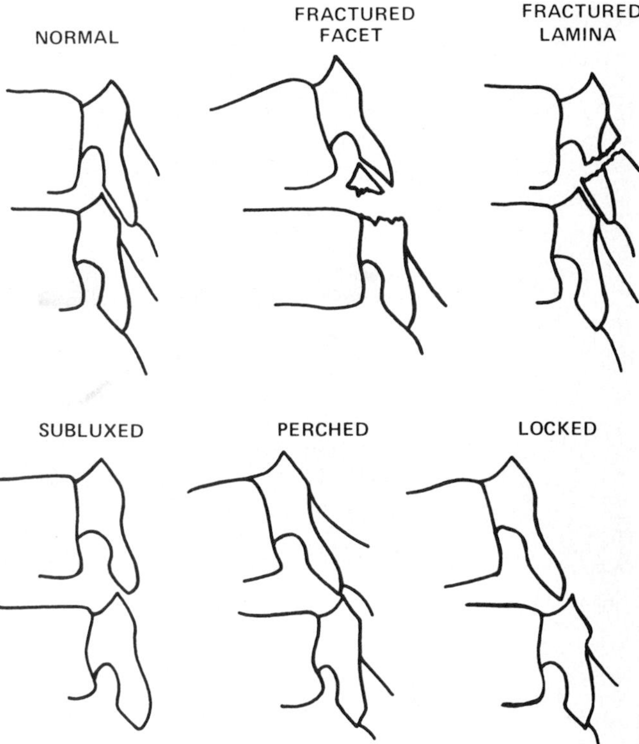

Figure 13–68. Types of disruption of facet joints and fractures of posterior elements encountered in vertebral fracture-dislocations. (From Rogers, L. F., Thayer, C., Weinberg, P. E., & Kim, K. S. [1980]. Acute injuries of the upper thoracic spine associated with paraplegia. A.J.R. Am. J. Roentgenol., *134*:67.)

three columns. The rotary fracture-dislocation is the most severe of all vertebral injuries.

All of these injuries, regardless of mechanism of origin, are associated with severe neurologic deficits.[35, 36] Those injuries occurring at the first through the eighth thoracic vertebrae (Fig. 13–69) are almost invariably associated with a complete motor and sensory deficit;[165] 60% to 70% of fracture-dislocations of the thoracolumbar junction are associated with a neurologic deficit.[93, 94] The most common site for a fracture-dislocation of the upper thoracic spine is at the level of T4–T5 and T5–T6[26, 85] (Fig. 13–70); most occur in motorcyclists.[40] The most frequent site of a dislocation of the thoracolumbar junction is at T11–L1[36, 52, 93] (Fig. 13–71). Fracture-dislocations at the lumbosacral junction are rare[37, 43, 77, 79] (Fig. 13–72). In adolescents, fracture-dislocations may occur through the ring apophysis of the vertebral body at any level[128] (Fig. 13–73).

Frequently, the fracture-dislocation is partially reduced by simply placing the patient supine with the shoulders in line with the pelvis. Accordingly, it is quite likely that the amount of displacement demonstrated on the radiographic examination is considerably less than that created at the time of injury.[52, 93, 163] The displacement may be so minimal that it is difficult to appreciate. MRI examination will invariably be performed and will show severe bone and soft tissue damage, as well as either transection of the spinal cord or cauda equina or internal damage to the cord itself[35, 36] (Fig. 13–74). A CT examination will display all the characteristic features of either a rotary or a shearing injury, however. As mentioned previously, rotary and shearing injuries are frequently confused with burst fractures because of the crush of the vertebral body and abnormalities of the posterior vertebral body line. It is imperative that the radiologist make this distinction, because, as mentioned, the treatment is significantly different for each injury. The hazard of not recognizing the type of injury and not treating it properly is illustrated in Figure 13–75.

Fracture-Dislocation of Upper Dorsal Spine

Mid-thoracic and upper thoracic fracture-dislocations may be difficult to demonstrate because of the minimal lateral displacement or rotation at the fracture site.[40] Furthermore, the neurologic deficit produced by the thoracic injury may be masked by an accompanying cerebral injury—a common combination in my experience. In many injuries in this region the paraspinous hematoma may be the first clue to the existence of the abnormality (Fig. 13–76). With injuries of the upper dorsal spine, the paraspinous hematoma may dissect over the apex of the lung, forming a pleural cap (see Fig. 13–9). The mediastinal hematoma associated with upper dorsal or lower cervical spinal fracture mimics that associated with an aortic rupture.[48] In most major Level I trauma centers, any

Text continued on page 514

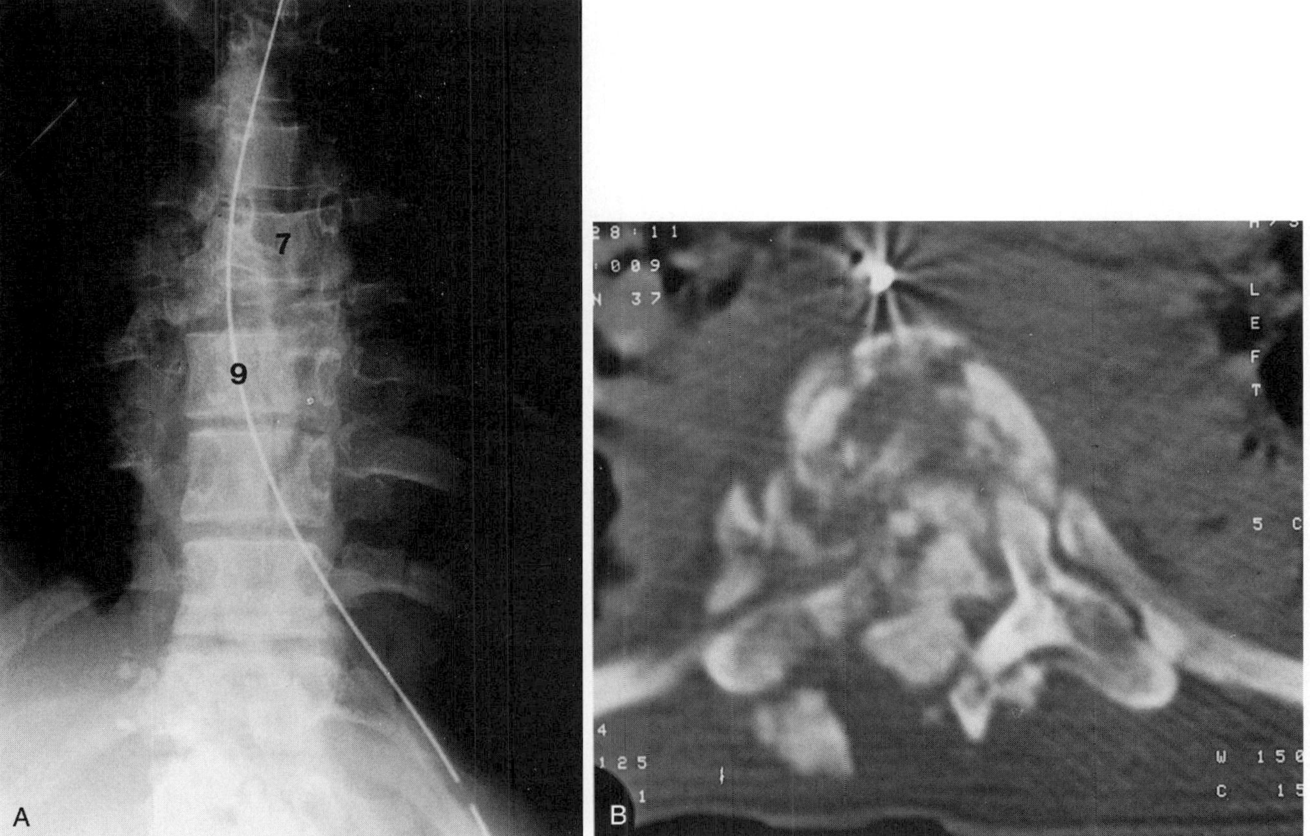

Figure 13–69. T7–T8 fracture-dislocation in a motorcyclist. *A*, Anteroposterior radiograph shows displacement of T7 to the left. T8 has been virtually disintegrated. Note the fractures at T12 and L1, as well as multiple rib fractures. *B*, CT image obtained through T8 shows the vertebra to be pulverized. The patient was, not surprisingly, paraplegic.

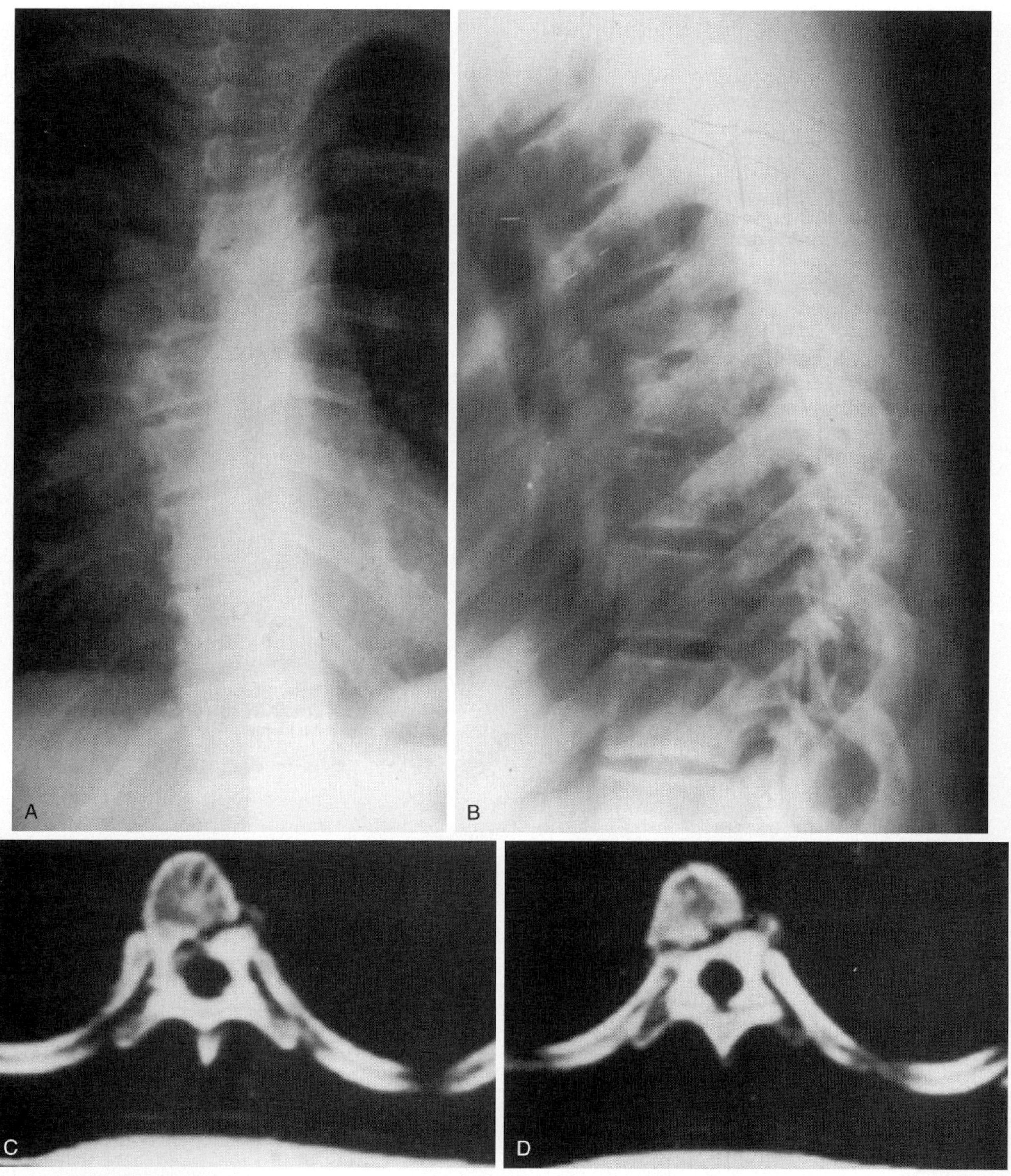

Figure 13–70. Severe upper thoracic fracture-dislocation in a motorcyclist. *A*, Anteroposterior radiograph demonstrates angulation of the mid-thoracic column, with fractures of multiple contiguous vertebrae. *B*, Lateral view shows fractures of multiple vertebral bodies and kyphotic angulation of the mid-thoracic region. *C* and *D*, CT images show coronally oriented fractures of the posterior vertebral bodies and pedicles that spare the vertebral canal. Despite the extent of the injury, the patient was, surprisingly, neurologically intact. (Case courtesy of Srikanta Siddalingappa, MD, Pontiac, Ill.)

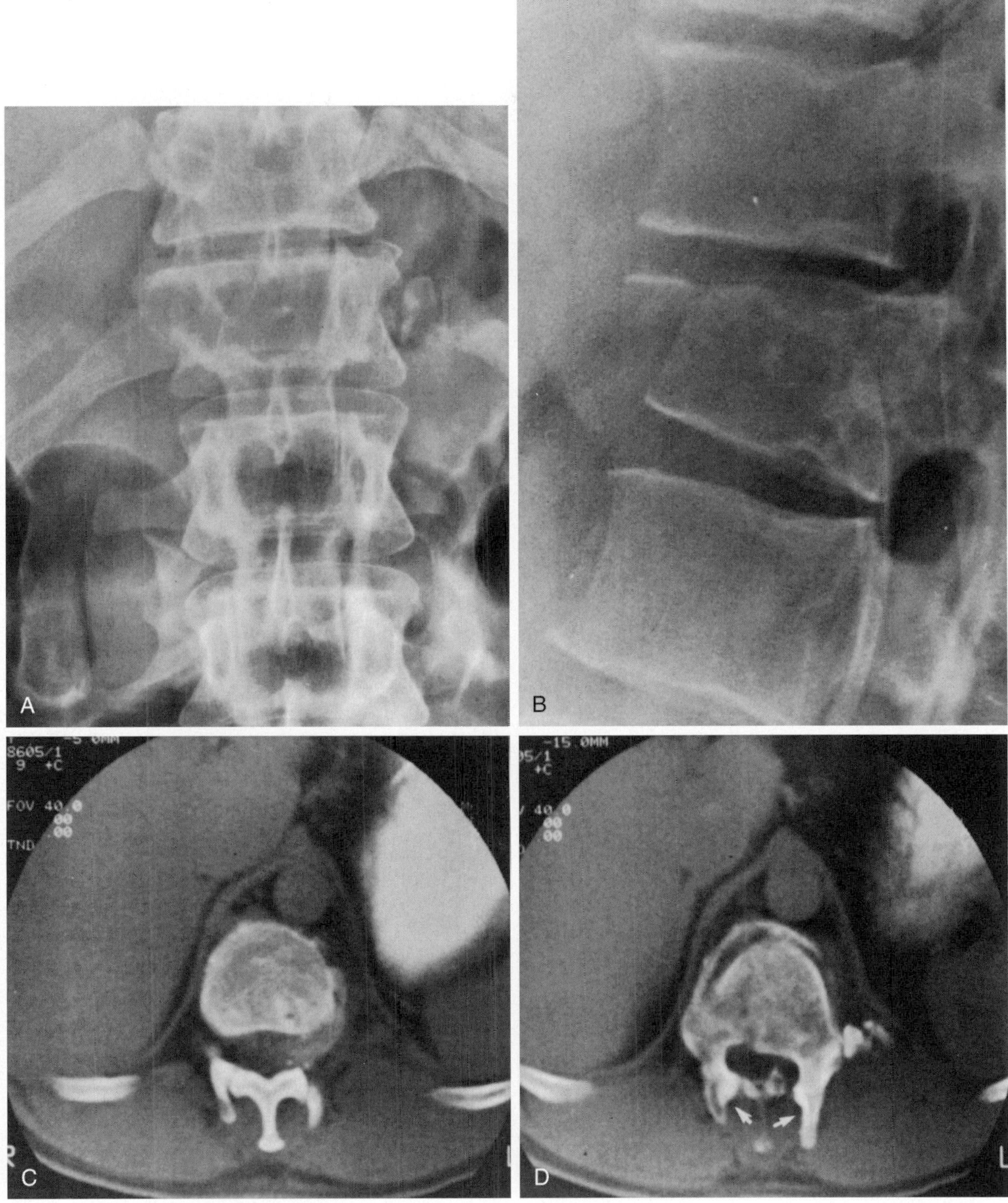

Figure 13–71. Rotary fracture-dislocation of T11–T12. *A*, Anteroposterior view demonstrates flattening of the body of T12, with widening of the interspinous distance between T11 and T12. There are obvious fractures of the lateral margins of the body and pedicle of T12 on the right. *B*, Lateral view confirms anterior dislocation with a "ripped can top" avulsed fragment from the superior margin of T12. The posterior vertebral body line is missing, indicating disruption of that structure. *C*, CT image obtained through the inferior aspect of T11 shows disruption of the facet joints, particularly on the left. *D*, CT image obtained through the upper portion of T12 shows fractures of the vertebral body in a circular array, fractured left transverse process, and naked facets *(arrows)*.

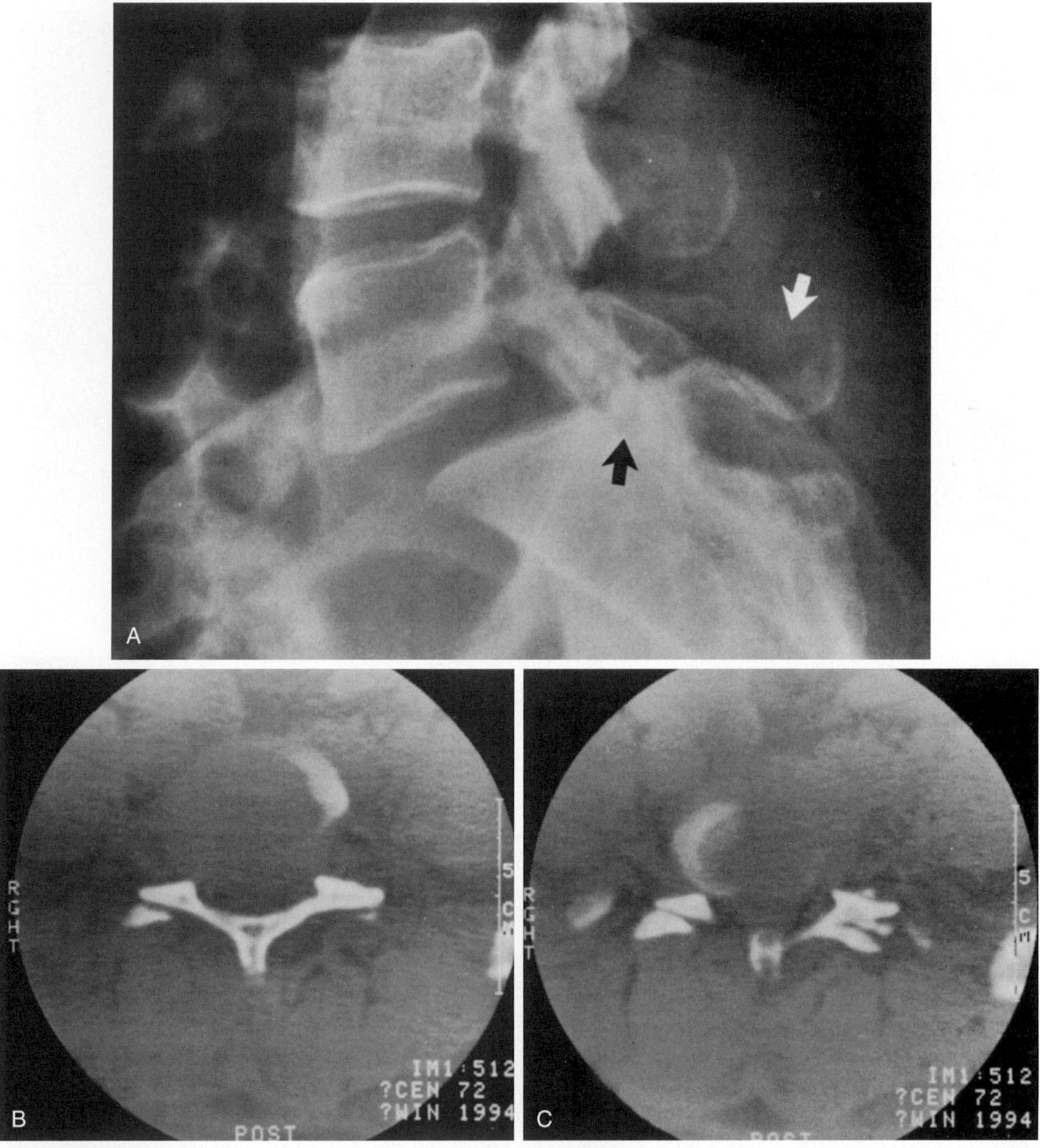

Figure 13–72. Dislocation of L5 on S1 with bilateral facet lock. *A*, Lateral radiograph shows the body of L5 displaced anteriorly and a fracture of the L5 spinous process *(white arrow)*; the appearance also suggests that the inferior facets of L5 lie anterior to the superior facets of S1 *(black arrow)*. *B*, CT image obtained through the L5–S1 interspace shows naked inferior facets of L5 lying anterior to the tips of the superior facets of S1. *C*, CT image obtained at a slightly lower level shows bilateral facet lock. On the left the superior facet of S1 is fractured.

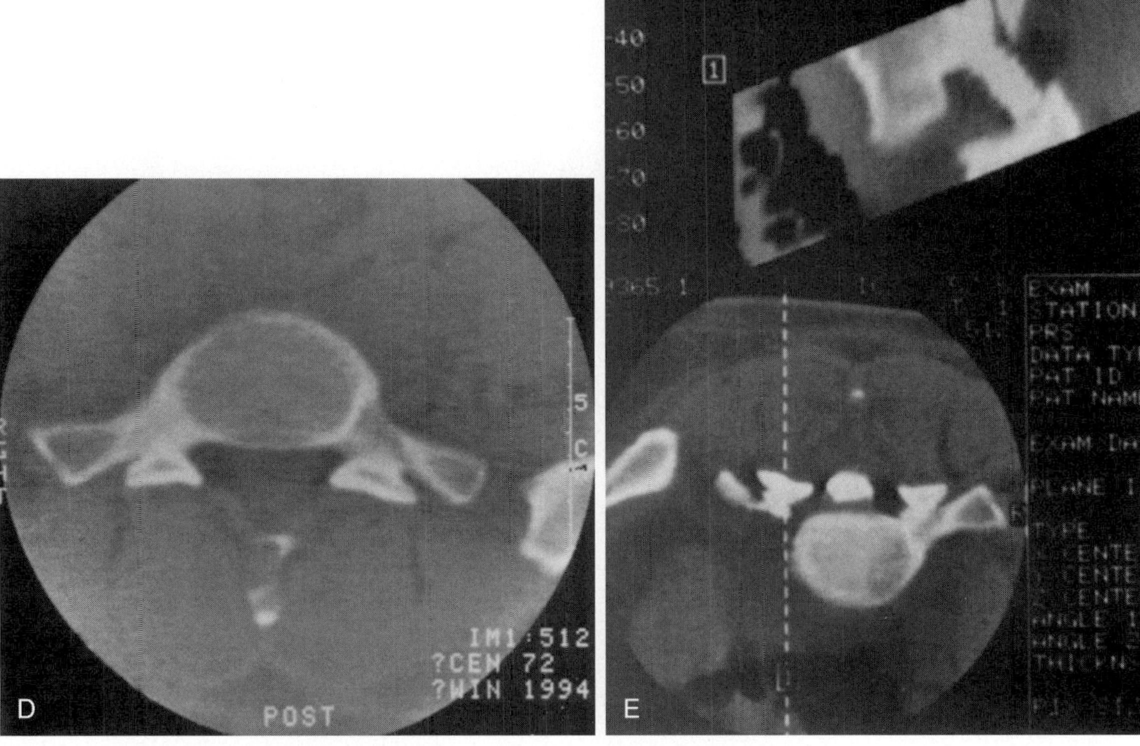

Figure 13–72 *Continued. D*, CT image obtained through the superior surface of S1 demonstrates naked facets. *E*, Sagittal reconstructed CT image shows facet lock.

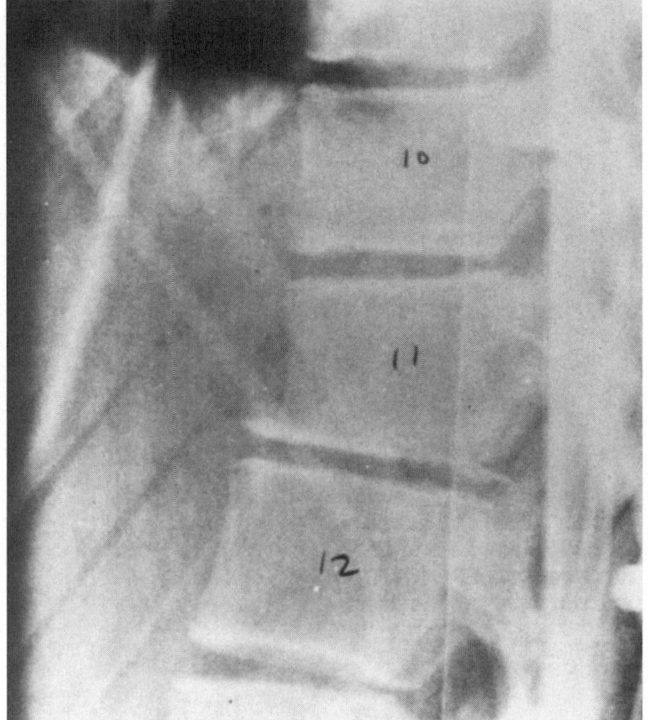

Figure 13–73. Fracture-dislocation through the ring apophysis of T11 in a 13-year-old. The inferior ring apophysis of T11 maintains its normal relationship with T12. The body of T11 is displaced posteriorly.

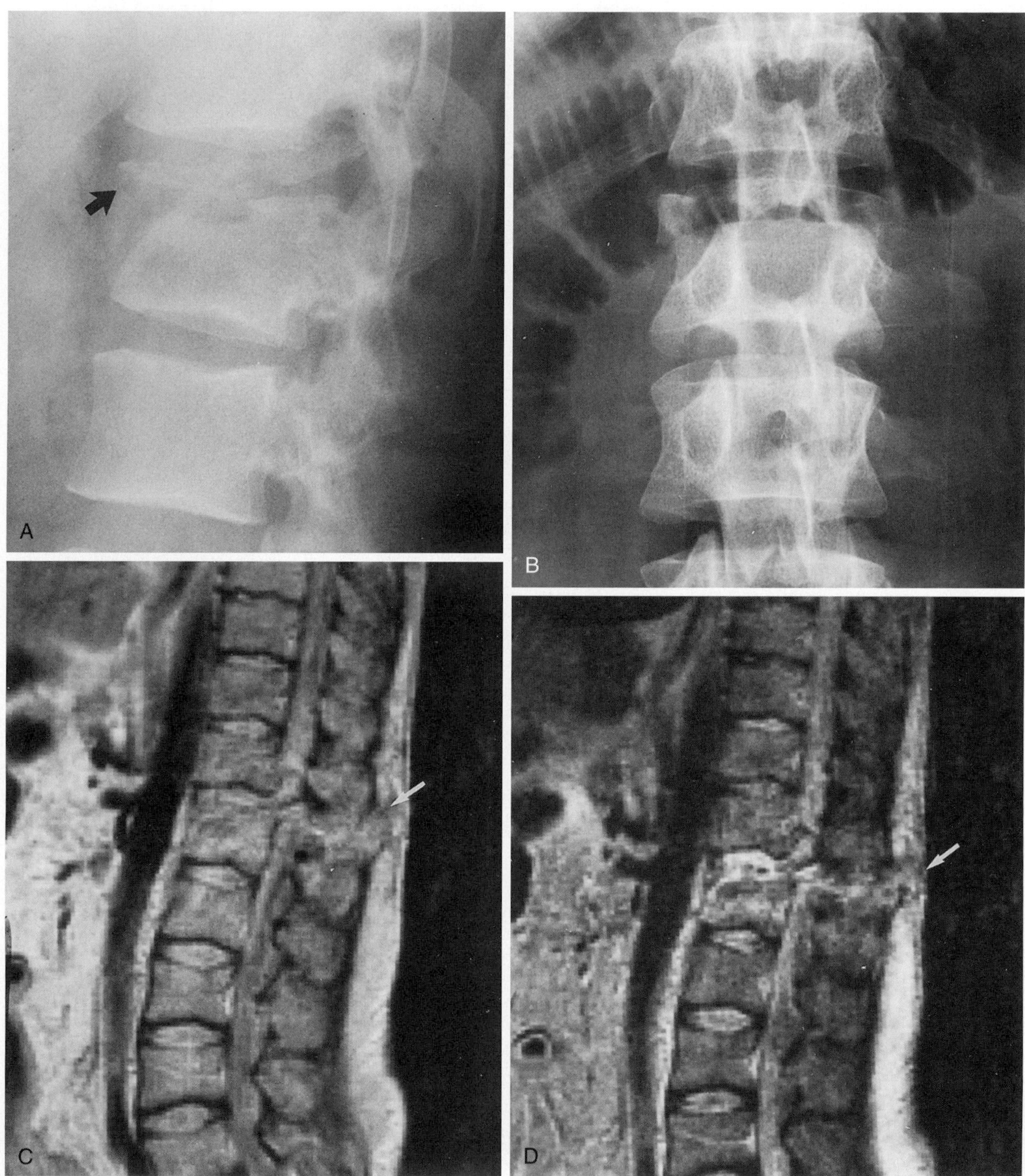

Figure 13–74. Rotary fracture-dislocation of T12–L1. *A* Lateral radiograph shows a horizontal fracture through L1 and minimal anterior displacement of T12 on L1. Note the "ripped can top" fragment *(arrow)*. *B*, Anteroposterior radiograph shows posterior distraction of T12 on L1, manifested as widening of the interspinous space and naked facets. The fracture of the top of L1 is faintly visible. Note also fractures of the transverse processes of L1 and L2 on the left. *C* and *D*, T_1-weighted and T_2-weighted sagittal MR images, respectively, show extensive anterior and posterior damage *(arrows)*. Note the transection of the thecal sac in *D*.

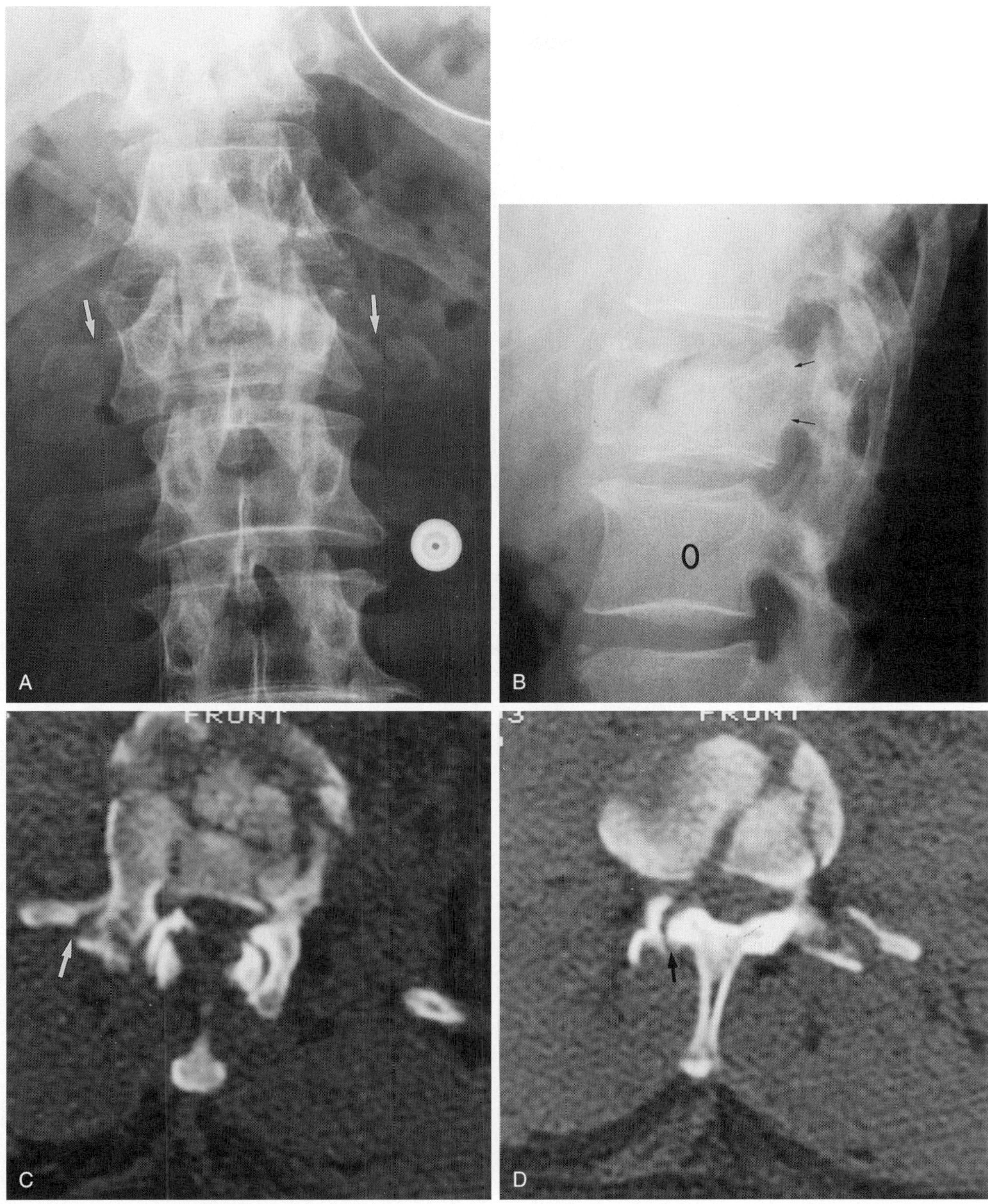

Figure 13–75. Importance of being able to differentiate a burst fracture from a rotary injury. *A*, Anteroposterior radiograph shows widening of the interpedicle distance and loss of the outline of the superior end plate of T1. Note the transverse process fractures of L1 *(arrows)*. *B*, Lateral radiograph shows a vertical fracture through the anterior body of L1 and posterior bowing of the posterior vertebral body line *(arrows)*. *C*, CT image shows severe comminution of the body of L1 as well as retropulsion of a bone fragment into the vertebral canal. Note the transverse process fracture on the right *(arrow)*. *D*, CT image slightly lower shows disruption of the right facet joint *(arrow)* as well as a transverse process fracture on the left.

Illustration continued on following page

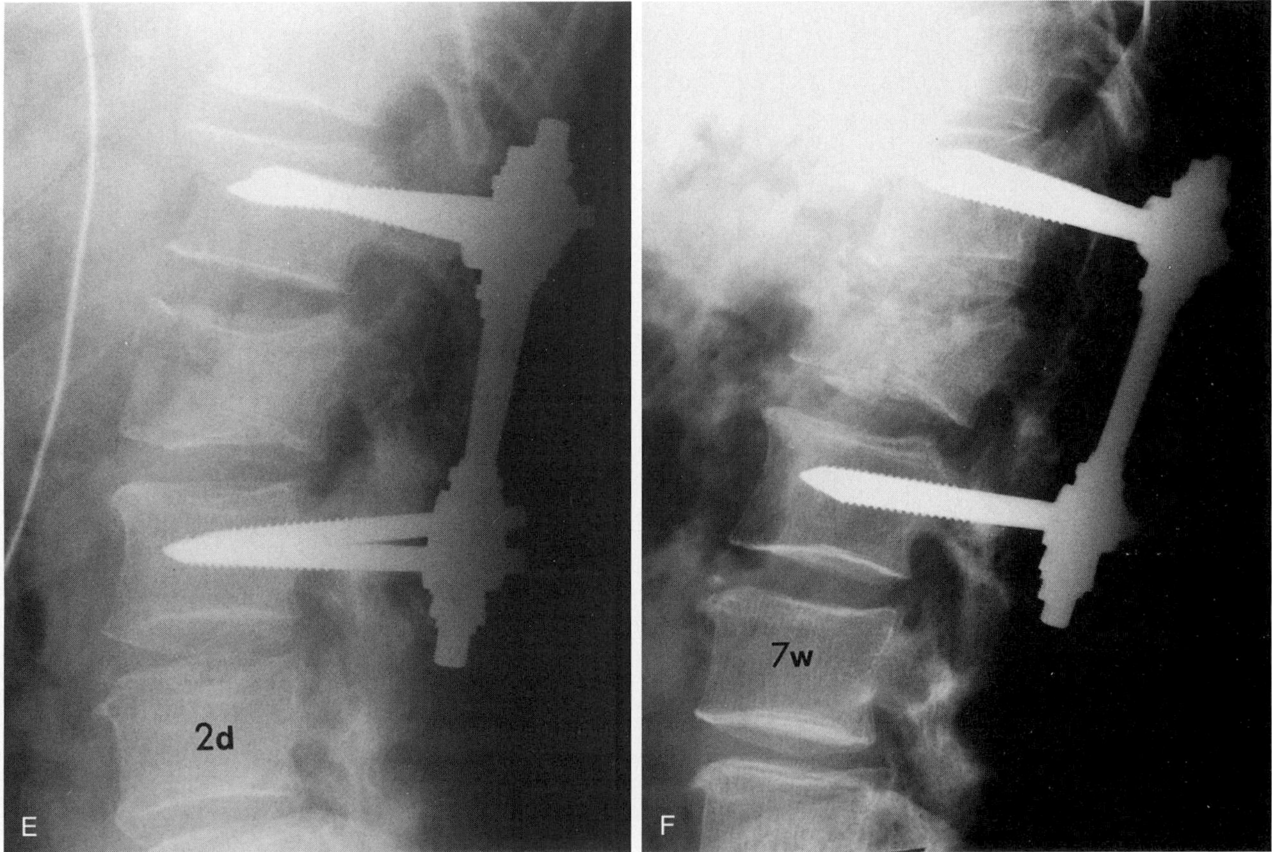

Figure 13–75 *Continued. E,* This lateral radiograph was obtained 2 days after the patient underwent surgical stabilization for a presumed burst fracture with pedicle screws and rods placed between T12 and L2. There was no stabilization for the rotary component of this highly unstable injury. *F,* Lateral radiograph obtained 7 weeks later shows collapse of L1 and retrolisthesis of T12 on L1. This injury resembled a burst fracture in most ways except for the fact that there were transverse process fractures—an unusual finding in burst injuries.

stable trauma victim with a wide mediastinum is likely to undergo a thoracic CT examination. This study is usually enough to rule out aortic or great vessel injury as the cause of mediastinal hematoma, as well as to demonstrate the thoracic vertebral injury. Fortunately, the combination of aortic rupture and upper thoracic fracture is rare. It is important to identify the presence of an upper thoracic injury because inadvertent manipulation of an unstable injury without a neurologic deficit may lead to a spinal cord injury.

Angulation in the sagittal plane may be identified on the frontal projection by an abrupt change in the projection of adjacent vertebrae. Below the level of dislocation the *vertebral bodies* may be seen in profile, whereas above this level the *laminae* may be identified in profile. Lateral displacement is characteristically minimal, and the lateral margins of the vertebrae must be scrutinized to determine the presence of displacement (Fig. 13–77). Similarly, the vertebral alignment can be determined by following the course of the spinous processes. These observations are particularly important because it is difficult to obtain a satisfactory radiograph of the mid-thoracic and upper thoracic spine in the lateral projection.

An unusual form of extensive fracture and dislocation occurs in the dorsal spine that, despite its radiographic appearance, is not accompanied by a neurologic deficit.[53, 167, 186] The injury involves multiple contiguous vertebrae. The dominant features are fractures in the coronal plane at the junction of the vertebral bodies and pedicles that separate the posterior elements from the vertebral bodies. This shearing is associated with lateral vertebral body compression and offset at the apex of the angulation. The separation of the posterior elements from the vertebral bodies results in decompression of the vertebral canal; thus, the cord is spared from injury. At the level of dislocation the vertebra above is commonly displaced inferiorly, by at least half the width of the vertebral body below. The coronal fracture of the pedicles is best demonstrated by CT.

The mediastinum may also be widened by hematomas caused by fractures of the sternum. Injuries of the sternum, particularly those involving the manubriosternal joint, have been reported to occur in association with fractures of the dorsal spine (Fig. 13–78), particularly of the mid-dorsal spine, but less commonly with fractures of the cervicothoracic or thoracolumbar junction.[76, 106, 108, 127, 134, 152] The combination of injury to the thoracic spine and to the sternum is usually due to flexion and compression of the trunk and infrequently occurs as the result of a simultaneous direct blow to the sternum. Spontaneous fractures of the sternum occur as the result of severe kyphotic deformities in the osteoporotic spine.[102]

Traumatic subarachnoid-pleural fistulas have been described as a source of persistent clear pleural effusion complicating fractures and fracture-dislocations of the thoracic spine.[23] Pneumorrhachis (air in the spinal canal) may occur because of jejunal entrapment within a fracture-dislocation of the lumbar spine.[174]

Minimal anterior or posterior subluxation may occur without associated fracture but with spinal cord injury. Traumatic paraplegia with injury levels in the upper dorsal spine may occur in the absence of fracture or dislocation. The mechanism is similar to that encountered in the cervical spine: A hyperextension injury results in compression of the cord between the ligamenta flava posteriorly and apposing margins of the vertebral bodies and intervertebral disc anteriorly, producing cord injury.

Fracture-Dislocations of Thoracolumbar Junction and Lumbar Spine

The typical fracture-dislocation at the thoracolumbar junction (see Figs. 13–11 and 13–71) is similar in appearance to that described elsewhere in the thoracic spine. However, there is usually less compression of the vertebral body below the level of dislocation.[163] The intervening facet joints are disrupted, with fractures of the superior facets of the vertebral body below the dislocation, or with locking or perching of the facets (Fig. 13–79; see also Fig. 13–71), similar to that seen in fracture-dislocation, as described previously.

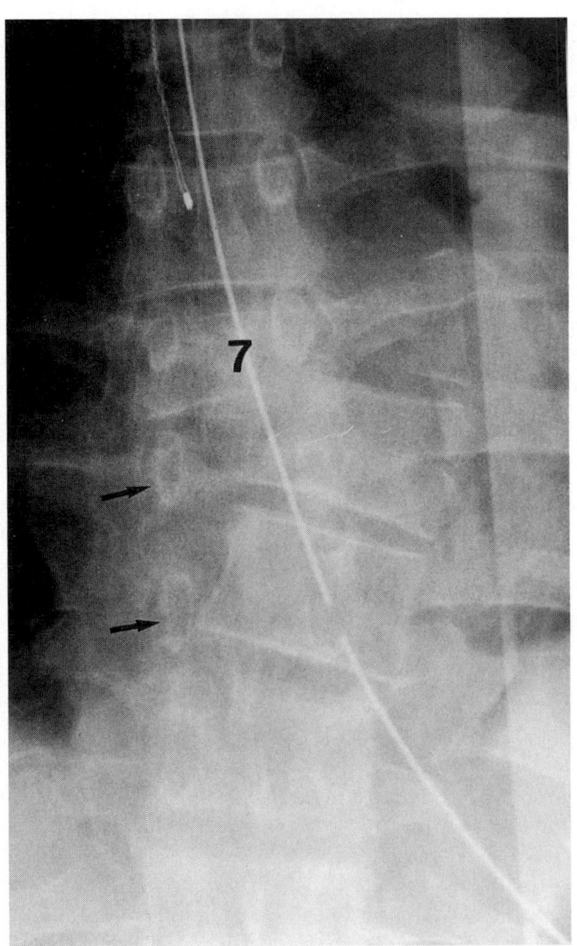

Figure 13–76. Fracture-dislocation of T7 on T8. This anteroposterior radiograph shows right laterolisthesis of T7 on T8 and a large bilateral paraspinal hematoma. The hematoma was the first abnormality noted on a chest radiograph (not shown). Although the bodies of T8 and T9 are displaced to the left, the pedicles *(arrows)* remain in their normal anatomic position. There was no neurologic deficit because the injury had decompressed the spinal cord.

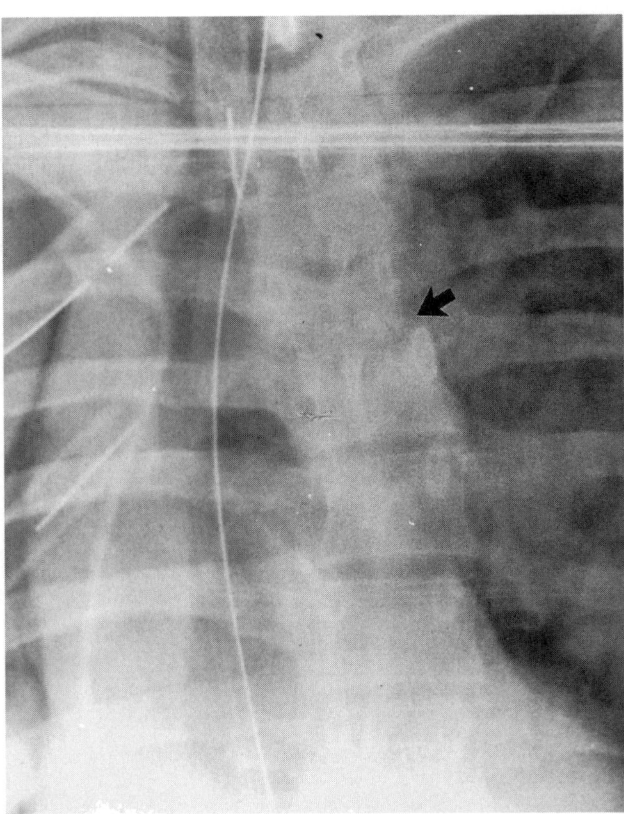

Figure 13–77. Fracture-dislocation of T4 on T5. Detail view of a chest film obtained by portable radiography shows minimal offset of T4 on T5 on the left *(arrow)*.

Commonly, a small triangular fragment is seen, as described previously (see Fig. 13–71*B*). This fragment is from an avulsion fracture, often ascribed to shearing by the anterior longitudinal ligament but more likely to be due to avulsion by the deeply embedded Sharpey fibers of the annulus fibrosis at the margin of the intervertebral disc. This injury is similar to the "slice fracture" described by Holdsworth.[93, 94] On radiographs the fragment may give the vertebra the appearance of a ripped can top, if accompanied by a more horizontal fragment of the vertebral end plate. On CT images this same fragment appears as an arc or crescent of bone anterior to the vertebral body. When a small triangular fracture is identified on the anterior superior margin of a vertebral body, the possibility of an unstable rotary injury must be considered, and further evaluation by CT to fully define the injury in the posterior column is warranted.

In some cases, the facets on one side are disrupted while the fracture line on the opposite side proceeds through the pedicle or pars interarticularis and then forward through a portion of the vertebral body.

Less commonly, fracture-dislocations are due to some combination of distraction, rotation, and shearing with little or no flexion component. Such combination injury is manifested as bilateral fractures of either the pedicle

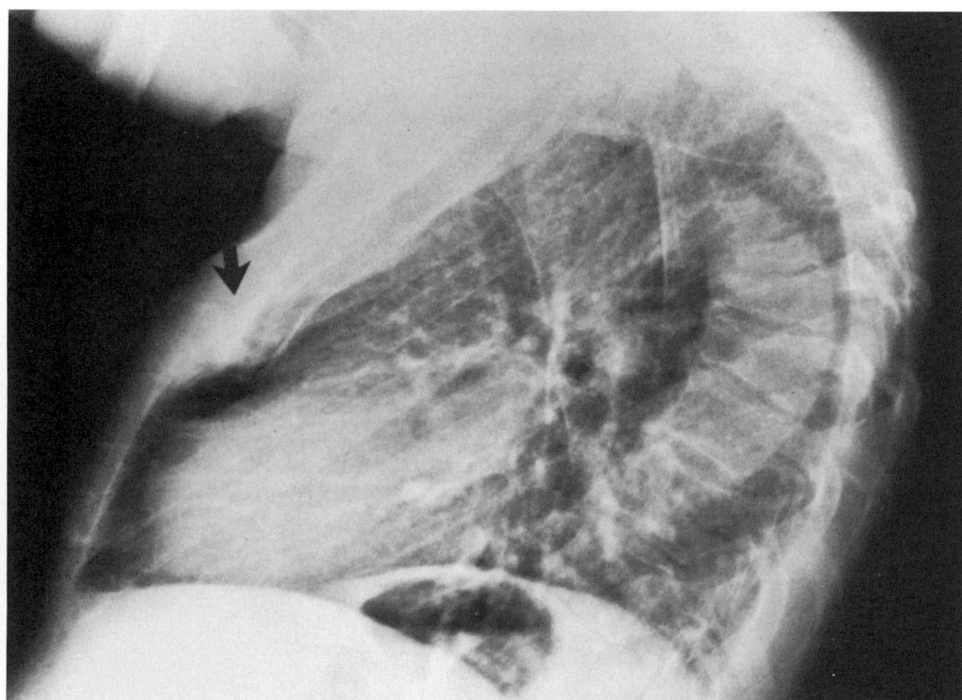

Figure 13–78. Thoracic vertebral fractures associated with a sternal dislocation. Note the extreme kyphosis of the upper thoracic column and posterior displacement of the sternum *(arrow)*.

or the pars interarticularis and anterior displacement of the vertebra associated with a disruption of the intervertebral disc; a very minimal compression fracture of the vertebral body may or may not be present below the level of dislocation.[159] Rarely, dislocation may be associated with ligamentous disruption posteriorly and disc disruption anteriorly without any accompanying fracture.

Pure lateral translational injuries occur more commonly in the lower lumbar spine or lumbosacral junction[144, 160] and less frequently in the upper lumbar spine. In some cases there is little or no displacement in the sagittal plane; therefore, dislocation or subluxation may not be evident on the lateral radiograph (see Fig. 13–79). On the lateral radiograph the injury is manifested as an apparent narrowing of the intervertebral disc without accompanying signs of degenerative disc disease, such as spur formation. The translational component of the injury is evident on the anteroposterior radiograph.

Lumbosacral dislocation is a rare, pure translational injury that is usually anterior and occasionally lateral,[144, 160] with little or no vertebral or sacral compression.[37, 43, 77] The facets are commonly dislocated bilaterally[79] and less often dislocated unilaterally,[14, 37] and may be locked (see Fig. 13–72). Lumbosacral junction injury may also occur in conjunction with an unstable pelvic injury.[124]

CT is useful for evaluating fracture-dislocations to (1) define the full extent of the injury, (2) identify canal compromise by displaced bone fragments, and (3) portray the injury in multiplanar (sagittal and coronal) format (Fig. 13–80). In the thoracic and lumbar regions, it is also useful for identifying fractured, perched, locked, or dislocated facets.

Although it may be difficult to appreciate displacement of vertebrae on axial CT images, several findings point to the presence of a dislocation.[147] Occasionally, two vertebrae will overlap and be displayed on the same axial image—the so-called *double vertebrae sign*, the most obvious CT sign of dislocation (Fig. 13–81). Compromise of the vertebral canal may also be demonstrated by a scissoring effect of overlapping posterior elements. On contiguous images two separate vertebrae may demonstrate a different axial orientation, representing an indirect sign of dislocation.

Facets are identified by the vertebral structures with which they are in continuity, the orientation of their joint surfaces with respect to the vertebral body, and the shape of their articular surface (Fig. 13–82*A*). Superior facets are projected in the same plane as that of the pedicles, and their articular surfaces are concave and directed posteromedially. Inferior facets are projected in the plane of the neural arch or laminae, and their articular surfaces are flat or convex and projected anterolaterally. Normal facet joints have the appearance of a hamburger bun, with flat inner surfaces and convex outer surfaces. With distraction injuries, the facet joints become completely disrupted, resulting in wide separation, perching, or locking of the facets. Complete dislocation of the superior facets from the inferior facets results in the *"naked facet" sign*[36, 147] (see Figs. 13–82*B* and 13–72*D*). A naked facet is a facet (superior or inferior) without an opposing facet. The number of intervening slices between the two facets depends upon the degree of distraction. When the inferior facet is projected just a level above the superior facet, the facets are said to be perched. Distraction can frequently be diagnosed on thoracic or abdominal CT images if naked facets are seen on more than one slice. Sagittal multiplanar reformatted images are better at portraying the relationship of the facets than are axial images (see Fig. 13–80).

Locking of the facets reverses the normal relationship of the facets.[125] This pathologic entity results in the "reverse hamburger bun" sign, in which the flattened sides

Text continued on page 521

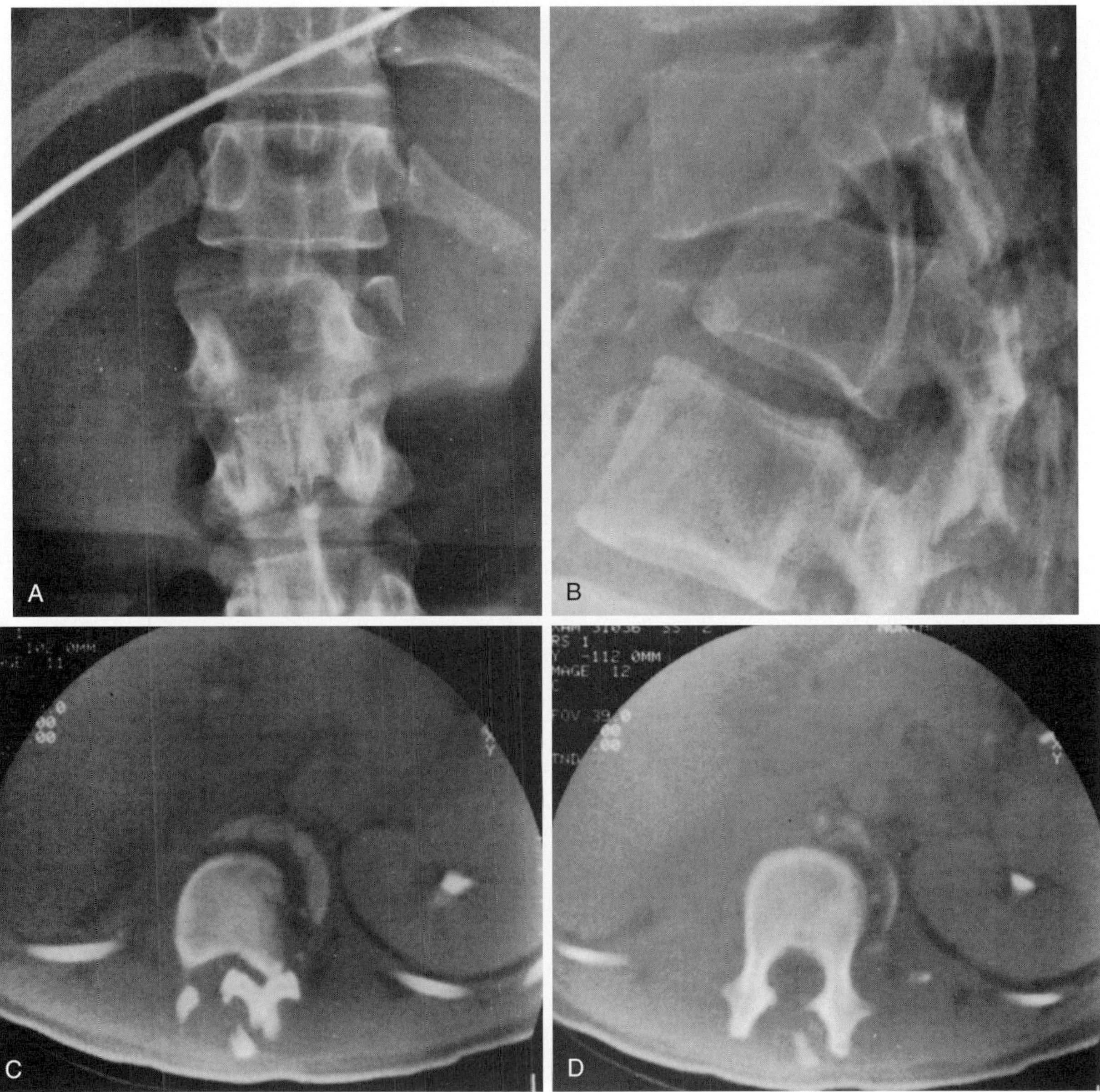

Figure 13–79. Combined rotary and shearing fracture-dislocation of T12–L1. *A*, Anteroposterior radiograph shows angulation and lateral dislocation at T12–L1. Note the avulsed fragment from the left lateral margin of L1 that accompanies T12. Note the naked facets, fractured transverse processes of L1, and fractured twelfth rib. *B*, Lateral radiograph demonstrates dislocation with an accompanying long, thin fragment from the superior margin of L1, the so-called slice fracture. This is analogous to the "ripped can top" appearance of a pure rotary injury. The facet joints are disrupted. *C*, CT image demonstrates characteristic features of lateral jumped facets, with the inferior facets of T12 lying to the left of the superior facets of L1. Because this is a combined rotational and shearing injury, the greater portion of the rim fragment arises from the lateral margin of the vertebra instead of from the anterior margin. *D*, CT image obtained through the midportion of L1 demonstrates naked facets.

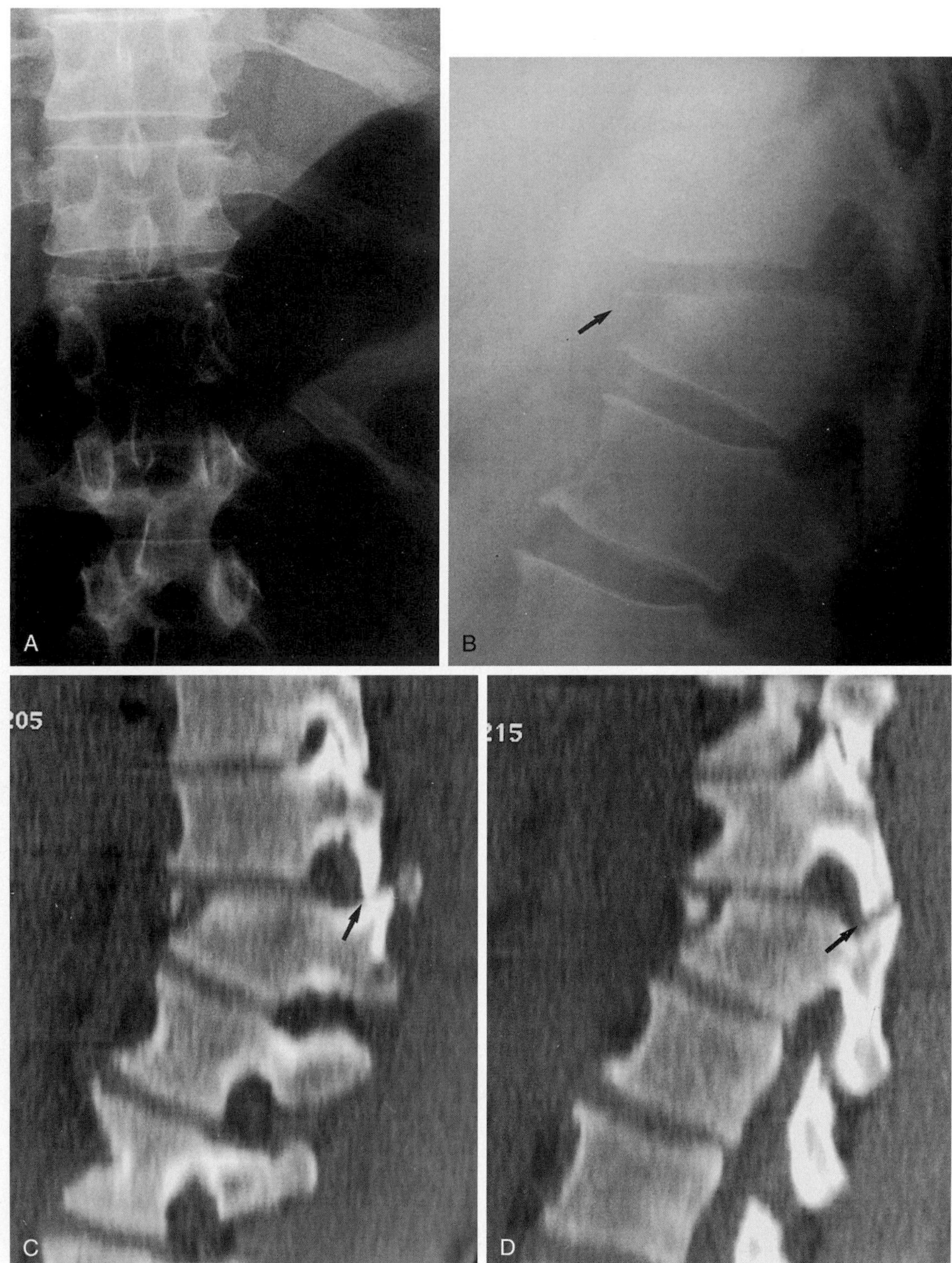

Figure 13–80. Fracture-dislocation of T11–T12 demonstrating the use of multiplanar imaging. *A*, Anteroposterior radiograph demonstrates widening of the interspinous space between T11 and T12 and naked facets. *B*, Lateral radiograph shows anterolisthesis of T11 on T12 and a small avulsed fragment from the top of the compressed T12 *(arrow)*. *C* and *D*, Sagittal reconstructed CT images show the jumped and locked facets *(arrows)*.

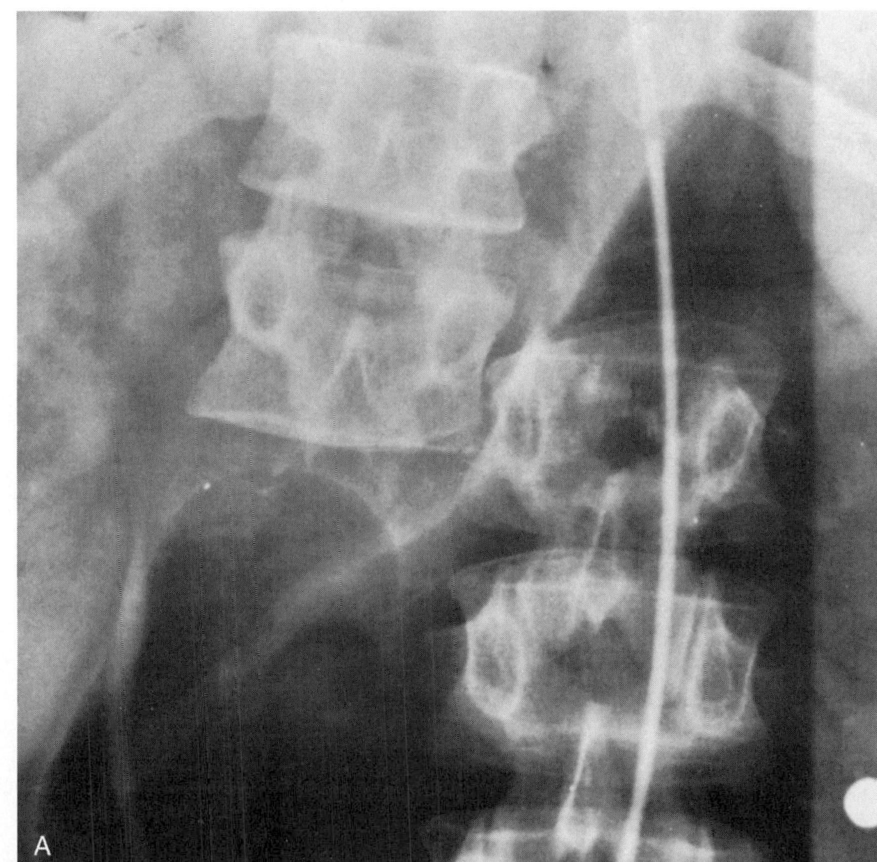

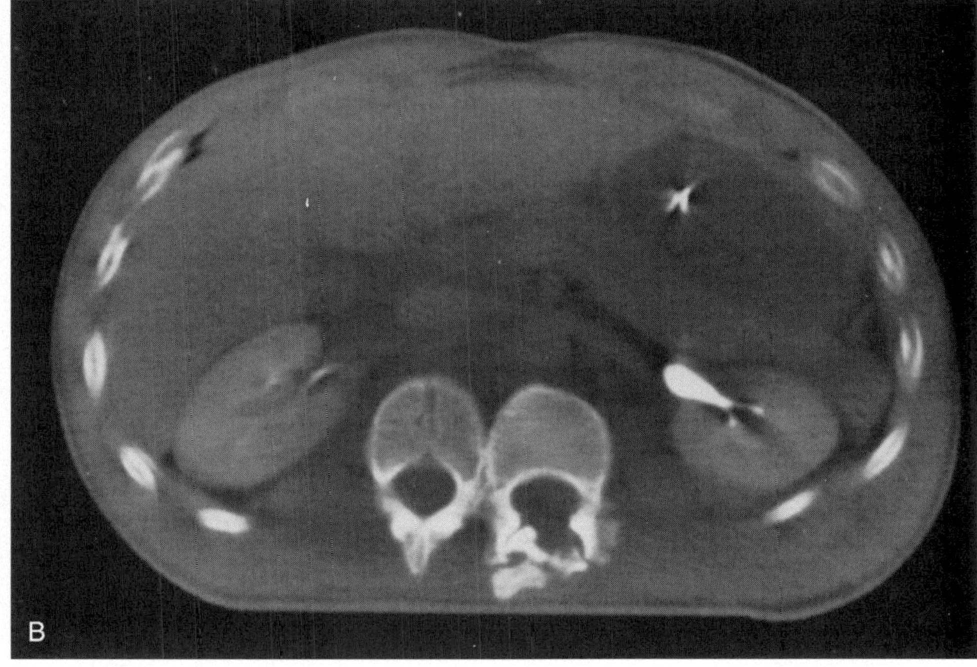

Figure 13–81. Lateral fracture-dislocation of L1–L2. *A*, Anteroposterior radiograph shows complete lateral displacement of L1 relative to L2. *B*, CT image shows both vertebrae side by side. L1 is on the right. Note the fractured inferior facets of L1 lying adjacent to the facets of L2. Injuries such as this one frequently produce aortic damage. In this case an aortogram (not shown) revealed no evidence of vascular injury.

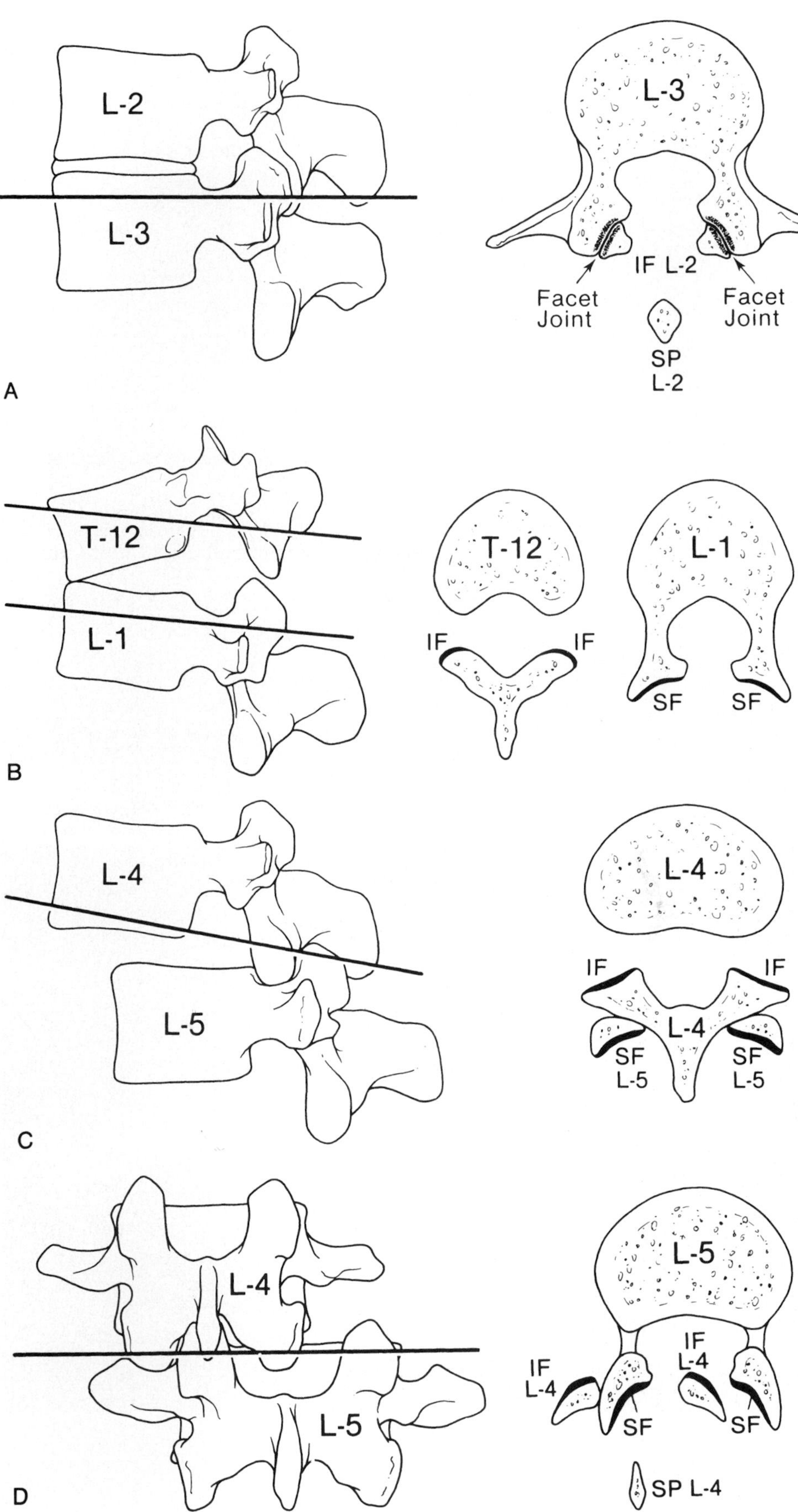

Figure 13–82. Drawings showing CT appearance of various facet abnormalities encountered in dislocation of the thoracolumbar spine. *A*, Normal facet alignment. Note that the inferior facets of L2 lie posteriorly and medially within the superior facets of L3. The joint surfaces of the inferior facets are slightly convex and the superior facets are slightly concave. *B*, "Naked facets." The facets are completely distracted. CT section through T12 demonstrates the characteristic convex appearance of the inferior facets unapposed by superior facets, whereas the section through L1 demonstrates the unapposed concave surface of the superior facets of L1. *C*, Facet lock. The inferior facets lie anterior to the superior facets. Note the characteristic configuration of the superior facets (convex anteriorly, with a slightly concave joint surface). The inferior facets at this level have a relatively straight joint surface. Note the resemblance to a reverse hamburger bun. *D*, Rotary, shearing, or lateral dislocations result in lateral jumping of the facets. This type of injury is characterized by a series of unapposed facets, with the inferior facets straddling the superior facets. Compare *C* with Figure 13–72 and *D* with Figure 13–79. (Adapted from Manaster, B. J. & Osborn, A. G. [1986]. CT patterns of facet fracture dislocations in the thoracolumbar region. A.J.N.R. Am. J. Neuroradiol., 7:1007.)

of the facets are anterior and posterior, with the curved convex sides together (see Figs. 13–72*B* and *C* and 13–82*C*).

The technique of open reduction and internal fixation is commonly employed in the treatment of fracture-dislocations of the spine.[107, 114, 139] This procedure is done principally to stabilize the spine and prevent further skeletal and neurologic damage. The neurologic status of those patients with complete loss of motor and sensory function is unlikely to change after surgery, but patients with incomplete motor or sensory lesions often improve.[11, 15, 45, 72] Paraplegia produces characteristic changes in the axial skeleton. Particularly noteworthy is the narrowing and obliteration of the sacroiliac joint.[2, 13]

Chance-Type Fractures (Pure Distraction Injuries)

In 1948 Chance described an unusual fracture of the vertebral body consisting of "horizontal splitting of the spine and neural arch, ending in an upward curve which usually reaches the upper surface of the body just in front of the neural foramen."[29] In his three cases there was very little wedging of the vertebral body. Since the advent of the automobile lap-type seat belt in the 1950s and its common usage in the 1960s, the Chance fracture has been found with increasing frequency as a result of injuries sustained while wearing it.[44, 176] Howland and associates in 1965 reported a case of a complete transverse fracture of the third lumbar vertebra in a 19-year-old man injured in an automobile accident while wearing a seat belt.[96] The authors theorized that "this injury was produced by the seat belt acting as a fulcrum over which the vertebral body was split transversely into two parts." The fracture was termed a *fulcrum fracture* of the lumbar spine. This theory was refined by Smith and Kaufer,[176] who described the more common variants of the injury Chance originally described. Thus, the term *Chance-type fracture* is used to describe this family of injuries in the same way that *Colles-type fracture* defines the family of wrist fractures.

In the usual hyperflexion injury of the spine, the compression forces generated are sustained by the anterior half of the vertebral body with the fulcrum in the middle column. In an accident victim wearing a seat belt, the fulcrum of the force is displaced anteriorly and lies at the seat belt on the abdominal wall. The entire spine is therefore posterior to the flexion axis, and all of its components are subjected to tension or distractive forces. The result is disruption of the ligaments of the posterior elements of the spine or, if the ligaments remain intact, a transverse or fission-type fracture of the posterior elements and, in some cases, the vertebral body. This same pattern has been seen in persons who were not wearing a seat belt but who fell or were thrown forward so that the anterior abdominal wall came in contact with some object (e.g., a tree limb or fence railing). This object serves as a fulcrum, as noted for the seat belt, forcing the body into acute flexion. I have seen several such cases in skiers who struck a fence or a tree.

Four basic injury patterns result from distraction injuries[147, 164] (Fig. 13–83):

1. Disruption of the posterior spinous ligaments, articular facets, and intervertebral discs. There may be associated avulsion of an articular facet or posterior inferior aspect of the vertebral body. The pedicles and spinous and transverse processes remain intact.
2. Transverse fracture involving the posterior elements with or without extension into the posterior superior or posterior inferior aspect of the vertebral body (Fig. 13–84; see also Fig. 13–40). The fracture line may involve one or both pedicles, the transverse processes, and the articular facets, as well as the lamina and spinous process. This type of injury is the classic Chance fracture.
3. Transverse fracture of the posterior elements with associated transverse fracture of the vertebral body (Fig. 13–85) as described by Howland and associates.[96] This fracture, which has been termed the *fulcrum fracture*, involves the spinous process, lamina, pedicles, and usually the transverse processes.
4. Transverse fracture of the vertebral body extending posteriorly through the pedicles, sparing the lamina and spinous process. This injury tears the interspi-

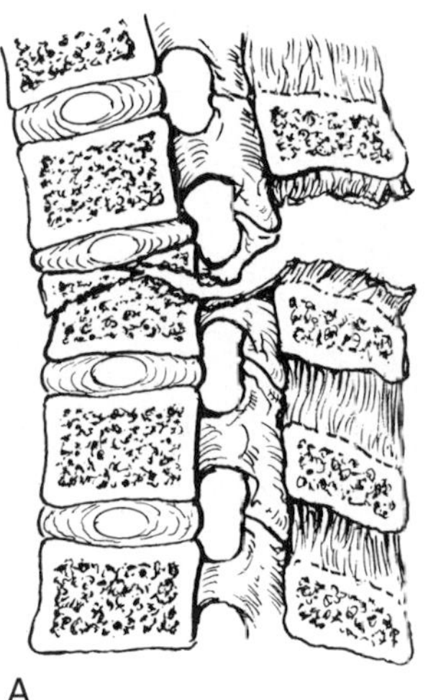
A

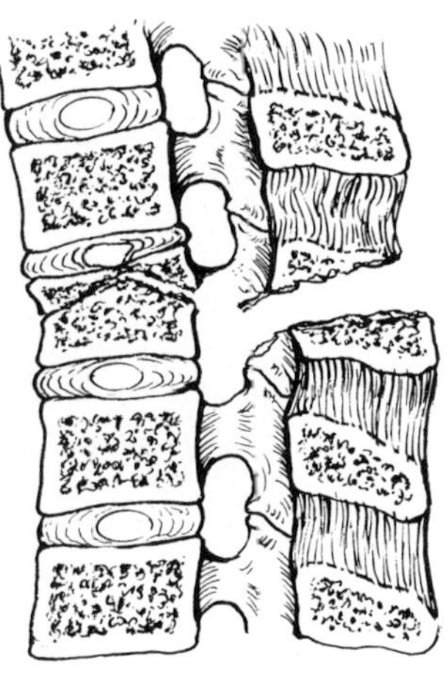
B

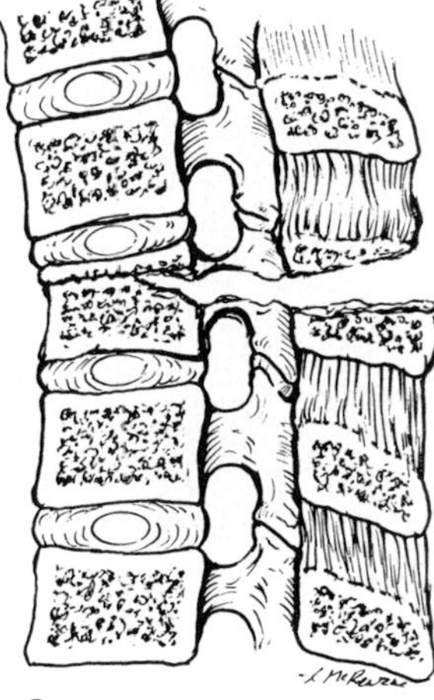
C

Figure 13–83. Pure distraction (Chance-type) flexion injuries. *A*, Smith fracture. *B*, Chance fracture. *C*, Horizontal fracture. See text for description.

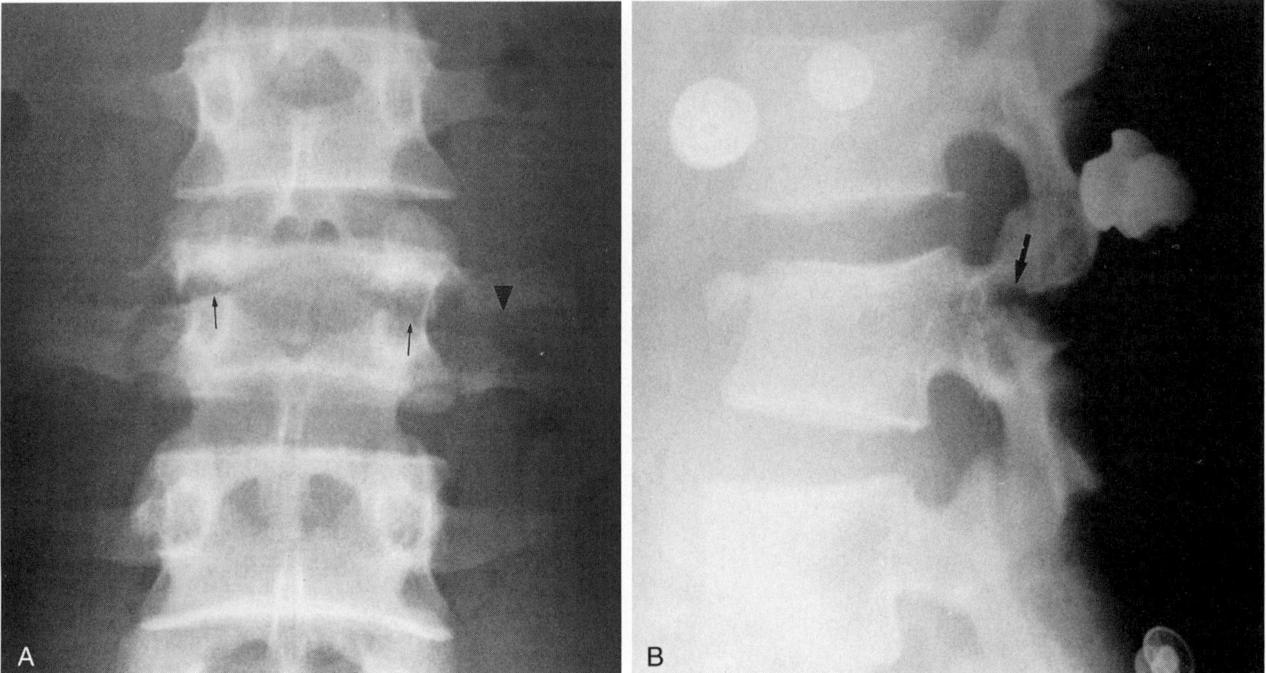

Figure 13–84. Chance fracture of L3 in a skier who hit a fence. *A*, Anteroposterior radiograph shows the fracture to involve both pedicles *(arrows)*, the lamina, and the left transverse process of L3 *(arrowhead)*. Note the increased interspinous distance between L2 and L3. *B*, Lateral radiograph reveals disruption of the posterior superior aspect of L2 that extends into the pedicle *(arrow)*.

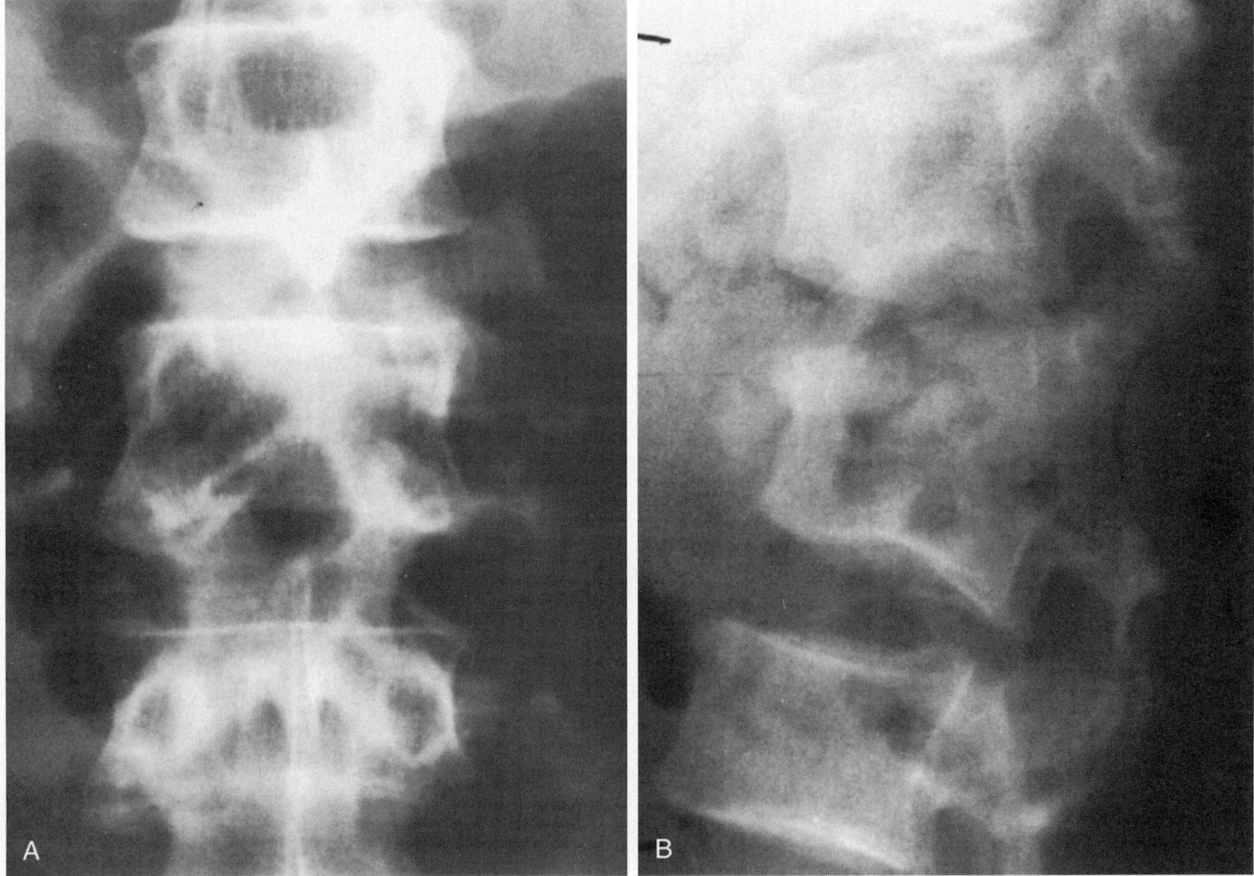

Figure 13–85. Transverse L2 fracture related to lap belt use. *A*, Anteroposterior view shows the fracture through both pedicles, the transverse processes, the lamina, and the spinous process. The widely separated fragments give rise to an empty or vacant appearance of the vertebral body. *B*, Lateral view shows angulation at the fracture and wide separation of the fragments at the level of the pedicles. The fracture extends through the inferior end plate of the vertebral body. (From Rogers, L. F. [1971]. The roentgenographic appearance of transverse or Chance fractures of the spine: The seat belt fracture. A.J.R. Am. J. Roentgenol., *111*:844.)

nous and supraspinous ligaments. This fracture is the classic Smith fracture (Fig. 13–86).

Chance-type injuries are readily visible on frontal radiographs.[4, 164] The involved vertebra appears elongated when compared with the ones above and below. Because of the posterior distraction there may be sufficient angulation of the superior fragment that a portion of the vertebral body is no longer overlain by the posterior elements (see Fig. 13–84*A*). Owing to this separation and elevation of the posterior elements, the vertebral body involved has an empty or vacant appearance; which is confirmed by noting an increased distance between two adjacent spinous processes. Another clue lies in recognition of a break in the continuity of the oval cortex of the pedicles or tear-shaped cortex of the spinous process, or both (see Fig. 13–84*A*). The fracture line may also be seen within the lamina (see Fig. 13–86*A*) or articular processes. A horizontal fracture of the transverse process creates an unusual bifid appearance (see Figs. 13–40*A* and 13–84*A*) of this structure. A similar horizontal fracture of the 12th rib has been reported.[4]

Confirmation rests with an adequately exposed and properly positioned lateral film (see Figs. 13–84*B* and 13–86*B*) that shows the line of fracture within the spinous process, pedicles, and vertebral body. If a pure ligamentous rupture has occurred, anterior angulation of the superior vertebra with separation of the posterior elements is demonstrated. The facets may be perched. Should the posterior elements be poorly defined because of overexposure or improper positioning, the presence of an avulsion fracture or irregularity of the posterior aspect of the superior or inferior plate of the vertebral body or anterior angulation may be a clue. When such a fracture or angulation is present, the frontal view should be carefully scrutinized for the presence of a horizontal fracture.[32]

Characteristically, there is minimal compression of the vertebral body. When present, it usually involves the anterior superior aspect. Lateral displacement or rotation of the fracture fragments does not occur with this type of injury. Anterior displacement of the superior vertebral body or the superior fragment is also unusual; when present, it is commonly associated with an injury to the spinal cord or cauda equina. A lateral flexion-distraction, Chance-type fracture has been described.[91]

Chance-type fractures or distraction injuries may be difficult to appreciate on axial CT images because they are transversely oriented in the axial plane. Some component of the fracture is likely to be lost with partial volume averaging. Reformatted images in the sagittal and coronal planes are required to fully define the injury (Fig. 13–87). Pluridirectional tomography, if available, may be helpful in these cases.

MRI of Chance-type fractures should be performed only if there are neurologic abnormalities. One consistent finding on MRI studies of these patients is the presence of marrow signal abnormalities in adjacent vertebrae, indicating that the energy expended to produce this injury involved more than one vertebra.

Transverse fractures of the lumbar vertebrae are often associated with significant visceral injuries. The term *seat belt syndrome* was coined by Garrett and Braunstein in 1962[66] to designate those injuries frequently encountered in persons wearing a lap-type seat belt. The syndrome

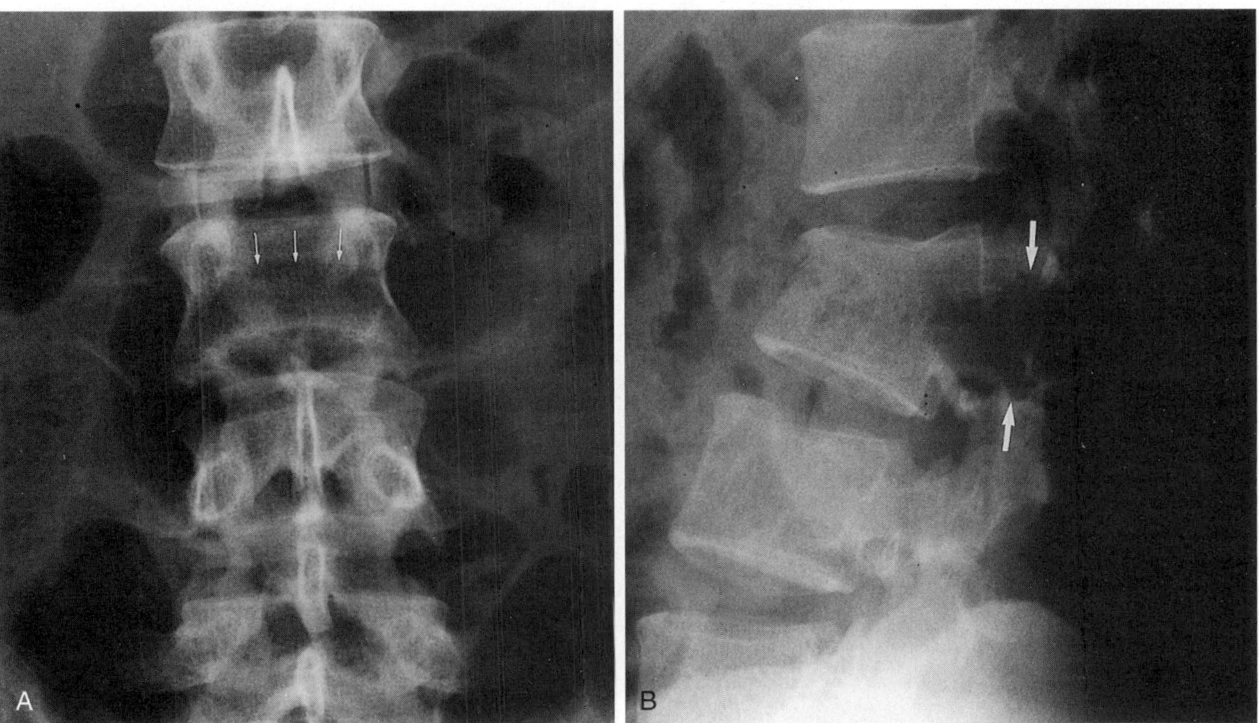

Figure 13–86. Smith fracture of L3 related to lap belt use. *A*, Anteroposterior view shows a vacant appearance of the body of L3. The fracture extends through the lower portion of the pedicles. The laminar involvement can be seen *(arrows)*. *B*, Lateral view shows the posterior distraction of the body and the involvement of the inferior pedicles *(arrows)*.

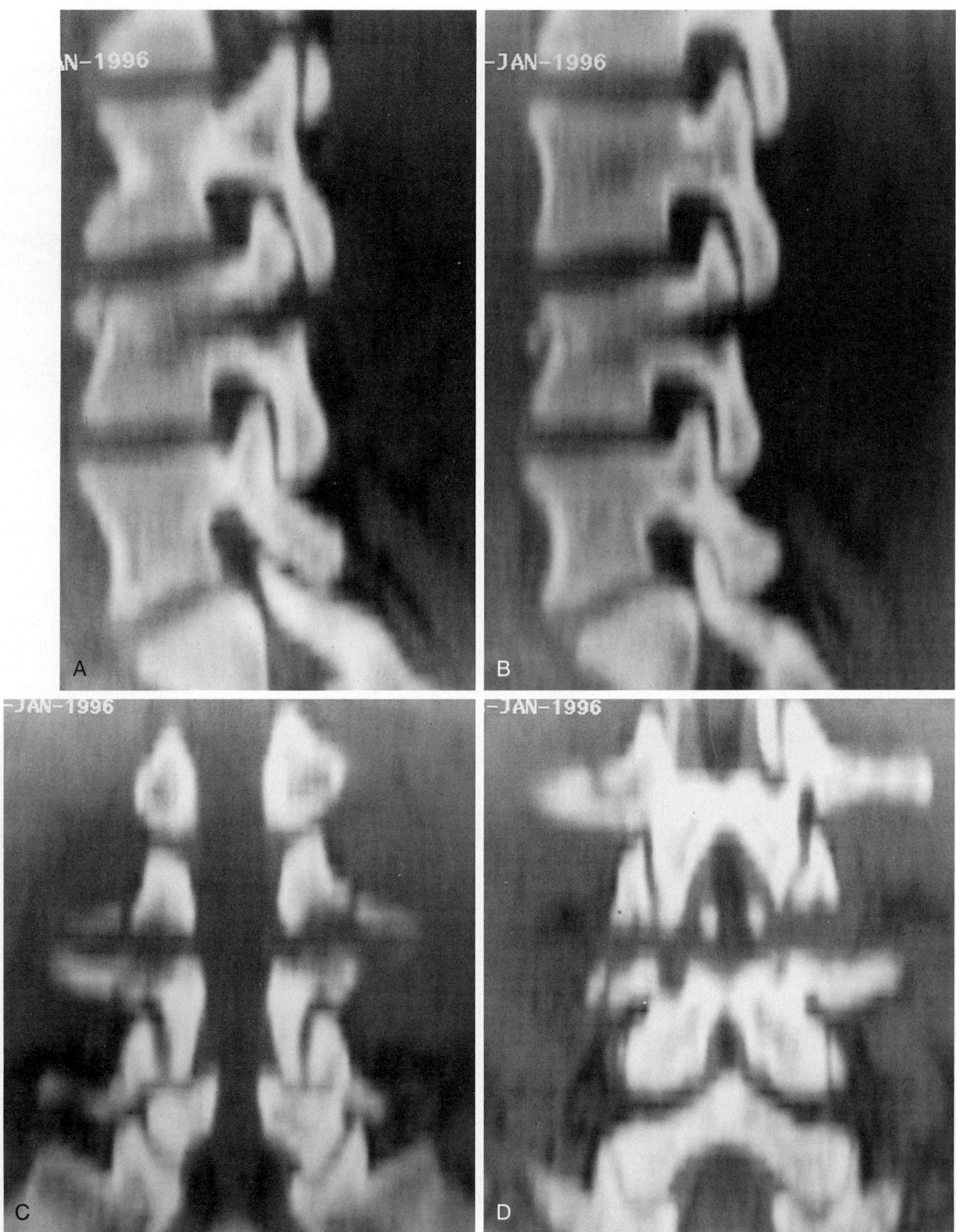

Figure 13–87. Chance fracture of L4 showing use of reformatted CT images. Sagittal *(A and B)* and coronal *(C and D)* reconstructions show the involvement of the pedicles. This patient is the same one as in Figure 13–21.

consists of one or more of the following injuries:[44, 66, 164] transverse abrasions of the lower anterior abdominal wall, outlining the position of the seat belt at the time of impact; ruptures of the anterior abdominal wall musculature; longitudinal lacerations of the small bowel, particularly on the antimesenteric border of the jejunum and ileum; tears of the mesentery; ruptures of the second or third portion of the duodenum,[99] spleen, stomach,[27] or pancreas; contusion of the abdominal aorta;[189] injuries to the cauda equina or spinal cord; and transverse fractures of the lumbar spine. Rupture of the gravid uterus also has been reported. A rare circumferential avulsion of the outer layers of the sigmoid colon, leaving the mucosa intact, has been described.[99] These injuries may be both clinically and radiologically obscure. When a transverse fracture is identified, the physician must be alert to the potential for associated abdominal visceral injury. Neurologic deficits occur in 15% of cases.[109, 164]

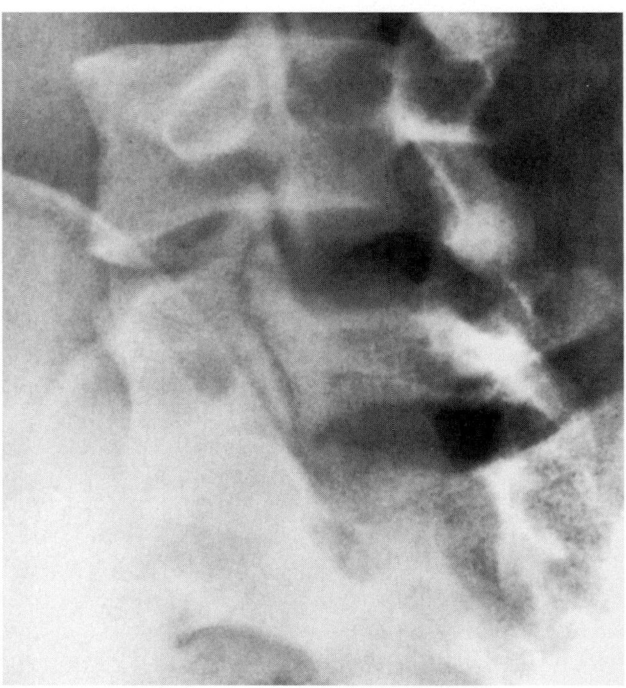

Figure 13–89. Fracture of the pars interarticularis and facets of L5 in a football player, due to an extension mechanism of injury. Oblique radiograph demonstrates a vertical fracture line extending from the inferior facet across the pars to the superior facet. There was a similar fracture on the contralateral side.

Fractures of the Posterior Elements

Isolated fractures of the transverse processes are common. These injuries result from pulls of the paraspinous muscles or occasionally from direct blows. Such fractures are frequently multiple (Fig. 13–88). The line of fracture is usually vertically or obliquely oriented. The vertebrae are otherwise intact. The fractures are often obscured by overlying gas and fecal material. Scoliosis, convex to the side of the fractures, may serve as a clue to an otherwise obscure injury (see Fig. 13–88).[73] The quadratus lumborum muscle inserts onto the transverse processes. With transverse process fracture, the effectiveness of this muscle on the side of fracture is reduced, and the unopposed action of the contralateral quadratus lumborum results in scoliosis convex to the side of the fracture.

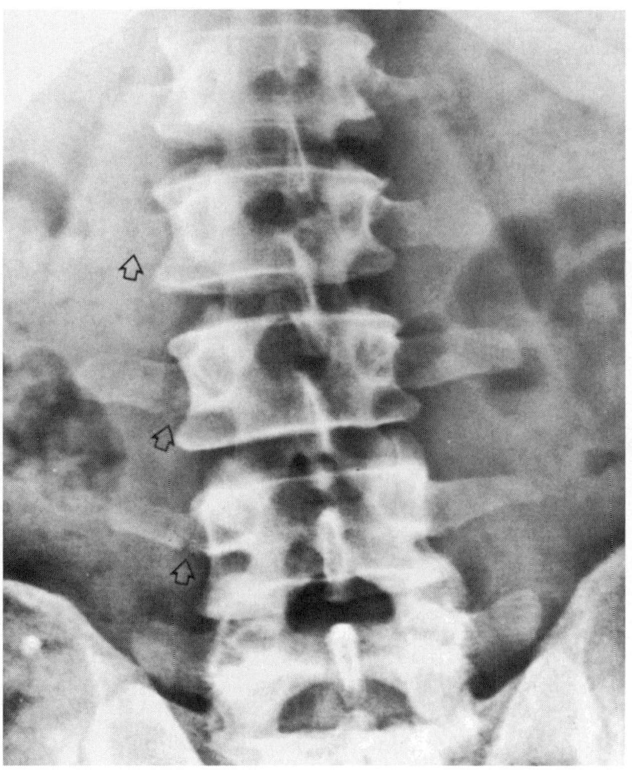

Figure 13–88. Fractures of the transverse processes *(arrows)* of L2 through L4 on the right. There is minimal displacement. Note the scoliosis convex toward the side of the fractures, which is characteristic of this type of injury.

Visceral injury is the only serious complication of isolated transverse process fractures and fulfills my own definition of a fracture as *a soft tissue injury in which a bone is broken*. In a large series of transverse process fractures, 21% were associated with injuries of the abdominal viscera, including hepatic, splenic, and colonic injuries. Hematuria was present in 55%.[179] No patient without hematuria incurred an injury of the urinary tract.

If the fracture line is horizontal, the other posterior elements should be scrutinized to exclude the possibility that this fracture represents a portion of a Chance-type fracture. Avulsion fractures of the fifth lumbar transverse process are frequently associated with pelvic fractures; in particular, the presence of such fractures serves as a useful clue to the presence of fractures of the sacral ala or disruption of the sacroiliac joint, which are often difficult to see on radiographs. Occasionally, the ossification center for the transverse process fails to unite with the vertebral body. This variation results in a vertical line of lucency between the vertebral body and the transverse process. The bony margins of this line are sharply defined by cortical bone and should not be mistaken for a fracture.

Isolated fractures of the remaining posterior elements are unusual. Fractures of the pars interarticularis (Fig. 13–89) or articular facets are occasionally encountered. Characteristically, there is very little displacement, and the fracture line is obscure. The mechanism of injury is probably acute hyperextension. The majority of pars defects encountered represent old stress fractures with sclerotic margins that are easily demonstrable on CT images. Acute fractures, in contrast, are associated with a specifically identifiable injury and frequently heal completely without residual defects.[193]

Isolated fractures of the spinous process or lamina may be encountered on occasion. These fractures are often difficult to visualize, and CT may be required. They are usually found in a patient who complains of persistent pain even though the radiographic appearance is normal.[67]

Stress Fractures of Posterior Elements

Stress fractures occur in the pars interarticularis, pedicles, and laminae. The majority are found in the pars interarticularis and are particularly common in gymnasts and football linemen; they are probably due to repeated hyperextension of the spine.[58, 178] Stress fractures of the pedicle have been reported in ballet dancers,[100] and fractures in the laminae, in runners[3] and other persons engaged in a variety of athletic pursuits.[103, 151] Patients commonly complain of low back pain, without radiation into the lower extremity, that is exacerbated by hyperextension and various twisting movements. Pain may be elicited by standing on one leg and hyperextending the spine, the so-called hyperextension test.[103] The radiographic appearance is frequently normal. The injury is identified by focal increases in radionuclide uptake on a bone scan[103, 151, 153] (Fig. 13–90). With healing, the scan returns to normal, and radiographs may never reveal any evidence of a lesion. In other cases, a distinct fracture line with marginal sclerosis is present. Lesions may also be identified by CT (Fig. 13–91).

Insufficiency or stress fractures of the pedicle or pars interarticularis may occur opposite the side of a preexisting spondylolysis.[178] These fractures are evidenced by a focal "hot spot" on a bone scan and often demonstrate bone hypertrophy involving the pedicle and margins of the fracture on the plain film. The diagnosis can be confirmed by CT (Fig. 13–92).

Lumbar Apophyseal Ring Fractures

Fractures of the lumbosacral apophyseal rings are rare but have distinctive radiographic features.[50, 51, 84, 115, 180, 183] The injuries are found in adolescents presenting with clinical features suggestive of acute herniation of intervertebral discs. Evidently the ring apophysis represents a site of focal weakness that allows the herniation to occur, carrying with it a portion of the inferior posterior margin of the apophyseal ring. The majority of these fractures have been reported at the posterior inferior margin of L4 and a lesser number at L5. A single case of fracture at the posterior superior margin of S1 has been reported.[64] The mechanism of injury is the same as that for the limbus vertebra.[132]

The radiographic findings are distinctive. A small bony spicule can be identified at the posterior inferior margin of the vertebral body projecting into the spinal canal (Fig. 13–93). CT is the best means of identifying the displaced segment of the apophysis and will show a characteristic arclike segment of bone protruding into the spinal canal.[42] MRI will show any herniated disc material.

Multiple-Level Vertebral Injuries

Fractures occur at multiple noncontiguous vertebral levels in approximately 4% to 20% of all patients with spinal injuries[8, 10, 26, 36, 116, 119, 170, 182] (Fig. 13–94). Multilevel vertebral injuries are extremely uncommon in patients who are neurologically intact, with the exception of primary injuries at the craniovertebral junction. Approximately 25% of craniovertebral injuries are associated with injuries at other locations,[121, 123, 169] most often in the lower cervical spine, less commonly in the thoracic spine, and infrequently in the lumbar spine. Second-level fractures are most commonly associated with mid-thoracic and upper thoracic fractures (Fig. 13–95), occurring in 17% of cases.[26, 36] A small percentage of cervical fractures are associated with fractures at the thoracolumbar junction, with fractures of L4 or L5.[26] These second fractures are important in explaining neurologic deficits or persistent pain and in determining definitive treatment plans. All patients who have sustained a single vertebral fracture or a spinal cord injury should undergo a total radiographic examination of the spine to determine whether additional fractures are present.[26, 36, 169] MRI is particularly useful for demonstrating multilevel injuries (Fig. 13–96).

Spinal Fractures in Rigid Spine Disease (Ankylosis)

Ankylosing Spondylitis

Vertebral fractures in patients with ankylosing spondylitis have a peculiar pattern of injury resulting from the rigidity of the fused segments and associated osteoporosis of the underlying vertebral bodies.[70, 78, 80, 142, 195] The ankylosed spine is rigid and functions much like a long bone or ceramic pipe. Therefore, a fracture, even seemingly minor, through such a spine is grossly unstable, is readily displaced, and in 55% to 70% of cervical injuries results in neurologic injury.[21, 92, 142, 150] In the thoracic and lumbar regions, the lower the location of the fracture, the less the incidence of neurologic deficit. The fractures are particularly common in the cervical spine, are often related to trivial trauma,[112] and are usually due to hyperextension forces.[157, 195] The fractures characteristically involve the posterior elements and an associated intervertebral disc space of the lower cervical spine. Similar fractures may occur anywhere within the spinal column, however. The wall of the aorta may become adherent to the anterior longitudinal ligament as a result of paraspinous inflammation, and fractures of the thoracolumbar spine may result in simultaneous lacerations of the adjacent aorta.[57, 168] Aortic laceration may occur in the absence of obvious dislocation. The fracture traverses the syndesmophytes (Figs. 13–97 and 13–98) at the involved interspace and characteristically spares the vertebral body.

Text continued on page 533

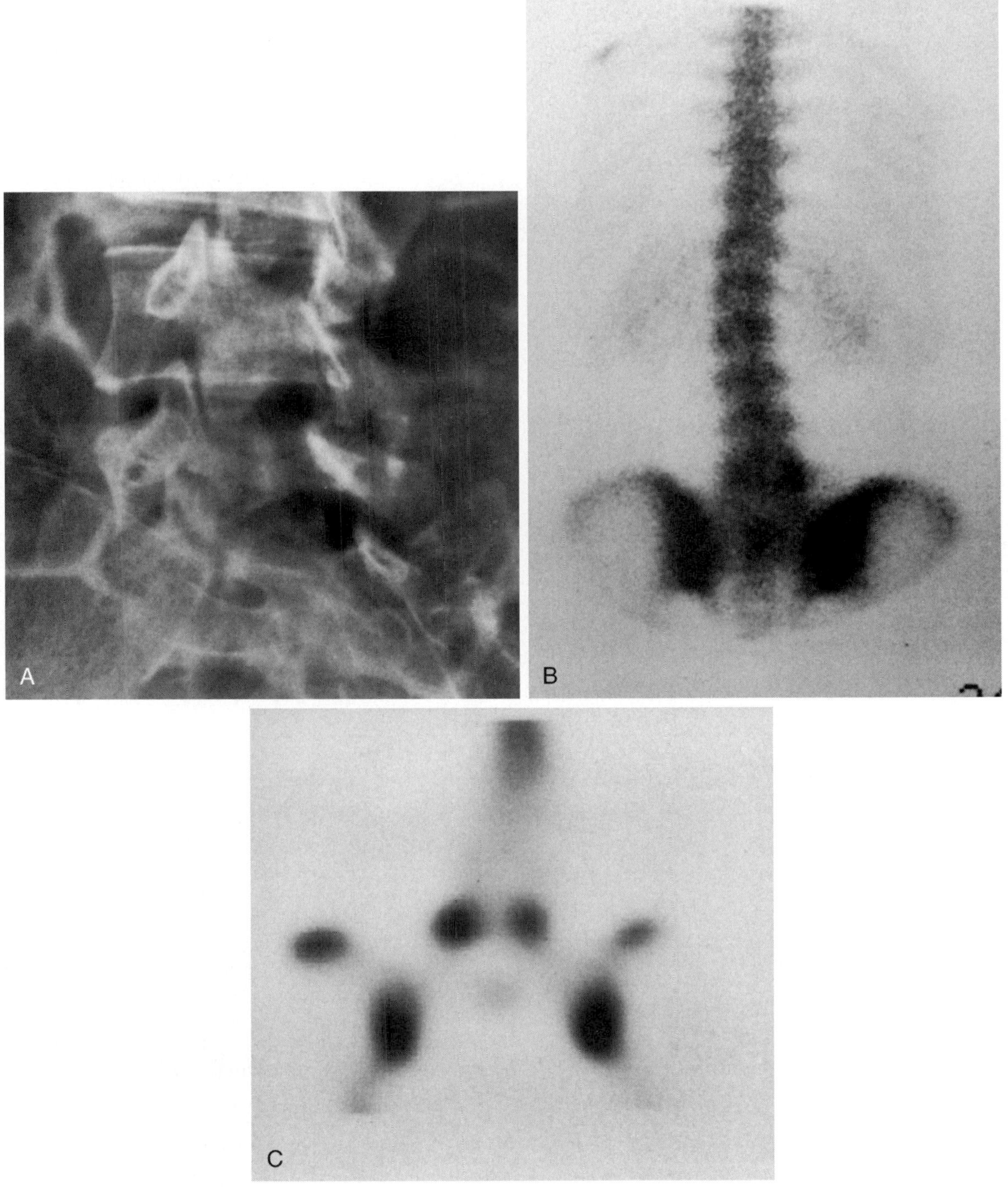

Figure 13–90. Bilateral stress fractures of the pars interarticularis. *A*, Oblique radiograph reveals no evidence of fracture or other abnormality of the pars. The contralateral oblique view was likewise normal. *B*, Posterior view from a radionuclide bone scan shows only slightly increased tracer activity in the region of the pars of L5. *C*, Coronal single-photon emission computed tomography (SPECT) image clearly demonstrates bilateral increased activity in the region of the pedicles and pars of L5—a finding strongly suggestive of an evolving stress fracture.

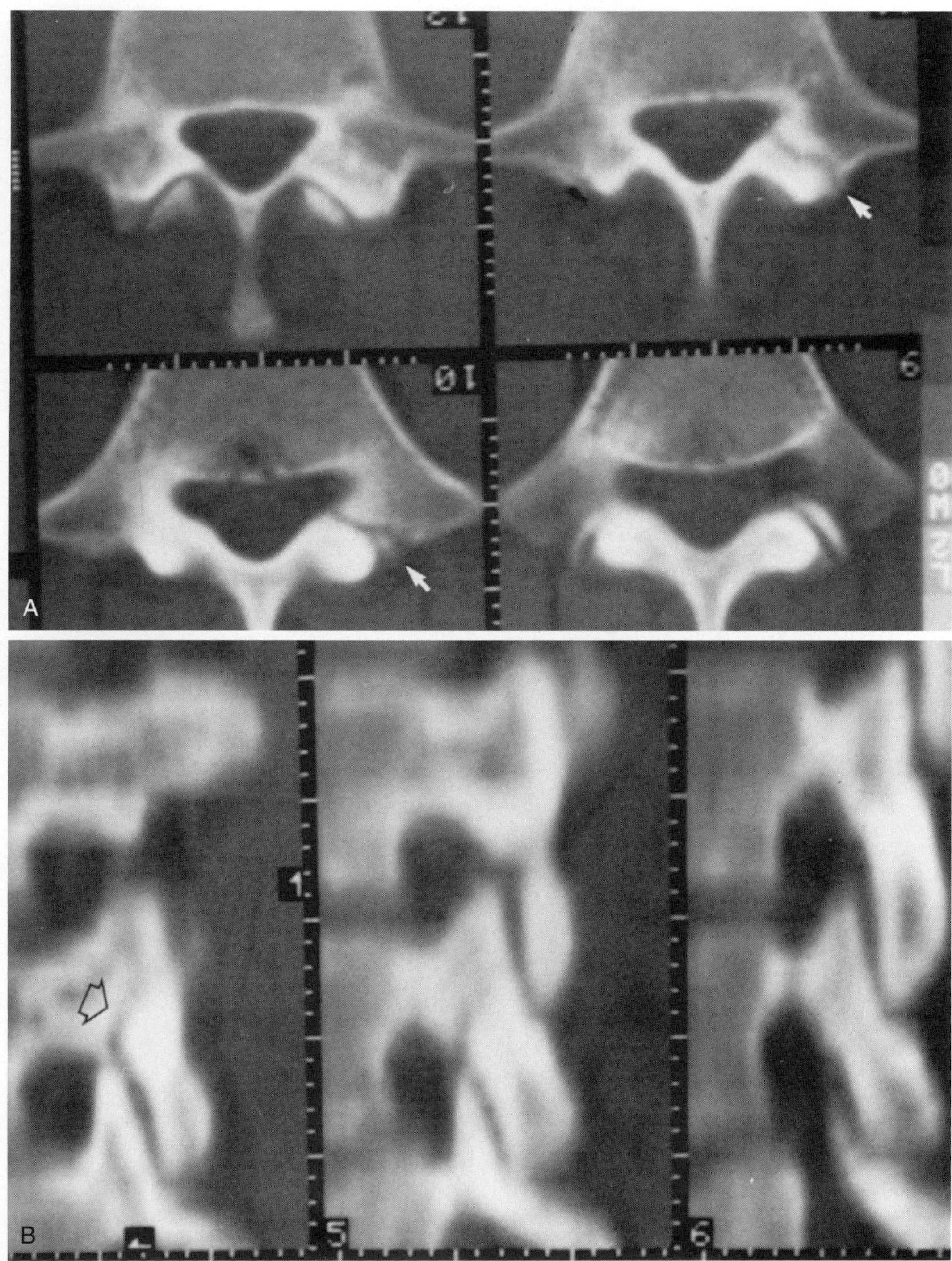

Figure 13–91. Pars interarticularis fracture in a basketball player with low back pain. *A*, Axial CT images demonstrate a fracture with surrounding sclerosis in the left pars interarticularis (*arrow* in *upper right* and *lower left* images). *B*, Parasagittal reconstructions clearly confirm the presence of a fracture (*arrow* in *left* image). Pars fractures are most likely to be discovered when CT examinations are performed for the evaluation of patients with back pain. (Case courtesy of Neil C. Chafetz, MD, and Clyde Helms, MD, San Francisco, Calif.)

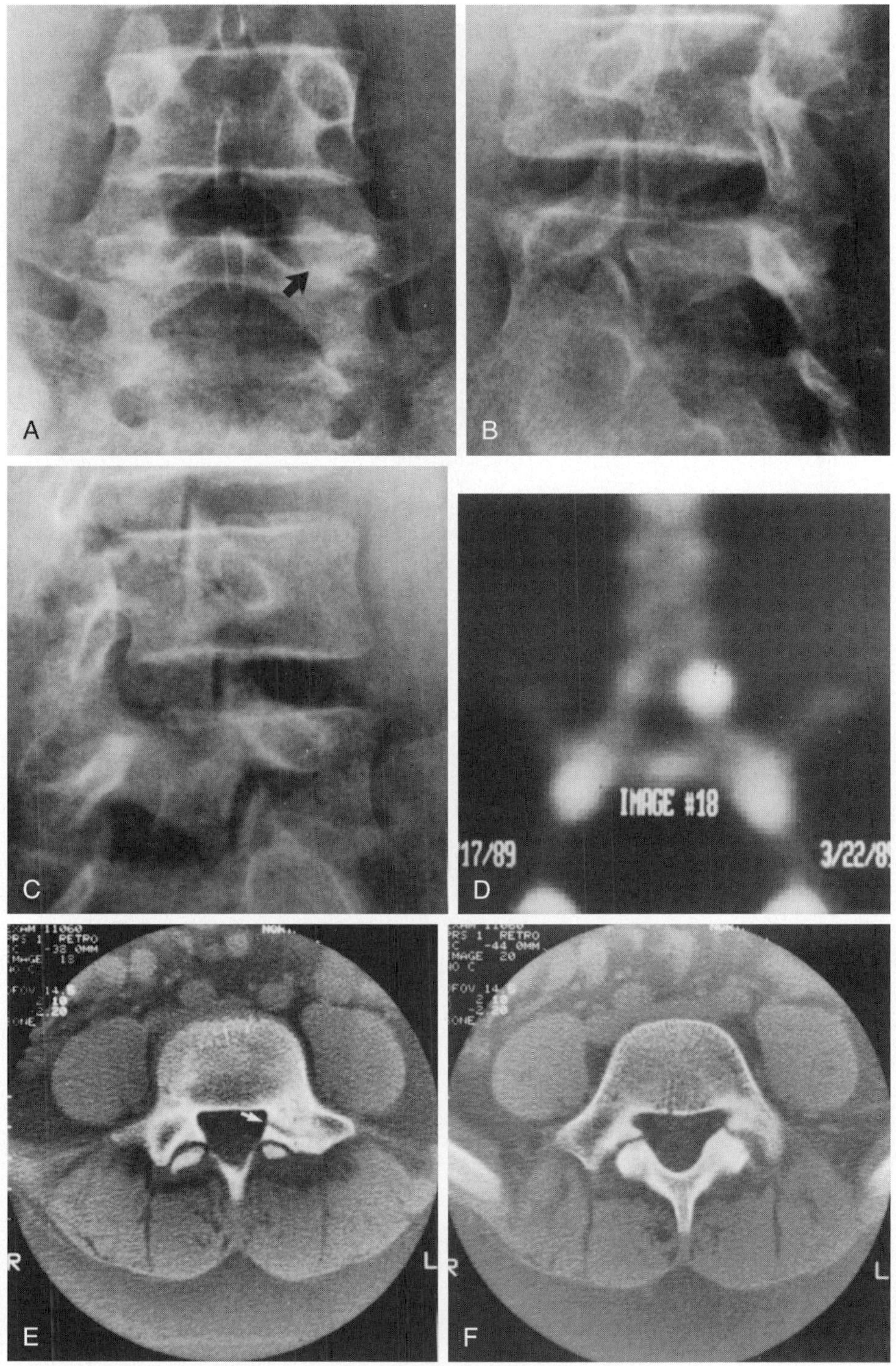

Figure 13–92. Spondylolysis of L5 on the right with subsequent fracture of the pars on the left in a 14-year-old boy. *A*, Anteroposterior view demonstrates bone hypertrophy in the left pedicle of L5 *(arrow)*. *B*, Right oblique view demonstrates a defect in the pars interarticularis of L5 on the right. *C*, Left posterior oblique demonstrates and confirms bone hypertrophy in the pedicle. The pars defect is not as clearly defined as it is on the right. *D*, Image from a radionuclide single-photon emission CT (SPECT) study demonstrates increased activity in the region of the pars of L5 on the left. *E*, CT image through the upper portion of L5 at the level of the L4–L5 facet joint demonstrates the fracture of the left pars *(arrow)*. *F*, At a more inferior level, a pars defect is identified on the right, and the more recent fracture of the left pars is visualized. Note the surrounding bony sclerosis and hypertrophy. It is presumed that there was an old fracture on the right that led to the pars defect, and that the more recent fracture on the left accounts for the patient's present symptoms. (Case courtesy of Ronald Krasner, MD, Chicago, Ill.)

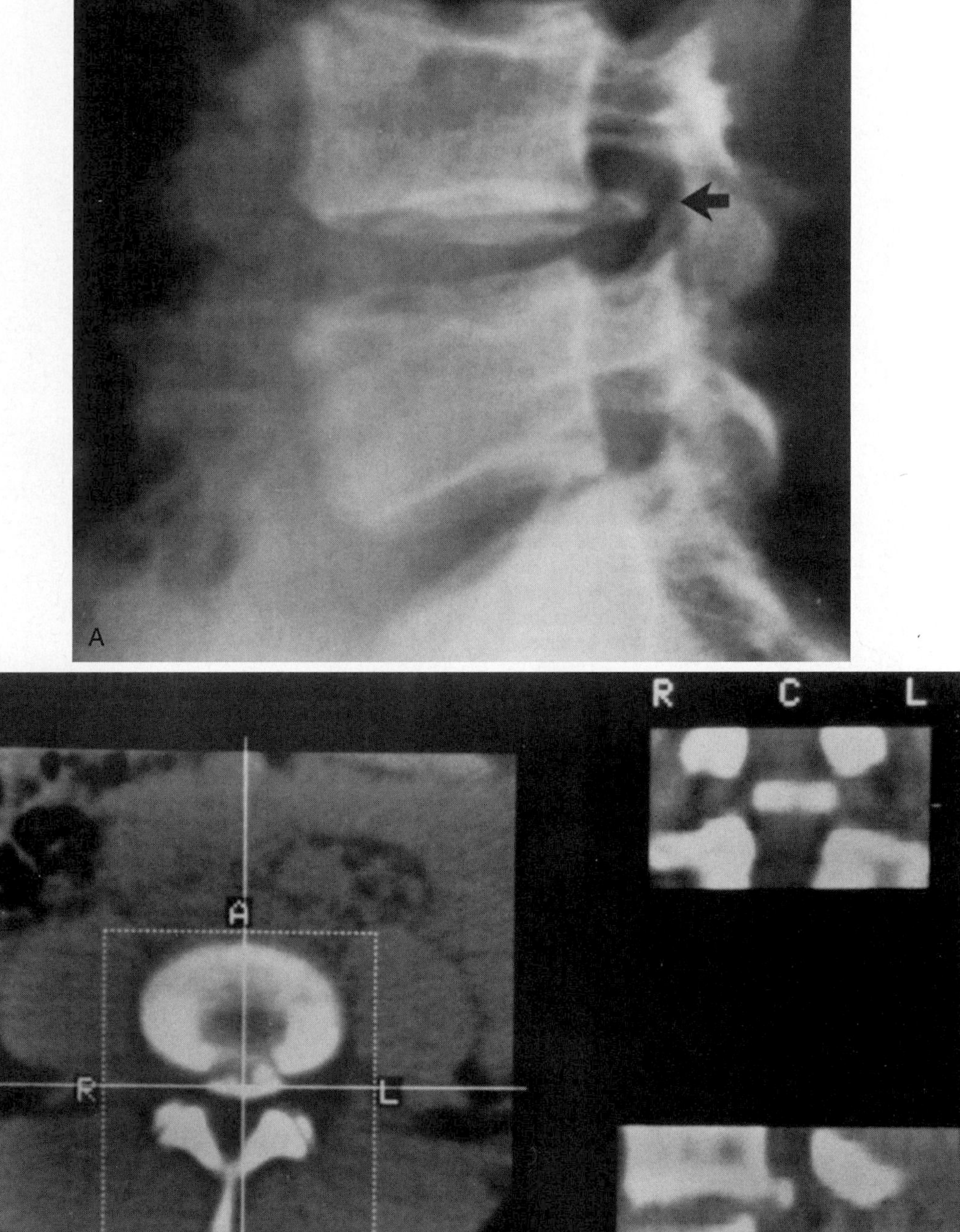

Figure 13–93. Acute herniation of the L4–L5 intervertebral disc, with associated fracture of the posterior rim apophysis of L4, in a teenage boy. A, Lateral view clearly demonstrates a bone fragment within the vertebral canal *(arrow)* opposite the inferior surface of L4. *B*, Axial CT image obtained through the inferior end plate of L4 demonstrates the displaced rim fragment of the apophysis that accompanies the herniated nucleus pulposus. Reconstructions in the coronal *(C)* and sagittal *(S)* planes clarify the injury. A, Anterior; L, left; P, posterior; R, right. (Case courtesy of Leland Holly II, MD, Muskegon, Mich.)

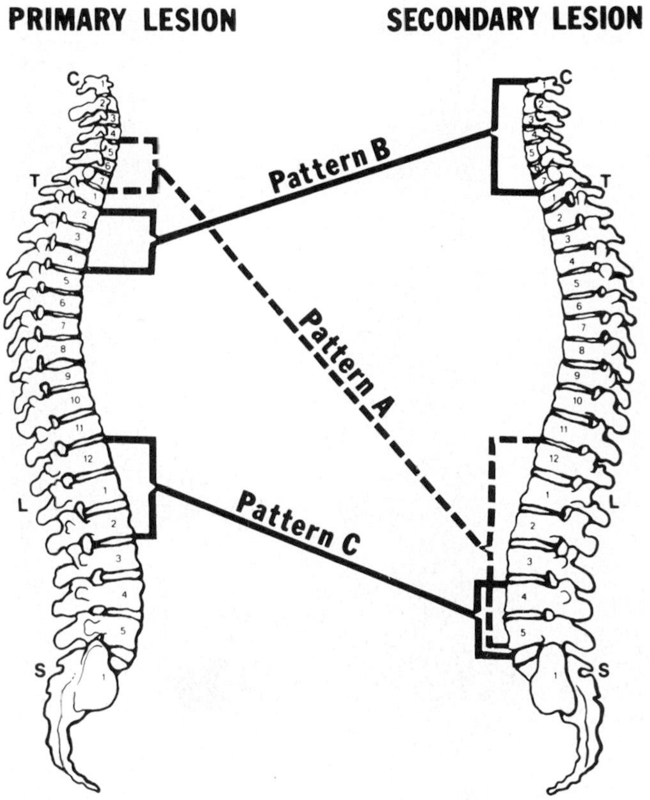

PRIMARY LESION SECONDARY LESION

Pattern B

Pattern A

Pattern C

Figure 13–94. Three major patterns of multiple-level injuries. Pattern A: primary lesion at C5–C7, with secondary lesion at T12 or lumbar spine. Pattern B: primary lesion at T2–T4, with secondary lesion in cervical spine. Pattern C: primary lesion at thoracolumbar junction, with secondary lesion at L4–L5. A fourth pattern, not demonstrated, consists of midthoracic fractures associated with cervical or thoracolumbar junction fractures. (From Calenoff, L., Chessare, J. W., Rogers, L. F. et al. [1978]. Multilevel spinal injuries: Importance of early recognition. A.J.R. Am. J. Roentgenol., *130*:665.)

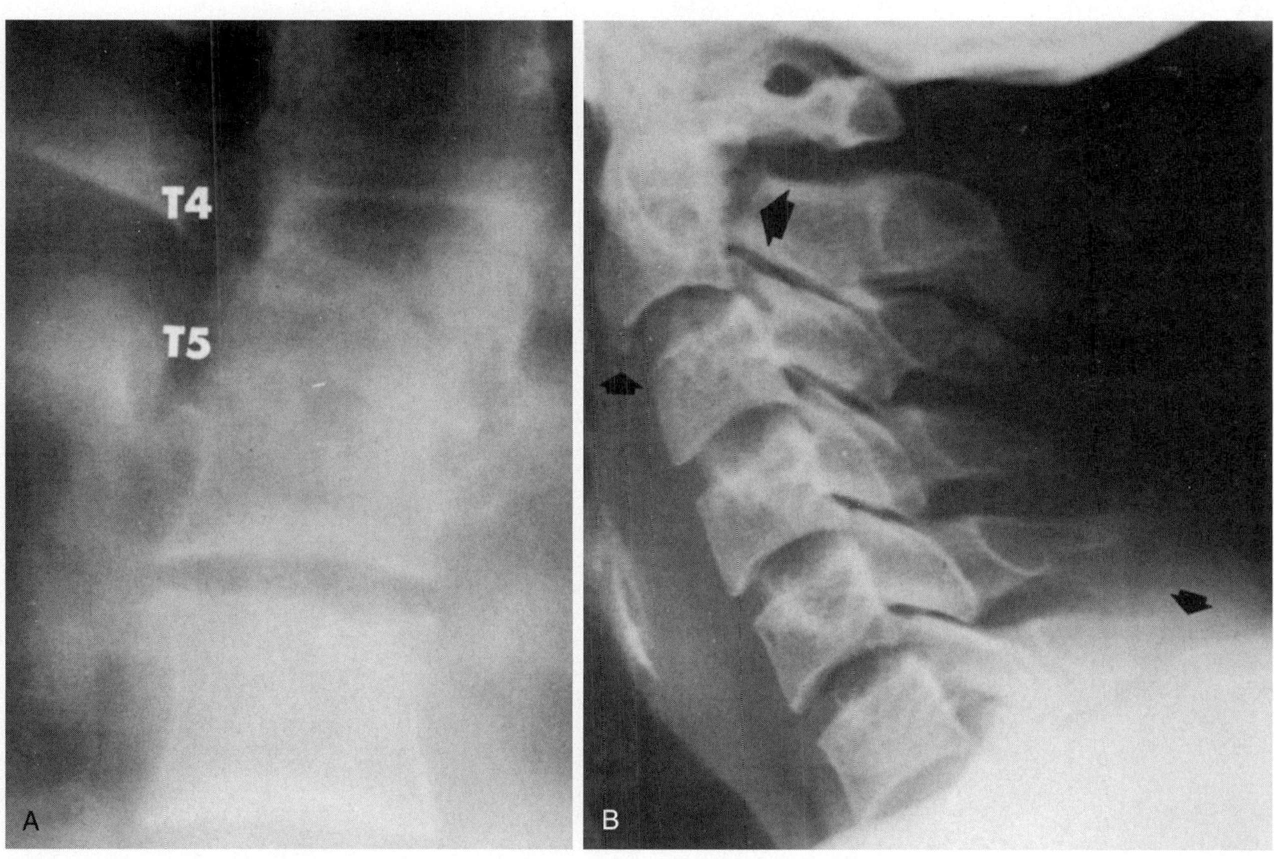

Figure 13–95. Multiple-level injury. *A*, The primary fracture-dislocation involved the bodies of T4 and T5. *B*, The second-level injury consisted of a hanged man fracture *(large arrow)* with a small avulsion from the body of C2 *(upper small arrow)* and a fracture of the spinous processes of C6 *(lower small arrow)*. (From Calenoff, L., Chessare, J. W., Rogers, L. F. et al. [1978]. Multilevel spinal injuries: Importance of early recognition. A.J.R. Am. J. Roentgenol., *130*:665.)

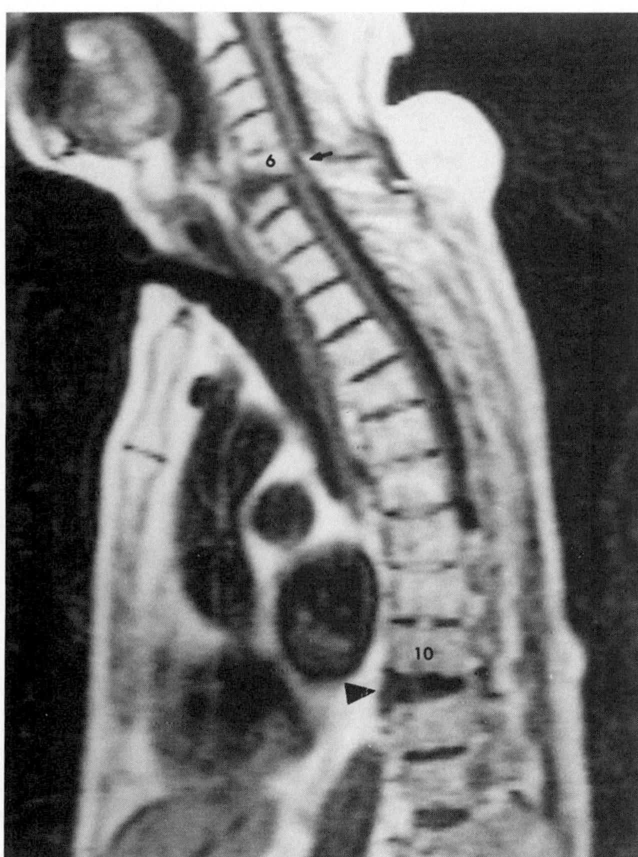

Figure 13–96. Sagittal T_1-weighted MR image showing extension injuries of C6 *(arrow)* and T10 *(arrowhead)* in a patient with ankylosing spondylitis. Note the wide disc space at each involved level.

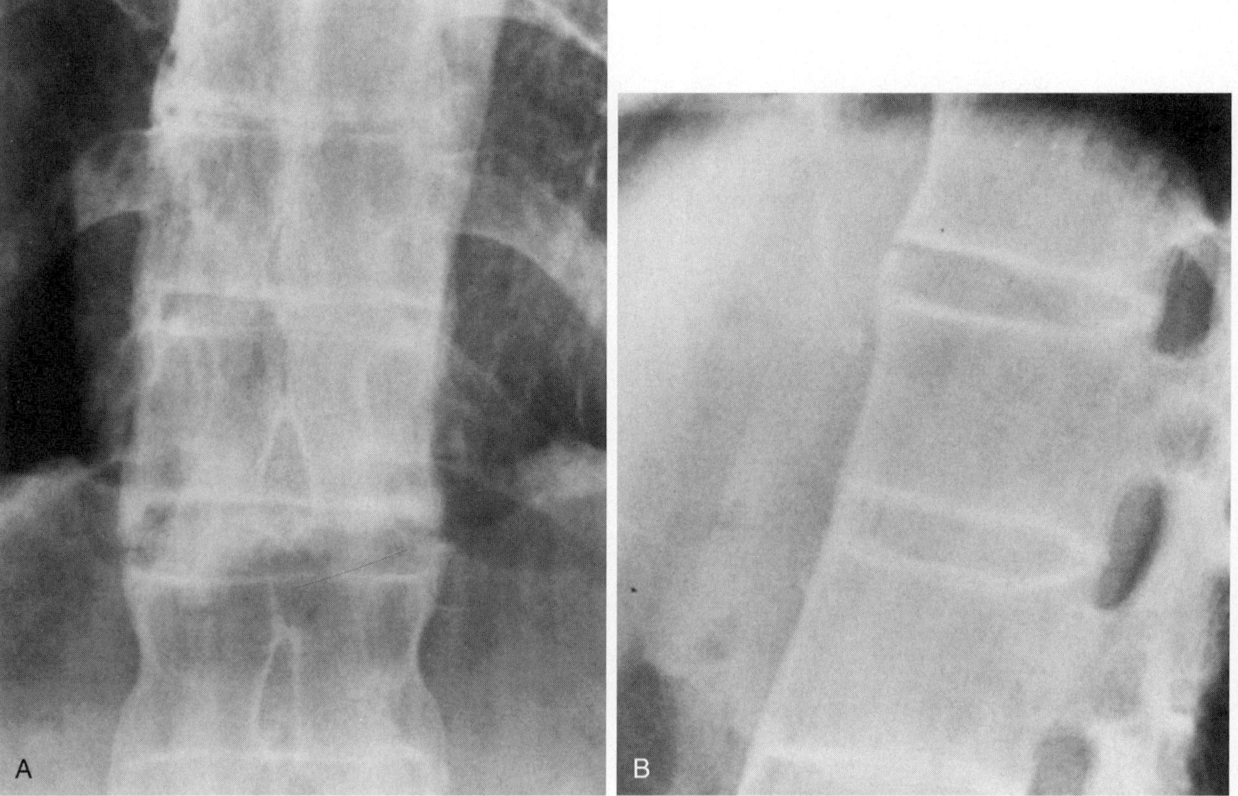

Figure 13–97. Fracture through the T12–L1 interspace sustained in a fall from a ladder. The patient was a man with ankylosing spondylitis. *A*, Anteroposterior view demonstrates cortical disruption through the syndesmophytes at the T12–L1 interspace. *B*, Lateral view shows that the fracture line is within the interspace and does not involve the vertebral body. There is no dislocation.

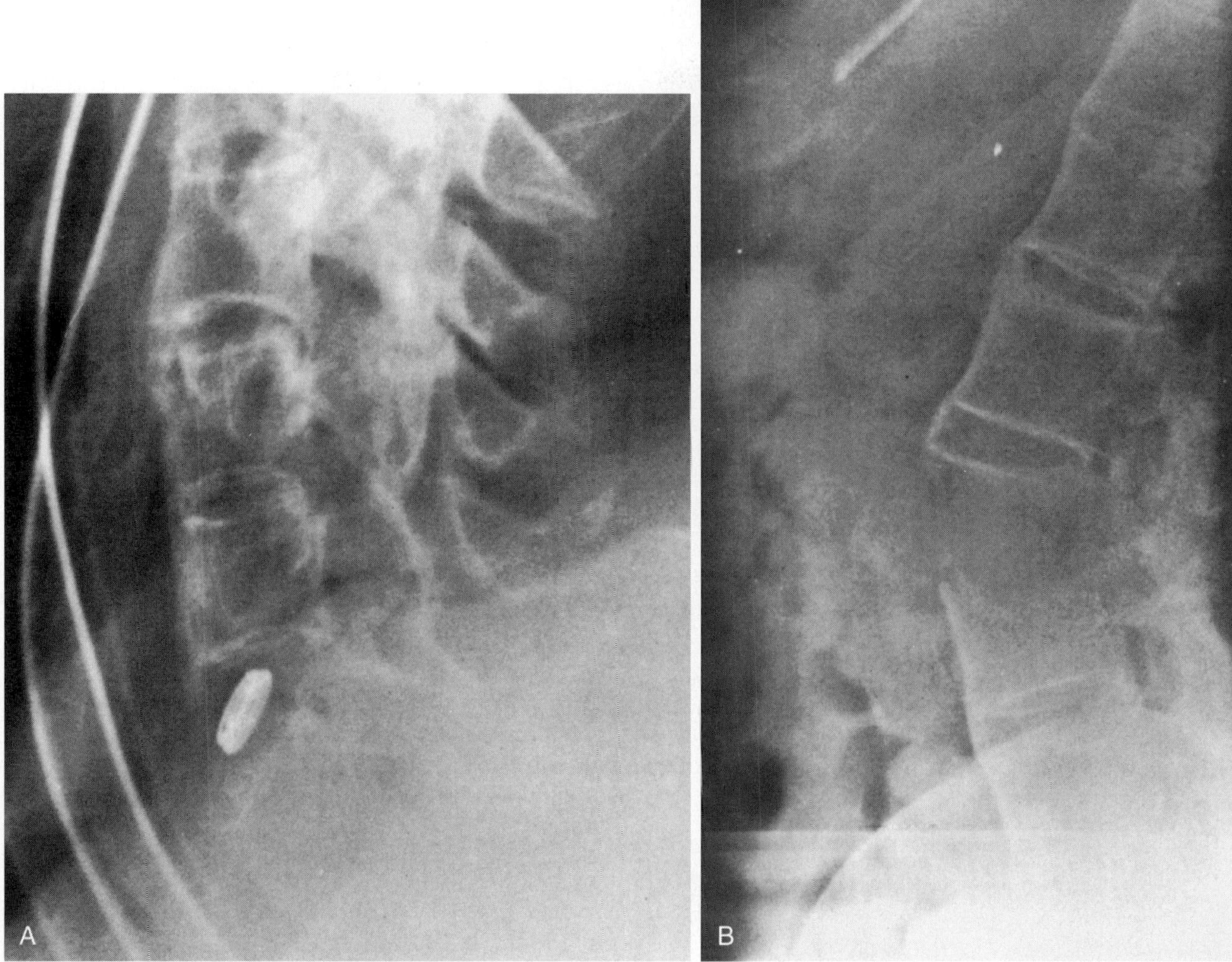

Figure 13–98. Hyperextension injuries at two levels of the spine in an elderly man with ankylosing spondylitis who fell down a short flight of stairs. *A*, Note extension fracture-dislocation of C6–C7, with posterior displacement of C6 upon C7 and markedly widened C7 intervertebral disc space. A snap on the patient's clothing is projected in this interspace. *B*, A transverse hyperextension fracture through the upper portion of the L3 vertebral body. Note the syndesmophytes characteristic of ankylosing spondylitis. Patient was quadriplegic with a transection of the spinal cord at the level of the cervical fracture-dislocation.

Healing occurs quickly after the application of a brace, body cast, or surgical instrumentation.

Fracture-dislocations occur with the fracture line located in the same position as that described previously.[80, 184] The degree of displacement and the resultant spinal cord injury are variable and in part dependent on the severity of the forces involved and the degree of compromise of the spinal canal. In their review, Woodruff and Dewing[195] found that the initial mortality from this fracture was 45%.

Delays in diagnosis of fracture are frequent.[166] A high index of suspicion is warranted to prevent displacement of the fracture. Sudden exacerbation of spinal pain or mild neurologic deterioration, even in the absence of trauma, in a patient with ankylosing spondylitis should suggest the possibility of spine fracture.[166, 184] Radiologic examination of the entire spine is indicated, because occasionally, multiple fractures occur simultaneously (see Fig. 13–96).

Evidence suggests that the locally destructive lesions arising at the interspace and involving the apposing surfaces of the vertebral bodies in ankylosing spondylitis are in fact due to stress fractures[196] or to healing fractures following minor trauma. These lesions have sometimes been referred to as destructive lesions or pseudarthrosis.[55] They are more frequently located in the thoracolumbar junction and the dorsal spine than are the acute fractures just described. Examination of material obtained at surgery has failed to demonstrate pannus or infection but has revealed bone fragmentation and proliferation of connective tissue and collagen. In many ways, the pathologic changes resemble those of neuropathic joints. The conclusion is that the destructive lesions in the rigid spine are initially stress or minor fractures of the posterior elements that, if they fail to heal or unite, result in a pseudarthrosis between the two adjacent vertebral bodies.[55]

Diffuse Idiopathic Skeletal Hyperostosis

Fractures occurring in association with diffuse idiopathic skeletal hyperostosis (DISH) were first described by Fardon[56] in 1978 and since then have been reported with increasing frequency.[12, 25, 90] As with an ankylosing spondylitis, they are more likely to occur in the lower cervical spine through the intervertebral disc space, with or without associated dislocation (Figs. 13–99 and 13–100). The cervical fractures, including dens fractures, are often due to hyperextension and result from minor falls. They may also occur in the thoracolumbar spine. Occasionally, transverse fractures involve the vertebral body. As with ankylosing spondylitis, pseudoarthrosis has also been reported to occur in patients with DISH.[156]

Open and Penetrating Wounds

Missile or gunshot wounds may injure the spine and spinal cord in several ways.[197] Direct passage of the missile through the spinal cord or nerve roots is not necessary to create a neurologic injury; the blast effect from nearby passage is sufficient. The missile may penetrate and remain within the spinal canal, penetrate and transit the canal, or ricochet off some component of the vertebral body. Various fractures of the vertebral body and posterior elements occur depending upon the caliber of the bullet and the force expended. The bullet and fragments will be identified on frontal and lateral radiographs. Localization to the vertebral canal requires that the object be seen within the canal on both projections. Often the course of transit is better defined by CT (Fig. 13–101).

Stab wounds are more likely in the thoracic spine and often result in the Brown-Séquard syndrome. They are occasionally accompanied by fractures of the posterior elements, which are disclosed more easily by CT.

Radiologic Assessment of Vertebral Stability

Throughout this chapter reference has been made to injuries that were considered stable and unstable. The stability of the vertebral column is dependent upon the integrity of both the bony and soft tissue elements. If an injury produces sufficient damage to allow abnormal motion at, above, or below the involved area, an unstable condition has been created.[35, 36] As a rule, disruption of any of the individual ligaments at a given vertebral level does not produce instability. However, isolated disruptions are the exception, rather than the rule, and a combination of abnormalities—the usual occurrence—will re-

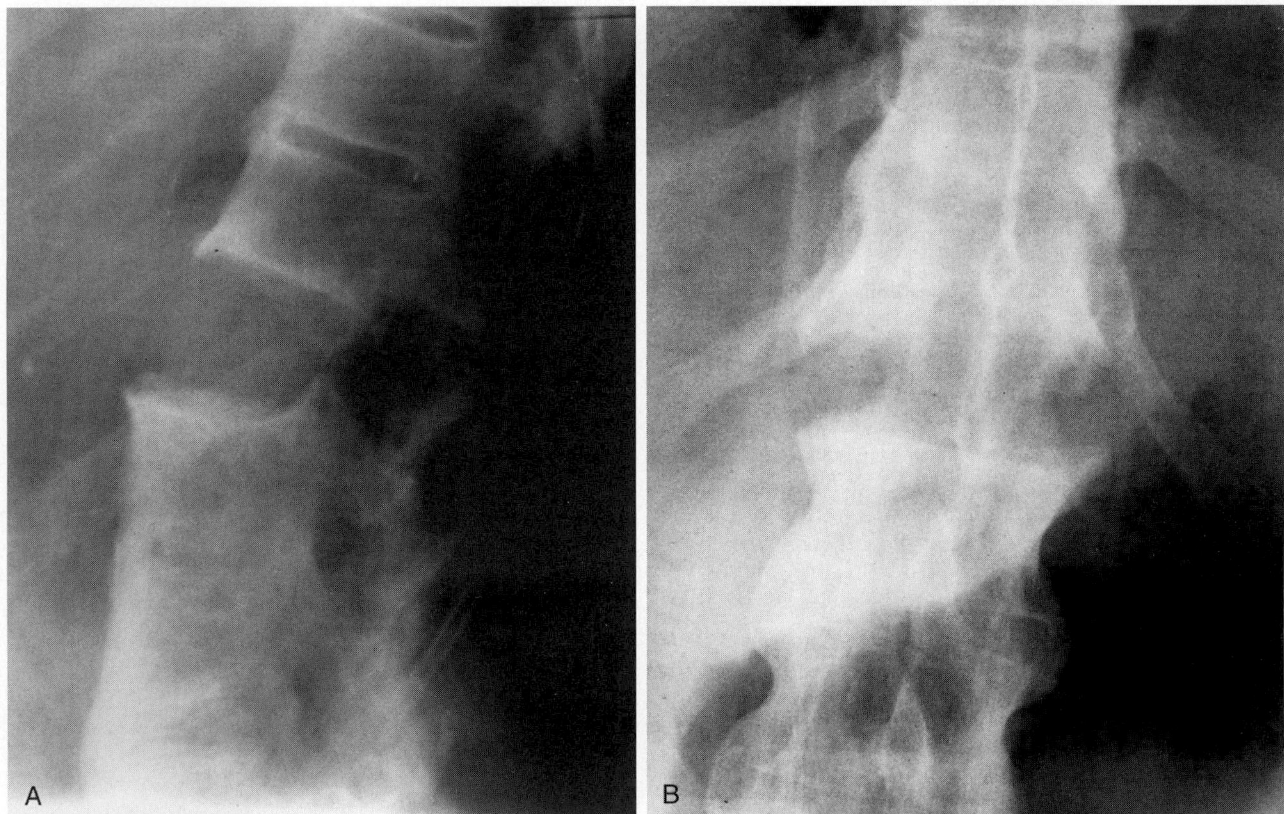

Figure 13–99. Extension fracture-dislocation in an elderly patient with diffuse idiopathic skeletal hyperostosis (DISH) who fell down stairs. *A*, Lateral view shows gaping anteriorly at the T12–L1 disc space. Note the firm ankylosis from syndesmophytes at all other levels. *B*, Anteroposterior view shows slight lateral malalignment in addition to the distraction.

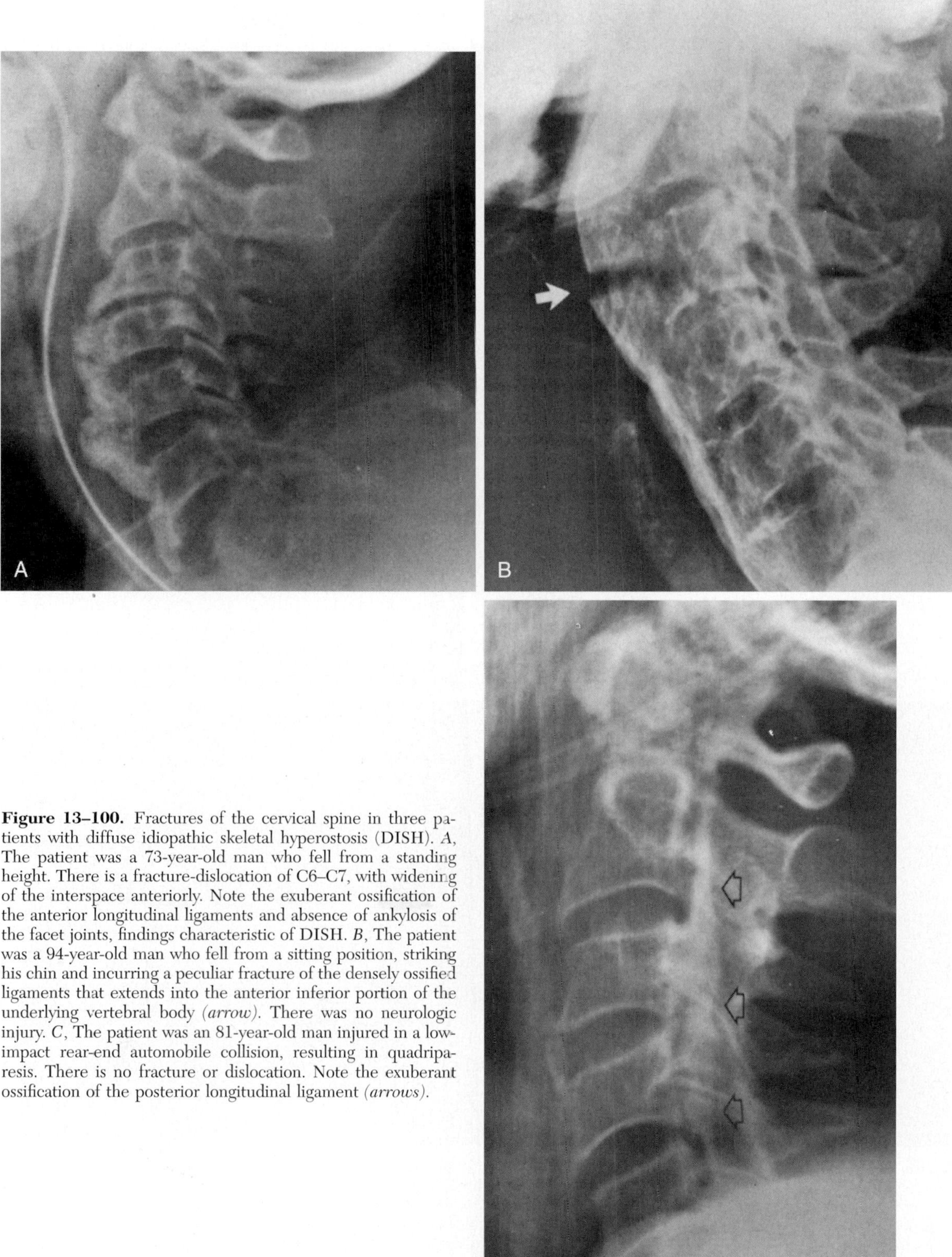

Figure 13–100. Fractures of the cervical spine in three patients with diffuse idiopathic skeletal hyperostosis (DISH). *A*, The patient was a 73-year-old man who fell from a standing height. There is a fracture-dislocation of C6–C7, with widening of the interspace anteriorly. Note the exuberant ossification of the anterior longitudinal ligaments and absence of ankylosis of the facet joints, findings characteristic of DISH. *B*, The patient was a 94-year-old man who fell from a sitting position, striking his chin and incurring a peculiar fracture of the densely ossified ligaments that extends into the anterior inferior portion of the underlying vertebral body *(arrow)*. There was no neurologic injury. *C*, The patient was an 81-year-old man injured in a low-impact rear-end automobile collision, resulting in quadriparesis. There is no fracture or dislocation. Note the exuberant ossification of the posterior longitudinal ligament *(arrows)*.

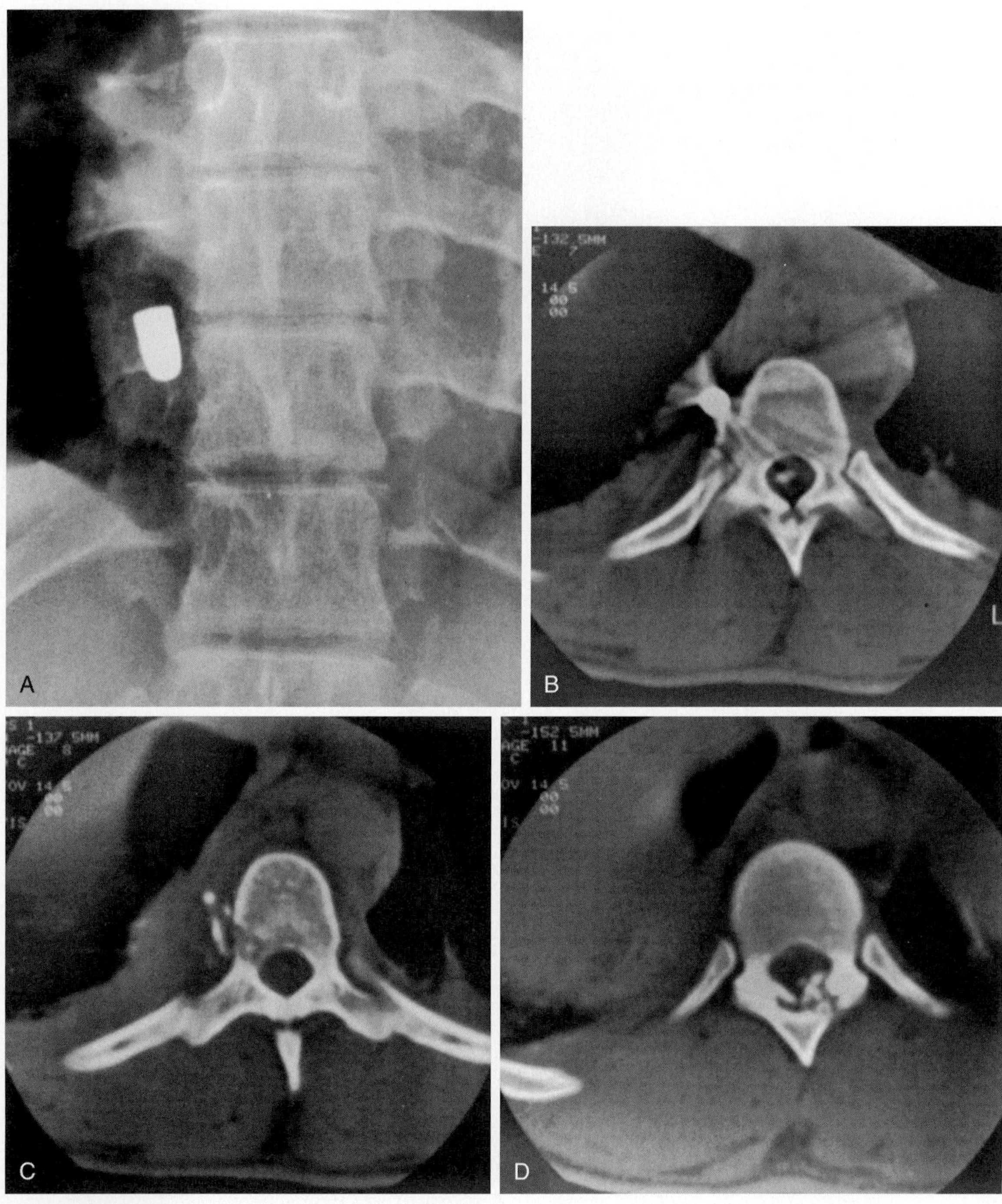

Figure 13–101. Gunshot wounds resulted in spinal cord transection in a 28-year-old man. *A*, Anteroposterior view demonstrates a bullet adjacent to T9, but the course of the bullet is not obvious. *B*, CT image obtained through the upper portion of T9 demonstrates the bullet. There is a small fragment of bone lying within the vertebral canal. *C*, CT image obtained at a slightly lower level in T9 demonstrates a fracture of the right pedicle. *D*, CT image obtained through T10 reveals fracture of the left lamina with multiple bone fragments. The course of the bullet is then clear, the bullet having entered inferiorly on the left and traversed the spinal canal to exit superiorly beneath the right pedicle of T9.

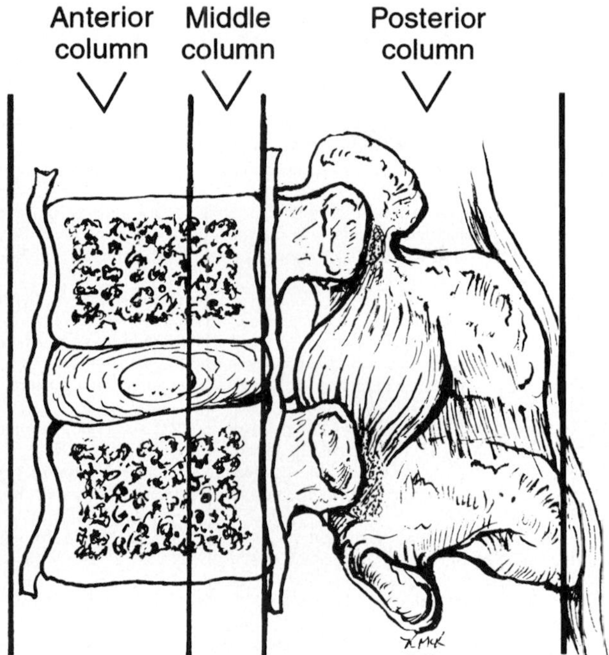

Figure 13–102. Denis' three-column concept of vertebral stability. See text for description.

sult in instability. From a clinical standpoint, unstable injuries are associated with the potential for increased skeletal deformity, for the production of neurologic damage, or for exacerbation of an existing neurologic deficit.[35, 36]

No subject has engendered more controversy than that of post-traumatic vertebral stability. Each surgeon will apply his or her own standards for management of the spine-injured patient. However, from a radiologic standpoint, it is possible to define the extent of injury and predict the probability of instability.[36, 38, 68, 148] In the thoracic region, the ribs provide a stabilizing influence in the T1–T8 region[148] that negate features of instability found in other areas of the spine.[36, 191]

Most authorities subscribe to Denis' three-column concept of the spine and its role in determining stability.[36, 38, 46] Denis divides the spine into three distinct functional columns. The anterior column extends from the anterior longitudinal ligament to a line drawn vertically from the junction of the middle and posterior thirds of the vertebral body. The middle column extends from this line to the posterior longitudinal ligament. The posterior column extends from the posterior longitudinal ligament to the supraspinous ligament (Fig. 13–102). According to Denis, the middle column is the most important one, and instability results whenever there is disruption to any two *contiguous* columns. For instability to occur, there must be damage to the posterior longitudinal ligament and the posterior third of the intervertebral disc.[35, 36, 46, 191]

There are five radiographic signs that indicate disruption of specific columns in the spine. Although the presence of only one of these signs is sufficient to indicate instability, as a rule two or more are often present in every unstable injury. The signs are (1) displacement greater than 2 mm, (2) widening of the interspinous space by greater than 2 mm, (3) widening of the facet joints, (4) widening of the interpedicle distance by more than 2 mm, and (5) disruption of the posterior vertebral body line.[36, 38, 68] Displacement disrupts all three columns (see Fig. 13–71). Widening of the interspinous distance and of the facet joints indicates that the middle and posterior columns have been violated by a severe posterior injury that has torn the supraspinous, interspinous, and interfacet ligaments, as well as the ligamentum flavum, the posterior longitudinal ligament, and the posterior third of the disc (see Fig. 13–39). Widening of the interpedicle distance indicates that the vertebral body has been fractured in the sagittal plane and that the lamina is fractured as well. Thus, all three columns have been disrupted (see Fig. 13–38). Finally, disruption of the posterior vertebral body line is direct evidence of middle column injury (see Fig. 13–62). This feature is found in bursting, rotary, and shearing injuries.[36, 38, 68]

When radiographic signs of instability are encountered, the findings should be communicated to the attending spine surgeon. As a rule, I never use the designations *stable* or *unstable* in an official radiographic report, because many injuries that appear unstable by radiographic criteria may be managed with nonoperative treatment. It is best for the radiologist to verbally express any concerns and allow the surgeon to make decisions on the basis of the clinical findings as well as the radiographic appearance. MRI may provide additional insight, because it can demonstrate the integrity of the various ligamentous structures or the lack of such integrity.[149]

References

1. Abel, M. S. (1983). Occult Traumatic Lesions of the Cervical and Thoracolumbar Vertebrae. 2nd Ed. Warren Green, St. Louis.
2. Abel, M. S. (1950). Sacroiliac joint changes in traumatic paraplegics. Radiology, 55:233.
3. Aland, C., Rineberg, B. A., Malberg, M. et al. (1986). Fracture of the pedicle of the fourth lumbar vertebra associated with contralateral spondylolysis. J. Bone Joint Surg. Am., *68*:1454.
4. Ashman, C. J., Yu, J. S., & Chung, C. B. (1997). The Chance fracture: Anteroposterior radiographic signs. Emerg. Radiol., *4*:320.
5. Atlas, S. W., Regenbogen, V., Rogers, L. F., & Kim, K. S. (1986). The radiographic characterization of burst fractures of the spine. A.J.R. Am. J. Roentgenol., *147*:575.
6. Baker, L. L., Goodman, S. B., Perkash, I. et al. (1990). Benign versus pathologic compression fractures of vertebral bodies: Assessment with conventional spin-echo, chemical shift, and STIR MR imaging. Radiology, *174*:595.
7. Baur, A., Stäbler, A., Brüning, R. et al. (1998). Diffusion-weighted MR imaging of bone marrow: Differentiation of benign versus pathologic compression fractures. Radiology, *207*:349.
8. Beldekos, A., Korres, D. S., & Nikolakakos, G. (1981). A Chance's fracture in a double level fracture of the spine. Injury, *13*:34.
9. Benson, D. R. (1988). Unstable thoracolumbar fractures, with emphasis on the burst fracture. Clin. Orthop., *230*:14.
10. Bentley, G., & McSweeney, T. (1968). Multiple spinal injuries. Br. J. Surg., 55:565.
11. Benzel, E. C., & Larson, S. L. (1986). Functional recovery after decompressive operation for thoracic and lumbar spine fractures. Neurosurgery, *19*:772.
12. Bernini, P. M., Floman, Y., Marvel, J. Jr., & Rothman, R. H. (1981). Multiple thoracic spine fractures complicating ankylosing hyperostosis of the spine. J. Trauma, *21*:811.
13. Bhata, D. V., Pizarro, A. J., Seitman, A., & Budiman, E. (1979). Axial skeletal changes in paraplegics. Radiology, *133*:55.
14. Boger, D. C., Chandler, R. W., Pearce, J. G. et al. (1983). Unilateral facet dislocation at the lumbosacral junction. Case report and literature review. J. Bone Joint Surg. Am., *65*:117.
15. Bohlman, H. H., Freehafter, A., & Dejak, J. (1985). The results of treatment of acute injuries of the upper thoracic spine with paralysis. J. Bone Joint Surg. Am., *67*:360.

16. Bohrer, S. P. (1965). Spinal fractures in tetanus. Radiology, *85*:1111.
17. Boukhris, R., & Becker, K. L. (1973). The inter-relationship between vertebral fractures and osteoporosis. Clin. Orthop., *90*:210.
18. Bretz, G. W., & Jenkins, R. G. (1981). Gas density in an ununited fracture of a vertebral body. J. Bone Joint Surg. Am., *63*:1183.
19. Brightman, R. P., Miller, C. A., Rea, G. L. et al. (1992). Magnetic resonance imaging of trauma to the thoracic and lumbar spine: The importance of the posterior longitudinal ligament. Spine, *17*:541.
20. Brinckmann, P., Johannleweling, N., Hilweg, D., & Biggemann, M. (1987). Fatigue fracture of human lumbar vertebrae. Clin. Biomech., *2*:94.
21. Broom, M. M., & Raycroft, J. R. (1988). Complications of fractures of the cervical spine in ankylosing spondylitis. Spine, *13*:763.
22. Brower, A. C., & Downey, E. F. Jr. (1981). Kümmell disease: Report of a case with serial monographs. Radiology, *141*:363.
23. Brown, W. H., Stothert, J. Jr. (1985). Traumatic subarachnoid-pleural fistula. J. Trauma, *25*:1105.
24. Buchanan, J. R., Myers, C. A., & Greer, R. B. (1988). A comparison of the risk of vertebral fracture in menopausal osteopenia and other metabolic disturbances. J. Bone Joint Surg. Am., *70*:704.
25. Burkus, J. K., & Denis, F. (1994). Hyperextension injuries of the thoracic spine in diffuse idiopathic skeletal hyperostosis. J. Bone Joint Surg. Am., *76*:237.
26. Calenoff, L., Chessare, J. W., Rogers, L. F. et al. (1978). Multilevel spinal injuries: Importance of early recognition. A.J.R. Am. J. Roentgenol., *130*:665.
27. Carragher, A. M., & Cranley, B. (1987). Seat-belt stomach transection in association with "Chance" vertebral fracture. Br. J. Surg., *74*:397.
28. Chakeres, D. W., Flickinger, F., Bresnahan, J. C. et al. (1987). MR imaging of acute spinal cord trauma. A.J.N.R. Am. J. Neuroradiol., *8*:5.
29. Chance, G. Q. (1948). A note on a type of flexion fractures of the spine. Br. J. Radiol., *21*:542.
30. Chiroff, R. T., & Sachs, B. L. (1976). Discontinuity of the spinous process on standard roentgenographs as an aid in the diagnosis of instable fractures of the spine. J. Trauma, *16*:313.
31. Cooper, K. L. (1988). Insufficiency fractures of the sternum: A consequence of thoracic kyphosis? Radiology, *167*:471.
32. Cope, R., Salmon, A., & Gaines, R. (1987). Association of a thoracic distraction fracture and an unusual avulsion fracture. Spine, *12*:943.
33. Crim, J. R., Bassett, L., Gold, R. H. et al. (1988). Spinal neuroarthropathy after traumatic paraplegia. A.J.N.R. Am. J. Neuroradiol., *9*:359.
34. Cuénod, C. A., Laredo, J.-D., Chevret, S. et al. (1996). Acute vertebral collapse due to osteoporosis or malignancy: Appearance on unenhanced and gadolinium-enhanced MR images. Radiology, *199*:541.
35. Daffner, R. H. (1998). Thoracic and lumbar vertebral injuries. Semin. Musculoskel. Radiol., *2*:45.
36. Daffner, R. H. (1996). Imaging of Vertebral Trauma. 2nd Ed. Philadelphia, Lippincott Raven.
37. Daffner, R. H. (1989). Dislocation at L-5–S-1 with unilateral facet lock. Skeletal Radiol., *18*:489.
38. Daffner, R. H., Deeb, Z. L., Goldberg, A. L. et al. (1990). The radiologic assessment of post-traumatic vertebral stability. Skeletal Radiol., *19*:103.
39. Daffner, R. H., Deeb, Z. L., & Rothfus W. E. (1987). The posterior vertebral body line: Importance in the detection of burst fractures. A.J.R. Am. J. Roentgenol., *148*:93.
40. Daffner, R. H., Deeb, Z. L., & Rothfus, W. E. (1987). Thoracic fractures and dislocations in motorcyclists. Skeletal Radiol., *16*:280.
41. Daffner, R. H., Deeb, Z. L., & Rothfus, W. E. (1986). Fingerprints of vertebral trauma—a unifying concept based on mechanisms. Skeletal Radiol., *15*:518.
42. Dake, M. D., Jacobs, R. P., & Margolin, F. R. (1985). Computed tomography of posterior lumbar apophyseal ring fractures. J. Comput. Assist. Tomogr., *9*:730.
43. Das De, S., & McCreath, S. W. (1981). Lumbosacral fracture-dislocation. A report of four cases. J. Bone Joint Surg. Br., *63*:58.
44. Dehner, J. R. (1971). Seatbelt injuries of the spine and abdomen. A.J.R. Am. J. Roentgenol., *111*:833.
45. De La Torre, J. C. (1981). Spinal cord injury. Review of basic and applied research. Spine, *6*:315.
46. Denis, F. (1983). The three column spine and its significance in the classification of acute thoracolumbar spinal injuries. Spine, *8*:817.
47. Denis, F., & Burkus, J. K. (1992). Shear fracture-dislocations of the thoracic and lumbar spine associated with forceful hyperextension (lumberjack paraplegia). Spine, *17*:156.
48. Dennis, L. N., & Rogers, L. F. (1989). Superior mediastinal widening from spine fractures mimicking aortic rupture on chest radiographs. A.J.R. Am. J. Roentgenol., *152*:27.
49. DeSmet, A. A., Robinson, R. G., Johnson, B. E., & Lukert, B. P. (1988). Spinal compression fractures in osteoporotic women: Patterns and relationship to hyperkyphosis. Radiology, *166*:497.
50. Dietemann, J. L., Runge, M., Badoz, A. et al. (1988). Radiology of posterior lumbar apophyseal ring fractures: Report of 13 cases. Neuroradiology, *30*:337.
51. Ehni, G., & Schneider, S. J. (1988). Posterior lumbar vertebral rim fracture and associated disc protrusion in adolescence. J. Neurosurg., *68*:912.
52. El-Khoury, G. Y., & Whitten, C. G. (1993). Trauma to the upper thoracic spine: Anatomy, biomechanics, and unique imaging features. A.J.R. Am. J. Roentgenol., *160*:95.
53. El Masri, W. S. (1983). Traumatic spondyloptosis of the dorsal spine with incomplete neurological deficit. Injury, *15*:35.
54. Falcone, S., Quencer, R. M., Green, B. A. et al. (1994). Progressive posttraumatic myelomalacic myelopathy: Imaging and clinical features. A.J.N.R. Am. J. Neuroradiol., *15*:747.
55. Fang, D., Leong, J. C. Y., Ho, E. K. W. et al. (1988). Spinal pseudarthrosis in ankylosing spondylitis. J. Bone Joint Surg. Br., *70*:443.
56. Fardon, D. F. (1978). Odontoid fracture complicating ankylosing hyperostosis of the spine. Spine, *3*:108.
57. Fazl, M., Bilbao, J. M., & Hudson, A. R. (1981). Laceration of the aorta complicating spinal fracture in ankylosing spondylitis. Neurosurgery, *8*:732.
58. Ferguson, R. J. (1974). Low-back pain in college football linemen. J. Bone Joint Surg. Am., *56*:1300.
59. Ferguson, R. J., & Allen, B. L. Jr. (1984). A mechanistic classification of thoracolumbar spine fractures. Clin. Orthop., *189*:77.
60. Ferrandez, L., Usabiaga, J., Curto, J. M. et al. (1989). Atypical multivertebral fracture due to hyperextension in an adolescent girl. Spine, *14*:645.
61. Fidler, M. W. (1988). Remodeling of the spinal canal after burst fracture. J. Bone Joint Surg. Br., *70*:730.
62. Flanders, A. E., Tartaglino, L. M., Friedman, D. P. et al. (1992). Magnetic resonance imaging in acute spinal injury. Semin. Roentgenol., *27*:271.
63. Frager, D., Elkin, C., Swerdlow, M., & Bloch, S. (1988). Subacute osteoporotic compression fracture: Misleading magnetic resonance appearance. Skeletal Radiol., *17*:123.
64. Fujita, K., Shinmei, M., Hashimoto, K., & Shimomura, Y. (1986). Posterior dislocation of the sacral apophyseal ring. A case report. Am. J. Sports Med., *14*:243.
65. Gallagher, J. C., Hedlund, L. R., Stoner, S., & Meeger, C. (1988). Vertebral morphometry: Normative data. Bone Mineral, *4*:189.
66. Garrett, J. W., & Braunstein, P. W. (1962). Seat belt syndrome. J. Trauma, *2*:220.
67. Garth, W. P. Jr., & VanPatten, P. K. (1989). Fractures of the lumbar lamina with epidural hematoma simulating herniation of a disc. J. Bone Joint Surg. Am., *71*:771.
68. Gehweiler, J. A. Jr., Daffner, R. H., & Osborne, R. L. Jr. (1981). Relevant signs of stable and unstable thoracolumbar vertebral column trauma. Skeletal Radiol., *7*:179.
69. Gellad, F. E., Levine, A. M., Joslyn, J. N. et al. (1986). Pure thoracolumbar facet dislocation: Clinical features and CT appearance. Radiology, *161*:505.
70. Gelman, M. I., & Umber, J. S. (1978). Fracture of the thoracolumbar spine in ankylosing spondylitis. A.J.R. Am. J. Roentgenol., *130*:485.
71. Gertzbein, S. D., & Court-Brown, C. M. (1988). Flexion-distraction injuries of the lumbar spine. Clin. Orthop., *227*:52.
72. Gertzbein, S. D., Court-Brown, C. M., Marks, P. et al. (1988). The neurological outcome following surgery for spinal fractures. Spine, *13*:641.
73. Gilsanz, V., Miranda, J., Cleveland, R., & Ulrich, W. (1980). Scoliosis secondary to fractures of the transverse processes of lumbar vertebrae. Radiology, *134*:627.
74. Goldberg, A. L., Deeb, Z. L., Rothfus, W. E., & Daffner, R. H. (1989). Magnetic resonance imaging in evaluation of acute spinal trauma. Spine: State of the Art Rev., *3*:339.
75. Goldberg, A. L., Rothfus, W. E., Deeb, L. et al. (1988). The impact of magnetic resonance on the diagnostic evaluation of acute cervicothoracic spinal trauma. Skeletal Radiol., *17*:89.
76. Gopalakrishnan, K. C., & El Masri, W. S. (1986). Fractures of the sternum associated with spinal injury. J. Bone Joint Surg. Br., *68*:178.
77. Graebe, R. P. (1988). Fracture-dislocation of the lumbosacral spine during a grand mal epileptic seizure. S. Afr. Med. J., *74*:129.
78. Graham, B., & Van Peteghem, P. K. (1989). Fractures of the spine in ankylosing spondylitis: Diagnosis, treatment, and complications. Spine, *14*:803.
79. Graves, V. B., Keene, J. S., Strother, C. M., & Bennett, L. N. (1988). CT of bilateral lumbosacral facet dislocation. A.J.N.R. Am. J. Neuroradiol., *9*:809.
80. Grisolia, A., Bell, R. L., & Peltier, L. F. (1967). Fractures and dislocations of the spine complicating ankylosing spondylitis. J. Bone Joint Surg. Am., *49*:339.
81. Guerra, J. Jr., Garfin, S. R., & Resnick, D. (1984). Vertebral burst fractures: CT analysis of the retropulsed fragment. Radiology, *153*:769.
82. Hackney, D. B., Asato, R., Joseph, P. M. et al. (1986). Hemorrhage and edema in acute spinal cord compression: Demonstration by MR imaging. Radiology, *161*:387.
83. Hall, H. E., & Robertson, W. W. Jr. (1985). Another Chance: A non–seatbelt related fracture of the lumbar spine. J. Trauma, *25*:1163.
84. Handel, S. F., Twiford, T. W. Jr., Reigel, D. H., & Kaufman, H. (1979). Posterior lumbar apophyseal fractures. Radiology, *130*:629.
85. Hanley, E. N., & Eskay, M. L. (1989). Thoracic spine fractures. Orthopedics, *12*:689.
86. Hazael, W. A. Jr., Jones, R. A., Morrey, B. F., & Stauffer, R. N. (1988). Vertebral fractures without neurological deficit. J. Bone Joint Surg. Am., *70*:1319.
87. Hedlung, L. R., & Gallagher, J. C. (1988). Vertebral morphometry in diagnosis of spinal fractures. Bone Mineral, 5:59.
88. Hedlung, L. R., Gallagher, J. C., Meeger, C., & Stoner, S. (1989). Change in vertebral shape in spinal osteoporosis. Calcif. Tissue Int., *44*:168.
89. Hegenbarth, R., & Ebel, K. D. (1976). Roentgen findings in fractures of the

vertebral column in childhood: Examination of 35 patients and its results. Pediatr. Radiol., 5:34.

90. Hendrix, R. W., Melany, M., Miller, R., & Rogers, L. F. (1994). Fractures of the spine in patients with ankylosis due to diffuse skeletal hyperostosis: Clinical and imaging findings. A.J.R. Am. J. Roentgenol., *162*:899.
91. Herron, L. D. (1987). Lateral flexion-distraction fracture. A variant of the seat-belt fracture. Spine, *12*:398.
92. Ho, E. K. W., & Leong, J. C. Y. (1987). Traumatic tetraparesis: A rare neurologic complication in ankylosing spondylitis with ossification of posterior longitudinal ligament of the cervical spine. Spine, *12*:403.
93. Holdsworth, F. W. (1970). Fractures, dislocations and fracture-dislocations of the spine. J. Bone Joint Surg. Am., *52*:1534.
94. Holdsworth, F. W. (1963). Fractures, dislocations and fracture-dislocations of the spine. J. Bone Joint Surg. Br., *45*:6.
95. Horal, J., Nachemson, A., & Scjeller, S. (1972). Clinical and radiological long term follow-up of vertebral fractures in children. Orthop. Scand., *4*:491.
96. Howland, W. J., Curry, J. L., & Buffington, C. B. (1965). Fulcrum fractures of lumbar spine. J.A.M.A., *193*:240.
97. Hubbard, D. D. (1976). Fractures of the dorsal and lumbar spine. Orthop. Clin. North Am., *7*:605.
98. Hubbard, D. D. (1974). Injuries of the spine in children and adolescents. Clin. Orthop., *100*:56.
99. Hudson, I., & Kavanagh, T. G. (1983). Duodenal transection and vertebral injury occurring in combination in a patient wearing a seat belt. Injury, *15*:6.
100. Ireland, M. L., & Mitcheli, L. J. (1987). Bilateral stress fracture of the lumbar pedicles in a ballet dancer. J. Bone Joint Surg. Am., *69*:140.
101. Isard, H. J. (1952). A roentgen evaluation of vertebral fractures resulting from convulsive shock therapy. A.J.R. Am. J. Roentgenol., *68*:247.
102. Itani, M., Evans, G. A., & Park, W. M. (1982). Spontaneous sternal collapse. J. Bone Joint Surg. Br., *64*:432.
103. Jackson, D. W., Wiltse, L. L., Dingeman, R. D., & Hayes, M. (1981). Stress reactions involving the pars interarticularis in young athletes. Am. J. Sports Med., *9*:304.
104. Jefferson, G. (1927–1928). Discussion on spinal injuries. Proc. Roy. Soc. Med., *21*:625.
105. Jelsma, R. K., Kirsch, P. T., Rice, J. R., & Jelsma, L. F. (1982). The radiographic description of thoracolumbar fractures. Surg. Neurol., *18*:230.
106. Jenyo, M. S. (1985). Post-traumatic fracture-dislocation of manubriosternal joint with a wedge fracture of the body of the fourth thoracic vertebra. J. Trauma, *25*:274.
107. Jodoin, A., Dupuis, P., Fraser, M., & Beaumont, P. (1985). Unstable fractures of the thoracolumbar spine: A 10-year experience at Sacre Coeur Hospital. J. Trauma, *25*:197.
108. Jones, H. K., McBride, G. G., & Mumby, R. C. (1989). Sternal fractures associated with spinal injury. J. Trauma, *29*:360.
109. Kachooie, A., Block, R., & Banna, M. (1985). Post-traumatic dorsal pseudomeningocele. J. Can. Assoc. Radiol., *36*:262.
110. Kanal, E., & Shellock, F. G. (1992). Policies, guidelines, and recommendations for MR imaging safety and patient management. J. Magn. Reson. Imaging, *2*:247.
111. Kaplan, P., Orton, D. F., & Asleson, R. J. (1987). Osteoporosis with vertebral compression fractures, retropulsed fragments, and neurologic compromise. Radiology, *165*:533.
112. Karasick, D., Schweitzer, M. E., Abidi, N. A., & Cotler, J. M. (1995). Fractures of the vertebrae with spinal cord injuries in patients with ankylosing spondylitis: Imaging findings. A.J.R. Am. J. Roentgenol., *165*:1205.
113. Keene, J. S. (1984). Radiographic evaluation of thoracolumbar fractures. Clin. Orthop., *189*:58.
114. Keene, J. S., Wackwitz, D. L., Drummond, D. S., & Breed, A. L. (1986). Compression-distraction instrumentation of unstable thoracolumbar fractures: Anatomic results obtained with each type of injury and method of instrumentation. Spine, *11*:895.
115. Keller, R. H. (1974). Traumatic displacement of the cartilaginous vertebral rim: A sign of intervertebral disc prolapse. Radiology, *110*:21.
116. Kewalramani, L. S., & Taylor, R. G. (1976). Multiple non-contiguous injuries to the spine. Acta Orthop. Scand., *47*:52.
117. Kilcoyne, R. F., Mack, L. A., King, H. A. et al. (1982). Thoracolumbar spine injuries associated with vertical plunges: Reappraisal with computed tomography. Radiology, *146*:137.
118. King, A. G. (1987). Burst compression fractures of the thoracolumbar spine. Pathologic anatomy and surgical management. Orthopedics, *10*:1711.
119. Korres, D. S., Katsaros, A., Pantazopoulos, T., & Hartofilakidis-Garofalidis, G. (1981). Double or multiple level fractures of the spine. Injury, *13*:147.
120. Kulkarni, M. V., Bondurant, F. J., Rose, S. L. et al. (1988). 1.5 Tesla magnetic resonance imaging of acute spinal trauma. Radiographics, *8*:1059.
121. Kumpan, W., Salomonowitz, E., Seidl, G., & Wittich, G. R. (1986). The intravertebral vacuum phenomenon. Skeletal Radiol., *15*:444.
122. Lawrason, J. N., Novelline, R. A., Rhea, J. T. et al. (1997). Early detection of thoracic spine fracture in the multiple trauma patient: Role of the initial portable chest radiograph. Emerg. Radiol., *4*:309.
123. Lee, C., Rogers, L. F., Woodring, J. H. et al. (1984). Fractures of the craniovertebral junction associated with other fractures of the spine: Overlooked entity? A.J.N.R. Am. J. Neuroradiol., *5*:775.
124. Leone, A., Cerase, A., Priolo, F., & Marano, P. (1997). Lumbosacral junction injury associated with unstable pelvic fracture: Classification and diagnosis. Radiology, *205*:253.
125. Levine, A. M., Boose, M., & Edwards, C. C. (1988). Bilateral facet dislocations in the thoracolumbar spine. Spine, *13*:630.
126. Levinthal, M. R. (1998). Fractures, dislocations, and fracture-dislocations of spine. pp. 2704–2790. In Canale, S. T. Ed.: Campbell's Operative Orthopaedics. 9th Ed. Mosby, St. Louis.
127. Louw, J. A., & Louw, J. A. (1987). Posterior dislocation of the sternoclavicular joint associated with major spinal injury. S. Afr. Med. J., *71*:791.
128. Lowrey, J. J. (1973). Dislocated lumbar vertebral epiphysis in adolescent children. J. Neurosurg., *38*:232.
129. Magerl, F., Aebi, M., Gertzbein, S. D. et al. (1994). A comprehensive classification of thoracic and lumbar injuries. Eur. Spine J., *3*:184.
130. Malcolm, B. W., Bradford, D. S., Winter, R. B., & Chou, S. N. (1981). Posttraumatic kyphosis. J. Bone Joint Surg. Am., *63*:891.
131. Manaster, B. J., & Osborn, A. G. (1986). CT patterns of facet fracture dislocations in the thoracolumbar region. A.J.N.R. Am. J. Neuroradiol., *7*:1007.
132. Martel, W., Seeger, J. F., Wicks, J. D., & Washburn, R. L. (1976). Traumatic lesions of the discovertebral junction in the lumbar spine. A.J.R. Am. J. Roentgenol., *127*:457.
133. Maruo, S., Tatekawa, F., & Nakano, K. (1987). Paraplegia resulting from vertebral compression fractures in senile osteoporosis. Z. Orthop., *125*:320.
134. Mayba, I. I. (1984). Hay balers fractures. J. Trauma, *24*:271.
135. McAfee, P. C., Yuan, H. A., Fredrickson, B. E., & Lubicky, J. P. (1983). The value of computed tomography in thoracolumbar fractures. An analysis of one hundred consecutive cases and a new classification. J. Bone Joint Surg. Am., *65*:461.
136. McGrory, B. J., VanderWilde, R. S., Currier, B. L., & Eismont, F. J. (1993). Diagnosis of subtle thoracolumbar burst fractures. A new radiographic sign. Spine, *18*:2228.
137. McHenry, M. C., Duchesneau, P. M., Keys, T. F. et al. (1988). Vertebral osteomyelitis presenting as spinal compression fracture. Arch. Intern. Med., *148*:417.
138. Melton, L. J. III, Kan, S. H., Frye, M. A. et al. (1989). Epidemiology of vertebral fractures in women. Am. J. Epidemiol., *129*:1000.
139. Meyer, P. R. Jr. (1989). Surgery of Spine Trauma. Churchill Livingstone, New York.
140. Miniaci, A., & McLaren, A. C. (1989). Anterolateral compression fracture of the thoracolumbar spine. A seat belt injury. Clin. Orthop., *240*:153.
141. Moulopoulos, L. A., Yoshimitsu, K., Johnston, D. A. et al. (1996). MR prediction of benign and malignant vertebral compression fractures. J. Magn. Reson. Imaging, *6*:667.
142. Murray, M. C., & Persellin, A. (1981). Cervical fracture complicating ankylosing spondylitis. A report of eight cases and review of the literature. Am. J. Med., *70*:1033.
143. Newbury, C. L., & Etter, L. E. (1955). Clarification of the problem of vertebral fractures from convulsive therapy. Arch. Neurol., *44*:479.
144. Nicholson, R. A. (1983). Lateral lumbosacral fracture dislocation: A case report. Injury, *15*:41.
145. Nicoll, E. A. (1949). Fractures of the dorso-lumbar spine. J. Bone Joint Surg. Br., *31*:376.
146. Obrant, K. J., Bengner, U., Johnell, O. et al. (1989). Increasing age-adjusted risk of fragility fractures: A sign of increasing osteoporosis in successive generations? Calcif. Tissue Int., *44*:157.
147. O'Callaghan, J. P., Ullrich, C. G., Yuan, B. A., & Kieffer, S. A. (1980). CT of facet distraction in flexion injuries of the thoracolumbar spine: The "naked facet." A.J.N.R. Am. J. Neuroradiol., *1*:97.
148. Oda, I., Abumi, K., Lu, D. et al. (1996). Biomechanical role of the posterior elements, costovertebral joints, and rib cage in the stability of the thoracic spine. Spine, *21*:1423.
149. Oner, F. C., van Gils, A. P. G., Dhert, W. J. A., & Verbout, A. J. (1999). MRI findings of thoracolumbar spine fractures: A categorisation based on MRI examinations of 100 fractures. Skeletal Radiol., *28*:433.
150. Osgood, C. P., Abbasy, M., & Mathews, T. (1975). Multiple spine fractures in ankylosing spondylitis. J. Trauma, *15*:163.
151. Papanicolaou, N., Wilkerson, R. H., Emans, J. B. et al. (1985). Bone scintigraphy and radiography in young athletes with low back pain. A.J.R. Am. J. Roentgenol., *145*:1039.
152. Park, W. M., McCall, I. W., McSweeney, T., & Jones, B. F. (1980). Cervicodorsal injury presenting as sternal fracture. Clin. Radiol., *31*:49.
153. Pennell, R. B., Maurer, A. H., & Bonakdarpour, A. (1985). Stress injuries of the pars interarticularis: Radiologic classification and indications for scintigraphy. A.J.R. Am. J. Roentgenol., *145*:763.
154. Petersilge, C. A., Pathria, M. N., Emery, S. E. et al. (1995). Thoracolumbar burst fractures: Evaluation with MR imaging. Radiology, *194*:49.
155. Post, M. J. D., & Green, B. A. (1983). The use of computed tomography in spinal trauma. Radiol. Clin. North Am., *21*:327.
156. Quagliano, P. V., Hayes, C. W., & Palmer, W. E. (1994). Vertebral pseudoarthrosis associated with diffuse idiopathic skeletal hyperostosis. Skeletal Radiol., *23*:253.
157. Rapp, G. F., & Kernek, C. B. (1974). Spontaneous fracture of the lumbar spine with correction of deformity in ankylosing spondylitis. J. Bone Joint Surg. Am., *56*:1277.
158. Reid, D. C., Hu, R., Davis, L. A., & Saboe, L. A. (1988). The nonoperative treatment of burst fractures of the thoracolumbar junction. J. Trauma, *28*:1188.

159. Rennie, W., & Mitchell, N. (1973). Flexion distraction injuries of the thoracolumbar spine. J. Bone Joint Surg. Am., *55*:386.
160. Resnik, C. S., Scheer, C. E., & Adelaar, R. S. (1985). Lumbosacral dislocation. J. Can. Assoc. Radiol., *36*:259.
161. Rigler, L. G. (1931). Kümmell's disease with report of a roentgenologically proved case. A.J.R. Am. J. Roentgenol., *15*:749.
162. Roaf, R. (1960). A study of the mechanics of spinal injuries. J. Bone Joint Surg. Br., *42*:810.
163. Roberts, J. B., & Curtiss, P. H. (1970). Stability of the thoracic and lumbar spine in traumatic paraplegia following fracture or fracture-dislocation. J. Bone Joint Surg. Am., *52*:1115.
164. Rogers, L. F. (1971). The roentgenographic appearance of transverse or Chance fractures of the spine: The seat belt fracture. A.J.R. Am. J. Roentgenol., *111*:844.
165. Rogers, L. F., Thayer, C., Weinberg, P. E., & Kim, K. S. (1980). Acute injuries of the upper thoracic spine associated with paraplegia. A.J.R. Am. J. Roentgenol., *134*:67.
166. Salathe, M., & Joehr, M. (1989). Unsuspected cervical fractures: A common problem in ankylosing spondylitis. Anethesiology, *70*:869.
167. Sasson, A., & Mozes, G. (1987). Complete fracture-dislocation of the thoracic spine without neurologic deficit. Spine, *12*:67.
168. Schaberg, F. J. Jr. (1986). Aortic injury occurring after minor trauma in ankylosing spondylitis. J. Vasc. Surg., *4*:410.
169. Scher, A. T. (1978). Double fractures of the spine—an indication for routine radiographic examination of the entire spine after injury. S. Afr. Med. J., *53*:411.
170. Shacked, I., Rappaport, Z. H., Barzilay, Z., & Ohri, A. (1983). Two-level fracture of the cervical spine in a young child. J. Bone Joint Surg. Am., *65*:119.
171. Shear, P., Hugenholtz, H., Tichard, M. T. et al. (1988). Multiple noncontiguous fractures of the cervical spine. J. Trauma, *28*:655.
172. Shuman, W. P., Rogers, J. V., Sicler, M. E. et al. (1985). Thoracolumbar burst fractures: CT dimensions of the spinal canal relative to postsurgical improvement. A.J.R. Am. J. Roentgenol., *145*:337.
173. Silberstein, M., Tress, B. M., & Hennessy, O. (1992). Prediction of neurologic outcome in acute spinal cord injury: The role of CT and MR imaging. A.J.N.R. Am. J. Neuroradiol., *13*:1597.
174. Silver, S. F., Nadel, H. R., & Flodmark, O. (1988). Pneumorrhachis after jejunal entrapment caused by a fracture dislocation of the lumbar spine. A.J.R. Am. J. Roentgenol., *150*:1129.
175. Slabaugh, P. B., & Smith, T. K. (1978). Neuropathic spine after spinal cord injury. J. Bone Joint Surg. Am., *60*:1005.
176. Smith, W. S., & Kaufer, H. (1969). Patterns and mechanisms of lumbar injuries associated with lap seatbelts. J. Bone Joint Surg. Am., *51*:239.
177. Sobel, J. W., Bohlman, H. H., & Freehafer, A. (1985). Charcot's arthropathy of the spine following spinal cord injury. J. Bone Joint Surg. Am., *67*:771.
178. Stanitski, C. L. (1982). Low back pain in young athletes. Physician Sports Med., *10*:77.
179. Sturm, J. T., & Perry, J. F. Jr. (1984). Injuries associated with fractures of the transverse processes of the thoracic and lumbar vertebrae. J. Trauma, *24*:597.
180. Takata, K., Inoque, S. I., Takahashi, K., & Ohtsuka, Y. (1988). Fracture of the posterior margin of a lumbar vertebral body. J. Bone Joint Surg. Am., *70*:589.
181. Tash, R. R., & Weitzner, I. Jr. (1986). Case report. Acute intervertebral gas following vertebral fracture: CT demonstration. J. Comput. Assist. Tomogr., *10*:707.
182. Tearse, D. S., Keene, J. S., & Drummond, D. S. (1987). Management of non-contiguous vertebral fractures. Paraplegia, *25*:100.
183. Techakapuck, S. (1981). Rupture of the lumbar cartilage plate into the spinal canal in an adolescent. A case report. J. Bone Joint Surg. Am., *63*:481.
184. Trent, G., Armstrong, G. W. D., & O'Neil, J. (1988). Thoracolumbar fractures in ankylosing spondylitis. High-risk injuries. Clin. Orthop., *227*:61.
185. Twomey, L. T., & Taylor, J. R. (1987). Age changes in lumbar vertebrae and intervertebral discs. Clin. Orthop., *224*:97.
186. Uriarte, E., Elguezabal, B., & Tovio, R. (1987). Fracture-dislocation of the thoracic spine without neurologic lesion. Clin. Orthop., *217*:261.
187. Vandemark, R. M. (1990). Radiology of the cervical spine in trauma patients: Practice, pitfalls, and recommendations for improving efficiency and communication. A.J.R. Am. J. Roentgenol., *155*:465.
188. Vernon-Roberts, B., & Pirie, C. J. (1973). Healing trabecular microfractures in the bodies of lumbar vertebrae. Ann. Rheum. Dis., *32*:406.
189. Warrian, R. K., Shoenut, J. P., Iannicello, C. M. et al. (1988). Seatbelt injury to the abdominal aorta. J. Trauma, *28*:1505.
190. Weinstein, J. N., Collalto, P., & Lehmann, T. R. (1988). Thoracolumbar "burst" fractures treated conservatively: A long-term follow-up. Spine, *13*:33.
191. White, A. A., & Panjabi, M. M. (1990). Clinical Biomechanics of the Spine. pp. 169–267. 2nd Ed. J. B. Lippincott, Co., Philadelphia.
192. Willén, J., Lindahl, S., Irstam, L. et al. (1984). The thoracolumbar crush fracture. An experimental study on instant axial dynamic loading: The resulting fracture type and its stability. Spine, *9*:624.
193. Wiltse, L. L., Widell, E. H., & Jackson, D. W. (1975). Fatigue fracture: The basic lesion in isthmic spondylolisthesis. J. Bone Joint Surg. Am., *57*:17.
194. Wirth, C. R., Jacobs, R. L., & Rolander, S. (1980). Neuropathic spinal arthropathy. A review of the Charcot spine. Spine, *5*:558.
195. Woodruff, F., & Dewing, S. B. (1963). Fracture of the cervical spine in patients with ankylosing spondylitis. Radiology, *80*:17.
196. Yao, A. C. M. C., & Chan, C. N. W. (1974). Stress fracture of the fused lumbo-dorsal spine in ankylosing spondylitis. J. Bone Joint Surg. Br., *56*:681.
197. Yashon, D., Jane, J. A., & White, R. J. (1970). Prognosis and management of spinal cord and cauda equina bullet injuries in sixty-five civilians. J. Neurosurg., *32*:163.
198. Yuh, W. T. C., Zachar, C. K., Barloon, T. J. et al. (1989). Vertebral compression fractures: Distinction between benign and malignant causes with MR imaging. Radiology, *172*:215.

Chapter 14

THE THORACIC CAGE

with Eric J. Stern, MD, and Eric K. Hoffer, MD

Blunt trauma to the chest may occur either as an isolated entity or as a component of multiple injuries. On initial patient presentation, fractures of the ribs and sternum are of secondary importance to accompanying injuries of the underlying lung, pleura, heart, great vessels, and upper abdominal viscera, except as markers of injury severity and kinetic energy absorption. Almost every multiply injured or unconscious patient should undergo chest radiography[8]; this examination is generally limited to a single anteroposterior view obtained with the patient supine. The ambulatory patient who has sustained isolated trauma to the chest can usually undergo a more extensive radiographic examination, including multiple views of the ribs and lateral radiographs of the chest.[40] Some authors consider special views of the ribs unwarranted,[26, 27] because standard posteroanterior and lateral radiographs of the chest disclose any associated pneumothorax and hemothorax, and because ordinarily the demonstration of rib fractures per se does not change the management of the patient. However, pain management may often be adjusted accordingly when rib fractures are shown. Furthermore, when the radiographic examination is limited to the chest film, as many as 20% of rib fractures will be missed. In our litigious society, such limited examination is considered unwise and ill advised.

Computed tomography (CT) scanning is four to five times more sensitive in detecting intrathoracic injury than conventional radiography.[6, 15, 16] In most cases, the demonstration by CT of abnormalities inapparent on the chest radiograph does not alter patient management. However, disclosure of a pneumothorax in patients who are to undergo general anesthesia or positive-pressure inhalation therapy is of importance because this finding may warrant placement of a chest tube to avoid the subsequent development of a tension pneumothorax.[21] Every CT scan of the abdomen in the trauma patient should include the diaphragm and base of the lungs to exclude an otherwise inapparent pneumothorax. For the same reason, it is of value to examine the lungs and diaphragm in every head-injured and every unconscious patient.

Bony Thorax

Rib Fractures

Fractures of the ribs are usually sustained in automobile accidents and falls and from direct blows to the chest.[13, 14, 22, 23] Gunshot wounds and pathologic fractures occur less commonly in most clinical practices. Fractures of the ribs are usually of secondary importance to any associated injuries of the lung and mediastinal structures.[14] The incidence of rib fractures associated with significant pulmonary trauma is approximately 50%,[9, 22, 36] whereas sternal, vertebral, scapular, and clavicular fractures are found in 3% to 8% of cases. In those patients who require hospitalization following trauma, 75% to 85% of rib fractures are associated with some manifestation of pulmonary injury.[24, 36] Fractures may lie any place along the course of the ribs but are somewhat more frequent in the posterior and middle thirds of the fourth through ninth ribs[3, 22, 36] laterally, away from the protection of the overlying chest wall musculature. The sixth, seventh, and eighth ribs are most commonly fractured, on the left slightly more often than on the right. In general, fractures of the upper ribs are accompanied by a larger number of other rib fractures and by more extensive intrathoracic and intra-abdominal injuries, with a corresponding increase in mortality.[1, 10]

The standard posteroanterior and lateral chest radiographs are inadequate for demonstration of rib fractures. The routine examination of the chest allows for an excellent view of the posterior portion of the ribs above the diaphragm, usually the first through the eighth or ninth ribs, and of the anterior portion of the ribs, but it does not allow adequate visualization of the lateral portion of the ribs between the anterior and posterior axillary lines. Fractures involving the lateral portion of the rib must be markedly displaced before they can be detected on routine chest radiographs. Furthermore, the posterior portions of the ribs lying below the diaphragms can be somewhat obscured, although less so with newer computed radiography systems. Rib fractures are best visualized when seen in profile. On the standard frontal view of the chest, the posterior and anterior portions of the ribs are seen in profile. To see the lateral portion of the ribs in profile, an oblique view of the ribs must be obtained (Fig. 14–1). Nondisplaced rib fractures often are visualized only as callus at the fracture site 10 to 14 days after injury (Fig. 14–2). Rib cartilage fractures or separations are not radiographically evident.

The standard radiographic examination for fractures of the ribs should consist of anteroposterior and oblique views of the chest wall and an additional anteroposterior view of the upper abdomen, utilizing higher kilovoltage to visualize the lower ribs. Because the lungs are not well

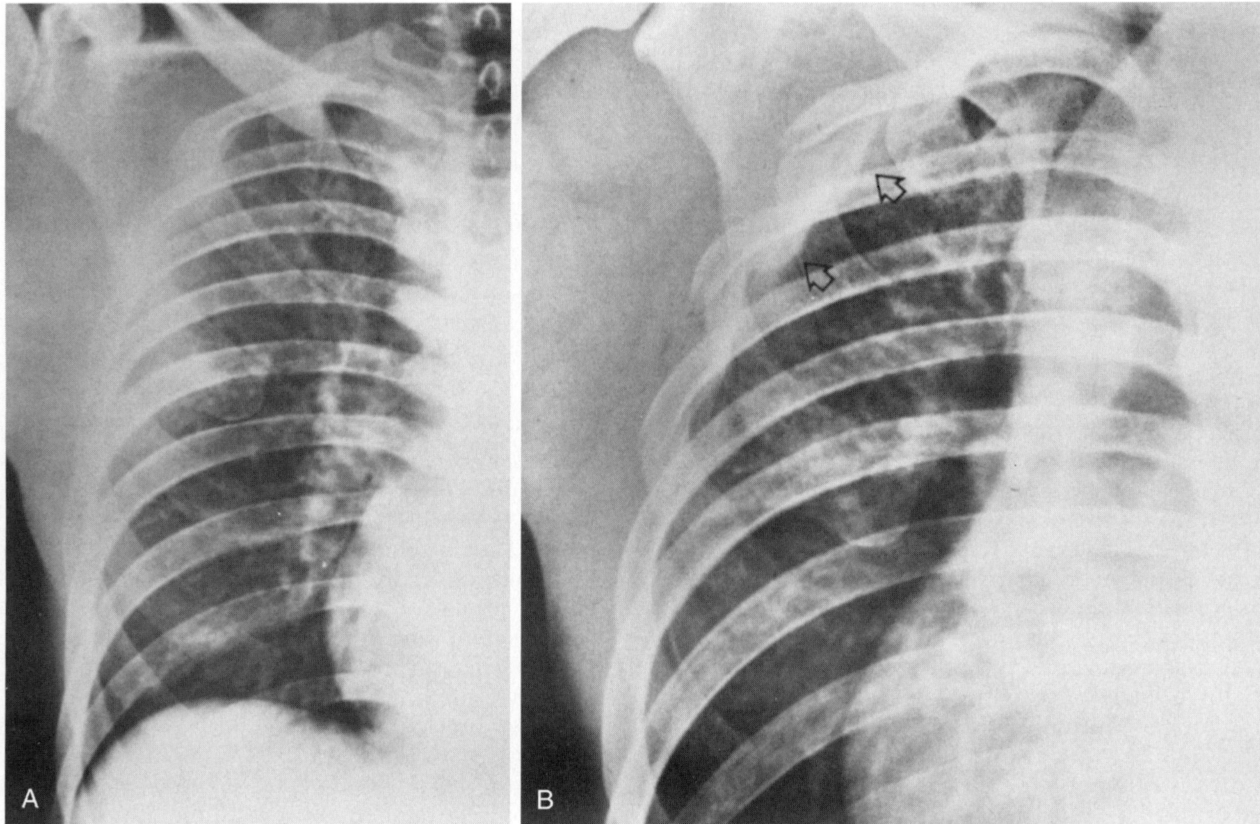

Figure 14–1. Fractures of the anterolateral aspect of the second through the fifth ribs. *A*, Anteroposterior view shows only minimal extrapleural density. The fractures are not demonstrated. *B*, Right posterior oblique view clearly shows the fractures of the second, third, fourth, and fifth right ribs, with a surrounding hematoma manifested by extrapleural density *(arrows)*.

visualized on these views, standard posteroanterior and lateral views of the chest should be obtained to evaluate the lung and mediastinum. It can be very helpful to place a lead "BB" over the point of the patient's pain.

Rib fractures may be detected by bone scanning.[33] Under unusual circumstances a bone scan may be warranted to disclose the source of obscure pain, especially when pain management is an important clinical concern, to delineate the full extent of injuries following trauma to the bony thorax, or to evaluate for pathologic fractures.

Sonography has been shown by some investigators to be much more sensitive than radiography in the detection of rib fractures.[19, 34, 45, 55] Sonography performed with a 9- or 12-MHz linear transducer showed 10 times as many fractures in 6 times as many patients as found by radiography.[34] These investigators found that 88% of patients presenting to the emergency department with suspected rib fracture had sustained a fracture. However, radiography detected only 8% of these fractures. In contrast with radiography, sonography can disclose fractures involving the costal cartilage and costochondral junction.

The ribs and costal cartilage are examined with the transducer aligned with the long axis of the rib, first focusing on the painful area and then surveying the entire length of the rib and costal cartilage. The anterior margin of the costal cartilage and bony rib is seen as a thin, continuous echogenic line (Fig. 14–3*A*), except at the costochondral junction, where there may be a slight discontinuity. The costal cartilage appears hypoechoic compared with the bony rib. Fractures of the rib, costochondral junction, and costal cartilages are seen as clear disruptions of the anterior echogenic margin, and a surrounding hematoma may be identified (see Fig. 14–3*B*).

Magnetic resonance imaging (MRI) is not used for evaluating rib fractures in the trauma setting.

On the initial examination, the fractures may be essentially undisplaced or minimally displaced and difficult to visualize. They are often more obvious on subsequent examinations[22] because of displacements at the fracture margins produced by respiratory motion (see Fig. 14–31). An undisplaced rib fracture is manifested as a vertical or obliquely oriented lucent line, usually accompanied by a slight offset that is more easily identified at the superior margin of the rib (see Fig. 14–13). With displacement, the offset of the fractured margins becomes more obvious. If the ends of the fracture overlap, they demonstrate a line of increased density (Fig. 14–4). Plastic bowing of the rib has been described in children[23] with Werdnig-Hoffmann disease and osteogenesis imperfecta but as yet has not been reported as a result of trauma. It seems logical that such fractures do occur, however.

Attention may be directed to minimally displaced or undisplaced fractures by the surrounding soft tissue density of the usually associated hematoma (Fig. 14–5; see also Fig. 14–1). This finding is an indirect radiographic sign that increases the yield of a directed search for rib fracture. The bleeding around the fractures displaces the parietal pleura toward the lung. This elevation of the

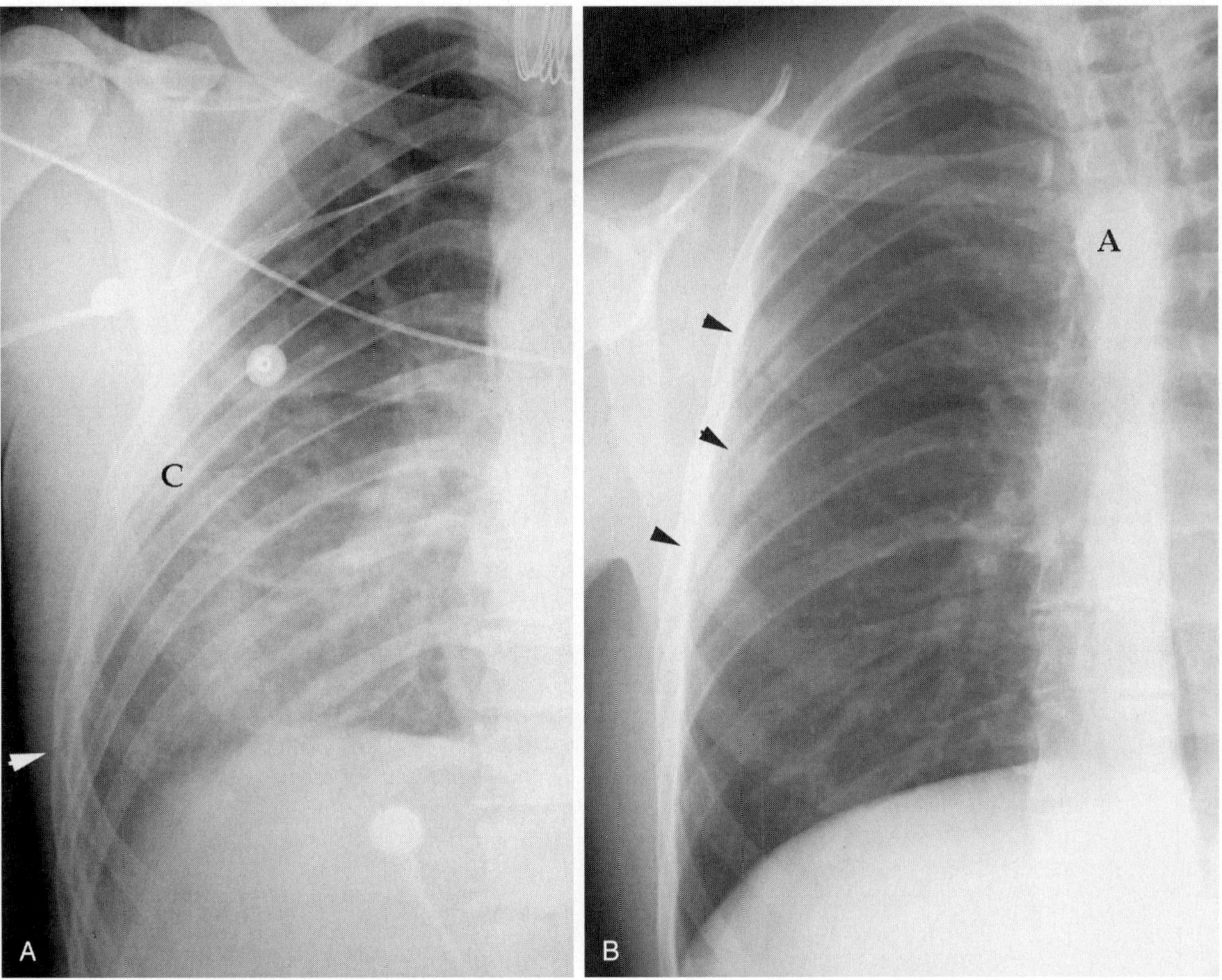

Figure 14–2. Nondisplaced rib fractures visualized only as callus forms at the fracture site, 17 days after injury. *A,* Initial chest radiograph, a coned-down anteroposterior view, shows a small nondisplaced fracture of the right eighth rib *(arrowhead)* and a peripheral opacity overlying the right midlung, typical for a contusion (C). *B,* At 17 days after injury, note callus formation around the anterolateral portions of the right fourth through sixth ribs *(arrowheads)* that was not evident on the initial examination but is certainly underneath the site of lung contusion. Note the incidental right aortic arch (A).

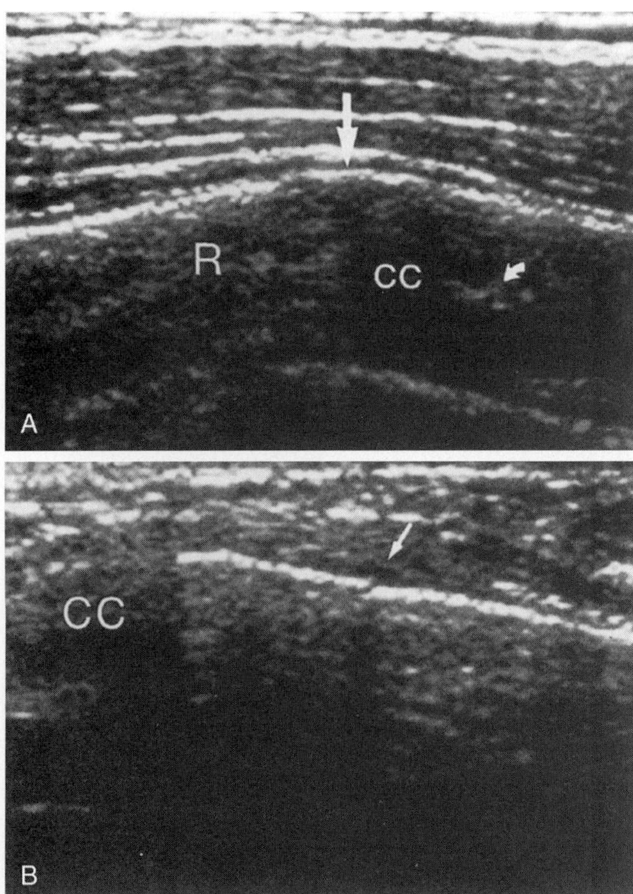

Figure 14–3. Sonography of rib fracture. *A,* Normal costochondral junction in an adult male. Transverse sonogram oriented along the long axis of the third costal cartilage (CC), costochondral junction *(straight arrow),* and rib (R) shows the anterior margin of the costal cartilage and rib as a thin, echogenic line. The line representing the anterior aspect of the rib is thicker than that representing the costal cartilage. Note costal cartilage calcification *(curved arrow). B,* Fracture of the fifth left rib in a 25-year-old man. Transverse sonogram shows undisplaced rib fracture *(arrow).* Note the small hematoma and the relatively hypoechoic costal cartilage (CC). (From Griffith, J.F., Rainer, T.H., Ching, A.S.C., et al. [1999]. Sonography compared with radiography in revealing acute rib fracture. A.J.R. Am. J. Roentgenol., *173:*1603.)

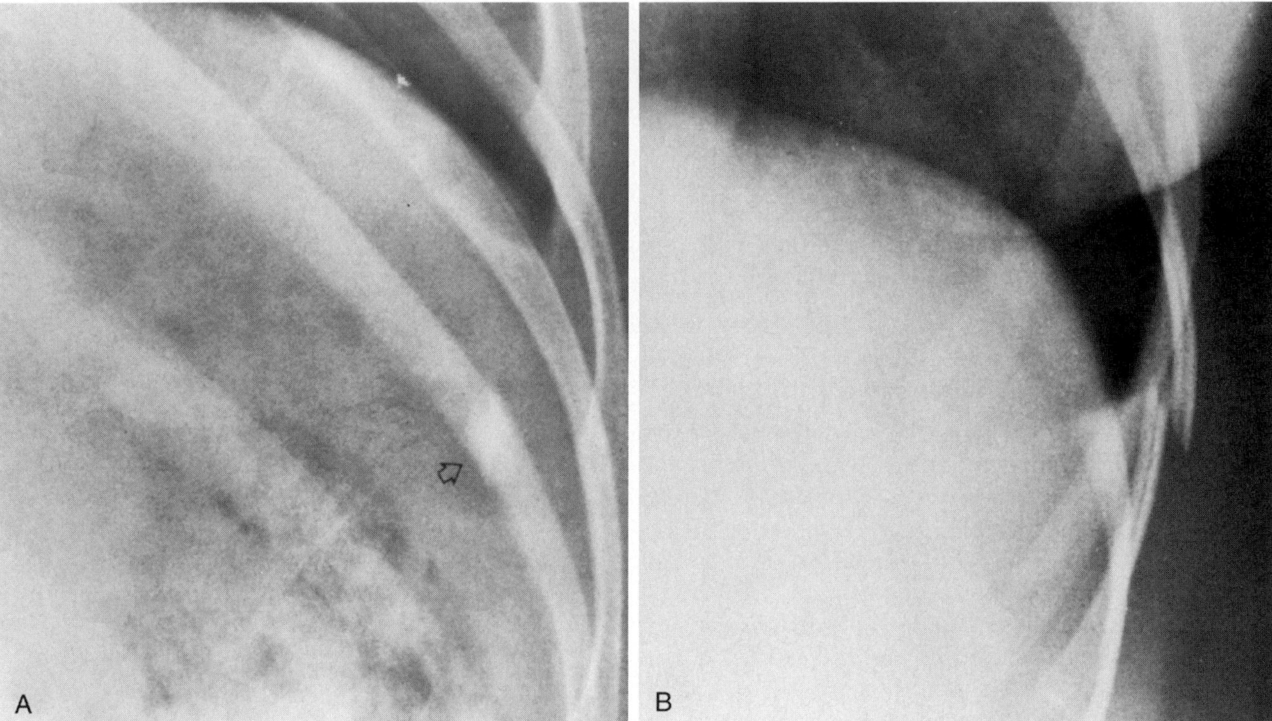

Figure 14–4. Fracture of the 10th left rib manifested by increase in bone density. *A,* Left posterior oblique view of the ribs shows an area of increased radiodensity in the 10th right rib *(arrow). B,* Anteroposterior view shows that the apparent increase in density is due to fracture of the rib with overlapping of the fracture fragments.

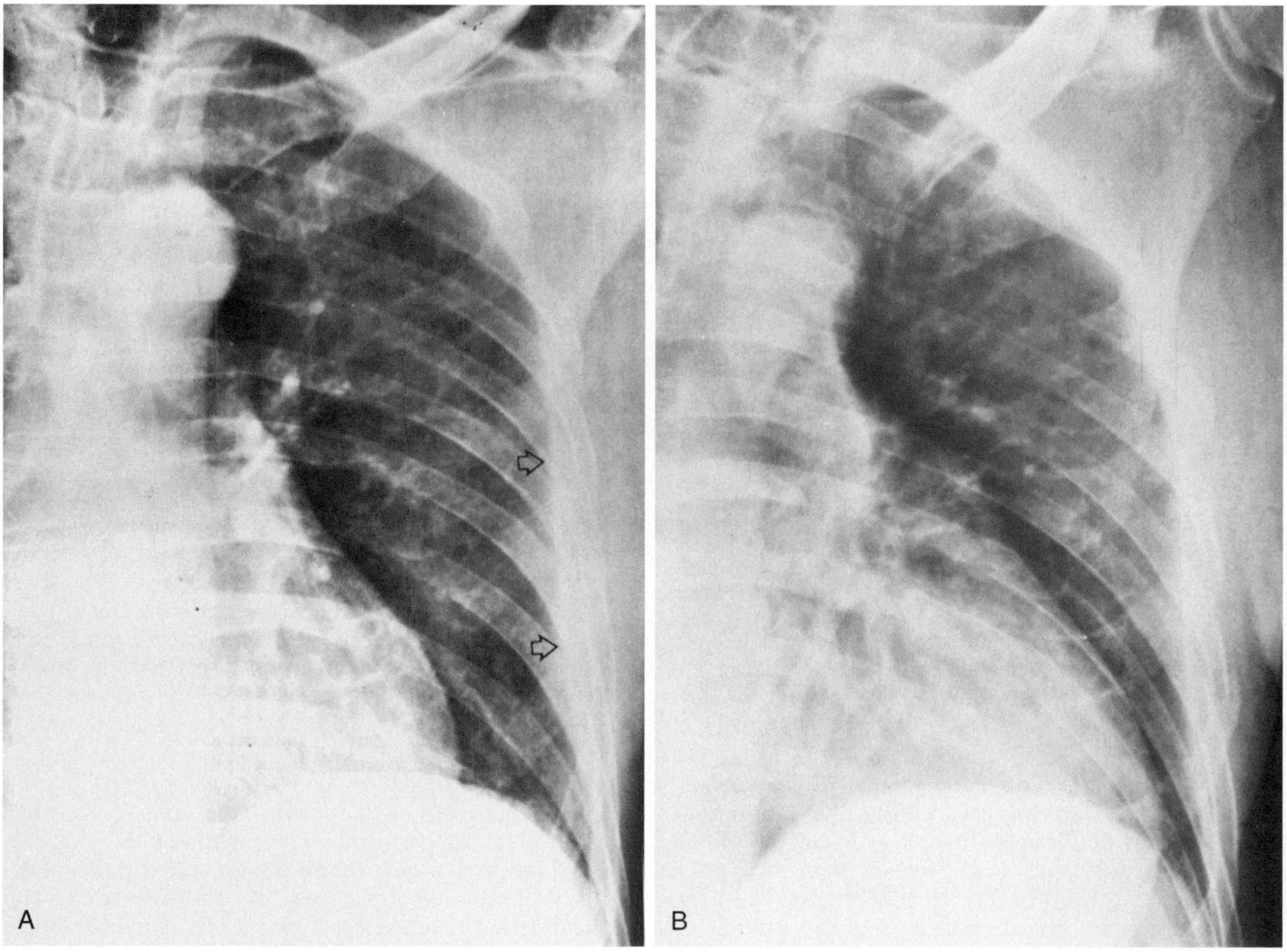

Figure 14–5. Fractures of the left ribs manifested by the extrapleural sign. *A,* A soft tissue density paralleling the lateral surface of the chest wall is sharply defined on its medial border *(arrows).* This finding represents an extrapleural hematoma. The underlying fractures are not visualized on this view. *B,* Left posterior oblique view clearly shows the fractures of the third, fourth, and fifth ribs, with a surrounding hematoma.

parietal pleura presents as a smooth soft tissue indentation at the margin of the lung, underlying the fractured rib. This extrapleural blood collection is frequently confused with free-flowing or loculated pleural fluid or blood, especially on radiographs obtained with the patient supine (Figs. 14–6 and 14–7). These hematomas are best seen when the fracture is visualized tangential to the central x-ray beam, accomplished by obtaining a view tangential to the site of maximum pain.

The presence of extrapleural blood should be suspected when the apparent pleural fluid does not clear with thoracostomy tube drainage and is intimately associated with one or more rib fractures. The chest wall outside the ribs can also contain large blood collections

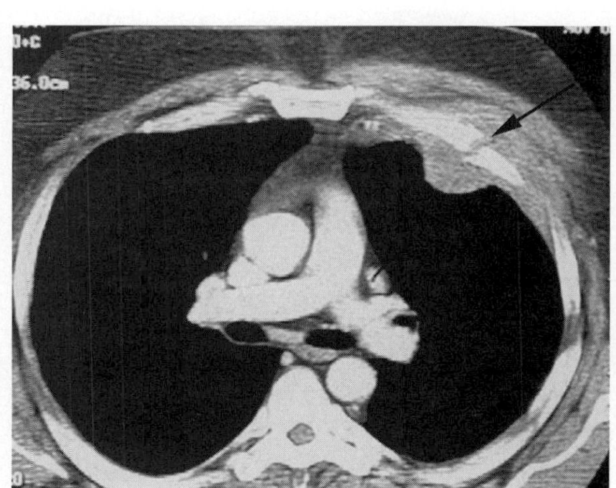

Figure 14–6. CT through the midchest shows an obvious *extra*pleural hematoma around an anterior rib fracture *(arrow).* A loculated pleural fluid collection is not distinguishable but would be very unlikely given the presence of the underlying rib fracture. (From Stern, E.J. & White, C.S. [1999]. Chest Radiology Companion. Lippincott Williams & Wilkins, Philadelphia.)

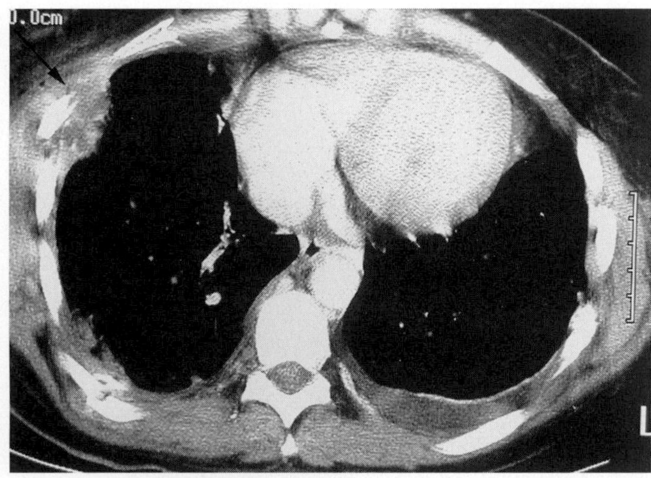

Figure 14–7. CT through the lower chest from a patient involved in a high-speed motor vehicle crash shows multiple right rib fractures *(arrow)* with associated *extra*pleural hematoma around each fracture. Also note a left pleural effusion.

associated with rib and soft tissue injuries. These soft tissue hematomas are most evident on CT scans (Fig. 14–8).

Rib fractures are coincidentally identified during the course of CT evaluation of the traumatized chest but are usually more readily visualized using standard radiographic techniques (Figs. 14–9 and 14–10). Fractures of the posterior aspects of the ribs and those involving the costovertebral articulations constitute an exception and may be better visualized by CT (see Fig. 14–9). Fractures of the sternum and scapula may also be more evident and readily appreciated on CT images than on routine chest radiographs (Fig. 14–11). In children, the chest can be markedly compressed, enough to cause pulmonary contusions, but without causing rib fractures (Fig. 14–12).

With high-energy injuries, there are frequently multiple fractures that usually involve adjacent ribs.[24, 36] They may result from direct blows or from indirect trauma produced by sudden movement of the thorax, such as that described in golfers.[49] The fractures involving adjacent ribs usually can be seen to lie along an imaginary vertical or oblique line (Fig. 14–13; see also Figs. 14–9 and 14–48A). Additional, less obvious fractures are often found on close examination of the ribs located proximally or distally along the course of these lines. Except in the most severely injured patients, fractures are less often bilateral.

A flail chest is the result of two separate fractures of the same rib (Fig. 14–14), creating a "free-floating" segment of rib. These segmental fractures usually involve multiple ribs. A true flail chest deformity severely compromises the efficiency of respiratory exchange, as well as the coughing mechanism, by allowing independent or paradoxical movement of the chest wall, especially when three or more ribs are involved. Often, the second fracture involves the costochondral junction or the chondrosternal junction, which cannot be identified radiographically. Combined fractures of the sternum and costochondral junction constitute a less common source of flail chest. The clinical manifestation of flail chest is paradoxical motion of the involved portion of the chest wall with respiration. Initially, paradoxical chest wall motion may not be clinically apparent because of muscle splinting, or it might be overlooked because of the patient's body habitus or other, more serious associated injuries.[2] A flail chest serves as a marker of high kinetic energy absorption but is not necessarily a marker for great vessel, tracheobronchial, or diaphragmatic injuries. Flail chest is frequently associated with pulmonary contusion or laceration, pneumothorax, and hemothorax,

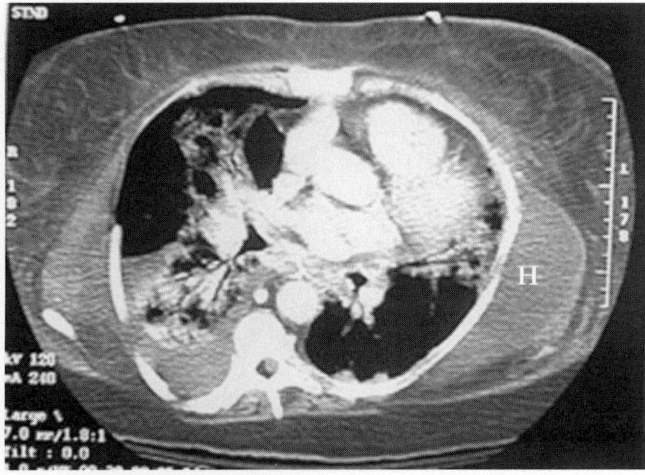

Figure 14–8. CT through the lower chest from a patient involved in a high-speed motor vehicle crash shows multiple left rib fractures, a right pleural effusion, diffuse lung injury, and a large hematoma in the left chest wall (H) resulting from blunt left chest wall trauma.

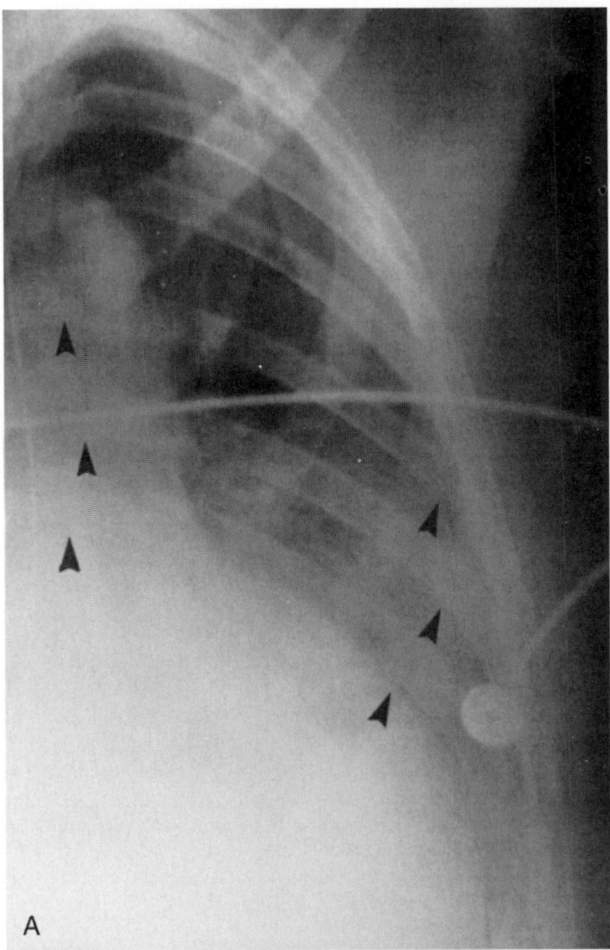

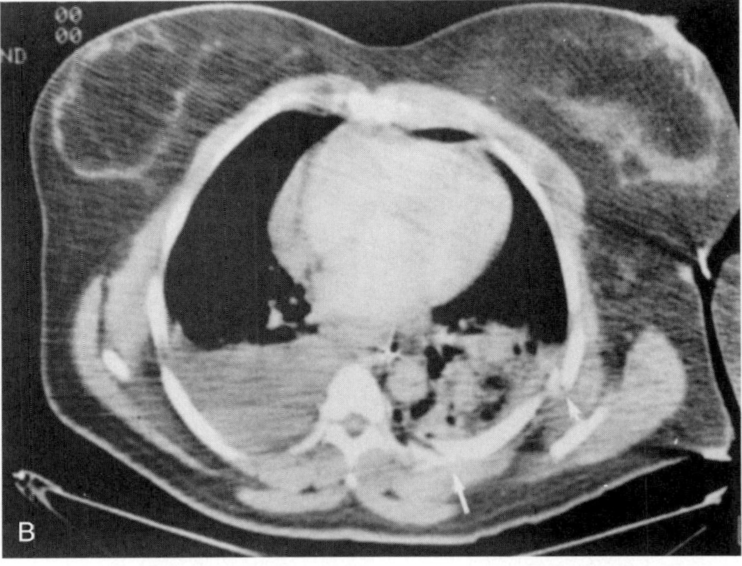

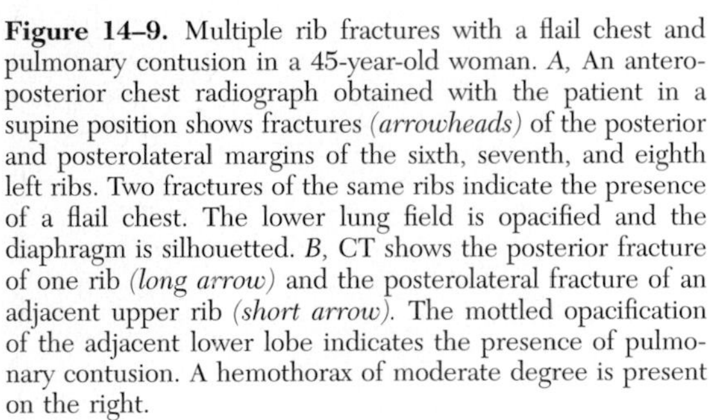

Figure 14–9. Multiple rib fractures with a flail chest and pulmonary contusion in a 45-year-old woman. *A,* An anteroposterior chest radiograph obtained with the patient in a supine position shows fractures *(arrowheads)* of the posterior and posterolateral margins of the sixth, seventh, and eighth left ribs. Two fractures of the same ribs indicate the presence of a flail chest. The lower lung field is opacified and the diaphragm is silhouetted. *B,* CT shows the posterior fracture of one rib *(long arrow)* and the posterolateral fracture of an adjacent upper rib *(short arrow).* The mottled opacification of the adjacent lower lobe indicates the presence of pulmonary contusion. A hemothorax of moderate degree is present on the right.

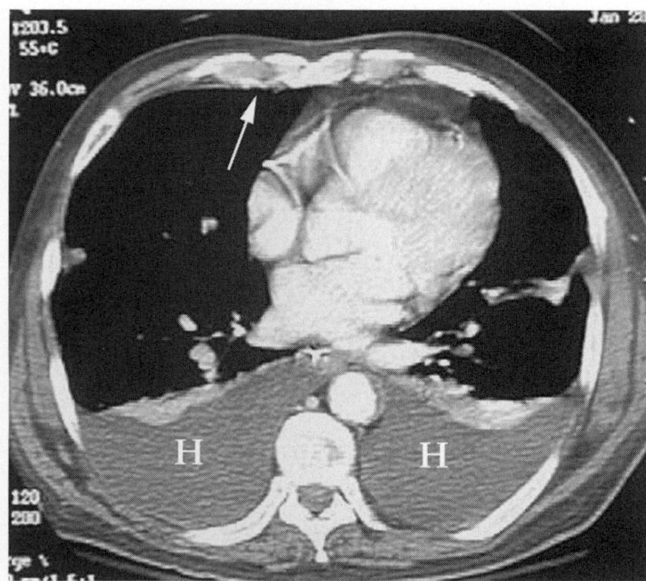

Figure 14–10. CT through the lower chest from a patient involved in a high-speed motor vehicle crash shows a fracture through the right costochondral junction anteriorly *(arrow)*. Bilateral hemothoraces (H) are also seen, the size of which was grossly underestimated on chest radiographs obtained with the patient in the supine position.

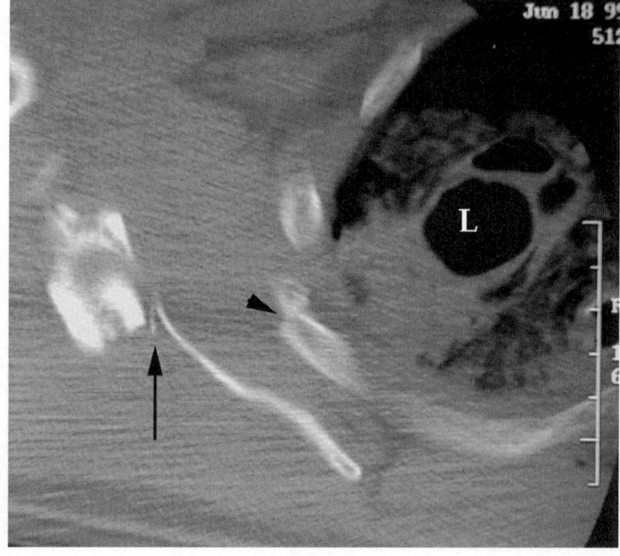

Figure 14–11. Close-up view from CT through the upper chest of a patient who fell from a ladder shows a fracture of the scapula *(arrow)* and right rib *(arrowhead)* and an underlying pulmonary laceration (L) with surrounding pulmonary contusion and hemorrhage. This is a common injury pattern that results from blunt trauma to the upper chest.

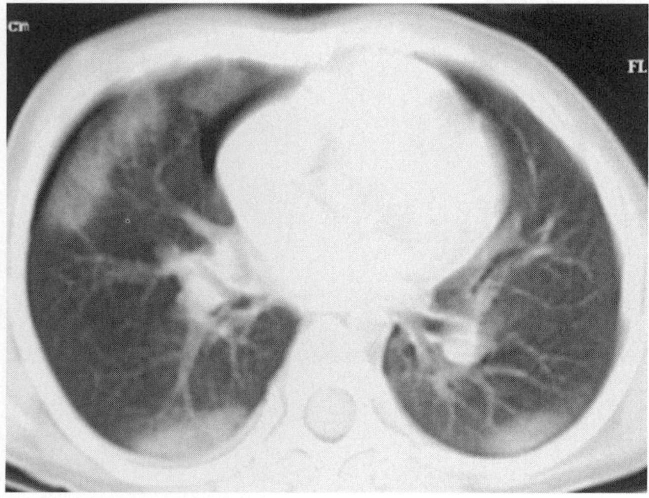

Figure 14–12. CT through the lower chest of an unrestrained 3-year-old boy involved in a motor vehicle crash shows typical findings of a pulmonary contusion in the right anterior lung. Note that this anterior lung opacity is peripheral and nonsegmental. Also evident is a right pneumothorax. The gravitationally dependent opacities in the caudal portions of both lungs are due to atelectasis and should not be confused with contusion.

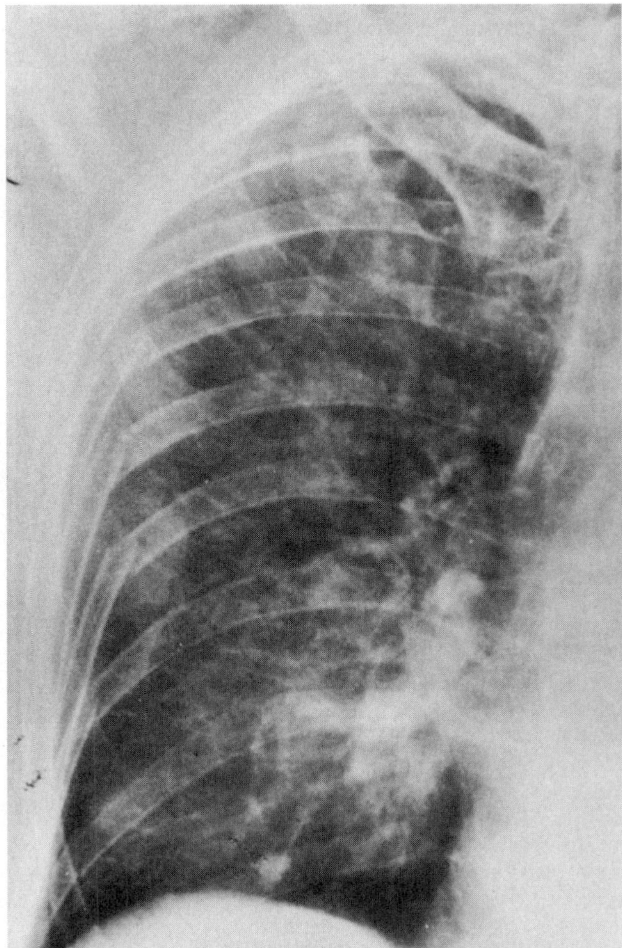

Figure 14–13. Fractures of the posterolateral aspect of the third through the ninth right ribs in a 65-year-old man. Note that the fractures lie in an approximately vertical line.

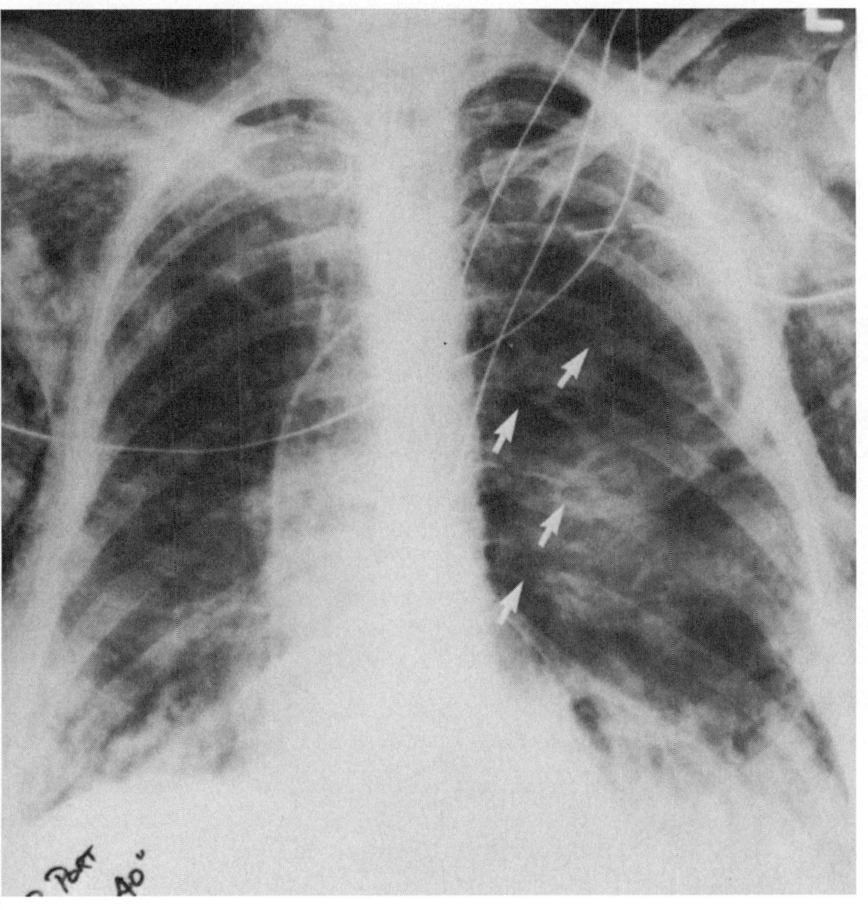

Figure 14–14. Flail chest with widely displaced fractures of the third through the ninth left ribs in a 60-year-old woman involved in an automobile accident. Fractures can be seen in both the posterior and posterior lateral aspects of several of these ribs *(arrows).* Pulmonary contusion is present in both lungs. There are fractures of the upper right ribs and of the right clavicle. Subcutaneous emphysema is present bilaterally.

especially with increasing numbers of rib fractures. Flail chest is also associated with clavicular and scapular fractures. Some patients with flail chest will require open reduction and internal fixation, with or without prolonged mechanical ventilation for management of respiratory failure. Therefore, flail chest is an important radiographic observation and should be communicated immediately to the physician responsible for the patient's care.

The indirect signs of rib fracture are pneumothorax, hemopneumothorax, hemothorax, and interstitial emphysema of the chest wall (Fig. 14–15). It is important to seek out these indirect signs to detect an underlying rib fracture. Any or all of these indirect signs may occur in the absence of rib fractures, however, especially in cases of penetrating trauma, and the presence of air, blood, or both within the pleural space is much more clinically important than the actual rib fracture. Interstitial emphysema is manifested radiographically as linear or ovoid lucencies within the soft tissues of the chest wall that dissect superiorly into the axilla and soft tissues of the neck (see Figs. 14–15 and 14–32). The dissection occurs in fascial and subcutaneous planes and is often found along muscle bundles outlining the course of muscles, particularly the pectoral muscles over the upper chest (see Fig. 14–46). Interstitial emphysema rarely occurs as a result of blunt trauma without an associated rib fracture. Close inspection of the radiographs will usually show one or more associated rib fractures. Interstitial emphysema without associated rib fracture or pneumothorax may occur as a result of a stab wound or may arise from a pneumomediastinum, with air dissecting out from the thoracic inlet.

Fractures of the upper ribs—particularly the first, second and third ribs[1, 4, 48, 54]—suggest that the patient has experienced a severe degree of trauma. The incidence of associated rupture of the aorta or brachiocephalic vessels has been variously reported as 8%,[56] 14%,[44] and 20%.[30] However, in patients without vascular injury, a similar incidence, location, and degree of displacement of fractures of the first rib have been noted.[30, 43, 44, 47]

Fractures of the anterolateral portions of the first three ribs are often difficult to detect. These fractures can be obscured by the adjacent ribs, clavicle, or scapula. Attention may be directed to the presence of a fracture[24] by the presence of a localized extrapleural hematoma at the fracture site (see Figs. 14–1, 14–3, and 14–5). Such extrapleural hematomas may be overlooked, or the radiographic abnormality may be dismissed as incidental pleural thickening representing the residua of previous inflammatory disease. The hematomas that accompany these fractures can be best seen in the oblique projection (see Fig. 14–1*B*). Displacement is rarely marked, and when it does occur the distal fragment is usually shifted directly backward so that there is no apparent separation

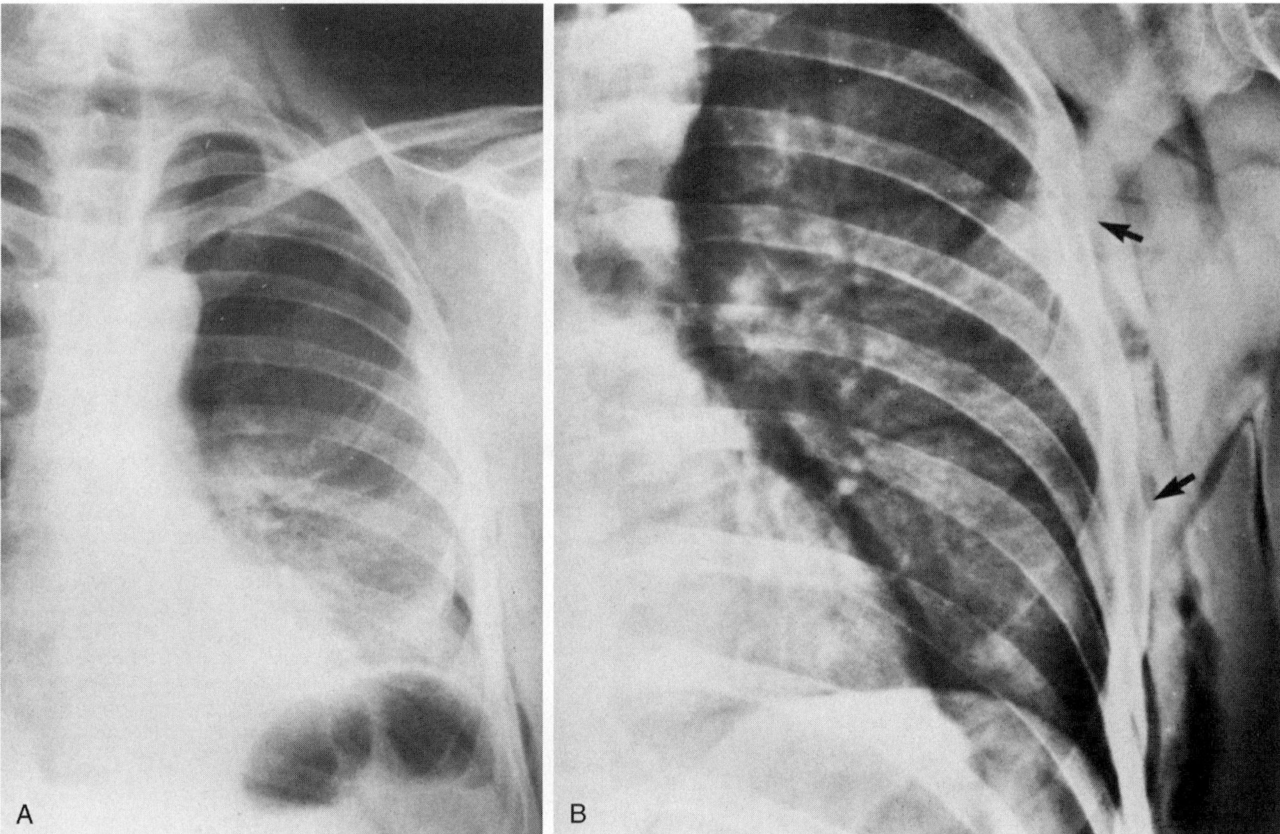

Figure 14–15. Fracture of the lateral margin of the fourth, fifth, and sixth left ribs associated with pneumothorax and subcutaneous emphysema. *A*, Chest radiograph shows the pneumothorax. Subcutaneous emphysema is present on the left within the chest wall. The fractures of the ribs are not clearly visualized. *B*, Posteroanterior view of the ribs shows fractures of the lateral margins of the fourth and sixth ribs *(arrows)*. The pneumothorax is not clearly demonstrated on this view.

or angulation on the standard frontal view. In some cases displacement is appreciated on the apical lordotic view, and certainly with CT scanning.

Fractures of the First Rib

Isolated fracture of the first rib is a peculiar injury associated with a significant degree of local complications.[37, 50] The first rib is well protected by surrounding anatomic structures, which suggests that a force of some magnitude is required to result in fracture. Five discrete mechanisms of injury for first rib fractures have been described: (1) posteriorly directed trauma to the upper thorax or shoulder girdle; (2) a direct blow to the sternum and anterior chest wall; (3) a blow fracturing the clavicle; (4) a strong sudden contraction of the scalenus anterior muscle; and (5) unknown mechanism of injury in which radiographic features of a first rib fracture are present without a history of trauma.[35] Isolated first rib fracture, regardless of mechanism of injury, is associated with a low incidence of major vascular injury (mean 3%), although with fracture fragment displacement, the incidence is higher. First rib fractures associated with concomitant head, thoracic, abdominal, or long bone trauma are associated with vascular injury in 24% of cases. Therefore, fracture of the first rib is in itself not an indication for arteriography. Arteriography should be performed only if specific features suggestive of vascular injury are present, such as mediastinal widening on chest radiographs, upper extremity pulse deficit, posteriorly displaced first rib fracture, anterior location of the fracture within the subclavian groove, brachial plexus injury, or expanding hematoma.[35]

The two most common sites of first rib fracture are at the subclavian sulcus and in the neck of the first rib near its articulation with the transverse process of the first thoracic vertebra posteriorly—the two weakest anatomic points in the ribs (Fig. 14–16*B*). The relationship of the scalenus muscles and the subclavian artery and vein plays an important role in the creation of fractures and concomitant vascular injury, a frequent complication. The scalenus anterior muscle arises from the transverse processes of the third to sixth cervical vertebrae and inserts on the scalene tubercle of the first rib between the subclavian artery and vein.[25, 29, 31] The scalene medius muscle inserts on the first rib posterior to the artery. The subclavian artery crosses the thoracic outlet in its groove over the first rib between the attachment of the two scalene muscles. The first rib is fixed by its attachment to the clavicle and manubrium anteriorly and the transverse process of the first thoracic vertebra posteriorly. These two points of firm attachment increase the vulnerability of the first rib to fracture at the subclavian groove as a result of a sudden contraction of the scalene muscle.

The rib may be fractured by direct trauma or indirectly through sudden strong contraction of the scalene muscles, as when the head is turned suddenly to the side; in status asthmaticus; or with violent coughing or sneezing.[29, 38] The neck of the rib[53] is usually fractured in association with fracture of the clavicle or separation of the acromioclavicular or sternoclavicular joint. Direct blows that result in isolated fracture of the first rib have frequently been associated with brachial plexus injuries and Horner's syndrome.[33, 47]

Injuries of the subclavian artery are common because of the frequent location of the fracture within the subclavian groove[29, 37] (Fig. 14–17). Often the arterial injury is not immediately apparent.[31, 36] Evidently, with the cyclic respiratory excursions of the thoracic cage, the fracture fragments of the first rib repeatedly impinge on and eventually lacerate the wall of the subclavian artery. A hematoma is formed about the laceration and is characteristically identified as an extrapleural mass on radiographs obtained 5 to 10 days after the initial trauma.[36] On occasion the fracture may result in thrombotic occlu-

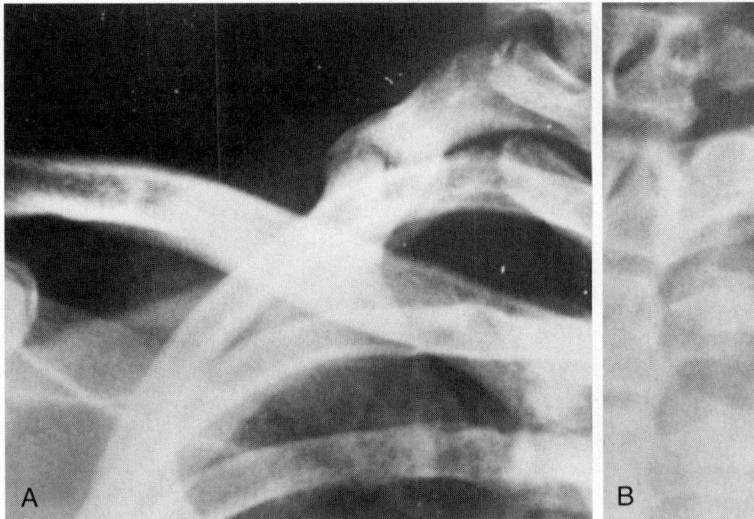

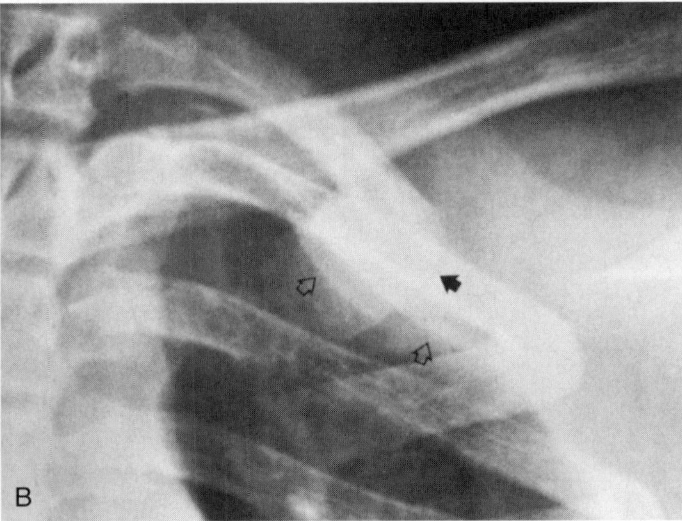

Figure 14–16. Fractures of the first rib. *A*, Stress fracture of the first rib in an 18-year-old professional right-handed baseball pitcher. He had recently experienced pain while pitching. Radiograph shows considerable callus formation about the midportion of the first rib. The site and appearance are typical of a stress fracture. (Case courtesy of Bert Sosnow, MD, Phoenix, Ariz.) *B*, Fracture of the first rib in a 17-year-old boy. The extrapleural hematoma *(open arrows)* about the first rib directs attention to the underlying fracture *(black arrow)*. Note that the hematoma extends over the apex of the lung. There were no associated injuries of the aorta or bronchus.

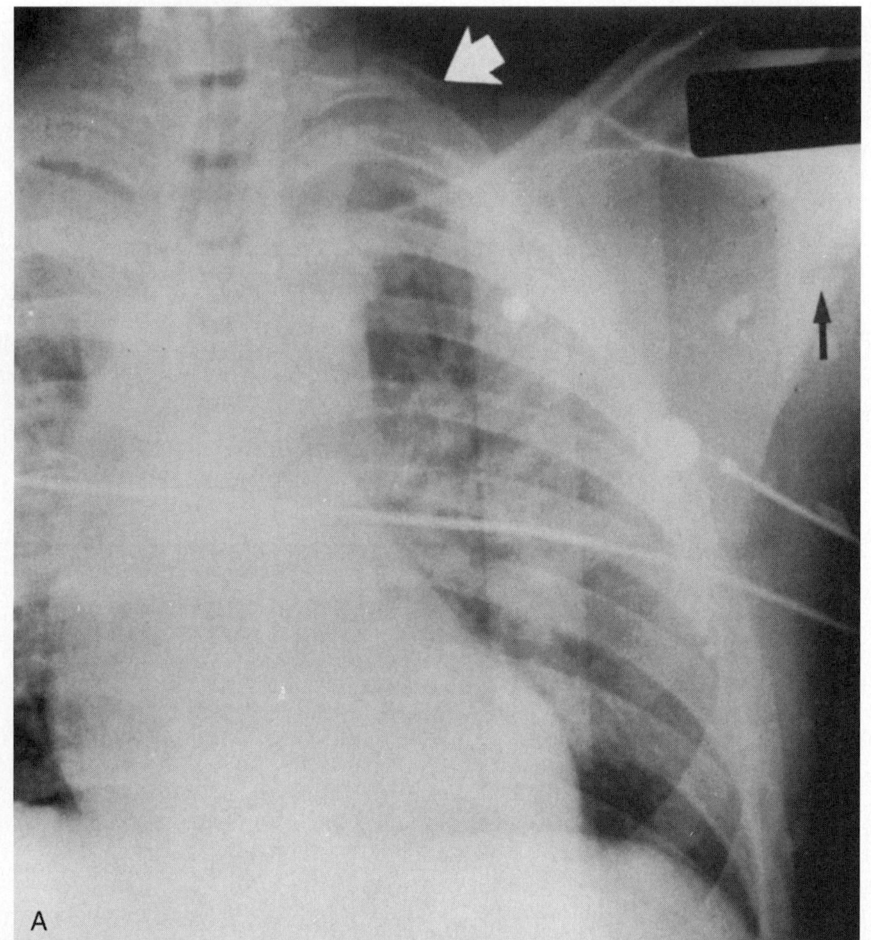

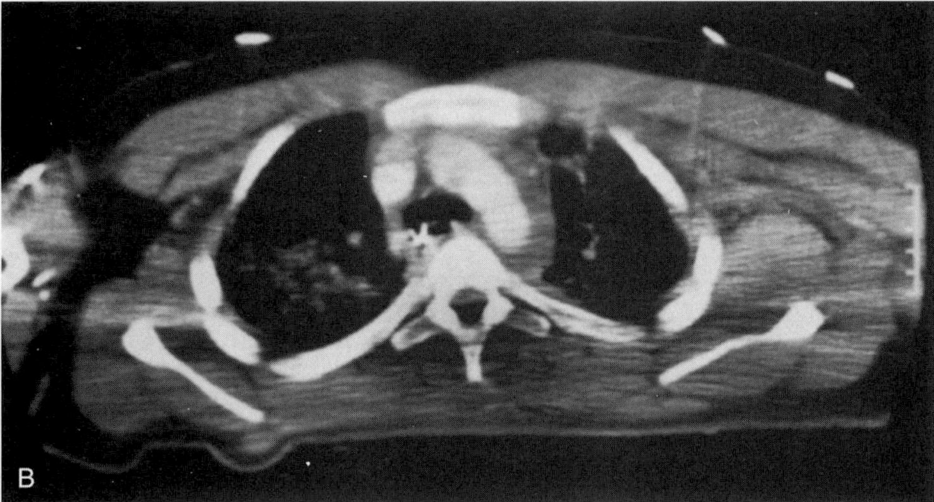

Figure 14–17. Fracture of the first rib and neck of the scapula associated with injury of the left subclavian artery, pulmonary contusion, and hemothorax in a 15-year-old boy. *A,* Anteroposterior view of the chest shows widening of the upper mediastinum, with a pleural cap extending over the left apex. There are fractures of the first left rib *(white arrow)* and neck of the scapula *(black arrow).* The upper lung is opacified. There is no obvious pleural effusion. An endotracheal tube is in place. *B,* Aortogram shows a normal arch with normal origin of the innominate and left common carotid arteries. There is reduced opacification in the left subclavian artery, and an intimal injury was identified.

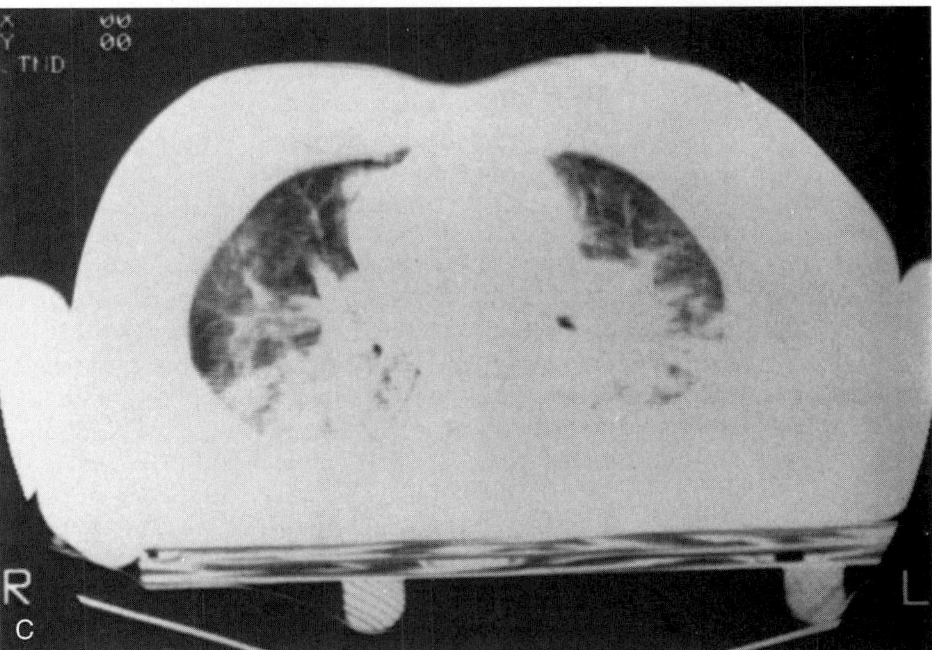

Figure 14–17 *Continued. C,* The bilateral pulmonary contusions are much better demonstrated on the lung window settings at a lower level.

sion of the subclavian artery, manifested clinically by absence of the radial arterial pulse.

Cases of thoracic outlet syndrome have also been described[46] as the result of fracture of the first rib. In these cases, callus that has formed about the first rib fracture compromises and compresses either the subclavian artery, the subclavian vein, or both. Surgical resection of the rib is required to alleviate symptoms of the syndrome. Both clinical and radiographic follow-up examinations are important to exclude the possibility of subclavian arterial injury whenever a fracture of the first rib is identified.

Approximately 2% of fractures of the first rib are associated with fractures of the bronchus. Like vascular ruptures, fractures of the bronchus[56] may also occur in the absence of rib fracture, particularly in young patients, but this is rather unlikely in patients older than 30 years of age. In an analysis of 90 cases, Burke[149] found that in 91% there was an associated fracture localized to the upper rib cage on the side of the ruptured bronchus.

The first costovertebral articulation is vulnerable to injury because of its exposed position at the top of the rib cage. The joints may be subluxated or dislocated with or without associated avulsion fractures of the transverse process[24] (Fig. 14–18). These injuries are often associated with clavicular injuries.

Bilateral fractures of the first rib may result from indirect trauma[28] and from shoulder straps of seat belt restraints[41] and airbags.[52]

Fractures of the lower ribs are associated with injury of the solid organs of the upper abdomen and retroperitoneum in approximately 6% to 8% of cases.[20] These injuries involve either the kidney or the liver on the right and the spleen (Figs. 14–19 and 14–20), kidney, or diaphragm on the left.[1, 20] When fractures of the lower ribs are found, some consideration must then be given to the possibility of associated visceral injuries. Ruptures of the spleen and liver result in free blood in the peritoneum, which is manifested by medial displacement of the colon in the paracolonic gutters, widening the paracolonic stripe and silhouetting or obliterating the inferior posterior margin of the liver (see Fig. 14–19). Subcapsular hematomas may occur, particularly in the spleen, which then presents as an enlarging mass in the left upper quadrant that displaces the stomach medially (see Fig. 14–20) and the

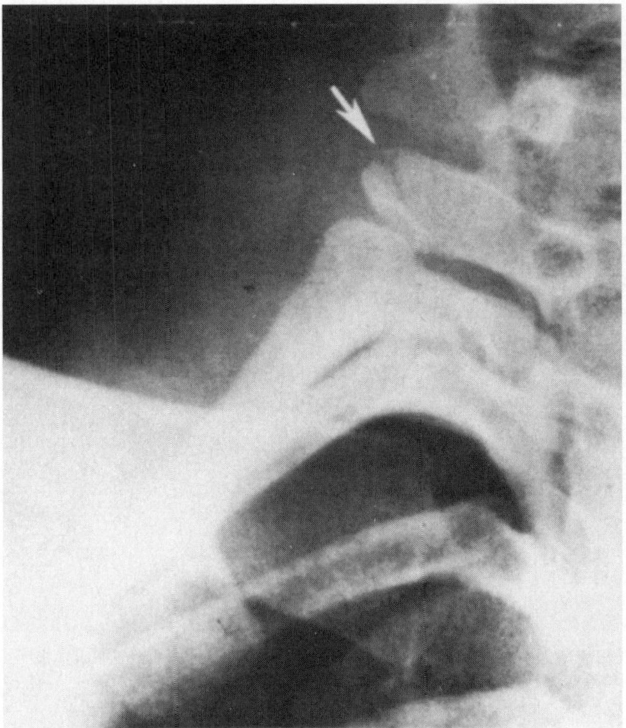

Figure 14–18. Avulsion fracture of the right transverse process of the first dorsal vertebra *(arrow).* The distance between the neck of the first rib and the transverse process of the first vertebra is widened. (From Christensen, E.E., & Dietz, G.W. [1980]. Injuries of the first costovertebral articulation. Radiology, *134:*41, with permission.)

splenic flexure inferiorly. Bleeding from a renal laceration or rupture obliterates the outline of the kidney. Abdominal visceral injuries are much more easily disclosed and better defined by ultrasonography or CT scanning than by conventional radiography (Figs. 14–21 and 14–22). Ruptures of the diaphragm are described below.

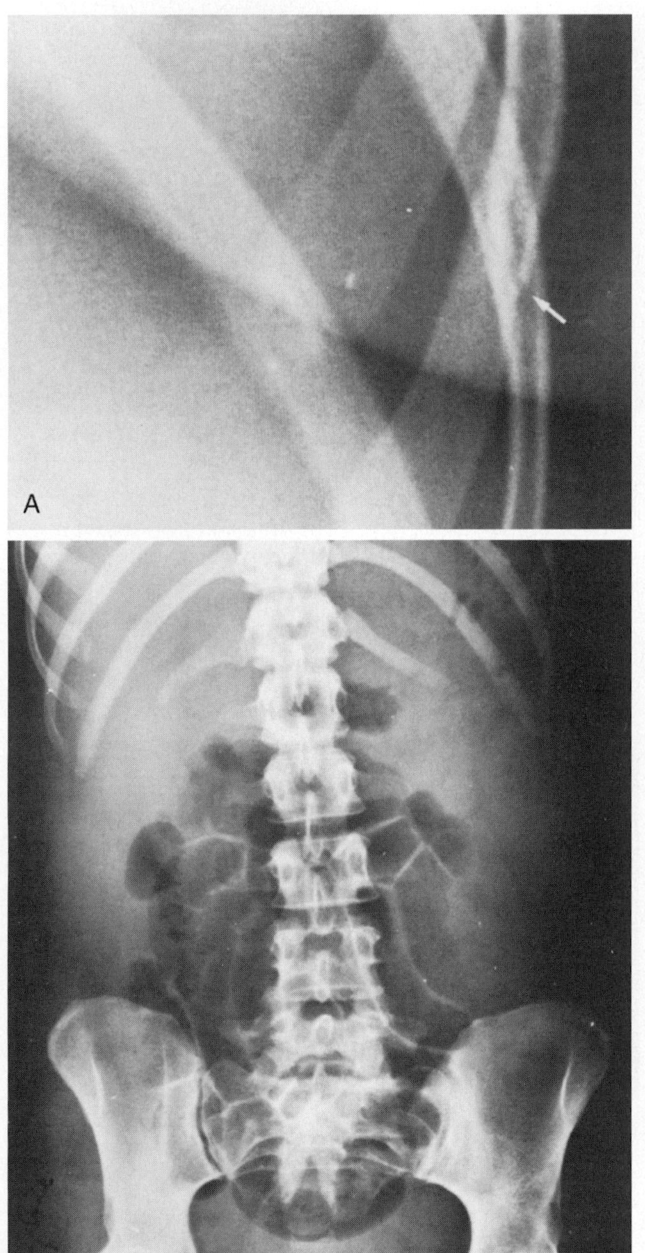

Figure 14–19. Fracture of the anterior lateral aspect of the eighth left rib associated with laceration of the left spleen. *A,* Close-up view of the left lower ribs shows a minimally displaced fracture of the anterior lateral aspect of the eighth rib *(arrow)*. *B,* The bowel loops are displaced centrally. The flanks are distended, and the medial margins of the paracolonic flank stripes are smooth. The bowel loops are displaced out of the pelvis. The findings indicate the presence of fluid—in this case, blood—within the abdomen. At surgery, a laceration of the spleen was identified, with free bleeding into the peritoneal cavity.

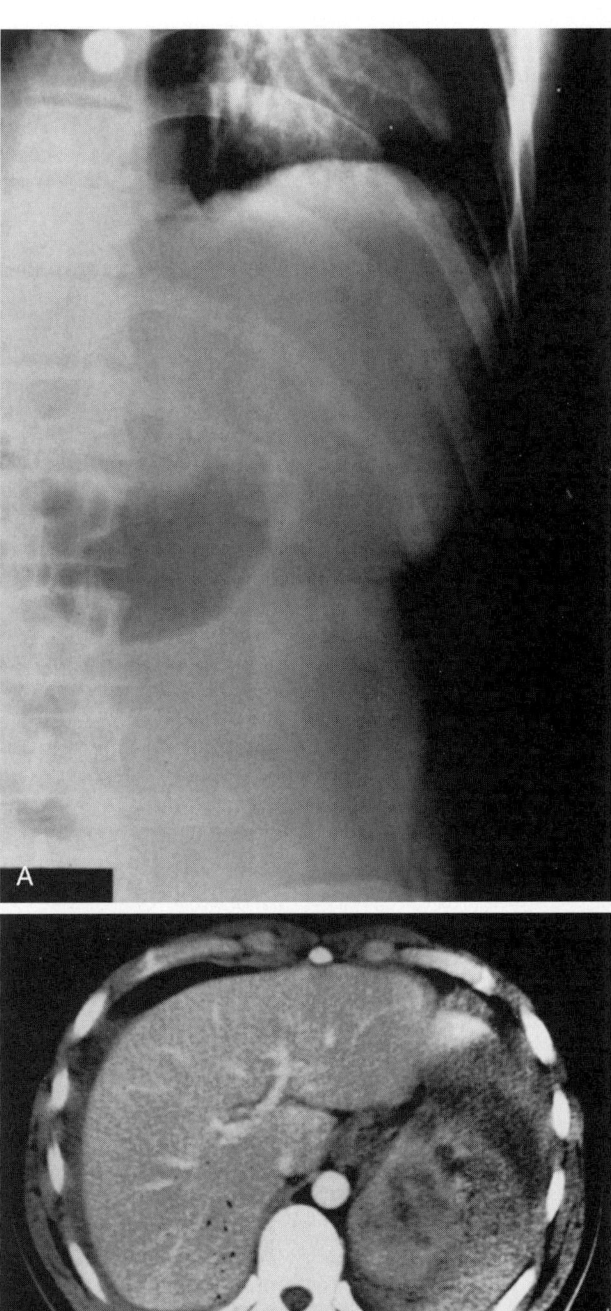

Figure 14–20. Rupture of the spleen without associated fractures of the ribs in a 36-year-old man. *A,* Radiograph of the lower left ribs shows no evidence of fracture, but a small hemothorax is present medially. A soft tissue mass is present in the left upper quadrant that displaces the stomach bubble medially and depresses the colon, consistent with a rupture of the spleen. *B,* CT of the upper abdomen shows a splenic rupture with surrounding hematoma. There is free blood within the peritoneum, as seen over the lateral margin of the liver on the right. (Case courtesy of M.G. Damm, MD, Madison, Wisc.)

In a study that examined 2080 children with blunt or penetrating trauma aged 0 to 14 years, Garcia and colleagues[32] found that children who had rib fractures were significantly more severely injured than children who had sustained blunt or penetrating trauma but without rib fractures. Child abuse accounted for 63% of the injuries to children younger than 3 years of age; pedestrian injuries predominated among older children. When compared with children without rib fractures, children with rib fractures had a higher mortality rate, but there was no statistically significant difference in morbidity. The mortality rate for the 18 children with both rib fractures and head injury was 71%.

Rib fractures, particularly of the posterior portion of the ribs, with a predilection for fracture near the costotransverse process, are a common skeletal manifestation of nonaccidental injury (NAI) in infants and young children and are generally considered to be highly specific for abuse. Nonaccidental rib fractures in young children with an unexplained history of injury in the absence of multiple trauma should alert the physician to the possibility of child abuse.

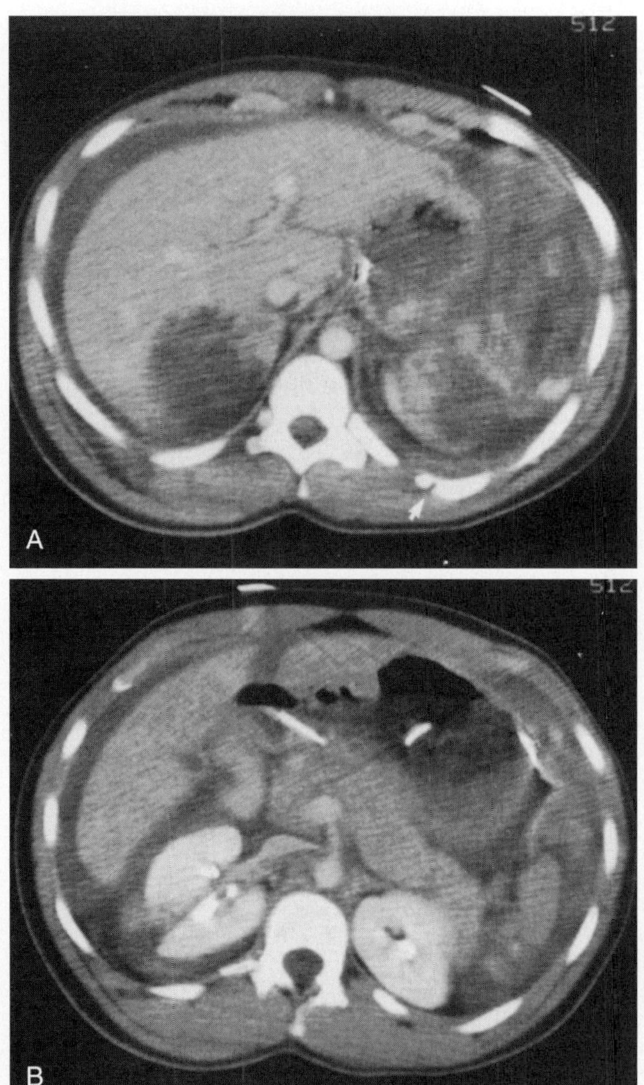

Figure 14–21. Rupture of the spleen, liver, and left kidney in a 20-year-old fire fighter crushed between two fire trucks. *A,* CT of the upper abdomen shows a minimally displaced fracture of the posterior aspect of a lower left rib *(arrow).* The spleen is shattered, as evidenced by the irregular, blotchy collections of the contrast in the left abdomen surrounded by blood. Blood is free within the peritoneum, located anterior and lateral to the liver. There is a low-density area in the posterior aspect of the right lobe of the liver, indicating a liver laceration with a hemorrhage. *B,* The right kidney has been transected and split into equal halves, both of which function. There is surrounding hemorrhage and free blood within the peritoneum.

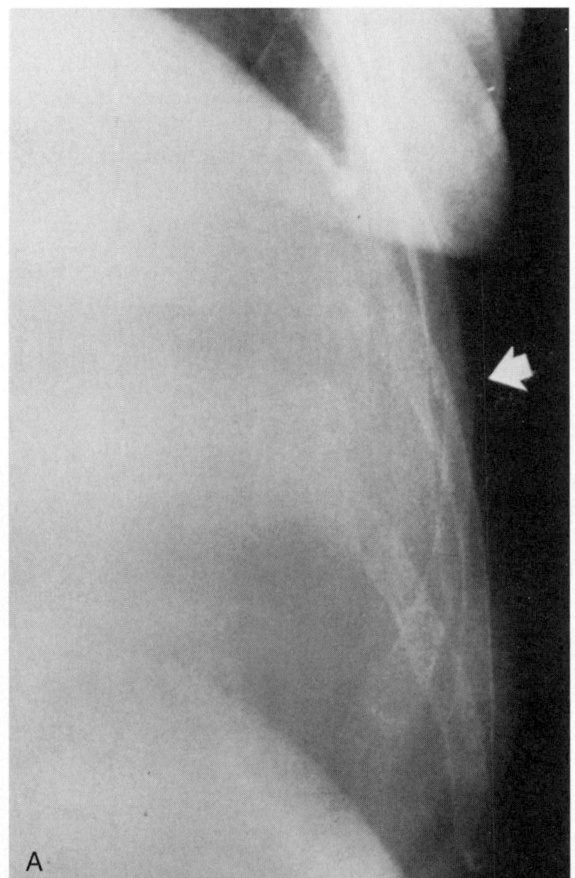

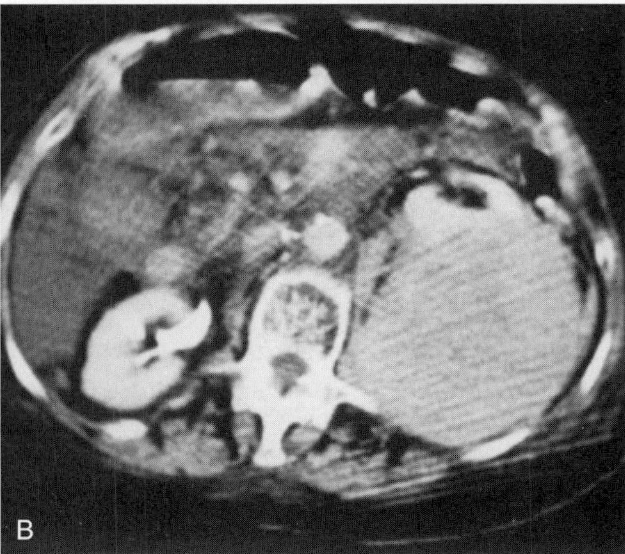

Figure 14–22. The patient was an 82-year-old woman who fell, sustaining a fracture of the anterior aspect of the ninth left rib and a laceration of the left kidney. *A,* Note the displaced fracture *(arrow)* of the lateral margin of the ninth left rib. *B,* CT shows the laceration of the left kidney, with a massive hematoma contained by Gerota's fascia. The CT was obtained after a paracentesis with saline.

Stress Fractures

Two types of stress fracture occur in the ribs. The cough fracture, or post-tussive fracture of Gooch, is a fracture of the anterior portion of the lower rib that occurs as a result of repeated coughing (Fig. 14–23). The fracture is usually found in association with chronic obstructive pulmonary disease, but it may also be associated with severe episodes of coughing in asthma, acute pneumonia, postnasal drip, or bronchitis. The fractures are often multiple and when associated with a chronic disease are found to vary in age. Thus, some fractures will be seen in the acute stage, and others will show various amounts of callus formation. Stress rib fractures have been described in elite rowers.[39] Fractures occur on the anterolateral to posterolateral aspects of ribs 5 through 9 and are typically associated with long-distance training and heavy load per stroke. The similarities between these stress fractures and fractures caused by cough suggest that in both cases, actions of the serratus anterior and external oblique muscles on the rib produce fracture through repetitive bending forces.

Stress fractures[29, 42] occur in the first rib, usually in the midportion or slightly anterior in the subclavian groove. These fractures are frequently the result of heavy lifting (as with the bench press) or carrying a heavy backpack; less often, they result from throwing, particularly in baseball pitchers (see Fig. 14–16A). When identified, the fractures are often associated with considerable callus formation. They may be bilateral.

Fractures of the Sternum

Injuries of the sternum[63] are caused either by direct kinetic energy absorption to the front of the chest occurring as the thorax rapidly decelerates against the steering wheel, shoulder belt, or airbag, in automobile accidents,[57, 58] or by indirect forces generated by flexion of the cervical and upper dorsal spinal segments (Fig. 14–24). The incidence of sternal fracture resulting from motor vehicle collisions is about 3%, although the incidence may decrease with the advent of supplemental restraint devices (airbags). A direct blow usually results in a transverse fracture of the body of the sternum (Fig. 14–25), with posterior displacement of the distal or lower fragment.

Indirect flexion compression forces characteristically produce an injury at or adjacent to the manubriosternal joint, with posterior displacement or depression of the manubrium relative to the body of the sternum[60, 62, 63]; the second rib remains attached to the manubrium. The most common injury is a fracture-dislocation of the manubriosternal joint. Less frequently there is a fracture of either the manubrium (Fig. 14–26) or the upper body of the sternum, with similar posterior displacement of the upper fragment; the anatomy of the joint determines the nature of the injury. In a majority of people the manubriosternal joint is of the cartilaginous type, similar to the pubic symphysis; however, in a third of the population the joint is of the synovial type. Dislocations are more likely to occur when the joint is synovial. Flexion of the neck and

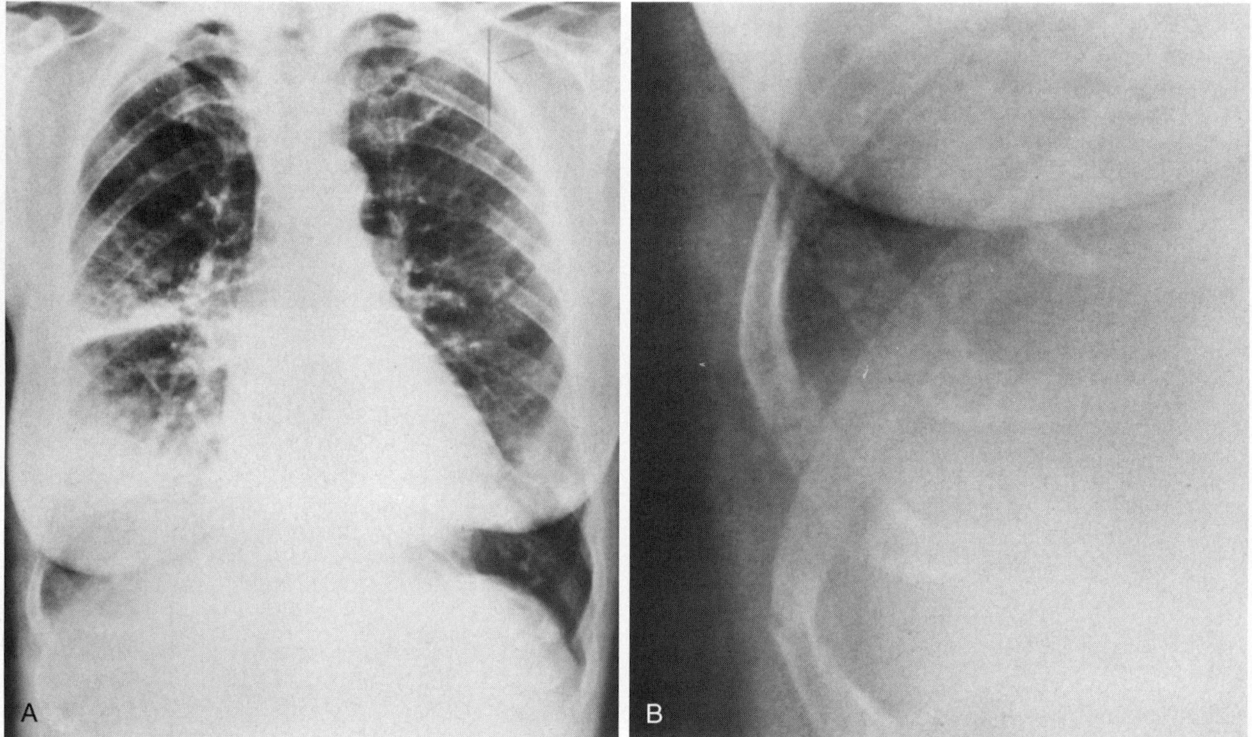

Figure 14–23. Stress fractures of the anterolateral margin of the ninth and tenth ribs in a 75-year-old woman with pneumonia. She had a febrile illness for 7 or 8 days with considerable coughing and experienced a "sticking" pain in the lower area of the chest for 3 days before this examination. *A,* Standard chest radiograph demonstrates the pneumonia within the right, mid-, and lower lung fields. *B,* Close-up view of the lower right ribs shows fractures of the anterior lateral margins of the eighth, ninth, and tenth ribs. There was no history of trauma, and these fractures are presumed to represent post-tussive fractures.

upper thoracic spine imparts a downward and backward movement to the upper ribs, particularly the upper two ribs. Flexion of the lumbar and thoracolumbar regions of the spine has no effect on the ribs until the abdominal contents push forward against the lower ribs. The sternum is then subjected to opposing forces: The manubrium is forced downward and backward by the upper two ribs, and the body of the sternum is forced upward and forward by the lower ribs. The sternum yields at its weakest point between these two forces, usually in the region of the manubriosternal joint. Pain and tenderness of the sternum are the most commonly reported symptoms.

Forty percent of the fractures of the sternum are associated with wedge compression fractures of the upper dorsal spine or, less commonly, the cervical or lumbar spine.[64, 67, 68, 71] Therefore, when a flexion-compression injury of the sternum is identified, it is important to exclude associated fractures of the spine. Flexion-compression fractures of the sternum have also been described in patients wearing a lap-and-shoulder combination seat belt[58] (see Fig. 14–26) and may result from seizures.[62] Usually fractures of the sternum are easily recognized, but in some cases they may be initially undisplaced and obscure. Attention can be directed to the fracture by a retrosternal hematoma (see Fig. 14–25); although this sign is specific for sternal fracture, it has a low sensitivity.[65] The hematoma is confined by the parietal pleura and therefore is seen as a smooth, elongated, rounded mass projecting into the mediastinum with its base on the sternum. The hemorrhage may be of sufficient magnitude to give the appearance of an enlarged, widening mediastinum on the frontal projection, mimicking the appearance of a mediastinal hematoma associated with aortic rupture.

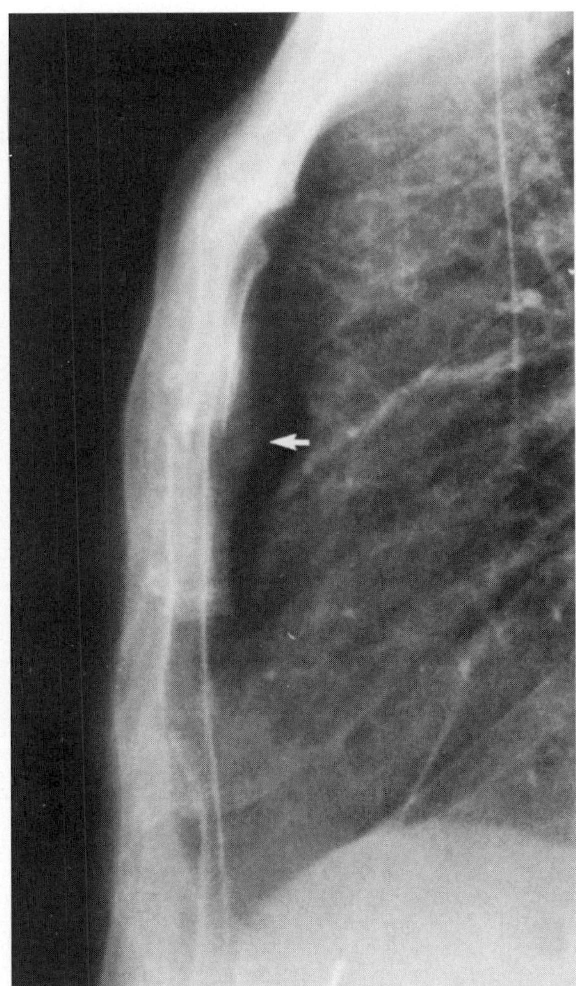

Figure 14–25. This transverse fracture of the sternum occurred during resuscitation of a 72-year-old man after cardiac arrest. The fracture is associated with a hematoma that displaces the underlying pleura *(arrow)*.

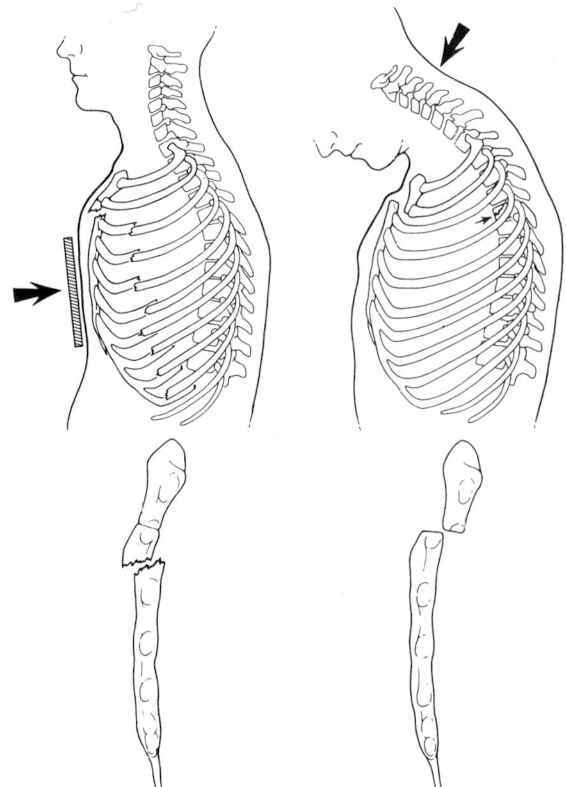

Figure 14–24. Fractures of the sternum. Direct blows create injuries that principally involve the body of the sternum *(left)* and are associated with posterior displacement of the distal fragment. Flexion compression injuries *(right)* are produced by flexion of the lower cervical and upper thoracic segments of the spine and result in fractures of the manubrium or dislocations of the manubriosternal joint, with characteristic posterior displacement of the manubrium. Note the associated compression fracture of the upper dorsal spine *(small arrow)*.

Characteristically, with these fractures the degree of offset is minimal, the two fragments being in apposition without significant separation. It is difficult, if not impossible, to visualize the fracture lines on the frontal chest radiograph because the fragments are in apposition, and the offset is characteristically in the sagittal plane—that is, either anterior or posterior, without significant lateral displacement or overlap to yield a double density. Because most injuries of the sternum are in the axial plane, they are difficult to identify by CT[66] unless multiplanar reconstruction is used. CT scanning may show the occasional sagittally oriented fracture of the body or separation of the sternocostal junction.[74]

Spontaneous fractures of the sternum have been identified in patients with a thoracic kyphosis resulting from severe osteoporosis[61] (Fig. 14–27) and can be accompa-

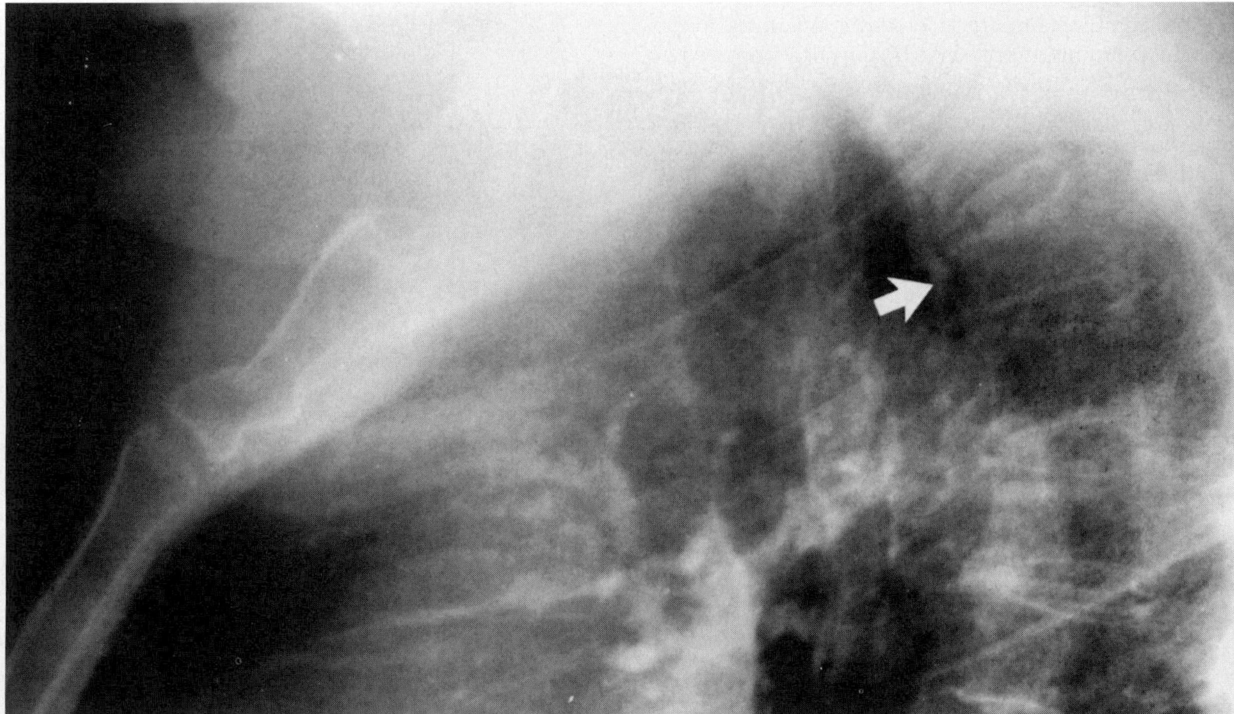

Figure 14–26. Flexion-compression fracture of the manubrium associated with a compression fracture of the third thoracic vertebra in a 79-year-old woman injured in an automobile accident. The patient was wearing a seat belt at the time of the accident. Note the fracture of the distal aspect of the manubrium, with surrounding hemorrhage. There is anterior wedging of the third thoracic vertebral body *(arrow)*.

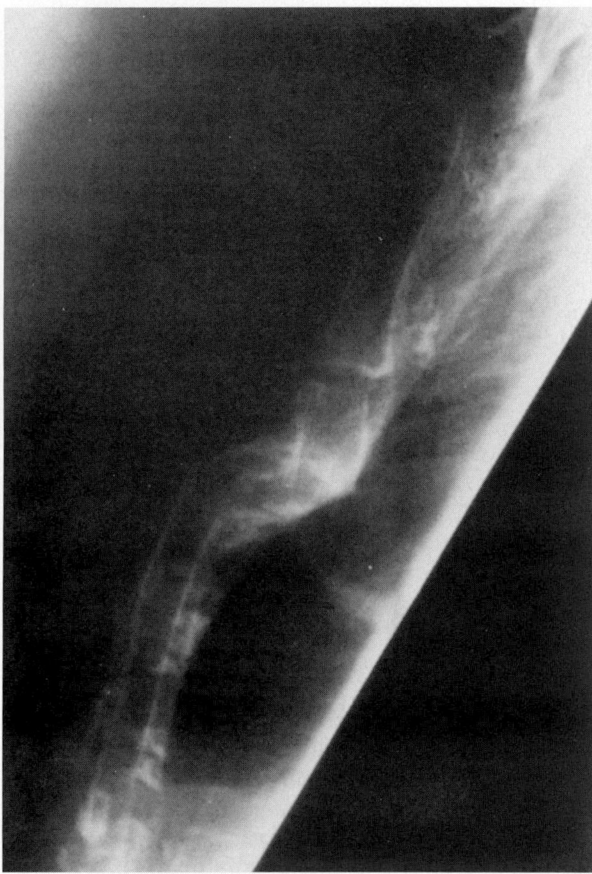

Figure 14–27. Spontaneous sternal collapse in a 61-year-old man with severe osteoporosis and progressive thoracic kyphosis resulting in spontaneous buckling of the sternum. Insufficiency fractures of the sternum and manubriosternal dislocations may be seen in association with osteoporosis. (Case courtesy of Donald D. Resnick, MD, and David J. Sartoris, MD, San Diego, Calif.)

nied by severe chest pain simulating myocardial infarction[73] or pulmonary embolism.[75] A spontaneous fracture of the sternum in a 16-year-old patient with cystic fibrosis has been described.[70]

A fracture of the sternum may be an indication of a severe crushing injury.[7] As might be anticipated, these fractures are associated with myocardial contusion[2, 54, 56] and other forms of cardiac injury and with rupture of the aorta, great vessels, diaphragm, trachea, and bronchi. Depressed, segmental sternal fractures have an increased association with myocardial lacerations. Manubrial fractures have a more frequent association with intrathoracic and upper mediastinal (especially great vessel) injuries. The outcome for patients with an isolated sternal fracture and normal electrocardiographic findings is very good.[65]

Most fractures of the sternum are treated conservatively and heal satisfactorily. Occasionally, open reduction with pin or wire fixation of the manubriosternal joint is required. Nonunion with pseudoarthrosis has been described.[64]

On occasion, gas (from the vacuum phenomenon) can be seen within the sternoclavicular joints on chest CT images.[72] Such gas is more frequently seen in patients who have sustained blunt chest trauma than in patients undergoing chest CT for other indications. Although the presence of gas suggests that the mechanism of injury involved significant distraction forces, thus serving as a marker of injury severity, this finding does not indicate a greater risk of significant mediastinal or thoracic injury.

Traumatic Lung Hernia

Lung hernias are classified by location and etiology. They occur through the lung apices, diaphragm, or chest wall and are either congenital or acquired secondary to trauma, chest wall neoplasms, or infection.[78] Spontaneous lung hernias have also been reported in weight lifters, wind instrument musicians, and patients with chronic cough. In the majority of cases, lung hernia is traumatic in origin and involves the thoracic wall as a delayed complication of blunt trauma.[11, 51] It occurs in either the intercostal space or the superclavicular region and is manifested clinically by a soft bulging of the chest wall that varies with respiration. The mass consists of a hernia of the underlying lung covered by parietal pleura.

Lung hernias are more common after rib resection, tube drainage, or penetrating wounds than after blunt trauma. Most patients are asymptomatic. The usual complaint is a bulging mass in the chest wall associated with coughing, straining, or lifting.

The diagnosis is radiographically confirmed by demonstration of a radiolucent area containing bronchovascular markings projecting beyond the confines of the thorax on tangentially oriented radiographs (Figs. 14–28 and 14–29). Because most hernias occur in the anterior or anterolateral chest wall, they are best demonstrated on a standard lateral or oblique view. Lung hernias may be missed unless the x-ray beam is oriented at a true tangent to the hernia. Fluoroscopy with spot films may be necessary to show a hernia to best advantage. CT scanning confirms the extent and anatomy of the injury (Fig. 14–30). The hernia can be accentuated with straining or coughing.

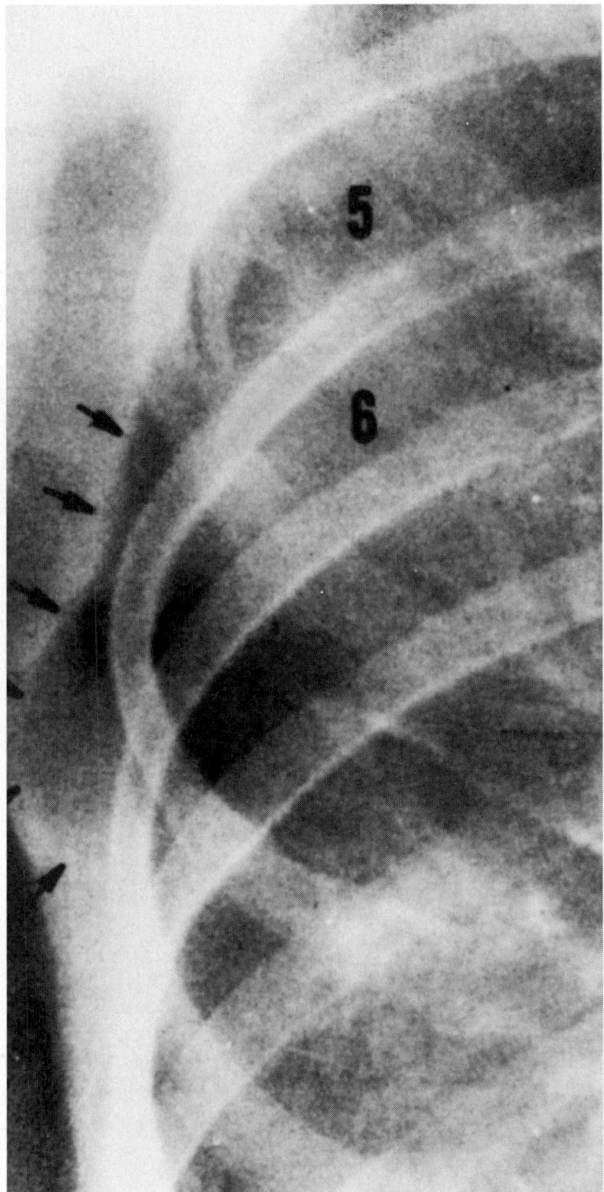

Figure 14–28. Lung hernia. This radiograph was obtained 3 years after a thoracotomy. The lung protrudes through the fifth and sixth intercostal spaces, along the course of the previous incision *(arrows)*. (From Reynolds, J., & Davis, J.T. [1966]. Injuries of the chest wall, pleura, pericardium, lungs, bronchi and esophagus. Radiol. Clin. North Am., *4*:383, with permission.)

In a small percentage of cases the hernia will regress spontaneously. A majority of the patients with lung hernia are asymptomatic, and in these cases management with a truss constitutes appropriate treatment. Surgical repair is indicated for cosmesis, persistent pain, incarceration, or strangulation. At present the preferred method of repair consists of closing the defect with a Gore-Tex patch.

Pleural Trauma

Injuries of the pleural surface result in effusion or pneumothorax, either of which may occur without associated rib fracture. The incidence of pneumothorax and

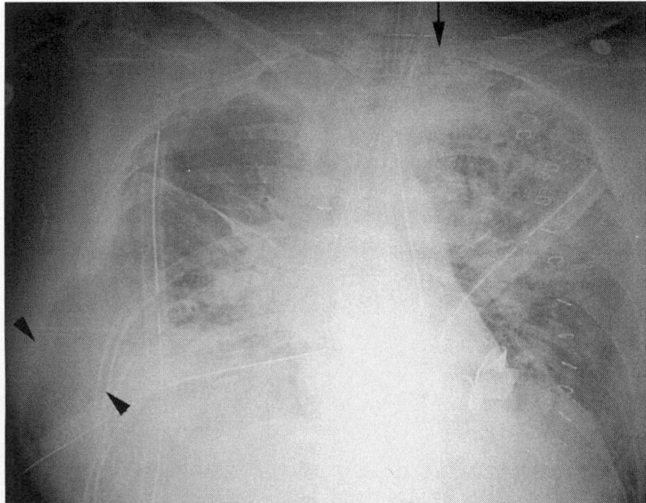

Figure 14–29. Lung hernia in a 41-year-old woman involved in a high-speed motor vehicle crash. A postoperative chest radiograph obtained with the patient in the supine position shows protrusion of the lung *(arrowheads)* through the fifth and sixth intercostal spaces, along the course of the recent thoracotomy incision. The patient also sustained a left sternoclavicular dislocation *(short arrow)*, as well as an aortic tear.

hemothorax varies with the severity of chest injury. In one study of rib fractures resulting from various degrees of chest trauma, there was a 13.6% incidence of hemothorax and a 9% incidence of pneumothorax.[92] However, in severe blunt chest trauma, the incidence of hemothorax and of pneumothorax was approximately 30% each.[95] Hemothorax is more likely to occur in patients with multiple or displaced rib fractures.

Hemothorax

Lacerations of the pleural surface and underlying chest wall or lung give rise to hemothoraces of small to moderate volume. With massive bleeding the most likely source of bleeding is in the chest wall or a major vessel at the hilus or in the mediastinum. Points of bleeding within the lung are tamponaded by the blood within the pleural space; therefore, massive bleeding from this source is unlikely. The radiographic findings associated with pleural fluid are well known, vary with patient position, and consist of blunting of the costophrenic angle, formation of a meniscus along the lateral chest wall on films obtained with the patient upright, and opacification of the hemithorax on films obtained with the patient supine (see Fig. 14–32*B*). The degree of opacification is dependent on the amount of fluid within the pleural space. On radiographs obtained with the patient supine, the amount of pleural fluid can be grossly underestimated (Fig. 14–31).

Blood does not clot within the pleural space. It is thought to be defibrinated by the respiratory motion of the lung and chest wall. Therefore, it is free to move into a dependent position. In cases of severe trauma the chest radiograph is obtained with the patient in the supine position; therefore, the fluid may lie posteriorly and appear as diffuse opacification of the entire lung. However, the pulmonary vessels and diaphragm remain identifiable. With the patient upright, the fluid may collect between the diaphragmatic surface of the lung and the diaphragm in the subpulmonic position.[79, 96] A characteristic distortion of the diaphragmatic silhouette results. There is a false appearance of diaphragmatic elevation, the apex of the diaphragm is shifted laterally, frequently the costophrenic angle is blunted, and on the lateral view the diaphragm appears somewhat flattened. If the patient's condition permits, a lateral decubitus view may be obtained to substantiate the subpulmonic location of the fluid. The fluid will then drain from the subpulmonic

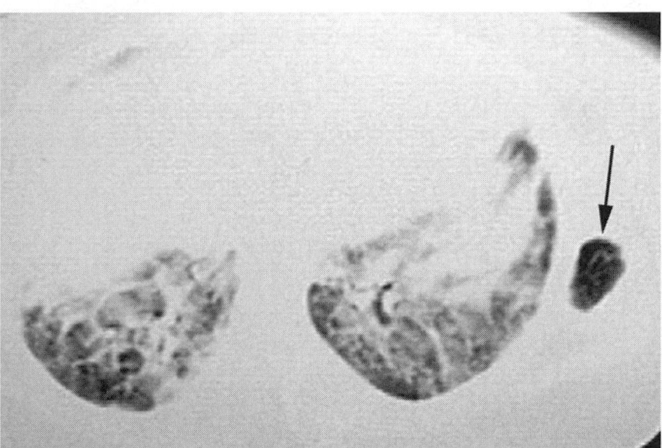

Figure 14–30. CT from a 71-year-old woman who suffered severe blunt trauma to the left side of her torso, resulting in a ruptured left hemidiaphragm, multiple left rib fractures, lung contusion, and splenic laceration. A routine chest radiograph (not shown) obtained 4 days after injury demonstrated a new lucency in the left lateral chest wall. CT obtained using lung window setting *(arrow)* shows normal lung tissue herniating through a post-traumatic intercostal space defect in the chest wall.

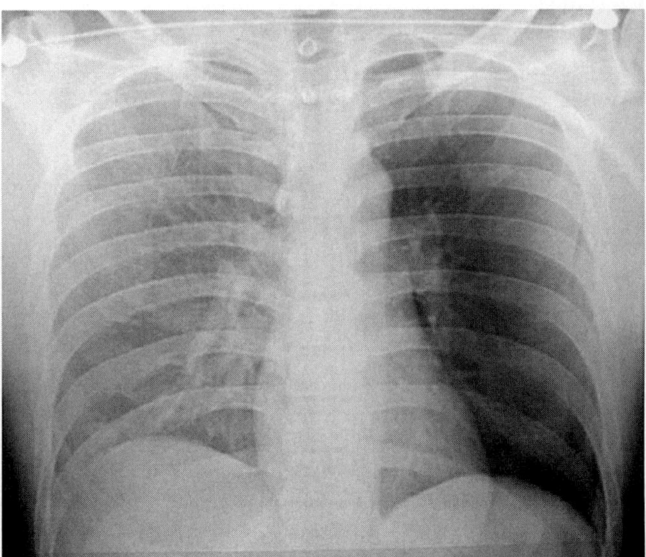

Figure 14–31. Hemothorax in a young patient who sustained blunt right chest trauma. A chest radiograph obtained with the patient supine shows an asymmetrically dense right hemithorax consistent with a hemothorax. Such supine radiographs can underestimate the size of pleural fluid collections. There proved to be 600 mL of blood in the pleural space.

position to the dependent portion of the chest along the lateral chest wall. CT scanning is more sensitive in showing hemothorax or other fluid collections such as chyle or stomach contents, as well as in determining whether they are free-flowing or loculated[105] (see Figs. 14–8, 14–10, and 14–12).

Hemothorax is not always evident on the initial radiographic examination of the chest.[92, 97] In a series reported by McLoughlin and associates,[92] only 47% of hemothoraces were evident on the day of injury. In the remainder of the cases, radiographic evidence of hemothorax was commonly delayed for 3 to 5 days but in some instances appeared as late as 4 weeks. In contrast, all pneumothoraces were evident on the day of injury.

Eosinophilic pleural effusions and eosinophilia have been reported[91] after chest trauma, and also with a wide variety of other disorders. The majority of these effusions are bloody. The pathogenesis is unknown, but they gradually clear without specific treatment.

Hemopneumothorax is manifested by an air-fluid level across the hemithorax (Fig. 14–32). Demonstration of an air-fluid level requires a radiograph obtained with a horizontal beam. Either the patient must be placed in the erect position, or a cross-table lateral view (see Fig. 14–37*B*) must be obtained to substantiate this diagnosis.

Chylous Effusion

Rupture of the thoracic duct caused by crushing injury of the chest occurs infrequently.[11] Although the diagnosis cannot be made from the radiographic appearance alone, characteristically the chylous effusion does not appear until 3 to 7 days following trauma (Fig. 14–33). Therefore, the delayed appearance of pleural effusion is highly suggestive. Evidently the chylous fluid is initially confined to the extrapleural space but eventually ruptures the parietal pleura and extends into the pleural space. The effusions are unilateral, and either side may be involved, but involvement of the right side is somewhat more frequent.

Pneumothorax

Pneumothorax exists when air is present inside the pleural cavity, outside the lung. The air usually enters the pleural space through a laceration of the visceral pleura. When pneumothorax is the result of blunt trauma to the chest, it is usually associated with fracture of one or more ribs (see Fig. 14–32), with the visceral pleura being punctured by the fractured rib. Pneumothorax resulting from blunt trauma may also occur without identifiable rib

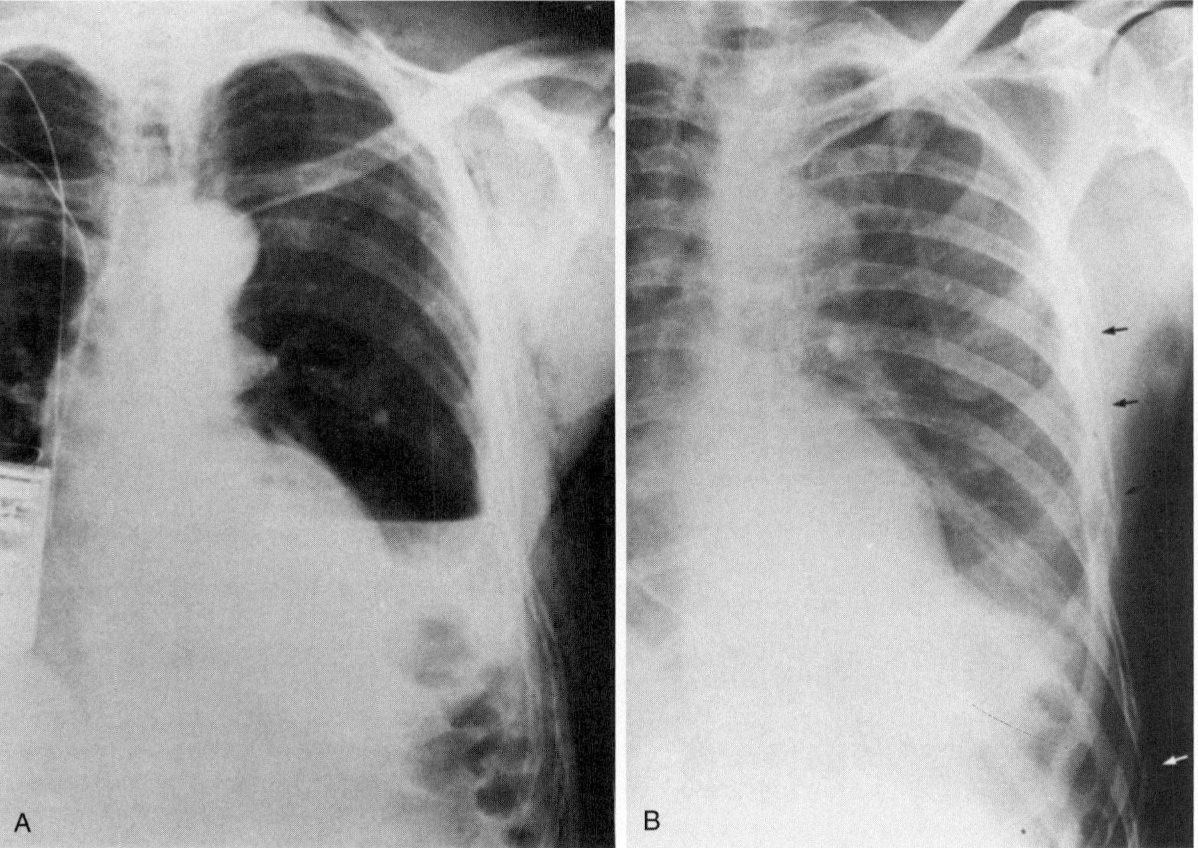

Figure 14–32. Fractures of the fourth through the ninth ribs associated with hemopneumothorax in a 73-year-old man. *A,* Standard chest radiograph shows a hemopneumothorax. There is an air-fluid level at the left base. Subcutaneous emphysema is present on the left in the chest wall. The seventh rib fracture is visualized, but no other fractures are obvious. *B,* Radiograph obtained 8 days later with the patient supine clearly shows fractures of the fourth through the ninth ribs *(arrows).* Pleural fluid, manifested as diffuse opacification, is present on the left. Note that the pulmonary vessels are still visualized. The fluid is layered posteriorly because of the patient's supine position for the examination.

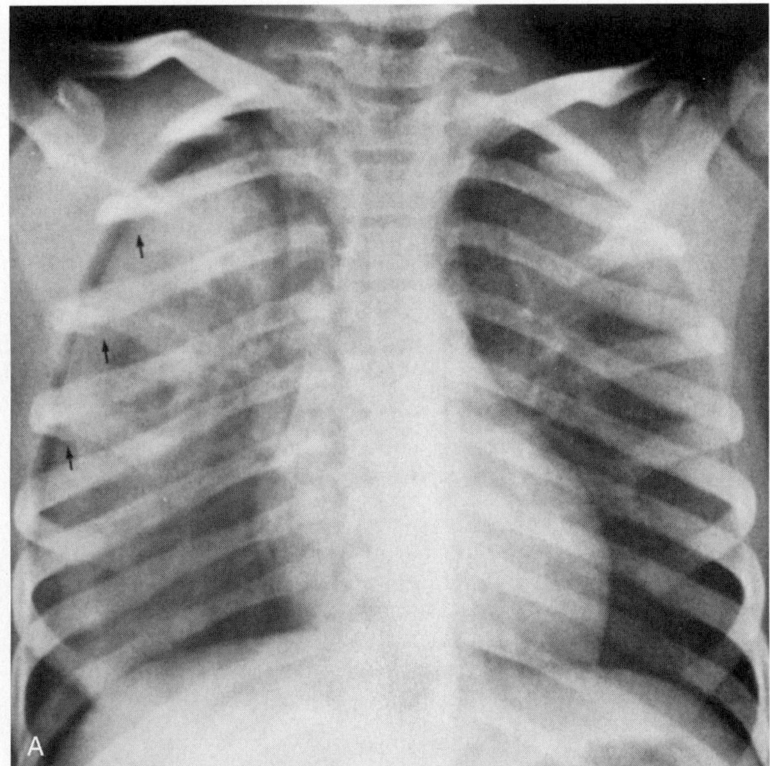

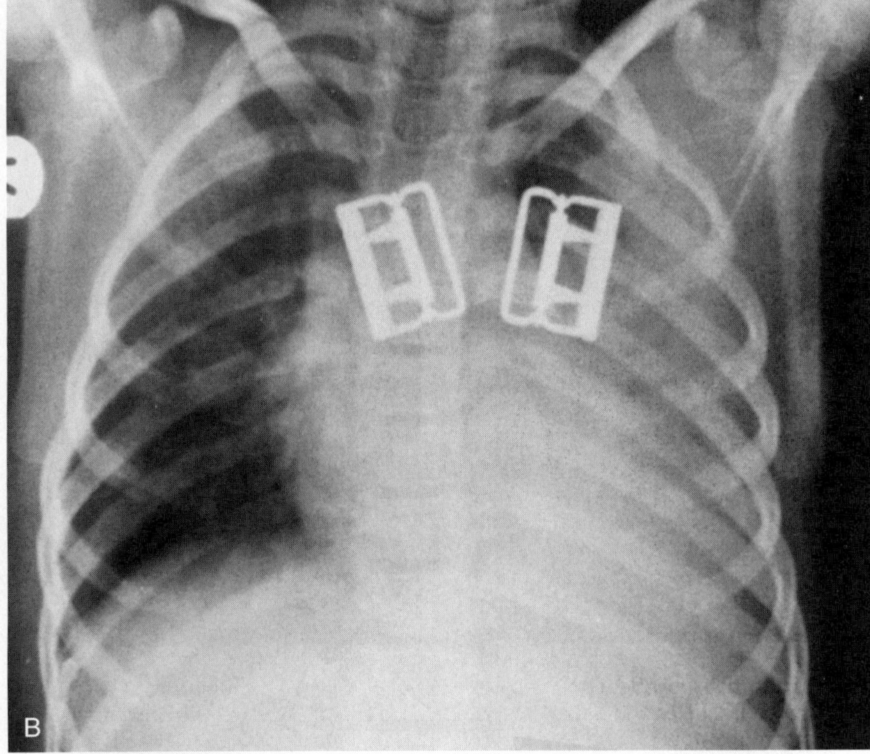

Figure 14–33. Fractures of the right ribs and clavicle with associated pneumothorax and subsequent chylous effusion. *A,* Initial radiograph obtained with the patient supine shows fractures of the anterior margin of the second, third, and fourth right ribs *(arrows)* and of the midclavicle, associated with pneumothorax. *B,* Repeat examination was performed 5 days later. A left pleural effusion noted at that time proved to be a chylous effusion. The delayed appearance is typical of chylous effusion.

fractures, especially if there is an underlying pulmonary laceration to suggest compression rupture of the lung (see Fig. 14–40). Pneumothorax is usually associated with some degree of bleeding from the lacerated pleural surface. In most cases the amount of bleeding is minimal, particularly in the absence of multiple displaced rib fractures.

Air may also enter the pleural space through an open wound in the chest wall. These wounds are known as "sucking wounds" and are usually obvious on clinical examination.

Radiographic identification of pneumothorax is dependent on visualization of the visceral pleura surface of the lung as it is displaced from the chest wall by the accumulation of air within the pleural space (Fig. 14–34). On the chest radiograph obtained with the patient upright, the visceral pleural surface of the lung is a thin, sharply defined line of radiodensity that parallels the chest wall. With moderate degrees of collapse there is no change in the density of the pulmonary parenchyma, presumably because of shunting of blood to the contralateral lung. There is increased radiolucency at the periphery of the lung lateral to the visceral pleural line, representing the air in the pleural space. The pulmonary

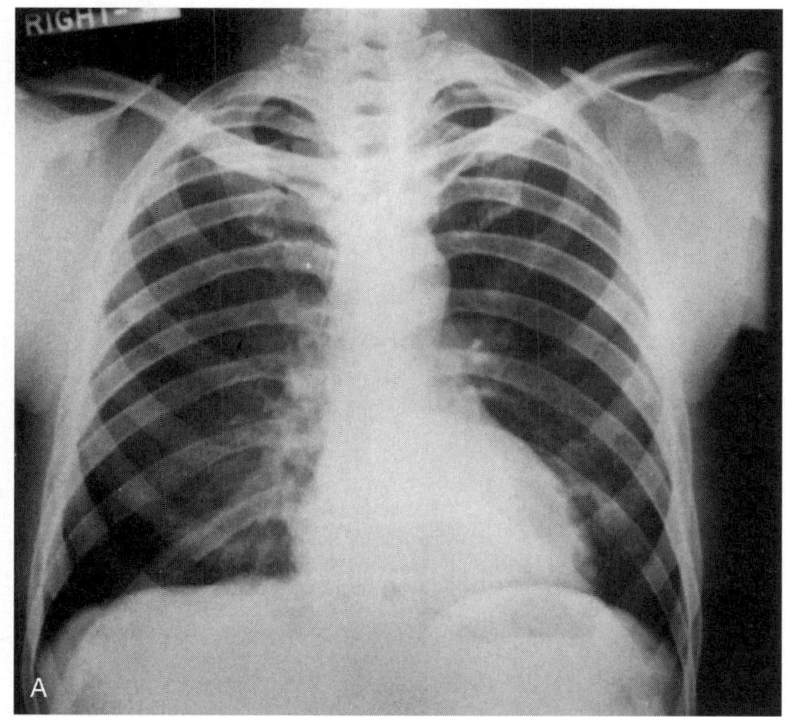

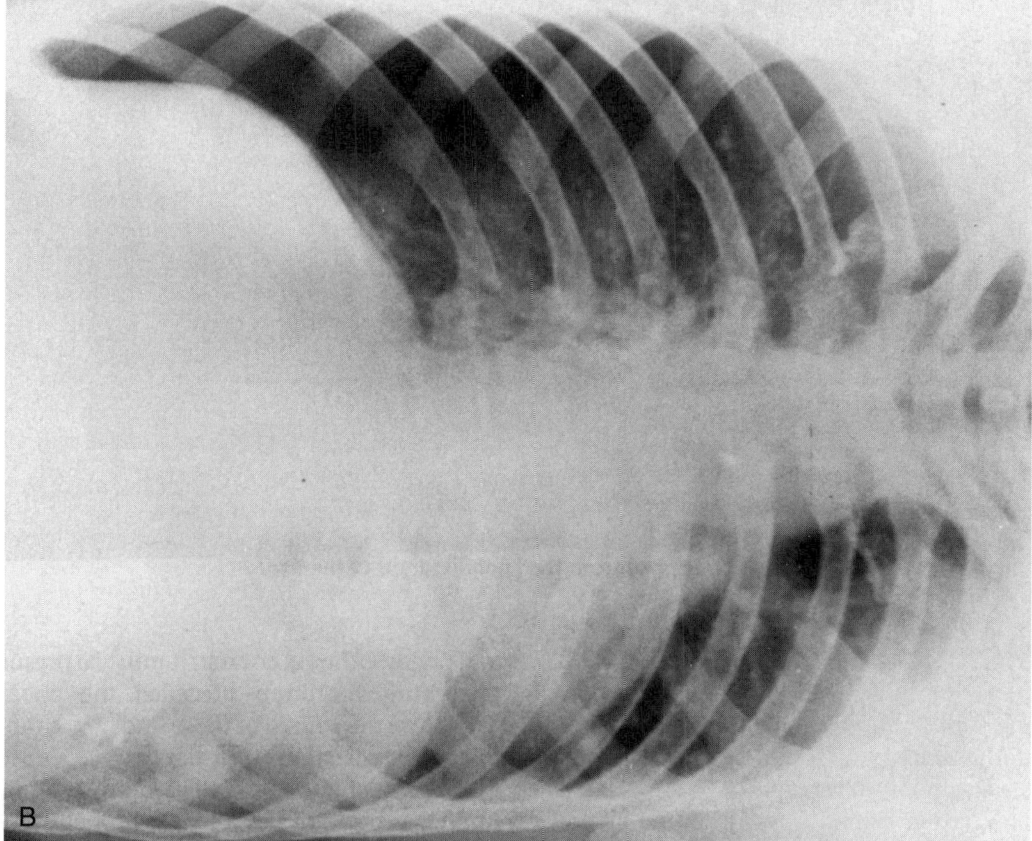

Figure 14–34. Pneumothorax following a stab wound. *A,* Standard chest radiograph shows a large pneumothorax with partial collapse of the lower right lobe. There are granulomas in the right upper lung field. The pneumothorax is best visualized at the right base. *B,* Decubitus view accentuates and clearly shows the pneumothorax.

vessels usually extend to the pleural line but not beyond it. The air is readily identified laterally and superiorly, but when loculated in the subpulmonic position or anteriorly it is more difficult to identify.

Pneumothorax is most easily demonstrated on a standard posteroanterior chest radiograph obtained with the patient in the erect position. The air-fluid level is identified in the costophrenic sulcus, representing the interface of blood and air. The exact position of the air-fluid level is, of course, dependent on the amount of accumulated blood and air.

When the pneumothorax is small, it may be very difficult to identify. Close examination of the lung parallel to the chest wall is necessary to identify the displaced visceral pleura. Although pneumothorax is accentuated in expiration (see Fig. 14–34), we do not recommend obtaining chest radiographs at end-exhalation. The very low lung volumes may make it somewhat easier to detect a very small pneumothorax but are more often misinterpreted as showing new congestive heart failure or pulmonary edema on comparison with the appearance on full-inspiration radiographs. We feel that any benefit deriving from use of this maneuver is not worth the possible confusion. A decubitus view obtained with the patient positioned with the affected side elevated allows the air to accumulate in the uppermost portion of the hemithorax, so that the pleural surface can be more easily recognized (see Fig. 14–34).

In the critically ill or injured patient, radiographic examination of the chest is performed with the patient supine. Air in the pleural space is less evident, or can easily defy detection, when the patient is supine. Air tends to accumulate anteriorly and medially and usually is either subpulmonic or is located in the anterior medial recess.[102, 103, 108] Subpulmonic air can be identified on the chest radiograph by the presence of basilar hyperlucency and the thin, sharp line of the visceral pleura elevated by the pneumothorax above the diaphragm, but these findings are not always evident. Other signs of pneumothorax include depression of the diaphragm, an unusually distinct cardiac apex, and visualization of the apical pericardial fat pad. These observations usually underestimate the actual size and extent of the pneumothorax. Anteromedial, posteromedial, and other localized pneumothoraces are best demonstrated by CT[102, 106] (Fig. 14–35). If unrecognized, a small pneumothorax may become a tension pneumothorax when the patient either undergoes general anesthesia or is placed on assisted ventilation. CT of the chest is of value to exclude a small pneumothorax when either of these procedures is contemplated.[104]

Because knowledge of patient positioning is essential for accurately detecting and determining the size of a pneumothorax, portable chest radiographs should always be marked with the relevant information. The technologist can mark the films by hand or can use one of several types of gravity/inclination markers available commercially.

With larger accumulations of air, the lung may collapse and become completely opacified (Fig. 14–36). When sufficient air accumulates within the pleural space, the intrapleural pressure may rise sufficiently to displace the mediastinal contents of the diaphragm. This condition is termed *tension pneumothorax*.[9] The tension is created by a flaplike or ball valve mechanism at the pleural surface that allows air to enter but not to exit from the pleural space. The result is acute respiratory embarrassment, which constitutes a true surgical emergency. The pressure must be relieved by drainage of the pleural space as soon as this condition is identified. Radiographically, tension pneumothorax is suggested by displacement of the heart and mediastinal contents to the contralateral side and depression of the diaphragm.[11] Because the physiologic consequences of a large pneumothorax can vary depending on underlying comorbid disease and cardiopulmonary reserve, the diagnosis of tension pneumothorax is clinical and only suggested by the radiographic appearance (Fig. 14–37; see also Figs. 14–36 and 14–40). Nonetheless, it is very important to routinely establish the

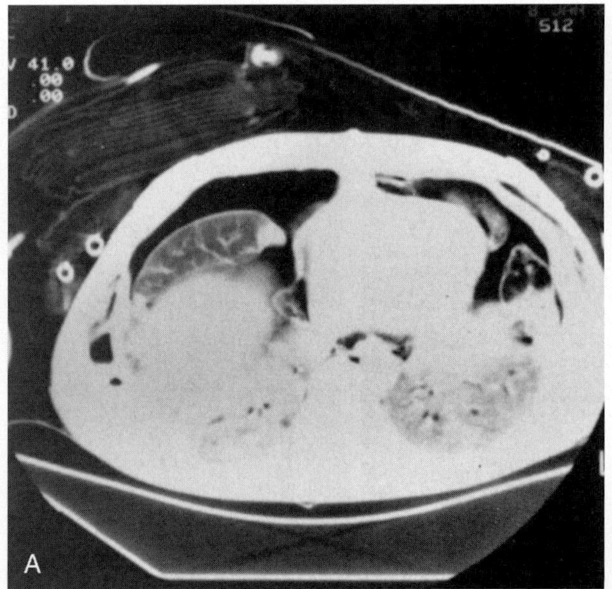

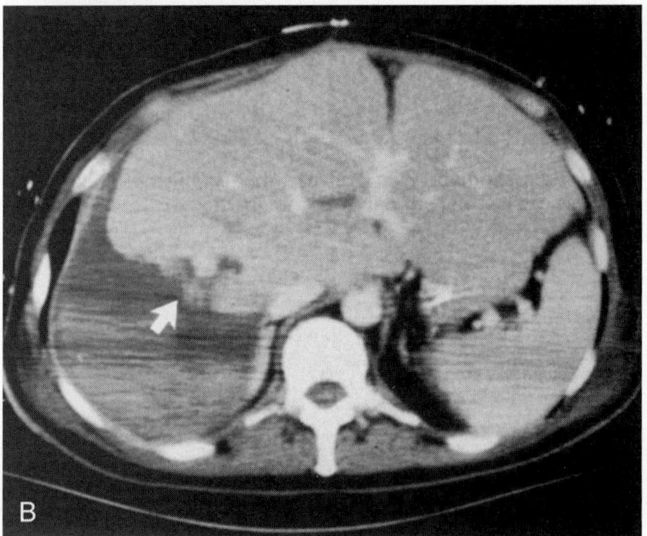

Figure 14–35. Pneumothorax and laceration of the liver in a 31-year-old man. *A,* Bilateral pneumothoraces are demonstrated anteriorly. Note the lung collapsed posteriorly. *B,* Liver laceration *(arrow)* with a massive subcapsular hematoma. The hemorrhage was contained by the capsule, and there was no free blood within the peritoneum. Note that the capsule is stripped from the lateral margin of the liver.

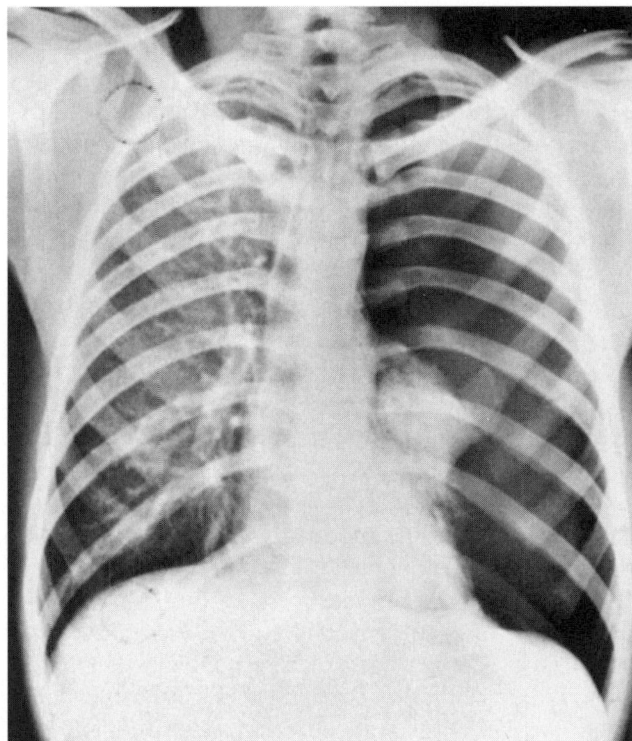

Figure 14–36. Tension pneumothorax in a young man. The left lung is completely collapsed against the hilus. The mediastinum is shifted to the left, and the diaphragm is depressed—findings strongly suggestive of a tension pneumothorax.

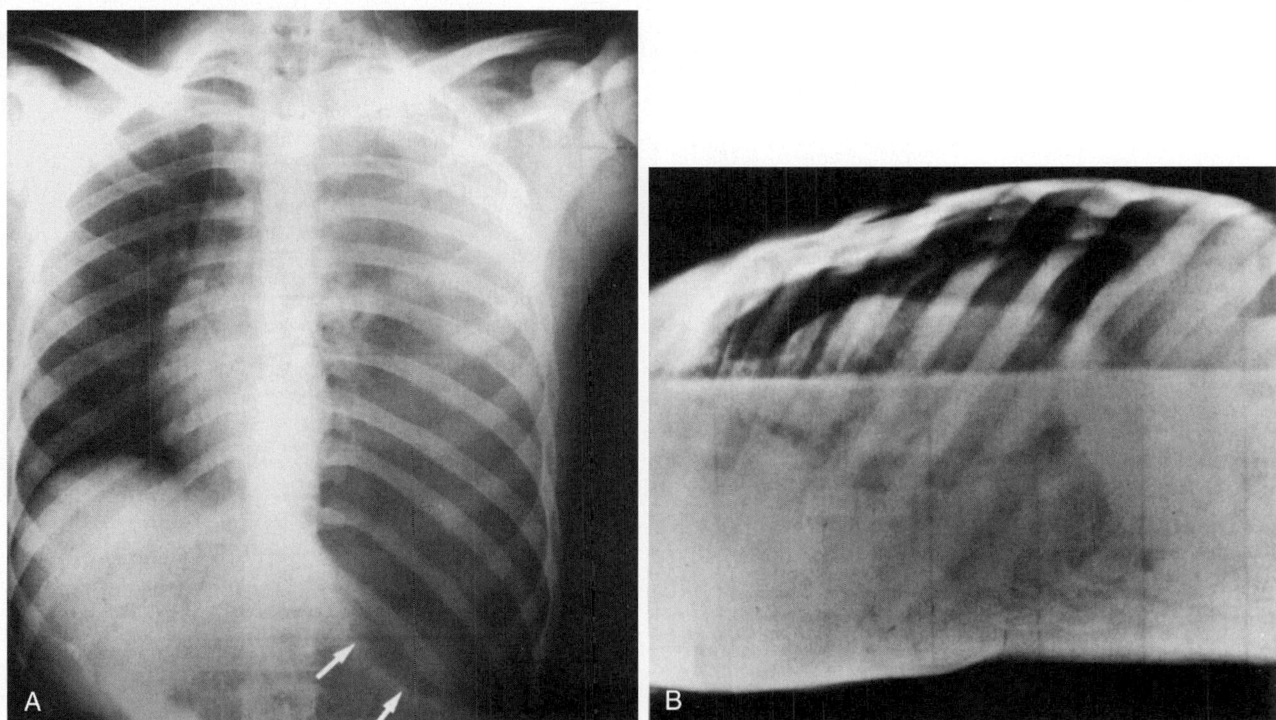

Figure 14–37. Tension hemothorax in a young man resulting from a gunshot wound. *A,* The anteroposterior chest radiograph was obtained with the patient in the supine position. A 22-caliber bullet overlies the spine. The left hemithorax is opacified, but note that the diaphragm is depressed *(arrows)* and that the mediastinal and cardiac silhouettes are shifted to the right hemithorax. *B,* Chest radiograph obtained as a cross-table lateral view shows the presence of a long air-fluid level in the left hemithorax. The large amount of blood in the pleural space opacified the hemithorax in the frontal projection. The tension is manifested by displacement of the mediastinum and diaphragm.

position of the mediastinum and diaphragm in every case of pneumothorax to either identify or exclude possible tension pneumothorax.

Pneumoperitoneum has been described as a complication of pneumothorax.[62, 76, 88] The pneumoperitoneum in such cases is benign and not associated with bowel injury. Presumably, air from the pleural space enters the abdomen by traversing fenestrations or dissecting along vascular sheaths within the diaphragm.

Traumatic pneumothorax is usually treated by insertion of a chest drainage tube. Most lacerations of the lung are sealed by the tube drainage. The lumen of a fractured bronchus cannot be sealed by this method. Failure of a pneumothorax to respond to tube drainage indicates a possible bronchopleural fistula. Progression of the pneumothorax despite drainage is highly suggestive of a ruptured bronchus.

It is possible to confuse a skin fold, bandages, or other extraneous material on the chest wall with pneumothorax. Such structures or objects present as linear radiodensities that may parallel the chest wall and mimic, in some respects, the thin line of radiodensity of the visceral pleural surface as seen in pneumothorax. A skin fold is the usual culprit (Fig. 14–38). On closer inspection the skin fold is seen to be thicker than the usual pleural surface and is not sharply defined medially but tends to fade into the lung. Vessels extend beyond it to the periphery of the intact lung. A fine line of radiolucency is identified at the periphery of the skin fold. This line is a *Mach band.* Although bandages and other material may be thinner than the skin fold, they usually do not parallel the pleural surface, and pulmonary vessels can be identified beyond the apparent pneumothorax.

Pneumomediastinum

Air does not enter the mediastinum from the pleural space; it does so only through the interstitium of the

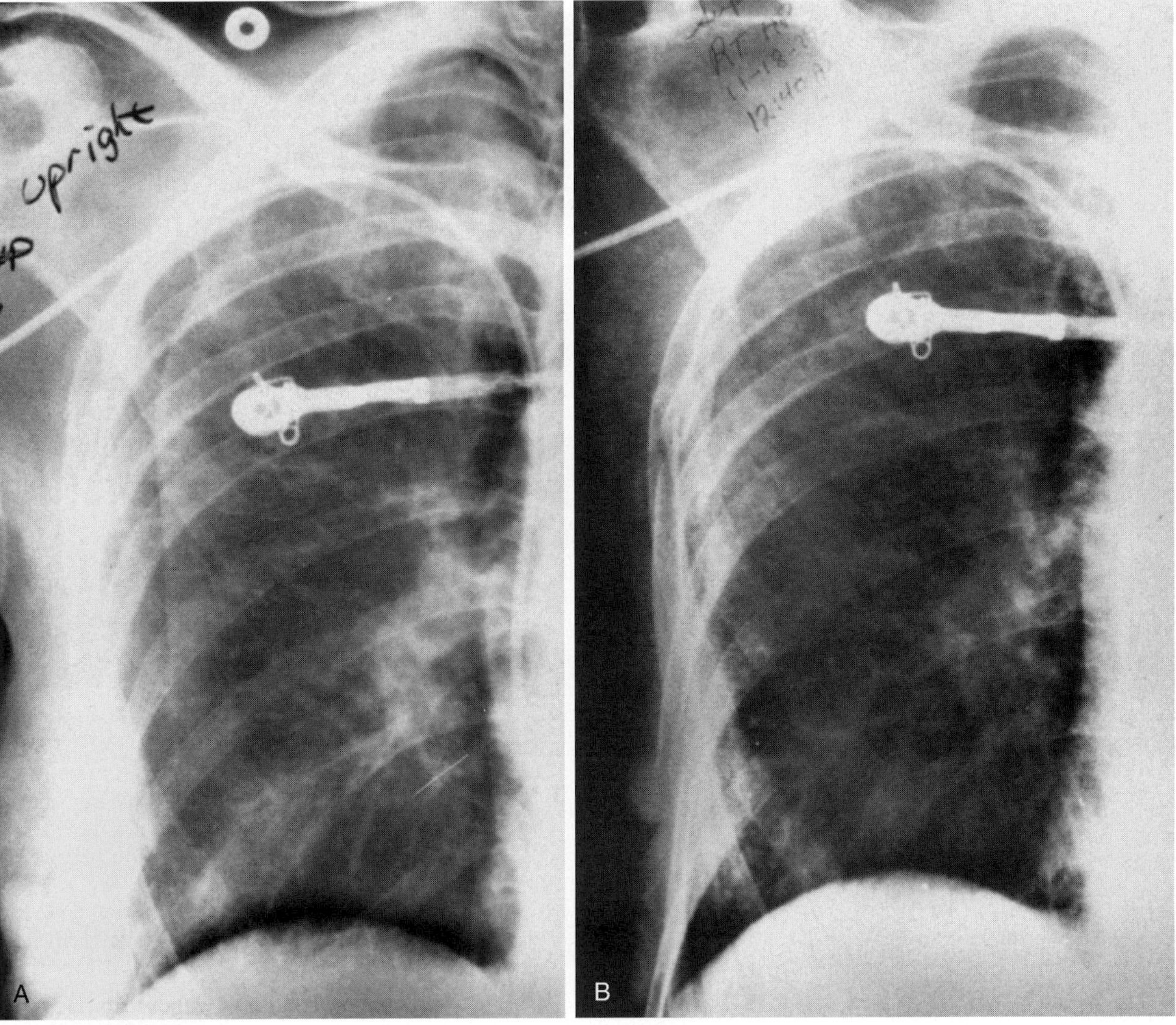

Figure 14–38. Rib fractures with a skin fold simulating pneumothorax in a 70-year-old woman. *A,* A portable chest radiograph shows multiple fractures of the lateral margins of the ribs. There is a density that parallels the rib cage, as is typical of a skin fold. Note the lung markings beyond this linear density. There is a slightly accentuated linear lucency at the outer margin of the density, representing a Mach effect. The density at the margin of the skin fold is broad, as opposed to the sharply defined line of visceral pleura seen in pneumothorax. *B,* Repeat radiograph shows no evidence of pneumothorax. The skin fold is no longer present.

lung.[12] In contrast, air from the mediastinum can enter the pleural space by disrupting the parietal pleural surface of the pleural space. When pneumomediastinum and pneumothorax coexist, it must be presumed that the pneumomediastinum preceded the pneumothorax.[12, 90] Therefore, the source of the radiographic changes is the cause of the pneumomediastinum. In the case of blunt trauma, the association of pneumomediastinum and pneumothorax implies rupture of the trachea, bronchus, or esophagus (see Fig. 14–55).

Trauma to the Pulmonary Parenchyma

The radiographic manifestations of trauma within the lung are variable. They are due to compressive forces created by the chest wall or shearing forces created by unequal displacement of the pulmonary parenchyma. Most injuries of the lung underlie the traumatized chest wall, but on occasion a contrecoup injury occurs in the opposite lung. CT scanning shows four to five times more pulmonary abnormalities than are evident by chest radiography.[15, 16]

Pulmonary Contusion

Pulmonary contusion usually results from blunt trauma to the chest wall. Contusions can also occur around the path of projectiles as well. This entity was first recognized during World War II by Zuckerman,[109] who studied the pulmonary injuries associated with blast injuries. Pathologically, the injury consists of arteriolar and capillary dilatation with exudation of fluid into the interstitial tissues and alveoli. Frank vascular rupture and hemorrhage are noted in more severe injuries, although the overall lung architecture is preserved. Before Zuckerman described the lesion, these findings were variously described as "traumatic pneumonitis" and "concussive pneumonia." There is no inflammatory component; therefore, these two terms are inappropriate.

Contusion is the most common traumatic injury of the lung. Only 75% of patients[101, 107] who sustain pulmonary contusion will have an associated rib fracture. Therefore, contusion usually occurs in the absence of rib fractures, especially in younger patients.[99]

The clinical signs and symptoms associated with a contusion are variable.[94, 99] Some patients with less severe injuries are asymptomatic, whereas others may have cough, hemoptysis, dyspnea, and chest pain. Alveolar hemorrhage and parenchymal destruction are maximal during the first 24 hours after injury and then usually resolve within 7 days. Physical examination frequently reveals decreased breath sounds and rales in the affected area. The patient can be febrile. Respiratory distress is common after lung trauma, with hypoxemia and hypercarbia greatest at about 72 hours. Although management of patients with pulmonary contusion is supportive, pneumonia and acute respiratory distress syndrome with long-term disability occur frequently.[180]

Radiographically, pulmonary contusion (Figs. 14–39 and 14–40; see also Figs. 14–9) is manifested by fluffy, patchy, ill-defined opacities that are not confined to lobar or segmental distribution,[99, 101, 105, 107] typically having a peripheral distribution under the point of chest wall injury.

The CT appearance with pulmonary contusion is similar to that on the chest radiograph, consisting of irregular, coarse nodular opacities that may be discrete or confluent[102] (see Figs. 14–9, 14–10, and 14–12). Again, these opacities are usually peripheral and not necessarily confined to the anatomic limits of pulmonary lobes and segments.

The opacities are frequently present on the initial chest radiograph but always appear within 6 hours of the injury.[99] Therefore, the initial radiographic appearance can be otherwise normal. Of equal importance, lung parenchymal opacities appearing after 6 hours are unlikely to be due to pulmonary contusion and are more likely to represent atelectasis, aspiration, or pneumonia. Parenchymal opacity may increase during the first 48 hours but does not progress after this time. Progression after 48 hours suggests a superimposed infection. Clearing usually begins within 48 to 72 hours, and resolution in uncomplicated pulmonary contusion is usually complete by 6 to 10 days after the injury. Superimposed pneumonia or atelectasis or the acute respiratory distress syndrome[82] is likely if the lesion progresses or fails to clear.

Pulmonary Laceration

Shearing forces within the lung lacerate the pulmonary parenchyma. There is frank disruption of lung tissue, causing a localized internal leak of air (pneumatocele) and blood (hematoma) in variable quantities. As air enters into the laceration, a spherical or elliptic cavity is formed, secondary to inherent lung elasticity, and bleeding occurs from the margins of the laceration.[84, 87] The injury is best described as a pulmonary laceration. These lesions are usually single, at times multilobulated, and on occasion multiple. Pulmonary lacerations are apparent on the initial radiograph as thin-walled cavities (Fig. 14–41), often containing an air-fluid level, usually 2 to 5 cm in diameter (up to 14 cm) (Figs. 14–42 and 14–43). The location of the laceration(s) depends upon the mechanism of injury. Four types of lacerations have been described on the basis of CT findings and mechanism of injury.[105] These types are (1) compression-rupture, the most common, usually located centrally within the pulmonary parenchyma (see Fig. 14–42*A*); (2) compression-shear (see Figs. 14–42 and 14–43); (3) rib penetration (Fig. 14–44), usually small and peripheral; and (4) the rare adhesion tears.

Pulmonary lacerations are present immediately after injury but are often masked by contusions (Fig. 14–45). On subsequent examinations, the wall of the pulmonary laceration is seen to become thicker because of edema formation or hemorrhage around the margin of the lesion. Initially, some lacerations are completely filled with blood, and the air-fluid level does not appear until 2 or 3 days after evacuation of a portion of the blood. The compression-shear type of laceration usually appears inferiorly in

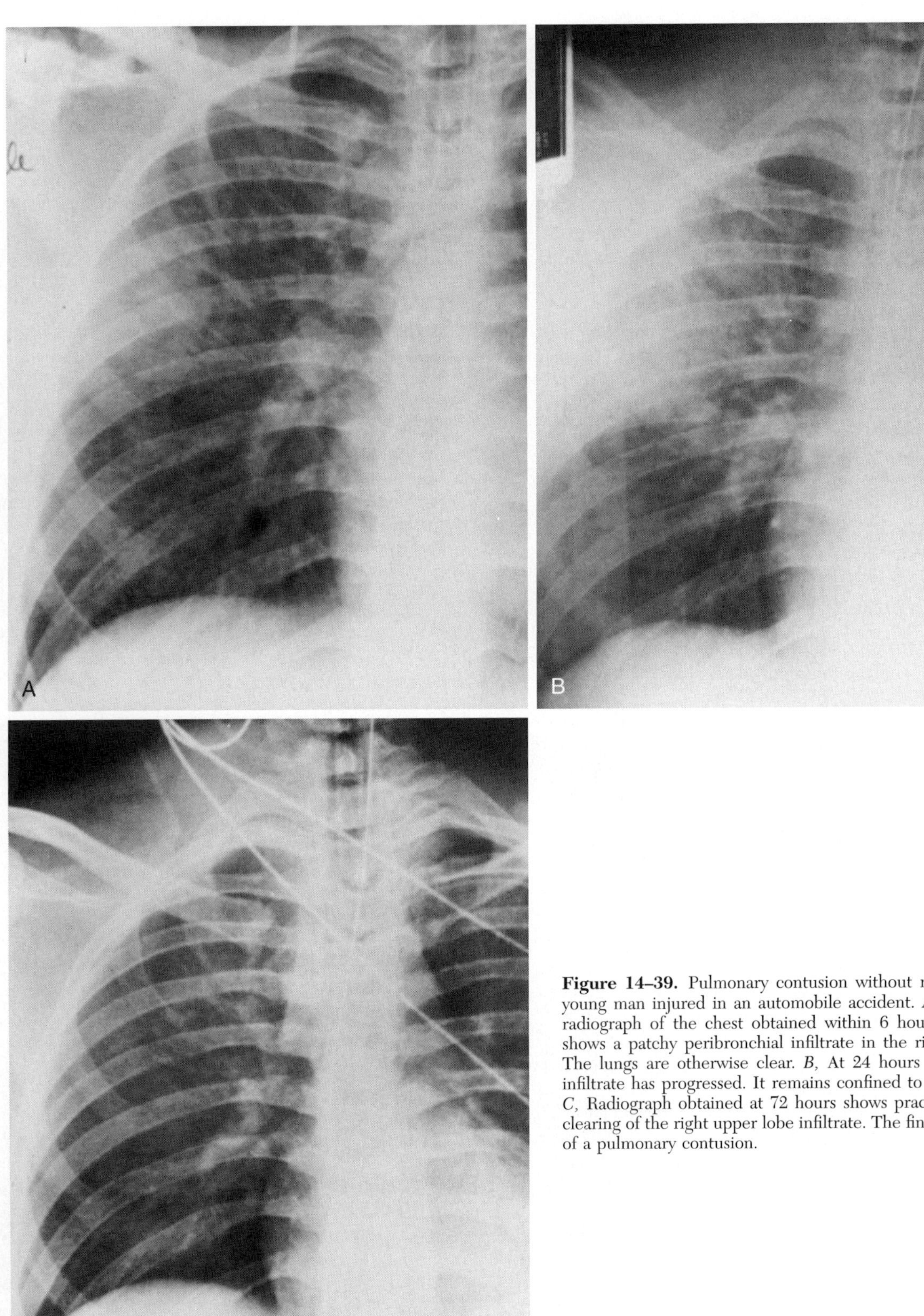

Figure 14–39. Pulmonary contusion without rib fracture in a young man injured in an automobile accident. *A,* Initial supine radiograph of the chest obtained within 6 hours of the injury shows a patchy peribronchial infiltrate in the right upper lobe. The lungs are otherwise clear. *B,* At 24 hours after injury the infiltrate has progressed. It remains confined to the upper lobe. *C,* Radiograph obtained at 72 hours shows practically complete clearing of the right upper lobe infiltrate. The findings are typical of a pulmonary contusion.

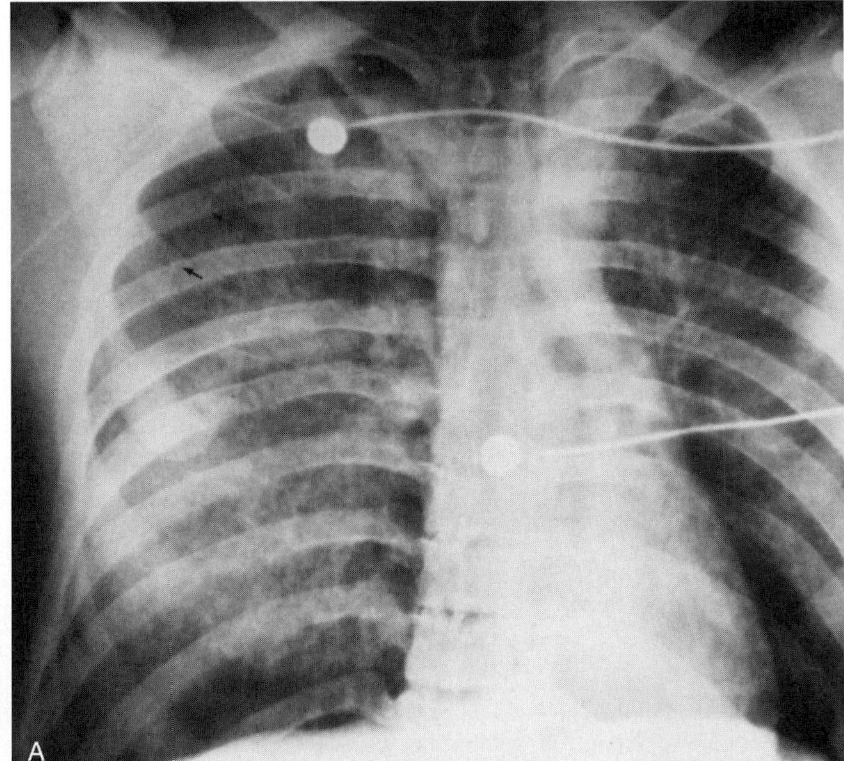

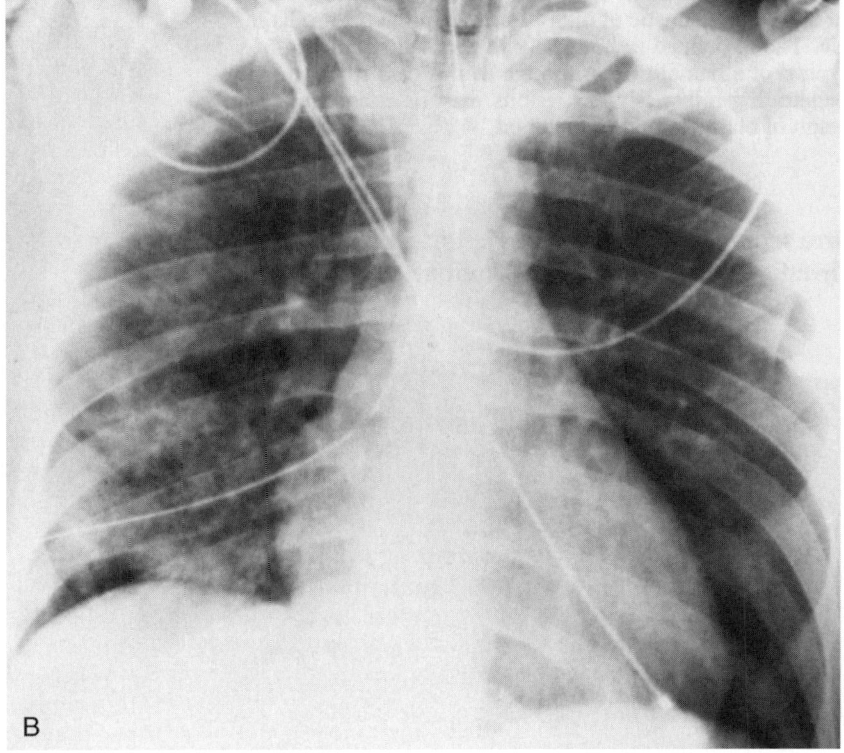

Figure 14–40. Pulmonary contusion with tension pneumothorax without rib fracture in a 24-year-old man. *A,* Initial radiograph shows a patchy infiltrate throughout the right lung. Note that the mediastinum and cardiac silhouette are shifted to the left, and the diaphragm is depressed. Closer inspection shows the presence of pneumothorax *(arrow).* The lung is not collapsed because of loss of compliance associated with the pulmonary contusion. *B,* Repeat radiograph obtained at 72 hours shows the chest drainage tube. Minimal pneumothorax is present in the apex, but there is no evidence of tension. The changes characteristic of pulmonary contusion are evident throughout the right lung. The contusion cleared completely within 7 days.

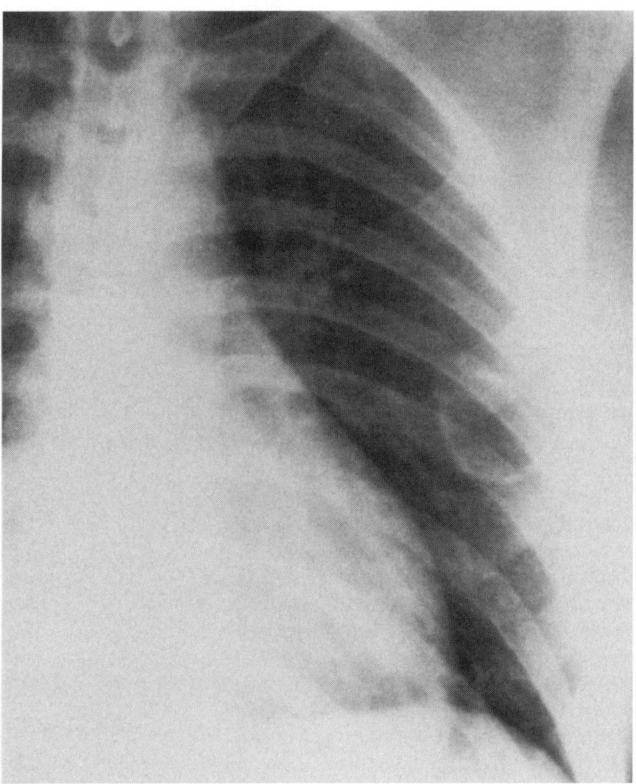

Figure 14–41. Traumatic lung cyst in a 26-year-old patient who sustained blunt chest trauma. A well-circumscribed, thin-walled cavity in the left midlung field is present on the initial chest radiograph. There is no rib fracture; however, there was a bruise on the left in the chest wall. The lesion cleared within 3 weeks without residua.

a paramediastinal location[83, 85, 86, 89, 100] as an elongated cavity extending from the region of the hilus to the diaphragm (see Fig. 14–43). Care should be taken not to confuse a lesion of this type with a loculated posterior medial pneumothorax.[100] An air-filled pulmonary laceration usually disappears in 1 to 3 weeks but occasionally will persist for a longer period. As would be expected, CT scanning shows many more pulmonary lacerations than those detected by chest radiography.[105]

The distinction between a pulmonary hematoma and a traumatic pneumatocele, both of which result from a pulmonary laceration, should not affect the care of the patient. It must be recognized that blunt chest trauma may result in solid or cystic lesions, both of which will resolve in time without medical or surgical intervention. Their true importance lies in the fact that they may be mistaken for some more ominous abnormality unrelated to chest trauma unless this possibility is kept in mind.

Pulmonary Hematoma

Hematoma of the lung is usually produced by a penetrating knife or missile wound and is less commonly associated with blunt trauma to the chest wall.[11, 17, 93] It results from laceration of the lung with hemorrhage into the pulmonary parenchyma. Radiographically, pulmonary hematoma (Fig. 14–46) presents as a smooth, round to ovoid mass of variable size. Initially, the hematoma itself may be obscured by the surrounding patchy infiltrates of pulmonary contusion, but as the contusion clears, a solid, more sharply defined, radiodense area appears. The lesion usually takes one of two courses: it may remain solid, or an air-fluid level may appear within the lesion as a result of partial evacuation of the blood. Rarely, a fibrin ball forms within the lesion and is manifested by a crescent of air on its superior surface—a radiographic appearance similar to that of a fungus ball within a cavity. In any case, the hematoma gradually shrinks and eventually disappears very slowly over several months—hence the lesion has been called a "vanishing lung tumor," which could be mistaken for a more sinister pulmonary abnormality if the treating physician fails to consider this possibility or is not aware of the history of trauma. The shrinking process may take 3 to 6 months or longer. Identification of the decrease in size of the lesion on serial films indicates resolution of the process and should allay any concern that this dense area represents a more serious lesion requiring medical investigation or surgical intervention.

Pulmonary opacification in the immediate and early postinjury period usually results from pulmonary contusion, hemorrhage, atelectasis, or aspiration pneumonia, or from all of the foregoing. Aspiration of blood clots or fractured teeth (see Fig. 12–11) may lead to a combination of pneumonia and atelectasis, with the radiographic changes generally having a lobar or segmental distribution. In the presence of facial fractures, the bronchi should be examined closely to identify fragments of teeth. At times it is impossible to distinguish among pulmonary contusion, hematoma, aspiration pneumonia, and atelectasis. Lung opacification due to contusion, although generally fluffy in appearance and irregular in contour, usually is not confined to a segmental or lobar distribution; however, on occasion, it may demonstrate a more consolidated appearance, with involvement of a lobe or a segment.

Bronchial rupture may lead to atelectasis of the involved portion of the lung, often associated with pneumo-

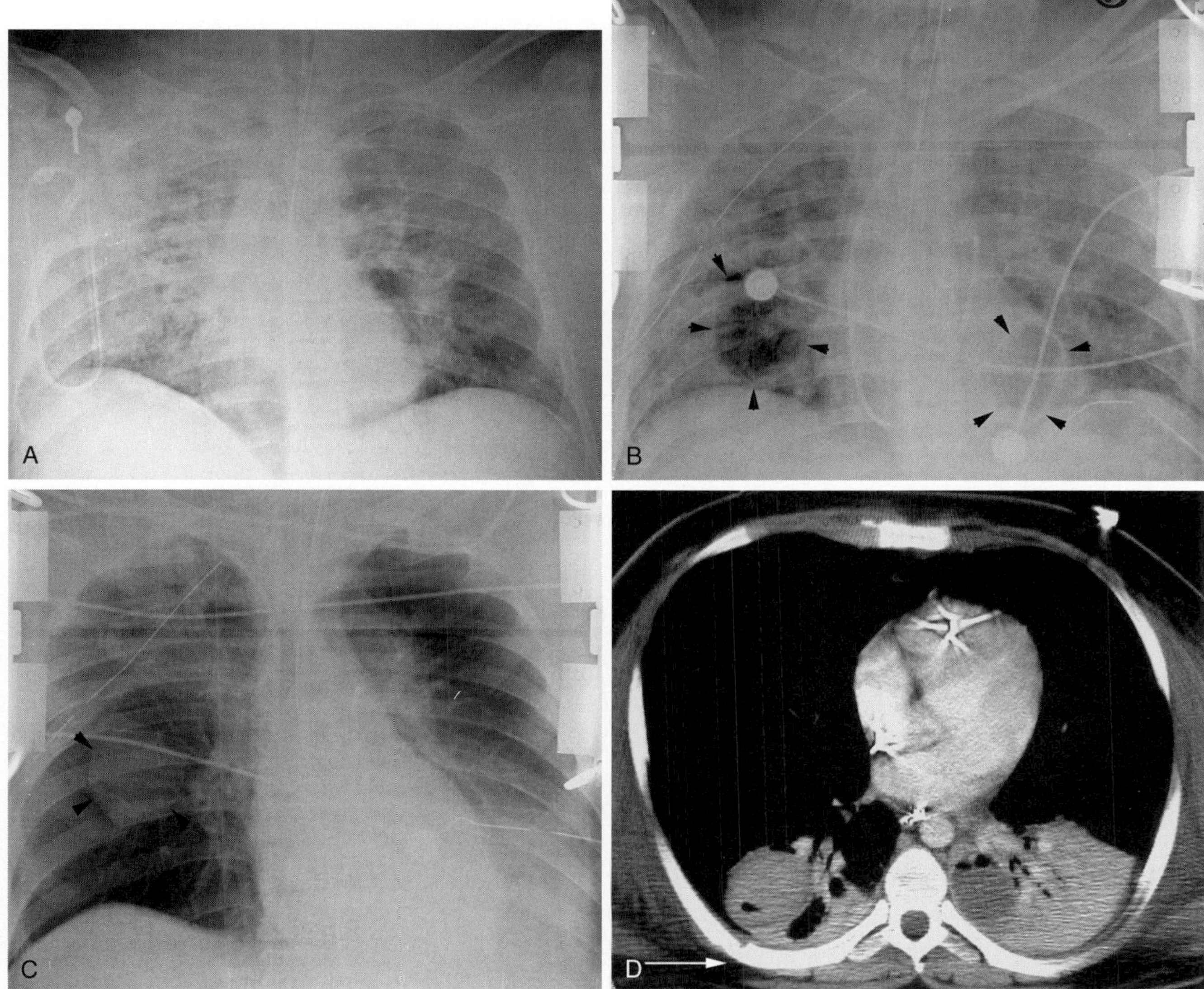

Figure 14–42. Pulmonary lacerations in a 27-year-old man involved in a high-speed motor vehicle crash. *A,* Initial chest radiograph shows nonspecific, diffuse bilateral lung opacification, probably representing a combination of contusion and volume overload. *B,* A subsequent chest radiograph obtained 48 hours after injury shows a 6-cm lucency in the middle right lung typical for a pulmonary laceration and a 5-cm lucency in the left lower lobe, also typical for a pulmonary laceration. These lacerations were not evident on the initial radiograph *(A)*. The patient is intubated. *C,* This radiograph, obtained 14 days after the original injury, shows that the right-sided laceration has now opacified by filling with blood. The underlying lung contusion and pulmonary edema have cleared, and the left lower lobe is collapsed, obscuring the laceration. *D,* CT scan through the lower chest, obtained at the same time as for *C,* again shows the bilateral pulmonary lacerations, both containing mostly blood. The laceration in the right lung is due to a puncture from a rib fracture *(arrow)*. The laceration in the left lung is a typical paravertebral, shearing-type laceration, in this case surrounded by extensive pulmonary hemorrhage and atelectasis that obscured its detection on radiographs.

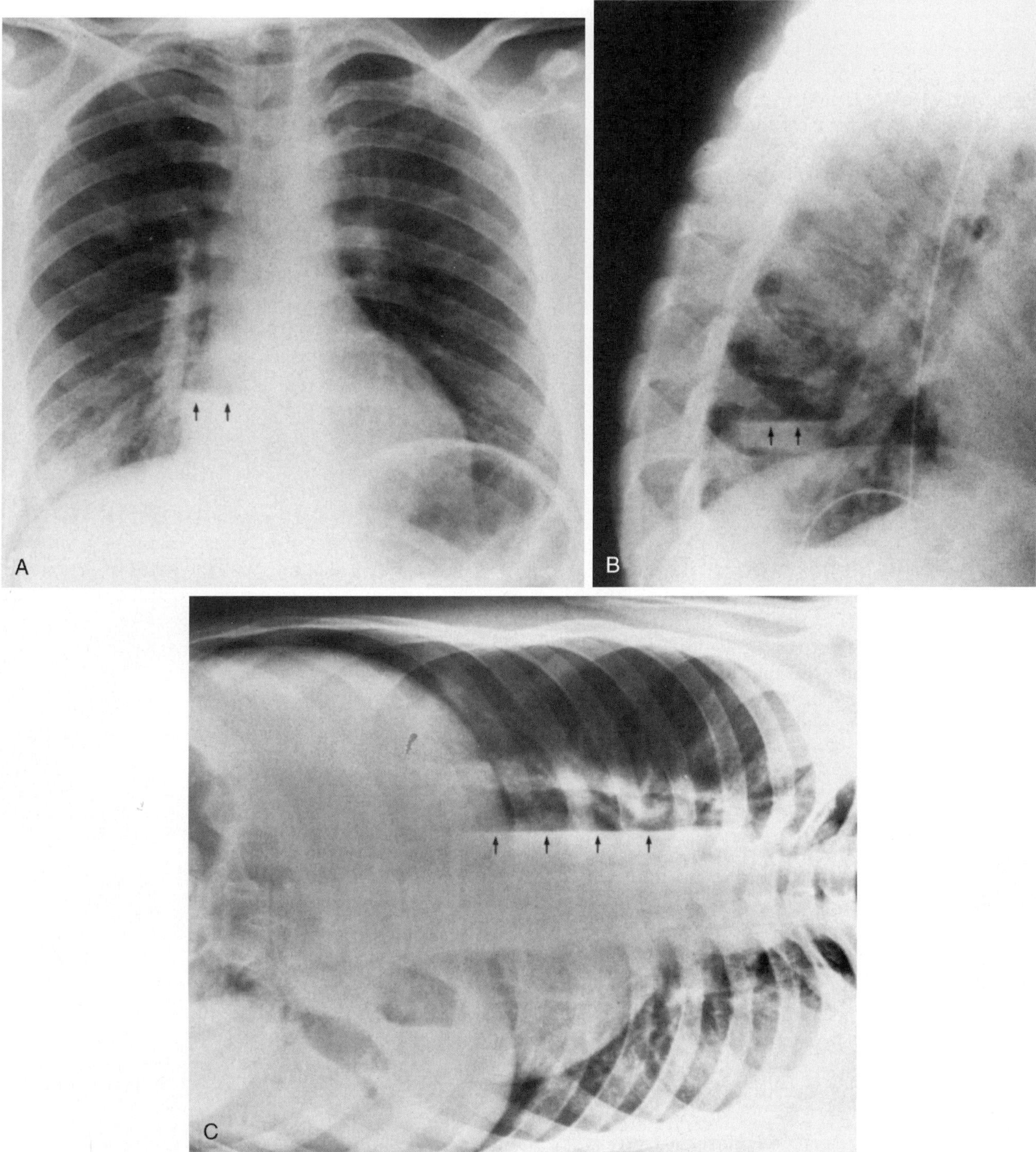

Figure 14–43. Paramediastinal traumatic lung cyst in a 19-year-old man who received blunt trauma to the chest in an automobile accident. *A*, Initial radiograph shows an air-fluid level *(arrows)* at the right base medially. The wall of the cyst is not well defined. An ill-defined infiltrate present laterally represents an area of pulmonary contusion. *B*, Lateral radiograph shows that the air-fluid level lies posteriorly *(arrows)*. *C*, Left lateral decubitus radiograph shows the margins of the cyst with a long air-fluid level *(arrows)*. The findings are typical of a paramediastinal type 2 (shearing-type) pulmonary laceration. The lesion resolved completely within 16 days.

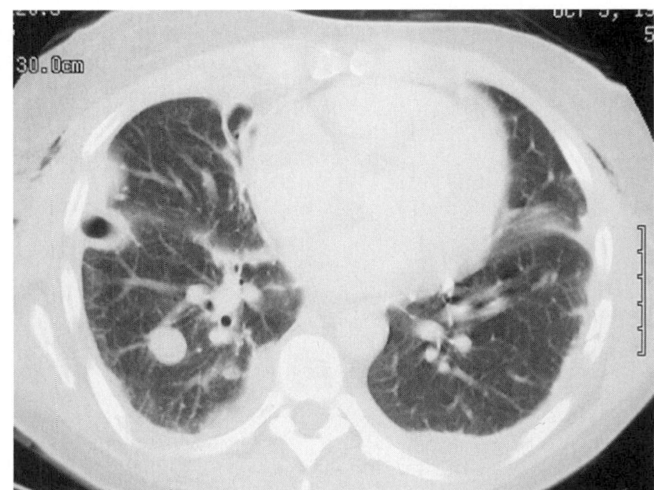

Figure 14–44. Pulmonary lacerations sustained in a high-speed motor vehicle crash. CT through the lower chest shows two pulmonary lacerations in the right lung, one filled with air (a so-called traumatic pneumatocele) and one filled with blood (a so-called pulmonary hematoma).

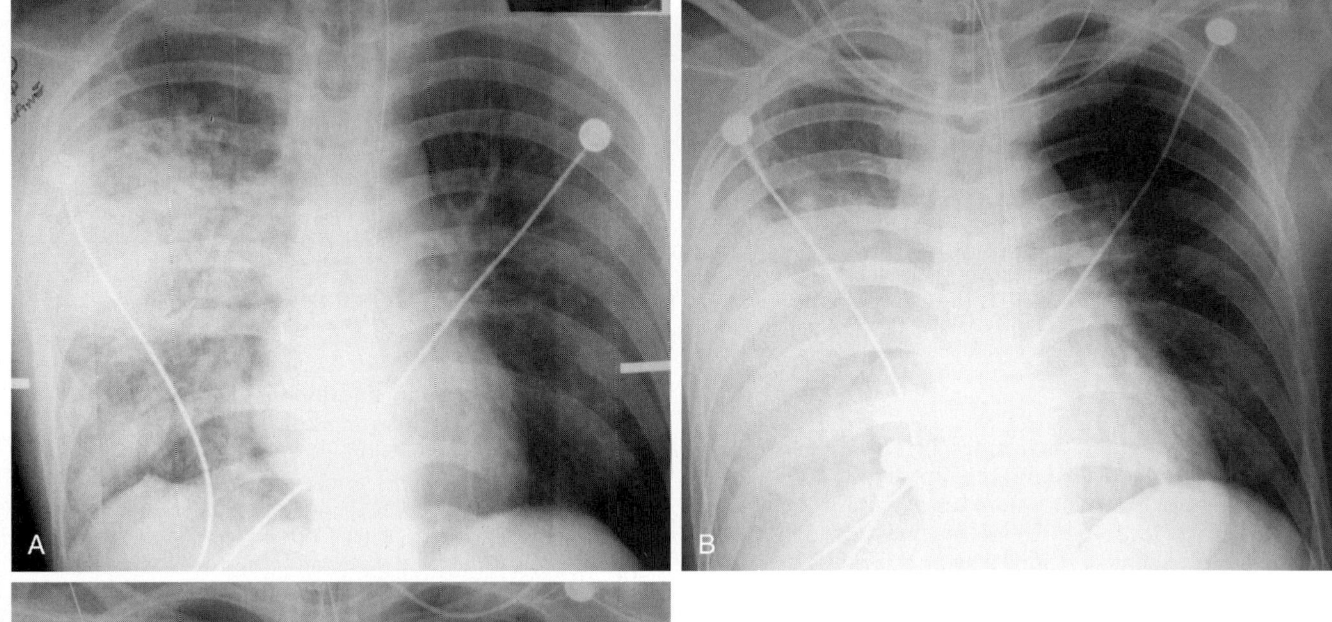

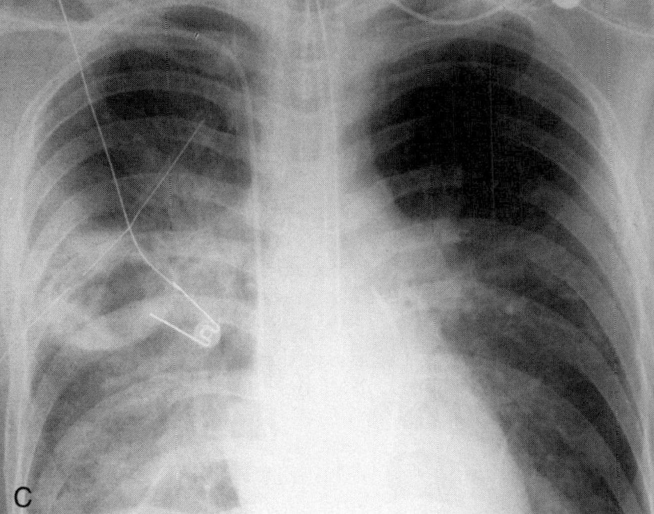

Figure 14–45. Lung contusion and laceration sustained in a high-speed motor vehicle crash. *A,* Initial chest radiograph obtained with the patient supine shows a dense peripheral opacification in the right midlung typical of a pulmonary contusion. No rib fractures were identified. *B,* Repeat examination 48 hours later shows increased opacification of the right lung. The causes of such progressive lung opacification often are multifactorial and include progressive contusion, hemorrhage, atelectasis, and hemothorax. *C,* Four days later, after thoracostomy tube drainage and clearing of contusion, a large pulmonary laceration with both air and fluid is now evident. This is a typical scenario in which the pulmonary laceration is obscured by contusion and hemothorax.

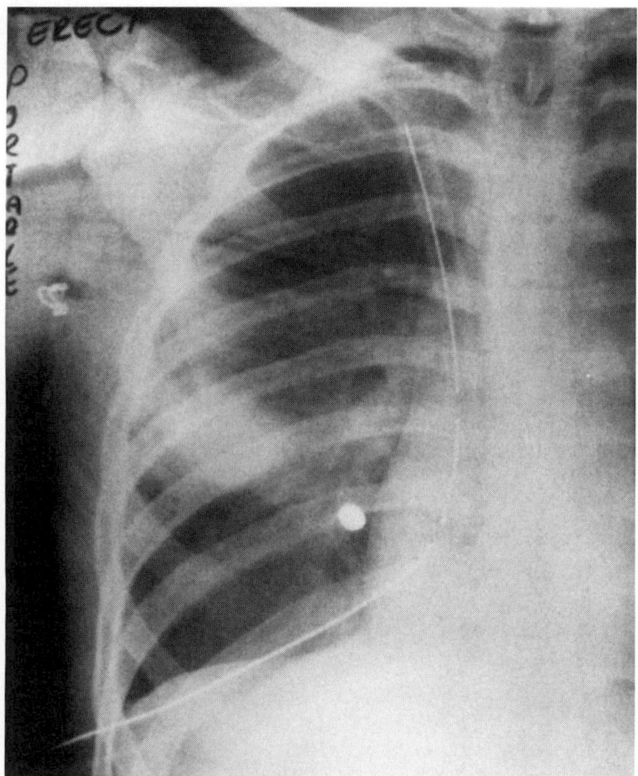

Figure 14–46. Pulmonary hematoma from a gunshot wound. A 22-caliber bullet is present in the right hemithorax. There is a chest drainage tube. Subcutaneous emphysema is present within the chest wall on the right. The alignment of the streaks of air is characteristic of dissection within the pectoralis muscle. The ill-defined radiodensity in the right midlung field is typical of hematoma. Although in this case it was due to a penetrating injury, similar lesions may be encountered as a result of blunt trauma to the chest.

thorax or pneumomediastinum. Certainly, when lobar consolidation is identified in the presence of either of these radiographic findings, bronchial rupture must be very strongly considered. Atelectasis may also be due to improper placement of endotracheal tubes. The optimal position of the distal tip of the endotracheal tube is just proximal to the carina. At times it may be passed beyond the carina, usually into the right main bronchus or even the intermediate bronchus. This placement results in atelectasis involving the left lung or, if the tube extends into the intermediate bronchus, atelectasis of the right upper lobe.

The problems of pulmonary infarction and pulmonary embolism are discussed in Chapter 9 (Complications of Fracture). The characteristic changes in these conditions are not present on the initial radiograph but appear subsequently. The fluffy, ill-defined diffuse small opacities of pulmonary fat embolism appear within 2 to 5 days, with onset generally lagging behind that of the clinical manifestations by 12 to 24 hours, and are associated with petechial hemorrhage and altered mental status when part of the fat embolism syndrome. Pulmonary infarction is a rare later event.

Traumatic Pulmonary Arteriovenous Fistula

Pulmonary arteriovenous fistula is a rare complication of penetrating trauma[77, 81] but as yet is undescribed as a complication of blunt chest trauma. The fistula becomes evident clinically when associated with left-sided heart failure or radiographically as a sharply defined mass in the lung intimately associated with a pulmonary vessel, appearing immediately after a penetrating injury or occasionally after a delay of several years.

Rupture of the Diaphragm

Rupture of the diaphragm is the result of penetrating or crushing injury to the lower area of the chest or epigastrium, or of simultaneous blunt injuries to both regions. In restrained passengers in motor vehicle crashes, a rather specific injury combination has been observed: diaphragmatic rupture, multiple costal fractures, and pelvic or vertebral fracture both above and below the diaphragm.[112] The left hemidiaphragm[116] is more commonly affected than the right. The ratio of left to right varies, ranging from 4:1[130, 139] to 9:1[125] in reported series. In those series in which diagnosis is based principally on abdominal exploration, the proportion of left-sided injuries is lower.[123, 131, 134] This finding suggests the possibility that lesions on the right may be clinically silent because they are tamponaded by the liver.[131]

The tear or rent tends to occur centrally in the dome or fibrous portion of the diaphragm, sparing the esophageal hiatus[118, 129, 136, 141] (Fig. 14–47). On rare occasions the gut is herniated into the pericardium.[96, 135, 137] As many as 50% of diaphragmatic ruptures are missed at the time of the initial evaluation.[111, 120, 122, 123, 125] The diagnosis is then established either during hospitalization or later because of incarceration of the herniated segment of the bowel.[116, 122] Associated injuries of the liver, spleen, and pancreas[117] and fractures of the long bones are the rule and easily direct attention away from and overshadow diaphragmatic injury. In approximately 50% of cases of traumatic rupture of the diaphragm, associated fractures of the lower ribs and pelvis[118, 124, 126, 130] (Fig. 14–48) reflect the crushing nature of the original injury. In view of this association, a chest radiograph should be obtained and examined closely in every case of pelvic fracture to exclude the possibility of an associated traumatic rent of the diaphragm. Compounding the difficulty is the subtle nature of the radiographic features coupled with the nonspecificity of the clinical findings. The diagnosis is frequently overlooked.[2, 122] In practice, it is often the combination of clinical suspicion of rupture of the diaphragm, based on physical examination and mechanism of injury, with compatible radiographic findings that leads to the correct diagnosis.

The cardinal radiographic features[113, 119, 121, 137, 139, 141, 144] that should suggest the possibility of diaphragmatic rupture is apparent elevation of the diaphragm on the initial chest radiograph (Figs. 14–49 through 14–51; see also Fig. 14–48). Pulmonary contusion (see Figs. 14–49 and 14–50), hemothorax,[142] or both are frequently associated. The apparent diaphragmatic elevation is caused by herniation of the abdominal contents through the rent in the diaphragm; the contents become interposed between the diaphragm and the lung. The stomach is most commonly involved and frequently is accompanied by a portion of the omentum.[124, 126, 136, 141] Less commonly, the spleen,

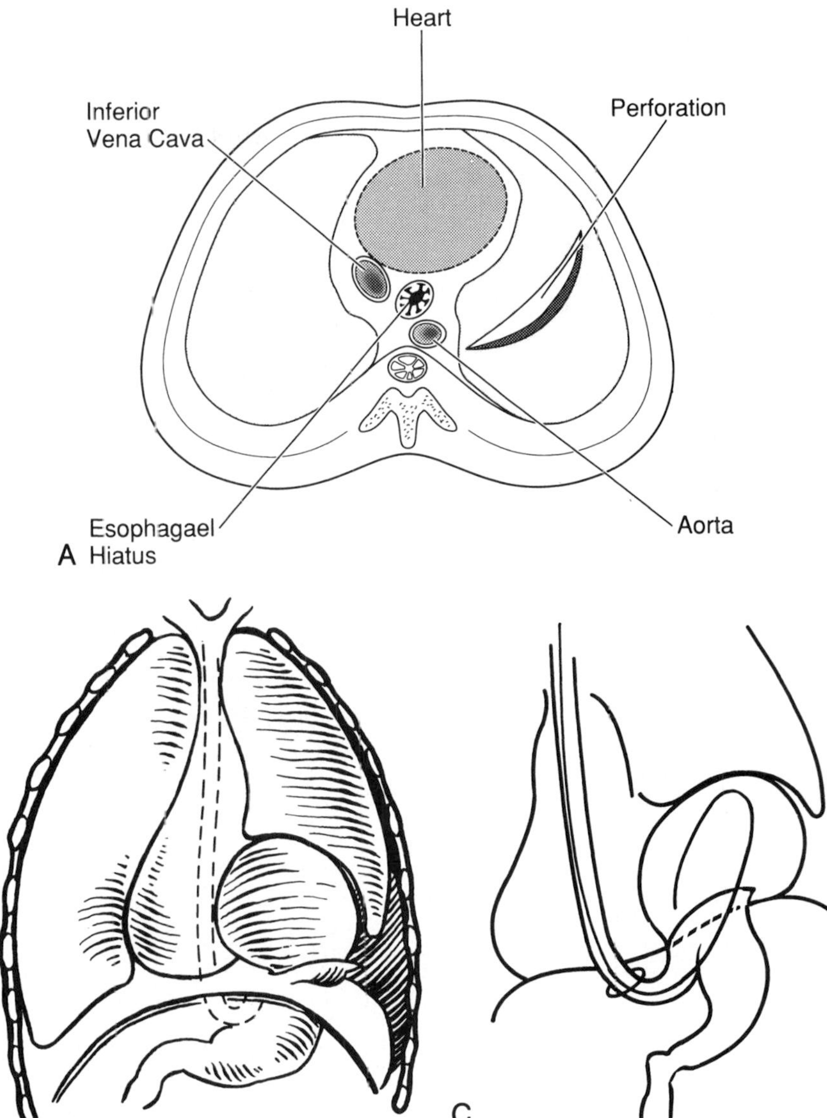

Figure 14–47. Traumatic rupture of the left hemidiaphragm. *A,* Schematic cross section of abdomen at the level of the diaphragm. A diaphragmatic tear usually occurs centrally and spares the esophageal hiatus. *B,* Schematic representation of the intrathoracic stomach protruding through a diaphragmatic rupture. The gastroesophageal junction occupies its normal anatomic position. *C,* Characteristic course of a nasogastric tube into a herniated fundus. (From Perlman, S.J., Rogers, L.F., Mintzer, R.A., & Mueller, C.F. [1984]. Abnormal course of nasogastric tube in traumatic rupture of left hemidiaphragm. A.J.R. Am. J. Roentgenol., *142:*85, with permission.)

colon, or small bowel is herniated, either alone or in combination with the stomach.

When a large rent is present, the stomach, colon, and a good portion of the small bowel may be herniated into the left side of the chest. The hernia is often of sufficient proportion to shift the cardiac and mediastinal contents into the right hemithorax[113, 119, 136, 141] (see Figs. 14–47, 14–48, and 14–50). When the hernia is large, the diagnosis is usually obvious because of the characteristic pattern of air within the herniated stomach and loops of colon and small bowel. However, when the major component of the hernia is the dilated air-containing stomach (see Fig. 14–50), the condition can mimic pneumothorax, aerated lung, or true diaphragm elevation secondary to partial left lung collapse.[118, 136, 141] With smaller herniated segments of bowel, the radiographic changes are very subtle, particularly when a portion of the fundus and body of the stomach rolls through the rent and is superimposed between the base of the lung and the diaphragm.

Often the diagnosis of rupture of the left hemidiaphragm is established after passage of a nasogastric tube[124, 134, 136, 139, 143] (see Figs. 14–47 through 14–50). The tube is seen to pass through the esophageal hiatus, located in its normal position, and then turn upward to coil within the herniated body and fundus of the stomach before returning inferiorly to enter the antrum and duodenal bulb.

On the right, either the liver or the kidney herniates through the diaphragmatic rent[131] (see Fig. 14–51*B*). Because these are solid organs, the diagnosis is much more difficult. Smaller hernias may suggest localized or partial eventration of the diaphragm, and larger, more complete hernias may mimic elevation of the right hemidiaphragm. Radioisotopic liver scans[111, 114, 127, 131, 138] may demonstrate a characteristic feature: elevation of a central portion of the right lobe surrounded by a bandlike, photon-deficient "collar" at the site of constriction of the hemidiaphragms at the site of herniation.

CT can also provide a specific diagnosis of diaphragmatic rupture.[125, 133] CT findings consistent with diaphragmatic injury include waistlike constriction of abdominal viscera, forming the "collar sign"; intrathoracic herniation of abdominal contents; and diaphragmatic discontinuity. CT findings are more evident on the left than on the

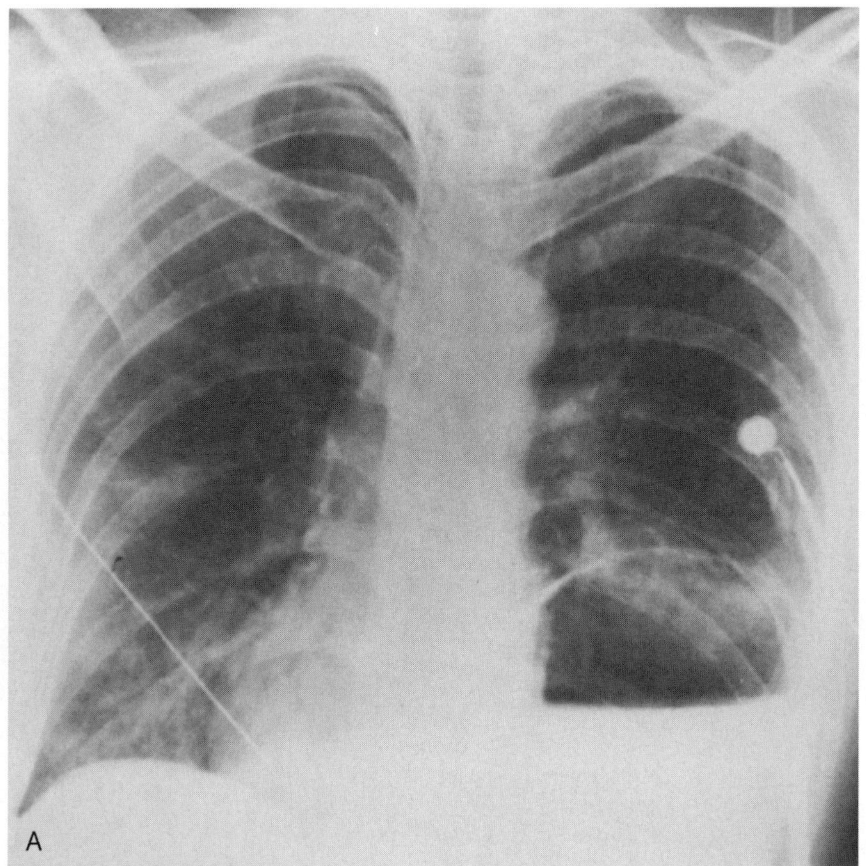

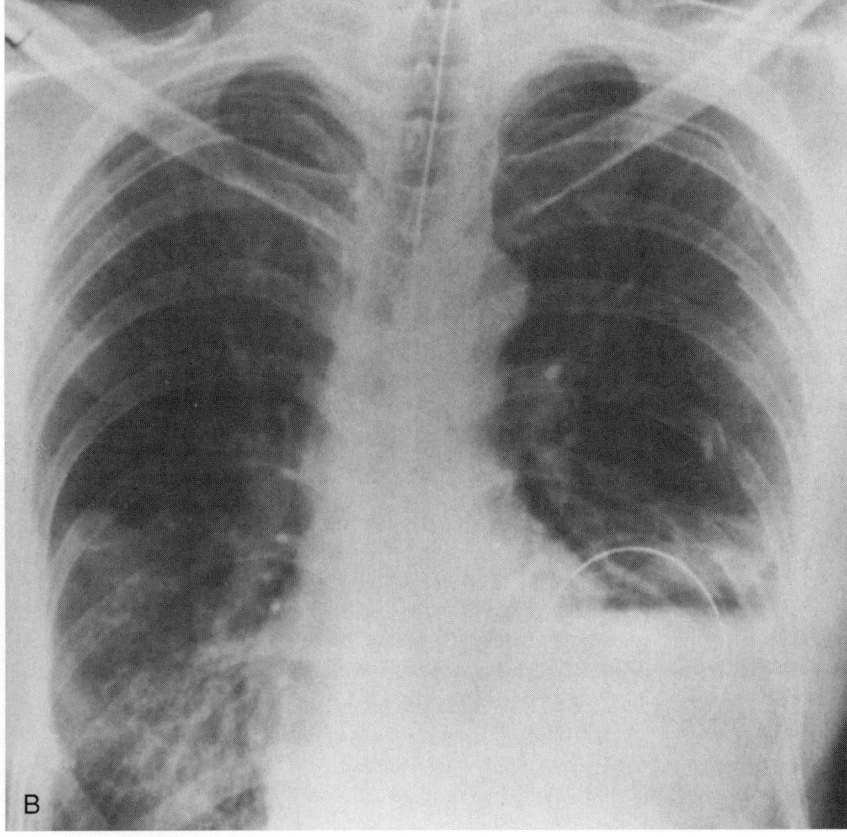

Figure 14–48. Traumatic rupture of the left hemidiaphragm associated with a pelvic fracture in a 38-year-old man involved in an automobile accident. *A,* Initial chest radiograph shows apparent elevation of the left hemidiaphragm. The long air-fluid level crossing the entire left hemithorax suggests that this is in fact the gastric fundus. The cardiac and mediastinal silhouettes are displaced into the right hemithorax. There are fractures of the posterior lateral margins of the fourth through the eighth left ribs. Hazy opacification of the right lower lung field is consistent with pulmonary contusion. *B,* Repeat examination after placement of a nasogastric tube shows that the tube is coiled within the gastric fundus in a position well above the diaphragm. The esophageal hiatus remains in a more inferior position. The course of the nasogastric tube definitely identifies the presence of traumatic rupture of the left hemidiaphragm, with displacement of the gastric fundus into the left hemithorax.

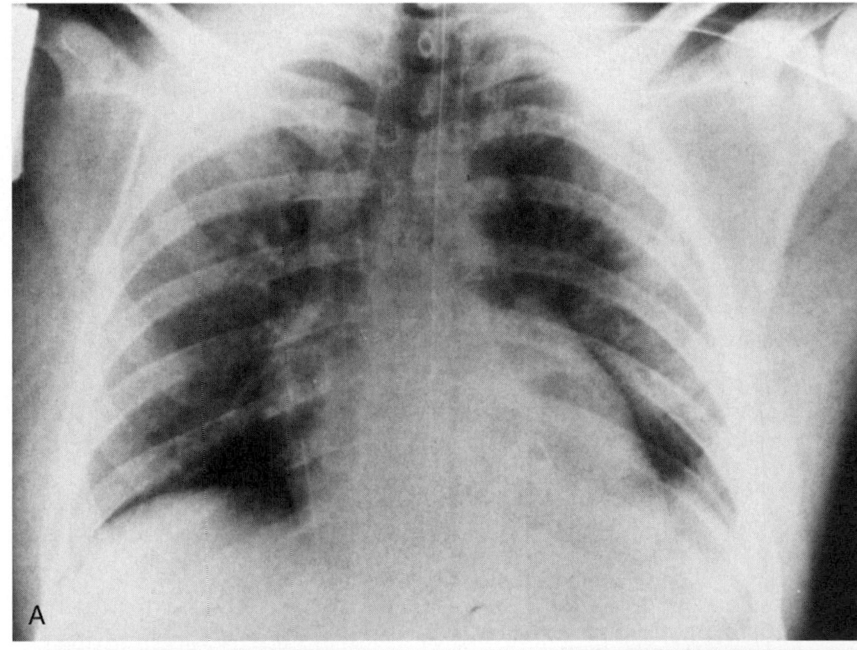

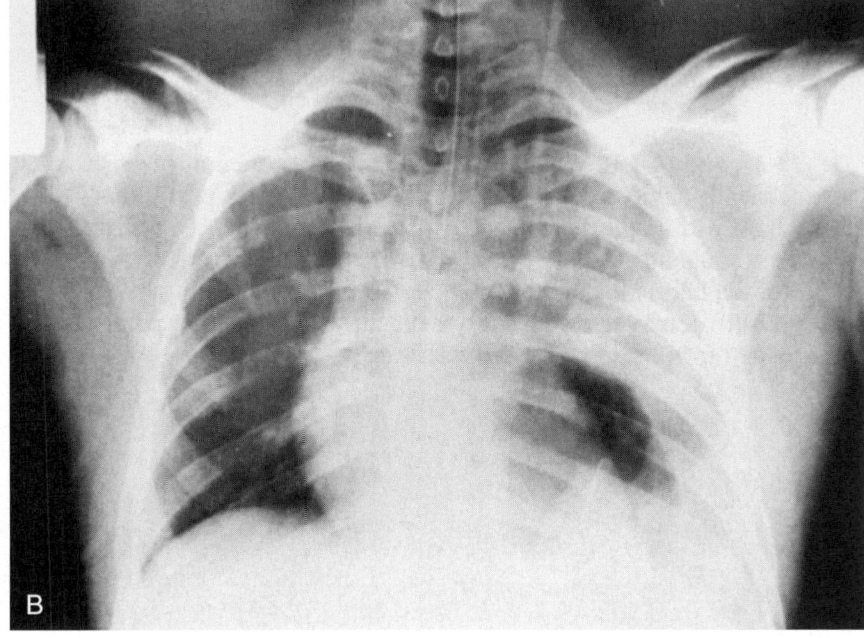

Figure 14–49. Traumatic rupture of the left hemidiaphragm. *A,* Initial radiograph obtained following passage of a nasogastric tube. The course of the tube strongly suggests the possibility of rupture of the left hemidiaphragm. Note that the diaphragm is poorly defined. There are no identifiable rib fractures. A hazy opacification of the left lung suggests pulmonary contusion. *B,* Another radiograph obtained 1 hour later, after injection of 50 mL of air into the nasogastric tube, clearly shows the displaced gastric fundus, establishing the diagnosis of traumatic rupture of the diaphragm. Note that in the 1-hour interval there has been an increase in opacification of the left lung, indicating progression of the pulmonary contusion.

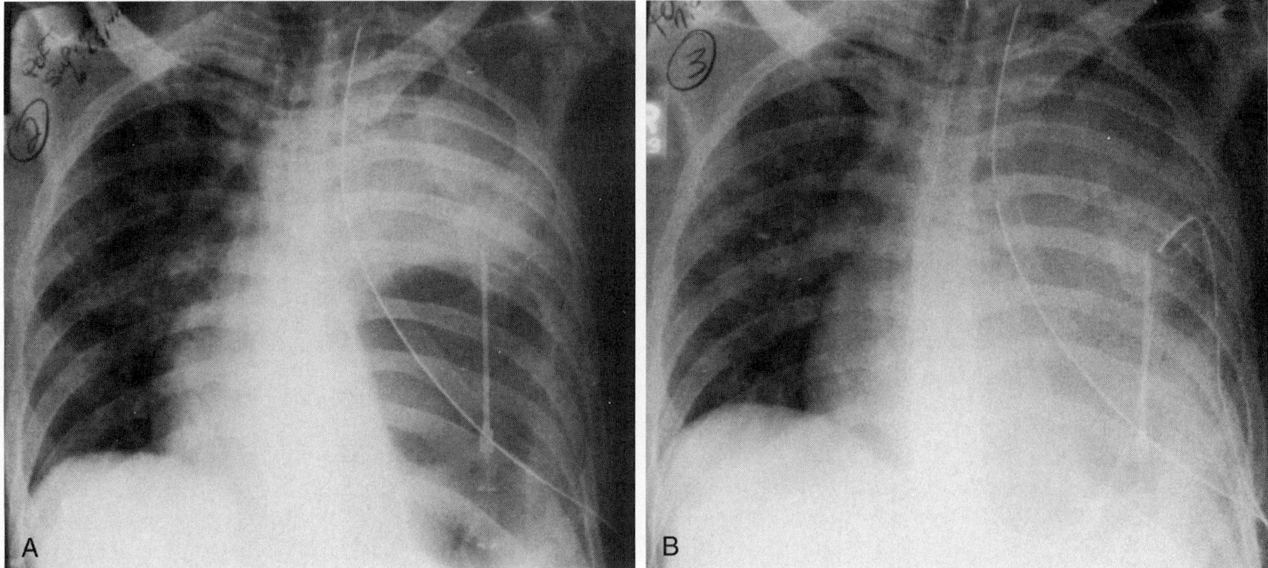

Figure 14–50. Traumatic rupture of the left hemidiaphragm. *A,* Examination of the chest with the patient supine shows the presence of a chest drainage tube and a central venous pressure catheter assembly overlying the left hemithorax. A pocket of gas filled the left inferior portion of the left hemithorax. The upper portion of the left side of the chest is opacified. The cardiac and mediastinal silhouettes are shifted into the right hemithorax. The right lung shows evidence of pulmonary contusion. There are no rib fractures. The chest drainage tube was placed before the initial radiographic examination. *B,* This examination was performed after the placement of a second chest drainage tube and a nasogastric tube. Note the course of the nasogastric tube, which is typical of traumatic rupture of the diaphragm with displacement of the stomach into the left hemithorax. On the initial radiograph, the pocket of gas has a configuration typical of the stomach. The stomach was evacuated after placement of the nasogastric tube; therefore, this gas is not evident on the second examination.

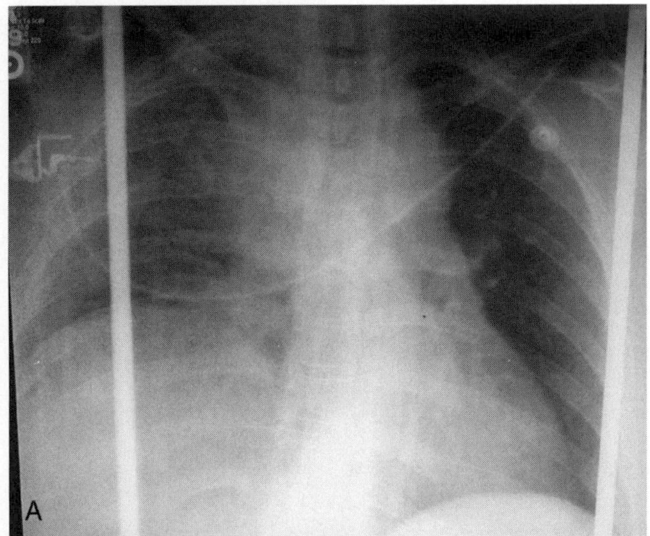

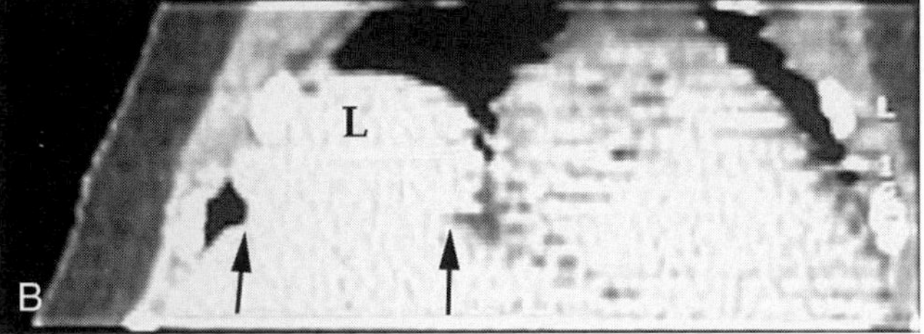

Figure 14–51. Traumatic rupture of the right hemidiaphragm. *A,* Often the only evidence of a rupture of the right hemidiaphragm is its apparent elevation. Other signs of right-sided torso injury such as lower right rib fractures are frequently present, although not in this case. In practice, it is often the combination of clinical suspicion of rupture of the diaphragm, based on physical examination and mechanism of injury, with compatible radiographic findings that leads to the diagnosis. *B,* Oblique sagittal reformated CT image obtained in a different patient with a rupture of the right hemidiaphragm shows the liver (L) protruding through the defect in the diaphragm *(arrows).* (From Stern, E.J. & White, C.S. [1999]. Chest Radiology Companion. Lippincott Williams & Wilkins, Philadelphia.)

right. Helical CT, especially with the aid of reformatted images (see Fig. 14–51*B*), is useful in the diagnosis of acute diaphragmatic rupture after blunt trauma, with detection rates of 78% of left-sided injuries and 50% of right-sided injuries.[132]

In rare cases, the diaphragmatic tear extends centrally to within the pericardium.[110, 137] The diagnosis is established by noting the herniation of bowel into the pericardium. The diaphragmatic tear can be limited to that segment beneath the heart, and the herniation of bowel is limited to the pericardium.

It is possible for a rupture to occur without immediate passage of abdominal contents through the rent.[120, 122, 125, 126, 129, 140] The appearance on the initial chest radiograph may be normal or at least may reveal no evidence of bowel within the chest despite laceration of the diaphragm. The absence of herniation may be more common in patients receiving mechanical ventilation with positive-pressure support. The rupture is present, but herniation is delayed until extubation, and the diagnostic features appear at subsequent examination of the chest.

If the diagnosis is not established initially, the patient may present later with partial obstruction or incarceration of the stomach or colon.[116] The herniated gut is obstructed, or at least restricted, at the point where it passes through the rent in the diaphragm. Either the proximal or the distal limb of the herniated bowel may be obstructed. Diagnosis is established by CT scanning or barium enema or barium swallow study.

Rupture of the Trachea and Major Bronchi

Rupture of the trachea and major bronchi is infrequent but is one of the most serious injuries due to crushing blows to the chest. The mortality rate is 30%,[150] diagnosis is often difficult to establish,[2, 17] and the morbidity associated with delays in diagnosis is appreciable.[17, 151, 156]

Injuries to the trachea (Fig. 14–52) usually occur in cervical segments outside the thorax (Fig. 14–53) and involve principally the cricoid and first two tracheal rings.[125] These injuries are discussed in Chapter 12.

Most bronchial fractures are within 2.5 cm of the carina.[148, 149, 155] Approximately 85% of bronchial injuries occur at the tracheal junction or within the main bronchi.[152, 159] Bilateral rupture of the main bronchi is found in 2%, and the remainder of these injuries are equally distributed between the upper lobe and lower lobe bronchi on each side. Overall, bronchial fracture occurs with approximately equal frequency on both sides.

The fractures (see Fig. 14–52) are usually transverse,[159] between the cartilaginous rings, and may be complete or incomplete. Occasionally the tears are longitudinal, involving the membranous posterior portion of the bronchus.[158, 159] Less commonly, a transverse fracture occurs that leaves the adventitial tissues about the trachea and bronchi intact. The mechanism of injury is presumed to be a shearing force that tears through the wall of the bronchus between the cartilaginous rings. This may be combined with increased intratracheal pressure created

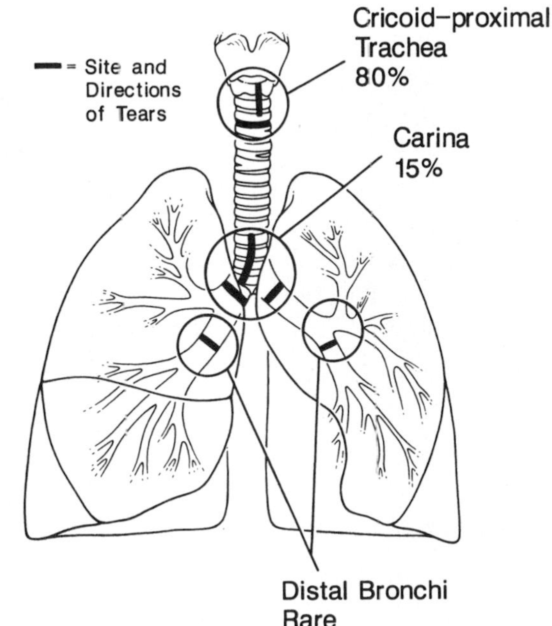

Figure 14–52. Locations of ruptures of the trachea and major bronchi.

by the simultaneous occurrence of a closed glottis and a crushing blow to the chest.

The classic signs and symptoms of bronchial injury[147, 149, 158] are cyanosis, dyspnea, hemoptysis, and subcutaneous emphysema. The classic radiographic triad consists of subcutaneous emphysema, with persistent or progressive pneumothorax, and pneumomediastinum (Figs. 14–54 and 14–55; see also Fig. 14–53). When these signs are present, the possibility of bronchial injury should be kept uppermost in mind; the diagnosis is readily established, and surgical repair is then performed. The classic signs and symptoms often are not present, however, and the diagnosis can be overlooked. About 10% of patients will have no radiographic or physical evidence of intrathoracic injury.[109, 148] As these bronchial tears heal, a stenotic cicatrix forms, which in a period of months or weeks leads to atelectasis of the affected lung, often associated with pneumonia and significant functional impairment.[156] Thus, even after surgical repair has been accomplished, some residual impairment can be anticipated.

Because they occur so frequently, subcutaneous emphysema and pneumothorax are not specific for large airway rupture. Of those patients with bronchial rupture, 50% are noted to have subcutaneous emphysema, particularly deep cervical emphysema,[153] and only 66%[145, 155, 160] have pneumothorax. Persistent pneumothorax despite thoracostomy tube drainage indicates a major airway leak and is highly suggestive of rupture of a bronchus.[147, 155] When the bronchus is completely transected, the lung may fall away from the mediastinum to the most dependent portion of the thorax.[157] On radiographs obtained with the patient in the upright position, the collapsed lung then appears as a soft tissue mass lying on the diaphragm well below the hilus—the so-called fallen lung sign.

Pneumomediastinum (see Figs. 14–53 through 14–55) has been identified in slightly less than half of all cases[160]

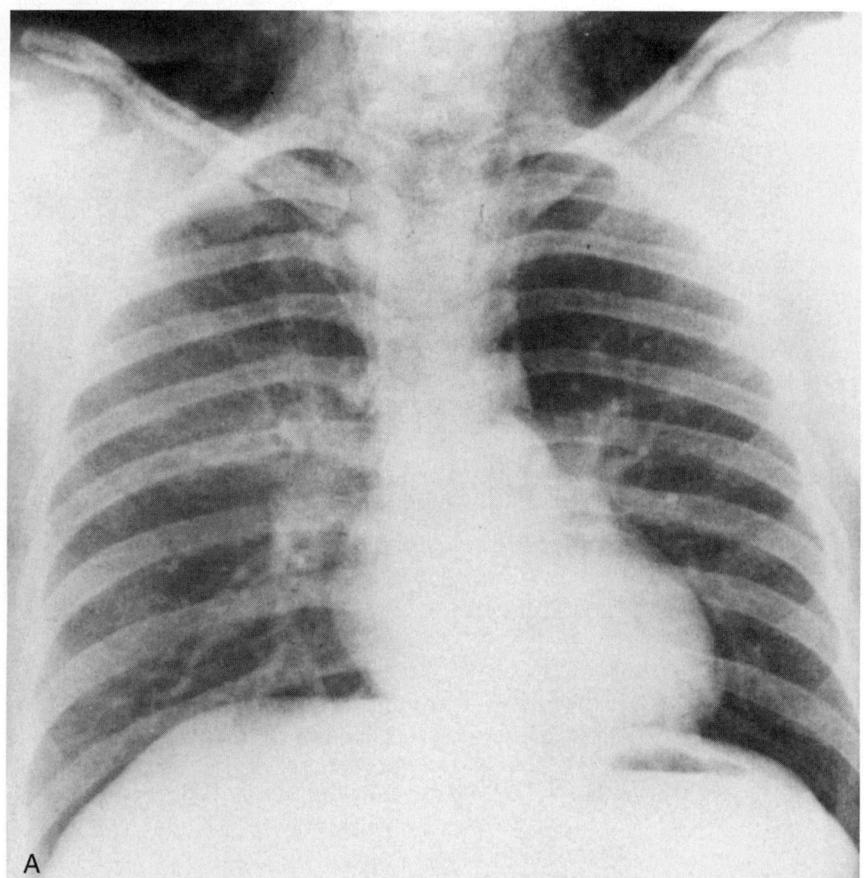

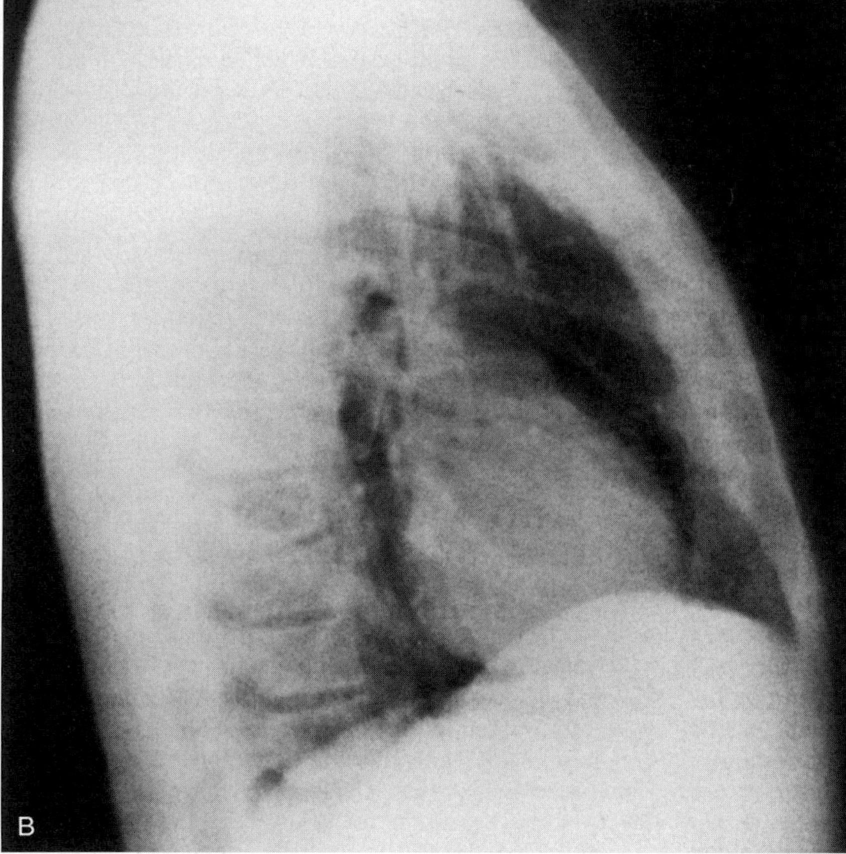

Figure 14–53. Rupture of the infracricoid portion of the trachea and posterior wall of the esophagus. *A*, Initial radiograph shows emphysema within the deep cervical soft tissues. Streaky radiolucencies present within the upper mediastinum and along the left cardiac border are indicative of pneumomediastinum. *B*, Lateral radiograph of the chest clearly shows the presence of air within the anterior mediastinum. Pneumomediastinum is usually more easily identified on the lateral radiograph. At operation there was a transverse laceration of the infracricoid portion of the trachea associated with a laceration of the posterior wall of the esophagus at the same level.

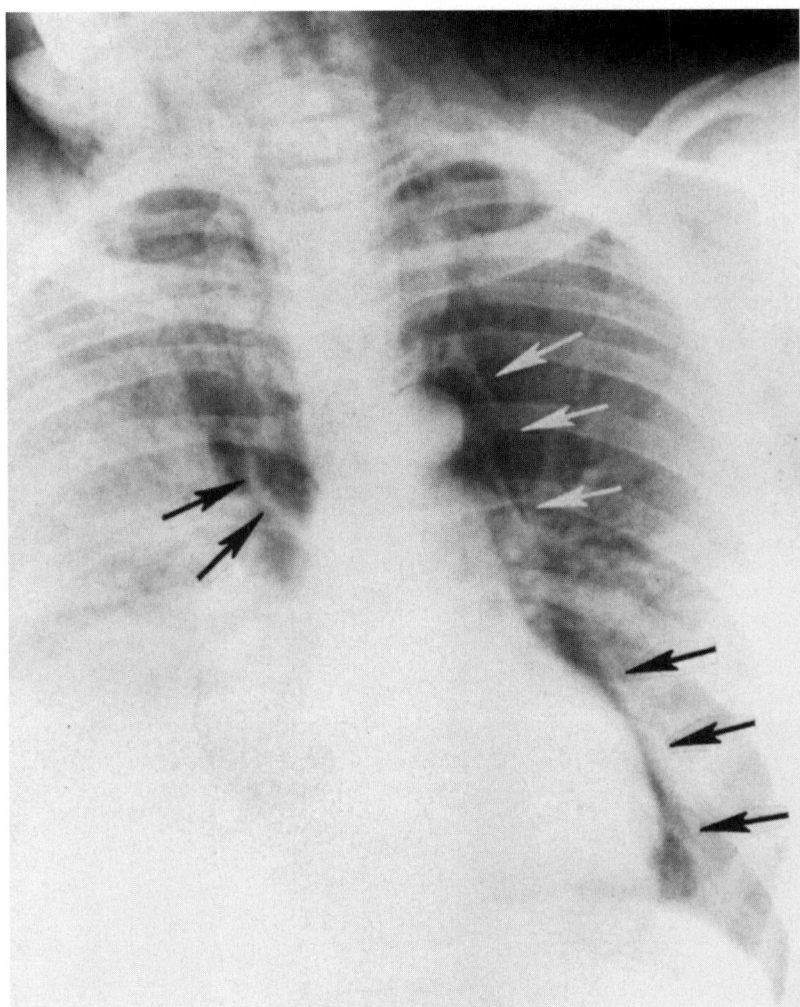

Figure 14–54. Transverse rupture of both main bronchi *(arrows)* in a 27-year-old man who sustained blunt trauma to the chest. Air is present within the fascial planes of the neck and within the mediastinum. (From Reynolds, J., & Davis, J.T. [1966]. Injuries of the chest wall, pleura, pericardium, lungs, bronchi and esophagus. Radiol. Clin. North Am., *4*:383, with permission.)

of airway rupture and rarely can occur as a result of remote injuries outside the thorax.[154] The air is seen as fine streaks overlying the hilus and along the aorta and extending into the upper mediastinum and the soft tissues of the neck.[153] It is more easily seen on the lateral view within the anterior mediastinum and about the base of the aorta (see Fig. 14–53*B*). CT is the most sensitive means of demonstrating air within the mediastinum (see Fig. 14–55).

The most specific indication of injury to the bronchus is fracture of the upper ribs. Burke[149] found that 91% of patients who had sustained bronchial rupture also had fractures of the first, second, or third rib, alone or in combination. He did not encounter rupture of the major bronchus without a fracture of an upper rib in a patient older than 30 years of age. Such fractures are less commonly associated with bronchial rupture in patients younger than 30 years.[56] Most authorities are in general agreement with Burke with regard to these findings. Although bronchial rupture sometimes occurs without associated fracture of the upper ribs in persons older than 30, these cases are by far a minority. Therefore, whenever fracture of an upper rib is identified in a patient older than 30, the diagnosis of bronchial rupture must receive serious consideration. The rupture is usually on the same side as that of the fracture. There are often five or more rib fractures contiguous with those of the upper rib. The suggestive signs of pneumomediastinum, pneumothorax, and subcutaneous emphysema should be sought whenever an upper rib fracture is identified.

Rupture of the Esophagus

Esophageal perforation from external blunt trauma is rare.[146] Together the cervical and the upper thoracic regions of the esophagus constitute the site of injury in greater than 80% of cases, and the remainder of the cases are evenly divided between the midesophagus and lower esophagus (Fig. 14–56). Delay in diagnosis is frequent and attendant with infectious complications. The perforations are longitudinal, and those of the upper esophagus are frequently associated with concomitant injuries of the larynx and upper trachea (see Fig. 14–53). Tracheoesophageal fistulas are infrequent. Pneumomediastinum and subcutaneous emphysema do not occur in every case.[146] In order to minimize delay in diagnosis, esophageal perforation should be considered as a possibility in every severe steering wheel injury of the chest, and the diagnostic evaluation directed accordingly.

Rupture of the lower esophagus is usually the result of vomiting, as in Boerhaave's syndrome, and has been

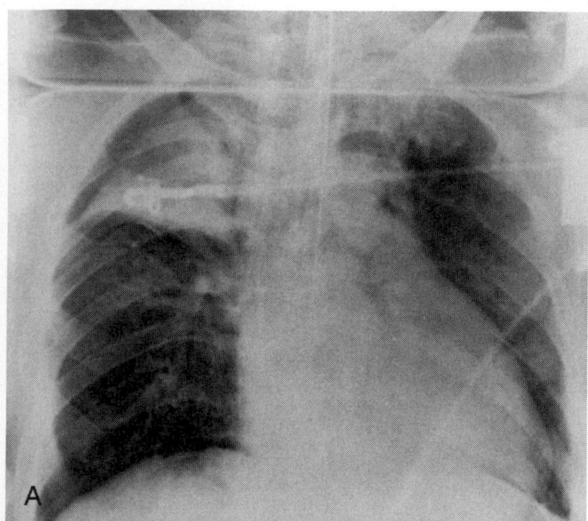

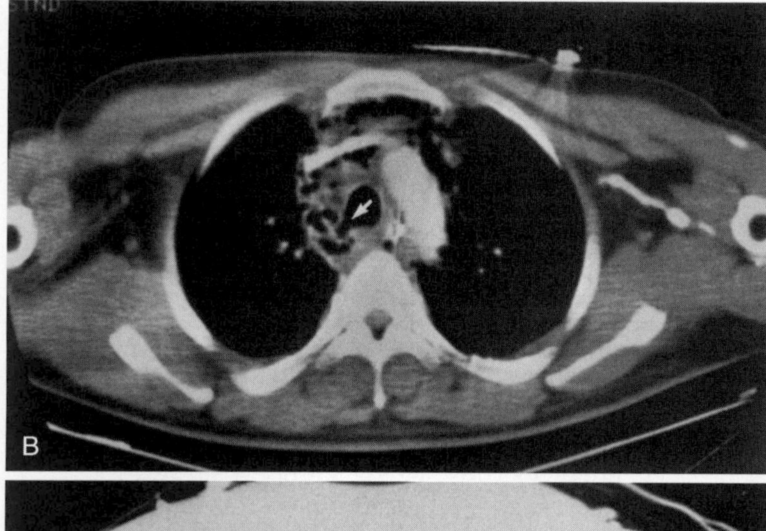

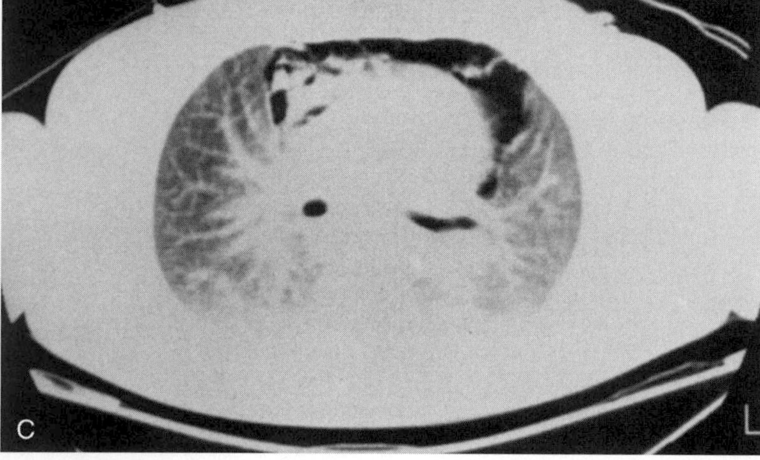

Figure 14–55. Rupture of the trachea in a 27-year-old man injured in an automobile accident. *A,* Pneumothorax is present on the right, with collapse of the right upper lobe as identified by opacification above the minor fissure. There are no definite streaks or bubbles of air to suggest pneumomediastinum. Opacification of the left lung is evident, representing areas of pulmonary contusion. *B,* CT clearly shows the bubbles of air within the mediastinum anterior and lateral to the aorta and about the right lateral margin of the trachea. Note the laceration of the posterior right lateral margin of the trachea *(arrow).* Lacerations of the trachea at this level are unusual. *C,* Lung window setting shows air anterior and lateral to the heart, indicating pneumomediastinum.

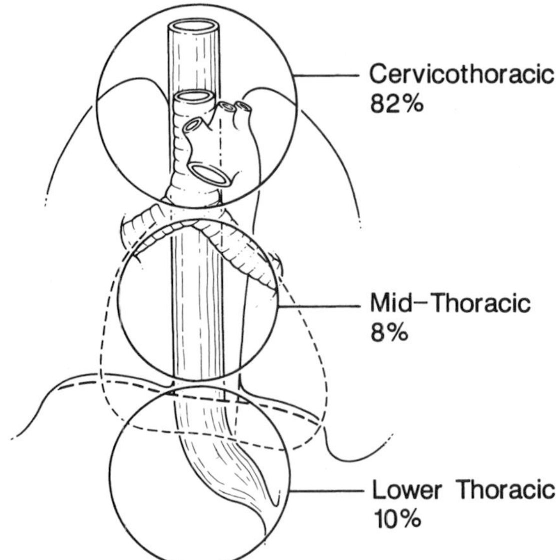

Figure 14–56. Locations of traumatic lacerations of the esophagus.

described in association with severe coughing, asthma, or defecation.[12] Rarely, rupture of the lower esophagus is the result of a severe crushing injury to the abdomen and epigastrium, as in a person who has been run over by a truck or tractor.[11, 12] The increased intra-abdominal pressure abruptly displaces the gastric contents into the esophagus. If the upper esophageal sphincter fails to relax, the intraesophageal pressure may rise precipitously, resulting in rupture of the esophageal wall. The tear usually occurs in the posterolateral wall of the esophagus just proximal to the diaphragm. This area is evidently a point of anatomic weakness. The gastric contents, both fluid and air, then flow freely into the adjacent mediastinum or pleural space. Clinically this event is associated with the onset of severe chest pain, dyspnea, and cyanosis, although on occasion the signs and symptoms may be much less severe in degree.

The radiographic findings are nonspecific, consisting of pneumomediastinum, located initially inferiorly about the esophagus but quickly dissecting proximally about the aorta and then into the neck, giving rise to subcutaneous emphysema. Pulmonary opacities appear in the basilar segments of the lower lobes, particularly on the left, and are often accompanied by pneumothorax, pleural effusions, or both. Irrespective of the location of the tear, the diagnosis is confirmed by a contrast swallow examination. A water-soluble contrast agent may be used, but occasionally the tear in the esophageal wall may be partially sealed and not demonstrated. Therefore, a two-phase contrast swallow examination is recommended. For the first phase a water-soluble contrast agent is given to permit identification of large tears. If the findings are unremarkable, barium is then given, as it is more readily visualized at fluoroscopy and has the theoretical advantage of penetrating partially sealed tears, which may be overlooked with the use of water-soluble contrast material.

Disruption of the Thoracic Aorta and Great Vessels

Disruption of the thoracic aorta is an often fatal injury, and although early repair may be lifesaving, prospective diagnosis is difficult because there are few diagnostic physical signs or symptoms.[166, 168, 178, 188] The challenge is to develop an imaging algorithm that is sensitive enough to identify all arch and great vessel injuries but specific enough to eliminate nontherapeutic thoracotomies.

The injury is most often due to high-speed motor vehicle accidents and is the cause of death in up to 30% of blunt trauma fatalities.[173, 185, 188] Death is immediate in 70% to 85% of cases, and of those patients who reach the hospital alive, 80% will die within 5 days if the aortic injury is not treated.[166, 168, 185, 188, 191] Although these patients often have other severe injuries that require immediate attention, the potentially fatal aortic injury requires early diagnosis and surgical repair to ensure survival.[168, 174, 195] The diagnostic and therapeutic dilemma exists because there is no rapid, inexpensive, and accurate screening examination for aortic injury. Although chest radiography is sensitive, abnormal findings are nonspecific; and the "gold standard" method of diagnosis, an angiogram of the aorta, is expensive in time and resources. Of those patients whose clinical and physical findings warrant an evaluation for aortic injury, only 0.8% will be found to have the injury.[167, 169]

The clinical findings of normal upper extremity pulses and decreased or absent lower extremity pulses (acute coarctation syndrome) can be diagnostic of aortic arch injury but are extremely rare. Owing to the variable historical, clinical, and radiographic findings, diagnosis requires a high level of suspicion and a highly sensitive screening examination. Patients subjected to rapid deceleration—that is, those involved in a motor vehicle crash, who have been ejected from a vehicle, or who have sustained a fall from a significant height—are at highest risk for aortic injury.

Multiple pathophysiologic explanations of aortic injury have been proposed. The shear stress of horizontal deceleration is most pronounced at the aortic isthmus or diaphragmatic hiatus, where the relatively mobile descending aorta is fixed.[173, 180, 188] Another theory postulates that the descending aorta remains fixed (by intercostal vessels and the ductus arteriosus) while the heart and ascending aorta swing forward or are displaced upward by an impact to the lower chest or abdomen, stretching and tearing the aorta at the fixed ductus.[164] The hydrostatic theory implicates pressure waves created by direct compression of the aorta. The compression force generated in the crash of a motor vehicle traveling at 40 miles per hour can create intraluminal pressures of up to 2500 mm Hg at the isthmus, which is sufficient to produce a laceration.[180] The "osseous pinch" model of acute thoracic compression suggests that the anterior osseous structures (manubrium, clavicle, and first rib) pivot to compress the aortic isthmus against the spine.[165]

Any or all of these mechanisms may be operative. All of the theories presented provide support for the isthmus of the aorta as a focal point for injury, which correlates with the 80% incidence of lesions at this location (Fig. 14–57; see also Fig. 14–59). Rates of occurrence for the less frequent sites of injury—5% to 6% of injuries for the ascending aorta at the root and 1% to 3% for the diaphragmatic aorta—support the deceleration mechanism, as these sites are relatively fixed. The great vessels are injured in 4% to 10%, and multiple sites of injury are evident in 2% to 3% of patients (Fig. 14–58).

Because of the large number of patients in whom the historical data are consistent with aortic injury and because of the lack of specificity of physical and chest radiographic findings, various algorithms have been suggested to diminish the number of negative angiographic procedures performed.

Chest radiography is the historical screening method of choice, with a sensitivity of 90% to 93% and a specificity of 10% to 45%.[162, 179, 182, 190, 196] The most strongly associated radiographic findings are widened mediastinum (greater than 8 cm at the level of the left subclavian origin), indistinct aortic contour, loss of the aortopulmonary window, widened right paratracheal stripe, and deviation of the trachea or nasogastric tube to the right (see Fig. 14–57). However, any or all of these signs may be absent in 6% to 12% of patients.[171]

The use of an abnormal appearance on the chest radiograph (or chest radiographic findings "indeterminate for aortic injury") as an indication for aortography results in the performance of this study in a large number of patients in whom the aorta is demonstrated to be normal. Because chest radiography is essentially a screening examination for mediastinal hematoma, the substitution of CT (a more sensitive and specific test owing to improved tissue characterization) has occurred as CT scanners have become more available and examination times shorter.[185] When used to identify the presence or absence of a mediastinal hematoma, CT scanning has nearly 100% accuracy[176, 185] (Figs. 14–59 and 14–60). Contrast CT scanning can diagnose aortic injury, but negative findings do not exclude aortic injury (i.e., the sensitivity is 85–95%)[20, 23, 24] or brachiocephalic artery injury.[172] The greater expense of CT as a screening test is offset by its increased specificity, which can result in a 50% to 80% reduction in the number of aortographic procedures performed.[167, 172, 190] CT findings of periaortic or diffuse mediastinal hematoma indicate the need for an aortogram (see Fig. 14–60). Aortography is also indicated for indeterminate CT findings, which can be caused by motion or streak artifact, partial volume averaging, or atelectasis adjacent to the mediastinal structures. The use of contrast-enhanced CT as a screening examination is controversial; if the contrast CT image demonstrates only mediastinal hematoma, further study is warranted.[176] Direct contrast CT findings of false aneurysm, linear lucency within the lumen due to myointimal flap, marginal irregularity of the lumen, intramural aortic hematoma, or dissection within the aortic wall establish a diagnosis of aortic injury (see Fig. 14–59). Although these direct findings may be sufficiently diagnostic for the patient to proceed to operation, an aortogram may still be indicated for further definition of great vessel injuries and anomalies before open operative or endovascular repair.

Angiography remains the gold standard modality for diagnosis of aortic and brachiocephalic artery injury, with a sensitivity of nearly 100%.[183] This position will be challenged as contrast-enhanced helical CT technology improves. In one study, the investigators found contrast-enhanced CT to be more sensitive than angiography; however, the small intimal flaps or filling defects that were identified resolved on follow-up scan without surgical repair and were therefore of debatable clinical significance.[167]

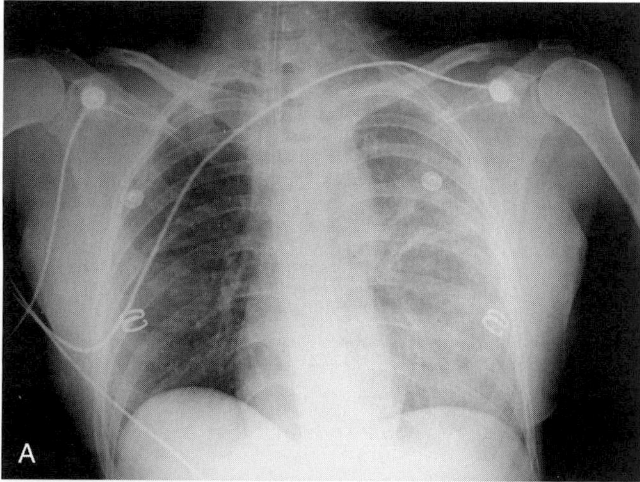

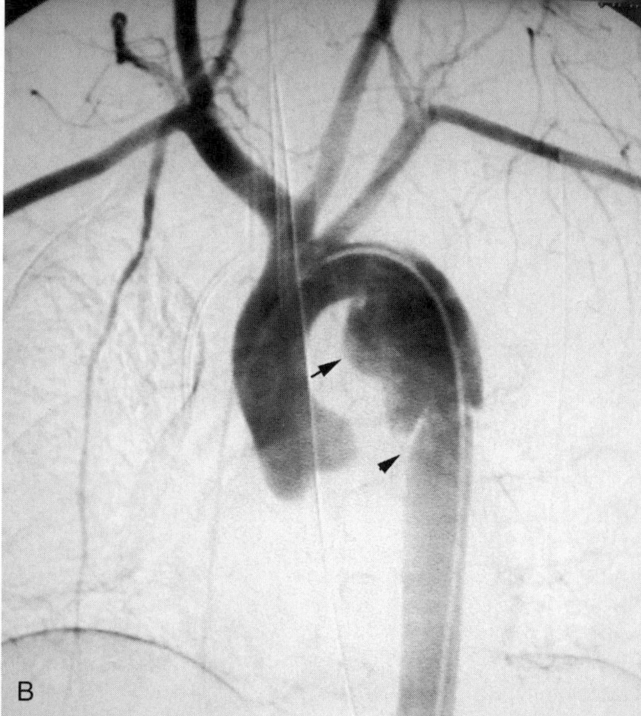

Figure 14–57. Traumatic rupture of the aorta in a young woman. *A*, Initial chest radiograph shows widening of the mediastinum with poor definition of an apparently enlarged aortic arch. The esophagus and trachea are displaced to the right, and the left main bronchus is depressed. The widening of the mediastinum extends over the apex of the left lung. There are no fractures of the ribs. The findings indicate a mediastinal hematoma and raise the suspicion of aortic rupture. *B*, Right posterior oblique projection of the digital subtraction percutaneous transfemoral angiogram shows the false aneurysm *(arrow)*, distal to the left subclavian artery. The retracted myointimal flaps are seen at the margins *(arrowhead)*.

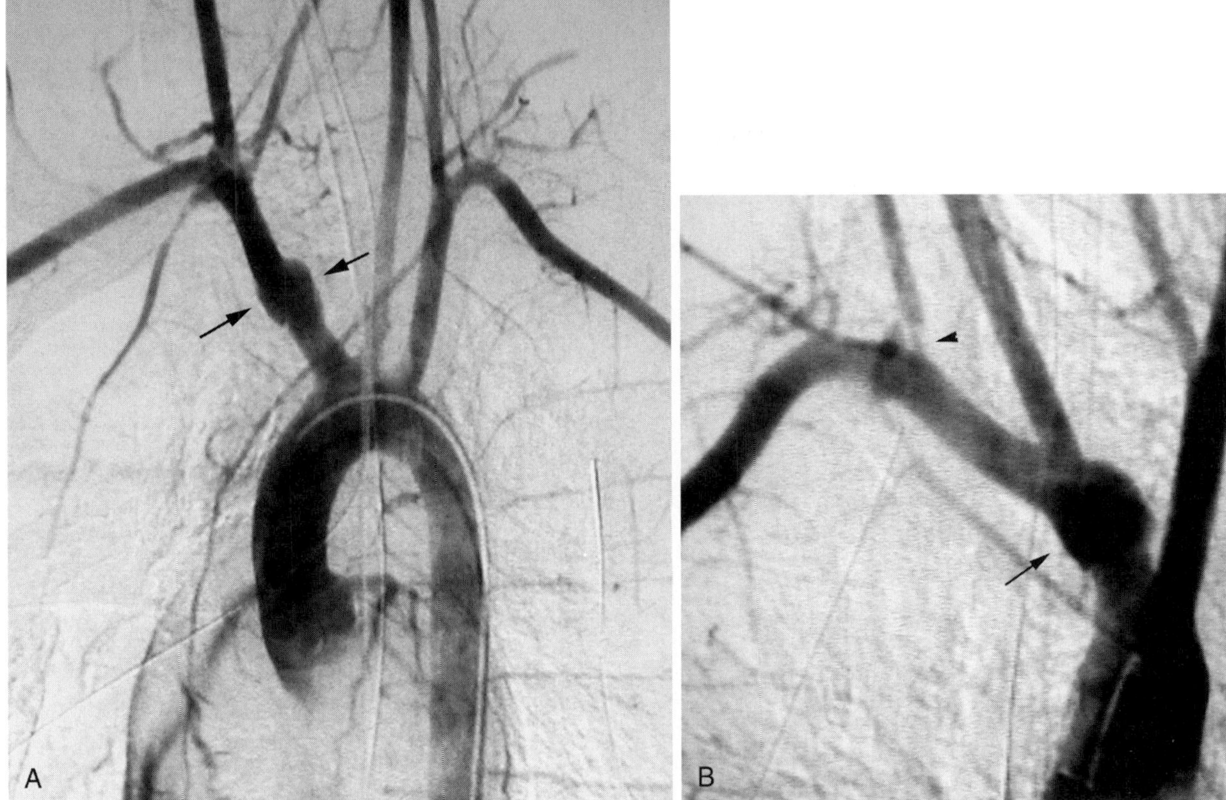

Figure 14–58. Right brachiocephalic artery transection in a young man after a seven-story fall. *A*, Right posterior oblique view on digital subtraction angiography demonstrates the right brachiocephalic artery false aneurysm *(arrows)*. *B*, Magnified left posterior oblique image demonstrates the full circumferential involvement of the brachiocephalic artery injury *(arrow)* and also depicts a right vertebral artery origin injury *(arrowhead)*.

Angiographic findings vary as the extent of the lesion varies. As increasing force is transmitted to the arterial wall, the layers fracture from the inside out.[161] Intimal injury may appear as a linear filling defect, or if clot has formed, it may appear as a thickened or irregular segment of luminal wall[175] (see Fig. 14–60). When the injury extends into the media (and possibly adventitia), the luminal contrast may extend beyond the normal contour of the aorta and is seen as a false aneurysm, often with linear filling defects representing retracted intimal-medial flaps at the proximal and distal edges. Complete disruption through the adventitia results in extravasation, which is seldom seen, as such disruption is usually a terminal event.

Angiography can yield indeterminate findings. A prominent ductus diverticulum, enlarged bronchial artery origin, or prominent aortic spindle may be confused with an injury.[184] An ulcer in an atherosclerotic plaque may be difficult to distinguish from a traumatic pseudoaneurysm.[187] In these cases, intravascular ultrasound or transesophageal echocardiography (TEE) may be useful to identify discontinuity in the intima or to demonstrate an intramural hematoma.

Although TEE is a useful adjunctive technique that can be performed intraoperatively or at the bedside, it is limited as a primary screening tool by its inability to identify brachiocephalic artery injuries and ascending aortic injuries (which together may account for up to 20% of injuries).[193] Injury cannot be excluded until the entire thoracic aorta and proximal great vessels have been studied.

Of patients whose clinical and physical findings indicate a need for screening for aortic injury, only 1% will be found to have such injury. The most cost-effective imaging approach depends on the pretest probability of aortic injury and the cost of the various methods of evaluation. A classification of clinical findings has been developed that can be used to determine a patient's probability of injury.[163] For this classification, composite predictors were identified that included the clinical factors of age greater than 50 years, unrestrained vehicle occupant, hypotension (any systolic pressure measurement of <90 mm Hg), and areas of injury grouped as thoracic injury, abdominopelvic injury, extremity long bone fracture, and head injury. For those patients with two or three of the composite predictors, risk of injury was between 0.5% and 5%, and CT of the chest was the best initial test.[163, 187] Those patients with fewer risk factors are best screened by chest radiography, and those with more than three risk factors are most effectively screened by angiography.

Once an injury is identified, immediate consideration by the surgical staff is the standard of care. The improved sensitivity of diagnostic imaging modalities (angiography, contrast-enhanced helical CT, TEE and intravascular ultrasonography [IVUS]) allows the identification of so-called minimal injury—that involving the intima only (see Fig. 14–60). If the limited extent of injury is confirmed by TEE or IVUS, nonoperative management may be

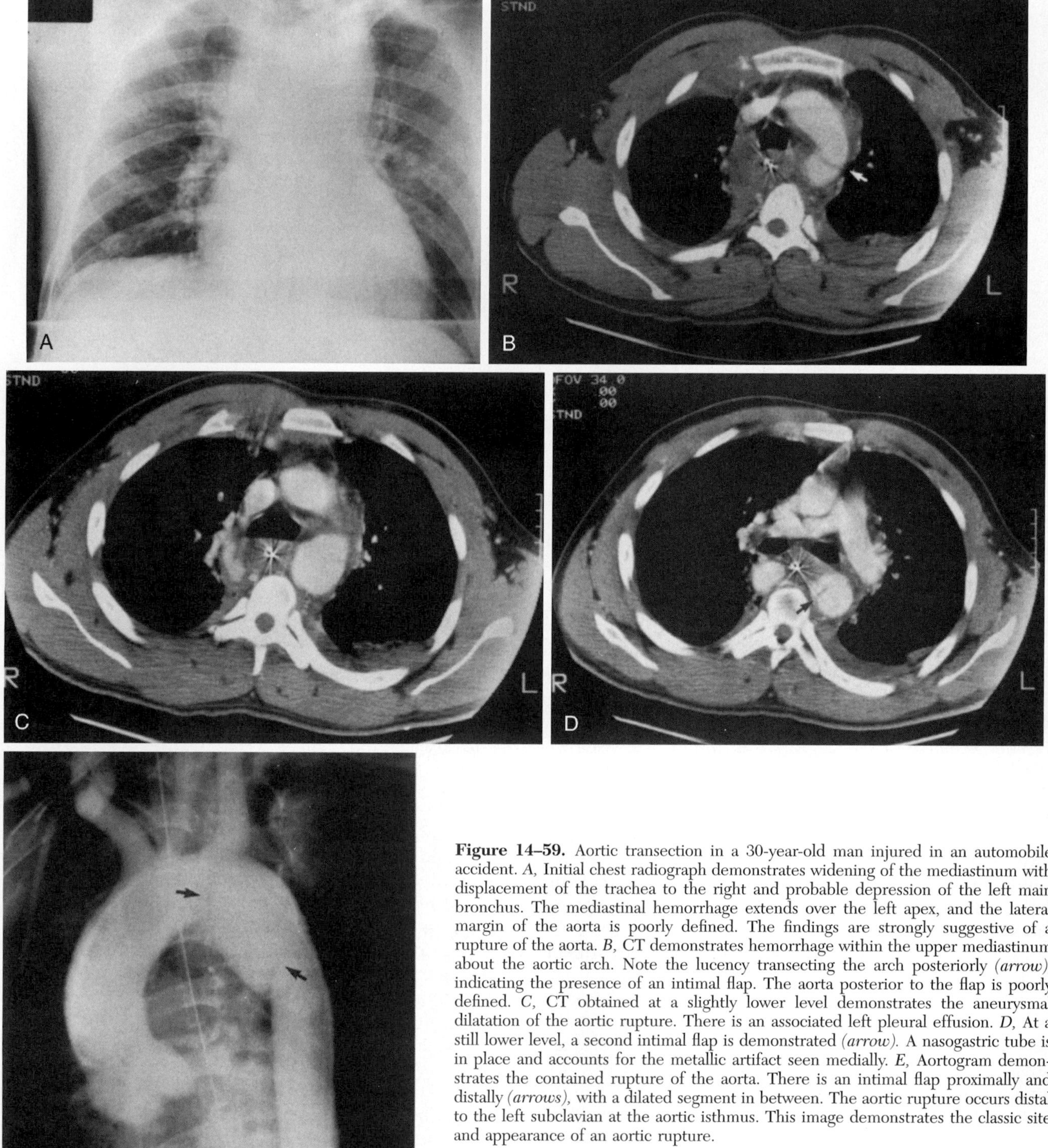

Figure 14–59. Aortic transection in a 30-year-old man injured in an automobile accident. *A,* Initial chest radiograph demonstrates widening of the mediastinum with displacement of the trachea to the right and probable depression of the left main bronchus. The mediastinal hemorrhage extends over the left apex, and the lateral margin of the aorta is poorly defined. The findings are strongly suggestive of a rupture of the aorta. *B,* CT demonstrates hemorrhage within the upper mediastinum about the aortic arch. Note the lucency transecting the arch posteriorly *(arrow),* indicating the presence of an intimal flap. The aorta posterior to the flap is poorly defined. *C,* CT obtained at a slightly lower level demonstrates the aneurysmal dilatation of the aortic rupture. There is an associated left pleural effusion. *D,* At a still lower level, a second intimal flap is demonstrated *(arrow).* A nasogastric tube is in place and accounts for the metallic artifact seen medially. *E,* Aortogram demonstrates the contained rupture of the aorta. There is an intimal flap proximally and distally *(arrows),* with a dilated segment in between. The aortic rupture occurs distal to the left subclavian at the aortic isthmus. This image demonstrates the classic site and appearance of an aortic rupture.

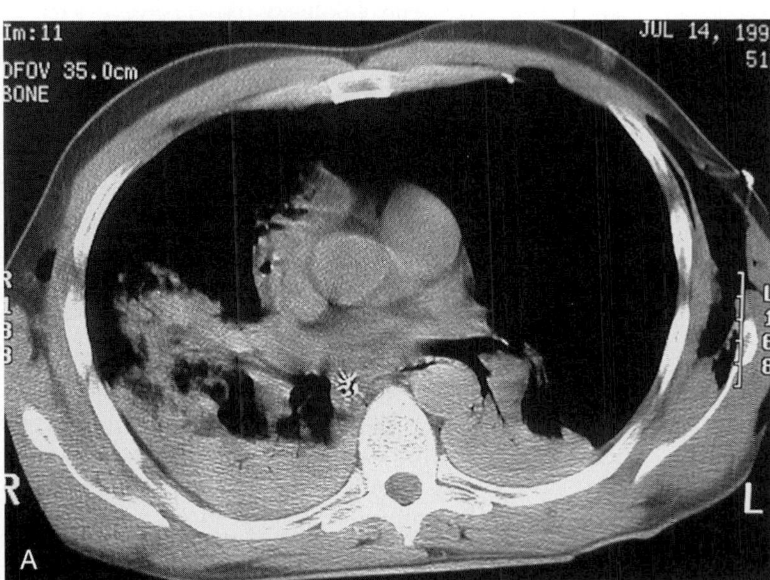

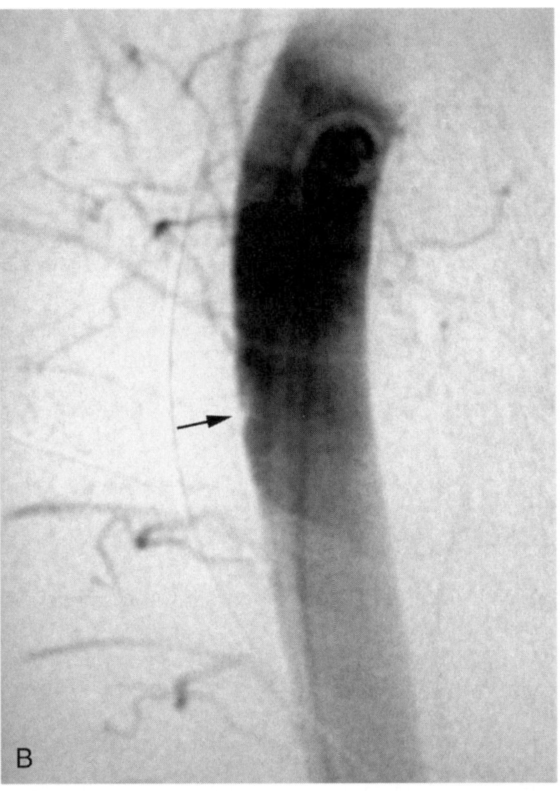

Figure 14–60. The patient was a logger who presented after a 50-foot fall with a pneumothorax and indeterminate mediastinum. *A,* CT shows soft tissue density adjacent to the expected contour of the aorta that becomes contiguous with atelectatic lung and pleural fluid. There is abnormal air within the mediastinum anteromedial to the aorta. Although not diagnostic of an aortic injury, these findings warrant further evaluation with an angiogram. *B,* On digital subtraction angiography, a left posterior oblique image of the descending aorta demonstrates a so-called minimal injury, consistent with a myointimal flap or subintimal hematoma *(arrow).* Transesophageal echocardiography did not identify an injury. Noninvasive management was elected, and a week later, appearance on a repeat angiogram was normal.

selected, as these injuries have been shown to heal spontaneously.[170, 192] These injuries require follow-up imaging until the abnormality has resolved.[175]

The presence of contrast beyond the normal confines of the aorta indicates significant compromise of the integrity of the aortic wall or a transmural injury, and immediate repair is indicated. However, if there is significant comorbidity, either preexisting (coronary artery disease, severe COPD) or concurrent injury (coagulopathy, intracranial injury with elevated intracranial pressure, or lung injury), the risk of operation and triage priorities may dictate a delay in the aortic repair to permit optimization of cardiopulmonary or coagulation status, or for treatment of acute hemorrhage.[186, 189] If there is a delay in diagnostic evaluation or repair, blood pressure should be controlled with administration of beta-adrenergic blocking agents and antihypertensive medications in a regimen that maintains the systolic pressure at less than 120 mm Hg.

Another, currently experimental option for repair of acute aortic or great vessel injury is placement of a graft-covered stent.[177, 181, 194] Initially developed for high-risk nontrauma patients, these devices may permit a less invasive, rapid repair of the injury. The endovascular approach may be particularly beneficial in patients with contraindications to immediate open operative repair.

Cardiac Injuries

Cardiac injuries are usually the result of penetrating injuries such as gunshot wounds or stab wounds or of blunt high-speed injuries such as those from skiing or motor vehicle crashes, particularly as the chest wall is crushed by a steering wheel[206]; such injuries have also been described in vehicle occupants who were restrained at the moment of collision.[203, 209] The resultant injury ranges in severity from myocardial contusion to myocardial lacerations to rupture of the ventricular or atrial wall, chordae tendineae, papillary muscle, valvular apparatus, intraventricular septum, or coronary arteries.[2, 199, 201, 206, 210–215] As a result of the bleeding associated with these injuries, blood collects within the pericardium; if the pericardium is intact, cardiac tamponade results. The tamponade is manifested clinically by dyspnea, cyanosis, paradoxical pulse, and shock. If the pericardium is also lacerated, the blood extravasates into the pleura, resulting in hemothorax.

Diagnosis of cardiac tamponade is established on clinical grounds. On the anteroposterior radiograph obtained in the emergency department with the patient supine, it is difficult to evaluate cardiac size and contour. Only 200 to 300 mL of blood will produce clinically evident cardiac tamponade, but this amount does not enlarge or distort the cardiac silhouette sufficiently to allow it to be recognized radiographically with any degree of certainty.[214] Given time, however, the pericardium has the capability to distend to accommodate large amounts of pericardial fluid, as seen in chronic pericardial effusion. The pericardium is not extremely elastic and therefore does not readily distend immediately in response to the fluid—in this case, blood within the pericardial space. Therefore, in the case of acute bleeding, cardiac tamponade may result from the presence of relatively small amounts of blood in the pericardium. The tamponade must be alleviated by immediate drainage of the pericardium. Lesser degrees of injury may not be associated with significant bleeding into the pericardium.

Myocardial contusions are diagnosed on the basis of electrocardiographic changes,[202] serial immunoassays, and radionuclide studies.[209] Myocardial contusion can also be diagnosed with transthoracic or transesophageal echocardiography. Only patients who develop cardiac complications benefit from echocardiography to exclude other potential injuries.[205] Cardioangiography is utilized for the evaluation of valvular injuries.[213, 215]

Cardiac injuries are frequently associated with fractures[2, 211] of the sternum[204, 212] and ribs, including flail chest, but these are of secondary importance and except for a fractured sternum, do not call attention directly to the possibility of myocardial injury. Ruptures of the myocardium and pericardium have been successfully repaired surgically.

Pneumopericardium is occasionally identified following blunt chest trauma and usually is of no significance.[198] It is the end result of dissection of air along the pulmonary veins following alveolar disruption caused by sudden compression of the chest wall and underlying lung. Rarely, this is sufficient to create a tension pneumopericardium, with the patient manifesting signs of acute cardiac tamponade.[200, 207, 208, 216] The diagnosis should be suspected on the basis of the chest radiograph when there is a large pneumopericardium or suggestion of decreasing cardiac size in the presence of a pneumopericardium. Tamponade is relieved by either percutaneous aspiration or surgical drainage of the pericardium.

Radiographs obtained in the morgue or emergency department in persons who have died in automobile accidents may demonstrate air within the heart (pneumocardia) (Fig. 14–61). This finding is the result of sucking open wounds, particularly about the head and neck. The air in the heart is associated with air in the major veins—the presence of which is, of course, incompatible with life.

Radiographic Evaluation of Chest Trauma

In general, the nature and severity of chest injuries are directly dependent on the nature and severity of the injuring force and on the amount of kinetic energy absorbed and the rate at which it is absorbed. Crushing chest injuries sustained in high-speed motor vehicle crashes frequently involve damage to multiple structures including the chest wall, lungs, pleura, and, less frequently, the thoracic aorta, major bronchi, and diaphragm. It is fortunate that life-threatening injuries of the bronchus, aorta, and diaphragm—those injuries with high morbidity—are infrequent, but it is unfortunate that the clinical and radiographic signs are often subtle and easily overlooked, obscured by more obvious abnormalities in the lungs or pleura, or overshadowed clinically by fractures of the long bones, spine, or pelvis and by head injuries.

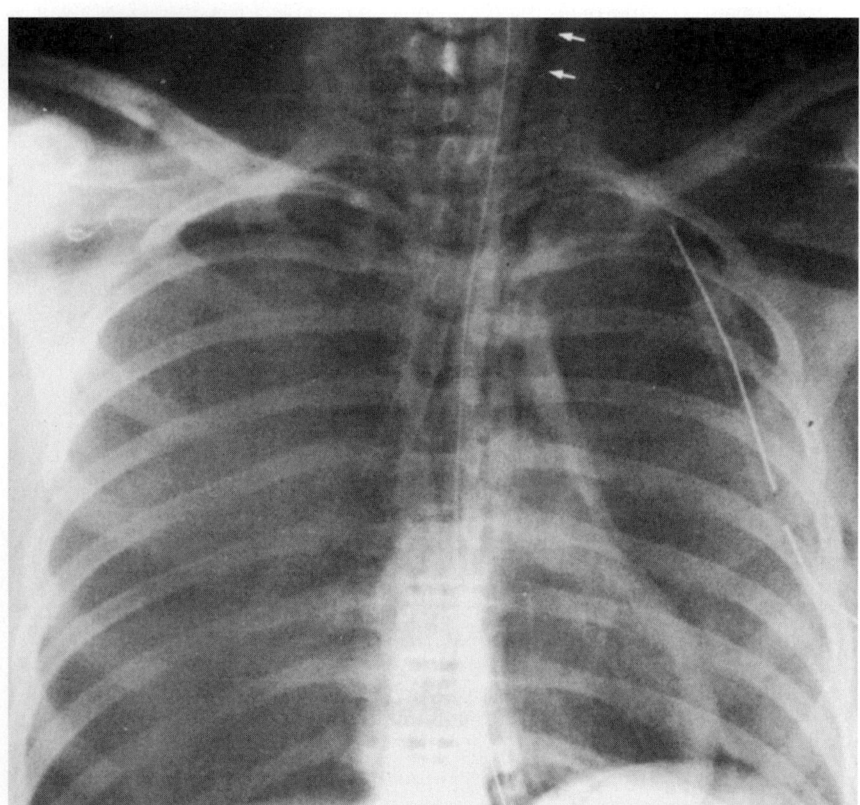

Figure 14–61. Pneumocardia. Chest radiograph, obtained at autopsy, is from a trauma victim who had sustained massive trauma including an open wound of the head and neck. Air was sucked into the circulatory system and is now present within the jugular vein *(arrows)* and cardiac chambers.

To decrease the chance that significant injuries will be overlooked, it is necessary to develop and maintain a disciplined search pattern in interpreting radiographs of the injured chest. There is a natural tendency to stop the search after identification of one abnormality or the source of several obvious abnormalities. To avoid errors, the search must continue until all possible forms of injury have been excluded; practically any combination of injuries is possible.

The examination should start with observation of the general contour of the chest and the position of the heart and mediastinum. Opacities in the lungs or pleural spaces are then identified. The subcutaneous tissues of the chest wall and base of the neck are examined for evidence of emphysema. The periphery of the lung is examined for evidence of pleural fluid or pneumothorax. This search usually starts with examining the contour of the costophrenic angle for blunting or a V sign indicating pneumothorax. If pneumothorax is identified, the position of the diaphragm and mediastinum must be observed to determine the presence or absence of tension. It should be emphasized that on radiographs obtained with the patient in the supine position, the size of pleural air or fluid collections can easily be underestimated, or the abnormalities may escape visualization entirely.

The position and contour of both hemidiaphragms should be identified, and any elevation or abnormal contour should be regarded with suspicion, especially when the mechanism of injury is consistent with such change. Scalloping or eventration is more common in older persons and is uncommon in the young. Abnormalities of the contour and position of the diaphragm suggest the possibility of diaphragmatic rupture.

The mediastinum is then evaluated. The width of the mediastinum, position of the trachea and nasogastric tube, if one is in place, and distinctness of the aortic arch and descending aorta are noted. Abnormality of any or all of these features suggests mediastinal hematoma with the possibility of aortic rupture. The mediastinum is also examined for evidence of emphysema, which when present suggests the possibility of rupture of the trachea, major bronchi, or esophagus, although less so if the patient is mechanically ventilated.

Finally, the ribs are searched for fractures, and the number and position of any fractures are noted. With multiple fractures, a search should be made for a second line of fracture within the same rib, which would indicate a flail chest deformity. It should be remembered that frequently the second rib injury consists of separation of the costochondral junction, so that the presence of flail chest may not be evident radiographically. If the fractures involve the first, second, or third rib, the mediastinum should be re-examined to exclude bronchial or aortic rupture, because these serious injuries are frequently associated with fractures of the upper ribs. If the fracture involves the lower ribs (i.e., the eighth or below), the diaphragm should be re-examined for evidence of rupture, and consideration should be given to possible abdominal visceral injury.

On serial radiographs, the position of the diaphragm should also be noted. As described, herniation of the abdominal viscera through a diaphragmatic rupture can be delayed. Very frequently, additional rib fractures are identified on subsequent examinations. They are made more obvious by displacement resulting from respiratory motion. These fractures are usually identified above or below and in line with previously identified fractures. Apparent increasing heart size should also be evaluated to exclude evolving hemopericardium.

References

General Thoracic Trauma

1. Bassett, J.S., Gibson, R.D., & Wilson, R.F. (1968). Blunt injuries to the chest. J. Trauma, *8*:418.
2. Blair, E., Topuzlu, C., & Davis, H.H. (1971). Delayed or missed diagnosis in blunt chest trauma. J. Trauma, *11*:129.
3. Conn, J.H., Hardy, J.D., Fain, W.R., & Netterville, R.E. (1963). Thoracic trauma: Analysis of 1022 cases. J Trauma, *3*:22.
4. Crawford, W.O. Jr. (1973). Pulmonary injury in thoracic and nonthoracic trauma. Radiol. Clin. North Am., *11*:527.
5. Dennis, L.N., & Rogers, L.F. (1989). Superior mediastinal widening from spine fractures mimicking aortic rupture on chest radiographs. A.J.R. Am. J. Roentgenol., *152*:27.
6. Goodman, P.C. (1986). CT of chest trauma. p. 168. In Federle, M.P. & Brant-Zwadzki, M. Eds.: Computed Tomography in the Evaluation of Trauma. 2nd Ed. Williams & Wilkins, Baltimore.
7. Kattan, D.R. (1978). Trauma of the bony thorax. Semin. Roentgenol., *13*:69.
8. Keen, G. (1974). Chest injuries. Ann. R. Coll. Surg. Engl., *54*:124.
9. Naclerio, E.A. (1971). Chest Injuries: Physiologic Principles and Emergency Management. Grune & Stratton, New York.
10. Poole, G.V. Jr., & Myers, R.T. (1981). Morbidity and mortality rates in major blunt trauma to the upper chest. Ann. Surg., *193*:70.
11. Reynolds, J., & Davis, J.T. (1966). Injuries of the chest wall, pleura, pericardium, lungs, bronchi and esophagus. Radiol. Clin. North Am., *4*:383.
12. Rogers, L.F., Puig, A.W., Dooley, B.N., & Cuellol, L. (1972). Diagnostic considerations in mediastinal emphysema. A.J.R. Am. J. Roentgenol., *115*:495.
13. Rossen, B., Laursen, N.O., & Just, S. (1987). Chest radiography after minor chest trauma. Acta Radiol., *28*:53.
14. Shorr, R.M., Rodriguez, A., Indeck, M.C. et al. (1989). Blunt chest trauma in the elderly. J. Trauma, *29*:234.
15. Toombs, B.D. (1987). Acute chest trauma. p. 11. In Toombs, B.D., & Sandler, C.M. Eds.: Computed Tomography in Trauma. W.B. Saunders Co., Philadelphia.
16. Toombs, B.D., Sandler, C.M., & Lester, R.G. (1981). Computed tomography of chest trauma. Radiology, *140*:733.
17. Wiot, J.F. (1975). The radiologic manifestations of blunt chest trauma. J.A.M.A., *231*:500.
18. Woodring, J.H., Lee, C., & Jenkins, K. (1988). Spinal fractures in blunt chest trauma. J. Trauma, *28*:789.

Fractures of the Ribs

19. Bitschau, R., Gehmacher, O., Kopf, A. et al. (1997). Ultrasound diagnosis of rib and sternum fractures. Ultraschall. Med. *18*:158.
20. Bodai, B.I., Hill, A., Smith, J.P. et al. (1984). Intraabdominal injury associated with rib fractures. J. Trauma, *24*:647.
21. Brasel, K.J., Stafford, R.E., Weigelt, J.A., et al. (1999). Treatment of occult pneumothoraces from blunt trauma. J. Trauma, *46*:987.
22. Cameron, D.A., O'Rourke, P.V., & Burt, C.W. (1949). An analysis of the management and complications of multiple (three or more) rib fractures. Am. J. Surg., *78*:668.
23. Caro, P.A., & Borden, S., IV. (1988). Plastic bowing of the ribs in children. Skeletal Radiol., *17*:255.
24. Christensen, E.E., & Dietz, G.W. (1980). Injuries of the first costovertebral articulation. Radiology, *134*:41.
25. Curran, J.P., & Kelly, D.A. (1966). Stress fracture of the first rib. Am. J. Orthop. Surg., *8*:16.
26. Danher, J., Eyes, B.E., & Kimar, K. (1984). Oblique rib views after blunt chest trauma: An unnecessary routine? Br. Med. J., *289*:1271.
27. Deluca, S.A., Rhea, J.T., & O'Malley, T. (1982). Radiographic evaluation of rib fractures. A.J.R. Am. J. Roentgenol., *138*:91.
28. Dwivedi, S.C., & Varma, A.N. (1983). Bilateral fracture of the first ribs. J. Trauma, *23*:538.
29. Fisher, R.D., & Rienhoff, W.F. (1966). Subclavian artery laceration resulting from fractured first rib. J. Trauma, *6*:579.
30. Fisher, R.G., Ward, R.E., Ben-Menachem, Y. et al. (1982). Arteriography and the fractured first rib: Too much for too little? A.J.R. Am. J. Roentgenol., *138*:1059.
31. Galbraith, N.F., Urschel, H.C., Wood, R.E., et al. (1973). Fracture of first

rib associated with laceration of subclavian artery. Report of a case and review of the literature. J. Thorac. Cardiovasc. Surg., *65:*649.

32. Garcia, V.F., Gotschall, C.S., Eichelberger, M.R. & Bowman, L.M. (1990). Rib fractures in children: A marker of severe trauma. J. Trauma, *30:*695.
33. Greenwald, L.V., Baisden, C.E., & Symbas, P.N. (1983). Rib fractures in coronary bypass patients: Radionuclide detection. Radiology, *148:*553.
34. Griffith, J.F., Rainer, T.H., Ching, A.S.C. et al. (1999). Sonography compared with radiography in revealing acute rib fracture. A.J.R. Am. J. Roentgenol., *173:*1603.
35. Gupta, A., Jamshidi, M., & Rubin, J.R. (1997). Traumatic first rib fracture: Is angiography necessary? A review of 730 cases. Cardiovasc. Surg., *5:*48.
36. Hinton, D., & Steiner, C.A.L. (1940). Fractures of the ribs. J. Bone Joint Surg., *22:*597.
37. Holmes, T.W., & Netterville, R.E. (1956). Complications of first rib fracture, including one case each of tracheoesophageal fistula and aortic arch aneurysm. J. Thorac. Surg., *32:*74.
38. Joshi, S.G., Panday, S.R., Parulkar, G.B. & Sen, P.K. (1965). Bilateral fracture of the first rib. J. Bone Joint Surg. Br., *47:*283.
39. Karlson, K.A. (1998). Rib stress fractures in elite rowers. A case series and proposed mechanism. Am. J. Sports Med., *26:*516.
40. Kattan, K.R. (1980). What to look for in rib fractures and how. J.A.M.A., *243:*262.
41. Kaye, J.R., Johnson, M., Sproed, R.P., et al. (1984). First rib fracture secondary to shoulder restraints. N. Engl. J. Med., *310:*1748.
42. Lankenner, P.A. Jr., & Micheli, L.J. (1985). Stress fracture of the first rib. J. Bone Joint Surg. Am., *67:*159.
43. Lee, J., Harris, J.H. Jr., Duke, J.H. Jr., & Williams, J.S. (1997). Noncorrelation between thoracic skeletal injuries and acute traumatic aortic tear. J. Trauma, *43:*400.
44. Livoni, J.P., & Barcia, T.C. (1982). Fracture of the first and second ribs: Incidence of vascular injury relative to type of fracture. Radiology, *145:*31.
45. Mariacher-Gehler, S., & Michel, B.A. (1994). Sonography: A simple way to visualize rib fractures [letter]. A.J.R. Am. J. Roentgenol., *163:*1268.
46. Mulder, D.S., Greenwood, F.A.H., & Brooks, C.E. (1973). Posttraumatic thoracic outlet syndrome. J. Trauma, *13:*706.
47. Philip, E.H., Rogers, W.F., & Gaspar, M.R. (1981). First rib fractures: Incidence of vascular injury and indications for angiography. Surgery, *89:*42.
48. Pierce, G.E., Maxwell, J.A., & Boggan, M.D. (1975). Special hazards of first rib fractures. J. Trauma, *15:*264.
49. Rasad, S. (1974). Golfer's fractures of the ribs. A.J.R. Am. J. Roentgenol., *120:*901.
50. Richardson, J.D., McElvein, R.B., & Trinkle, J.K. (1975). First rib fracture: A hallmark of severe trauma. Ann. Surg., *181:*251.
51. Saw, E.C., Yokoyama, T., Lee, B.C., & Sargent, E.N. (1976). Intercostal pulmonary hernia. Arch. Surg., *11:*548.
52. Stoneham, M.D. (1995). Bilateral first rib fractures associated with driver's air bag inflation: Case report and implications for surgery. Eur. J. Emerg. Med., *2:*60.
53. Weiner, D.S., & O'Dell, H.W. (1969). Fractures of the first rib associated with injuries to the clavicle. J. Trauma, *9:*412.
54. Wilson, J.M., Thomas, A.X., Goodman, P.C., & Lewis, F.R. (1978). Severe chest trauma. Morbidity implication of first and second rib fracture in 120 patients. Arch. Surg., *113:*846.
55. Wischofer, E., Fenkl, R., & Blum, R. (1995). Ultrasound detection of rib fractures for verifying fracture diagnosis: A pilot project. Unfallchirurg., *98:*296.
56. Woodring, J.H., Fried, A.M., Hatfield, D.R. et al. (1982). Fractures of first and second ribs: Predictive value for arterial and bronchial injury. A.J.R. Am. J. Roentgenol., *138:*211.

Fractures of the Sternum

57. Blacksin, M.J. (1993). Patterns of fracture after airbag deployment. J. Trauma, *35:*840.
58. Breederveld, R.S., Patka, P., & VanMourik, J.C. (1988). Fractures of the sternum. Netherlands J. Surg., *40:*133.
59. Buckman, R., Trooskin, S.Z., Flancbaum, L., & Chandler, J. (1987). The significance of stable patients with sternal fractures. Surgery, *164:*261.
60. Cameron, H.U. (1980). Traumatic disruption of the manubriosternal joint in the absence of rib fractures. J. Trauma, *20:*892.
61. Cooper, K.L. (1988). Insufficiency fractures of the sternum: A consequence of thoracic kyphosis? Radiology, *167:*471.
62. Dastgeer, G.M., & Mikolich, D.J. (1987). Fracture-dislocation of manubriosternal joint: An unusual complication of seizures. J. Trauma, *27:*91.
63. Fowler, A.W. (1957). Flexion-compression injury of the sternum. J. Bone Joint Surg. Br., *393:*487.
64. Gopalakrishnan, K.C., & El Masri, W.S. (1986). Fractures of the sternum associated with spinal injury. J. Bone Joint Surg. Br., *68:*178.
65. Hills, M.W., Delprado, A.M., & Deane, S.A. (1993). Sternal fractures: Associated injuries and management. J. Trauma, *35:*55.
66. Huggett, J.M., & Roszler, M.H. (1998). CT findings of sternal fracture. Injury, *29:*623.
67. Jenyo, M.S. (1985). Post-traumatic fracture-dislocation of manubriostemal joint with a wedge fracture of the body of the fourth thoracic vertebra. J. Trauma, *25:*274.
68. Jones, H.K., McBride, G.G., & Mumby, R.C. (1989). Sternal fractures associated with spinal injury. J. Trauma, *29:*360.
69. Mayba, I.I. (1985). Non-union of fractures of the sternum. J. Bone Joint Surg. Am., *67:*1091.
70. Mitchell, E.A., & Elliott, R.B. (1980). Spontaneous fracture of the sternum in a youth with cystic fibrosis. J. Pediatr., *97:*789.
71. Park, W.M., McCall, I.W., McSweeney, T., & Jones, B.F. (1980). Cervicodorsal injury presenting as sternal fracture. Clin. Radiol., *31:*49.
72. Patten, R.M., Dobbins, J., & Gunberg, S.R. (1999). Gas in the sternoclavicular joints of patients with blunt chest trauma: Significance and frequency of CT findings. A.J.R. Am. J. Roentgenol., *172:*1633.
73. Rutledge, D.I. (1962). Spontaneous fracture of the sternum simulating myocardial infarction. Postgrad. Med., *32:*502.
74. Stark, P., & Jaramillo, D. (1986). CT of the sternum. A.J.R. Am. J. Roentgenol., *147:*72.
75. Vassallo, L. (1969). Spontaneous fracture of the sternum simulating pulmonary embolism. Br. J. Clin. Pract., *23:*388.

Pulmonary and Pleural Trauma

76. Andrew, T.A., & Milne, D.D. (1980). Pneumoperitoneum associated with pneumothorax or pneumopericardium: A surgical dilemma in the injured patient. Injury, *11:*65.
77. Arom, K.V., & Lyons, G.W. (1975). Traumatic pulmonary arteriovenous fistula. J. Thorac. Cardiovasc. Surg., *70:*918.
78. Bhalla, M., Leitman, B.S., Forcade, C. et al. (1990). Lung hernia: Radiographic features. A.J.R. Am. J. Roentgenol., *154:*51.
79. Bryk, D. (1976). Infrapulmonary effusion. Radiology, *120:*33.
80. Cohn, S.M. (1997). Pulmonary contusion: Review of the clinical entity. J. Trauma, *42:*973.
81. Ekstrom, D., Weiner, M., & Baier, B. (1978). Pulmonary arteriovenous fistula as a complication of trauma. A.J.R. Am. J. Roentgenol., *130:*1178.
82. Ellis, D. (1978). The adult respiratory distress syndrome (ARDS). p. 1. In Tuddenham, W.J. Ed.: Contemporary Diagnostic Radiology. Williams & Wilkins, Baltimore.
83. Ellis, R. (1976). Traumatic lung cysts. J.A.M.A., *236:*1976.
84. Fagan, C.J. (1966). Traumatic lung cyst. A.J.R. Am. J. Roentgenol., *97:*186.
85. Fagan, C.J., & Swischuk, L.E. (1976). Traumatic lung and paramediastinal pneumatoceles. Radiology, *120:*11.
86. Friedman, P.J. (1985). Adult pulmonary ligament pneumatocele: A loculated pneumothorax. Radiology, *155:*575.
87. Ganske, J.G., Dennis, D.L., & Vanderveer, J.B. (1981). Traumatic lung cyst: Case report and literature review. J. Trauma, *21:*493.
88. Glauser, F.L., & Bartlett, R.H. (1974). Pneumoperitoneum in association with pneumothorax. Chest, *66:*536.
89. Hyde, E. (1971). Traumatic para-mediastinal air cysts. Br. J. Radiol., *44:*380.
90. Jantz, M.A., & Pierson, D.J. (1994). Pneumothorax and barotrauma. Clin. Chest Med., *15:*75.
91. Kumar, U.N., Varkey, B., & Mathai, G. (1975). Post-traumatic pleural-fluid and blood eosinophilia. J.A.M.A., *234:*625.
92. McLoughlin, R., Mulcahy, R., Kent, P. et al. (1987). Haemothorax after rib fracture—incidence, timing and prediction. Irish J. Med. Sci., *156:*117.
93. Milne, E., & Dick, A. (1961). Circumscribed intrapulmonary haematoma. Br. J. Radiol., *34:*587.
94. Parham, A.M., Yarbrough, D.R., & Redding, J.S. (1978). Flail chest syndrome and pulmonary contusion. Arch. Surg., *113:*900.
95. Ross, R.M., & Cordoba, A. (1986). Delayed life-threatening hemothorax associated with rib fractures. J. Trauma, *26:*576.
96. Schwarz, M.I., & Marmorstein, B.L. (1975). A new radiologic sign of subpulmonic effusion. Chest, *67:*176.
97. Singh, N.K., & Singh, R.J. (1984). Delayed haemothorax in chest injury. J. Indian Med. Assoc., *82:*399.
98. Sorsdahl, O.A., & Powell, J.W. (1965). Cavitary pulmonary lesions following non-penetrating chest trauma in children. A.J.R. Am. J. Roentgenol., *95:*118.
99. Stevens, E., & Templeton, A.W. (1965). Traumatic nonpenetrating lung contusion. Radiology, *85:*247.
100. Stulz, P., Schmitt, H.E., Hasse, J., & Gradel, E. (1984). Traumatic pulmonary pseudocysts and paramediastinal air cyst: Two rare complications of blunt chest trauma. J. Trauma, *24:*850.
101. Ting, Y.M. (1966). Pulmonary parenchymal findings in blunt trauma to the chest. A.J.R. Am. J. Roentgenol., *98:*343.
102. Tocino, I.M. (1985). Pneumothorax in the supine patient: Radiographic anatomy. Radiographics, *5:*557.
103. Tocino, I.M., Miller, M.H., & Fairfax, W.R. (1985). Distribution of pneumothorax in the supine and semirecumbent critically ill adult. A.J.R. Am. J. Roentgenol., *144:*901.
104. Tocino, I.M., Miller, M.H., Frederick, P.R., et al. (1984). CT detection of occult pneumothorax in head trauma. A.J.R. Am. J. Roentgenol., *143:*987.
105. Wagner, R.B., Crawford, W.O. Jr., & Schimpf, P.P. (1988). Classification of parenchymal injuries of the lung. Radiology, *167:*77.
106. Wall, S.D., Federle, M.P., Jeffrey, R.B., & Brett, C.M. (1983). CT diagnosis of unsuspected pneumothorax after blunt abdominal trauma. A.J.R. Am. J. Roentgenol., *141:*919.
107. Williams, J.R., & Stembridge, V.A. (1964). Pulmonary contusion secondary to nonpenetrating chest trauma. A.J.R. Am. J. Roentgenol., *91:*284.

108. Ziter, F.J. Jr., & Westcott, J.L. (1981). Supine subpulmonary pneumothorax. A.J.R. Am. J. Roentgenol., *137*:699.
109. Zuckerman, S. (1940). Experimental study of blast injuries to the lungs. Lancet, *2*:219.

Rupture of the Diaphragm

110. Alexander, D.C., & Torrance, D.J. (1971). Traumatic intrapericardial herniation of the transverse colon masquerading as a pericardial effusion on the scan. Case report. Radiology, *98*:627.
111. Ball, T., McCrory, R., Smith, J.O., & Clements, J.L. Jr. (1982). Traumatic diaphragmatic hernia: Errors in diagnosis. A.J.R. Am. J. Roentgenol., *138*:633.
112. Bergqvist, D., Dahlgren, S., & Hedelin, H. (1978). Rupture of the diaphragm in patients wearing seatbelts. Trauma, *18*:781–783.
113. Bernatz, P.W.E., Burnside, A.F. Jr., & Clagett, O.T. (1958). Problem of the ruptured diaphragm. J.A.M.A., *168*:877.
114. Blumenthal, D.H., Raghu, G., Rudd, T.G., & Herman, C.M. (1984). Diagnosis of right hemidiaphragmatic rupture by liver scintigraphy. J. Trauma, *24*:536.
115. Buckman, R.F. Jr., Piano, G., Dunham, C.M. et al. (1988). Major bowel and diaphragmatic injuries associated with blunt spleen or liver rupture. J. Trauma, *28*:1317.
116. Carter, B.N., Giuseffi, J., & Felson, B. (1951). Traumatic diaphragmatic hernia. A.J.R. Am. J. Roentgenol., *65*:56.
117. Cox, C.L., Anderson, J.N., & Guest, J.L. (1977). Bronchopancreatic fistula following traumatic rupture of the diaphragm. J.A.M.A., *237*:1461.
118. Desforges, G., Strieder, J.W., Lynch, J.P., & Madoff, I.M. (1957). Traumatic rupture of the diaphragm. Clinical manifestations and surgical treatment. J. Thorac. Surg., *34*:779.
119. Drews, J.A., Mercer, E.C., & Benfield, J.R. (1973). Acute diaphragmatic injuries. Ann. Thorac. Surg., *16*:67.
120. Ebert, P.A., Gaertner, R.A., & Zuidema, G.D. (1967). Traumatic diaphragmatic hernia. Surg. Gynecol. Obstet., *125*:59.
121. Esrera, A.S., Platt, M.R., & Mills, L.J. (1979). Traumatic injuries of the diaphragm. Chest, *75*:306.
122. Feliciano, D.V., Cruse, P.A., Mattox, K.L. et al. (1988). Delayed diagnosis of injuries to the diaphragm after penetrating wounds. J. Trauma, *28*:1135.
123. Gourin, A., & Garzon, A.A. (1974). Diagnostic problems in traumatic diaphragmatic hernia. J. Trauma, *14*:20.
124. Grage, T.B., MacLean, L.D., & Campbell, G.S. (1959). Traumatic rupture of the diaphragm. Surgery, *46*:669.
125. Graivier, L., & Freeark, R.J. (1963). Traumatic diaphragmatic hernia. Arch. Surg., *86*:363.
126. Griswold, F.Q., Warden, H.E., & Gardner, R.J. (1972). Acute diaphragmatic rupture caused by blunt trauma. Am. J. Surg., *124*:359.
127. Harman, P.K., Mentzer, R.M. Jr., Weinberg, A.C. et al. (1981). Early diagnosis by liver scan of a right-sided traumatic diaphragmatic hernia. J. Trauma, *21*:489.
128. Heiberg, E., Wolverson, M.K., Hurd, R.N. et al. (1980). CT recognition of traumatic rupture of the diaphragm. A.J.R. Am. J. Roentgenol., *135*:369.
129. Hill, L.D. (1972). Injuries of the diaphragm following blunt trauma. Surg. Clin. North Am., *52*:611.
130. Hood, R.M. (1971). Traumatic diaphragmatic hernia. Ann. Thorac. Surg., *12*:311.
131. Jarrett, F., & Bernhardt, L.C. (1978). Right-sided diaphragmatic injury. Rarity or overlooked diagnosis? Arch. Surg., *113*:737.
132. Killeen, K.L., Mirvis, S.E., & Shanmuganathan, K. (1999). Helical CT of diaphragmatic rupture caused by blunt trauma. A.J.R. Am. J. Roentgenol., *173*:1611.
133. Morgan, A.S., Flancbaum, L., Esposito, T., & Cox, E.F. (1986). Blunt injury to the diaphragm: An analysis of 44 patients. J. Trauma, *26*:565.
134. Noon, G.P., Beall, A.C., & DeBakey, M.E. (1966). Surgical management of traumatic rupture of the diaphragm. J. Trauma, *6*:344.
135. Ory, P.A., & Stern, E.J. (1997). Strangulated hernia through a prior pericardial window. Radiologic case-of-the-month. Appl. Radiol., *26*:36.
136. Perlman, S.J., Rogers, L.F., Mintzer, R.A., & Mueller, C.F. (1984). Abnormal course of nasogastric tube in traumatic rupture of left hemidiaphragm. A.J.R. Am. J. Roentgenol., *142*:85.
137. Rodriguez-Morales, G., Rodriguez, A., & Shatney, C.H. (1986). Acute rupture of the diaphragm in blunt trauma: Analysis of 60 patients. J. Trauma, *26*:438.
138. Salomon, N.W., & Zukoski, C.F. (1979). Isolated rupture of the right hemidiaphragm with eventration of the liver. J.A.M.A., *241*:1929.
139. Schreiber, M.H., & Brown, F.E. Jr. (1979). Traumatic diaphragmatic hernia. Curr. Probl. Diag. Radiol., *7*:6.
140. Schwindt, W.D., & Gale, J.W. (1967). Late recognition and treatment of traumatic diaphragmatic hernias. Arch. Surg., *94*:330.
141. Sutton, J.P., Carlisle, R.B., & Stephenson, S.E. (1967). Traumatic diaphragmatic hernia. A review of 25 cases. Ann. Thorac. Surg., *3*:136.
142. Tribble, J.B., Julian, S., & Myers, R.T. (1989). Rupture of the liver and right hemidiaphragm presenting as right hemothorax. J. Trauma, *29*:116.
143. van der Werken, C., Lubbers, E.J.C., & Goris, R.J.A. (1983). Rupture of the diaphragm by blunt trauma as a marker of injury severity. Injury, *15*:149.
144. Ward, R.E., Flynn, T.C., & Clark, W.P. (1981). Diaphragmatic disruption secondary to blunt abdominal trauma. J. Trauma, *21*:35.

Rupture of the Esophagus, Trachea, and Major Bronchi

145. Battersby, J.S., & Kilman, J.W. (1964). Traumatic injuries of the tracheobronchial tree. Arch. Surg., *88*:644.
146. Beal, S.L., Pettmeyer, E.W., & Spisso, J.M. (1988). Esophageal perforation following external blunt trauma. J. Trauma, *28*:1425.
147. Beesinger, D.E., Grover, F.L., & Trinkle, J.K. (1974). Tracheobronchial injuries secondary to blunt thoracic trauma. Tex. Med., *70*:74.
148. Bertelsen, S., & Howitz, P. (1972). Injuries of the trachea and bronchi. Thorax, *27*:188.
149. Burke, J.F. (1962). Early diagnosis of traumatic rupture of the bronchus. J.A.M.A., *181*:682.
150. Chesterman, J.T., & Satsangi, P.N. (1966). Rupture of the trachea and bronchi by closed injury. Thorax, *21*:21.
151. Deslauriers, J., Beaulieu, M., Archambault, G. et al. (1982). Ann. Thorac. Surg., *33*:32.
152. Ecker, R.R., Libertini, R.V., Rea, W.J., et al. (1971). Injuries of the trachea and bronchi. Ann. Thorac. Surg., *11*:289.
153. Eijgelaar, A., & Van der Heide, J.N.H. (1970). A reliable early symptom of bronchial or tracheal rupture. Thorax, *25*:116.
154. Flood, T.R. (1988). Mediastinal emphysema complicating a zygomatic fracture: A case report and review of the literature. Br. J. Oral Maxillofac. Surg., *26*:141.
155. Hood, R.M., & Sloan, H.E. (1959). Injuries of the trachea and major bronchi. J. Thorac. Cardiovasc. Surg., *38*:458.
156. Hurwitz, S.S., Conlan, A.A., & Nicoloau, N. (1982). Traumatic rupture of the right main bronchus. S. Afr. Med. J., *61*:248.
157. Kumpe, D.A., Oh, K.S., & Wyman, S.M. (1970). A characteristic pulmonary finding in unilateral complete bronchial transection. Am. J. Roentgenol., *110*:704.
158. Neugebauer, M.K., Fine, J.B., & Hoyt, T.W. (1974). Traumatic rupture of the trachea and right main stem bronchus. J. Trauma, *14*:265.
159. Ramzy, A.I., Rodriguez, A., & Turney, S.Z. (1988). Management of major tracheobronchial ruptures in patients with multiple system trauma. J. Trauma, *28*:1353.
160. Silbiger, M.L., & Kushner, L.N. (1965). Tracheobronchial perforation: Its diagnosis and treatment. Radiology, *85*:242.

Disruption of the Thoracic Aorta and Great Vessels

161. Amato, J.J., Rich, N.M., Billy, L.J. et al. (1971). High-velocity arterial injury: A study of the mechanism of injury. J. Trauma, *11*:412.
162. Ayella, R.J., Hankins, J.R., Turney, S.Z., & Cowley, R.A. (1977). Ruptured thoracic aorta due to blunt trauma. J. Trauma, *17*:199.
163. Blackmore, C.C., Zweibel, A., & Mann, F.A. (2000). Determining risk of traumatic aortic injury: How to optimize imaging strategy. A.J.R. Am. J. Roentgenol., *174*:343.
164. Coermann, R., Dotzauer, G., Lange, W., & Voigt, G.E. (1972). The effects of the design of the steering assembly and the instrument panel on injuries (especially aortic rupture) sustained by car drivers in head-on collision. J. Trauma, *12*:715.
165. Cohen, A.M., Crass, J.R., Thomas, H.A. et al. (1992). CT evidence for the "osseous pinch" mechanism of traumatic aortic injury. A.J.R. Am. J. Roentgenol., *159*:271.
166. Eddy, A.C., Rusch, V.W., Marchioro, T. et al. (1990). Treatment of traumatic rupture of the thoracic aorta. A 15-year experience. Arch. Surg., *125*:1351.
167. Fabian, T.C., Davis, K.A., Gavant, M.L. et al. (1998). Prospective study of blunt aortic injury: Helical CT is diagnostic and antihypertensive therapy reduces rupture. Ann. Surg., *227*:666.
168. Fabian, T.C., Richardson, J.D., Croce, M.A. et al. (1997). Prospective study of blunt aortic injury: Multicenter Trial of the American Association for the Surgery of Trauma. J. Trauma, *42*:374.
169. Fenner, M.N., Fisher, K.S., Sergel, N.L. et al. (1990). Evaluation of possible traumatic thoracic aortic injury using aortography and CT. Am. Surg., *56*:497.
170. Fisher, R.G., Oria, R.A., Mattox, K.L. et al. (1990). Conservative management of aortic lacerations due to blunt trauma. J. Trauma, *30*:1562.
171. Gammie, J.S., Shah, A.S., Hattler, B.G. et al. (1998). Traumatic aortic rupture: Diagnosis and management. Ann. Thorac. Surg., *66*:1295.
172. Gavant, M.L., Menke, P.G., Fabian, T. et al. (1995). Blunt traumatic aortic rupture: Detection with helical CT of the chest. Radiology, *197*:125.
173. Greendyke, R.M. (1966). Traumatic rupture of aorta; special reference to automobile accidents. J.A.M.A., *195*:527.
174. Hartford, J.M., Fayer, R.L., Shaver, T.E. et al. (1986). Transection of the thoracic aorta: Assessment of a trauma system. Am. J. Surg., *151*:224.
175. Hoffer, E.K., Sclafani, S.J.A., Herskowitz, M.M., & Scalea, T.M. (1997). The natural history of arterial injuries diagnosed by arteriography. J. Vasc. Interv. Radiol., *8*:43.
176. Hunink, M.G., & Bos, J.J. (1995). Triage of patients to angiography for detection of aortic rupture after blunt chest trauma: Cost-effectiveness analysis of using CT. A.J.R. Am. J. Roentgenol., *165*:27.
177. Kato, N., Dake, M.D., Miller, C. et al. (1997). Traumatic thoracic aortic aneurysm: Treatment with endovascular stent-grafts. Radiology, *205*:657.

178. Kirsh, M.M., Behrendt, D.M., Orringer, M.B. et al. (1976). The treatment of acute traumatic rupture of the aorta: A 10-year experience. Ann. Surg., *184:*308.
179. Kram, H.B., Appel, P.L., Wohlmuth, D.A. et al. (1989). Diagnosis of traumatic thoracic aortic rupture: A ten-year retrospective analysis. Ann. Thorac. Surg., *47:*282.
180. Londevall, J. (1966). The mechanism of traumatic rupture of the aorta. Acta Pathol. Microbiol. Scand., *62:*34.
181. Marin, M.L., Veith, F.J., Panetta, T.F. et al. (1994). Transluminally placed endovascular stented graft repair for arterial trauma. J. Vasc. Surg., *20:*466.
182. Mirvis, S.E., Bidwell, J.K., Buddemeyer, E.U. et al. (1987). Value of chest radiography in excluding traumatic aortic rupture. Radiology, *163:*487.
183. Mirvis, S.E., Bidwell, J.K., Buddemeyer, E.U. et al. (1987). Imaging diagnosis of traumatic aortic rupture. A review and experience at a major trauma center. Invest. Radiol., *22:*187.
184. Mirvis, S.E., Pais, S.O., & Shanmuganathan, K. (1994). Atypical results of thoracic aortography performed to exclude aortic injury. Emerg. Radiol., *1:*24.
185. Mirvis, S.E., Shanmuganathan, K., Miller, G.H. et al. (1996). Traumatic aortic injury: Diagnosis with contrast-enhanced thoracic CT—five-year experience at a major trauma center. Radiology, *200:*413.
186. Moar, J.J. (1985). Traumatic rupture of the thoracic aorta. An autopsy and histopathological study. S. Afr. Med. J., *67:*383.
187. Morse, S.S., Glickman, M.G., Greenwood, L.H. et al. (1988). Traumatic aortic rupture: False-positive aortographic diagnosis due to atypical ductus diverticulum. A.J.R. Am. J. Roentgenol., *150:*793.
188. Parmley, L.F., Thomas, W.M., Manion, W.C., & Jahnke, E.J. (1958). Nonpenetrating traumatic injury of the aorta. Circulation, *17:*1086.
189. Pezzela, A.T., Todd, E.P., Dillon, M.L. et al. (1978). Early diagnosis and individualized treatment of blunt thoracic aortic trauma. Am. Surg., *44:*699.
190. Raptopoulos, V., Sheinman, R.G., Phillips, D.A. et al. (1992). Traumatic aortic tear: Screening with chest CT. Radiology, *182:*667.
191. Sturm, J.T., Billiar, T.R., Dorsey, J.S. et al. (1985). Risk factors for survival following surgical treatment of traumatic aortic rupture. Ann. Thorac. Surg., *39:*418.
192. Wigle, R.L., & Moran, J.M. (1991). Spontaneous healing of a traumatic thoracic aortic tear: Case report. J. Trauma, *31:*280.
193. Willens, H.J., & Kessler, K.M. (2000). Transesophageal echocardiography in the diagnosis of diseases of the thoracic aorta. Part II. Atherosclerotic and traumatic diseases of the aorta. Chest, *117:*233.
194. Williams, D.M., Andrews, J.C., Chee, S.S. et al. (1994). Canine model of acute aortic rupture: Treatment with percutaneous delivery of a covered Z-stent—work in progress. J. Vasc. Interv. Radiol., *5:*797.
195. Williams, J.S., Graff, J.A., Uku, J.M., & Steining, J.P. (1994). Aortic injury in vehicular trauma. Ann. Thorac. Surg., *57:*726.
196. Woodring, J.H., & King, J.G. (1989). The potential effects of radiographic criteria to exclude aortography in patients with blunt chest trauma: Results of a study of 32 patients with proved aortic or brachiocephalic arterial injury. J. Thorac. Cardiovasc. Surg., *97:*456.
197. Woodring, J.H., Pulmano, C.M., & Stevens, R.K. (1982). The right paratracheal stripe in blunt chest trauma. Radiology, *143:*605.

Cardiac Injuries

198. Cimmino, C.V. (1967). Some radiodiagnostic notes on pneumomediastinum, pneumothorax, and pneumopericardium. Va. Med. Monthly, *94:*205.
199. Crow, N.E., & Brogdon, B.G. (1959). Interventricular septal defect secondary to nonpenetrating injury. Arch. Intern. Med., *103:*791.
200. Cummings, R.G., Wesly, R.L.R., Adams, D.H., & Lowe, J.E. (1984). Pneumopericardium resulting in cardiac tamponade. Ann. Thorac. Surg., *37:*511.
201. DiMarco, R.F., Layton, T.R., Manzetti, G.W., & Pellegrini, R.V. (1983). Blunt traumatic rupture of the right atrium and the right superior pulmonary vein. J. Trauma, *23:*353.
202. Flancbaum, L., Wright, J., & Siegel, J.H. (1986). Emergency surgery in patients with post-traumatic myocardial contusion. J. Trauma, *26:*795.
203. Glock, Y., Roux, D., Dalous, P., & Puel, P. (1986). Embrochage ventriculaire gauche sur fracture de côte après traumatisme ferme thoracique. Ann. Chir., *40:*98.
204. Harley, D.P., & Mena, I. (1986). Cardiac and vascular sequelae of sternal fractures. J. Trauma, *26:*553.
205. Karalis, D.G., Victor, M.F., Davis, G.A. et al. (1994). The role of echocardiography in blunt chest trauma: A transthoracic and transesophageal echocardiographic study. J. Trauma, *36:*53.
206. Lo, A.M., & Van Stiegmann, G. (1973). Cardiac rupture secondary to blunt trauma. Ill. Med. J., *143:*250.
207. Lynn, R.B. (1983). Delayed post-traumatic pneumopericardium producing acute cardiac tamponade. Can. J. Surg., *26:*62.
208. Mirvis, S.E., Indeck, M., Schorr, R.M., & Diaconis, J.N. (1986). Posttraumatic tension pneumopericardium: The "small heart" sign. Radiology, *158:*663.
209. Muwanga, C.L., Cole, R.P., Sloan, J.P. et al. (1986). Cardiac contusion in patients wearing seat belts. Injury, *17:*37.
210. Noon, G.P., Boulafendis, D., & Beall, A.C. (1971). Rupture of the heart secondary to blunt trauma. J. Trauma, *11:*122.
211. O'Sullivan, M.J., Spagna, P.M., Bellinger, S.B., & Doohen, D.J. (1972). Rupture of the right atrium due to blunt trauma. J. Trauma, *12:*208.
212. Parmley, L.F., Manion, W.C., & Mattingly, T.W. (1958). Nonpenetrating traumatic injury of the heart. Circulation, *18:*371.
213. Primm, R.K., Karp, R.B., & Schrank, J.P. (1979). Multiple cardiovascular injuries and motor vehicle accidents. J.A.M.A., *241:*2540.
214. Soulen, R.L., & Freeman, E. (1971). Radiologic evaluation of traumatic heart disease. Radiol. Clin. North Am., *9:*285.
215. Werne, C., Sagraves, S.G., & Costa, C. (1989). Mitral and tricuspid valve rupture from blunt trauma sustained during a motor vehicle collision. J. Trauma, *29:*113.
216. Westaby, S. (1977). Pneumopericardium and tension pneumopericardium after closed-chest injury. Thorax, *32:*91.

INDEX

Note: Page numbers followed by f indicate illustrations; those by a t, tables.

Abbreviated Injury Scale, 172, 173t–174t
Abdomen
  bleeding within, computed tomography of, 160, 161f, 161t
  trauma to
    computed tomography of, 159–160, 160t, 161f, 161t
    nonoperative management of, 162–163, 162t, 163f, 163t
    peritoneal lavage in, 158
    screening evaluation of, 158–160, 160t
    sonographic assessment of, 158–160, 160t, 161t
Abscess, clostridial, 236
Acetabulum, 979–1002
  anatomy of, 979, 980f–981f
  anterior (iliopubic) column of, 979, 980f–982f
    fracture of, 988, 989f, 991f–993f
  associated fracture of, 986, 988, 989f
  both column fracture of, 986f–987f, 991, 999f
  central fracture-dislocation of, 986, 988f
  computed tomography of, 938, 939f, 982, 984f–987f, 986
  elementary fracture of, 986, 988, 989f
  fracture of, 979–1002, 1069f
    bone fragment trapping in, 982, 986
    classification of, 986, 988, 989f
    complications of, 1002, 1004f
    computed tomography of, 89–90, 93f, 941, 942f, 1037–1038, 1039f
    pediatric, 1007, 1007f–1010f, 1009
    radiography of, 91f
    Salter-Harris type 2, 1007, 1007f–1010f, 1009
    three-dimensional reconstruction of, 939
    treatment of, 1002
      computed tomography in, 982, 986f–987f
  fracture-dislocation of, central T-shaped, 1004f
  ilioischial line on, 979, 982f
  iliopectineal (arcuate) line on, 979, 982f
  insufficiency fracture of, 1002
  obturator oblique projection of, 982, 983f
  occult fracture of, 995, 1000, 1000f–1002f, 1002
    computed tomography of, 1002, 1002f
    obturator internus sign in, 995, 1000, 1001f
    vs. hip fracture, 1000, 1002, 1002f
  pathologic fracture of, 1002, 1003f, 1004f
  posterior (ilioischial) column of, 979, 980f–982f
    fracture of, 985f, 988, 989f, 990f, 991, 994f, 1074f
Acetabulum *(Continued)*
    in posterior hip dislocation, 1072, 1076f, 1077f
  quadrilateral surface of, 979
  radiography of, 979, 982, 982f, 983f
  roof of, 979, 982f
  sciatic buttress of, 979, 980f
  stress fracture of, 1002
  superolateral margin of, accessory ossification center at, 941, 944f
    vs. fracture, 1039, 1041
  transverse fracture of, 991, 995, 995f–999f
    central dislocation with, 995, 996f
    complex, 995, 998f, 999f
    computed tomography of, 995, 997f
    posterior rim fracture with, 984f, 985f, 995, 997f, 1001f
    T-shaped, 995, 998f, 999f
  triradiate cartilage fracture of, 935f–936f
  T-shaped fracture of, 983f
  undisplaced fracture of, 1001f
  wall fracture of, 988, 989f, 990f
Achilles tendon
  in calcaneal tuberosity beak fracture, 1337–1338, 1339f
  magnetic resonance imaging of, 96f, 1238f
  rupture of, 1284–1285, 1284f–1286f
    magnetic resonance imaging of, 1284–1285, 1284f, 1285f
    pre-Achilles triangle in, 1230
Acromioclavicular joint
  anatomy of, 604
  injury to, 604–607
    radiography of, 597, 604–605, 606f–608f
    Rockwood classification of, 605, 609f
    treatment of, 607
    types of, 605, 609f, 610f
  pseudodislocation of, 605, 611f
  sprains of, 605, 609f, 610f
  sternoclavicular dislocation with, 607
  subluxation of, 605
Acromioclavicular ligament, 599f
  injury to, 605, 606f
Acromion process, fracture of, 626, 627f
Adductor aponeurosis, in ulnar collateral ligament tear, 916–917
Adductor brevis, avulsion of, pediatric, 1012
Adductor longus, avulsion of, pediatric, 1012
Aerocele, subgaleal, 305
Aging
  bone strength effects on, 19
  in fracture, 26–28, 26f, 27f
Alveolar process, fracture of, 358–359, 359f
Amphiarthrosis, 12, 13, 14f
Amputation, traumatic, open fracture in, 41, 43f
Angulation, 18, 18f
Anisotropy, 18
Ankle, 1222–1314
  abduction of, 1236
  adduction of, 1236
    talar dome osteochondral fracture from, 1289, 1292f
  anatomy of, 1223–1225, 1223f–1225f
  bimalleolar fracture of, 1249
    supination–external rotation and, 1258f
    treatment of, 1280
  computed tomography of, 1231, 1234f–1236f
  dislocation of, 1281
  disuse osteoporosis of, 214f
  dorsiflexion of, 1236
  epiphyseal injury to, 1296–1297, 1297f–1300f, 1301, 1302f–1305f
    classification of, 1312–1313
    mechanism of, 1296
    pediatric, 1296
    treatment of, 1313–1314
  epiphyseal-ligament relationships of, pediatric, 1289, 1295f
  eversion of, 1236
  external rotation of, 1236
    injury pathomechanics in, 1238–1239, 1239f
    proximal fibular fracture and, 1161
  fracture of
    pre-Achilles triangle in, 1230, 1231f
    tension injury in, 1240, 1240f
    transverse forces in, 20
    types of, 1240–1254
  fracture-dislocation of, 1249
    in proximal tibiofibular joint dislocation, 1164
    transverse-oblique, 44f
    trimalleolar, 1242f
  greenstick fracture of, 1289, 1295f
  injury to
    angular/rotary force in, 1240
    classification of, 1254–1279
    Danis-Weber (AO) classification of, 1254–1255, 1255t, 1267, 1269, 1269f
    displacement, 1249, 1252f
    hemorrhage in, 1230, 1231f
    history of, 1222–1223
    Lauge-Hansen classification of, 1255–1270, 1256t
      Dupuytren's fracture in, 1270, 1274f
      key to, 1269–1270
      Maisonneuve's fracture in, 1270, 1275f–1278f
      pilon (pestle) fracture in, 1270, 1271f–1273f
      pronation-abduction in, 1267, 1267f–1269f

Ankle *(Continued)*
pronation-dorsiflexion in, 1267
pronation–external rotation in, 1263, 1265f, 1266f, 1267
supination-adduction in, 1256, 1257f
supination–external rotation in, 1257, 1259f–1264f, 1263
mechanism of, 1236, 1239–1240
pediatric, 1289–1314
radiography of, 78, 78t
interpretation of, 1279–1280
soft tissue features in, radiography of, 1230, 1230f, 1231f
stable, 1239, 1239f
tension force in, 1240, 1240f
treatment of, 1279–1280
unstable, 1239, 1239f
instability of, osteoarthritis from, 1381
inversion of, 1236
joint capsule of, ligaments and, 1224–1225, 1225f
la ligne claire in, 1225, 1226f, 1227
lateral clear space in, 1225, 1226f, 1227
levers of, 1238–1239, 1239f
ligamentous injury to, 1380–1381, 1383f
arthrography of, 1231
radiography of, 1230, 1230f, 1231f, 1249, 1252f
ligaments of, epiphysis and, in children, 1289, 1295f
magnetic resonance imaging of, 1231, 1236, 1237f, 1238f
medial clear space of, 1227
mortise of, talus and, 1238
neuropathic fracture of, in diabetes, 1282, 1283f, 1284
plantar flexion of, 1236
radiography of, 1225, 1226f–1233f, 1227, 1229–1231
anteroposterior projection in, 1225, 1226f
45-degree oblique views in, 1229, 1229f
full-length tibia/fibula views in, 1229–1230
internal oblique projection in, 1225, 1226f, 1227, 1228f
interpretation of, 1230, 1230f, 1231f
lateral view in, 1227, 1227f
mortise view in, 1227
"poor" ("off"-) lateral view in, 1227, 1229, 1229f
pre-Achilles triangle in, 1230, 1231f
stress views in, 1230–1231, 1232f, 1233f
as ring, 1239, 1239f
sprain fracture of, 1240f
sprains of, 1249, 1254, 1254f, 1255f
reflex dystrophy syndrome from, 254f
stenosing synovitis from, 1384
toddler's fracture of, 1289, 1295f
transverse fracture of, 1240f
trimalleolar fracture of, 1249
tibial spiral fracture with, 1282, 1283f
trimalleolar fracture-dislocation of, 1261f
Ankylosing spondylitis, vertebral fracture in, 526, 532f, 533–534, 533f
Annular ligament, 684
Anterior drawer sign, in lateral collateral ligament rupture, 1230–1231, 1233f, 1254, 1255f
Anterolisthesis, cervical spine, 436
Anticoagulants, in fracture healing, 209
Aorta, disruption of, 583–587
angiography of, 584–585, 584f, 585f
chest radiograph in, 584, 584f
computed tomography of, 584, 586f, 587f
diagnosis of, 583
great vessel injury in, 584, 585f

Aorta *(Continued)*
imaging of, 152, 153f, 155f
isthmus in, 583–584, 584f
pathophysiology of, 583–584
repair of, 585, 587
transesophageal echocardiography of, 585
Apophysis, 12, 13f
pelvic, avulsion fracture of, 1009, 1010f–1014f, 1012
separation of, 117, 120, 121f, 128
vs. avulsion fracture, 127, 127f
Arteriovenous fistula, traumatic pulmonary, 574
Artery(ies). *See also specific artery.*
of bone, 9, 9f
injury to
arteriography of, 232–234, 234f
fracture and, 231–234, 232f–234f
knee dislocation and, 1187, 1191
mechanism of, 231–232
signs/symptoms of, 232
sites for, 231
treatment of, 233–234
spasm of, 231
Arthritis
degenerative, 263, 265f, 266
after tibial plateau fracture, 1149
cervical spine, 440
retrolisthesis with, 436
neurotrophic
in diabetes, 1282, 1283f, 1284
insufficiency fracture in, 73, 74f
Arthropathy, lead, 266, 266f, 268
Articular cartilage, 13, 16, 16f
nutritional status of, 16
tidemark of, 49
Articular disc, 13
Athletics, femoral neck stress fracture from, 1052, 1053f
Atlantoaxial dislocation, 412, 415–416, 415f, 416f
with odontoid process fracture, 411
posterior, 416, 416f
rotary, 417–418
computed tomography of, 418, 421f
radiography of, 418, 419f, 420f
torticollis type, 417, 419f
traumatic, 417, 420f
traumatic, 415, 415f
V-shaped predens space in, 415, 415f
Atlantoaxial ligaments, in rotary atlantoaxial dislocation, 417
Atlantoaxial subluxation, in Down's syndrome, 415
Atlanto-occipital articulation, 394–418
dislocation of, 416–417, 417f, 418f
anatomic relationships in, 416–417
soft tissue swelling in, 416, 417f
traumatic, 416, 418f
X-line method for, 417, 418f
Atlas (C1), 394, 395f
anterior arch of
horizontal fracture of, 398
segmental fracture of, 398
arches of, developmental defects of, 400, 403, 405f
fracture of, 398–403
associated fractures with, 397, 397f, 398f
neurologic injury in, 418
Jefferson's fracture of, 398, 400, 401f–404f, 403
lateral mass of, medial fracture of, 398
neural arch of
fracture of, 398, 399f, 400f
vertical fracture of, 398, 399f
pseudospread of, upon axis, 400, 404f

Atrophy, disuse. *See* Disuse atrophy.
Austin-Moore prosthesis, osteomyelitis after, 249f
Automobile accidents, pediatric pelvic fracture in, 1002, 1005, 1005f
Autonomic neuropathy, 1384
Avascular necrosis
in femoral neck fractures, 1056–1057
of humeral head, 639
Avulsion, Sharpey's fibers in, 16
Avulsion fracture
calcaneal, 1333, 1335f, 1338, 1339f, 1340f
cervical vertebral body, 440–441
cuboidal, 1369, 1375f
distal humeral, 693f
fifth metatarsal, 1319–1320, 1393, 1394f, 1403, 1403f
fovea capitis, 1069, 1071f
greater femoral trochanter, 1063, 1064f
in hangman's fracture, 403, 407f
lesser femoral trochanter, 1063, 1065f, 1066f
malleolar, 1246, 1246f
peroneal tendon dislocation in, 1246, 1248f
with subtalar joint dislocation, 1358, 1360f
metacarpal head, 897, 898f
patellar, 1164, 1167, 1169
pelvic, 971–972
apophyseal, pediatric, 1009, 1010f–1014f, 1012
phalangeal
foot, 1388f
hand, 876f
proximal humeral, 635f
proximal tibial, 1154–1157, 1156f, 1157f
scaphoidal, 829
scapular, 625, 627f
Sharpey's fibers in, 46
talar, 1354, 1354f
talonavicular, 1364
tibial, 1154–1157, 1156f, 1157f
of anterior apophysis, 1180, 1181f
of anterior tubercles, 1246, 1248, 1249f, 1250f
of intercondylar eminence, 1152–1154, 1154f, 1155f
lateral, 1157–1158, 1158f, 1159f
tibial spine, 1131f, 1152–1153, 1154f–1156f
transverse process, in first rib fracture, 553, 553f
ulnar coronoid process, 708, 709f
ulnar olecranon, posteromedial elbow dislocation with, 710f
uncinate process, 440–441
volar plate, 876f
vs. apophyseal separation, 127, 127f
Axillary artery, injury to
in anterior shoulder dislocation, 658
in proximal humerus fractures, 638
Axis (C2), 394, 395f
anterior inferior margin of, fracture of, 412, 414f
body of, fracture of, 410, 411–412, 413f
fracture of, 403, 406f–414f, 408–412
associated fractures with, 397, 397f, 398f
neurologic injury in, 418
hangman's fracture of, 403, 406f–409f, 408. *See also* Hangman's fracture.
hypertension teardrop fracture of, 412, 414f
neural arch of, fracture of. *See* Hangman's fracture.

Bankart lesion, 671
with shoulder dislocation, 654

Barton's fracture, 789, 792f
Baseball, humeral shaft fracture in, 648f, 649
Baseball finger, 880, 881f, 882, 882f
  swan neck deformity with, 880, 882f
Basic multicellular unit, in fracture healing, 205
Battered child syndrome, 132–137
  bone scans in, 137
  bucket handle fracture in, 132, 135, 136f, 137f
  clinical findings in, 132
  corner fracture in, 132, 135, 136f
  diaphyseal fracture in, 132
  differential diagnosis of, 137
  metaphyseal fracture in, 132, 133f, 134f, 135, 136f
  radiography of, 132, 133f, 134f
  rib fractures in, 132, 135, 135f
  shaking in, 135
  skull fracture in, 135, 136f
Beak fracture, of calcaneal tuberosity, 1337–1338, 1339f
Bending, 18, 18f
Bennett's fracture, 911–912, 913f, 914f
  pediatric, 923
Biceps tendon, rupture of, 727, 729f
Bifurcate ligament, calcaneal avulsion fracture at, 1337
Biomechanics, 17–24
  of fracture, 17–19, 17f–19f
Birth
  clavicular fracture in, 599, 603f
  distal humeral epiphyseal separation in, 754, 755f
  epiphyseal separation in, 125–126, 126f
  ossification centers at, 11–12
  proximal femoral epiphyseal separation in, 1088, 1091f
  proximal humeral epiphyseal separation in, 642, 647f
Bladder, injury to, pelvic fracture and, 1015, 1018f–1023f
Bleeding. *See* Hemorrhage.
Bone
  accessory, fracture of, 49
  cancellous, 7
  cartilaginous, endochondral ossification in, 9
  characteristics of, 6
  classification of, 6–7, 6f
  compact, 7–9, 8f
  composition of, 7–9
  compression strength of, 19
  density of
    fracture risk and, 34, 36–37, 36f
    in osteoporosis, 33–34
    therapy monitoring and, 37
  fatigue of, 18–19
  fibered, 10
  flat, 7, 7f
    fracture of, 49
  formation of. *See* Ossification.
  fragmentation of, crush injuries and, 23
  growth of, vascular supply of, 11, 11f
  healing of, 203–229
    biochemical events in, 203
    histologic stages of, 203–204, 203f
  heterotopic formation of, 258–259, 260f
  hypertrophy of, in forearm valgus stress fracture, 722, 724f
  irregular, 7, 8f
    fracture of, 49
  lamellar, 8f, 9, 19, 19f
  lengthening of, external fixation for, 194–195, 197
  long, 6, 6f, 7
    fracture of. *See* Fracture, long bone.
Bone *(Continued)*
  mature, 7, 8f
    vs. osteoporotic, 29, 30f
  microcracking of, 18–19, 19f
  porosity of, in children vs. adults, 111, 112f
  radiograph of, 6
  resorption of, 255, 256f
  short, fracture of, 49
  spongy, 7
  strength of
    aging effects on, 19
    osteons in, 19
  stress response of, 1330
  subchondral
    in bone bruises, 54
    in osteochondral fracture, 52
  tensile strength of, 19
  trabecular, 7, 8f
  tubular, 7
  vascular supply of, 9, 9f
  woven, 10
    formation of, 11
Bone bruise, 52–54, 53f, 54f
  femoral/tibial, magnetic resonance imaging of, 1124, 1125f–1127f, 1126–1127
  foot, 1331–1332
  magnetic resonance imaging of, 52–54, 53f, 54f, 94, 95f
  with osteochondral fracture, 53f
  patellar, 1167, 1169f
Bone cyst
  aneurysmal, post-traumatic, 268, 268f
  pediatric, pathologic fracture with, 137, 138f
Bone grafting, 197–199
  allograft, 197–198
  autograft, 198
  cancellous, 198–199, 199f
  cortical, 198, 198f
  material for, 197
Bone morphogenetic protein, 204
Bosworth fracture, juvenile, 1310, 1312
Boutonnière deformity, 885, 886f, 887f
Bowel injury
  computed tomography of, 163–164, 164f
  in pelvic fracture, 1024f, 1025, 1025f
Bowing fracture, 114–115, 116f, 117f
  pediatric, 84f, 766–767
Boxer's fracture, 888, 894, 894f–896f
Brachial artery, injury to, 231, 684
  pediatric elbow dislocation and, 765
  posterior elbow dislocation and, 711–712
Brachial plexus, injury to, 439f
  in proximal humeral fractures, 638
Brachiocephalic artery, transection of, 585f
Brain, in head injury, 273–275, 274f
Breast cancer, pathologic fracture in, 80f, 81f
Bronchus, rupture of, 579, 579f–582f, 581
  in first rib fracture, 553
Brown tumors, insufficiency fracture in, 70, 72f
Brown-Séquard syndrome, 443
Bucket handle fracture, in battered child syndrome, 132, 135, 136f, 137f
Bunk bed fracture, 1400, 1401f
Burst fracture
  cranial, 306
  lower cervical spine, 422, 423f
  lumbar spine. *See* Lumbar spine, burst fracture of.
  thoracic spine. *See* Thoracic spine, burst fracture of.
Buttonhole deformity, 885, 886f, 887f

C1. *See* Atlas (C1).
C2. *See* Axis (C2).
Calcaneal ligament, injury to, 1383f
Calcaneocuboid joint, dislocation of, 1371, 1377f
Calcaneofibular ligament, 1224, 1224f
  anterior, avulsion of, 1381, 1383f
  magnetic resonance imaging of, 1237f
  rupture of, 1254
    supination-adduction in, 1256
Calcaneus, 1319f, 1332–1348
  anatomy of, 1332–1333, 1333f
  anterior process of
    avulsion fracture of, 1337, 1337f
    fracture of, 1333, 1335, 1336f, 1337
      cuboid compression fracture with, 1369
      forefoot abduction and, 1337, 1339f
      magnetic resonance imaging of, 1337, 1338f
  avulsion fracture of, 1333, 1335f, 1337, 1337f
  comminuted fracture of, 1341, 1343
  compression fracture of, 86f, 1338, 1340–1341, 1341f–1345f, 1343, 1345
    centrolateral depression type, 1340, 1341f, 1343f
    computed tomography of, 1346f–1348f
    fragment position in, 1340–1341, 1341f
    joint depression type, 1340, 1341f
    residuals of, 1346, 1349f
    split, 1341, 1344f
    tongue type, 1340, 1341f, 1346f–1348f
  computed tomography of, 1326f, 1329f
  fracture of
    Boehler's angle in, 1332–1333, 1333f, 1343, 1345
    complications of, 1346, 1349f
    computed tomography of, 89, 1343, 1344f–1345f, 1345–1346, 1347f–1349f
    distribution of, 1333, 1334f
    healing of, computed tomography of, 226, 226f
    navicular tuberosity fracture with, 1364, 1367f
    pediatric, 1400
    peroneal tendons in, 1346, 1350f
    pre-Achilles triangle in, 1230, 1231f
    soft tissue swelling in, 1333
    spinal fracture with, 1333, 1334f
    stenosing synovitis from, 1384
    treatment of, 1346, 1348
  insufficiency fracture of, 1348, 1352f
  noncompressive fracture of, 1333, 1335, 1335f–1340f, 1337–1338
  occult fracture of, 1331, 1332f
    pediatric, 1400, 1400f
  radiography of, 1324–1325, 1325f
  stress fracture of, 58, 59f, 63, 1329, 1348, 1351f
    magnetic resonance imaging of, 1331, 1331f, 1332f
    radiography of, 1330
  toddler's fracture of, 1400, 1400f
  tongue-type fracture of, 1332f
  tuberosity of
    avulsion fracture of, 1338, 1339f, 1340f
    beak fracture of, 1337–1338, 1339f
    vertical fracture of, 1333, 1335f
Calcar femorale, 1031, 1032f
Callus
  in fracture healing, 205, 218
  in fracture union, 216
  in internal fixation, 248
  periosteal, in stress fracture, 58, 58f
  radiography of, 209, 210f, 211f
Calvaria
  comminuted fracture of, 289

Calvaria (Continued)
depressed fracture of, 289–290, 292, 292f–294f
blow-in, 290, 292f
dural tear in, 290
ping-pong, 290, 293f, 294f
diastatic fracture of, 289, 290f, 291f
fracture of, 287–292
old vs. recent, 288–289
linear fracture of, 287–289
computed tomography of, 288
vs. cranial sutures, 288, 289f
multiple fracture of, 289
Canal of Guyon, computed tomography of, 821, 823f
Canaliculi, in haversian system, 8f, 9
Canthal ligament, medial, in naso-orbital-ethmoidal fracture, 353, 356
Capitate, 813
avascular necrosis of, 846
computed tomography of, 821, 822f
coronal fracture of, 846
45-degree pronation oblique view of, 818, 819f
fracture of, 827, 843–846, 844f
associated fractures with, 844, 846f
mechanism of, 844, 846f
perilunate dislocation with, 844, 846f
proximal fragment with, 844, 844f–845f, 846
scaphoid dislocation with, 844, 845f
scaphoid fracture with, 834
head of, fracture of, 844, 846f
with lunate dislocation, 854, 858f
lateral view of, 818, 818f
waist of, fracture of, 844, 845f, 846f
Capitellum, fracture of, radiography of, 685
Capitolunate joint
disruption of, in perilunate dislocation, 851, 852f
instability of, 866
lateral view of, 818
Cardiac tamponade, 587–588
Carotid artery, injury to
imaging of, 164, 166
in transverse sphenoid fracture, 298, 299f
Carpal instability, 855, 857, 859–861, 859f–863f
axis alignment measurement in, 857, 859, 860f
dorsal, 860, 860f–862f
forms of, 859–860, 863, 866
link joint concept in, 857, 859f
longitudinal axes in, 860–861
palmar, 860, 863f
perilunar, 860, 863f
radiography of, 857
treatment of, 861
Carpal ligament, transverse, 821
Carpal tunnel
computed tomography of, 819, 821, 821f–823f
radiography of, 818
Carpal tunnel syndrome, computed tomography of, 821, 823f
Carpometacarpal joint
dislocation of, 904–909
diagnosis of, 907
distribution of, 905, 907
dorsal, 908f
hamate fracture with, 907, 909, 912f
mechanism of, 907
in metacarpal base fracture, 897
metacarpal shaft fracture in, 909
multiple, 909f
radiography of, 904, 905f
Carpometacarpal joint (Continued)
fifth, dislocation of, 907f, 908f, 909
first, dislocation of, 920, 921f, 922f
fracture-dislocation at, posterior, 909, 910f
movements of, 879
Carpus, 7, 813–867
accessory ossification centers in, 827, 828f, 829
anatomy of, 813–814, 814f, 815f
axial dislocation of, 855, 859f
dislocation of, 850
classification of, 852
radial rim fracture with, 789, 792f
radiography of, 854–855
distal row of, 813, 814
fracture of, 826–867
diagnosis of, 827
frequency of, 826–827
magnetic resonance imaging of, 821, 826, 826f
vs. tendon calcification, 827, 828f
injury to
arthrography of, 826, 827f
bone scans of, 819, 820f
computed tomography of, 819, 821, 821f–825f
prayer position in, 821, 821f
fracture-dislocation patterns in, 814–815
magnetic resonance imaging of, 821, 826, 826f
pathomechanics of, 814–815, 816f
posteroanterior view of, 815, 817f
radiography of, 815–819, 817f–820f
carpal tunnel view in, 818, 820f
45-degree oblique views in, 818, 819f
lateral view in, 818, 818f
magnification view in, 818–819
stages of, 815
tomography of, 819
zone of vulnerability in, 814, 815, 816f
instability of, 855, 857, 859–861, 859f–863f
ligamentous structures of, 813, 814f
as link joint, 857, 859f
mid-
fracture-dislocation of, 852, 854f
instability of, 866
parallel arcs of, 817, 817f
proximal row of, 813, 814
subluxation of
dorsal, 866
palmar, 866
volar ligaments of, 813, 814f
Cartilage
articular, 13, 16, 16f
nutritional status of, 16
tidemark of, 49
formation of, 11
hyaline, 13, 16, 16f
secondary centers of ossification and, 11, 13f
Cartilaginous growth plate, 10f, 11
histologic zones of, 117, 119f
Cast
as brace, 180, 182, 183f
cutting of, 180, 181f, 182f
fiberglass, 182
history of, 180
plaster-of-Paris, 180, 181f
radiopacity of, 180, 181f
splint with, 180, 181f
wedging of, 180, 182f
Cataract, traumatic, 342
Cellulitis, anaerobic, 236
Central cord syndrome, 440, 442–443
quadriplegia with, 427f
Cephalhydrocele, 306
Cerebral contusion, computed tomography of, 275, 277, 279f, 280f
Cerebral palsy, pathologic fracture in, 142
Cerebrospinal fluid otorrhea
skull fracture and, 305–306, 305f
temporal bone fracture and, 302
Cerebrospinal fluid rhinorrhea, skull fracture and, 305–306, 305f
computed tomographic cisternography of, 306
Cervical spine, 376–498
anterolisthesis of, 436
articular pillars of, fracture of, 441–442
compression fracture of, 421f
convex lines of, 390, 391f
degenerative arthritis of, retrolisthesis with, 436
delayed dislocation of, 435
dislocation of, in hyperflexion strain, 436
extension injury to, 378f, 379, 532f
facet locking of, 422, 427f–432f, 432
bilateral, 422, 427f
computed tomography of, 432, 432f
fracture with, 431f–432f, 432
fracture-dislocation with, 422, 428f, 432
unilateral, 422, 427f, 429f, 432, 433f
facets of, fracture of, 441–442
fracture of, 384–394
in ankylosing spondylitis, 526, 533–534, 533f
computed tomography of, 391, 394
in diffuse idiopathic skeletal hyperostosis, 534, 535f
distribution of, 376–377, 376f
hematoma in, 386
incidence of, 385f
intervertebral disc space in, 389
lateral translation, 388f
magnetic resonance imaging of, 391, 394
malalignment in, 389, 390f–394f, 391
multiple-level injury in, 526
nasopharyngeal soft tissue swelling in, 386
neurologic deficit in, 376–377
prevertebral fat stripe in, 389
radiography of, 384–386, 385f–389f, 389, 391
retropharyngeal soft tissue swelling in, 385–386, 389, 389f
spinous processes in, 391
swimmer's view of, 384, 387f
vertebral body height abnormalities in, 391
fracture-dislocation of, 170f, 387f, 388f
hematoma of, 385f
hyperextension injury to, 436–442
with fracture, 437f, 438f
fracture-dislocation in, 441
with spondylosis, 440f, 441
strain type, 439–440, 440f
types of, 436, 439, 440f
hyperflexion strain of, 381f, 432, 434f–436f, 435–436
injury to
classification of, 379–380, 380t
compression forces in, 378f, 379
computed tomographic myelography of, 384
computed tomography of, 381, 382f–383f, 383–384
in degenerative arthritis, 440
distraction forces in, 378f, 379
distribution of, 376, 376f
flexion forces in, 378–379, 378f
imaging of, 380–384
incidence of, 376, 376f

Cervical spine *(Continued)*
magnetic resonance imaging of, 384, 384f, 385f
neurologic injury with, 442–443
pathomechanical classification of, 379–380, 380t
pathomechanics of, 378–379, 378f
radiography of, 380–381, 381f
rotational forces in, 378f, 379
second-level injuries in, 168, 171f, 172f
shearing forces in, 378f, 379
soft tissue status in, 380
in spondylosis, 440
stability of, 380
without obvious fracture, 442, 443f
intervertebral disc herniation of, 385f
laminae of, fracture of, 442
lower, injury to, 418, 421f–443f, 422–443
classification of, 418
radiography of, 418
normal radiographic appearance of, 392f–393f
polytrauma to, imaging studies of, 148–150, 148f–149f, 150t
posterior elements of, fracture of, 441–442
pseudosubluxation of, 394f
radiography of, oversights in, 168, 170f
retrolisthesis of, 436
spinous processes of, fracture of, 441
spondylosis of, 426, 427f
retrolisthesis with, 436
teardrop fracture of, 384f, 422, 424f, 425f
transverse processes of, fracture of, 442
vertebral body of
avulsion fracture of, 440–441
vertical split of, 422
whiplash injury to, 436
Cervicothoracic junction, flexion injuries to, 397, 398f
Chance-type fracture, lumbar spine. *See* Lumbar spine, Chance-type fracture of.
Charcot foot, 1384
Charcot joint, spinal, vs. Kümmell phenomenon, 495
Chest trauma, radiography of, 588–589
Child abuse
first rib fracture in, 554–555
skull fracture in, 307, 308f, 309f
Children
ankle injury in, 1289–1314
anterior tibial spine avulsion fracture in, 1152
apophyseal separation in, 117
battered, 132–137. *See also* Battered child syndrome.
bone porosity in, 111, 112f
bow fracture in, 114–115, 116f, 117f
bowing forearm fracture in, 84f, 714, 766–767
depressed calvaria fracture in, 290, 292, 293f, 294f
distal femoral epiphyseal injury in, 1209–1212, 1209f–1214f, 1215
distal humeral epiphyseal injury in, 752, 753f–756f, 754, 757
distal radial fracture in, 804–813
distal ulnar fracture in, 804–813
elbow dislocation in, 763–765, 764f
elbow injury in, 730–771
elbow traction injury in, 722, 726
epiphyseal injury in, 116–132. *See also* Epiphyseal injury.
facial fracture in, 315
fat pad sign in, in elbow injuries, 687
femoral intertrochanteric fracture in, 1088–1089, 1092f
Children *(Continued)*
femoral neck fracture in, 1088–1089, 1092f
first rib fracture in, 554–555
foot fracture in, 1400–1401, 1400f–1403f
forearm fractures in, 730–771
fracture in, 111–142
classification of, 111, 113f
joint effusion in, 111, 113f
radiography of, 111
Galeazzi fracture in, 770–771
greenstick fracture in, 111, 112, 114f, 115f, 806, 808f
growing skull fracture in, 306–307, 307f
hand dislocations in, 923, 925
hand fractures in, 920–921, 922f–926f, 923
head injury in, 274
hip dislocation in, 1089–1090, 1093f
hip injuries in, 1086–1090
humeral shaft fracture in, 649
infrapatellar tendon rupture in, 1178
knee injury in, frequency of, 1130
lead pipe fracture in, 113, 115f
lumbar spine injury in, 453
mandibular fracture in, 368, 372
medial epicondylar injury in, 744–752
Monteggia fracture in, 767, 768f–770f, 770
odontoid process fracture in, 410, 412f
olecranon fracture in, 761, 762f, 763, 763f
olecranon stress fracture in, 707
pathologic fracture in, 137–142
after radiation therapy, 142
in β-thalassemia, 138, 141f
bone cyst and, 137–142
in cerebral palsy, 142
compression, 138, 139f
in idiopathic juvenile osteoporosis, 138
in myelomeningocele, 138, 142, 142f
nonossifying fibroma and, 137, 139f
osteogenesis imperfecta and, 138, 140f
in renal osteodystrophy, 138, 141f
in rickets of prematurity, 138
pelvic fracture in, 1002, 1005–1012
proximal femoral epiphyseal injury in, 1086–1088, 1088f–1091f
proximal femoral epiphysiolysis in, 1087, 1089f
proximal humeral epiphyseal injury in, 642, 647f
proximal tibial epiphyseal injury in, 1209–1212, 1209f–1214f, 1215
pulled elbow in, 765, 765f
pulmonary contusion in, 546, 548f
radial fracture in, 765–772
radial head/neck fracture in, 757, 758f–761f, 761
spinal fracture-dislocation in, 507, 511f
splenic trauma in, nonoperative management of, 162, 162t
thoracic spine injury in, 453
tibial fracture in, 1196–1197, 1197f
toddler's fracture in, 115–116, 117f, 118f
torus fracture in, 112–113, 114f, 115f
ulnar fracture in, 765–772
vertebral bone density in, 111, 112f
vertebral compression fracture in, 489, 491f
voluntary shoulder dislocation in, 651
Chip fracture, 47. *See also* Avulsion fracture.
Chondral fracture, knee, 1180, 1182, 1185–1187
Chondroblasts, in fracture healing, 205
Chopart's joint, 1371, 1376f
dislocation of, 1371, 1376f, 1377f
Choroid, hemorrhage within, 342, 346f
Choroid plexus, calcification of, in head trauma, 287
Chylous effusion, thoracic duct rupture and, 561, 562f
Ciprofloxacin, in fracture healing, 209
Clavicle
anatomy of, 594, 596–597, 599f
epiphysis of, 596–597
fracture of, 597, 599, 601f–603f, 603–604
age in, 27
during birth, 599, 603f
complications of, 603–604
medial third, 599, 603f
mid-, 603
middle third, 597, 599, 601f
outer third, 599, 602f
pseudarthrosis of, 224f
radiography of, 597, 600f
medial epiphysis of
closure of, 11
in sternoclavicular dislocation, 610, 612f
metaphysis of, 596
osteolysis of, 256f
post-traumatic osteolysis of, 604
stress fracture of, 63, 599, 603
Clivus, fracture of, vascular injury in, 299f
Clostridium, in gas gangrene, 236–237
Coccyx, 931, 932f
fracture of, 955, 958f
Collagen, in bone, 7
Collateral ligament, 878, 878f
injury to
bone bruise with, 53
at metacarpophalangeal joint, 888, 890f
lateral, 1112f, 1113, 1224, 1224f
avulsion of, 1155
magnetic resonance imaging of, 1123, 1124f
rupture of, 1241
without fracture, 1253f
sprain of, 1249, 1254, 1254f, 1255f
anterior drawer sign in, 1230–1231, 1233f, 1254, 1255f
stress views of, 1230–1231, 1232f, 1233f
medial, 1112f, 1113, 1224, 1224f
avulsion of, 1155, 1240, 1241
injury to, 1156f
fibular head fracture with, 1161
magnetic resonance imaging of, 1122–1123, 1124f, 1237f
rupture of, 1270
in epiphyseal injury, 1210–1211, 1212f, 1214f
in lateral malleolus fracture, 1227
pronation-abduction and, 1267, 1267f–1269f
pronation–external rotation and, 1263, 1265f, 1266f
supination–external rotation and, 1257, 1262f, 1263f
in tibial plateau fracture, 1145, 1151f
without fracture, 1253f
stress radiography of, 1116
radial, 684, 685f, 813, 814f
avulsion of, 917, 920f, 921f
rupture of, 1240f
treatment of, 1280
tibial, magnetic resonance imaging of, 1122–1123
ulnar, 813, 814f
avulsion by, 795
injury to, 727
medial, 684, 685f
medial epicondyle, 744
tear of, 916–917, 917f–919f
valgus stress injury to, 726, 726f
Colles' fracture, 784–785, 786f–790f, 787–788
carpal instability from, 855
carpal tunnel syndrome after, 787–788

Colles' fracture *(Continued)*
elbow fracture with, 787
hip fracture with, 785, 786f
mechanism of, 785, 786f
in older population, 785
osteoporosis and, 32, 32f
proximal radial fractures with, 699
radiography of, 785, 787f–790f
reverse, 788
scaphoid fracture with, 834
treatment of, 787
Colliculus
anterior, 1223, 1223f, 1225
fracture of, 1242f
transverse fracture of, 1240, 1241f
posterior, 1223, 1223f, 1225
fracture of, 1240–1241, 1241f, 1242f
transverse fracture of, 1240, 1241f
Comminuted fracture, 20, 20f, 21, 41, 42f, 103
bone density in, 84
calcaneal, 1341, 1343
distal humeral, butterfly fragment with, 48f
femoral, 1090, 1093, 1094f, 1095f
fibular
cast for, 181f
degenerative arthritis after, 265f
first metacarpal, 912, 914f, 915f
humeral, compression plate fixation of, 212f
humeral head, 638, 642f
markedly, 41
metacarpal head, 897, 897f
moderately, 41, 42f
proximal femoral, 42f, 43f
proximal humeral, 636f
scapular, 619, 619f
severely, 41, 42f
skull, 285f
slightly, 41
thumb, 912, 914f, 915f
tibial, 51f
degenerative arthritis after, 265f
external fixation for, 196f–197f
open, 181f
osteomyelitis in, 247f
tibial plafond, 1231, 1236f
ulnar coronoid process, with anterior elbow subluxation, 707, 707f
Compartment syndrome, 234–236
lateral, of knee, 1161
tibial fracture in, 1197–1198, 1198f
Compression, 18, 18f
bone resistance to, 19
in epiphyseal injury, 120
osteoporotic, vertebral body, 492, 493f
in spinal cord injury, 378f, 379
Compression fracture, 49, 51f
bone density in, 84
calcaneal. *See* Calcaneus, compression fracture of.
cervical spine, 421f
cuboidal, navicular tuberosity fracture with, 1369, 1376f
femoral, with posterior hip dislocation, 1079, 1081, 1082f, 1083f
humeral head, 669
in shoulder dislocation, 658, 661f
lumbar spine, 172f, 460, 489, 491–492, 491f, 492f
simple, 480f
vs. wedge fracture, 466
pathologic, pediatric, 138, 139f
pelvic
anterior, 972, 974f, 975, 975f
imaging of, 940f–941f
lateral, 975, 976f, 977, 977f, 1022f, 1023f
Compression fracture *(Continued)*
spinal
bone scans of, 98
osteoporotic, 471, 475f, 491f, 492–493, 493f–496f
magnetic resonance imaging of, 493, 495f, 496f
vs. pathologic, 471, 474f, 492, 493f
pediatric, 138, 489, 491f
stress, femoral neck, 1053–1054
thoracic spine, 459f, 460, 489, 491–492, 491f, 492f
vs. wedge fracture, 466
thoracolumbar junction, 453
vertebral body, 49, 51f
wedge, spinal, 484
Compression plates, 185, 188, 188f
Computed tomography
of abdominal trauma, 159–160, 160t, 161f, 161t
of acetabular fracture, 89–90, 93f, 941, 942f, 982, 984f–987f, 986, 1037–1038, 1039f
of acetabulum, 938, 939f
of ankle, 1231, 1234f–1236f
of aortic disruption, 584, 586f, 587f
of atlantoaxial rotary dislocation, 418, 421f
of bowel injury, 163–164, 164f
of calcaneal compression fracture, 1346f–1348f
of calcaneal fracture, 89, 1343, 1344f–1345f, 1345–1346, 1347f–1349f
of calcaneal fracture healing, 226, 226f
of calcaneus, 1326f, 1329f
of calvaria fracture, 288
of canal of Guyon, 821, 823f
of capitate, 821, 822f
of carpal tunnel, 819, 821, 821f–825f
of carpal tunnel syndrome, 821, 823f
of cerebral contusion, 275, 277, 279f, 280f
of cerebral hematoma, 275, 280f
of cervical spine facet locking, 432, 432f
of cervical spine injuries, 381, 382f–383f, 383–384, 391, 394
of Chance-type fracture, 523, 524f
of cuboid bone, 1326f, 1329f
of cuneiform bone, 1327f, 1329f
of depressed skull fracture, 277, 282f, 283f
of diaphragmatic injury, 155, 158f, 159f, 575, 578f, 579
of distal tibial complex fracture, 1231, 1236f
of distal tibial epiphyseal triplane fracture, 1309f, 1310
of elbow injury, 689
of epidural hematoma, 275, 277, 278f, 279f
of epiphyseal injury, 127
of extensor carpi ulnaris tendon, 821
of extensor pollicis tendon, 821
of extra-axial hematoma, 275, 277
of facial fracture, 89, 315, 316, 323, 323f–326f, 325, 325t, 327t
of femoral condyles, 1118
of femoral head fracture, 1038, 1039f
of femoral neck fracture, 1040f
of first metatarsal, 821, 822f
of flexor hallucis longus tendon, 1326f
of foot, 1326–1327, 1326f–1329f
of forearm injury, 689, 795
of fracture, 88–90, 91f–93f, 93
of fracture healing, 225–226, 225f–229f
of glenohumeral joint dislocation, 652, 669, 670f, 671f
of hangman's fracture, 403, 407f
of head injury, 272–273, 273t, 275, 275f–284f, 277
helical, 89
Computed tomography *(Continued)*
of Hill-Sachs defect, 672f
of hip dislocation, 1069, 1073f–1075f
of hip fracture, 89, 92f, 1037–1038, 1039f–1041f
of hip posterior dislocation, 1073f, 1078f, 1079
of hook of hamate fracture, 819, 821, 822f, 848, 849f
of iliac wing fracture, 938, 938f
image reformatting in, 89
of insufficiency fracture, 68f, 69
of intertrochanteric femoral fracture, 1041f
of intracranial pneumocephalus, 303, 305f
of laryngeal fracture, 444–445, 445f
of lesser trochanter femoral fracture, 1040f
of liver trauma, 162–163, 163f, 163t
of lumbar spine fracture, 463, 464f–470f, 465–466
of lumbar spine fracture-dislocation, 516, 518f–520f
of lunate, 821, 822f
of malleolus, 1231, 1234f–1235f, 1326f, 1328f
of mandibular fractures, 369, 369f, 370f
of mediastinal polytrauma, 150, 152, 153f, 155f
of mesenteric trauma, 163–164, 164f
of midfoot fracture, 89
of nasal fracture, 353, 355f
of naso-orbital-ethmoidal fracture, 355f, 356–357, 356f
of navicular, 1326f, 1327f, 1329f
of navicular stress fracture, 1330
of occult acetabular fracture, 1002, 1002f
of odontoid process (dens) fracture, 410
of orbital blow-out fracture, 333f, 334f, 335, 335f
of patellofemoral joint, 1118
of pelvic fracture, 89, 91f
of pelvic insufficiency fracture, 960f–963f, 964
of pelvic open book anterior compression injury, 940f–941f
of pelvis, 934, 937–939, 938f–943f, 941
of penetrating abdominal trauma, 164, 166f
of peroneal tendons, 1326f, 1328f
of pilon (pestle) fracture, 226, 227f, 1270, 1272f, 1273f
of pisiform, 821, 822f
of pisotriquetral joint, 819, 821, 821f–823f
of pneumothorax, 564, 564f
of polytrauma, 147, 148
of posterior shoulder dislocation, 669, 670f, 671f
of proximal humerus, 634, 635f
quantitative, bone density measurement with, 34, 35f
of radioulnar dislocation, 802, 803f
of radioulnar joint, 819
of rib fractures, 546, 546f–548f
of sacral fracture, 967
of sacroiliac joint, 938, 939, 939f, 941
of sacrum, 938, 939f
of scaphoid fracture, 225f, 226, 821, 822f, 831
of scapular injuries, 620, 624f
of shoulder injuries, 594, 595f, 652, 671, 672f
of skull, 272–273, 273t
of skull base fracture, 89, 298
of skull fracture, 275, 275f–284f, 277, 298
of splenic trauma, 162, 162t
of sternal fracture, 89
of sternoclavicular joint dislocation, 612, 615f–617f, 617

Computed tomography *(Continued)*
  of stress fracture, 63–64
  of subdural hematoma, 275, 276f, 277, 277f, 281f
  of subtalar joint, 1326f
  of sustentaculum tali, 1329f
  of talocalcaneal joint, 1329f
  of talus, 1231, 1234f–1235f, 1328f
  of tarsal stress fracture, 1330
  of tarsus, 1326, 1326f–1327f, 1327
  of temporal bone fracture, 301, 302f
  of thoracic spine fracture, 463, 464f–470f, 465–466
  of thoracic spine polytrauma, 150, 151f
  three-dimensional, 89, 93
  of thromboembolism, 240
  of tibial fracture healing, 229f
  of tibial fracture nonunion, 228f
  of tibial plateau fracture, 1118, 1119f, 1143
  of tibiofibular joint, 1118, 1231, 1234f–1235f
  of transverse acetabular fracture, 995, 997f
  of trapezium, 821, 822f
  of trapezium fracture, 819
  of trapezoid, 821, 822f
  of triquetrum, 821, 822f
  of vertebral fracture, 89
  of zygomatic complex fracture, 348, 349f, 351f
Connective tissue, in synovial joint, 13
Conoid ligament, 594, 596
Contracture, Volkmann's, 234–236
Contusion, pulmonary, in rib fracture, 546, 548f
Cooley's anemia, pathologic fracture in, 138, 141f
Coracoclavicular ligament, 594, 596, 599f
  injury to, 605, 606f
Coracoid process, scapular
  fracture of, 605, 610f, 626–627, 628f, 629f
  stress fracture of, 63
Corner fracture, in battered child syndrome, 132, 135, 136f
Corner sign, in epiphyseal injury, 126
Coronal suture, diastasis of, 289, 290f, 291f
Coronoid process, ulnar
  avulsion fracture of, 708, 709f
  comminuted fracture of, with anterior elbow subluxation, 707, 707f
  fracture of, 707f–709f, 708
    with posterolateral elbow dislocation, 711, 712f
Cortex, bony, 6–7
Corticosteroids, in fracture healing, 209
Costoclavicular ligament, 607, 610, 612f
Cough fracture, 556, 556f
Cranial bones, developmental fissures of, vs. linear calvaria fractures, 288
Cranial fossa
  anterior, fracture of, cerebrospinal fluid rhinorrhea in, 305
  floor of, fracture of, 292, 294, 297f
Cranial sutures
  coronal, diastasis of, 289, 290f, 291f
  as fibrous joints, 12, 14f
  lambdoid, interdigitation of, 289f
  sagittal, diastasis of, 289, 290f, 291f
  vs. linear calvaria fractures, 288, 289f
Craniovertebral junction, 394–418
  dislocation/subluxation of, 412, 415–418, 415f–421f
  extension injuries to, 397, 398f
  fracture of
    associated fractures with, 397, 397f, 398f
    bony relationships in, 397
    forces causing, 395–396
Craniovertebral junction *(Continued)*
    ligamentous structure of, 394
    multiple-level, 526
    neurologic deficit in, 397–398, 418
    radiography of, 395, 395f, 396–397, 396f
    soft tissue swelling with, 397
Cranium
  burst fracture of, 306
  extension of, 394–395
  flexion of, 394–395
  foreign bodies in, 292, 294f–296f
  growing fracture of, 306
Cruciate ligament, 1111, 1112f
  anterior, 1112f, 1113
    avulsion of, in epiphyseal injury, 1211–1212
    insertion of, avulsion at, 1154–1155, 1156f
    magnetic resonance imaging of, 1121–1122, 1122f
    radiography of, 1116
    in Segond fracture, 1158f, 1159f
    tear of, 1152–1153, 1154f, 1155f
      bone bruise with, 53
      deep notch sign with, 1160, 1160f
      drawer sign in, 1116
      hemarthrosis in, 1128
    in tibial plateau fracture, 1145
  posterior, 1112f, 1113
    insertion of, avulsion at, 1155, 1155f
    magnetic resonance imaging of, 1122, 1123f
    radiography of, 1116
    tear of, 1153–1154, 1156f
      drawer sign in, 1116
      magnetic resonance imaging of, 1124, 1125f
Crush injuries, bone fragmentation in, 23
Cubital tunnel, 685, 685f
Cuboid bone, 1319f
  avulsion fracture of, 1369, 1375f
  compression fracture of, navicular tuberosity fracture with, 1369, 1376f
  computed tomography of, 1326f, 1329f
  fracture of, 1369
    navicular tuberosity fracture with, 1364, 1367f
  ligaments of, 1371
  stress fracture of, 1369
    radiography of, 1330
  toddler's fracture of, 1369
Cuneiform bone, 1319f
  computed tomography of, 1327f, 1329f
  dislocation of, with navicular crush fracture, 1366, 1371f
  fracture of, 1369, 1376f
    radiography of, 1321, 1323f
  ligaments of, 1371
  stress fracture of, 1369
    radiography of, 1330
Cuneonavicular joint, dislocation of, 1371, 1378f
Curved fracture, 20–21, 20f
Cyst
  aneurysmal bone, post-traumatic, 268, 268f
  bone, pediatric pathologic fracture with, 137, 138f
  leptomeningeal, 306
  traumatic lung, 570f, 572f

Dancer's fracture, 1385f, 1386, 1393–1394, 1394f
Death
  by age, 1, 2f
Death *(Continued)*
  motor vehicle accidents and, 1, 1f
  from trauma, 1, 1f, 2f
Deformation, force and, 18
Degenerative arthritis, 263, 265f, 266
  after tibial plateau fracture, 1149
  cervical spine
    injury in, 440
    retrolisthesis with, 436
Deltoid ligament, 1224, 1224f
Deltoid muscle, 645
Denis' three-column concept, of vertebral stability, 537, 537f
Depressed fracture, 23–24, 24f, 49
  calcaneal, 1340, 1341f, 1342f
  calvaria, 289–290, 292, 292f–294f
  metacarpal head, 897, 898f
  skull, 277, 282f, 283f
Diabetes mellitus
  neuroarthropathy in, 1384, 1385f
    fractures in, 1282, 1283f, 1284
  osteoarthropathy in, metatarsal stress fracture in, 1396, 1398f
Diaphragm
  evaluation of, in chest trauma, 589
  eventration of, imaging of, 155, 157f
  injury to
    computed tomography of, 155, 158f, 159f
    false-positive causes of, 155, 157f
    imaging diagnosis of, 152, 155, 156f–159f, 158
    magnetic resonance imaging of, 155, 159f
  penetrating injury to, computed tomography of, 155, 158, 159f
  rupture of, 574–575, 575f–577f, 579
    computed tomography of, 575, 578f, 579
    injuries associated with, 574, 576f
    nasogastric tube in, 575, 575f–578f
    pelvic fracture and, 1021
    pulmonary contusion with, 574, 577f, 578f
    radiography of, 574–575, 576f–578f
    traumatic, 155, 156f
Diaphysis, 6, 6f
  fracture of, in battered child syndrome, 132
  proximal, in Jones fracture, 1394, 1397f, 1398f
Diarthroses, 12, 14f
Diastasis, 55, 56f
Diffuse idiopathic skeletal hyperostosis
  epidural hematoma in, thoracic fracture-dislocation with, 473f
  fractures in, 534, 534f, 535f
Digit(s). *See also* Phalanx (phalanges).
  extensor mechanism of, 878–879, 879f
  injury to, radiography of, 875, 876f
Disc space, in spinal fracture, 455, 459f
Dislocation, 54–55, 55f–57f
  description of, 105
  epiphyseal separation in, 117
Distraction injury
  cervical spine, 378f, 379
  lumbar spine, 458f
Disuse atrophy
  cortical changes in, 214
  in fracture healing, 211, 214, 214f–217f, 216
  hyperemia in, 216
  osteoporosis in, 211, 214
  radiographic patterns in, 211
  resorption in, 211, 216f, 217f
  site involvement in, 211, 214f, 215f
  stress fracture from, 214, 216, 218f
  translucent bands in, 214
Dolan's lines, 330, 330f, 331f
Double vertebrae sign, 516, 519f
Dowager's hump, 492, 493f

Down's syndrome
atlantoaxial dislocation with, 412
atlantoaxial subluxation in, 415
Dual x-ray absorptiometry, bone density measurement with, 34
Dupuytren's fracture, 1252f, 1270, 1274f
pronationnexternal rotation and, 1263, 1266f
talus in, 1274f
Duverney's fracture, 954–955, 955f, 956f

Elastic modulus, 17, 17f
Elbow, 683–773
anatomy of, 683–685, 684f, 685f
anterior dislocation of, vs. Monteggia fracture, 716, 718f
anterior fracture-dislocation of, 705, 707, 707f
vs. Monteggia fracture, 767
anterior subluxation of, with ulnar coronoid process comminuted fracture, 707, 707f
arteries of, 684–685, 685f
condylar fracture of, pediatric, 738
dislocation of, 708, 709f–712f, 711–712
brachial artery injury with, 711–712
classification of, 708
fractures associated with, 711, 712f
joint instability with, 711
mechanism of, 711
median nerve entrapment with, 711
myositis ossificans with, 712
pediatric, 763–765, 764f
posterolateral, 708, 709f
posteromedial, 708, 710f
proximal radial fracture with, 699
divergent fracture-dislocation of, 708, 711f
effusion of
fat pad sign in, 686f, 687, 687f, 688f
pediatric, fat pad sign in, 730–731, 730f
fat pads of, 684, 686f, 688f
fracture of, in Colles' fracture, 787
fracture-dislocation of, wires for, 186f
injury to, 683–773
arthrography of, 689
associated injuries with, 771, 772f, 773
capitellum view of, 685, 686f
computed tomography of, 689
fat pad sign in, 686–687, 686f–688f
frequency of, 690
lipohemarthrosis in, 687, 689
magnetic resonance imaging of, 689–690
olecranon bursa hemorrhage in, 689, 689f
pathomechanics of, 690
pediatric, 730–771
anterior humeral line in, 731, 731f
arthrography of, 733
frequency of, 734
magnetic resonance imaging of, 733–734, 733f
radiocapitellar line in, 731–732, 731f, 732f
radiography of, 684f–689f, 685–689
supinator fat plane in, 689
intra-articular body in, 722, 726f
joint capsule of, 684, 686f, 688f
lateral condylar fracture of, pediatric, 739, 739f–744f, 744
complications of, 744
impaction, 739, 743f
mechanism of, 739, 741f
oblique view of, 739, 743f
Salter-Harris type 4, 739, 741f, 742f
treatment of, 744
triplane, 744
types of, 739, 739f, 740f

Elbow *(Continued)*
undisplaced, 739, 742f, 744f
lateral dislocation of, 708, 710f
pediatric, 763, 764f
ligaments of, 684, 685f
medial, traction injury to, 722, 726
medial dislocation of, pediatric, 764–765
myositis ossificans of, 258, 260f
nerves of, 684–685, 685f
ossification centers of, 732–733, 733f
pulled, 765, 765f
supracondylar fracture of, pediatric, 734–736, 734f–738f, 738
anterior humeral line in, 735–736, 738
Baumann's angle in, 734, 735f
complete vs. incomplete, 734–735
complications of, 738
differential diagnosis of, 738
displaced complete, 736, 736f
epiphyseal separation in, 738
mechanism of, 734, 734f
plastic bowing type, 736, 738f
reduction of, 734, 735f
torus, 736, 737f
undisplaced, 736, 737f
translocation of, 708, 711
traumatic synovitis of, 689
Embolus, fat, 239
Emphysema
interstitial, in rib fracture, 550, 550f
soft tissue, 236–237, 238f, 239f
subcutaneous, in bronchial rupture, 579, 580f, 581f
Ender rods, 189, 190f, 192
Enophthalmos, in orbital blow-out fracture, 335
Epicondylitis, medial, 726–727, 727f
Epiphora, in orbital rim fracture, 337
Epiphyseal artery, 1033
Epiphyseal injury, 116–132
after radiation therapy, 142
age incidence in, 120, 120f, 132
ankle, 1296–1297, 1297f–1300f, 1301, 1302f–1305f, 1312–1314
anterior cruciate ligament avulsion in, 1211–1212
birth injury and, 125–126, 126f
blood supply in, 117–118, 120f
classification of, 120–121, 122f–125f, 123, 125
compression force in, 120
computed tomography of, 127
corner sign in, 126
in dislocation, 117
distal femoral, 1209–1212, 1209f–1214f, 1215
distal humeral, 752, 753f–756f, 754, 757
distal radial, 805, 806, 808, 809f–811f, 813
distal tibial, osteochondritis dissecans in, 1302f–1303f
distal ulnar, 805, 806, 808, 809f–811f, 813
growth arrest after, 132
hand, 923f
histology of, 117, 119f
knee. *See* Knee, epiphyseal injury to.
lamellar sign in, 126
magnetic resonance imaging of, 127, 132
medial collateral ligament rupture in, 1210–1211, 1212f, 1214f
metacarpal, 923, 926f
metatarsal, 1400, 1401f
occult, of distal phalanges, 1401, 1401f, 1402f
open reduction/fixation of, 128, 130f
pathologic
in myelomeningocele, 138, 142, 142f, 1087–1088, 1090f

Epiphyseal injury *(Continued)*
in renal osteodystrophy, 138, 141f
pathway in, 118, 120
phalangeal
foot, 1400–1401, 1401f
hand, 925f
prognosis for, 128–129, 130f, 131f, 132
proximal femoral, 1086–1088, 1088f–1091f
proximal humeral, 639, 642, 643f–647f, 647f
proximal radial, 757, 758f, 760f, 761, 761f
proximal tibial, 1209–1212, 1209f–1214f, 1215
radiography of, 126–127, 127f
remodeling after, 128, 128f, 129f
Salter-Harris classification of, 105, 120–125
type 1, 121, 122f
type 2, 121, 122f, 123
type 3, 123, 123f
type 4, 123, 124f
growth disturbance in, 128, 129f
type 5, 123, 125, 125f
shortening after, 128–129, 130f
sites for, 120, 121f
in supracondylar pediatric elbow fracture, 738
treatment of, 128, 128f, 129f
valgus deformity after, 129, 131f
varus deformity after, 129
vector of force in, 118, 120
Epiphyseal line, 10f, 11
histologic zones of, 117, 119f
Epiphysiolysis, proximal femoral, 1087, 1089f
Epiphysis
blood supply of, 11, 11f, 117, 120f
clavicular, 596–597
distal tibial, triplane fracture of, 1301, 1306f–1310f, 1310
phalangeal, vs. epiphyseal fracture, 1320
pressure, 12, 13f
traction, 12, 13f
types of, 12, 13f
Esophagus
laceration of, 446
rupture of, 581, 583, 583f
Essex-Lopresti fracture, 800f, 801
Ethmoid sinus
fracture of, 292, 297f, 353, 354f
cerebrospinal fluid rhinorrhea in, 305
orbital plate of, in blow-out fracture, 333, 334f
Extension injury
cervical spine, 378f, 379, 532f
craniovertebral junction, 397, 398f
lumbar spine, 459f, 484, 489f
spinal cord, 378f, 379
thoracic spine, 478f, 484, 489f
Extensor carpi ulnaris tendon, computed tomography of, 821
Extensor digitorum brevis, calcaneal avulsion fracture at, 1337, 1337f
Extensor pollicis tendon, computed tomography of, 821
Extensor tendinopathy, 727, 728f
Extensor tendon
central slip of, rupture of, 885, 886f
distal phalangeal, avulsion of, 880, 881f, 882, 882f
entrapment of, with Smith's fracture, 789, 791f
tear of, 727, 728f
External auditory canal, bleeding from, in temporal bone fracture, 302
External fixation. *See* Fixation, external.
Extraocular muscles, entrapment of, in orbital blow-out fracture, 335, 336f
Eye, anatomy of, 321f

Fabella
fracture of, 1191
vs. free joint body, 1130, 1134f
Face, 315–372
anatomy of, 316, 317f–320f, 320
fracture of, 315–372. *See also specific area, e.g.,* Mandible.
anatomy in, 320–321, 322f
areas of strength in, 321, 322f
causes of, 315
chest radiograph in, 316
computed tomography of, 89, 315, 316, 323, 323f–326f, 325, 325t, 327t
distribution of, 315
facial struts in, 321, 322f
forces in, 315
fragment in, 315
imaging of, 316, 320–332
injuries associated with, 316
LeFort, 359–360, 360f–365f, 365–366
classification of, 320, 321, 322f, 359–360, 360f
type I, 360, 360f, 361f, 364f, 365
type II, 362f, 365, 365f
type III, 363f, 366
pediatric, 315
pneumomediastinum with, 316
radiography of, 325, 327, 328f–331f, 329–332
base view in, 328f–329f, 331, 331f
Caldwell view in, 328f–329f, 330–331
cortical bone appearance in, 327
lateral view in, 328f–329f, 331, 331f
orbital emphysema in, 329
penetrating injury and, 329
soft tissue appearance in, 327
Towne's view in, 328f–329f, 331–332
views for, 329
Water's view in, 328f–330f, 329–330
regions involved in, 320–321
smash, 366, 367f, 368f
soft tissue injuries with, 325, 325t
vs. normal bone discontinuities, 325, 327t
Facet joint
cervical, locking of, 422, 427f–432f, 432
bilateral, 422, 427f
computed tomography of, 432, 432f
fracture with, 431f–432f, 432
fracture-dislocation with, 422, 428f, 432
unilateral, 422, 427f, 429f, 432, 433f
in lumbar spine fracture, 455, 458f, 465, 468f
in lumbar spine fracture-dislocation, 506, 506f, 516, 520f, 521
in thoracic spine fracture, 465, 468f
in thoracolumbar junction fracture-dislocation, 515, 517f
Facial nerve, injury to, in temporal bone fracture, 300, 302–303, 302f
Failure point, 18
Falls
fracture from, 28, 29f
hip fracture in, 36–37
Fascial planes, in fracture, 84
Fat embolism syndrome, 237–239
arterial oxygen findings in, 238
femur fracture and, 1099
onset of, 238
pathophysiology of, 238–239
radiography of, 238, 241f
treatment of, 239
Fat pad sign, elbow, 686–687, 686f–688f
pediatric, 730–731, 730f
Fat pads, prefemoral, in joint effusion, 1128, 1129f
Fatigue, 18–19, 19f
Fatigue fracture, 57
Femoral artery
deep, 1033
superficial, 1033
injury to, 231, 233f, 234f
pseudoaneurysm from, 235f
Femur, 1030–1105
anatomy of, 1030–1031, 1032f
bone bruise of, magnetic resonance imaging of, 1124, 1125f
comminuted fracture of, 1090, 1093, 1094f, 1095f
condyles of, 1111, 1112f
bone bruise of, magnetic resonance imaging of, 1124, 1126, 1126f
computed tomography of, 1118
contusion of, with patellar dislocation, 1172, 1175f
fracture of, 1135, 1135f, 1140f, 1141f
irregular calcification on, 1130, 1134f
kissing contusions of, 1160, 1160f
lateral
configuration of, 1175
contusion of, 1186f
osteochondral fracture of, 1183f–1185f
medial, stress fracture of, 1204
normal variants in, 1128, 1130
radiography of, 1116
secondary ossification center on, vs. osteochondritis dissecans, 1130
distal
anatomy of, 1111, 1112f
epiphysis of
injury to, 1209–1215
prognosis of, 1212, 1215
Salter-Harris type 2 injury to, 1209, 1209f
Salter-Harris type 3 injury to, 1209, 1210, 1210f, 1213f, 1214f
Salter-Harris type 4 injury to, 1209, 1210f
Salter-Harris type 5 injury to, 1209, 1211f, 1212
stress fracture of, 1212
fracture of, 1134–1135, 1135f–1139f
Y-shaped intercondylar fracture of, 50f
epiphysis of
normal variants in, 1130
separation of, birth injury and, 125
fracture of, 1030–1104, 1090
age in, 27
arterial supply in, 1032f, 1033
bone mineral density and, 36f
bowing, 1093, 1096f
classification of, 1090, 1093
complications of, 1099–1100
Ender rod fixation of, 190f
epidemiology of, 1030, 1031f, 1090
fat embolism in, 1099
healing of, 213f
with hip fracture-dislocation, 167, 169f
with hip/knee injury, 1094, 1096f–1100f
interlocking nails for, 1098, 1099f
intramedullary nails for, migration of, 1100
intramedullary rod fixation of, 192f
magnetic resonance imaging of, 96f
oblique, 1090, 1094f
osteomyelitis in, 245, 246f
pediatric, treatment of, 1099, 1100f
with posterior hip dislocation, 1081, 1084f, 1085f
posterior hip dislocation with, 1096f
proximal, 1090, 1094f
Schneider nail for, 189f
treatment of, 1098–1099, 1099f, 1100f
Femur *(Continued)*
vascular injury in, 1099
greater trochanter of, 1030–1031, 1032f
avulsion fracture of, 1063, 1064f
head of, 1030, 1032f
compression fracture of, with posterior hip dislocation, 1079, 1081, 1082f, 1083f
fracture of, 1065, 1069, 1069f–1071f
anterior hip dislocation with, 1084–1085
computed tomography of, 1038, 1039f
fragment in, 1074f–1075f
medial displacement of, in acetabular anterior column fracture, 988, 992f
osteonecrosis of, 264f
posterior subluxation of, in acetabular posterior rim fracture, 988, 990f
shear fracture of, 1071f
with posterior hip dislocation, 1079, 1081f–1083f
spurring at, vs. impacted fracture, 1047, 1051f
insufficiency fracture of, 72f, 1101
intercondylar notch of, 1111, 1112f
intertrochanteric region of, 1030–1031, 1032f
fracture of, 1058–1063
classification of, 1058, 1060, 1060f
comminuted, 1058, 1059f, 1060f
complications of, 1062–1063, 1063f
computed tomography of, 1041f
four-part, 1058, 1060f
fracture line in, 1058, 1059f
incomplete, 1060–1061
nail fixation of, 192–193, 192f
osteomyelitis in, 245
pediatric, 1088–1089, 1092f
reverse diagonal fracture line in, 1061, 1061f
Richard compression screw and plate for, 193, 193f
three-part, 1058, 1059f
treatment of, 1062–1063, 1063f
two-part, 1061, 1062f
unstable, 1060, 1060f
lateral, notch in, 1158–1160, 1160f
lesser trochanter of
avulsion fracture of, 1063, 1065f, 1066f
fracture of, computed tomography of, 1040f
neck of, 1030, 1032f
avascular necrosis of, 1056–1057
basicervical fracture of, 1044, 1044f
complications of, 1056–1058
fracture of, 1041–1058
classification of, 1047, 1052, 1052f
computed tomography of, 1040f
healing of, 1058
intracapsular pressure in, 1058
in osteoarthritis, 1047
osteonecrosis after, 259, 262f
pediatric, 1088–1089, 1092f
prosthesis for, osteomyelitis after, 249f
with shaft fracture, 1094, 1098f
insufficiency fracture of, 1052–1058
in elderly, 1052, 1056f
pelvic insufficiency fracture with, 1054
presentation of, 1052–1053
sclerosis in, 1053, 1056f
subcapital, 1053, 1055f, 1056f
intracapsular fracture of, 1044–1052
mechanisms of, 1044
pseudofracture of, 1047, 1051f
radiography of, 1034, 1034f
stress fracture of, 63, 1052–1058

Femur *(Continued)*
athletics and, 1052, 1053f
basicervical, 1053, 1053f, 1054f
complications of, 1056–1058
compression, 1053–1054
in elderly, 1052, 1055f
magnetic resonance imaging of, 1054, 1057f
presentation of, 1052–1053
radiography of, 1054–1055
renal disease and, 1052, 1054f
sclerosis in, 1053, 1056f
treatment of, 1055–1056, 1058f
subcapital fracture of, 1044–1047, 1044f
classification of, 1047, 1052, 1052f
complete, 1046, 1046f
disimpacted, 1046, 1049f
displaced, 1045–1046, 1045f
foreshortening in, 1046
impacted, 1046, 1046f–1050f
incomplete, 1046
valgus displacement in, 1047f
varus displacement in, 1046–1047, 1047f, 1050f
transcervical fracture of, 1044, 1044f, 1047, 1051f
treatment of, 1055–1056, 1058f
open fracture of, 41
pathologic fracture of, 75, 81f, 1102–1103
physeal stress injury to, 126
proximal
comminuted fracture of, 42f, 43f
epiphyseal injury to, 1086–1088, 1088f–1091f
birth and, 1088, 1091f
pathologic, 1087–1088, 1090f
with pelvic fracture, 1006f
Salter-Harris type 1, 1086, 1088f
epiphysiolysis of, 1087, 1089f
extracapsular fracture of, 1044
fracture of
epidemiology of, 1041–1042, 1044
magnetic resonance imaging of, 1038, 1042f
osteoporosis and, 1042
tibial/fibular fracture with, 1191, 1194
types of, 1044
insufficiency fracture of, magnetic resonance imaging of, 1042f–1044f
intracapsular fracture of, 1044
osteoporotic fracture of, 32
pseudofracture of, 1102, 1103f
radiography of, 1033
anteroposterior view in, 1036–1037, 1037f–1038f
lateral view in, 1036–1037, 1037f
refracture of, 1100
segmental fracture of, 49f, 1093, 1096f
shaft of, 1030–1105
spiral fracture of, 1094f
wires for, 187f
stress fracture of, 64f, 1100–1102, 1101f, 1102f
magnetic resonance imaging of, 1102, 1102f
vs. malignant disease, 1102
subtrochanteric fracture of, 1063, 1065, 1067f, 1068f
classification of, 1065, 1068f
in elderly, 1065, 1068f
pathologic, 1065, 1067f
supracondylar fracture of, 1134–1135, 1135f–1139f
arteries in, 1116–1118
comminuted, 183f
with shaft fracture, 1094, 1097f

Femur *(Continued)*
transverse fracture of, 1090, 1093, 1095f, 1097f
blade plate for, 189f
healing of, 210f
as tubular bone, 7
Fetus, primary centers of ossification in, 9–10
Fibroma, nonossifying, pediatric pathologic fracture with, 137, 139f
Fibula, 1111–1215
anatomy of, 1113
bending fracture of, pronation-abduction and, 1267, 1269f
boot-top fracture of, 1194f
bowing fracture of, 1197, 1197f
comminuted fracture of
cast for, 181f
degenerative arthritis after, 265f
distal
epiphysis of
Salter-Harris type 1 injury to, 1296–1297, 1297f, 1300f
Salter-Harris type 2 injury to, 1297, 1298f
greenstick fracture of, 1297, 1300f
insufficiency fracture of, 1285, 1287f, 1288f, 1289, 1290f–1291f
posterior dislocation of, 1281–1282, 1282f
stress fracture of, 1285, 1286f
transverse fracture of, 42f, 1241, 1244f, 1245f
fracture of, 1191–1208
ankle trauma and, 1241, 1244f
arteries in, 1116–1118
disuse osteoporosis in, 217f
external fixation for, 186f, 1199f
hip fracture-dislocations with, 1191, 1194, 1195f
incomplete, 1191, 1195f
interlocking nails for, 1200f
in lateral malleolar fracture, 1227
location of, 1191, 1194f
mechanism of, 1191
nonunion of, osteomyelitis in, 244f
pronation-dorsiflexion and, 1270, 1271f, 1272f
pronation–external rotation and, 1270, 1274f
proximal ipsilateral femoral fracture with, 1191, 1194
radiography of, 1191, 1192f
tibial plateau fracture with, 1191, 1194, 1196f
tibiofibular syndesmosis disruption in, 1249, 1252f
treatment of, 1198–1199, 1199f, 1200f
greenstick fracture of, 1197, 1197f
head of
avulsion of, vs. Segond fracture, 1158
displacement of, in proximal tibiofibular joint dislocation, 1161, 1164, 1165f
fracture of, 1161, 1191, 1192f
in tibial plateau fracture, 1145, 1151f
neck of, fracture of, 1161
in tibial plateau fracture, 1145
oblique fracture of, pronation-abduction and, 1267, 1268f
pathologic fracture of, 1198
physeal stress injury to, 126
proximal
avulsion fracture of, 1161
fracture of, 1161, 1162f, 1163f, 1270, 1275f
Maisonneuve's fracture of, 1270, 1275f–1278f
stress fracture of, 1199, 1204, 1207f

Fibula *(Continued)*
radiography of, 1116, 1117f, 1229–1230
spiral fracture of, pronationnexternal rotation and, 1263, 1266f
stress fracture of, 1206
styloid process of, 1113
avulsion of, 1155, 1161
transverse fracture of, 48f
Fibular notch, 1223, 1223f
Finger, extensor mechanism of, 878–879, 879f
Fistula
arteriovenous, traumatic pulmonary, 574
subarachnoid-pleural, thoracic fracture-dislocation and, 514–515
urethra-hip, acetabular fracture-dislocation and, 1002, 1004f
Fixation, 180
appliance migration in, 252–253
external, 180, 193–197
bone lengthening with, 194–195, 197
compression/distraction with, 195, 197
devices for, 182, 186f
Ilizarov apparatus in, 194–195, 197
indications for, 194
pins in, 193–194, 196f–197f
internal, 180, 184–193
callus formation in, 248
complications of, 193, 195f
compression plates in, 185, 188, 188f, 189f
failure of, in nonunion, 221, 224f, 225
fracture healing in, 209, 212f
indications for, 184–185
intramedullary rods and nails in, 188–189, 189f–192f, 191–193
plates in, 185
osteomyelitis with, 244, 244f, 245f
screws in, 185, 188f, 189f
wires in, 185, 186f, 187f
Flail chest, 546, 549f, 550
Flat bone fracture, 49
Flexion injury
cervicothoracic junction, 397, 398f
in motorcycle accidents, 475, 479f
seat belts and, 475, 480
spinal, 475, 479f, 480
burst, 480, 481f, 482f
dislocation, 480, 484f
distraction, 480, 483f
simple, 480, 480f
spinal cord, 378–379, 378f
Flexion-distraction injury, spinal, 462f, 487, 490f, 495, 497, 499f
Flexor carpi radialis tendon, 821
Flexor carpi ulnaris tendon, calcification of, 827, 828f
Flexor digitorum longus tendon, magnetic resonance imaging of, 1237f, 1238f
Flexor digitorum profundus tendon, avulsion of, 882–883, 883f
Flexor hallucis longus tendon
in calcaneal fracture, 1346
computed tomography of, 1326f
os trigonum impingement by, 1355, 1357f
Flexor pollicis longus tendon, 821
Flexor profundus digitorum tendon
entrapment of, in interphalangeal dislocation, 901
fifth, 821
Flexor tendinopathy, 727
Flexor-pronator tendon
tearing of, at medial epicondyle, 726–727, 727f
traction from, in pediatric medial epicondylar avulsion, 744, 745f, 746
Floating elbow, 691

Foot, 1319–1403
abduction of, 1320
accessory ossification centers of, vs. fracture, 1319–1320, 1320f, 1321f
adduction of, 1320
anatomy of, 1319–1320, 1319f–1321f
bone bruise of, 1331–1332
computed tomography of, 1326–1327, 1326f–1329f
disuse osteoporosis of, 214f
dorsiflexion of, 1320
eversion of, 1320
fracture of, pediatric, 1400–1401, 1400f–1403f
injury to, radiography for, 78, 78t
inversion of, 1320
ligament injuries to, 1380–1381, 1383f
magnetic resonance imaging of, 1327
metatarsal fractures of, 1386, 1387f–1398f, 1393–1394, 1396
neuropathy in, 1384, 1385f, 1386, 1386f
occult fracture of, 1331–1332, 1332f
phalangeal fractures of, 1386, 1387f–1398f, 1393–1394, 1396
plantar flexion of, 1320
pronation of, 1236, 1238, 1320
radiography of, 1320–1321, 1322f–1325f, 1324–1325
stress fracture of, 1329–1330
fatigue-type, 1329–1330
magnetic resonance imaging of, 1330, 1331, 1331f, 1332f
marrow edema in, 1331, 1331f
radiography of, 1330
sites of, 1329, 1330f
supination of, 1236, 1238, 1320
Foramina transversarium, 394
Force, 17
angulation (bending), 18, 18f
compression, 18, 18f
rotation (torsion), 18, 18f
shear, 18, 18f
tension, 18, 18f
Forearm, 683–773. *See also* Radius; Ulna.
anatomy of, 683–685, 684f, 685f
bowing fracture of, 714
pediatric, 766–767, 766f
dislocation of, 708, 754
distal, 779–813
anatomy of, 779, 780f, 781f
fracture of
computed tomography of, 795
magnetic resonance imaging of, 799–800, 799f
soft tissue complications in, 795, 799
magnetic resonance imaging of, 783, 784t
radiography of, 779–781, 780f, 782f, 783, 783f
fracture of
age in, 27
anatomic features in, 713
associated injuries with, 771, 772f, 773
cast for, 181f
complications of, 714, 715f
compression plates for, 188f
diagnosis of, 713–714, 714f
pediatric, 730–771
arthrography of, 733
magnetic resonance imaging of, 733–734, 733f
plate fixation of, refracture after, 258, 258f
radial tuberosity and, 713–714, 714f
remodeling in, 220f
synostosis after, 714, 715f
greenstick fracture of, 765, 766f
Forearm *(Continued)*
injury to, 683–773
arthrography of, 689
computed tomography of, 689
frequency of, 690
magnetic resonance imaging of, 689–690
pathomechanics of, 690
radiography of, 684f–689f, 685–689
Monteggia fracture of, pediatric, 767, 768f–770f, 770
radioulnar fracture in, 712–714, 713f, 714f
stress fracture of, 722, 723f–730f, 726–727, 730
soft tissue injury in, 727, 728f–730f, 730
torus fracture of, pediatric, 805–806, 806f, 807f
valgus stress injury to, 722, 724f–727f, 726–727
bone hypertrophy and, 722, 724f
throwing motion and, 722
Forefoot, 1319, 1319f, 1320f
Foreign body
cranial, 292, 294f–296f
intraorbital, 342, 346, 347f
wooden, 292, 296f
Fovea capitis femoris
avulsion of, 1069, 1071f
vs. hip fracture, 1041
Fracture, 41–105. *See also specific anatomic site, e.g.,* Acetabulum, fracture of.
accessory bone, 49
activity and, 28–29, 29f
age in, 26–28, 26f, 27f
aneurysmal bone cyst after, 268, 268f
angulation of, 103–104
arterial injury in, 231–234, 232f–234f
arthrography of, 99
avulsion, 47
description of, 104
vs. apophyseal separation, 127, 127f
biologic factors in, 19
bone density in, 84, 86f, 87f
bone scan of, 97–98, 98f
bow, 114–115, 116f, 117f
bucket handle, in battered child syndrome, 132, 135, 136f, 137f
butterfly fragment in, 21
"chip," 47
chondral, 49, 52, 52f
classification of, 41, 104–105
closed, 41
osteomyelitis in, 245
comminuted, 20, 20f, 21, 41, 42f, 103
bone density in, 84
markedly, 41
moderately, 41, 42f
severely, 41, 42f
slightly, 41
compartment syndrome in, 234–236
complete, 41
complications of, 231–268
delayed, 259–268
immediate, 231–244
intermediate, 244–259
compound, 41
compression, 49, 51f
bone density in, 84
computed tomography of, 88–90, 91f–93f, 93
corner, in battered child syndrome, 132, 135, 136f
cortex irregularity in, 83, 86f
crush injuries and, 21
curved, 20–21, 20f
degenerative arthritis after, 263, 265f, 266
depressed, 23–24, 24f, 49
Fracture *(Continued)*
description of, 102–105, 104f
detection of
anatomic variants in, 99–102, 101f
factors in, 99–102, 101f
lines of junction in, 101
normal structures in, 99–102, 101f
secondary ossification centers in, 101–102
sesamoids in, 101–102
vascular channels in, 100–101, 101f
visual perception in, 102
digital imaging of, 102
distribution of, 26–29
effects of, 204–205
epidemiology of, 26–37
eponyms for, 105
fat embolism syndrome after, 237–239
fatigue, 57
fixation of, migrating appliances in, 252–253
flat bone, 49
fluoroscopy of, 98
force types in, 18, 18f
fragmentation in, 104
crush injuries and, 23
overlapping of, 216
frequency factors in, 26–29
gas gangrene from, 236–237, 237f
gender in, 26–28, 26f, 27f
greenstick, 111, 112, 114f, 115f
gunshot wounds and, 22f, 23
hangman's, 56f
healing of, 203–229
basic multicellular unit in, 205
biologic failure of, 218, 220
bone loss in, 206, 208f
bone scans of, 97
callus formation in, 205
computed tomography in, 225–226, 225f–229f
delayed union in, 220–221, 222f
delays in, 206t
disuse atrophy in, 211, 214, 214f–217f, 216
factors in, 206–209, 206t, 207f, 208f
fibrinolysis and, 208–209
fragment separation in, 206, 208f
granulation tissue formation in, 205
hormonal influences in, 209
infection in, 207
inflammatory phase of, 204f
magnetic resonance imaging in, 226
malunion in, 218, 221f
modeling in, 205
nonunion in, 221, 222f–224f, 225
in open reduction/internal fixation, 209, 210f, 211, 211f
osteomyelitis in, 247
pathologic conditions and, 208
pharmacologic agents in, 209
phases of, 204–205, 204f
problems in, 218, 220–221, 222f–224f, 225
radiography of, 209, 210f, 211, 211f, 225
remodeling phase of, 204f, 205, 220f
reparative phase of, 204f
stages of, 203–204, 203f
technical failure of, 218
transforming growth factor-beta in, 204
treatment choices in, 206–207
ultrasonography in, 229, 229f
union in, 74, 216, 219f, 220f
vascularity in, 206, 207f
imaging of, 83–99
impaction, 49
incomplete, 41, 41f
insufficiency. *See* Insufficiency fracture.

Fracture *(Continued)*
intra-articular, 49, 50f, 51f
healing of, fibrinolysis and, 208–209
irregular bone, 49
of joint surface, 16
lead arthropathy after, 266, 266f, 268
location of, 103
long bone, 41, 44–49
avulsion, 46–47, 47f
butterfly fragment in, 47, 48f
comminuted, 47, 48f, 49
division of thirds in, 44
fracture line direction in, 44
horizontal, 44
location of, 44
longitudinal, 44
oblique fracture line in, 44, 45f
segmental, 47, 49f
spiral fracture line in, 44, 46, 46f
T, 49
teacup, 46, 47f
transverse fracture line in, 44, 44f, 45f
vertical, 44, 46, 47f
Y, 49
magnetic resonance imaging of, 93–94, 95f, 96f
mechanism of injury and, 94, 97t
Malgaigne, 965–966, 965f–967f
radiography of, 90f
mechanical definition of, 17
mechanical factors in, 17–19, 17f–19f
myositis ossificans after, 258–259, 260f
nightstick, 21, 21f
oblique, 20f, 21
occult intraosseous, 53f
open. *See* Open fracture.
osteoarthritis after, 263, 265f, 266
osteochondral. *See* Osteochondral fracture.
osteolysis after, 255, 256f
osteomyelitis in, 244–245, 244f–252f, 247–248, 251–252
osteonecrosis in, 259–263, 262f–264f
in osteoporosis, 29–37. *See also* Osteoporosis.
osteoporosis after, 266f, 267f, 268
parry, 21, 21f
pediatric, 111–142. *See also under* Children.
penetrating injury and, 23–24, 23f, 24f
position of, 103
post-traumatic reflex dystrophy syndrome in, 253, 254f, 255, 255f
production of, 20–24
angulation in, 20, 20f
angulation-compression forces in, 20–21, 20f
bending in, 20, 20f
compressive force in, 20, 20f
direct forces in, 21, 22f–24f, 23–24
indirect forces in, 20–21, 21f
rotational force in, 20, 20f
tension in, 20, 20f
pseudoaneurysm in, 234, 235f
race in, 26–28
radiography of, 83–84, 84f–90f, 88
Mach effect in, 102
stress views in, 99, 100f
views in, 83, 84f, 85f
radiology report for, 104–105
radiolucency in, 83, 84f, 85f
risk of, bone density and, 34, 36–37, 36f
rotation in, 104, 104f
short bone, 49
simple, 41
skeletal system and, 29
soft tissue changes in, 84
soft tissue emphysema in, 236–237, 238f, 239f

Fracture *(Continued)*
solitary, associated fracture with, 88, 89f, 90f
sonography of, 99
spiral, 20, 20f
stress. *See* Stress fracture.
subchondral, magnetic resonance imaging of, 52, 53f
Sudeck's atrophy in, 253, 255
synostosis with, 259, 262f
tapping, 21
thromboembolism in, 239–244, 243f
"thrower's," 48f
toddler's, 115–116, 117f, 118f
tomography of, 99
torus, 112–113, 114f, 115f
transverse, 20, 20f
pathologic, 75, 77f
transverse-oblique, 20–21, 20f
treatment of, 180–201. *See also* Fixation; Reduction.
bone grafting in, 197–199, 198f, 199f
casts in, 180, 181f–183f, 182
electrical stimulation in, 199, 200f
external fixation of, 193–195, 195f–196f, 197
open reduction/internal fixation in, 184–193
pins-and-plaster technique in, 182, 184f, 186f
postreduction radiographs in, 200–201
Steinmann pins in, 182, 184f, 186f
traction in, 182, 184f, 186f
ultrasound stimulation in, 199–200
union of, 74, 216, 219f, 220f
vocabulary for, 41–55
Volkmann's ischemic contracture in, 234–236
Fracture-dislocation, 55, 56f
Freiberg's disease, vs. fracture, 1386, 1387f, 1391f, 1392f
Frontal bones, 317f
Frontal sinus, fracture of, 292, 294, 297, 297f, 357–358, 357f–359f
Fulcrum fracture, 521
Funny bone, 685, 685f

Galeazzi fracture, 719, 720f, 721f, 722
pediatric, 770–771
Gamekeeper's thumb, 916–917, 917f–919f
Gas gangrene, 236–237, 237f
Gastrocnemius muscle, fabella in
fracture of, 1191
vs. free joint body, 1130, 1134f
Gender, in fracture, 26–28, 26f, 27f
Glasgow Coma Scale, 172, 174t
Glass, in orbit, 347f
Glenohumeral joint, 633
anatomy of, 633
anterior dislocation of, 652, 654, 655f–661f, 658, 661
anterior glenoid rim fracture with, 654, 656f
arm abduction in, 654, 655f
diagnosis of, 654
greater tuberosity fracture with, 654, 655f
Hill-Sachs defect in, 654, 657f, 658, 659f–661f
humeral head defect with, 654, 657f, 658, 659f
labrocapsular complex tear with, 654
neurovascular injury with, 658
recurrent, 658
rotator cuff injury with, 658, 661f

Glenohumeral joint *(Continued)*
treatment of, 658
dislocation of, 638, 650–651
computed tomography of, 652
Grashey projection in, 652, 653f
magnetic resonance imaging of, 652
Moloney's arch in, 652, 653f, 654f
radiography of, 651f–654f, 652
scapular Y view in, 652, 653f
scapulohumeral arch in, 652, 653f, 654f
transthoracic view in, 652, 653f, 654f
intrathoracic fracture-dislocation of, 658, 661
luxatio erecta of, 661–662, 662f, 663f
posterior dislocation of, 651, 662, 664
computed tomography of, 669, 670f, 671f
humeral head in, 662
radiography of, 664, 666f–668f, 669, 670f
seizure and, 662, 664
radiography of, 633–634, 634f
simultaneous bilateral dislocation of, 651–652
subcoracoid anterior dislocation of, 651, 651f
subglenoid anterior dislocation of, 651, 652f
superior dislocation of, 662, 664f
voluntary dislocation of, 651
Glenohumeral ligament, humeral avulsion of, 671
Glenoid joint
anterior, fracture of, 620, 623f
fracture of, 627, 630f, 631f
Glenoid labrum ovoid mass, 671
Glenoid rim
fracture of, 654, 656f
posterior, in posterior shoulder dislocation, 664, 667f, 668f, 671f
Glenolabral articular disruption, 671
Globe, rupture of, orbital trauma and, 342, 344f
Gorham's disease, vs. post-traumatic osteolysis, 255
Gracilis muscle, avulsion of, pediatric, 1012
Granulation tissue, in fracture healing, 205
Great toe
distal phalanx of
fracture of, 1324, 1324f
occult epiphyseal separation of, 1401, 1401f, 1402f
injuries to, 1389f
interphalangeal dislocation of, 1386
phalanx of, epiphysis of, vs. epiphyseal fracture, 1320
proximal phalanx of, stress fracture of, 1396
radiography of, 1324, 1324f
seasmoid fracture and, 1396, 1398f
Greenstick fracture, 111, 112, 114f, 115f
ankle, 1289, 1295f
distal fibular, 1297, 1300f
distal radial/ulnar, 805, 806, 808f
intercondylar vertical humeral, 757
pediatric, 111, 112, 114f, 115f, 757, 806, 808f
Growth plate, 10f
cartilaginous, 10f, 11
histologic zones of, 117, 119f
distal radial
normal appearance of, 813, 813f
stress injury to, in gymnasts, 812f, 813
fracture of, magnetic resonance imaging of, 94
injury to, nail bed disruption and, 923, 925f
proximal humeral, 639, 644f
stress injury to, 126, 127f
Gunshot wound
fracture in, 22f, 23

Gunshot wound *(Continued)*
lead arthropathy from, 266, 266f, 268
open fracture in, 41, 43f
Guyon's canal, in hook of hamate fracture, 849, 850f
Gymnasts, distal radius growth plate stress injuries in, 812f, 813

Half-moon overlap, 669
Hamate, 813
45-degree pronation oblique view of, 818, 819f
dislocation of, 849
dorsal surface of, fracture of, 847f, 848
fracture of, 827, 846–849
carpometacarpal dislocation with, 907, 909, 912f
hook of
computed tomography of, 821, 822f
fracture of
bone scan of, 819, 820f
computed tomography of, 819, 848, 849f
magnetic resonance imaging of, 848–849, 850f
mechanism of, 848
radiography of, 820f, 848, 848f, 849f
radiography of, 846, 848
secondary ossification center of, 849
posteroanterior view of, 817
Hand, 874–927
anatomy of, 874, 878–879, 878f, 879f
dislocation of, 898–909
pediatric, 923, 925
treatment of, 879
epiphyseal separations of, 923f
fracture of
pediatric, 920–921, 922f–926f, 923
treatment of, 879
radiography of, 874, 875f–877f
Hangman's fracture, 56f, 403, 406f–409f, 408
avulsion in, 403, 407f
classification of, 403, 408, 408f
computed tomography of, 403, 407f
mechanism of, 408
neurologic injury in, 408, 418
unilateral, 408, 409f
vs. synchondrosis, 408
Hard palate, fracture of, in sagittal plane, 366, 366f
Haversian system, 8f, 9
atypical, 10
Head injury
child abuse and, 307, 308f, 309f
choroid plexus calcification in, 287
computed tomography of, 275, 275f–284f, 277
indications for, 272–273, 273t
imaging of, 275–287
indirect imaging signs of, 286–287, 287f, 288f
magnetic resonance imaging of, 281, 285f, 286
pathomechanics of, 273–275, 274f
pediatric, 274
pineal gland calcification in, 287
pneumocephalus in, 287, 288f
radiography of, 277, 281, 284f
indications for, 272–273, 273t
sinus opacification in, 286, 288f
Hearing loss
conductive, in temporal bone fracture, 300, 302, 302f
neurosensory, inner ear fracture and, 302
Heart, injuries to, 587–588, 588f
Hemarthrosis
in intra-articular knee injury, 1127–1128, 1129f
with olecranon fracture, 687f
Hematocrit effect, vs. lipohemarthrosis, 1128, 1133f
Hematoma
anterior talofibular ligament tear and, 1381
cerebral
in battered child syndrome, 135
computed tomography of, 275, 280f
in cervical spine fracture, 386
epidural
computed tomography of, 275, 277, 278f, 279f
in lumbar/thoracic spine fracture, 471, 473f
extra-axial, computed tomography of, 275, 277
extrapleural, in rib fracture, 542, 545–546, 545f, 546f, 550–551
fracture and, 204
in head trauma, 286
mediastinal
imaging of, 152, 154f
in upper thoracic fracture-dislocation, 507, 514, 515f
paraspinous
in lumbar/thoracic fracture, 455, 459f–462f, 460
in upper thoracic fracture-dislocation, 507, 515f
perioptic, 342, 346f
pulmonary, vs. traumatic pneumatocele, 570
retrosternal, in sternum fracture, 557, 557f
subdural
in battered child syndrome, 135
in children vs. adults, 274–275
computed tomography of, 275, 276f, 277, 277f, 281f
isodense, 277
posterior interhemispheric, child abuse and, 307, 309f
Hematomyelia, 440
Hematuria, posterior element fracture and, 525
Hemipelvectomy, traumatic, 978, 978f
Hemopneumothorax, rib fracture and, 550, 550f, 561, 561f
Hemorrhage
abdominal, computed tomography of, 160, 161f
in ankle injury, 1230, 1231f
external ear, in temporal bone fracture, 302
mediastinal, thoracic polytrauma and, 150, 152, 152f
orbital, 342, 345f, 346f
in pelvic fracture, 945, 945f, 946f, 1012–1013, 1015, 1015f, 1016f
Hemothorax, 560–561, 560f
Hernia, traumatic lung, 559, 559f, 560f
Hill-Sachs defect
with anterior shoulder dislocation, 654, 657f, 658, 659f–661f
with anterior subcoracoid dislocation, 659f
computed tomography of, 672f
magnetic resonance imaging of, 672f, 675f
Stryker notch view of, 658, 660f
Hindfoot, 1319, 1319f
Hip, 1030–1104
anatomy of, 1030–1031, 1032f, 1033
anterior dislocation of, 1084–1086, 1086f, 1087f
complications of, 1085–1086
treatment of, 1085
Hip *(Continued)*
dislocation of, 1069, 1072–1086
computed tomography of, 1069, 1073f–1075f
fracture fragments in, 1069, 1073f, 1074f
intra-articular gas bubble in, 1069, 1075f
mechanisms of, 1069
pediatric, 1089–1090, 1093f
simultaneous bilateral, 1069, 1072f
three-dimensional reconstruction in, 1069, 1075f
fracture of, 1030–1104
arterial supply in, 1032f, 1033
Colles' fracture with, 785, 786f
computed tomography of, 89, 92f, 1037–1038, 1039f–1041f
epidemiology of, 28, 1030, 1031f
falls and, 36–37
magnetic resonance imaging of, 1038–1039, 1042f–1044f
in osteoporosis, 36–37
radiography of, 92f, 1033–1036
anteroposterior view in, 1033–1035, 1034f
fat planes of, 1035
groin lateral view in, 1035–1036, 1036f
oblique (frog-leg) view in, 1032f, 1035
obturator internus fascial plane in, 1035
shoot-through-hip view in, 1035–1036, 1036f
soft tissue clues in, 1035
sciatic nerve in, 1033
tomography of, 1039
vs. occult acetabular fracture, 1000, 1002, 1002f
fracture-dislocation of
femoral fracture with, 167, 169f
tibial/fibular fracture with, 1191, 1194, 1195f
injury to
in femoral fracture, 1094
pediatric, 1086–1090
joint surface congruity in, 1035
myositis ossificans of, 258, 261f
normal variants of, 1039, 1041
posterior dislocation of
chronic, 1079f
classification of, 1081
computed tomography of, 1073f, 1078f, 1079
delay in, 1081, 1084
femoral fracture with, 1081, 1084f, 1085f, 1096f
femoral head compression fracture with, 1079, 1081, 1082f, 1083f
femoral head position in, 1072, 1078f, 1079f
femoral head shear fracture with, 1079, 1081f
forces in, 1072
fracture fragment in, 1072, 1079, 1080f
fractures associated with, 1072
open reduction of, 1079
posterior acetabular fracture in, 1072, 1076f, 1077f
vs. anterosuperior dislocation, 1072
posterior fracture-dislocation of, 1073f, 1076f
width of, measurement of, 1035
Hormones, in fracture healing, 209
Hospital Trauma Index, 172, 175f
Humeroradial joint, 683
Humeroulnar joint, 683
Humerus, 593–676
anatomy of, 683

Humerus *(Continued)*
condyles of, intra-articular fracture of, 50f
distal
anterior line of, pediatric, 731, 731f
avulsion fracture of, 693f
capitellum of, fracture of, 694, 694f–696f
classification of, 692, 692f
comminuted fracture of, butterfly fragment with, 48f
condylar fracture of, 691, 693f, 694f
epiphyseal injury to, 752, 753f–756f, 754, 757
fracture of, 690–696
treatment of, 696
ossification centers of, 732–733, 733f
Salter-Harris type 1 injury to, 754f
sideswipe fracture of, 691
supracondylar fracture of, 696, 697f
pediatric, 730f
transcondylar fracture of, 696, 697f
T-shaped condylar fracture of, 691, 692f
Y-shaped condylar fracture of, 691, 692f
epiphyseal separation of, birth injury and, 125, 126f
fracture of
age in, 27
Ender rod fixation of, 190f
osteoporosis after, 266f, 268
osteoporosis and, 32, 32f
radiography of, 84f
greater tuberosity of, nondisplaced fracture of, 594, 596f
greenstick fracture of, 757
head of
avascular necrosis of, 639
comminuted fracture of, 638, 642f
compression fracture of, 669
in shoulder dislocation, 658, 661f
defects of, in anterior shoulder dislocation, 654, 657f, 658, 659f
displacement of, with rotator cuff tear, 658, 661f
fracture of
fragment location in, 771
osteonecrosis after, 259, 263f
radial head fracture with, 705
fracture-dislocation of, 638
intrathoracic dislocation of, 658, 661
ossification center of, 639, 643f
osteochondral fracture of, 722, 725f, 771, 773
pediatric, 770f, 771
posterior dislocation of, 664
posterior fracture of, 635f
radiography of, 634, 635f
lateral condylar fracture of, 50f
pediatric, vs. distal humeral epiphyseal separation, 757
medial condylar fracture of, pediatric, 751–752, 752f
medial epicondyle of
avulsion injury to, 745f, 746
dislocation associated with, 746, 750–751, 750f
entrapment injury to, 746, 747f–749f
ossification center of, treatment and, 750–751
pediatric injuries to, 744–752
physeal stress injury to, 126
proximal
anatomic neck fracture of, 636–637, 637f
anatomy of, 632–633
avulsion fracture of, 635f
comminuted fracture of, 636f
computed tomography of, 634, 635f
epiphyseal injury to, 639, 642, 643f–647f

Humerus *(Continued)*
four-part fracture of, 637, 640f, 641f
fracture of, 632, 633f, 634, 636–638, 636f–642f
complications of, 638–639, 642f
myositis ossificans in, 639, 642f
Neer classification of, 637–638, 639f–642f
fracture-dislocation of, 636, 640f, 641f
greater tuberosity fracture of, 636, 636f, 637, 637f
with anterior shoulder dislocation, 654, 655f
growth plate of, 639, 644f
lesser tuberosity fracture of, 637, 638f
lipohemarthrosis and, 634, 635f
nondisplaced fracture of, 636, 637f
radiography of, 633–634, 634f, 635f
surgical neck fracture of, 636, 636f
three-part fracture of, 637
two-part fracture of, 637, 639f
shaft of, 593–676
anatomy of, 645, 649f
comminuted fracture of, compression plate fixation of, 212f
fracture of, 642, 645, 648f
complications of, 649–650
diagnosis of, 645–646
displacement direction in, 646
floating elbow in, 646, 649
pediatric, 649
throwing motion and, 648f, 649
treatment of, 650
types of, 646, 648f–651f, 649
oblique fracture of, 646, 648f
pathologic fracture of, 649, 650f
spiral fracture of, 646, 648f
transverse fracture of, 646, 648f
stress fracture of, 63
as tubular bone, 7
Hyaline cartilage, 13, 16, 16f
Hyoid bone, fracture of, 445–446, 446f
Hyperemia, in disuse atrophy, 216
Hyperextension injury
cervical spine, 436–442, 437f, 438f, 440f
interphalangeal joint, 923
Hyperflexion injury, cervical spine, 381f, 432, 434f–436f, 435–436
Hyperparathyroidism, insufficiency fracture in, 72f
Hypoxemia, in fat embolism syndrome, 238, 239
Hysteresis, 18, 18f

Iliac artery, in pelvic fracture, 1013, 1015f
Iliac crest, avulsion of, pediatric, 1009, 1012, 1013f
Iliac spine, avulsion of, pediatric, 1009, 1011f
Iliac wing
fracture of, 954–955, 955f, 956f
computed tomography of, 938, 938f
radiography of, 938, 938f
torus fracture of, 956f
Iliolumbar ligament, 933, 933f
Ilium, 931, 931f
fracture of, 965f, 966, 966f
in posterior acetabular column, 979
stress fracture of, 955, 958
Y vascular groove of, 941, 944f
Infection, soft tissue, 236–237, 238f, 239f
Infrapatellar fat pad, 1112f
Infrapatellar tendon
radiography of, 1116
in recurrent patellar subluxation, 1175, 1177f

Infrapatellar tendon *(Continued)*
rupture of, 1178, 1179f
Infraspinatus muscle, strain of, magnetic resonance imaging of, 596f
Injury. *See* Polytrauma; Trauma.
Injury Severity Score, 172, 176f
Inner ear, fracture in, neurosensory hearing loss from, 302
Innominate bone, pelvic, 7f, 930–931, 931f
Insufficiency fracture, 57, 64–73
acetabular, 1002
after irradiation, 70, 73f
bone scans of, 64, 68f, 98
in brown tumors, 70, 72f
calcaneal, 1348, 1352f
computed tomography of, 68f, 69
in congenital disease, 69–70, 71f
distal tibial/fibular, 1285, 1287f, 1288f, 1289, 1290f–1291f
disuse atrophy and, 214, 216, 218f
femoral, 72f, 1101
femoral neck, 1052–1058, 1055f, 1056f
in hyperparathyroidism, 72f
magnetic resonance imaging of, 69, 94, 96f
in neurotrophic arthritis, 73, 74f
in osteogenesis imperfecta, 69–70, 71f
in osteopetrosis, 70, 71f
in osteoporosis, 64, 66f–68f, 68, 69, 266f, 268, 959, 959f–963f, 1285, 1287f, 1348, 1352f
in Paget's disease, 69, 70f
in paraplegia, 73, 73f
pelvic, 64, 66f–68f, 68, 958–964, 958f–963f
proximal femoral, 1042f–1044f
proximal phalangeal, 71f
in pyknodysostosis, 70, 72f
in quadriplegia, 73, 73f
in renal osteodystrophy, 64, 70, 72f
in rheumatoid arthritis, 64, 69, 1285, 1288f
sacral, 963, 963f
after pelvic irradiation, 70, 73f
in β-thalassemia, 73
tibial plateau, 1149, 1152, 1152f
transversely oriented, 69, 70f
Interclavicular ligament, 607, 609–610, 612f
Intercondylar notch, radiographic view of, 1116, 1118f
Internal fixation. *See* Fixation, internal.
Interosseous ligament, 1225, 1225f
injury to, anterior talofibular ligament rupture with, 1270
pediatric, 1289, 1295f, 1296
Interosseous membrane, pediatric, 1289, 1295f, 1296
Interphalangeal joint
foot
dislocation of, 1386, 1389f, 1390f
irreducible injuries to, 1386
pseudodislocation of, 1386, 1391f
subluxation of, 1386, 1391f
great toe, dislocation of, 1386
hand
complex dislocation of, 898
dislocation of, 900–903
pediatric, 923, 925
treatment of, 898, 900
types of, 898, 899f
volar plate rupture in, 900–901
dorsal dislocation of, 55f, 900, 901, 901f
dorsolateral dislocation of, 898, 899f
fracture-dislocation of, 901
irreducible dislocation of, 901, 925
lateral subluxation of, 902f, 903
multiple dislocation of, 900, 901f
proximal
in boutonnière deformity, 885

Interphalangeal joint *(Continued)*
extensor mechanism of, 878–879, 879f
lateral subluxation of, 898, 900f
Salter-Harris type 4 fracture-dislocation of, 925f
volar lateral subluxation of, 898, 900f
Salter-Harris type 1 fracture-dislocation of, 925f
simple dislocation of, 898
swelling of, radiography of, 874
volar dislocation of, 902–903
thumb, dislocation of, 56f, 917
Intervertebral disc, 377, 377f
herniation of
in lumbar apophyseal ring fracture, 526, 530f
in lumbar/thoracic spine fracture, 465, 466f, 471, 474f
Intervertebral disc space, in cervical spine fracture, 391
Intrapatellar tendon, 1113
Ischial ramus
single fracture of, 947, 948f, 949f
stress fracture of, 63
Ischial tuberosity, apophyseal avulsion of, pediatric, 1009, 1011f, 1012f
Ischiopubic synchondrosis, 941
Ischium, 931, 931f
in posterior acetabular column, 979

Jefferson's fracture, 398, 400, 401f–404f, 403
neural arch fracture with, 398
neurologic injury in, 418
stable, 400, 402f–403f
Jewett nail, 192f
Joint(s), 12–16
air in, in fracture-dislocation, 238f
cartilaginous, 12, 13, 14f, 16, 16f
classification of, 12, 14f
diarthrodial, 13, 14f
osteoarthritis of, 263
effusion of
in fracture, 84
knee, 1127–1128, 1129f
in pediatric fracture, 111, 113f
fibrous, 12, 14f
floating, in segmental fracture, 47
fractures of, open reduction for, 185
in intra-articular fracture, 49
meniscus in, 13, 15f
open injury to, 55, 57f
soft tissue injury around, radiography of, 3
synovial, 12, 13, 14f
Joint capsule, elbow, 684
Jones fracture, 1393–1394, 1394f
in proximal diaphysis, 1394, 1397f, 1398f
Jumper's knee, 1176, 1177f

Kidney(s). *See also* Renal *entries.*
diseases of, femoral neck stress fracture in, 1052, 1054f
rupture of, in first rib fracture, 553, 555f
Kienböck's disease, 839–840, 840f
Kirschner wire, 193, 194f
Knee, 1111–1215
anatomy of, 1111, 1112f, 1113, 1114f
angiography of, 1116–1118
apophyseal injury to, 1209–1212, 1209f–1214f, 1215
arteries of, 1113, 1114f
chondral fracture of, 1180, 1182, 1185–1187
magnetic resonance imaging of, 1127

Knee *(Continued)*
dislocation of, 1187, 1189f, 1190f, 1191
anterior, 1187, 1189f
arterial injury in, 1187, 1191
lateral, 1187, 1189f
medial, 1187, 1189f
posterior, 1187
posterolateral, 1187, 1190f, 1191
rotary, 1187, 1190f, 1191
effusion of, in intra-articular injury, 1127–1128, 1129f
epiphyseal injury to, 1209–1212, 1209f–1214f, 1215
diagnosis of, 1210
ligamentous injury with, 1209–1212, 1213f, 1214f
Salter-Harris type 2, 1209f, 1210, 1212f
Salter-Harris type 3, 1210, 1212f–1214f
Salter-Harris type 5, 1212
undisplaced, 1210, 1212f–1214f
valgus stress ligament injury with, 1210
extensor mechanism of, 1176, 1177f–1180f, 1178
fracture of, cast for, 180, 182, 183f
injury to, 1180–1191
arteries in, 1116–1118
in femoral fracture, 1094
frequency of, 1130
radiography of, 78, 79t
intra-articular fracture of
frequency of, 1130
hemarthrosis in, 1127–1128, 1129f
lipohemarthrosis in, 1128, 1130f–1133f
jumper's, 1176, 1177f
ligamentous injury to
in femoral fracture, 1094
stress radiography of, 1116
magnetic resonance imaging of, 15f, 1118, 1120–1124, 1121f–1124f
occult intraosseous injury to, magnetic resonance imaging of, 1124, 1125f–1127f, 1126–1127
osteochondral fracture of, 52f, 1180, 1182, 1182f–1187f, 1185–1187
articular bone in, 1186
fragments in, 1182, 1183f, 1184f
impaction and, 1186, 1186f
magnetic resonance imaging of, 1181, 1185, 1185f
mechanism of, 1180, 1182, 1182f
patellar dislocation and, 1180, 1182, 1182f, 1185, 1186, 1186f
radiodensity in, 1187
undisplaced shorn fragments in, 1185–1186
vs. osteochondritis dissecans, 1186, 1187f
vs. secondary ossification center, 1186–1187, 1188f
radiography of, 1113–1116
anteroposterior view in, 1114–1115, 1115f
lateral view in, 1115–1116, 1115f
normal variants in, 1128, 1130, 1134f
notch view in, 1116, 1117f
oblique projection in, 1115f, 1116
soft tissue clues in, 1127–1128, 1129f–1133f, 1130
suprapatellar bursa of, radiography of, 1116
Kümmell phenomenon, 493–495, 498f
Kuntscher nails, 188
osteomyelitis with, 251f
Kyphosis, spontaneous sternal fracture in, 557–558, 558f
in osteoporosis, 492–493

Labrocapsular complex, tear of, with shoulder dislocation, 654

Labrum, 13
Laceration
fracture with, 23, 24f
pulmonary, 567, 570, 570f–573f
Lacrimal bone, 316
Lacunae, in haversian system, 8f, 9
Lambdoid suture, interdigitation of, 289f
Lamellae, in haversian system, 8f, 9
Lamellar sign, in epiphyseal injury, 126
Larynx, fracture of, 443–446
cause of, 444
classification of, 444
computed tomography of, 444–445, 445f
radiography of, 444, 444f, 445f
symptoms of, 444
Lateral margin, stress fracture of, 63
Latissimus dorsi muscle, 593
Lead, retained, arthropathy from, 266, 266f, 268
Lead pipe fracture, pediatric, 113, 115f
LeFort fractures, 359–366
classification of, 320, 321, 322f, 359–360, 360f
type I, 360, 360f, 361f, 364f, 365
type II, 362f, 365, 365f
type III, 363f, 366
Lens
dislocation of, 342, 345f
injury to, orbital trauma and, 342, 344f, 345f
subluxation of, 342, 344f
Lifting fracture, ulnar, 722, 723f
Ligament(s), 13
avulsion of, bone scans of, 97
in epiphyseal injury, 117
tears of, 16
in transverse fracture, 44
Ligamentum flavum, 377
Lipohemarthrosis
in elbow injuries, 687, 689
in fracture, 84, 86
in intra-articular knee fractures, 1128, 1130f–1133f
in lateral tibial plateau fracture, 1143, 1145f
vs. hematocrit effect, 1128, 1133f
Lisfranc's joint, 1371, 1376f, 1379f
fracture-dislocation of
diabetic neuroarthropathy and, 1384, 1385f
divergent, 1380, 1380f, 1382f
forms of, 1380, 1380f
fracture types in, 1380, 1382f
homolateral, 1380, 1380f–1382f
mechanism of, 1376, 1380, 1380f
in neurotrophic arthritis, 73, 74f
ligaments of, 1371
injuries to, 1380–1381, 1383f
neuroarthropathy of, 1384
normal radiograph of, 1371, 1379f
tendon injuries in, 1384, 1384f
Little League elbow, 722, 726, 746
Liver, trauma to
classification of, 162–163, 163t
computed tomography of, 162–163, 163f, 163t
nonoperative management of, 162–163
pelvic fracture and, 1021
rib fracture and, 553, 555f
Longitudinal ligament
anterior, 377, 377f
posterior, 377, 377f
Low back pain, in posterior element stress fracture, 526, 528f
Lumbar spine, 453–537
apophyseal rings of, fracture of, 526, 530f
burst fracture of, 382f–383f, 457f, 497, 500f–506f, 504, 506

Lumbar spine *(Continued)*
canal compromise in, 467f
epidural hematoma in, 473f
flexion injury and, 480, 481f, 482f
fragment configuration in, 497, 500f
fragment retropulsion in, 497, 503f, 504
stable, 484, 506
unstable, 484, 487
vertebral body height in, 497, 502f
vertebral body sagittal fracture in, 497
vs. rotary injury, 504, 505f, 506, 507, 513f
vs. shearing injury, 504, 506, 506f, 507, 513f
vs. simple wedge compression fracture, 497, 504, 504f
Chance-type fracture of, 480, 483f, 487, 521–525
computed tomography of, 523, 524f
fulcrum fracture in, 521
injury patterns in, 521, 521f–523f, 523
magnetic resonance imaging of, 523
radiography of, 523
Smith fracture in, 521, 523, 523f
transverse, 521, 522f
vs. flexion-distraction fracture, 497
compression fracture of, 172f, 460, 489, 491–492, 491f, 492f
osteoporotic vs. pathologic, 471, 474f, 492, 493f
simple, 480f
contiguous fracture of, 464f
distraction injury to, 458f
extension injury to, 459f, 484, 489f
flexion injury to, 475, 479f, 480
burst, 480, 481f, 482f
dislocation, 480, 484f
distraction, 480, 483f
simple, 480, 480f
flexion-distraction injury to, 462f, 487, 490f, 495, 497, 499f
fracture of
alignment abnormalities in, 454–455, 456f, 457f, 471, 474f
anatomic abnormalities in, 454–455, 456f, 457f
in ankylosing spondylitis, 526, 532f, 533–534
bone integrity abnormalities in, 455
cartilage abnormalities in, 455, 458f, 459f
Chance-type injury in, 466, 470f
computed tomography of, 463, 464f–470f, 465–466
in diffuse idiopathic skeletal hyperostosis, 534, 534f
disc herniation in, 465, 466f, 471, 474f
disc space abnormalities in, 455, 459f
epidural hematoma with, 471, 473f
evaluation approach to, 454
facet joint integrity in, 465, 468f
interpedicle space in, 455, 457f
interspinous space in, 455, 457f
joint space abnormalities in, 455, 458f, 459f
magnetic resonance imaging of, 466, 471, 471f–478f, 475
osteoporotic collapse in, 471, 475f
pedicle injury in, 465, 468f
posterior element status in, 460, 462f
posterior vertebral body line in, 454–455, 456f
radiography of, 453–454, 455f–463f, 460, 463
soft tissue abnormalities in, 455, 459f–461f, 460
spinal cord contusion in, 471, 477f
spinal cord hemorrhage in, 471, 472f, 477f

Lumbar spine *(Continued)*
spinal cord injury with, 471, 471f, 472f
spinal cord status in, 466, 469f
vertebral canal compromise in, 465, 467f
vertebral canal fragments in, 471, 476f
wedge vs. compression, 466
fracture-dislocation of, 506–521
computed tomography of, 516, 518f–520f
double vertebrae sign in, 516, 519f
facet joint abnormalities in, 506, 506f, 516, 520f, 521
lateral translational injury in, 516
magnetic resonance imaging of, 507, 512f
neurologic deficit in, 507, 507f–511f
posterior element fracture in, 506, 506f
reduction of, 521
thecal sac tear with, 469f
injury to, 453–537
biomechanics of, 453–454
classification of, 475, 479f–490f, 480–481, 484, 487, 489
distribution of, 453–454, 454f
incidence of, 453–454
mechanism of, 475, 479f–490f, 480–481, 484, 487, 489
pediatric, 453
wedge deformity in, 491–492
lateral fracture-dislocation of, 456f
limbus vertebra of, 489, 491, 491f, 492f
open wounds of, 534, 536f
osteoporotic compression fracture of, 491f, 492–493, 493f–496f
pathologic fracture of, 493, 497f
penetrating trauma to, 534, 536f
posterior elements of
fracture of, 495, 497, 499f, 525–526, 525f
stress fracture of, 526, 527f–529f
post-traumatic vertebral body collapse in, 493–495, 498f
rotary (grinding) injury to, 480–481, 485f, 486f
vs. burst fracture, 504, 505f, 506, 507, 513f
shearing injury to, 481, 487f, 488f
vs. burst fracture, 504, 506, 506f, 507, 513f
Smith fracture of, pedicle fracture with, 468f
translation (dislocation) injury to, 487
vertebral edge separation of, 489, 491, 491f, 492f
wedge compression fracture of, 484
Lumbosacral junction, fracture-dislocation at, 507, 510f
Lunate, 813
anterior dislocation of, 852, 854f
computed tomography of, 821, 822f
dislocation of, 849–855
with capitate fracture, 844, 846f
capitate head fracture with, 854, 858f
cortical arcs/lines in, 851–852, 851f
displacement in, 852
fracture with, 851, 854, 857f
mechanism of, 849–850
radiography of, 851, 852f
treatment of, 855
triangular appearance in, 852, 854, 857f
dorsal dislocation of, 850, 851f
fracture of, 827
injury to, 839–840, 839f, 840f
lateral view of, 818
posterior dislocation of, 851, 853f
posteroanterior view of, 816, 817f
synostosis of, 818
vascular patterns of, 840
volar dislocation of, 850, 851, 851f, 853f

Lunatomalacia, 839–840, 840f
Lunatotriquetral ligament, disruption of, 863, 865f
Lung(s)
contusion of, 573f
in diaphragm rupture, 574, 577f, 578f
laceration of, 567, 570, 570f–573f
parenchyma of, trauma to, 567–574
traumatic arteriovenous fistula of, 574
traumatic hernia of, 559, 559f, 560f

Mach effect
in fracture radiography, 102
in odontoid process fractures, 410–411, 412f
Magnetic resonance arthrography
of shoulder injury, 594, 598f
of shoulder instability, 671, 674f, 675
Magnetic resonance imaging
of Achilles tendon, 96f, 1238f
of Achilles tendon rupture, 1284–1285, 1284f, 1285f
of ankle, 1231, 1236, 1237f, 1238f
of anterior cruciate ligament, 1121–1122, 1122f
of anterior tibiofibular ligament, 1237f
of bone bruise, 52–54, 53f, 54f, 94, 95f, 1124, 1125f–1127f, 1126–1127
of calcaneal anterior process fracture, 1337, 1338f
of calcaneal stress fracture, 1331, 1331f, 1332f
of calcaneofibular ligament, 1237f
of carpal fracture, 821, 826, 826f
of cervical spine injury, 384, 384f, 385f, 391, 394
of Chance-type fracture, 523
of chronic neuroarthropathy, 1386, 1386f
of diaphragmatic injury, 155, 159f
of distal forearm, 783, 784t
of distal forearm fracture, 799–800, 799f
of elbow injury, 689–690
pediatric, 733–734, 733f
of epiphyseal injury, 127, 132
of femoral bone bruise, 1124, 1125f, 1126, 1126f
of femoral fracture, 96f
of femoral neck stress fracture, 1054, 1057f
of femoral stress fracture, 1102, 1102f
of fibular stress fracture, 1206
of flexor digitorum longus tendon, 1237f, 1238f
of foot, 1327
of foot stress fracture, 1330, 1331, 1331f, 1332f
of forearm injury, 689–690
pediatric, 733–734, 733f
of fracture, 93–94, 95f, 96f, 97t
of fracture healing, 226
of glenohumeral dislocation, 652
of growth plate fracture, 94
of head injury, 281, 285f, 286
of Hill-Sachs defect, 672f, 675f
of hip fracture, 1038–1039, 1042f–1044f
of hook of hamate fracture, 848–849, 850f
of infraspinatus muscle strain, 596f
of insufficiency fracture, 69, 94, 96f
of knee, 15f, 1118, 1120–1124, 1121f–1124f
of knee osteochondral fracture, 1181, 1185, 1185f
of lateral collateral ligament, 1123, 1124f
of lumbar spine fracture, 466, 471, 471f–478f, 475
of lumbar spine fracture-dislocation, 507, 512f

Magnetic resonance imaging *(Continued)*
of medial collateral ligament, 1122–1123, 1124f, 1237f
of meniscus, 1118, 1120–1121, 1121f
of metatarsal stress fracture, 1331, 1332f
of occult intraosseous knee injury, 1124, 1125f–1127f, 1126–1127
of osteochondral fracture, 94
of osteonecrosis, 94, 260–263, 264f
of patellar dislocation, 1172, 1174f, 1175f
of patellar tendon, 1123–1124
of pelvic insufficiency fracture, 963f, 964
of peroneal tendon, 1237f, 1238f
of peroneal tendon fibrosing synovitis, 1346, 1350f
of peroneal tendon subluxation, 1346, 1350f
of polytrauma, 147, 148
of posterior cruciate ligament, 1122, 1123f
of posterior cruciate ligament tear, 1124, 1125f
of posterior tibial tendon, 1237f, 1238f
of posterior tibiofibular ligament, 1237f
of proximal femoral fracture, 1038, 1042f
of proximal femoral insufficiency fracture, 1042f–1044f
of proximal tibial stress fracture, 63, 65f
of quadriceps tendon, 1123–1124
of quadriceps tendon rupture, 1178, 1180f
of scaphoid fracture, 826f–827f, 831, 832f
of scaphoid fracture nonunion, 226
of scapholunate dissociation, 863, 864f, 865f
of shoulder dislocation, 652
of shoulder injury, 594, 596f–599f
of shoulder instability, 671, 672f–675f
of skull base fracture, 285f
of skull fracture, 281, 285f, 286
of soft tissue, 94, 95f
of spinal compression fracture, 493, 495f, 496f
of stress fracture, 63, 65f, 94, 96f
of subchondral fracture, 52, 53f
of supraspinatus tendon tear, 596f
of temporal bone fracture, 301–302
of thoracic spine fracture, 466, 471, 471f–478f, 475
of thoracic spine fracture-dislocation, 507, 512f
of tibial bone bruise, 1124, 1125f, 1126, 1127f
of tibial collateral ligament, 1122–1123
of tibial condylar crack, 1124, 1127f
of tibial plateau (plafond) bone bruise, 1124, 1126f
of tibial plateau (plafond) fracture, 1145, 1148f–1150f
of tibial stress fracture, 1206, 1208f
of transverse tibiofibular ligament, 1237f
of trauma, 94
of triangular fibrocartilage complex injury, 866, 867f
of wrist, 783, 784t
Maisonneuve's fracture, 1270, 1275f–1278f
pronationnexternal rotation and, 1263
radiography of, 1230
Malar eminence, 316
fracture of, 346
Malgaigne fracture, 965–966, 965f–967f
radiography of, 90f
Malleolus
avulsion fracture of, 1246, 1246f
computed tomography of, 1231, 1234f–1235f, 1326f, 1328f
fracture of
in diabetic neuroarthropathy, 1283f, 1284
radiography of, internal oblique view in, 1227, 1228f
Malleolus *(Continued)*
tibial spiral fracture with, 1282, 1283f
lateral
avulsion fracture of, peroneal tendon dislocation in, 1246, 1248f
fracture of, 1241, 1244f
talus in, 1227
vs. proximal fifth metatarsal fracture, 1393
oblique fracture of, 44f
radiography of, 1225, 1226f
spiral fracture of
with posterior distal fibular dislocation, 1281
supination–external rotation and, 1257, 1259f
transverse fracture of, 1241, 1245f, 1246, 1270, 1272f
supination-adduction and, 1256–1257, 1257f, 1258f
medial, 1223, 1223f
avulsion fracture of
posterior tibial tendon injury with, 1246, 1248f
with subtalar joint dislocation, 1358, 1360f
comminuted fracture of, 1241, 1241f, 1242f
fracture of, 1270, 1278f
stability of, 1240
treatment of, 1280
oblique fracture of, 1240, 1240f, 1241, 1243f, 1270, 1272f
pronation-dorsiflexion and, 1270, 1271f
pronation–external rotation and, 1270, 1274f
radiography of, 85f, 1225, 1226f, 1227, 1229, 1229f
transverse fracture of, 44f, 1240, 1240f, 1241f
pronation-abduction and, 1267, 1267f–1269f
pronation–external rotation and, 1263, 1265f, 1266f
supination–external rotation and, 1257, 1261f, 1262f
posterior, 1222
fracture of, 1248–1249, 1251f, 1275f
supination–external rotation and, 1263, 1264f
fracture-dislocation of, pronation–external rotation and, 1270, 1274f
sprain fracture of, 1230, 1230f, 1246, 1246f
vs. secondary ossification centers, 1246, 1247f
Mallet finger, 880, 881f, 882, 882f
Mallet thumb, 917
Malocclusion, in mandibular fracture, 371
Malunion, 218, 221f
Mandible, 316, 317f, 320
condyles of
dislocation of, 369
fracture of, 371
sagittal splitting fracture of, 368, 370f
coronoid process of, fracture of, 371
fracture of, 366–372
computed tomography of, 369, 369f, 370f
distribution of, 368, 368f
fracture lines in, 371
healing of, 372
malocclusion in, 371
mechanisms of, 366
panoramic view of, 371f
pediatric, 368
pharyngeal air in, 371
radiography of, 369, 370f, 371, 371f
Mandible *(Continued)*
teeth displacement in, 371
temporomandibular joint in, 368
treatment of, 372
multiple fracture of, 368, 369f, 370f
triple fracture of, 371–372
Manubrium, flexion-compression fracture of, 556–557, 558f
March fracture, 1394
Mass, paraspinous, in lumbar/thoracic fracture, 455, 459f
Mastoid, fracture of, 298, 300–303
direction of, 298, 300f
location of, 302–303
signs/symptoms of, 302–303
Mastoid air cells, in head trauma, 286, 288f
Materials
brittle, 18
ductile, 18
Maxilla, 316, 317f
fracture of, 356, 358–366
in sagittal plane, 366, 366f
frontal process of, fracture of, 353, 354f
Maxillary sinus, 319f
Mechanical factors, in fracture, 17–19, 17f–19f
Median nerve, 821
entrapment of
after Colles' fracture, 787–788
elbow dislocation and, 711
pediatric elbow dislocation and, 765
radius greenstick fracture and, 766
injury to, 684
humeral shaft fracture and, 649
Mediastinum
evaluation of, in chest trauma, 589
great vessels of, 610, 613f
hematoma of
imaging assessment of, 152, 154f
upper thoracic fracture-dislocation and, 507, 514, 515f
hemorrhage of, thoracic polytrauma and, 150, 152, 152f
polytrauma to, computed tomography of, 150, 152, 153f, 155f
widening of, sternal fracture and, 514, 516f
Medullary cavity, 6, 6f
Mendosal sutures, vs. linear calvaria fractures, 288
Meningeal artery, in linear calvaria fractures, 288
Meniscus, 13, 15f, 1111, 1112f
magnetic resonance imaging of, 1118, 1120–1121, 1121f
medial, injury to, 1156f
deep notch sign in, 1158, 1160f
Mesentery, trauma to, computed tomography of, 163–164, 164f
Metacarpal(s), 879
base of
avulsion of, 896
dorsal dislocation of, 907, 909f
fracture of, 894, 896f, 897, 897f
volar dislocation of, 906f–908f, 907
boxer's fracture of, 888, 894, 894f–896f
fifth, 904–905
torus fracture of, 920, 922f
first
comminuted fracture of, 912, 914f, 915f
dorsal subluxation of, 912, 914f
extra-articular fracture of, 912, 916f
fracture of, 911, 913f
Salter-Harris type 2 epiphyseal injury to, 923, 926f
fourth, 904–905
fracture of, 888, 894, 894f–896f, 909
incidence of, 879

Metacarpal(s) *(Continued)*
head of
avulsion fracture of, 897, 898f
comminuted fracture of, 897, 897f
depressed fracture of, 897, 898f
epiphyseal injury to, 923
fracture of, 897–898, 897f, 898f
oblique fracture of, 894, 895f, 896f
radiography of, 874, 877f
Salter-Harris type 2 injury to, 924f
second, 904
third
lateral view of, 818, 818f
styloid process of, 904
transverse fracture of, 894, 894f
as tubular bone, 7
volar dislocation of, 908f
Metacarpohamate joint
disruption of, hamate fracture with, 907, 909, 912f
fifth, dislocation of, 905, 906f–909f, 907
Metacarpophalangeal joint, 879
collateral ligament injury at, 888, 890f
complex dislocation of, 898, 900f, 903–904, 904f
complex fracture-dislocation of, 904, 905f
dislocation of, 902f–905f, 903–904
pediatric, 923, 925
treatment of, 898, 900
types of, 898
irreducible dislocation of, 925
lateral subluxation of, 904
ligamentous injury at, 916–917, 917f–921f
simple dislocation of, 898, 900f, 903, 903f
simultaneous dislocation of, 902f, 903
thumb, 909, 911
dislocation of, 920
volar dislocation of, 904
Metacarpotrapezoid joint, injury to, 911f
Metal, in orbit, 347f
Metaphysis, 6, 6f
blood supply of, 11, 11f, 117–118, 120f
fracture of, in battered child syndrome, 132, 133f, 134f, 135, 136f
Metastasis
pathologic femoral fracture in, 1102–1103
pathologic fracture in, 75
spinal, fracture in, 493, 497f
Metatarsal(s)
accessory ossification center of, 1371, 1376, 1379f
epiphyseal injury to, 1400, 1401f
fifth
base of
apophysis of
vs. avulsion fracture, 1319–1320
vs. fracture, 1401, 1402f, 1403
avulsion fracture of, 1393, 1394f, 1403, 1403f
fracture of, 1393, 1394f
pediatric injury to, 1401, 1402f, 1403, 1403f
fracture of, vs. ankle fracture, 1227, 1227f
proximal
stress fracture of, 1396, 1397f
transverse fracture of, 1393–1394, 1394f
first
base of
epiphyseal separation of, 1400, 1401f
stress fracture of, 1396
computed tomography of, 821, 822f
fracture of, 1386, 1387f
pediatric, 1400, 1401f
ligaments of, 1371
march fracture of, 1394

Metatarsal(s) *(Continued)*
radiography of, 1321
second, stress fracture of, 58f
stress fracture of, 63, 1329, 1394, 1395f–1398f, 1396
diabetic osteoarthropathy and, 1396, 1398f
magnetic resonance imaging of, 1331, 1332f
nonunion of, 1397f
radiography of, 1330
third, stress fracture of, 59f, 1396f, 1397f
Metatarsophalangeal joint
foot, dislocation of, 1386, 1389f, 1390f
great toe, dislocation of, 1389f
injuries to, 1386
Metatarsotarsal joint, fracture-dislocation of, 1389f
Methotrexate, in fracture healing, 209
Microfracture, in bone bruise, 53
Middle ear, fracture of, cerebrospinal fluid otorrhea in, 302
Midface, LeFort fracture of
classification of, 315
with naso-orbital-ethmoidal fracture, 356
Midfoot, 1319, 1319f
fracture of, computed tomography of, 89
Midtarsal joint, dislocation of, 1371, 1376f, 1377f
Mineralization, in fracture healing, 205
Modified Injury Severity Scale, 172, 174t
Monteggia fracture, 716, 717f–719f, 718–719
diagnosis of, 718
mechanism of, 716, 718
pediatric, 767, 768f–770f, 770
treatment of, 718–719
types of, 716, 717f, 718f
vs. elbow fracture/dislocation, 716, 718f, 767
Motion, in joint cartilage health, 13
Motor neuropathy, 1384
Motor vehicle accidents
death from, 1, 1f
fracture from, 28
Motorcycle accidents
flexion injury in, 475, 479f
polytrauma in, 145
thoracic fracture-dislocation in, 507, 508f
Muscle, stress response of, 1330
Musculoskeletal system
macroscopic components of, 17
microscopic components of, 17
Myelomeningocele
pathologic epiphyseal injury in, 138, 142, 142f
proximal femoral epiphyseal separation in, 1087–1088, 1090f
Myocardium, contusions of, 588
Myonecrosis, in gas gangrene, 236, 237f
Myositis ossificans, 258–259, 260f
elbow dislocation and, 712
in proximal humeral fracture, 639, 642f

Nail(s), intramedullary, 188–189, 189f–192f, 191–193
dynamic, 191
locking, 191–192, 191f
nonlocking, 191
osteomyelitis in, 244–245, 246t
reamed, 189, 191, 191f
retrograde, 191, 192f
static, 191
unreamed, 189, 190f
Nail bed, disruption of, growth plate injuries and, 923, 925f

Naked facet sign, in thoracolumbar junction fracture-dislocation, 516, 520f
Nasal bones, 316, 317f
Nasal cartilage, displacement of, 354f
Nasal fracture, 353–357
computed tomography of, 353, 355f
radiography of, 353, 353f, 354f
Nasal spine fracture, 353f
Naso-orbital-ethmoidal fracture, 353, 354f–356f, 356–357
bilateral, 355f, 356, 356f
classification of, 356
computed tomography of, 355f, 356–357, 356f
injuries associated with, 356
unilateral, 355f, 356
Nasopharyngeal soft tissue, swelling of, in cervical spine fractures, 386
Navicular, 1319f, 1364, 1366–1369
avulsion injury of, 1355
body of, fracture of, 1364, 1366, 1368f–1370f
computed tomography of, 1326f, 1327f, 1329f
crush fracture of, cuneiform dislocation with, 1366, 1371f
dislocation of, body fracture with, 1364, 1366, 1370f
horizontal fracture of, 1364, 1368f
stress fracture of, 1329, 1330, 1366, 1369, 1372f–1374f
synchondrosis of, 1364, 1368f
tuberosity of, fracture of, 1364, 1367f
cuboid compression fracture with, 1369, 1376f
vs. accessory ossification center, 1364, 1368f
vertical fracture of, 1364, 1369f, 1370f
dislocation with, 1364, 1366, 1370f
Navicular fat stripe, posteroanterior view of, 817, 817f
Naviculocuneiform joint, dislocation of, 1364, 1370f, 1371, 1378f
Necrosis, avascular
in femoral neck fractures, 1056–1057
of humeral head, 639
Nelson's X, 732–733, 733f
Neural arch, 377, 377f
Neuroarthropathy, 1384
chronic, magnetic resonance imaging of, 1386, 1386f
diabetic, 1384, 1385f
fractures in, 1282, 1283f, 1284
Neuropathy, peripheral, 1384, 1385f, 1386, 1386f
Neurotrophic arthritis
diabetic, 1282, 1283f, 1284
insufficiency fracture in, 73, 74f
Nicotine, in fracture healing, 209
Nightstick fracture, 21, 21f
distal ulnar, 716, 716f
Nonunion, 221, 222f–224f, 225
appliance failure in, 221, 224f, 225
atrophic, 221
fibular, osteomyelitis in, 244f
in fracture healing, 221, 222f–224f, 225
hypertrophic, 221, 222f, 223f
in internal fixation failure, 221, 224f, 225
of metatarsal stress fracture, 1397f
of odontoid process (dens) fracture, 411
osteomyelitis in, 244f
of scaphoid fracture, 223f, 226, 779, 836–837, 837f
of supracondylar fracture, pseudarthrosis with, 219f
of tibial fracture, 219f, 222f, 228f, 244f, 1194

Nonunion *(Continued)*
of ulnar fracture, 223f, 224f
Nutcracker fracture, 1369
Nutrient artery, 11, 11f

Obturator artery, bleeding of, pelvic fracture and, 1016f
Obturator internus muscle, in pelvis injury, 941, 945
Occipital condyle, fracture of, 298, 299f, 300f, 412
Occipital fissure, vs. linear calvaria fractures, 288
Occult fracture
acetabular, 995, 1000, 1000f–1002f, 1002
computed tomography of, 1002, 1002f
obturator internus sign in, 995, 1000, 1001f
vs. hip fracture, 1000, 1002, 1002f
calcaneal, 1331, 1332f
pediatric, 1400, 1400f
foot, 1331–1332, 1332f
intraosseous, 53f
knee, magnetic resonance imaging of, 1124, 1125f–1127f, 1126–1127
phalangeal epiphyseal
foot, 1401, 1401f, 1402f
great toe, 1401, 1401f, 1402f
scaphoid, bone scan of, 831, 833f
stress, 63
talar, 1331
Odontoid process (dens), 394
fracture of, 399f, 408–411
anteroposterior open-mouth projection of, 409, 410f
classification of, 408–410, 409f
computed tomography of, 410
diagnosis of, 410–411
Mach effect in, 410–411, 412f
nonunion of, 411
pediatric, 410, 412f
type II, 396f
type III, 397f
vs. normal variants, 410
transverse fracture of, vs. os odontoideum, 410
Olecranon
apophysis of, separation of, 761, 763f
displaced fracture of, 706f
fracture of, 705, 706f, 707–708, 707f
hemarthrosis with, 687f
pediatric, 757, 760f, 761, 762f, 763, 763f
incomplete fracture of, 41, 41f
oblique fracture of, 705, 706f
torus fracture of, 762f
Olecranon bursa, hemorrhage into, elbow injuries and, 689, 689f
Open fracture, 41, 42f
classification of, 182, 182t, 184
comminuted, tibial, cast for, 181f
distal tibial, 42f
femoral, 41
gunshot wounds and, 41, 43f
of joints, 55, 57f
lumbar spine, 534, 536f
osteomyelitis in, 244–245
pelvic, 967, 969, 969f, 970f
proximal tibial, popliteal artery transection with, 169f
radial, 41
tibial, 41
traumatic amputation and, 41, 43f
treatment of, 182, 184
ulnar, 41
Open fracture *(Continued)*
osteomyelitis after, 248f
Optic nerve, hemorrhage into, 342, 346f
Orbicular ligament, 684
Orbit, 319f, 320f
blow-in fracture of, 290, 292f, 337, 338f–340f
blow-out fracture of, 332–335, 332f–336f, 337
buckling mechanism of, 332f, 333, 334–335
computed tomography of, 333f, 334f, 335, 335f
extraocular muscle entrapment in, 335, 336f
hydraulic mechanism of, 332f, 333–334, 335
radiography of, 335, 337
soft tissue injury with, 335, 336f
floor of, 316
blow-out fracture of, 333, 333f, 335
fracture of, 339–340
foreign body in, 342, 346, 347f
fracture of, 332–342
imaging of, 332
soft tissue injuries with, 325, 325t
hemorrhage within, 342, 345f, 346f
innominate line of, 330
lateral, fracture of, with zygomatic complex fracture, 348
lateral oblique line of, 330
medial, fracture of, 353, 354f, 356
rim of, 316
blow-in fracture of, 337
blow-out fracture of, 333
fracture of, 337, 339, 340f, 341f
in Water's view, 330
roof of
blow-in fracture of, 338f, 339f
fracture of, 341
soft tissue injury to, 342, 344f–347f, 346
wall of
blow-in fracture of, 339f
blow-out fracture of, 333, 334f
fracture of, 340–341
Orbital apex, fracture of, 341–342, 342f, 343f
Orbital compartment syndrome, 337, 342
Orbital space, 316
Os acetabuli, 941, 944f
vs. fracture, 1041
Os acromiale, vs. acromion process fracture, 626
Os calcaneus secundarius, 1320f
Os calcis, calcaneal apophysis on, 1319
Os intermetatarseum, 1320f, 1371, 1376, 1379f
Os odontoideum, vs. transverse odontoid process fracture, 410
Os peroneum, 1319, 1320f, 1321f
fracture of, with peroneus longus tendon rupture, 1369, 1375f
vs. cuboid fracture, 1369
vs. metatarsal base transverse fracture, 1394
Os supranaviculare, 1319, 1320f
vs. talonavicular avulsion fracture, 1364, 1366f
Os supratalare, 1319, 1320f
Os tibiale externum, 1319, 1320f, 1321f
Os trigonum, 1319, 1320f
avulsion of, 1355, 1356f
flexor hallucis tendon impingement by, 1355, 1357f
vs. posterior talar tubercle fracture, 1355, 1356f, 1357f
Os vesalianum, 1319, 1320f
vs. cuboid fracture, 1369
Os vesalianum *(Continued)*
vs. metatarsal base transverse fracture, 1394
Osgood-Schlatter disease
anterior tibial apophysis ossification centers in, 1130
vs. anterior tibial tubercle fracture, 1180
Ossicles
disruption of, in temporal bone fracture, 300, 302, 302f
fracture of, 49
Ossification, 9–12
ages at, 11, 12f
endochondral, 9, 10f, 11
intracartilaginous, 9
intramembranous, 9
periosteal, 10
Ossification centers
accessory
acetabular, 941, 944f
vs. fracture, 1039, 1041
carpal, 827, 828f, 829
foot, vs. fracture, 1319–1320, 1320f, 1321f
metatarsal, 1371, 1376, 1379f
patellar, 1167, 1170f
vs. navicular tuberosity fracture, 1364, 1368f
at birth, 11–12
distal humeral, 732–733, 733f
distal tibial, 1296, 1296f
elbow, 732–733, 733f
humeral head, 639, 643f
medial epicondylar, treatment and, 750–751
in Osgood-Schlatter disease, 1130
pelvic, 931, 931f
primary, 9–10
scapular, 620, 620f
secondary, 10–12, 10f–12f
appearance of, 11, 12f
closure of, 10–11
in fracture detection, 101–102
of hook of hamate, 849
knee, vs. osteochondral fracture, 1186–1187, 1188f
patellar, 1128
pelvic, 931
trauma and, 11
types of, 12, 13f
vs. malleolar sprain fracture, 1246, 1247f
vs. osteochondritis dissecans, 1130
Osteitis pubis, traumatic, 1012, 1014f
Osteoarthritis, 263, 265f, 266
ankle instability and, 1381
femoral fracture in, 1047
tibial stress fracture in, 1204
Osteoarthropathy, diabetic, metatarsal stress fracture in, 1396, 1398f
Osteoblasts, in fracture healing, 205
Osteochondral fracture, 49, 52
bone bruise with, 53f
glenoid fossa, 761
humeral head, 722, 725f, 771, 773
pediatric, 770f, 771
knee. *See* Knee, osteochondral fracture of.
lateral femoral condylar, 1183f–1185f
magnetic resonance imaging of, 94
in patellar dislocation, 1180, 1182, 1182f, 1185
subchondral bone in, 52
talar
with Dupuytren fracture, 1266f
in subtalar joint dislocation, 1363, 1364f
talar dome, 1289, 1292f–1294f
types of, 52f
ultrasonography of, 52
vs. osteochondritis dissecans, 1186, 1187f

Osteochondritis dissecans
of capitellum, 770f, 771
talar dome, in type 2 distal tibial epiphyseal injury, 1302f–1303f
vs. femoral secondary ossification center, 1130
vs. osteochondral fracture, 1186, 1187f
Osteodystrophy, renal
epiphyseal separations in, 138, 141f
insufficiency fracture in, 64, 70, 72f
pathologic fracture in, 138, 141f
Osteogenesis
electrical stimulation of, 199, 200f
ultrasound stimulation of, 199–200
Osteogenesis imperfecta
insufficiency fracture in, 69–70, 71f
recurring fracture in, 138, 140f
Osteoid, 9
Osteoid matrix, 7
Osteolysis, post-traumatic, 255, 256f
clavicular, 604
Osteomalacia, pathologic femoral fracture in, 1102, 1103
Osteomyelitis, 244–252
bone destruction in, 248, 248f, 250f
bone scan of, 248
chronic, 251, 251f, 252
definition of, 244
diagnosis of, 248, 248f–252f, 251–252
incidence of, 244–245
in intramedullary nails, 244–245, 246t
in open reduction, 244–245, 244f–246f
organisms in, 247
pain in, 247
pathogenesis of, 245, 247–248, 247f
pathologic fracture in, 75, 78f
periosteal bone formation in, 248, 249f
in plate fixation, 244, 244f, 245f
radiography of, 248, 248f–252f, 251–252
sclerosis in, 251, 251f
sesamoid, 1399
sinography of, 251–252, 251f
sites for, 245
tomography of, 251, 252f
treatment of, 252
vertebral, 492
Osteonecrosis, 259–263, 262f–264f
clinical manifestations of, 260
magnetic resonance imaging of, 94, 260–263, 264f
radiography of, 260, 262
revascularization in, 259–260
sclerotic mechanisms in, 260
sites for, 259, 262f, 263f
Osteons, 8f
in bone strength, 19
primary, 10
woven bone from, 11
Osteopathy, neurotrophic, 1384, 1386
Osteopetrosis, insufficiency fracture in, 70, 71f
Osteoporosis
age-related, 30
bone densitometry in, 33–34, 35f
bone mass loss in, 29, 30, 30f
bone mineral density in, 34
bone resorption in, 29
classification of, 30
diagnosis of, 33–34, 35f, 36–37, 36f
distal tibial insufficiency fracture in, 1285, 1287f
disuse, 214f, 215f, 216f
in disuse atrophy, 211, 214
fracture in, 29–37
incidence of, 30, 32
risk for, 34, 36–37, 36f
sites for, 32, 32f

Osteoporosis *(Continued)*
idiopathic juvenile, metaphyseal fractures in, 138
impact of, 37
insufficiency fracture in, 266f, 268, 1348, 1352f
kyphosis in, spontaneous sternal fracture in, 492–493
pelvic insufficiency fracture in, 64, 66f–68f, 68, 959, 959f–963f
postmenopausal, 30
Colles' fracture in, 785
post-traumatic, 266f, 267f, 268
in proximal femoral fractures, 1042
radiography of, 33, 33f
in reflex dystrophy syndrome, 253, 255
senile, insufficiency fracture in, 69
spinal compression fracture in, 471, 475f, 491f, 492–493, 493f–496f
magnetic resonance imaging of, 493, 495f, 496f
spontaneous sternal fracture in, 557–558, 558f
steroid-related, 959–960, 962f–963f
trabecular fracture in, 30, 30f, 31f
treatment of, bone mineral density monitoring of, 37
vacuum vertebra in, 492, 494f
Otorrhea, cerebrospinal fluid
skull fracture and, 305–306, 305f
temporal bone fracture and, 302

Paget's disease
insufficiency fracture in, 69, 70f
pathologic femoral fracture in, 1102, 1103
Panner's disease, 722
Paranasal sinuses, fracture of, pneumocephalus in, 303
Paraplegia, insufficiency fracture in, 73, 73f
Parry fracture, 21, 21f
Pars interarticularis
fracture of, 525–526, 525f
stress fracture of, 526, 527f, 528f
spondylolysis with, 526, 529f
Patella
accessory ossification centers of, 1167, 1170f
anatomy of, 1111, 1112f, 1113
avulsion fracture of, 1164, 1167, 1169
bone bruise of, 1167, 1169f
comminuted fracture of, 1164–1165
dislocation of, 1169, 1172–1173
chondral fracture with, 1169, 1172, 1175f
femoral condylar contusion with, 1172, 1175f
with horizontal rotation, 1173, 1176f
impaction fracture with, 1172, 1172f
magnetic resonance imaging of, 1172, 1174f, 1175f
mechanism of, 1172, 1173f
osteochondral fracture with, 1169, 1172, 1172f, 1180, 1182, 1182f, 1185
recurrent, 1172f, 1173, 1175, 1177f
with vertical rotation, 1173
fracture of, 1164, 1166f–1170f, 1167, 1169
classification of, 1164, 1166f
sunrise projection of, 1167, 1169f
treatment of, 1169
lateral dislocation of, 1169, 1171f, 1173f
pathologic fracture of, 1167
radiography of, axial (sunrise) view in, 1116, 1119f
secondary ossification center in, 1128
separated fracture of, 1164, 1167
stellate fracture of, 1164, 1167f

Patella *(Continued)*
stress fracture of, 1204
transverse fracture of, 20, 1164–1165, 1166f, 1167, 1167f
with femur fracture, 1094, 1097f
undisplaced fracture of, 1164, 1167f, 1169
vertical fracture of, 1164, 1168f
Patella alta, identification of, 1175, 1177f
Patella cubiti, fracture of, 707
pediatric, 763
Patellar tendon, magnetic resonance imaging of, 1123–1124
Patellofemoral groove, 1111, 1112f
Patellofemoral joint, computed tomography of, 1118
Pathologic fracture, 57, 73–76
acetabular, 1002, 1003f, 1004f
in breast cancer, 80f, 81f
in cerebral palsy, 142
in Cooley's anemia, 138, 141f
femoral, 75, 81f, 1102–1103
proximal, 1087–1088, 1090f
subtrochanteric, 1065, 1067f
in systemic disease, 1102, 1103
fibular, 1198
humeral, 649, 650f
metastases and, 73, 75, 76f
in myelomeningocele, 138, 142, 142f
in osteomyelitis, 75, 78f
patellar, 1167
pediatric, 137–142. *See also under* Children.
in pediatric bone cyst, 137, 138f
in pediatric β-thalassemia, 138, 141f
phalangeal, 879
in sarcoidosis, 79f
radiography of, 73, 75, 76f–81f
in renal osteodystrophy, 138, 141f
in sarcoidosis, 75, 79f
tibial, 1198
transverse, 75, 77f
tumors and, 77f
vertebral, 75, 80f, 493, 497f
vs. osteoporotic compression fracture, 471, 474f, 492, 493f
Patient record, in fractures, 102–105, 104f
Pectoral girdle, injuries to, 593
Pectoralis major muscle, 594, 633
Pellegrini-Stieda disease, 1130, 1134f
Pelvic ring, 930, 930f
Pelvis, 930–1026
anatomy of, 930–933, 930f–933f
anterior arch of, 930, 930f
anterior compression injury of, 972, 974f, 975, 975f
apophyseal avulsion fracture of, 1009, 1010f–1014f, 1012
arches of, 930, 930f
avulsion fracture of, 971–972
bucket handle fracture of, 975
coccyx of, 931, 932f
complex fracture of, 969, 971f, 977–978, 977f
computed tomography of, 934, 937–939, 938f–943f, 941
dislocation of, 967, 968f
double fracture of, 964–969
double vertical fracture-dislocation of, 964–967, 965f–967f
femorosacral arch of, 930, 930f
fracture of, 930, 945–979
arteriography in, 1015, 1015f, 1016f
biomechanical classification of, 969, 971f
bladder rupture in, 1015, 1018f–1023f
bowel injury in, 1024f, 1025, 1025f
classification of, 945–946, 947f
computed tomography of, 89, 91f

Pelvis *(Continued)*
external fixation of, 978, 978f
hemorrhage in, 945, 945f, 946f, 1012–1013, 1015, 1015f, 1016f
incidence of, 945–946
pediatric, 1002, 1005, 1005f
injury associated with, 1012–1013, 1015–1025
instability in, 969, 971–972
mortality in, 946
pediatric, 1002, 1005–1012
classification of, 1007
distribution of, 1007
proximal femoral epiphyseal separation with, 1086
Salter-Harris type 1, 1007
Salter-Harris type 2, 1007, 1007f–1010f
through Y cartilage, 1007
peripheral nerve injury in, 1021, 1023f, 1025
screw-plate fixation of, 978–979, 979f
stability concept in, 969, 971–972
stable, 945–946, 947f
treatment of, 978–979, 978f, 979f
unstable, 945, 946, 947f
urethral injury in, 1015–1016, 1017f, 1021, 1021f, 1022f
urinary tract injury in, 1015–1016, 1017f–1021f, 1021
visceral injury in, 1021, 1022f
vs. ischiopubic synchondrosis, pediatric, 1005, 1006f, 1007
ilium of, 931, 931f
injury to, 930
hemorrhage in, 945, 945f, 946f
obturator internus muscle in, 941, 945
soft tissue clues to, 941, 945, 945f, 946f
innominate bones of, 7f, 930–931, 931f
insufficiency fracture of, 64, 66f–68f, 68, 958–964, 958f–963f
computed tomography of, 960f–963f, 964
femoral neck insufficiency fracture with, 1054
healing of, 964
magnetic resonance imaging of, 963f, 964
in osteoporosis, 959, 959f–963f
presentation of, 958–960
sclerosis in, 959f–961f, 960, 964
ischium of, 931, 931f
lateral compression injury to, 975, 976f, 977, 977f, 1022f, 1023f
ligaments of, 931, 933, 933f
Malgaigne fracture of, 965, 965f–967f
normal variants of, 941, 944f
open book anterior compression injury to, 940f–941f
open book injury of, 972, 974f, 975, 975f
open fracture of, 967, 969, 969f, 970f
ossification centers of, 931, 931f
posterior arch of, 930, 930f
fracture of, 966–967, 966f, 967f
radiography of, 933–934, 935f–937f
angled view of, 934, 936f
anteroposterior view in, 934, 935f–937f, 1033–1035, 1034f
Judet view of, 934
oblique view in, 934, 937f, 1036
sacrum of, 930–931, 931f, 932f
secondary ossification centers of, 931
single fracture of, 946–964
straddle fracture of, 967, 968f
stress fracture of, 955, 958, 958f
tie arch of, 930, 930f
unstable bucket handle fracture of, 965, 965f
vertical shearing injury of, 972, 972f, 973f

Pelvis *(Continued)*
windswept, 977–978, 977f
Pericardial tamponade, polytrauma and, 150, 151f
Perichondrium, periosteum from, 9–10
Perilunate dislocation, 849–855
bilateral, 850
capitate fracture with, 844, 845f, 854, 858f
capitolunate joint disruption in, 851, 852f
cortical arcs/lines in, 851–852, 851f
displacement in, 852
dorsal, 850
fractures associated with, 851, 852, 855f, 856f
mechanism of, 849–850
posterior, 852
radiography of, 851, 852f
with scaphoid fracture, 834
spontaneous reduction of, 855
transcapitate, fracture fragment in, 854, 858f
transscaphoid, 850, 852f
irreducible, 855
treatment of, 855
Perilunate fracture-dislocation, 850
Periosteal sleeve, anterior labroligamentous avulsion of, 671
Periosteum
in epiphyseal injury treatment, 128
from perichondrium, 9–10
tears of, bone scans of, 97
Peripheral nerves, injury to, pelvic fracture and, 1021, 1023f, 1025
Peripheral neuropathy, 1384, 1385f, 1386, 1386f
Peritendinitis calcarea, vs. hip fracture, 1041
Peritoneal lavage, 158
Peritoneum, bleeding into, 158
Peroneal nerve, 1113
injury to, proximal fibular fracture and, 1161
Peroneal tendons
in calcaneal fracture, 1346
computed tomography of, 1326f, 1328f
dislocation of, 1384
in lateral malleolar avulsion fracture, 1246, 1248f
fibrosing synovitis of, magnetic resonance imaging of, 1346, 1350f
magnetic resonance imaging of, 1237f, 1238f
rupture of, with os peroneum fracture, 1369, 1375f
split of, 1384, 1384f
subluxation of, magnetic resonance imaging of, 1346, 1350f
tear of, 1384
Petrous pyramid, fracture of, 298, 300–303
Phalanx (phalanges)
distal
dorsal dislocation of, 55f
vertical fracture of, 46, 47f
foot
dislocation of, 1390f
distal
bipartite, 1400, 1401f
epiphyseal separation of, 1400–1401, 1401f
fracture of, 1388f
pediatric fracture in, 1400–1401, 1401f
fracture of, 1386, 1388f
pediatric, 1400
radiography of, 1386, 1388, 1392f–1393f, 1393
proximal
avulsion fracture of, 1388f

Phalanx (phalanges) *(Continued)*
fracture of, 1388f, 1392f–1393f
stress fracture of, 1396
radiography of, 1321, 1324, 1324f
great toe, epiphysis of, vs. epiphyseal fracture, 1320
hand
distal
condyles of, fracture of, 888, 893f
epiphyseal injury to, 925f
extensor tendon insertion on, avulsion of, 880, 881f, 882, 882f
fracture of, 879–880, 881f
with flexor digitorum profundus tendon avulsion, 882–883, 883f
treatment of, 885, 887f
growth plate of, disruption of, 923, 925f
volar plate avulsion at, 883, 884f–886f
fracture of, 879–888
classification of, 879
incidence of, 879
pediatric, 920–921, 922f–926f, 923
power saws and, 879, 880f
middle, fracture of, 883
neck of, fracture of, pediatric, 920, 922f
pathologic fracture of, 879
proximal
fracture of, 885–886, 886f–891f, 888
impacted fracture of, 886, 889f
insufficiency fracture of, 71f
intra-articular fracture of, 886, 888, 890f–892f
oblique fracture of, 886, 887f
Salter-Harris type 1 fracture of, 920, 921, 923, 925f
Salter-Harris type 2 fracture of, 920–921, 923f, 924f
Salter-Harris type 3 fracture of, 920, 923, 925f
Salter-Harris type 4 fracture of, 920, 925f
transverse fracture of, 886, 888f
vascular channels of, vs. fracture, 874, 878f
volar plate at, avulsion fracture of, 876f
sarcoidosis of, pathologic fracture in, 79f
as tubular bone, 7
Pilon (pestle), fracture of, 1231, 1236f, 1249
computed tomography of, 1270, 1272f, 1273f
healing of, computed tomography of, 226, 227f
Pineal gland, calcification of, in head trauma, 287
Ping-pong fracture, 290, 293f, 294f
Pins
in external fixation, 193–194, 196f–197f
migration of, 252–253
osteomyelitis after, 250f
Pisiform, 813
computed tomography of, 821, 822f
45-degree oblique views of, 818, 819f
dislocation of, 842
fracture of, 827, 841–842, 842f
posteroanterior view of, 816–817
Pisohamate ligament, 841
Pisometacarpal ligament, 841
Pisotriquetral joint
computed tomography of, 819, 821, 821f–823f
45-degree supination oblique view of, 818, 819f
Plates, 185
blade, 188, 189f
compression, 185, 188, 188f

Plates *(Continued)*
osteomyelitis with, 244, 244f, 245f
refracture after, 258, 258f
Pleura, trauma to, 559–567
Pleural effusion, eosinophilic, 561
Pneumocephalus
computed tomography of, 303, 305f
in head trauma, 286, 287, 288f
mechanism of, 303
onset of, 303, 304f
in skull fracture, 303, 304f, 305, 305f, 310–311
in temporal bone fracture, 301
tension, 303, 305f
Pneumolabyrinth, in temporal bone fracture, 301, 302f
Pneumomediastinum, 566–567
in bronchial rupture, 579, 580f–582f, 581
with facial fracture, 316
Pneumopericardium, 588, 588f
Pneumoperitoneum, 566
Pneumothorax, 561–566
in bronchial rupture, 579, 580f, 581f
computed tomography of, 564, 564f
radiography of, 562–564, 563f
in rib fracture, 550, 550f, 561, 562f
tension, 564, 565f, 566
pulmonary contusion with, 569f
traumatic, 566, 566f
Polytrauma, 145–176. *See also* Trauma.
Abbreviated Injury Scale for, 172, 173t–174t
abdominal, 158–164
bowel injury in, 163–164, 164f, 164t
vs. increased central venous pressure, 164, 165f
vs. pneumoperitoneum, 164, 165f
vs. shock bowel, 164, 166f
hemorrhage in, computed tomography of, 160, 161f
nonoperative management of, 162–163, 162t, 163t, 164f
penetrating, computed tomography of, 164, 166f
screening evaluation in, 158–160, 160t
age distribution in, 145
care systems in, 145–147
carotid artery injury in, 164, 166
causes of, 145
cerebrovascular injury in, 164, 166–167
cervical spine
imaging studies of, 148–150, 148f–149f, 150t
radiographic oversights in, 168, 170f
computed tomography of, 147, 148
definition of, 145, 146f
diagnostic oversights in, 167–168, 168f
fracture distribution in, 145, 147f
Glasgow Coma Scale in, 172, 174t
imaging in, 147–148, 167
injury severity in, coding systems for, 168, 172, 173t–174t, 175f, 176, 176f
Injury Severity Score in, 172, 176f
magnetic resonance imaging of, 147, 148
Modified Injury Severity Scale for, 172, 174t
physical examination of, 167, 169f
radiography of, 147
shock in, 145
spinal cord, second-level injuries in, 168, 171f, 172f
thoracic spine, 150–158. *See also under* Thoracic spine.
vertebral artery injury in, 166
Popliteal artery, 1113, 1114f
angiography of, 1116–1118
complete occlusion of, 231, 233f
Popliteal artery *(Continued)*
injury to, 231, 232f, 233f
partial occlusion of, 231, 232f
transection of, in proximal tibial fracture, 169f
Porencephaly, post-traumatic, 306
Post-tussive fracture of Gooch, 556, 556f
Power saws, phalangeal fracture from, 879, 880f
Pre-Achilles triangle, 1230, 1231f
Pregnancy, symphysis pubis separation in, 964, 964f
Pronation, foot, 1236, 1238, 1320
Pronation-abduction, in fibular bending fracture, 1267, 1269f
Pronation-dorsiflexion
in anterior tubercular tibial fracture, 1270, 1271f
in fibular fracture, 1270, 1271f, 1272f
in medial malleolar oblique fracture, 1270, 1271f
in tibial plateau (plafond) fracture, 1270, 1272f, 1273f
Pronation–external rotation
in ankle injury, 1263, 1265f, 1266f, 1267
in Dupuytren's fracture, 1263, 1266f
in fibular fracture, 1270, 1274f
in fibular spiral fracture, 1263, 1266f
in Maisonneuve's fracture, 1263
in medial collateral ligament rupture, 1263, 1265f, 1266f
in medial malleolar oblique fracture, 1270, 1274f
in medial malleolar transverse fracture, 1263, 1265f, 1266f
in posterior malleolar fracture-dislocation, 1270, 1274f
Pronator quadratus, 779, 780f
in distal radial epiphyseal displacement, 808
in distal radial fractures, 781, 782f, 783, 783f
in transverse distal radial fracture, 795, 796f
Pseudarthrosis, supracondylar fracture nonunion with, 219f
Pseudoaneurysm, 234
aortic, 152, 153f
ultrasonography of, 234, 235f
Pseudofracture, vs. shin splints, 59
Pseudogout, tibial stress fracture in, 1204
Psoas stripe, in lumbar/thoracic fracture, 455, 459f
Pubic ramus
fracture of, 947, 948f–953f, 1069f
lateral compression and, 975, 977f
vs. acetabular fracture, 1002
insufficiency fracture of, 960, 962f–963f, 963
stress fracture of, 63, 954, 954f
unilateral fracture of, 946–947, 948f–953f, 954
Pubis, 931, 931f
insufficiency fracture of, 963, 963f
Pulmonary contusion, 567, 568f, 569f, 573f
in diaphragm rupture, 574, 577f, 578f
in rib fracture, 546, 548f
Pulmonary embolism, 240, 242. *See also* Thromboembolism.
Pulmonary laceration, 567, 570, 570f–573f
adhesion tear, 567
compression-rupture, 567, 571f
compression-shear, 567, 570, 571f, 572f
rib penetration, 567, 573f
Pulmonary parenchyma, trauma to, 567–574
Pulse, in arterial injury, 231
Pyknodysostosis, insufficiency fracture in, 70, 72f
Quadriceps tendon, 1112f, 1113
magnetic resonance imaging of, 1123–1124
radiography of, 1116
rupture of, 1176, 1178, 1178f
magnetic resonance imaging of, 1178, 1180f
Quadriplegia
with central cord syndrome, 427f
insufficiency fracture in, 73, 73f

Race, in fracture, 26–28
Radial nerve, in humeral shaft fractures, 645, 649
Radiation therapy
insufficiency fracture after, 70, 73f
pediatric epiphyseal separation after, 142
Radiculopathy, cervical, in articular pillar fracture, 442
Radiocapitate ligament, 813, 814f
Radiocapitellar line, 731–732, 731f, 732f
Radiocarpal joint, dislocation of, 793, 793f, 794f
in Colles' fracture, 785, 790f
Radiocarpal ligament
dorsal, 813–814, 814f
volar, 813, 814f
Radiography
diagnosis with, 3
errors in, 79, 82f, 83
exposure for, 79, 82f
postreduction, 200–201
procedure for, 79, 83
satisfaction of work in, 168
skeletal, 6
with splints, 2, 2f, 3f
in trauma, 2–3, 2f, 3f, 76, 78–79, 78t, 79t
views in, 83
Radiology report, in fractures, 104–105, 104f
Radionuclide bone scan
in battered child syndrome, 137
of carpal injury, 819, 820f
of fracture, 97–98, 98f
of fracture healing, 97
of hook of hamate fracture, 819, 820f
of insufficiency fracture, 64, 68f, 98
of ligament avulsion, 97
of occult scaphoid fracture, 831, 833f
of osteomyelitis, 248
of periosteum tears, 97
of rib fracture, 541
of scaphoid fracture, 98f, 819, 831, 833f
of spinal compression fracture, 98
of stress fracture, 63, 64f, 98
of trapezium fracture, 819
of traumatic synovitis, 97
Radioscaphoid ligament, 813, 814f
Radiotriquetral ligament, 813, 814f
Radioulnar joint, 683
anterior dislocation of, 802
computed tomography of, 819
dislocation of
in Colles' fracture, 785, 790f
computed tomography of, 802, 803f
diagnosis of, 802
distal radial fracture with, 801
treatment of, 802, 804
distal, 779, 780f
dislocation of, 800–802, 801f, 803f–805f, 804
with Galeazzi fracture, 719, 720f, 721f
proximal migration of, 699, 704f, 705f
partial dislocation of, 802, 805f
posterior dislocation of, 802, 804f
proximal translocation of, 763

Radioulnar joint *(Continued)*
rotational subluxation of, 802
Radius
anatomy of, 683
anterior rim of, fracture of, carpus dislocation with, 789, 792f
dislocation of, 708
distal
Colles' fracture of, 784–785, 786f–790f, 787–788
capitellum fracture with, 771, 772f
complete fracture of, 805, 805f
epiphyseal injury to, 805, 806, 808, 809f–811f, 813
Salter-Harris type 1, 806, 810f, 811f
Salter-Harris type 2, 806, 809f, 811f
volar displacement in, 806, 811f
fracture of, 784–813
carpal instability from, 855
classification of, 784, 785f
elbow fracture with, 787
hip fracture with, 785, 786f
pediatric, 804–813
sites for, 804–805
pronator quadratus in, 781, 782f, 783, 783f
with radioulnar joint dislocation, 801
scapholunate dissociation in, 861
soft tissue injury with, 795, 799–800, 800f
types of, 784, 784f
ulnar styloid process fracture and, 795, 797f
greenstick fracture of, 805, 806, 808f
growth plate of
normal appearance of, 813, 813f
stress injuries to, 812f, 813
incomplete fracture of, 86f
intra-articular fracture of, 799f, 800f
lateral view of, 818
Smith's fracture of, 788–789, 791f
stress fracture of, 795, 798f
torus fracture of, 781, 782f, 783, 783f
pediatric, 805–806, 806f, 807f
transverse fracture of, 793, 795, 796f, 797f
dorsal, fracture of, 700f
fracture of, 719, 720f, 721f, 722
osteoporosis and, 32, 32f
pediatric, 765–772
ulnar fracture with, 712–714, 713f, 714f
Galeazzi fracture of, 719, 720f, 721f, 722
pediatric, 770–771
head of
dislocation of
in Monteggia fracture, 767, 768f–770f, 770
pediatric, 764, 764f
ulnar fracture with, 772
Essex-Lopresti fracture of, 699, 704f, 705f
fracture of, 696, 698f–701f, 699, 704f, 705f
capitate fracture with, 844, 846f
classification of, 696
fat pad sign in, 688f
pediatric, 757, 758f–761f, 761
scaphoid fracture with, 834
Galeazzi fracture-dislocation with, 722
humeral head fractures with, 694, 696f
nondisplaced fracture of, 701f
length of, 779–780, 780f
metaphyseal fracture of, pediatric, 757, 759f
neck of
displaced fracture of, 757, 761
fracture of, 696, 699, 700f, 702f, 703f, 705

Radius *(Continued)*
pediatric, 757, 758f–761f, 761
synostosis after, 714, 715f
impaction fracture of, 699, 702f
open fracture of, 41
physeal stress injury to, 126, 127f
posterior rim of, fracture of, carpus dislocation with, 789, 792f
proximal
epiphyseal injury to, 757, 758f, 760f, 761, 761f
fracture of, 696, 698f–705f, 699, 705
line bisecting, 731–732, 731f, 732f
refracture of, 257f
shaft of, fracture of, 712–730
stress fracture of, 63, 722
styloid process of
carpal instability from, 855
fracture of, 793, 795f
with scaphoid fracture, 834
Rectus muscle, inferior, in orbital floor fracture, 339–340
Reduction, 180
closed, 180
external, 180
open, 180, 184–193
fracture healing in, 209, 212f
indications for, 184–185
radiographs after, 200–201
Reflex dystrophy syndrome
osteoporosis in, 253, 255
post-traumatic, 253, 254f, 255, 255f
Refracture, 255, 257f–259f, 258
Renal osteodystrophy
epiphyseal separations in, 138, 141f
insufficiency fracture in, 64, 70, 72f
pathologic fracture in, 138, 141f
Resorption, in disuse atrophy, 211, 216f, 217f
Retrolisthesis, cervical spine, 436
Retropharyngeal soft tissue, swelling of, in cervical spine fractures, 385–386, 389, 389f
Rheumatoid arthritis
atlantoaxial dislocation with, 412
distal tibial/fibular insufficiency fractures in, 1285, 1288f
insufficiency fracture in, 64, 69
tibial stress fracture in, 1204
Rhinorrhea, cerebrospinal fluid, skull fracture and, 305–306, 305f
computed tomographic cisternography of, 306
Rhomboid fossa, 596
Rib(s)
evaluation of, in chest trauma, 589
first, fracture of, 551, 551f–555f, 553–555
bronchus fracture in, 553
costovertebral articulation injury in, 553, 553f
mechanisms of, 551
pediatric, 554–555
sites of, 551, 551f
subclavian artery injury in, 551, 552f, 553
thoracic outlet syndrome in, 553
transverse process fracture in, 553, 553f
visceral injury in, 553–554, 554f, 555f
fracture of, 541–556
anterolateral, 550
in battered child syndrome, 132, 135, 135f
bone density in, 542, 544f
bone scans of, 541
bronchial rupture in, 581
callus in, 541, 543f
cardiac injuries in, 588
computed tomography of, 546, 546f–548f
extrapleural hematoma in, 542, 545–546, 545f, 546f, 550–551

Rib(s) *(Continued)*
hemopneumothorax from, 561, 561f
incidence of, 541
indirect signs of, 550, 550f
multiple, 546, 549f
nondisplaced, 541, 542, 543f
oblique view of, 541, 542f
pneumothorax with, 561, 562f
pulmonary contusion in, 546, 548f, 568f
pulmonary injury with, 541
radiography of, 541–542, 542f, 543f, 546, 547f, 548f
skin fold in, vs. traumatic pneumothorax, 566, 566f
sonography of, 541, 544f
vascular injury in, 550
stress fracture of, 63, 556, 556f
Richard compression screw and plate, 193, 193f
Rickets, prematurity and, fracture in, 138
Rim sign, 664, 667f, 668f, 671f
Rods, intramedullary, 188–189, 189f–192f, 191–193
fatigue fracture of, 258, 259f
Rolando's fracture, 912, 914f, 915f
Rotary injury
in atlantoaxial dislocation, 418, 421f
in knee dislocation, 1187, 1190f, 1191
in scaphoid subluxation, 859–860, 864f
spinal, 480–481, 485f, 486f
vs. burst fracture, 504, 505f, 506, 507, 513f
in thoracolumbar junction fracture-dislocation, 517f
Rotation, 18, 18f
Rotator cuff, injury to, in anterior shoulder dislocation, 658, 661f
Rush rod and wire, 186f, 192

Sacroiliac joint, 930f, 931
in anterior pelvic compression injury, 972, 974f, 975f
computed tomography of, 938, 939, 939f, 941
diastasis of, in posterior pelvic fracture, 966, 966f
separation of, 967, 968f
Sacroiliac ligament
anterior, 933, 933f
interosseous, 933, 933f
posterior, 933, 933f
in anterior pelvic compression injury, 972, 974f, 975f
Sacrospinous ligament, 933, 933f
Sacrotuberous ligament, 933, 933f
Sacrum, 930–931, 931f, 932f
computed tomography of, 938, 939f
fracture of, 955, 956f, 957f, 966–967, 967f
computed tomography of, 967
neurologic deficits in, 1025
insufficiency fracture of, 963, 963f
after pelvic irradiation, 70, 73f
midline longitudinal fracture of, 955
transverse fracture of, 955, 957f
traumatic fracture of, 86f
Sagittal suture, diastasis of, 289, 290f, 291f
Salter-Harris epiphyseal injury, 120–125
classification of, 105
proximal humeral, 642, 645f, 646f
type 1, 121, 122f
distal fibular, 1296–1297, 1297f, 1300f
distal humeral, 754f
distal radial, 806, 810f, 811f
distal tibial, 1297, 1298f, 1299f, 1301, 1310, 1312

Salter-Harris epiphyseal injury *(Continued)*
interphalangeal joint, 925f
pelvic, 1007
proximal femoral, 1086, 1088f
proximal phalangeal, 920, 921, 923, 925f
proximal tibial, 1180, 1181f, 1209, 1210
type 2, 121, 122f, 123
acetabular, 1007, 1007f–1010f, 1009
distal femoral, 1209, 1209f
distal fibular, 1297, 1298f
distal radial, 806, 809f, 811f
distal tibial, 1297, 1300f, 1301, 1302f–1303f, 1313, 1313f
knee, 1209f, 1210, 1212f
metacarpal, 923, 924f, 926f
pelvic, 1007, 1007f–1010f
proximal phalangeal, 920–921, 923f, 924f
proximal tibial, 1209, 1210, 1212f
type 3, 123, 123f
distal femoral, 1209, 1210, 1210f, 1213f, 1214f
distal tibial, 1301, 1304f, 1305f, 1310, 1312f
knee, 1210, 1212f–1214f
proximal phalangeal, 920, 923, 925f
type 4, 123, 124f
distal femoral, 1209, 1210f
distal tibial, 1310, 1311f, 1312f
growth disturbance in, 128, 129f
lateral condylar, 739, 741f, 742f
medial condylar, 751–752, 752f
proximal Interphalangeal, 925f
proximal phalangeal, 920, 925f
type 5, 123, 125, 125f
distal femoral, 1209, 1211f, 1212
knee, 1212
proximal tibial, 1212
tibial fracture and, 1196
Sarcoidosis, pathologic fracture in, 75, 79f
Scalenus muscles, in first rib fracture, 551
Scalp, swelling of, 286, 287f
Scaphocapitate syndrome, 844, 846f
Scaphoid, 813
aseptic necrosis of, disuse osteoporosis in, 216f
avulsion fracture of, 829
computed tomography of, 821, 822f
45-degree pronation oblique view of, 818, 819f
dislocation of, 838–839, 838f
with capitate fracture, 844, 845f
fracture of, 829–837
arthrography of, 837
aseptic necrosis from, 834, 836f
associated fractures with, 834
blood supply in, 829f
bone scan of, 98f, 819, 831, 833f
Colles' fracture with, 789
computed tomography of, 831
delayed examination of, 831, 834, 834f
delayed union of, 222f, 829, 834, 835f
diagnosis of, 829, 830f–832f
distribution of, 829, 829f
frequency of, 827
healing of, 211f, 829, 837
computed tomography of, 225f, 226
magnetic resonance imaging of, 826f–827f, 831, 832f
mechanism of, 829
nonunion of, 223f, 829, 836–837, 837f
magnetic resonance imaging of, 226
pediatric, 837, 837f
perilunate dislocation with, 851
proximal radial fractures with, 699
pseudarthrosis in, 837
radiography of, 829–830, 830f–832f
Scaphoid *(Continued)*
anteroposterior view in, 831, 833f
soft tissue clues in, 830–831
tenderness in, 830
union assessment in, 837
ununited, 834, 835f, 836f
injury to, computed tomography of, 821
lateral view of, 818
magnification views of, 819
occult fracture of, bone scan of, 831, 833f
posteroanterior view of, 816, 817f
proximal pole of, 829
fracture of, 829, 832f
rotary subluxation of, 859–860, 864f
stress fracture of, 63, 837
transverse fracture of, 837, 837f
tuberosity of, fracture of, 829, 830f
waist of
fracture of, 816f
capitate fracture with, 844, 846f
radiography of, 829, 831f, 833f
pseudofracture of, 833f
Scaphoid fat stripe, posteroanterior view of, 817, 817f
Scapholunate dissociation, 859–863
magnetic resonance imaging of, 863, 864f, 865f
mechanism of, 861, 864f
radiography of, 861–863, 864f, 865f
symptoms of, 861
Terry Thomas sign in, 863
Scapholunate ligament, 779, 781f
injury to, 861
Scapula
acromion process of, fracture of, 626, 627f
anatomy of, 619–620, 620f
avulsion fracture of, 625, 627f
body of, fracture of, 621f, 625, 625f, 626f
comminuted fracture of, 619, 619f
complex fracture of, 624f
coracoid process of
fracture of, 605, 610f, 626–627, 628f, 629f
stress fracture of, 63
dislocation of, 627
fracture of, 625–626, 625f–627f
associated injuries with, 632
treatment of, 632
glenoid of, fracture of, 627, 630f, 631f
horizontal fracture of, 625, 626f
injury to, 619–632
apical oblique view of, 620, 622f, 623f
computed tomography of, 620, 624f
diagnosis of, 619
radiography of, 620, 621f–624f
Y view of, 620, 622f
neck of, fracture of, 625, 625f
ossification centers of, 620, 620f
stress fracture of, 625
vertical fracture of, 625
Scapulothoracic dislocation, 627
Scapulothoracic dissociation, 627, 632, 632f
Sciatic nerve, injury to, pelvic fracture and, 1021, 1023f, 1025
Sclerosis
endosteal, in stress fracture, 58
osteomyelitis with, 251, 251f
Screws
lag (cancellous), 185, 189f
machine (cortical), 185, 188f
Seat belt syndrome, 523, 525
Seat belts
Chance-type fracture from, 521
flexion injury with, 475, 480
Segond fracture, 1156, 1157–1158, 1158f, 1159f
Seizure
fracture from, 28–29
posterior shoulder dislocation from, 662, 664
Sensory neuropathy, 1384
Sesamoid bone, 7, 100
bipartite, 1396, 1398f, 1399, 1399f
forefooot, 1319, 1319f, 1320f
in fracture detection, 101–102
fracture of, 49, 1396, 1398f, 1399, 1399f
in irreducible dorsal interphalangeal dislocation, 901
osteomyelitis of, 1399
stress fracture of, 1396
radiography of, 1330
thumb, fracture of, 916, 917f
Sesamoid tibiale anterius, 1320f
Shaking, in battered child syndrome, 135
Sharpey's fibers, 16
in avulsion fracture, 46
Shear, 18, 18f
Shearing injury
pelvic, 972, 972f, 973f
spinal, 378f, 379, 481, 487f, 488f
vs. burst fracture, 504, 506, 506f, 507, 513f
in thoracolumbar junction fracture-dislocation, 517f
Shin splints, 1204, 1204f
in stress fracture, 59, 60f
Shock, in polytrauma, 145
Shoulder, 593–676
anterior dislocation of, 652, 654, 655f–661f, 658, 661
anterior glenoid rim fracture with, 654, 656f
arm abduction in, 654, 655f
diagnosis of, 654
greater tuberosity fracture with, 654, 655f
Hill-Sachs defect in, 654, 657f, 658, 659f–661f
humeral head compression fracture in, 658, 661f
humeral head defect with, 654, 657f, 658, 659f
labrocapsular complex tear with, 654
neurovascular injury with, 658
recurrent, 658
rotator cuff injury with, 658, 661f
treatment of, 658
dislocation of, 650–651, 651f, 652f
computed tomography of, 652
Grashey projection in, 652, 653f
magnetic resonance imaging of, 652
Moloney's arch in, 652, 653f, 654f
radiography of, 651f–654f, 652
scapular Y view in, 652, 653f
scapulohumeral arch in, 652, 653f, 654f
transthoracic view in, 652, 653f, 654f
injury to
computed tomography of, 594, 595f
Grashey view of, 594, 594f
magnetic resonance arthrography of, 594, 598f
magnetic resonance imaging of, 594, 596f–599f
radiography of, 593–594, 593f, 594f
instability of, 669, 671–675
computed tomography of, 671, 672f
magnetic resonance arthrography of, 671, 674f, 675
magnetic resonance imaging of, 671, 672f–675f
posterior, 675
intrathoracic fracture-dislocations of, 658, 661

Shoulder (*Continued*)
posterior dislocation of, 651, 662, 664
computed tomography of, 669, 670f, 671f
humeral head in, 662
radiography of, 664, 666f–668f, 669, 670f
recurrent, 670f
seizure and, 662, 664
simultaneous bilateral dislocation of, 651–652
subcoracoid anterior dislocation of, 651, 651f
subglenoid anterior dislocation of, 651, 652f
superior dislocation of, 662, 664f–665f
voluntary dislocation of, 651
Sinus tarsi, 1348, 1352
Sinuses
ethmoid
fracture of, 292, 297f, 353, 354f
cerebrospinal fluid rhinorrhea in, 305
orbital plate of, in blow-out fracture, 333, 334f
frontal, fracture of, 292, 294, 297, 297f, 357–358, 357f–359f
opacification of, in head trauma, 286, 288f
sphenoid, fracture of, 292
cerebrospinal fluid rhinorrhea in, 305, 305f
Skeleton
anatomy of, 6–16
appendicular, 6
axial, 6
pediatric, 111, 112f
secondary centers of, fusion of, ages at, 11, 12f
Skull, 272–310
basiliar fracture of, 297–298, 298f–300f
carotid artery involvement in, 298, 299f
computed tomography of, 298
comminuted fracture of
frontal sinuses in, 297f
magnetic resonance imaging of, 285f
computed tomography of, after head trauma, 272–273, 273t
depressed fracture of, computed tomography of, 277, 282f, 283f
fracture of, 272–310
in battered child syndrome, 135, 136f
bone density in, 84
child abuse and, 307, 308f, 309f
complications of, 303–307
computed tomography of, 275, 275f–284f, 277
growing, 306–307, 307f
imaging of, 275–287
indirect imaging signs of, 286–287, 287f, 288f
intracerebral injury in, 307, 310, 310f
linear, computed tomography of, 277, 284f
magnetic resonance imaging of, 281, 285f, 286
pathomechanics of, 273–275, 274f
pneumocephalus in, 303, 304f, 305, 305f, 310–311
radiography of, 277, 281, 284f
indications for, 272
signs/symptoms of, 307, 310, 310f
radiography of, after head trauma, 272–273, 273t
Skull base, fracture of, 297–298, 298f–300f
carotid artery involvement in, 298, 299f
computed tomography of, 89, 298
direction of, 297, 298f
magnetic resonance imaging of, 285f
Smash fracture, 366, 367f, 368f
Smith's fracture, 521, 523, 523f, 788–789, 791f
Smith's fracture (*Continued*)
classification of, 788–789
pedicle fracture with, 468f
Soccer, pediatric pelvic avulsion injury in, 1012
Soft tissue
in ankle injury, 1230, 1230f, 1231f
in cervical spine injury, 380
cranial, swelling of, 286, 287f
in distal radial fracture, 795, 799–800, 800f
emphysema of, 236–237, 238f, 239f
in facial fracture, 325, 325t, 327
in forearm fracture, 795, 799
in forearm stress fracture, 727, 728f–730f, 730
in fracture, 84
in hip fracture, 1035
in joint injury, 3
in knee radiography, 1127–1128, 1129f–1133f, 1130
in lumbar spine fracture, 455, 459f–461f, 460
magnetic resonance imaging of, 94, 95f
nasopharyngeal, swelling of, in cervical spine fractures, 386
in orbital blow-out fracture, 335, 336f
in orbital fracture, 325, 325t
in orbital injury, 342, 344f–347f, 346
in pelvic injury, 941, 945, 945f, 946f
in reflex dystrophy syndrome, 253, 254f
retropharyngeal, swelling of, in cervical spine fractures, 385–386, 389, 389f
in scaphoid fracture, 830–831
swelling of
in atlanto-occipital dislocation, 416, 417f
in calcaneal fracture, 1333
in craniovertebral fracture, 397
in thoracic spine fracture, 455, 459f–461f, 460
Space of Poirier, 813, 814f
Sphenoid bone
fracture of, 292, 297–298, 298f
cerebrospinal fluid rhinorrhea in, 305, 305f
vascular injury with, 298, 299f
greater wing of, 316
pterygoid processes of, 318f
Spinal cord
contusion of, in lumbar/thoracic spine fracture, 471, 475, 477f
hemorrhage of, in lumbar/thoracic spine fracture, 471, 472f, 477f
injury to
compression forces in, 378f, 379
distraction forces in, 378f, 379
extension forces in, 378f, 379
flexion forces in, 378–379, 378f
fracture-dislocation and, 442–443
pathomechanical classification of, 379–380, 380t
pathomechanics of, 378–379, 378f
rotational forces in, 378f, 379
second-level injuries in, 168, 171f, 172f
shearing forces in, 378f, 379
spondylosis in, 426f, 427f
transection of, 471
gunshot wounds and, 534, 536f
thoracic spine dislocation and, 471f
Spinal shock, in polytrauma, 145
Spine
anatomy of, 377, 377f
biomechanics of, 377–378
cervical. *See* Cervical spine.
columnar concept of, 377–378
compression fracture of, bone scans of, 98
Spine (*Continued*)
fracture of
computed tomography of, 89
multiple level, 526, 531f, 532f
osteoporosis and, 32
lumbar. *See* Lumbar spine.
sacrum in. *See* Sacrum.
stability of, radiography of, 534, 537, 537f
thoracic. *See* Thoracic spine.
three-column concept of, 537, 537f
Spinous process
in cervical spine fracture, 391
fracture of, 526
Spiral fracture, 20, 20f
anteroinferior tibiofibular ligament, supination–external rotation and, 1257, 1259f
femoral, 1094f
wires for, 187f
fibular, pronation–external rotation and, 1263, 1266f
humeral, 646, 648f
lateral malleolar
with posterior distal fibular dislocation, 1281
supination–external rotation and, 1257, 1259f
long bone, 44, 46, 46f
posteroinferior tibiofibular ligament, supination–external rotation and, 1257, 1260f
tibial, 89f
malleolar fracture with, 1282, 1283f
Spleen, trauma to
computed tomographic classification of, 162, 162t
first rib fracture and, 553, 554f, 555f
grading system for, 162, 162t
nonoperative management of, 162, 162t
pelvic fracture and, 1021
Splint
with cast, 180, 181f
radiography with, 2, 2f, 3f
Split peroneus brevis syndrome, 1384, 1384f
Spondylolysis, in pars interarticularis stress fracture, 526, 529f
Spondylosis, cervical spine, 426f, 427f
hyperextension injury with, 440, 440f, 441
retrolisthesis with, 436
Sprain
acromioclavicular joint, 605, 609f, 610f
ankle, 1249, 1254, 1254f, 1255f
reflex dystrophy syndrome from, 254f
stenosing synovitis from, 1384
anterior talofibular ligament, 1249, 1254, 1254f, 1255f
lateral collateral ligament, 1249, 1254, 1254f, 1255f
anterior drawer sign in, 1230–1231, 1233f, 1254, 1255f
stress views of, 1230–1231, 1232f, 1233f
Staphylococcus aureus, in osteomyelitis, 247
Steinmann pins, 182, 184f, 186f
osteomyelitis after, 250f
Sternoclavicular joint
anatomy of, 607, 609–610, 612f–613f
anterior dislocation of, 613, 615f, 618f
dislocation of, 607–619
acromioclavicular dislocation with, 607
complications of, 617, 619
computed tomography of, 612, 615f–617f, 617
diagnosis of, 612
Heining projection of, 613
mechanism of, 610, 612, 614f
medial clavicular epiphysis in, 610, 612f
radiography of, 612–613, 614f–617f, 617
Rockwell projection of, 613, 614f, 615f, 617

Sternoclavicular joint *(Continued)*
treatment of, 617, 618f
types of, 610, 612, 613f
mediastinal vessels of, 610, 613f
posterior dislocation of, 613, 614f, 616f, 617f
Sternoclavicular ligaments, 607, 609, 612f
Sternocleidomastoid muscle, 594
Sternum
fracture of, 556–559
cardiac injuries in, 588
computed tomography of, 89
mechanism of, 556, 557f
mediastinal widening from, 514, 516f
retrosternal hematoma in, 557, 557f
spontaneous fracture of, 557–558, 558f
in osteoporotic kyphosis, 492–493
transverse fracture of, resuscitation and, 556, 557f
Straddle fracture, 967, 968f
Strain, 17
elastic, 17, 17f
plastic, 17
repetitive, in stress fracture, 57, 58f
Streptococcus, soft tissue infection by, 236, 237f
Stress, 17
bone response to, 1330
energy dissipation in, 18
Stress fracture, 56–64
acetabular, 1002
acromion process, 626
bone scans of, 63, 64f, 98
calcaneal, 58, 59f, 63, 1329, 1348, 1351f
magnetic resonance imaging of, 1331, 1331f, 1332f
radiography of, 1330
clavicular, 63, 599, 603
computed tomography of, 63–64
cuboid, 1330, 1369
cuneiform, 1330, 1369
distal femoral epiphyseal, 1212
distal fibular, 1285, 1286f
distal radial, 795, 798f
distal tibial, 1289, 1290f–1291f
disuse atrophy and, 214, 216, 218f
femoral, 64f, 1100–1102, 1101f, 1102f
magnetic resonance imaging of, 1102, 1102f
vs. malignant disease, 1102
femoral neck. *See* Femur, neck of, stress fracture of.
fibular, 1206
foot, 1329–1330
magnetic resonance imaging of, 1330, 1331, 1331f, 1332f
marrow edema in, 1331, 1331f
radiography of, 1330
sites of, 1329, 1330f
forearm, 722, 723f–730f, 726–727, 730
humeral, 63, 126
ilial, 955, 958
ischial ramus, 63
location of, 59, 63
lumbar spine, 63, 526, 527f–529f
magnetic resonance imaging of, 63, 65f, 94, 96f
medial femoral condylar, 1204
metatarsal, 58f, 59f, 63, 1329, 1394, 1395f–1398f, 1396
diabetic osteoarthropathy and, 1396, 1398f
magnetic resonance imaging of, 1331, 1332f
nonunion of, 1397f
radiography of, 1330

Stress fracture *(Continued)*
navicular, 1329, 1330, 1366, 1369, 1372f–1374f
occult, 63
pars interarticularis, 526, 527f, 528f, 529f
patellar, 1204
pelvic, 954, 954f, 955, 958, 958f
posterior element, 526, 527f–529f
proximal fibular, 1199, 1204, 1207f
proximal phalangeal, 1396
proximal tibial, 59, 61f–63f, 1199, 1201f–1202f, 1212
in arthritic conditions, 1204
magnetic resonance imaging of, 63, 65f
radial, 63, 722
radiography of, 57–59, 58f–64f
repetitive strains in, 57, 58f
rib, 63, 556, 556f
scaphoid, 63, 837
scapular, 63, 625
sesamoid, 1330, 1396
shin splints as, 59, 60f
talar, 1330
tarsal, 63, 1329, 1330
tibial, 1199, 1203f, 1204, 1204f, 1206f, 1329
complete fracture progression of, 1206, 1207f
locations for, 1206
longitudinal, 1204, 1205f
magnetic resonance imaging of, 1206, 1208f
tibial plateau, 58, 59f, 1149
ulnar, 63, 707
Wolff's law in, 1330
Stress-strain curve, 17, 17f
hysteresis in, 18, 18f
loading in, 18, 18f
mineral component in, 19
unloading in, 18, 18f
Styloid process, 779, 780f
radial
carpal instability from, 855
fracture of, 793, 795f
with scaphoid fracture, 834
third metacarpal, 904
ulnar, fracture of, 795, 798f
Subarachnoid space, pneumocephalus in, in head trauma, 287, 288f
Subclavian artery, injury to, in first rib fracture, 551, 552f, 553
Subgaleal aerocele, 305
Subluxation, 55, 56f
Subtalar joint, 1332
in calcaneal compression fracture, 1340
computed tomography of, 1326f
dislocation of, 1358, 1359f–1365f, 1363
osteochondral fracture with, 1363, 1364f
reduction of, 1363
spectrum of, 1363
talar fractures with, 1355, 1358, 1359f, 1361f
vs. Chopart's dislocation, 1371
lateral dislocation of, 1358, 1362f
medial dislocation of, 1358, 1360f
with talar fracture, 1361f
swivel dislocation of, 1363, 1365f
Subtrochanteric fracture, Jewett nail fixation of, 192f
Sudeck's atrophy, 253, 255
Supination, foot, 1236, 1238, 1320
Supination-adduction
in ankle injury, 1256, 1257f
in anterior talofibular ligament rupture, 1256, 1257f
in calcaneofibular ligament rupture, 1256
in lateral malleolar transverse fracture, 1256–1257, 1257f, 1258f

Supination-adduction *(Continued)*
in tibial plateau (plafond) vertical fracture, 1257, 1257f, 1258f
Supination–external rotation
in ankle injury, 1257, 1259f–1264f, 1263
in anteroinferior tibiofibular ligament spiral fracture, 1257, 1259f
in bimalleolar ankle fracture, 1258f
in lateral malleolar spiral fracture, 1257, 1259f
in medial collateral ligament rupture, 1257, 1262f, 1263f
in medial malleolar transverse fracture, 1257, 1261f, 1262f
in posterior malleolar fracture, 1263, 1264f
in posterior tibial tubercle fracture, 1257, 1260f–1262f, 1263, 1264f
in posteroinferior tibiofibular ligament spiral fracture, 1257, 1260f
in talar subchondral fracture, 1289
talus response to, 1261f
in Tillaux fracture, 1257
Supracondylar process, fracture of, 645, 649f
nonunion of, with pseudoarthrosis, 219f
Suprapatellar bursa
in joint effusion, 1128, 1129f, 1131f
in lipohemarthrosis, 1128, 1130f
Suprapatellar fat pad, 1112f
Suprapatellar tendon, rupture of, 1176, 1178
Supraspinatus tendon
in anterior shoulder displacement, 658, 661f
tear of, magnetic resonance imaging of, 596f
Sustentaculum tali, computed tomography of, 1329f
Swan-neck deformity, in baseball finger, 880, 882f
Swivel dislocation
subtalar, 1363, 1365f
vs. Chopart's dislocation, 1371
Symphysis, 13
Symphysis pubis
adductor avulsive injury near, pediatric, 1012, 1014f
in anterior pelvic compression injury, 972, 974f, 975, 975f
diastasis of, anterior bladder herniation in, 1021
insufficiency fracture of, 960, 962f–963f, 963
separation of, 967, 968f
in pregnancy, 964, 964f
urinary tract injury in, 1015, 1017f
Synarthrosis, 12, 14f
Synchondrosis, 13
separation of, 410, 412f
vs. hangman's fracture, 408
Syndesmosis, 13
Synostosis, 259, 262f
Synovial membrane, 13
Synovialis, suprapatellar plica, 1128
Synovitis, traumatic, bone scans of, 97
Syringomyelia, thoracic, 475, 478f

Talocalcaneal joint, 1332
computed tomography of, 1329f
dislocation of, 1358, 1360f
Talofibular ligament
anterior, 1224, 1224f
avulsion of, 1381, 1383f
rupture of
with interosseous ligament injury, 1270
supination-adduction in, 1256, 1257f
sprain of, 1249, 1254, 1254f, 1255f

Talofibular ligament *(Continued)*
posterior, 1224, 1224f
posteroinferior, rupture of, 1270
Talonavicular joint
avulsion fracture of, 1364
dislocation of, 1358, 1360f, 1361f, 1371, 1377f
Talus, 1223f, 1224, 1319f, 1348, 1352–1363
anatomy of, 1348, 1352, 1353f
arterial supply of, 1348, 1352
avulsion fracture of, distribution of, 1354
body of, 1348
fracture of, 1354–1355, 1354f
posterior dislocation of, 1355
in calcaneal compression fracture, 1340, 1341f
computed tomography of, 1231, 1234f–1235f, 1328f
dislocation of, 1358, 1360f
fractures with, 1358, 1361f
dome of
osteochondral fracture of, 1289, 1292f–1294f, 1358
osteochondritis dissecans of, 1302f–1303f
in Dupuytren's fracture, 1274f
fracture of
distribution of, 1352, 1354–1355, 1354f–1359f, 1358
pediatric, 1400
fracture-dislocation of, distribution of, 1354
head of, avulsion fracture of, 1354
in lateral collateral ligament tear, 1230, 1232f
in lateral malleolar fracture, 1227
medial displacement of, 1281
neck of, 1348
avulsion fracture of, 1354, 1354f
fracture of
classification of, 1355, 1358
subtalar dislocation with, 1355, 1358, 1359f, 1361f
vertical fracture of, 1355, 1357f, 1358f
occult fracture of, 1331
osteochondral fracture of
with Dupuytren fracture, 1266f
in subtalar joint dislocation, 1363, 1364f
posterior process of, 1355
fracture of, 1355, 1355f
vs. os trigonum, 1355, 1356f, 1357f
radiography of, 1227, 1227f, 1352, 1353f
stress fracture of, 1330
subchondral fracture of, supinationnexternal rotation and, 1289
in supinationnexternal rotation ankle injury, 1261f
trochlea of, 1348
Tarsometatarsal joint, 1371, 1379f
diabetic neuroarthropathy of, 1384, 1385f
dislocation of, cuneiform fracture with, 1369
fracture-dislocation of
divergent, 1380, 1380f, 1382f
forms of, 1380, 1380f
fracture types in, 1380, 1382f
homolateral, 1380, 1380f–1382f
mechanism of, 1376, 1380, 1380f
ligaments of, 1371
normal radiograph of, 1371, 1379f
tendon injuries in, 1384, 1384f
Tarsus, 7
computed tomography of, 1326, 1326f–1327f, 1327
fracture of
pediatric, 1400
vs. ankle fracture, 1227
stress fracture of, 63, 1329
Tarsus *(Continued)*
computed tomography of, 1330
Teardrop fracture
hypertension, of axis, 412, 414f
of lower cervical spine, 422, 424f, 425f
Technetium 99m, in radionuclide bone scanning, 97
Tegmen tympani
disruption of, in temporal bone fractures, 300, 302f
fracture of, cerebrospinal fluid otorrhea in, 302
Telecanthus, in naso-orbital-ethmoidal fracture, 356
Temporal bone, petrous pyramid of
fracture of
air space opacification in, 301, 302f
computed tomography of, 301, 302f
direction of, 298, 300f
facial nerve injury in, 300, 302f
hearing loss in, 300–301, 302f
longitudinal, 298, 300, 301f
magnetic resonance imaging of, 301–302
ossicular chain disruption in, 300, 302f
pneumocephalus in, 301
pneumolabyrinth in, 301, 302f
signs/symptoms of, 302–303
vascular injury in, 298, 299f
oblique fracture of, 300
transverse fracture of, 298, 301, 301f, 302f
Temporomandibular joint
dislocation of, 369
in mandibular fractures, 368
Tendons
avulsions of, 16
of joints, 13
in transverse fracture, 44
Tennis elbow, 727
Tension, 18, 18f
Terry Thomas sign, in scapholunate dissociation, 863
β-Thalassemia
insufficiency fracture in, 73
pediatric, pathologic fracture in, 138, 141f
Thoracic cage, injury to, 541–589
Thoracic duct, rupture of, chylous effusion from, 561, 562f
Thoracic outlet syndrome, in first rib fracture, 553
Thoracic spine
burst fracture of, 461f, 476f, 497, 500f–506f, 504, 506
fragment configuration in, 497, 500f
fragment retropulsion in, 497, 503f, 504
sagittal, 497
stable, 484, 506
unstable, 484, 487
vertebral body height in, 497, 502f
vs. rotary injury, 504, 505f, 506, 507, 513f
vs. shearing injury, 504, 506, 506f, 507, 513f
vs. simple wedge compression fracture, 497, 504, 504f
Chance-type fracture of, 480, 483f, 487, 521–525
computed tomography of, 523, 524f
fulcrum fracture in, 521
injury patterns in, 521, 521f–523f, 523
magnetic resonance imaging of, 523
radiography of, 523
Smith fracture in, 521, 523, 523f
transverse, 521, 522f
vs. flexion-distraction fracture, 497
compression fracture of, 459f, 460, 489, 491–492, 491f, 492f
osteoporotic vs. pathologic, 471, 474f, 492, 493f
Thoracic spine *(Continued)*
dislocation of, facet lock with, 468f
extension injury to, 478f, 484, 489f
flexion injury to, 475, 479f, 480
burst, 480, 481f, 482f
dislocation, 480, 484f
distraction, 480, 483f
simple, 480, 480f
flexion-distraction injury to, 487, 490f, 495, 497, 499f
fracture of
alignment abnormalities in, 454–455, 456f, 457f, 471, 474f
anatomic abnormalities in, 454–455, 456f, 457f
in ankylosing spondylitis, 526, 532f, 533–534
bone integrity abnormalities in, 455
cartilage abnormalities in, 455, 458f, 459f
Chance-type injury in, 466
computed tomography of, 463, 464f–470f, 465–466
in diffuse idiopathic skeletal hyperostosis, 534, 534f
disc herniation in, 465, 466f, 471, 474f
disc space abnormalities in, 455, 459f
epidural hematoma with, 471, 473f
evaluation approach to, 454
facet joint integrity in, 465, 468f
interpedicle space in, 455, 457f
interspinous space in, 455, 457f
joint space abnormalities in, 455, 458f, 459f
magnetic resonance imaging of, 466, 471, 471f–478f, 475
osteoporotic collapse in, 471, 475f
pedicle injury in, 465, 468f
posterior element status in, 460, 463, 463f
posterior vertebral body line in, 454–455, 456f
radiography of, 453–454, 455f–463f, 460, 463
second-level fractures in, 526, 531f
soft tissue abnormalities in, 455, 459f–461f, 460
spinal cord contusion in, 471, 475, 477f
spinal cord hemorrhage in, 471, 472f, 477f
spinal cord injury with, 471, 471f, 472f
spinal cord status in, 466, 469f
vertebral canal compromise in, 465, 467f
vertebral canal fragments in, 471, 476f
wedge vs. compression, 466
fracture-dislocation of, 171f, 172f, 460f, 462f, 463f, 506–521
facet joint disruption in, 506, 506f
magnetic resonance imaging of, 507, 512f
neurologic deficit in, 507, 507f–511f
pediatric, 507, 511f
posterior elements fracture in, 506, 506f
upper dorsal, 507, 514–515, 515f, 516f
hematoma in, 507, 515f
paraplegia in, 515
subarachnoid-pleural fistulas in, 514–515
vertebral bodies in, 514, 515f
injury to, 453–537
biomechanics of, 453–454
classification of, 475, 479f–490f, 480–481, 484, 487, 489
distribution of, 453–454, 454f
incidence of, 453–454
mechanism of, 475, 479f–490f, 480–481, 484, 487, 489
pediatric, 453

Thoracic spine *(Continued)*
wedge deformity in, 491–492
limbus vertebra of, 489, 491, 491f, 492f
open wounds to, 534, 536f
osteoporotic compression fracture of, 491f, 492–493, 493f–496f
pathologic fracture of, 493, 497f
penetrating trauma to, 534, 536f
polytrauma to
aortic injury in, 152, 153f
diaphragmatic injury in, 152, 155, 156f–159f, 158
imaging studies of, 150–158
mediastinal hematoma in, 152, 154f
mediastinal hemorrhage in, 150, 152, 152f
pericardial tamponade in, 150, 151f
screening computed tomography in, 150, 151f
posterior elements of, fracture of, 495, 497, 499f, 525–526
post-traumatic vertebral body collapse in, 493–495, 498f
rotary (grinding) injury to, 480–481, 485f, 486f
vs. burst fracture, 504, 505f, 506, 507, 513f
shearing injury to, 481, 487f, 488f
vs. burst fracture, 504, 506, 506f, 507, 513f
syringomyelia of, 475, 478f
translation (dislocation) injury to, 487
vertebral edge separation of, 489, 491, 491f, 492f
wedge compression fracture of, 484
Thoracolumbar junction
compression fracture of, 453
dislocation of, 507, 509f
fracture-dislocation of, 515–521
computed tomography of, 516, 518f–520f
facet joints in, 515, 516, 517f, 520f, 521
fragment in, 515
reduction of, 521
rotary/shearing injury in, 517f
injury to, biomechanics of, 453
Thromboembolism, 239–244
chest radiograph of, 242, 243f
computed tomography of, 240
computed tomograpic angiography of, 242, 244
diagnosis of, 241
lung scanning of, 242, 243f
nuclear medicine evaluation of, 240
pathogenesis of, 241–242
pulmonary, 240–241
signs/symptoms of, 240
ultrasonography of, 240
venography of, 240
Thrombosis, 231
Throwing
fracture in, 48f
valgus stress fracture in, 722
Thumb
abduction of, trapezium fracture in, 842, 843f
Bennett's fracture of, 911–912, 913f, 914f
carpometacarpal dislocation in, 920, 921f, 922f
comminuted fracture of, 912, 914f, 915f
dislocation of, 917, 920
extra-articular fracture of, 912, 916f
first metacarpal fracture of, 911, 913f
gamekeeper's injury to, 916–917, 917f–919f
injury to, 909–920
interphalangeal joint of
dislocation of, 917
Thumb *(Continued)*
hyperextension of, pediatric, 923
posterior dislocation of, 56f
metacarpophalangeal dislocation in, 920
radiography of, 874, 875f, 909, 911, 913f
Rolando's fracture of, 912, 914f, 915f
sesamoid of, fracture of, 916, 917f
traumatic amputation of, open fracture in, 43f
Thurston-Holland fragment, 126
Thyroid cartilage, fracture of, 445, 445f
Tibia, 1111–1215
anterior cortex of, stress fracture of, 1204, 1206f
anterior eminence of, avulsion fracture of, 1154–1155, 1156f
anterior tubercle of, 1223, 1223f
avulsion fracture of, 1246, 1248, 1249f, 1250f
fracture of, 1180, 1181f, 1182f, 1241, 1243f, 1249, 1251f
pronation-dorsiflexion and, 1270, 1271f
radiography of, 1229, 1229f
apophysis of
avulsion fracture of, 1180, 1181f
normal variants in, 1130
bone bruise of, magnetic resonance imaging of, 1124, 1125f
boot-top fracture of, 1194f
comminuted fracture of
degenerative arthritis after, 265f
external fixation for, 196f–197f
osteomyelitis in, 247f
condyles of, 1111, 1112f
bone bruise of, magnetic resonance imaging of, 1124, 1126, 1127f
crack of, magnetic resonance imaging of, 1124, 1127f
distal, 1223–1224, 1223f
anatomy of, 1111, 1112f
comminuted fracture of, 51f
complex fracture of, computed tomography of, 1231, 1236f
epiphysis of
fusion of, 1296, 1296f
injury to, 1296
neglected Salter-Harris type 3 injury to, 1310, 1312f
ossification center of, 1296, 1296f
Salter-Harris type 1 injury to, 1297, 1298f, 1299f, 1301
external rotation in, 1310, 1312
Salter-Harris type 2 injury to, 1297, 1300f, 1301, 1302f–1303f
external rotation in, 1313, 1313f
Salter-Harris type 3 injury to, 1301, 1304f, 1305f
Salter-Harris type 4 adduction injury to, 1310, 1311f, 1312f
Tillaux fracture of, 1301, 1305f
triplane fracture of, 1231, 1301, 1306f–1310f, 1310
computed tomography of, 1309f, 1310
four-fragment, 1301
three-fragment, 1301, 1306f, 1310f
two-fragment, 1301, 1306f–1309f
fracture of
pre-Achilles triangle in, 1230
in proximal tibiofibular joint dislocation, 1164
insufficiency fracture of, 75f, 1285, 1287f, 1288f, 1289, 1290f–1291f
longitudinal stress fracture of, 1289, 1290f–1291f
oblique fracture of, 45f, 88f
Tibia *(Continued)*
open transverse fracture of, 42f
teacup fracture of, 46, 47f
vertical nondisplaced fracture of, 46, 47f
fracture of, 1191–1208
age in, 27
compartment syndrome with, 1197–1198, 1198f
delayed union of, 1194
disuse osteoporosis in, 217f
external fixation for, 89f, 186f
healing of, 1194
computed tomography of, 229f
hip fracture-dislocations with, 1191, 1194, 1195f
incomplete, 1191, 1195f
interlocking nail fixation of, 90f, 191f
location of, 1191, 1194f
mechanism of, 1191
nonunion of, 219f, 222f, 1194
computed tomography of, 228f
osteomyelitis in, 244f
osteomyelitis in, 245, 245f
pediatric, 1196–1197, 1197f
proximal ipsilateral femoral fracture with, 1191, 1194
radiography of, 1191, 1192f
Salter-Harris type 5 injury and, 1196
tibial plateau fracture with, 1191, 1194, 1196f
toddler's, 1197, 1197f
treatment of, 1198–1199, 1199f, 1200f
intercondylar eminence of, avulsion fracture of, 1152–1154, 1154f, 1155f
lateral, avulsion fracture of, 1157–1158, 1158f, 1159f
midshaft
stress fracture of, 1199, 1203f, 1204, 1204f
transverse fracture of, 44f
open comminuted fracture of, cast for, 181f
open fracture of, 41
pathologic fracture of, 1198
peroneal groove of, 1225, 1226f
physeal stress injury to, 126
posterior tubercle of, 1223, 1223f
fracture of, 1248–1249, 1251f, 1270, 1278f
radiography of, 1227, 1229, 1229f
supination–external rotation and, 1257, 1260f, 1261f, 1262f, 1263, 1264f
isolated fracture of, 1270, 1279, 1279f
proximal
epiphysis of
injury to, 1209–1215
prognosis of, 1215
Salter-Harris type 1 injury to, 1180, 1181f, 1209, 1210
Salter-Harris type 2 injury to, 1209, 1210, 1212f
Salter-Harris type 5 injury to, 1212
stress fracture of, 1212
fracture of, 1135, 1142–1161
arteries in, 1116–1118
injury to, deep notch sign in, 1158, 1160, 1160f
intercondylar fracture of, 1152, 1153f
intra-articular avulsion fracture of, 1154–1157, 1156f, 1157f
medial collateral ligament injury at, 1211
metaphyseal fracture of, 1194, 1197
open fracture of, popliteal artery transection with, 169f
periarticular avulsion fracture of, 1154–1157, 1156f, 1157f
segmental fracture of, 48f

Tibia *(Continued)*
stress fracture of, 59, 61f–63f, 1199, 1201f–1202f
in arthritic conditions, 1204
magnetic resonance imaging of, 63, 65f
subcondylar fracture of, 1152, 1153f
transcondylar fracture of, 1152, 1153f
radiography of, 1116, 1117f, 1229–1230
refracture of, 1194, 1196
segmental fracture of, 1191, 1193f
spiral fracture of, 1191, 1192f
malleolar fracture with, 1282, 1283f
radiography of, 89f
stress fracture of, 1329
complete fracture progression of, 1206, 1207f
locations for, 1206
longitudinal, 1204, 1205f
magnetic resonance imaging of, 1206, 1208f
supramalleolar fracture of, 1280–1281, 1281f
transverse fracture of, 23
with butterfly fragment, 45f
Tibial artery, 1113, 1114f
Tibial ligament, meniscal, avulsion of, 1156, 1157f
Tibial plateau (plafond), 1223f, 1224
avulsion from, 1156–1157
comminuted fracture of, 1231, 1236f
depression fracture of, with lipohemarthrosis, 87f
fracture of, 1135, 1142–1143, 1142f–1151f, 1145, 1149
anatomy in, 1135, 1142
anterior cruciate ligament injury in, 1145
classification of, 1142, 1142f
computed tomography of, 1118, 1119f, 1143
considerations in, 1135
degenerative arthritis after, 1149
fibular fracture in, 1145, 1151f
frequency of, 1130
incidence of, 1142, 1142f
ligamentous injuries in, 1145, 1151f
lipohemarthrosis in, 1132f
magnetic resonance imaging of, 1145, 1148f–1150f
mechanism of, 1142
medial collateral ligament injury in, 1145, 1151f
pronation-dorsiflexion and, 1270, 1272f, 1273f
tibial/fibular fracture with, 1191, 1194, 1196f
treatment of, 1145, 1149
insufficiency fracture of, 1149, 1152, 1152f
lateral
bone bruise of, magnetic resonance imaging of, 1124, 1126f
fracture of, 1142, 1143, 1145f
fibular head fracture with, 1161
lipohemarthrosis in, 1143, 1145f
radiography of, 1143
split-depression type, 1142–1143, 1143f–1147f
stress fracture of, 58, 59f, 1149
vertical fracture of, supination-adduction and, 1257, 1257f, 1258f
Tibial spine
anterior, avulsion fracture of, 1152–1153, 1154f, 1155f
suprapatellar effusion in, 1131f
posterior, avulsion fracture of, 1153–1154, 1156f
Tibial tendon, posterior
magnetic resonance imaging of, 1237f, 1238f
rupture of
ankle fracture and, 1280
in malleolar avulsion fracture, 1246, 1248f
Tibiofemoral joint, dislocation of, 1187, 1189f, 1190f, 1191
Tibiofibular joint, 1113
computed tomography of, 1231, 1234f–1235f
distal, 1225, 1225f
inferior, as fibrous joints, 12–13
proximal
computed tomography of, 1118
dislocation of, 1161, 1164, 1164f, 1165f
anterolateral, 1161, 1165f
classification of, 1161, 1164f
mechanism of, 1161
posteromedial, 1161, 1164
Tibiofibular ligament
anterior
avulsion fracture at, 1248, 1249f
magnetic resonance imaging of, 1237f
rupture of, with posterior tibial tubercular fracture, 1270, 1279f
anteroinferior, 1225, 1225f
spiral fracture of, supination–external rotation and, 1257, 1259f
pediatric, 1295f, 1296
posterior, magnetic resonance imaging of, 1237f
posteroinferior, 1225, 1225f
spiral fracture of, supination–external rotation and, 1257, 1260f
transverse, magnetic resonance imaging of, 1237f
Tibiofibular syndesmosis, 1224–1225, 1224f, 1225f
diastasis of, 56f
injury to, 1249, 1253f
ligaments of, pediatric, 1295f, 1296
rupture of, pronation-abduction and, 1267
Tibiotalar joint, dislocation of, 1281
Tidemark, 13
Tillaux fracture, 1248, 1249f, 1250f
juvenile, 1301, 1305f
supination–external rotation and, 1257
Toddler's fracture, 115–116, 117f, 118f
ankle, 1289, 1295f
calcaneal, 1400, 1400f
cuboid, 1369
tibial, 1197, 1197f
Toe
fifth, interphalangeal joint of, subluxation of, 1391f
great. *See* Great toe.
Tooth (teeth)
in alveolar process fracture, 358–359, 359f
in mandibular fracture, 371
Torticollis, 417, 419f
Torus fracture
distal radial, 781, 782f, 783, 783f
pediatric, 805–806, 806f, 807f
elbow, supracondylar, pediatric, 736, 737f
fifth metacarpal, 920, 922f
iliac wing, 956f
olecranon, 762f
pediatric, 112–113, 114f, 115f
Trabecula, 6, 6f, 7
fracture of, in osteoporosis, 30, 30f, 31f
Trachea, rupture of, 579, 579f–582f, 581
Traction, 182, 184f, 186f
Transforming growth factor-β, in fracture healing, 204
Transverse ligament, 394
inferior, 1225, 1225f
Transverse process
avulsion fracture of, in first rib fracture, 553, 553f
fracture of, 525–526, 525f
Trapezium, 813
computed tomography of, 821, 822f
45-degree pronation oblique view of, 818, 819f
dislocation of, 843
fracture of, 827, 842, 843f
volar tubercle of, fracture of, 842, 843f
bone scan of, 819
computed tomography of, 819
Trapezius muscle, 593
Trapezoid, 813
computed tomography of, 821, 822f
45-degree pronation oblique view of, 818, 819f
fracture of, 827, 843
Trapezoid ligament, 594, 596
Trauma, 1. *See also* Polytrauma; *at anatomic site, e.g.,* Spleen, trauma to; *specific trauma, e.g.,* Fracture.
amputation in, open fracture from, 41, 43f
assessment of, 2–3
biologic factors in, 17
biomechanics of. *See* Biomechanics.
chest, radiography of, 588–589
as leading cause of death, 1, 1f, 2f
magnetic resonance imaging of, 94
mechanism of, biologic-mechanical interaction in, 17
nonaccidental, 307, 308f, 309f
patterns of, 3
penetrating, fracture from, 23–24, 23f, 24f
radiography in, 2–3, 2f, 3f
indications for, 76, 78–79, 78t, 79t
secondary ossification centers and, 11
Triangular fibrocartilage complex, 779, 780f, 801
injury to, 866, 866f, 867f
in distal radial fracture, 800
magnetic resonance imaging of, 866, 867f
Triangular ligament, 779, 781f
Triceps muscle, scapular insertion of, avulsion of, 625–626
Triceps tendon, rupture of, 727, 730, 730f
Trimalar fracture, 346
Trimalleolar fracture, 1222
Triplane fracture, distal tibial epiphyseal, 1301, 1306f–1310f, 1310
computed tomography of, 1309f, 1310
two-fragment, 1301, 1306f–1309f
three-fragment, 1301, 1306f, 1310f
four-fragment, 1301
Tripod fracture, 346
Triquetropisiform space, widening of, 818
Triquetrum, 813
computed tomography of, 821, 822f
45-degree pronation oblique view of, 818, 819f
fracture of, 816f, 841, 841f
capitate fracture with, 844, 846f
frequency of, 827
with scaphoid fracture, 834
lateral view of, 818
posteroanterior view of, 816–817
synostosis of, 818

Tumors, pathologic fracture in, 77f
Turf toe, 1386

Ulna, 712–730
  anatomy of, 683
  Colles' fracture of, capitellum fracture with, 771, 772f
  coronoid process of
    avulsion fracture of, 708, 709f
    comminuted fracture of, with anterior elbow subluxation, 707, 707f
    fracture of, 707f–709f, 708
      with posterolateral elbow dislocation, 711, 712f
  dislocation of, 708
  distal, 780–781
    Colles' fracture of, 784–785, 786f–790f, 787–788
    eminence of, 779, 780f
    epiphyseal injury to, 805, 806, 808, 809f–811f, 813
    fracture of, 784–813
      pediatric, 804–813
        sites for, 804–805
      types of, 784, 784f
    greenstick fracture of, 805, 806, 808f
    nightstick fracture of, 716, 716f
  fracture of, 714, 716, 716f–719f, 718–719
    in Monteggia fracture, 767, 768f–770f, 770
    nonunion of, 223f, 224f
    pediatric, 765–772
    pseudarthrosis of, 223f
  glenoid fossa of, osteochondral fracture of, 761
  head of, 779, 780, 780f
  length of, 779–780, 780f
  lifting fracture of, 722, 723f
  midshaft, oblique fracture of, 45f
  Monteggia fracture of, 716, 717f–719f, 718–719
    diagnosis of, 718
    mechanism of, 716, 718
    treatment of, 718–719
    types of, 716, 717f, 718f
    vs. anterior elbow dislocation, 716, 718f
  nightstick fracture of, 21, 21f
  olecranon of
    avulsion fracture of, posteromedial elbow dislocation with, 710f
    fracture of, 705, 706f, 707–708, 707f
    stress fracture of, 707
  open fracture of, 41
    osteomyelitis after, 248f
  physeal stress injury to, 126, 127f
  proximal, fracture of, 705, 706f–709f, 707–708
  stress fracture of, 63
  styloid process of, 780, 780f
    fracture of, 795, 798f
  traction spur of, 726
  translocation of, 863
  variance of, 780
Ulnar nerve
  entrapment of, 726
  in hook of hamate fracture, 849, 850f
  injury to, 684
Ulnar nerve *(Continued)*
    humeral shaft fracture and, 649
Ulnar notch, 779, 780f
Ulnolunate ligament, 813, 814f
Ulnotriquetral ligament, 813, 814f
Ultrasonography
  of fracture healing, 229, 229f
  of osteochondral fracture, 52
  of pseudoaneurysm, 234, 235f
  of thromboembolism, 240
Ultrasound, osteogenesis stimulation by, 199–200
Ultrasound index, quantitative, bone density measurement with, 34
Uncinate process, avulsion fracture of, 440–441
Union, 74, 216, 219f, 220f
  delayed, 220–221, 222f
    in tibial fracture, 1194
  fluoroscopy of, 216
  in scaphoid fracture, 837
  stress film of, 216, 220f
Urethra, injury to, pelvic fracture and, 1015–1016, 1017f, 1021, 1022f
Urinary tract, injury to, pelvic fracture and, 1015–1016, 1017f–1021f, 1021

Vacuum vertebra, osteoporotic compression and, 492, 494f
Valgus deformity, after epiphyseal injury, 129, 131f
Valgus stress injury
  forearm, 722, 724f–727f, 726–727
    bone hypertrophy in, 722, 724f
  to knee, 1210
  to medial collateral ligament, 726, 726f
  throwing and, 722
Varus deformity
  after epiphyseal injury, 129
  after femoral supcapital neck fracture, 1046–1047, 1047f, 1050f
Vascular channels, in fracture detection, 100–101, 101f
Vastus lateralis, 1112f, 1113
Vastus medialis, 1112f, 1113
Vertebrae
  anatomy of, 377, 377f
  compression fracture of, pediatric, 138, 139f
  fracture of
    bone mineral density and, 36f
    in calcaneal fracture, 1333, 1334f
    epidemiology of, 27–28
  osteomyelitis of, 492
  pathologic fracture of, 75, 80f
  stability of, radiography of, 534, 537, 537f
  stress fracture of, 63
Vertebral artery, trauma to, 166
Vertebral body, 377, 377f
  in ankylosing spondylitis, 533
  cervical
    avulsion fracture of, 440–441
    in hyperflexion strain, 435
    subluxation of, 56f
    vertical split of, 422
  compression fracture of, 49, 51f
  height of
    in burst fracture, 497, 502f
Vertebral body *(Continued)*
    in cervical spine fractures, 391
  in lumbar spine fracture, 454–455, 456f
  osteoporotic compression of, 492, 493f
  post-traumatic collapse of, 493–495, 498f
  in upper dorsal fracture-dislocation, 514, 515f
Vertebral canal, in lumbar/thoracic spine fracture, 465, 467f
Viscoelasticity, 18
Vitreous, hemorrhage within, 342, 345f
Volar ligaments, 813, 814f
Volar plate, 878, 878f
  avulsion fracture of, at phalangeal base, 876f, 883, 884f–886f
  rupture of, interphalangeal joint dislocation and, 900–901
Volkmann's canals, 8f
Volkmann's ischemic contracture, 234–236

Wagstaffen-LeFort fracture, 1248, 1249f, 1257, 1260f
Walther's fracture, 988, 989f, 991, 994f
Whiplash injury, 436
Windswept pelvis, 977–978, 977f
Wires, 185, 186f, 187f
  appliance migration in, 252–253
  Kirschner, 193, 194f
Wolff's law, in stress fracture, 1330
Wood
  in cranium, 292, 296f
  in orbit, 347f
Wrist, 779–868
  anatomy of, 779, 780f, 781f
  arthrography of, 826, 827f
  calcific tendinitis of, vs. fracture, 827, 828f
  cortical arcs/lines of, 851, 851f
  magnetic resonance imaging of, 783, 784t
  radiography of, 779–781, 780f, 782f, 783, 783f
  ulnar deviation of, 814, 815f
Wryneck, 417, 419f

X-ray, 2

Zone of elastic deformation, 17, 17f
Zone of plastic deformation, 17
Zygoma, 316, 317f
  orbital plate of, 316
Zygomatic arch, fracture of, 348, 351f, 352f, 353
  components involved in, 320
  LeFort II fracture with, 362f, 365
  posterior displacement of, 348
Zygomatic complex, fracture of, 315, 346, 348, 348f–351f
  components of, 348
  computed tomography of, 348, 349f, 351f
  orbital floor fracture with, 339
  radiography of, 348, 350f
  surgery for, 348, 351f
Zygomaticofrontal suture, separation of, 348

ISBN 0-443-06563-2